BASIC CLINICAL LAB COMPETENCIES FOR RESPIRATORY CARE

AN INTEGRATED APPROACH

FOURTH EDITION

BASIC CLINICAL LAB COMPETENCIES FOR RESPIRATORY CARE

AN INTEGRATED APPROACH

FOURTH EDITION

Gary C. White, MEd, RRT, RPFT
Spokane Community College
Spokane, Washington

THOMSON

DELMAR LEARNING

Australia Canada Mexico Singapore Spain United Kingdom United States

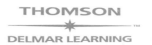

Basic Clinical Lab Competencies for Respiratory Care:
An Integrated Approach
Fourth Edition
by Gary C. White

Executive Director, Health Care Business Unit:
William Brottmiller

Executive Editor:
Cathy L. Esperti

Acquisitions Editor:
Rhonda Dearborn

Developmental Editor:
Deb Flis

Editorial Assistant:
Natalie Wager

Executive Marketing Manager:
Dawn F. Gerrain

Channel Manager:
Jennifer McAvey

Project Editor:
Shelley Esposito

Production Coordinator:
Nina Lontrato

Art & Design Coordinator:
Connie Lundberg-Watkins

For permission to use material from this text or product, contact us by
Tel   (800) 730-2214
Fax   (800) 730-2215
www.thomsonrights.com

Library of Congress Cataloging-in-Publication Data
White, Gary C., 1954–
    Basic clinical lab competencies for respiratory care: an integrated approach / Gary C. White.—4th ed.
        p. cm.
Includes bibliographical references and index.
ISBN 0-7668-2532-9 (soft cover)
    1. Respiratory therapy—Laboratory manuals.
    [DNLM: 1. Respiratory Therapy—methods—Examination Questions. 2. Respiratory Therapy—methods—Laboratory Manuals 3. Clinical Competence—standards—Examination Questions. 4. Clinical Competence—standards—Laboratory Manuals. WB 342 W584b 2003] I. Title.
RC735.15 W47 2003
615.8'36—dc21   2002004188

NOTICE TO THE READER

Publisher does not warrant or guarantee any of the products described herein or perform any independent analysis in connection with any of the product information contained herein. Publisher does not assume, and expressly disclaims, any obligation to obtain and include information other than that provided to it by the manufacturer.

The reader is expressly warned to consider and adopt all safety precautions that might be indicated by the activities herein and to avoid all potential hazards. By following the instructions contained herein, the reader willingly assumes all risks in connection with such instructions.

The Publisher makes no representation or warranties of any kind, including but not limited to, the warranties of fitness for particular purpose or merchantability, nor are any such representations implied with respect to the material set forth herein, and the Publisher takes no responsibility with respect to such material. The Publisher shall not be liable for any special, consequential, or exemplary damages resulting, in whole or part, from the reader's use of, or reliance upon, this material.

CONTENTS

LIST OF PERFORMANCE EVALUATIONS

DEDICATION

To my wife Carolyn and my two sons "A^2" Andrew (age 16) and Austin (age 12), who were often neglected in the preparation of this revision.

PREFACE

FOURTH EDITION

Basic Clinical Lab Competencies for Respiratory Care continues to be a very popular book in the discipline of respiratory care. The integration of theoretical knowledge and psychomotor skills is unique in a text of this type. The combination has proved to be very popular and has facilitated students' learning and retention of this material. The text is more than a laboratory manual. It reinforces the rationale for therapy, typically learned in a didactic class, and applies it to the laboratory or clinical setting.

The American Association for Respiratory Care has undertaken a significant and valuable project in the development and release of Clinical Practice Guidelines for the respiratory care discipline. These guidelines are included, where appropriate, throughout the text to further expand students' understanding of indications, contraindications, hazards and complications, and monitoring appropriate for the various procedures.

Existing chapters have been expanded and updated to reflect changes in the scope of practice. Many educators have suggested that additional topics and procedures be added to the new edition. Six new chapters have been added to help this text stay current with changes in the scope of clinical practice. New chapters include Radiologic Assessment, Documentation and Goals Assessment, Bronchial Hygiene Therapy, Chest Tubes, Noninvasive Positive-Pressure Ventilation, and Wave Form Analysis. Along with the new chapters, nine additional performance evaluations have been included in this edition.

The text has been divided into four major sections: Section I: Patient Assessment (Chapters 1–10); Section II: Therapeutics (Chapters 11–19); Section III: Emergency Management (Chapters 20–24); and Section IV: Ventilation (Chapters 25–29). These sections follow in a logical sequence, building from simple to complex skills and tasks. The division of the text into sections also facilitates the ease of finding specific procedures related to each section.

This text is designed to provide a concise, integrated approach to laboratory and clinical instruction. Its intent is to prepare the student rapidly for entry into the clinical setting. The content provides the student with the basis required for proficient and safe practice in the clinical setting. A student who possesses a foundation in basic skills may progress very quickly in the clinical setting, focusing on problem solving and modification of therapy.

Last, I have continued to listen to my own students and other students who use this text. Many individuals have shared with me how they enjoy the ability to read the book and understand it the first time. I have strived to maintain a student-friendly reading style with sound educational andragogy to assist the reader in the assimilation of this important subject material.

Gary C. White, MEd, RRT, RPFT

INTRODUCTION TO THE TEXT

The approach of this textbook is to integrate the theory and the psychomotor skills required to perform a therapeutic procedure safely and effectively. The theory concepts include the principles of equipment operation, troubleshooting, physiological effects, and hazards and complications of the therapeutic modality. Only by thoroughly understanding both aspects of a therapeutic modality can the student be flexible, adapting to changes in technology and patient management.

Begin by reading the introduction to the chapter you wish to study. Try to form an image in your mind, visualizing what is contained in the chapter.

Study the objectives. The objectives outline what you will be expected to know after you study the chapter. You will be held accountable for the knowledge on a written self-evaluation post test and a performance evaluation demonstrating the therapeutic modality. Refer to the objectives frequently as you study the chapter.

Read the theory portion of the text. If the equipment being discussed is available, keep it handy so you can refer to it as you read the text. Following the completion of the theory portion, study the theory objectives again. Ask yourself whether you understand every objective listed. If you do, take the self-evaluation post test to assess your knowledge.

Read the procedure portion of the text. Following completion of this section, perform the practice activities with a laboratory partner. Become familiar with all of the equipment. Understand how to set up, test, troubleshoot, and correctly apply all of the equipment discussed in the chapter.

With a laboratory partner, practice the check list for the chapter. Your partner may role-play the part of the patient while you perform the therapeutic modality. You will be expected to perform the skills on this check list during a performance evaluation conducted by your instructor. Practice the skills until they become second nature and flow smoothly from one step to the next.

Have one of your peers evaluate your skills using the performance evaluation and filling in the PEER column. When you are confident and prepared, have your instructor evaluate you.

ACKNOWLEDGMENTS

I would like to thank all of the educators who have provided input and suggestions as to how this book could continue to be improved. Many educators have spoken to me personally, telephoned, or written to me with comments, suggestions, and encouragement. The reviewers who painstakingly reviewed the third edition manuscript and offered further suggestions also contributed to the strengths of this new edition. The reviewers are:

Ann M. Allen, RRT
Clinical Coordinator
Respiratory Care
Piedmont Technical College
Greenwood, South Carolina

Lynn W. Capraun, MS, RRT
Program Director, Respiratory Care
Valencia Community College
Orlando, Florida

Ralph C. Lucki, MA, RRT
Professor and Program Director of Respiratory Care
West Virginia Northern Community College
Wheeling, West Virginia

Marcus Stowe, MS, RRT
Assistant Professor/Program Director
Respiratory Care
Ivy Tech State College
Indianapolis, Indiana

I would also like to thank my students. This book was written for you. Your suggestions and comments have continued to influence my writing and the many decisions that must be made whenever a new edition is produced.

I owe much to my wife, Carolyn, who has continued to support my technical writing efforts, now approaching nearly 20 years. Her support, encouragement, understanding, and occasional prodding are a big part of my success. Without her support, I would not be able to devote the time, energy, and effort required to produce a book such as this.

CONTRIBUTORS

David A. Field, RRT, RPFT
Perinatal/Pediatric Respiratory Care Specialist
Spokane Respiratory Consultants
Spokane, Washington

Kelly P. Jones, RRT
Perinatal/Pediatric Respiratory Care Specialist
Sacred Heart Medical Center
Spokane, Washington

Stephen S. Pitts, RRT, NREMT-P
Spokane Community College
Spokane, Washington

Darren Powell, RCVT
Instructor, Invasive Cardiovascular Technology
Spokane Community College
Spokane, Washington

CHAPTER 1
BASICS OF ASEPSIS

INTRODUCTION

The patient who is hospitalized is at increased risk for infection. The illness or surgery that has necessitated hospitalization frequently has weakened the body's natural defense mechanisms, and the hospital setting provides the perfect setting for the growth of many "super bugs," which are resistant to standard antimicrobial agents.

Health care workers are frequently the agents for contact transmission of microorganisims between patients. There is some risk to the hospital worker as well, particularly if personal health and resistance are not carefully maintained. The respiratory care practitioner may come in contact with many patients over the course of a day. It is essential for all health care workers to maintain an awareness of aseptic technique to protect themselves and the patient.

The incidence of nosocomial (hospital-acquired) infection is quite high. Such infections result in complications, extended hospital stays, and even death (Feingold, 1970). Through the practice of careful aseptic technique, the incidence of nosocomial infections can be reduced. Diseases such as hepatitis can put any hospital worker who has contact with secretions at risk for infection.

This chapter reviews the basic principles of infection transmission and simple techniques to prevent the spread of microorganisms.

KEY TERMS

- Airborne transmission
- Asepsis
- Contact transmission
- Cross-contamination
- Droplet transmission
- HEPA mask
- Pathogen
- Sterility
- Vector transmission
- Vehicle transmission
- Virulence

OBJECTIVES

At the end of this chapter, you should be able to:

- Define the following terms:
  — Asepsis
  — Sterile
  — Nosocomial
  — Cross-contamination
  — Infection
  — Microorganism
  — Pathogen
- Explain the following mechanisms of microorganism transmission:
  — Direct contact
  — Airborne transmission
  — Vehicle
  — Vector
- Explain the importance of handwashing and when handwashing should be performed.
- Explain the purpose of gloving and gowning.
- Understand the concept and purpose of universal blood and body fluid precautions:

  — Body fluids requiring precautions
  — Precaution measures recommended
  — Precautions to be taken for drawing blood
  — Safe practices of syringe handling
- Explain the purpose and indication for each of the following types of isolation, and describe the precautions and what procedures are required:
  — Strict
  — Contact
  — Airborne precautions
  — Droplet precautions
  — Tuberculosis isolation (acid-fast bacilli [AFB] isolation)
  — Enteric
  — Drainage/secretion
  — Blood/body fluid
- Explain what procedures may be used in the care of severely compromised patients and burn-injury patients.

Maintaining asepsis is an essential part of the practice of respiratory care. Before you can learn the various techniques and skills of asepsis, you must first review some basic concepts regarding microorganisms, infection, contamination, and how microorganisms are transmitted.

Microorganisms are microscopic life forms that are present in every environment. Some of the microorganisms are beneficial and others are not. Microorganisms that are capable of causing disease in humans are termed *pathogens*. Pathogenic microorganisms vary in *virulence*, or ability to cause disease. Some are more virulent than others.

The practice of asepsis is an attitude as well as a skill. As a practitioner, you must always remain aware of the microorganisms that exist in the environment. You must prevent transmission of microorganisms by handwashing, keeping dirty equipment and supplies in plastic bags while transporting them, keeping clean and dirty equipment physically separated, and many similar practices. Only by vigilance and using aseptic techniques can the incidence of nosocomial infections be reduced.

Asepsis

Asepsis is defined as the absence of disease-producing microorganisms. Microorganisms may include bacteria, mycoplasmas, fungi, and viruses. The concept of asepsis is generally distinguished from sterility. Total absence of disease-producing microorganisms, termed *sterility*, is difficult and expensive to sustain for a long period. Asepsis is adequate for much of the equipment and procedures in the hospital, except for so-called invasive procedures. Such procedures may adversely affect the body's natural protective defenses against infection. Respiratory care equipment is usually aseptic because it is too difficult and costly to keep sterile.

Sterility

Sterility is defined as the complete absence of all forms of microorganisms. In the hospital environment, it is not always necessary for items to be sterile. They need only be free of pathogens, or aseptic. The operating room, however, requires sterility, owing to the invasive nature of surgery.

It is difficult to obtain and maintain sterility. Instruments or other equipment that are required to be sterile must be able to withstand the rigors of the sterilization process. Sterilization is accomplished by the use of heat or chemical agents that destroy all microorganisms.

Nosocomial Infections

Nosocomial infections are hospital-acquired infections. That is, the patient acquires an infection while in the hospital and did not have the infection before hospital admission. Nosocomial infections result in countless complications, additional expenses, and deaths (Feingold, 1970).

Cross-contamination

Cross-contamination is the transmission of microorganisms between places or persons. Pathogens can be spread from an infected patient to a noninfected patient through mutual contact with health care personnel or with clinical equipment. For example, microorganisms can build up on frequently used items such as stethoscopes. Periodic cleansing of the diaphragm and bell of your stethoscope with alcohol or other antiseptic will help to prevent cross-contamination (Wilkens, 1990).

Pathogens

A *pathogen* is defined as a microorganism capable of causing disease in humans. A virulent organism is one that can produce disease very easily in many individuals. In addition to virulence, the ability of a pathogen to produce disease is dependent on the ability of the body to fight infection. Patients in the hospital are frequently infected by microorganisms not normally pathogenic to a person in good health. Many of these microorganisms are present in everyday environments but do not generally make healthy people ill because the body's defense mechanisms are adequate to prevent infection.

Microorganisms may exist in great numbers in the hospital. Patients in intensive care units (ICUs) are at risk from nearly any microorganism. Burn victims, for example, have such poor ability to resist infection that nearly everything entering their environment must be sterile. Patients receiving immunosuppressive drugs do not have the ability to resist infection and therefore are also at risk.

MICROORGANISM TRANSMISSION

Microorganisms can be transmitted in many ways. They may be transmitted by direct contact, by air currents, by vehicles, or by vectors.

Contact Transmission

Contact transmission is direct transmission of microorganisms via physical contact between one person and another. This method is the most common means of microorganism transmission and the most common cause of nosocomial infections. For example, a practitioner who has a cold or mild flu symptoms and who does not use proper handwashing technique may transmit pathogens to patients, or to other health care workers in contact with patients. Handwashing is an important way of minimizing this form of disease transmission. Limiting contact with potentially contaminated surfaces is also important. Do not sit on the patient's bed, lean on the bed rails, or lay your stethoscope on the bed or bedside table.

Airborne Transmission

Air currents can transport microorganisms from one area to another. Because these organisms are microscopic and very light, air currents may carry them for quite a distance. The bacterium that causes tuberculosis is commonly transmitted in this way. Patients requiring isolation should have the door closed. Laminar air flow (air flow without turbulence) in the ICU, emergency department, and surgery suite is intended to minimize *airborne transmission*.

Droplet Transmission

Droplet transmission of microorganisms is a form of contact transmission via droplets that are larger than 0.5 micrometer (μm). (This unit of measure was formerly called a micron.) Droplets of this size may be generated by coughing, sneezing, or talking or in performing procedures such as assisting with bronchoscopy, suctioning artificial airways, or changing a ventilator circuit. These droplets do not travel far or remain suspended for long; therefore, special rooms with laminar flow or negative pressure are not required.

Vehicle Transmission

Vehicle transmission is the transmission of microorganisms via inanimate objects. It may involve instruments, contaminated water or food, soil, or other objects. Vehicle transmission is important to recognize in respiratory care because some equipment may be used in the care of more than one patient. Examples of items implicated in vehicle transmission are portable respirometers, intermittent positive-pressure breathing (IPPB) equipment, ultrasonic nebulizers, and stethoscopes.

Vector Transmission

Vector transmission is not very common in the hospital. It involves an intermediate host. The host can be an insect, animal, or plant. One disease transmitted in this manner is Rocky Mountain spotted fever, which is carried by a tick.

CENTERS FOR DISEASE CONTROL AND PREVENTION GUIDELINES

The Centers for Disease Control and Prevention (CDC) has revised its isolation guidelines to synthesize elements from the previous two recommendations: *universal precautions* and *body substance isolation* (Garner & Hospital Infection Control Practices Committee, 1996). The new guidelines have been divided into two major parts: *standard precautions* and *transmission-based precautions*. These new guidelines are based on routes of transmission of microorganisms (airborne, droplet, and contact transmission) rather than disease-specific or body substance isolation as in the previous system of universal precautions and body substance isolation.

Standard Precautions

Use of standard precautions is strongly recommended for all hospitals (Centers for Disease Control, 1996). Standard precautions require that the health care worker make informed decisions about the likelihood of coming into contact with moist body fluids. On the basis of this knowledge, the health care worker must then decide which infection control procedures are most appropriate for the immediate situation. Standard precautions include guidelines for handwashing; the use of gloves, mask, eye protection (or face shield), and gown; for handling of patient care equipment, patients' linens, sharps, and mask to mouth ventilation devices; and for patient placement.

Importance of Handwashing

Handwashing is the most important way to prevent the transmission of microorganisms via the contact route of transmission. Different techniques may be used in various areas of the hospital. You should wash your hands thoroughly when you arrive at the hospital for work.

The 30-second scrub is the most common handwashing protocol used in the hospital setting. It is performed between patients, before preparing medications, before and after eating, and after contact with contaminated equipment. It is also performed after use of the rest room and any other time the hands come in contact with body secre-

tions. Even when wearing gloves, discard the gloves following patient or body fluid contact and wash your hands.

The 10-minute scrub is performed prior to surgery and before entry into specialized areas such as the newborn ICU or burn unit. It may also be required before working with particularly high-risk patients. The arms from the elbow down are scrubbed, as are the wrists and hands. In the surgery suite, sterile towels are used to dry the hands. The hands are then immediately inserted into sterile gloves.

The 3-minute scrub should be performed on arriving at work in the hospital and on leaving the facility at the end of the day. The lower forearms, wrists, and hands are thoroughly scrubbed.

Use of Gloves

The use of disposable gloves (latex or vinyl) is advised when procedures necessitate contact with blood, body fluids, secretions, and excretions and contaminated items. Gloves should also be worn before contact with mucous membranes or broken or nonintact skin. If you come in contact with a patient's body fluids, change gloves between tasks or procedures when working with the same patient. This measure will help to prevent the spread of microorganisms via the contact route of transmission. Prior to touching other surfaces in the room (environmental surfaces), patient care equipment, and other noncontaminated items, remove your gloves and wash your hands. Always remove your gloves and properly dispose of them, washing your hands between patients. If you have a latex allergy, hypoallergenic gloves are available.

Use of Mask, Eye Protection, or Face Shield

When you as a health care provider believe that you may be at risk for being splashed or sprayed by blood, body fluids, secretions, or excretions, you should protect your mouth and eyes with a mask and goggles or a face shield. The combination of a mask and eye protection (goggles with side shields) will prevent body fluids from splashing or spraying your mouth and eyes. A face shield serves the same purpose, only it covers both the mouth and eyes as one barrier device, rather than two. In the practice of respiratory care, you are at risk for this event during trauma resuscitation, airway aspiration, ventilator circuit changes, and bronchoscopy assisting.

Use of a Cover Gown

The use of a cover gown is indicated to protect your skin and soiling of your clothing during procedures or patient care situations that may produce splashes or sprays of blood, body fluids, secretions, or excretions. In some cases, a disposable paper gown is adequate for protection. Other situations (bronchoscopy assisting and trauma resuscitation) may require a waterproof gown. As soon as practicable following the procedure or patient care, properly dispose of the gown and wash your hands to prevent the spread of microorganisms via the contact transmission route.

Handling of Patient Care Equipment

Handling patient care equipment soiled with blood, body fluids, secretions, or excretions requires the same precautions as patient care situations in which you may come in contact with these secretions. The use of gloves is required, and mask/eye protection and use of a cover gown may also be required if you determine that you may be splashed or sprayed. All permanent equipment soiled with body fluids should be decontaminated with appropriate cleaning products prior to use in the care of another patient. All disposable equipment should be properly disposed of and handled with other contaminated waste.

Handling of Patient Linen

Linen supplies used in the care of patients that have been soiled by blood, body fluids, secretions, or excretions should be handled in a way that prevents contact with your skin, mucous membranes, and clothing. This requires the use of gloves and may also require the use of a cover gown and mouth and eye protection if the linens are heavily soiled.

Sharps Precautions

The use of sharps—needles, scalpels, and other sharp instruments—requires special care and handling to prevent skin punctures when you handle them following patient use. Special puncture-proof containers are provided for the disposal of these items. Do not ever attempt to recap a needle—this is the most frequent cause of needle sticks.

Do not attempt to remove discarded needles or syringes from sharps containers or attempt to force a needle or sharp instrument into an already full container. Exercising caution and common sense will prevent you from injuring yourself with a sharp instrument already contaminated with a patient's blood or body fluids.

Use of Mask to Mouth Ventilation Devices

Mask to mouth ventilation devices are designed to allow a rescuer to perform pulmonary resuscitation without direct contact with the patient's mucous membranes (Figure 1-1). The mask to mouth device provides a barrier between the patient and the caregiver. The availability of these devices is warranted in any area where resuscitation may be predicted or imminent.

Specific Transmission Precautions

Use of transmission precautions is recommended to address specifically the prevention of microorganism transmission via the various routes. These routes include airborne, droplet, and contact transmission.

Airborne Transmission

Airborne transmission involves microorganism transmission via small aerosolized particles of 5 μm or smaller in size. In addition to the standard precautions described previously, the following precautions are also recommended.

Patient Placement. The patient should be placed in a private room with negative air pressure (relative to ambient pressure and the surrounding environment) and undergoing at least 6 to 12 air changes per hour. The door should remain closed at all times. If another patient is infected with the same microorganism and has no other infections, two patients may be placed in the same room (a practice termed *cohorting*).

This precaution is most commonly employed in the care of patients who have *mycobacterium tuberculosis*. Other diseases placed into this category include varicella and measles.

Respiratory Protection. Caregivers entering the patient's room should wear additional respiratory protection consisting of a high efficiency particulate air mask (*HEPA mask*) approved by the Occupational Safety and

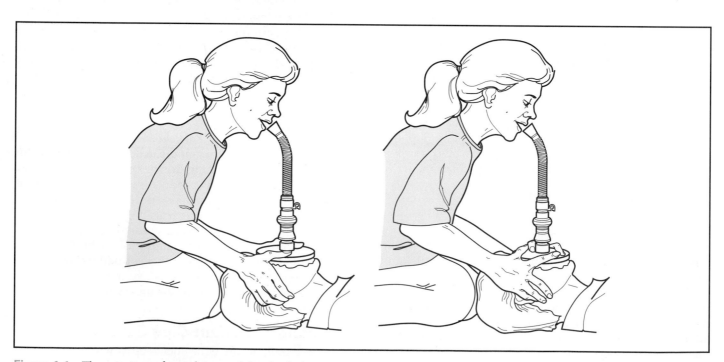

Figure 1-1   *The correct use of a mask to mouth barrier device*

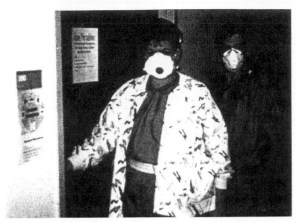
Figure 1-2 *Two different types of HEPA filter masks*

Health Administration (OSHA) (Figure 1-2) or other OSHA-approved respiratory filtration device.

Health care providers who are immune to varicella and measles may enter the hospital room without wearing HEPA protection when caring for patients infected with these conditions.

Patient Transport. Avoid transporting patients who are infected with TB, varicella, and measles within the hospital unless for specific essential purposes only. During transport, have the patient wear a simple surgical mask or a HEPA mask. This will help to prevent the transmission of droplet nuclei.

Droplet Precautions

Droplet precautions are precautions taken when transmission of microorganisms by droplets larger than 5 µm is likely. Droplets of this size can be generated by sneezing, coughing, or talking or in the performance of patient care procedures including bronchoscopy, suctioning, and ventilator circuit changes.

Patient Placement. The patient should be placed in a private room. The door should remain closed at all times. If another patient is infected with the same microorganism and has no other infections, two patients may be placed in the same room (cohorting).

Respiratory Protection. Caregivers who enter the patient's room should wear a mask when working within 3 feet of the patient. In some clinical facilities, all personnel who enter the patient's room may be required to wear a mask for all practical purposes, rather than strictly adhering to the 3-foot distance recommendation.

Patient Transport. Avoid transporting patients who are confined with droplet precautions within the hospital unless for specific essential purposes only. During transport, have the patient wear a simple surgical mask. This is sufficient to prevent the spread of droplets.

Contact Precautions

Contact precautions are employed when transmission of pathogenic microorganisms is likely through direct patient contact. Direct contact could occur through wound care, skin contact, contact with environmental surfaces, or patient care items in the patient's room.

Patient Placement. The patient should be placed in a private room. If another patient is infected with the same microorganism and has no other infections, two patients may be placed in the same room (cohorting).

Gloves and Handwashing. The use of gloves for patient contact is required. As discussed earlier, changing gloves between procedures on the same patient and before leaving the patient's room is required. Thorough handwashing should be performed when you enter and leave the patient's room. The use of antimicrobial agents or a waterless antiseptic agent is advised.

Use of a Gown. You should wear a cover gown if you anticipate that your clothing may have substantial contact with the patient, the patient care equipment (soiled), or other soiled environmental surfaces. The gown should be properly disposed of before you leave the patient's room.

Patient Transport. Transport of the patient within the hospital should be limited to essential purposes only. During transport, exercise caution such that contact transmission is minimized to other patients or environmental surfaces.

Patient Care Equipment. Permanent equipment should be dedicated to the care of patients confined by contact precautions. Avoid sharing equipment between patients. It is important to properly disinfect equipment after removing it from the patient's room and before using it for other patients.

OBJECTIVES

At the end of this chapter, you should be able to:
* Demonstrate the technique used for a 3-minute handwashing protocol.
* Demonstrate how to glove and gown for isolation, including the following:
  — Wash hands.
  — Apply cap to cover hair.
  — Apply mask covering mouth and nose.
  — Correctly apply gown.
* Demonstrate how to aseptically apply surgical gloves.
* Demonstrate how to aseptically double-bag equipment being removed from isolation.
* Demonstrate how to remove gloves, cap, mask, and gown when leaving isolation.

HANDWASHING

As discussed in the theory portion of this chapter, handwashing is essential in the prevention of the transmission of microorganisms. Like other procedures in respiratory care, handwashing requires a special technique. There is a correct way to do it.

Remove Jewelry, Including Your Watch

Jewelry has small crevices that can harbor microorganisms. Sweat, dead skin, and dirt combine with a warm semimoist environment to facilitate microbial growth. Removal of jewelry and watches will enable you to thoroughly wash your hands and wrists.

Never Contact the Sink with Your Hands or Body

Moisture or water is one of the requirements for microbial growth; therefore, the sink provides an excellent area for microbial growth. In many hospitals, a variety of bacteria may be cultured from the sinks on a regular basis. *Pseudomonas aeruginosa* is a common microorganism found in the vicinity of sinks (Johnson, 1982). Transmission may result from contact with your hands or clothing. *P. aeruginosa* may be a virulent pathogen for debilitated patients in ICUs.

Adjust the Water Flow and Temperature

Adjust the water flow and temperature prior to actually washing your hands. Warm or cold water is better than hot water. The hot water is not hot enough to kill pathogens anyway, and tends to open the pores of your skin, facilitating removal of the skin's oil. Use of hot water leads to chapped skin much more quickly than use of warm or cool water. Chapped skin, which cracks, allows for bacterial growth and infection. Adjust the flow so that it is brisk but not strong enough to cause splashing.

Wet Your Forearms, Wrists, and Hands

Hold your hands under the running water with the forearms more elevated than the fingertips. The fingers are considered to be the most contaminated, while the arms are less contaminated. Water should flow from the clean to the dirty area.

Liberally Apply Soap

Always use liquid soap from the dispenser. Special disinfectant soap is provided in the hospital. The exception is in specialty areas, such as the newborn ICU or a surgical suite, where individual disposable scrub pads are used. Never use bar soap, particularly if it is sitting in a puddle of water. Bar soap may harbor microorganisms.

Wash Palms with Strong Friction

Soap, friction, and running water are the keys to removal of microorganisms. Begin by rubbing the palms and backs of the hands, thoroughly cleaning the area.

Wash between the Fingers

Fingers may be washed individually or may be interlaced, creating sufficient friction. Be sure to clean the interdigital spaces and the knuckles.

Wash the Wrists with a Rotary Motion

The rotary motion ensures thorough cleansing due to friction.

Scrub under the Nails and around the Cuticles

Ideally, nails should be kept short and free of polish to facilitate thorough cleansing. The nails and nailbeds provide another good environment for microbial growth. Use a nail brush to completely clean under the fingernails. The same instrument may be gently applied to the cuticle area.

Rinse Hands without Touching the Sink

Rinse your hands using the same technique as you used when you first wet them.

Obtain Towels Aseptically

Carefully remove the disposable paper towels from the dispenser without contacting it with your hands. Most hospital dispensers are designed so that aseptic removal is possible.

Dry Your Hands Using Separate Towels

Dry your hands from the wrist or forearm toward the fingertips. Use a clean towel for each hand.

Turn Off the Water with a Clean, Dry Towel

When you have finished, use a clean, dry towel to handle the faucet when turning off the water flow. Obtain several more towels and aseptically clean up any splashes in the vicinity.

ASEPTIC GOWNING

Gowning may be required before entering certain isolation situations. It is important to know how to apply and remove isolation clothing. Isolation attire should not be worn anywhere other than in the patient's room. Be sure to assemble all needed supplies before preparing to enter the room.

Application of the Cap and Mask

The purpose of the cap is to contain hair, dust, and microorganisms and prevent their distribution in the room as well as to prevent contamination of your hair by dust and microorganisms. The cap is applied first. Cover all of your hair completely. If long hair requires manipulation to insert it into the cap, wash your hands again for 30 seconds after applying the cap.

Apply the mask over your nose and mouth with the strap behind the neck. If an adjustable bridge piece is provided, adjust it to the contours of your nose by pinching the mask.

Once the mask becomes saturated with moisture from your exhaled air, it is no longer effective and should be changed. Never reuse a mask.

Application of the Gown

Begin by grasping the gown by the neck and unrolling or unfolding it at arm's length, or by removing it from its hanger or hook. Insert your hands into the sleeves and pull them through the cuffs without contacting the outside of the gown (Figure 1-3).

Fasten the tie at the neck. Use a bow knot to facilitate the removal of the gown later.

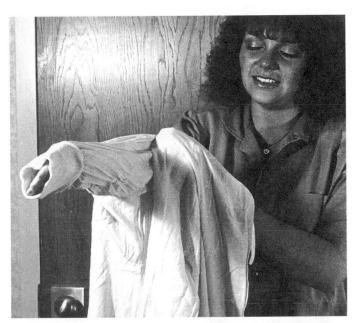

Figure 1-3 *Applying an isolation gown*

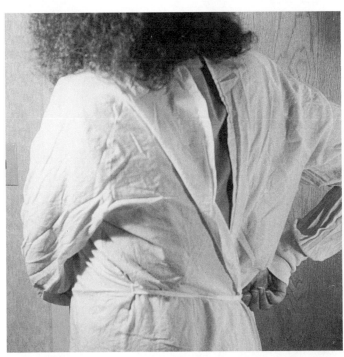

Figure 1-4 *Closing the back of an isolation gown*

Close the gown completely in the back and fasten the waist tie (Figure 1-4). Again, the use of a bow knot will simplify removal later. The back is considered dirty, as well as those areas below the waist.

ASEPTIC APPLICATION OF SURGICAL LATEX GLOVES

Open the Package, Forming a Sterile Field

Open the package lengthwise and open the inner package by grasping the flaps and folding it flat (Figure 1-5).

Aseptically Apply the Gloves

Begin by picking up one glove by the cuff, touching only the surface that will contact the skin when the cuff is turned back. Insert your hand into the glove, taking care to properly align the thumb and fingers.

Grasp the other glove with your gloved hand, only touching the outside surface. This can be done by slipping your gloved fingers between the rolled cuff and the glove (Figure 1-6). Insert your hand into the glove, aligning your thumb and fingers. If minor adjustments are required in the fingers, you may make them now by gently manipulating the gloves.

Remember that touching *anything* with the gloves defeats their purpose.

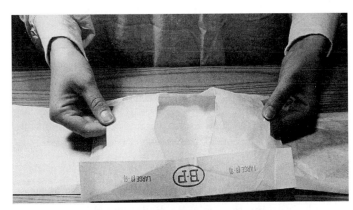

Figure 1-5 *Opening a sterile glove package*

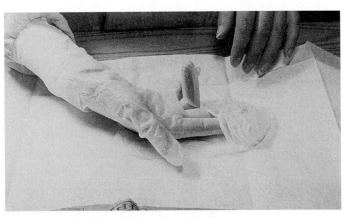

Figure 1-6 *Applying the second sterile glove*

DOUBLE-BAGGING OF EQUIPMENT AND SUPPLIES

All equipment and supplies leaving an isolation area must be double-bagged in nonporous plastic bags. The equipment is first bagged inside the room by a person in isolation attire. A second person then opens a separate bag outside the room. The person in isolation attire drops the bagged equipment or supplies into the second bag without touching it. The second person then ties off the second bag and removes it to the appropriate decontamination area. The bag should be labeled, showing that it is from an isolation area, the contents, the patient's name, and the room number. Labeling may vary from one institution to another and adherence to local policies should be observed.

ASEPTIC REMOVAL OF ISOLATION ATTIRE

Aseptic removal of isolation attire is just as important as aseptical application. The clothing may be removed inside or outside the room, depending on the type of isolation. Strict and contact isolation necessitates the removal of the attire inside of the patient's room. If removal is done improperly, contact transmission is possible. Used isolation attire should not be reused.

Removal of Cap and Mask

The cap and mask are removed first. Under some circumstances (such as isolation for virulent respiratory infection), it may be desirable to remove the cap and mask last. Remove these without touching your hair or face with your gloved hands.

Remove Your Gloves

Gloves are easily removed by grasping the cuff and turning them inside out. Do not touch your skin when removing your gloves. The second glove may be removed over the first, and then both may be discarded together.

Remove the Gown

Begin by untying the waist tie. Following this, wash your hands. The area from the waist down is considered dirty.

Untie the neck tie and shrug your shoulders forward so that the gown slips off your body down your arms. Insert one index finger between the cuff and your wrist and pull your hand inside the sleeve. With your hand inside the one sleeve, remove the other sleeve (Figure 1-7).

Allow the gown to slip down so that it can be grasped inside at the neck of the gown. Fold the gown inside out and dispose of it appropriately.

Handwashing

Wash your hands inside the room for 30 seconds before leaving. Outside of the room, wash your hands for 3 minutes before seeing other patients.

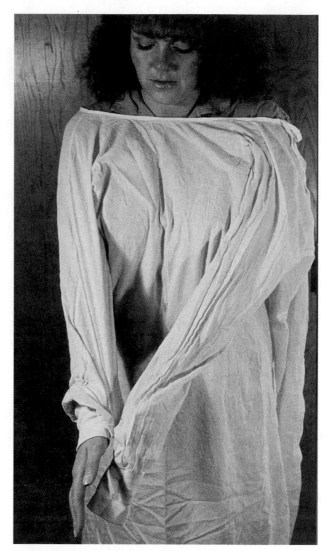

Figure 1-7 *Removing an isolation gown aseptically*

References

Centers for Disease Control. (1996). *Guideline for isolation precautions in hospitals.* Atlanta: Author.

Feingold, D. S. (1970). Hospital acquired infections. *New England Journal of Medicine, 283,* 1384–1391.

Garner, J. S., & the Hospital Infection Control Practices Committee. (1996). Guideline for isolation precautions in hospitals. *American Journal of Infection Control, 24*(2), 24–52.

Johnson, W. G. (1982). Infectious complications of respiratory therapy. *Respiratory Care, 27*(4), 445–452.

Wilkens, R. L. (1990). *Clinical assessment in respiratory care.* St. Louis, MO: Mosby.

Additional Resources

Eubanks, D. H., & Bone, R. C. (1991). *Comprehensive respiratory care* (2nd ed.). St. Louis, MO: Mosby.

Garner, J. S., & Simmons, B. P. (1983). *CDC guideline for isolation precautions in hospitals.* Atlanta: Centers for Disease Control.

Kozier, B., Erb, G. L., & Marcus, W. (1983). *Fundamentals of nursing concepts and procedures* (2nd ed.). Reading, MA: Addison-Wesley.

Practice Activities: Basics of Asepsis

1. Practice washing your hands for the 3-minute scrub. Include the following in your practice:
   a. Remove jewelry and watch.
   b. Adjust water flow and temperature.
   c. Wet forearms and hands.
   d. Apply soap liberally.
   e. Wash the following with strong friction:
      (1) Palms
      (2) Between digits
      (3) Under fingernails and around cuticles
   f. Wash for the appropriate length of time.
   g. Never touch the sink with your hands or body.
   h. Rinse from the forearm to the fingertips.
   i. Obtain towels aseptically.
   j. Dry hands individually using separate towels.
   k. Turn off water using a clean dry towel.

2. Practice applying and removing an isolation cap, mask, and gown. Include the following in your practice:
   a. Wash your hands.
   b. Apply cap covering all of your hair.
      (1) If required, wash your hands again.
   c. Apply a mask covering your nose and mouth.
   d. Apply the gown.
      (1) Pick it up by the neck.
      (2) Place the hands inside sleeves and slip the hands through the cuffs.
      (3) Fasten the neck tie.
      (4) Close the back and fasten the waist tie.

3. While wearing an isolation cap, mask, and gown, practice applying sterile gloves. Include the following in your practice:
   a. Open the package, creating a sterile field.
   b. Pick up the first glove by the inside of the cuff.
   c. Slip your hand into the glove, aligning your fingers and thumb.
   d. Pick up second glove by sliding your gloved fingertips under the turned cuff.
   e. Slip your other hand into the glove.
   f. Adjust the fingers as required.

4. Practice removing isolation attire aseptically:
   a. Remove cap and mask.
   b. Remove and discard gloves appropriately.
   c. Untie waist tie on the gown.
   d. Wash your hands.
   e. Untie the neck tie.
   f. Slip gown off your shoulders.
   g. Slip a finger between cuff and your wrist and pull sleeve partially off.
   h. Using sleeve as protection, pull other sleeve off.
   i. Fold gown inside out and dispose of it properly.

5. Practice double-bagging equipment or supplies with a laboratory partner.

Check List: Basics of Asepsis

HANDWASHING

_____ 1. Remove jewelry and watch.
_____ 2. Adjust the water flow and temperature.
_____ 3. Wet your forearms and hands.
_____ 4. Apply disinfectant soap liberally.
5. Wash the following with strong friction:
_____ a. Palms
_____ b. Between digits
_____ c. Under fingernails and around cuticles
_____ 6. Wash for the appropriate length of time.
_____ 7. Never touch the sink with your hands or body.
_____ 8. Rinse from the forearm to the fingertips.
_____ 9. Obtain towels aseptically.
_____ 10. Dry hands individually using separate towels.
_____ 11. Turn off the water using a clean, dry towel.

ISOLATION PROCEDURES

_____ 1. Wash your hands.
2. Apply a cap covering all of your hair.
_____ a. If required, wash your hands again.
3. Apply a mask covering your nose and mouth.
4. Apply the gown:
_____ a. Pick it up by the neck.
_____ b. Place your hands inside sleeves and slip your hands through the cuffs.
_____ c. Fasten the neck tie.
_____ d. Close the back and fasten the waist tie.
5. Apply the sterile gloves aseptically:
_____ a. Open the package, creating a sterile field.
_____ b. Pick up the first glove by the inside of the cuff.

_____ c. Slip your hand into the glove, aligning your fingers and thumb.

_____ d. Pick up the second glove by sliding your gloved fingertips under the turned cuff.

_____ e. Slip your other hand into the glove.

_____ f. Adjust the finger as required.

_____ 6. Double-bag equipment and supplies with a laboratory partner for removal from isolation.

7. Remove isolation attire aseptically:

_____ a. Remove the cap and mask.

_____ b. Remove and discard the gloves appropriately.

_____ c. Untie the waist tie on the gown.

_____ d. Wash your hands.

_____ e. Untie the neck tie.

_____ f. Slip the gown off your shoulders.

_____ g. Slip a finger between the cuff and your wrist and pull the sleeve partially off.

_____ h. Using the sleeve as protection, pull the other sleeve off.

_____ i. Fold the gown inside out and dispose of it properly.

_____ 8. Wash your hands before leaving the room.

_____ 9. Wash your hands again after leaving the room.

Self-Evaluation Post Test: Basics of Asepsis

1. Asepsis is defined as:
   a. the absence of all living things.
   b. the absence of disease-producing microorganisms.
   c. the absence of all forms of microorganisms.
   d. the absence of viruses.

2. Sterility is defined as:
   a. the absence of all living things.
   b. the absence of disease-producing microorganisms.
   c. the absence of all forms of microorganisms.
   d. the absence of viruses.

3. A disease may be transmitted from one patient to another by a health care practitioner. This mode of disease spread is termed:
   a. septic.
   b. contamination.
   c. vector transmission.
   d. cross-contamination.

4. A microorganism capable of producing disease in humans is termed a(n):
   a. bacterium.
   b. virus.
   c. pathogen.
   d. infection.

5. Nosocomial infections are _____ infections.
   a. community-acquired
   b. hospital-acquired
   c. nasally introduced
   d. medication-related

6. Airborne transmission precautions include which of the following?
   I. Donning a HEPA mask on entering the room
   II. Placement of patient in private room with negative pressure or laminar air flow
   III. Use of gloves
   IV. Handwashing before entering and after leaving the patient's room
   a. I
   b. I, II
   c. I, II, III
   d. I, II, III, IV

7. Microorganism transmission may occur by:
   I. contact transmission.
   II. airborne transmission.
   III. resistance transmission.
   IV. vehicle transmission.
   V. vector transmission.
   a. I, II, III, IV
   b. II, III, IV, V
   c. I, II, IV, V
   d. III, IV, V

8. When working with nonisolated patients, you should wash your hands for _____ between patients.
   a. 30 seconds
   b. 1 minute
   c. 2 minutes
   d. 3 minutes

9. Standard precautions should be employed:
   a. for all health care providers working with patients.
   b. only when you are touching the patient.
   c. only by a nurse who remains in the room for extended time periods.
   d. by physicians only.
   e. by the respiratory care practitioner.

10. Droplet transmission requires:
    I. a private room for the patient.
    II. use of a filter mask for working within 3 feet of the patient.
    III. use of gloves
    IV. use of a protective gown if soiling of clothing is likely.
    a. I
    b. I, II
    c. I, II, III
    d. I, II, III, IV

PERFORMANCE EVALUATION: HANDWASHING

Date: Lab _____ Clinical _____ Agency _____

Lab: Pass _____ Fail _____   Clinical: Pass _____ Fail _____

Student name _____ Instructor name _____

No. of times observed in clinical _____

No. of times practiced in clinical _____

PASSING CRITERIA: Obtain 90% or better on the procedure. Tasks indicated by * must receive at least 1 point, or the evaluation is terminated. Procedure must be performed within designated time, or the performance receives a failing grade.

SCORING:
2 points — Task performed satisfactorily without prompting.
1 point — Task performed satisfactorily with self-initiated correction.
0 points — Task performed incorrectly or with prompting required.
NA — Task not applicable to the patient care situation.

TASKS:			PEER	LAB	CLINICAL
*	1.	Removes jewelry and watch	☐	☐	☐
*	2.	Does not contact the sink with clothing or body	☐	☐	☐
	3.	Adjusts the water flow and temperature	☐	☐	☐
	4.	Wets forearms and hands thoroughly	☐	☐	☐
*	5.	Applies soap liberally	☐	☐	☐
	6.	Washes hands with strong friction			
*		a. Palms	☐	☐	☐
*		b. Wrists	☐	☐	☐
*		c. Between fingers	☐	☐	☐
*		d. Under nails and around cuticles	☐	☐	☐
*	7.	Washes for appropriate length of time	☐	☐	☐
*	8.	Does not touch faucets, sides, or bottom of sink with hands or fingers	☐	☐	☐
*	9.	Rinses thoroughly from wrists to fingertips	☐	☐	☐
*	10.	Obtains paper towels without contaminating hands	☐	☐	☐
*	11.	Dries hands and wrists thoroughly using a separate towel for each, drying from wrists to fingertips	☐	☐	☐
*	12.	Turns off water with clean, dry paper towel	☐	☐	☐

SCORE:
Peak   Peer   _____ points of possible 30; _____%

Lab   _____ points of possible 30; _____%

Clinical   _____ points of possible 30; _____%

TIME: _____ out of possible 5 minutes

STUDENT SIGNATURES   INSTRUCTOR SIGNATURES

PEER: _____   LAB: _____

STUDENT: _____   CLINICAL: _____

PERFORMANCE EVALUATION: ISOLATION PROCEDURES

Date: Lab _____ Clinical _____ Agency _____

Lab: Pass _____ Fail _____   Clinical: Pass _____ Fail _____

Student name _____ Instructor name _____

No. of times observed in clinical _____

No. of times practiced in clinical _____

PASSING CRITERIA: Obtain 90% or better on the procedure. Tasks indicated by * must receive at least 1 point, or the evaluation is terminated. Procedure must be performed within designated time, or the performance receives a failing grade.

SCORING:
2 points — Task performed satisfactorily without prompting.
1 point — Task performed satisfactorily with self-initiated correction.
0 points — Task performed incorrectly or with prompting required.
NA — Task not applicable to the patient care situation.

TASKS:		PEER	LAB	CLINICAL
*	1. Obtains appropriate apparel	☐	☐	☐
	2. Washes hands	☐	☐	☐
*	3. Applies mask and cap, covering hair	☐	☐	☐
	4. Washes hands again if required	☐	☐	☐
	5. Aseptically applies gown			
	a. Picks up gown at the neck	☐	☐	☐
	b. Places hands inside sleeves, working hands through the cuffs	☐	☐	☐
	c. Fastens the ties at the neck	☐	☐	☐
	d. Closes gown in the back, tying waist ties	☐	☐	☐
	6. Aseptically applies sterile gloves			
*	a. Opens the package without contamination, forming a sterile field	☐	☐	☐
*	b. Picks up the first glove by the inside of the turned cuff, sliding hand in	☐	☐	☐
*	c. Picks up the second glove by sliding the gloved fingers under the turned cuff	☐	☐	☐
*	d. Applies the second glove	☐	☐	☐
	7. Enters the room and removes the articles by double-bagging	☐	☐	☐
	8. Removes isolation attire before leaving			
*	a. Removes cap and mask	☐	☐	☐
*	b. Removes gloves, turning them inside out	☐	☐	☐
	c. Unties the waist of the gown	☐	☐	☐
	d. Washes hands	☐	☐	☐
	e. Removes gown by			
	(1) Untying neck	☐	☐	☐

         (2) Pulling one sleeve off by reaching inside the cuff
               with a finger

         (3) Using one hand inside the sleeve to pull off second sleeve

         (4) Folding the gown inside out

         (5) Disposing of the gown appropriately

*   9. Washes hands before leaving room

*   10. Washes hands again outside the room

SCORE: Peer   _____ points of possible 48; _____%

              Lab   _____ points of possible 48; _____%

              Clinical   _____ points of possible 48; _____%

TIME: _____ out of possible 5 minutes

STUDENT SIGNATURES

PEER: _____

STUDENT: _____

INSTRUCTOR SIGNATURES

LAB: _____

CLINICAL: _____

CHAPTER 2
BASIC PATIENT ASSESSMENT: VITAL SIGNS AND BREATH SOUNDS

INTRODUCTION

Basic patient assessment is an important aspect of respiratory care. The basic assessment skills—taking vital signs and auscultating breath sounds—provide clinical means for the examination and diagnosis of the patient. Frequently, these skills are utilized to measure the effects of medication or therapy being administered. These skills are easily learned and require little practice to maintain proficiency.

In this chapter you will learn the significance of the various vital signs and how to measure them, normals, and causes of abnormal findings. You will also learn the theory of sound, the construction and use of the stethoscope, the various breath sounds and how they are produced, and how to auscultate the chest in a systematic way.

KEY TERMS

- Abnormal breath sounds
- Auscultation
- Bradycardia
- Bradypnea
- Diastolic
- Hypertension
- Hyperthermia
- Hypotension
- Hypothermia
- Normal breath sounds
- Systolic
- Tachycardia
- Tachypnea

OBJECTIVES

At the end of this chapter, you should be able to:

VITAL SIGNS
- Explain the significance of measuring body temperature.
- State the normal temperature range, in degrees Fahrenheit and Celsius, for adults and for children.
- List the causes of an abnormal body temperature.
- Explain the significance of the pulse and give the normal range for adults and for children.
- List the causes of an abnormal pulse.
- Explain what is meant by *rhythm* and *strength* of the pulse.
- Describe the significance of the respiratory rate and give the normal rate for adults and for children.
- Explain what is meant by the terms *tachypnea* and *bradypnea*.
- Describe the various factors that influence blood pressure:
  — Pumping action of the heart
  — Resistance in the cardiovascular system
  — Elasticity of the vessel walls
  — Viscosity of the blood
- Describe what is meant by the terms *systolic blood pressure* and *diastolic blood pressure*.
- State the normal ranges for blood pressure.
- List the following causes of abnormal blood pressure:
  — Hypertension
    — Cardiovascular disorders
    — Hormonal imbalance
    — Exercise

    — Stimulants
    — Emotional stress
  — Hypotension
    — Shock
      Hormonal imbalance
    — Depressants

SOUND GENERATION
- Define *sound* and identify its characteristics and physical properties.
- Explain how density affects sound conduction and transmission.

STETHOSCOPES
- Identify the two most common types of stethoscopes and their advantages and disadvantages:
  — Sprague–Rappaport stethoscope
  — Single tube stethoscope
- Discuss the importance of proper earpiece fit when using the stethoscope.

BREATH SOUNDS
- Identify the following four major classifications of normal breath sounds and their characteristics, location, and relevant theory of sound production.
  — Vesicular
  — Bronchial
  — Bronchovesicular
  — Tracheal
- Discuss the importance of a systematic method of auscultating the chest.

(Continued)

- Describe and identify the anatomical landmarks used in auscultating the chest.
- Explain the importance of proper patient positioning for auscultation and under what circumstances the optimal positioning may be modified.
- For the following abnormal breath sounds, describe their characteristics, duration, and relevant theory of sound production:
  — Crackles
  — Wheezes
  — Rhonchi
  — Pleural rub

BODY TEMPERATURE

The body, when in a normal state of balance between heat production and heat loss, is often referred to as being homeostatic. The normal metabolic heat-producing process is controlled primarily by the hypothalamus in the brain. The hypothalamus, when regulating temperature by controlling the sympathetic nervous system, causes vasoconstriction or dilation, sweating, shivering, and the production of epinephrine and norepinephrine.

The normal temperature range for adults is 96.0 to 99.5°F, equivalent to 35.5 to 37.5°C. The normal values for both temperature scales are 98.6°F and 37.0°C, respectively.

Children have a slightly faster metabolic rate than adults, causing their temperature to be slightly higher. The temperature in a newborn ranges from 36.1 to 37.7°C, or 97 to 99.9°F. A newborn's temperature regulation mechanism is not fully developed, allowing the temperature to fluctuate in response to the environment more than in an adult. A normal temperature of a 2-year-old should be about 37.2°C, or 98.9°F. A child's temperature will not be fully regulated until puberty, at which time it will be the same as an adult's.

Abnormal Body Temperature

An abnormally low body temperature is termed *hypothermia* and an abnormally high body temperature is termed *hyperthermia*. Abnormalities in body temperature may be caused by many different factors. Table 2-1 is a listing of some of the causes of an abnormal body temperature.

TABLE 2-1: Causes of an Abnormal Body Temperature

CONDITION	CAUSES
Hypothermia	Exposure Increased heat loss Diaphoresis Blood loss Hypothalamus injury Hormonal imbalance
Hyperthermia	Increased environmental temperature Decreased heat loss (clothing) Drug or medication reaction Hormonal imbalance Infection/illness

PULSE

The pulse is a direct indicator of the heart's actions. The pulse rate is an indication of the heart rate. The pulse rhythm is an indicator of the heart's rhythm, and its contour reflects the characteristics of the heart ejecting blood, blood pressure, and the presence of aortic stenosis.

The normal heart rate for adults ranges from 60 to 90 beats per minute. Children's pulses range from 90 to 120 beats per minute.

Abnormal Heart Rates

An abnormally low heart rate is termed *bradycardia* and an abnormally high heart rate is termed *tachycardia*. Several disorders or conditions may cause an abnormal heart rate. Table 2-2 is a partial listing of the causes of bradycardia and tachycardia.

Rhythm

The rhythm is the regularity of the heartbeat. Normally, the heartbeat is regular and rhythmic. Abnormalities in the rhythm may result from cardiac arrhythmias or changes in the vascular system affecting blood flow.

Two types of altered pulse rhythms are a bounding pulse and a plateau pulse. With a bounding pulse, there are both a rapid upstroke and a rapid downstroke, with a maximum point of intensity between them (Figure 2-1). This may be caused by an abnormally high blood pressure (hypertension) or exercise.

With a plateau pulse, there are both a gradual upstroke and a gradual downstroke, as illustrated in Figure 2-2. This may be caused by aortic stenosis, which is a narrowing of the aorta that causes a decrease in blood flow.

TABLE 2-2: Causes of Bradycardia and Tachycardia

CONDITION	CAUSES
Bradycardia	Hypothermia Infection Heart abnormalities Depressant drugs
Tachycardia	Hypoxemia Fever Emotional stress Heart abnormalities Blood volume loss

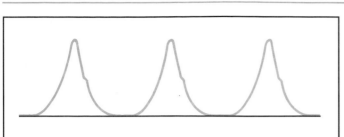

Figure 2-1   *A graph illustrating a bounding pulse*

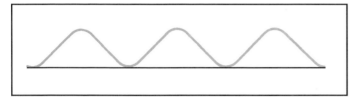

Figure 2-2   *A graph illustrating a plateau pulse*

RESPIRATORY RATE

The respiratory rate is the number of breaths taken by a patient in a 1-minute time interval. The respiratory rate normally varies depending on physical condition and level of activity. The normal rate for adults is between 12 and 20 and for children between 20 and 40 per minute.

It is important to determine rate as well as depth (volume of air inspired, indicated by chest wall excursion), pattern, and rhythm of respirations. Irregularities of rhythm and pattern are discussed in Chapter 3, "Advanced Patient Assessment." A patient's ability to oxygenate the blood adequately may diminish when the depth becomes too shallow. This may result from the effects of depressant drugs or anxiety from pain.

Tachypnea and Bradypnea

Tachypnea and *bradypnea* refer to abnormalities in respiratory rate. *Tachypnea* is a faster than normal respiratory rate. Tachypnea can result from anxiety, exercise, fever, and hypoxemia. Frequently, tachypnea is observed as a sign of impending respiratory failure. *Bradypnea* is a lower than normal respiratory rate. Bradypnea may be caused by certain pharmacologic agents (narcotics), head injuries, or hypothermia.

BLOOD PRESSURE

Blood pressure is the measurement of the pressure within the arterial system. Several factors influence blood pressure. These include the pumping action of the heart, resistance in the cardiovascular system, elasticity of the vessel walls, blood volume, and the viscosity of the blood.

Systolic and Diastolic Pressures

The *systolic* pressure is the pressure measured at the time the ventricles are contracting. During this period, the arteries momentarily expand to accommodate the increase in pressure from the blood volume ejected by the heart.

TABLE 2-3: Causes of Hypotension and Hypertension	
CONDITION	**CAUSES**
Hypotension	Shock Hormonal imbalances Depressant drugs Postural (positioning) Fluid loss
Hypertension	Cardiovascular imbalances Hormonal imbalances Exercise Stimulant drugs Emotional stress Renal failure/fluid retention

The *diastolic* pressure is the pressure in the arterial system when the ventricles are at rest. During this period, the aortic valve closes, causing a wave of pressure throughout the arterial system. This wave propels the blood through the arterial system. The diastolic pressure is considered to be the more critical in that it is the lowest pressure to which the arterial system and heart are subjected.

Normal Ranges

The normal range for blood pressure in adults is 100/60 to 140/90 mm Hg. The fractional representation is the systolic pressure over the diastolic pressure. Range in children will vary depending on the child's age. A neonate may have a blood pressure of 60/30 to 90/60 mm Hg. As the child becomes older, the blood pressure increases until it is equal to an adult's.

Abnormal Blood Pressure

An abnormally low blood pressure is termed *hypotension* and an abnormally high blood pressure is termed *hypertension*. Many factors may cause a lowered or elevated blood pressure. Table 2-3 is a partial listing of some of the common causes of hypertension and hypotension.

SOUND

Sound is produced by vibrations that alternately compress air into a wave form. The wave form enters the ear and causes the tympanic membrane (eardrum) to vibrate. The inner ear then conducts and converts these vibrations to nervous impulses, which we perceive as sound.

If wave forms could be perceived visually, they would be similar to the wave action observed in a pond. If a small object is dropped into a body of still water, it produces waves or ripples on the surface radiating from the point of impact. Sound waves travel in a similar way, radiating through the air in all directions from the source.

Sound has three main characteristics or properties: frequency, amplitude, and duration. Figure 2-3 illustrates these three properties using a graphic format.

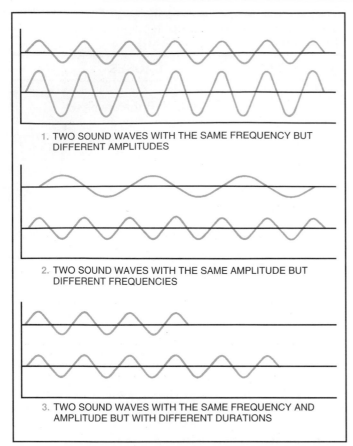

1. TWO SOUND WAVES WITH THE SAME FREQUENCY BUT DIFFERENT AMPLITUDES

2. TWO SOUND WAVES WITH THE SAME AMPLITUDE BUT DIFFERENT FREQUENCIES

3. TWO SOUND WAVES WITH THE SAME FREQUENCY AND AMPLITUDE BUT WITH DIFFERENT DURATIONS

Figure 2-3 *A graph representing the properties of sound: (1) amplitude, (2) frequency, and (3) duration*

A low-pitched sound is low in frequency, and a high-pitched sound is higher in frequency. Human hearing detects sounds with frequencies ranging roughly from 16 to 16,000 hertz (Hz), or vibrations per second. Although human hearing has a broad frequency range, acute hearing has a more narrow frequency band ranging from 1000 to 2000 Hz.

The amplitude of a sound wave determines its intensity. The greater the amplitude, the higher the intensity of the sound wave. If you were to pluck a string on an electric guitar and simultaneously increase the volume on the amplifier, the frequency would remain relatively constant while the amplitude or intensity would increase dramatically.

Duration relates to the length of time a sound continues. A sound of long duration is perceived for a longer period of time than one of short duration.

The Effects of Density on Sound Production and Conduction

Sound vibrations may be conducted through mediums other than air, such as solid matter or fluid. The nature of the medium may affect the distance over which a sound can be carried. The denser a material is, the more easily it can conduct sound vibrations. This concept is important from a physiological standpoint. In our bodies, sound produced in the lungs is conducted through tissue, bone,

fluid, and air. All of these structures and materials have different properties and densities. Furthermore, some disease states cause a change in the tissue density, further increasing the conduction of sound or transmitting sounds not normally heard from one location to another. *Auscultation* (listening for sounds) allows detection of changes that may indicate disease states.

Stethoscopes

Since its invention in 1816 the stethoscope has remained essentially the same, with just a few changes and refinements. With the advances in technology, stethoscope design has been improved, resulting in greater performance, comfort, and convenience.

Parts of the Stethoscope

There are several parts that make up a stethoscope. All parts must be functioning properly for the instrument to perform well.

The chest piece is one of the more critical elements of the stethoscope. The chest piece may consist of a diaphragm, a bell, or a diaphragm-bell combination. The diaphragm is usually made from a thin semirigid polymer and has a relatively large surface area with a diameter of approximately 2 inches. The diaphragm allows the transmission of high-pitched sounds and filters out the low-pitched sounds. The diaphragm is most suited to listening to breath sounds. The bell chest piece is smaller in diameter than the diaphragm and conical in shape. The bell filters high-frequency sounds and allows the transmission of low-frequency sounds. The bell is most suited to listening to heart tones and other low-pitched sounds.

The chest piece is connected to the binaurals, or earpieces, by one or two short pieces of tubing. Shorter tubing is preferred for better transmission or passage of the sounds free of artifact. Longer tubing tends to pick up external sounds and also has the tendency to rub or bump into bed frames or other objects, creating further distractions and artifact.

The binaurals should fit comfortably into the ear canals and be canted anteriorly, matching the angle of the ear canal. It is often helpful to have a lab partner or other clinician help you fit your stethoscope precisely to the angle of your auditory canals. The earpieces must be comfortable and yet seal the canal well. Comfort is very important in reducing fatigue and allowing the maximum attenuation (lessening) of unwanted sounds.

Several major types of stethoscopes are available. Each type has its limitations and advantages for clinical use. The two common types of stethoscopes are the single tube nurse scope and the Sprague-Rappaport stethoscope.

Single Tube Stethoscope

The single tube stethoscope consists of a diaphragm or diaphragm-bell combination chest piece attached to the binaurals with a single flexible tube. Figure 2-4 shows a good-quality stethoscope. A single tube stethoscope can be a very satisfactory instrument for the respiratory care practitioner. It is important that you purchase the highest-quality stethoscope you can afford. Prices for this type

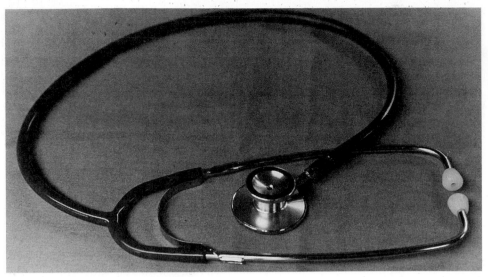

Figure 2-4   *A single tube stethoscope*

of stethoscope range from $30 to $200. A medium-quality stethoscope of this type will cost approximately $70.

One indicator of quality is the thickness of the tubing wall. The thicker the wall, the better it will attenuate sounds not produced by the diaphragm or bell. Stethoscopes having thin wall tubing tend to pick up sounds from the room more easily.

The advantages of this stethoscope are its size and easy portability. Having only one piece of connecting tubing, it can easily be coiled and stuffed into a lab coat pocket.

Sprague-Rappaport Stethoscope

A Sprague-Rappaport stethoscope consists of a bell-diaphragm or diaphragm-diaphragm chest piece attached directly to the binaurals by two pieces of flexible tubing. Figure 2-5 shows a medium-quality Sprague-Rappaport stethoscope. This type of stethoscope has been favored in clinical practice over the nurse scope. It has been shown that the training of the listener is more important than the type of stethoscope used in the auscultation of breath sounds (Kindig, Beeson, Campbell, Andrics, & Tavel, 1982).

The construction of this stethoscope is generally of more durable materials, and therefore it tends to survive the rigors of clinical practice a little better. It is also larger and a little more awkward to carry easily in the pocket compared with the single tube stethoscope. Prices range from around $30 to $200. A good-quality stethoscope manufactured in Japan can be purchased in the lower spectrum of the price range. Some of these Japanese stethoscopes have a rotating chest piece. Frequently (once per week) check the screw at the center of the pivot for tightness (Figure 2-6). With repeated use of the stethoscope, the screw may work loose and be lost, along with the springs and ball bearings that lock the chest piece into position.

Breath Sounds

The sounds you hear when auscultating the chest have been described and classified into normal and abnormal sounds. Various descriptive terms have evolved over the years since these sounds were first described by Läennec. In the clinical setting, you may hear physicians describing sounds using any of numerous descriptive terms or classification systems.

In recent years, the American Thoracic Society (ATS) has recommended a descriptive system to standardize the

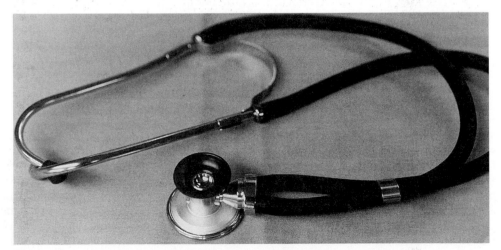

Figure 2-5   *A Sprague-Rappaport stethoscope*

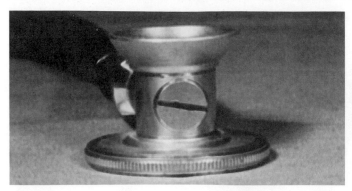

Figure 2-6 *The pivot screw that requires periodic inspection for tightness*

way breath sounds are described. In this chapter, the ATS system is used in the description of breath sounds.

Normal Breath Sounds

Normal breath sounds have been divided into four major classifications: vesicular, bronchial, bronchovesicular, and tracheal. Each sound has unique characteristics, and a different mechanism of sound production has been theorized for each type. Normal sounds may be heard over specific areas of the chest. If these sounds are heard elsewhere, they are then classified as abnormal.

Vesicular Breath Sounds. Vesicular breath sounds are relatively low-pitched soft sounds. They have been described as whispering or rustling in nature. The inspiratory phase is longer in duration than the expiratory phase. There is no pause between inspiration and expiration. This sound is heard over the majority of the lung periphery except over the right apex anteriorly.

Vesicular sounds are thought to be generated by turbulent air flow in the lobar and segmental bronchi. It has been theorized that the turbulent flow generates vibration in these anatomical structures, resulting in the production of sound.

Bronchial Breath Sounds. Bronchial breath sounds are loud and generally of higher pitch. The expiratory phase is longer than the inspiratory phase, with a short pause between phases. This sound is often described as similar to the sound generated by blowing through a tube. It is normally heard over the upper portion of the sternum, or the manubrium.

This sound is thought to be generated by turbulent air vibrating in the trachea and right and left mainstem bronchi. This vibration ultimately produces an audible sound that can be heard when using a stethoscope.

Bronchovesicular Breath Sounds. As the name suggests, bronchovesicular sounds are characterized by the combination of bronchial and vesicular sounds. They are somewhat muted, without a pause between inspiration and expiration. The inspiratory and expiratory phases are roughly equal in length. These sounds are normally heard over the sternum at around the second intercostal space, between the scapulae and over the right apex of the lung.

Sound production is again thought to arise from turbulent air flow.

Tracheal Breath Sounds. As the name implies, tracheal sounds are characteristically heard over the trachea. Above the clavicular notch, they are very harsh and quite high-pitched, with the expiratory phase lasting a little longer than the inspiratory phase.

Tracheal sounds are produced by the high-velocity, turbulent air as it passes through the trachea.

Abnormal Breath Sounds

Abnormal breath sounds are often referred to as *adventitious sounds*. Keep in mind, though, that normal breath sounds heard in an uncharacteristic location are also abnormal. The transmission of normal sounds to remote areas may be a result of consolidation or other changes affecting the transmission of that sound.

The ATS has recommended that adventitious sounds be classified as crackles, wheezes, rhonchi, and rubs.

Crackles. Crackles are abnormal sounds described as coarse or fine. The quantity (few or many) can also be noted. The phase in which such sounds occur—inspiratory or expiratory—should be indicated. It is also important to describe the location on the chest where crackles are heard. These may be almost anywhere. This finding might be charted as "coarse inspiratory crackles heard over the right middle lobe."

These sounds are thought to be produced by the sudden opening of alveoli or sections of the lung. The resultant sudden change in pressure generates the sound.

Wheezes. Wheezes are high-pitched sounds. Wheezes may also be described as continuous sounds in that they continue without interruption.

It is thought that these sounds are generated by air passing through a narrowed lumen. The passage of this air causes the lumen to vibrate much like a double reed on an oboe or bassoon.

When describing this sound, indicate its location, when it occurs with respect to inspiration or expiration, its pitch, and its intensity.

Rhonchi. Rhonchi are also continuous sounds but are quite low-pitched. Rhonchi are sometimes described as similar to the sounds produced by blowing into a milkshake through a straw. Often these sounds are described as being "wet." Rhonchi are thought to be produced by fluid or secretions vibrating in the airways. They may be heard throughout the lung fields.

When describing this sound, indicate its location, pitch, and intensity. The patient can be asked to cough; rhonchi may frequently clear following a vigorous cough.

Pleural Rub. A pleural rub occurs when the two pleural layers rub together with more friction than normal. An increase in friction may be caused by irritation or inflammation. The resulting sound is often described as "creaking leather," similar to the sound produced when riding a horse using a well-worn saddle.

Anatomical Positions for Auscultation

Air exchange and movement in the lungs are influenced by patient position. To optimize air flow, the patient should be sitting in an upright position to allow for good chest expansion. In the hospital, the patient who has no physical limitations should sit on the side of the bed (dangling position). In some instances, because of poor physical condition, the patient may be unable to sit unassisted in the upright position. As long as the patient will not be physically compromised, have someone assist you in holding the patient in a high Fowler's position to allow auscultation of the posterior chest. Have the patient roll the shoulders forward to separate the scapulae.

Figures 2-7 and 2-8 show the anterior and posterior positions for auscultating the chest. It is important when auscultating the chest that you move from one segment of the lung to the corresponding segment on the opposite side of the chest. Humans are bilateral mammals, making comparison of one side with the other a relatively informative and easy task.

When auscultating the chest, have the patient breathe slowly and a bit more deeply than normal through the mouth. Listen carefully to each segment. Compare one side with the other. Progress from the superior segments to the inferior segments when auscultating either posteriorly or anteriorly.

Environmental Considerations

During auscultation of the chest, your patient's privacy may be compromised. If possible, close the door and dis-

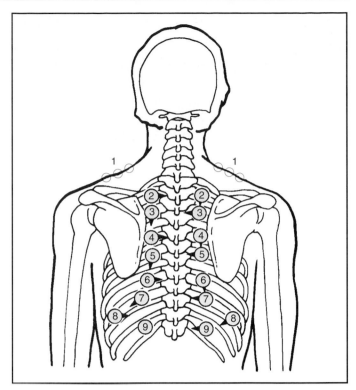

Figure 2-8 *Posterior positions used in auscultating the chest*

miss any visitors prior to beginning your examination. The temperature of the room should be comfortable and not too cold. Turn off any radios, televisions, or appliances that may be distracting while auscultating the chest. The sounds you are trying to hear are often faint and somewhat muffled.

The stethoscope should be used on bare skin. Contact of the stethoscope with the patient's clothing or gown may cause artificial sounds to be produced, confusing the examiner about what is real and what is not. Hair on a male patient's chest will often cause slight movement against the diaphragm of the stethoscope, producing the sound of crackles. Wet the hair slightly so that it will stick to the skin and not produce this unwanted distraction.

The female patient with large breasts presents an additional challenge in the auscultation of breath sounds. If the patient is alert and cooperative, ask her to move her breast to one side to facilitate your use of the stethoscope. If the patient is unable to do so, you may be required to move the breast yourself while preserving the patient's dignity.

The Case for a Systematic Method

Learning to recognize breath sounds requires considerable practice. The more you listen to the different sounds, the sooner you will be able to distinguish among them. It is important that you develop a systematic method of auscultating the chest early in your training. If you consistently use the same technique for all patients, the mechanics will soon become second nature. You will then be able to concentrate on recognizing the sounds. Only by learning to discriminate among the sounds will you be able to become a skilled examiner.

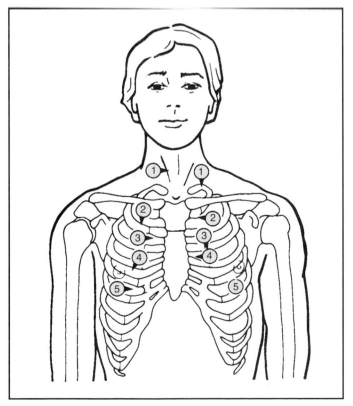

Figure 2-7 *Anterior positions used in auscultating the chest*

PROFICIENCY OBJECTIVES

At the end of this chapter, you should be able to:

VITAL SIGNS
- Using a laboratory partner, locate the three most common sites for measuring body temperature.
- Using a laboratory partner, correctly measure the oral temperature.
- Using a laboratory partner, locate the most common sites to measure the pulse.
- Using a laboratory partner, measure the pulse and describe the following:
  — Rate
  — Rhythm
  — Normalcy

- Using a laboratory partner, measure the respiratory rate, determining whether the rate and rhythm are normal.
- Using a laboratory partner, correctly measure the blood pressure.

BREATH SOUNDS
- Demonstrate the proper preparation of the stethoscope for use, with emphasis on aseptic technique.
- Demonstrate how to test the stethoscope for function and how to troubleshoot the instrument when it does not function properly.
- Demonstrate how to auscultate the chest in a systematic way.

MEASURING BODY TEMPERATURE

The three most common sites used for measuring body temperature are oral, rectal, and axillary.

The oral temperature is taken by having the patient open the mouth, inserting the thermometer under the tongue, and having the patient close the mouth. The rectal temperature is taken by having the patient lie on his or her side and inserting the thermometer into the rectum.

The axillary temperature is measured by placing the thermometer within the armpit and holding the arm down snugly against the patient's side.

Tympanic temperatures may be taken using an electronic thermometer. A probe is inserted into the ear canal, sealing it. Once the temperature stabilizes, the thermometer beeps, signaling that the temperature has been measured. This thermometer is quick and accurate and, with use of disposable probe covers, minimizes the risk of cross-contamination.

The rectal temperature is 1 degree higher than the oral temperature, and the axillary temperature is 1 degree lower.

MEASURING ORAL TEMPERATURE

Equipment

A thermometer and alcohol prep pads are all that is required to measure a patient's temperature.

Preparation for Use

When using a mercury thermometer, first cleanse it with an alcohol prep pad and then shake it down. To shake down a thermometer, hold it by the end opposite the bulb and briskly shake it, using a snapping motion of the wrist. This will force the mercury into the bulb. The temperature should read no higher than 95°F, or 35°C.

Checking the Patient

Ask whether the patient can breathe through the nose without difficulty. Also ask whether the patient has had any food or liquids or has smoked in the past 10 minutes, as these can affect the oral temperature.

The patient should be alert and able to follow directions. If this is not the case, consider taking rectal or axillary temperatures.

Placement of the Thermometer

Ask the patient to open the mouth, and place the thermometer under the tongue. Ask the patient to close the mouth and not bite on the thermometer. Leave the thermometer in place for 3 minutes.

Reading the Thermometer

After 3 minutes have passed, remove the thermometer by holding the end opposite the bulb. Never touch the portion of the thermometer that was inside the patient's mouth. Immediately after removing the thermometer, read and record the temperature.

MEASURING THE PULSE

Common Sites

The four most common sites to measure the pulse are over the radial, brachial (shown in Figure 2-9), femoral, and carotid arteries.

The femoral pulse is felt immediately lateral to the pubic bone in the pelvis. Palpate the pubic bone. In the male, the pubic bone is immediately superior to the penis, and in the female, it is immediately superior to the pudendum. On moving laterally into the area of the groin, the femoral pulse should be immediately evident.

The carotid pulse is felt lateral to the larynx on either side of the neck.

Assessment of the Pulse

The pulse should be measured for one full minute at the radial site. Measuring the pulse for a shorter time interval will compromise your ability to assess for arrhythmias or irregularities.

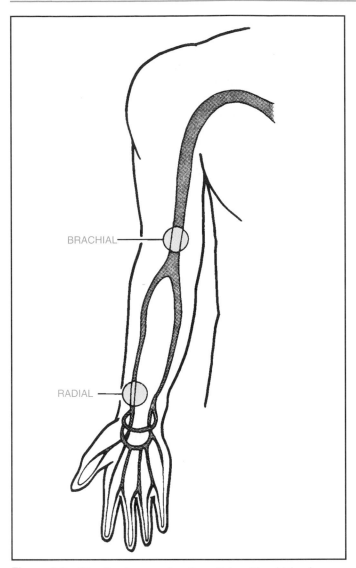

Figure 2-9 *The sites for assessing the radial and brachial pulses*

MEASURING RESPIRATORY RATE

It is often difficult to assess the respiratory rate without the patient's becoming aware of it. If the patient becomes aware of what you are doing, the rate may be adversely affected. Therefore, it is beneficial not to disclose that the respiratory rate will be measured.

A way to measure the respiratory rate without the patient's awareness is to pretend you are measuring the pulse by palpating the radial artery while actually counting the respirations.

In some patients, the respiratory excursions are very small. It may be necessary to place a hand on the patient's abdomen in order to perceive these excursions.

ASSESSING BLOOD PRESSURE

Equipment

The equipment required for assessing blood pressure is a stethoscope and a sphygmomanometer (blood pressure cuff).

To measure blood pressure, the diaphragm of the stethoscope is used. The diaphragm is placed over the brachial artery.

Sphygmomanometer Placement

The sphygmomanometer is placed on the arm approximately 1 inch above the antecubital space. Palpate the brachial artery and then apply the cuff in proper position. The sphygmomanometer is commonly closed by self-fasteners (Velcro) or hooks.

Measuring Blood Pressure by Palpation

Palpate the brachial artery. Once the artery is located, slowly inflate the sphygmomanometer. When the artery becomes totally occluded, the pulse will no longer be felt. At this point, measure the reading on the pressure gauge. This is the systolic blood pressure. Continue to inflate the sphygmomanometer another 30 mm Hg. Immediately measure the blood pressure by auscultation.

Measuring the Blood Pressure by Auscultation

Using your stethoscope, place the diaphragm over the brachial artery. Deflate the sphygmomanometer slowly, while auscultating for the blood pressure. When sound is first heard in the artery, note the reading on the pressure gauge. Continue deflating the cuff and note the reading at which all sound ceases. The point at which the sound is first heard is the systolic measurement; the point where all sound stops is the diastolic measurement.

AUSCULTATION OF BREATH SOUNDS

Preparation of the Stethoscope

If you have recently purchased a stethoscope and have not adjusted it for your anatomy, now is the time to do so. Have a laboratory partner assist you. Adjust the binaurals so that they fit snugly in your auditory canals but not so tight that they cause discomfort. This may be accomplished by spreading or compressing the leaf spring on which the binaurals are attached until the fit is comfortable and snug. Next, have your partner assist you in adjusting the angle of the binaurals so that the tips are each pointing into your auditory canals. Now your stethoscope is properly fitted to you and you alone.

Preparation and Cleaning

If the stethoscope you are using is one commonly used by others, such as those found at a nurses' station, take the time to prepare the instrument for use. Using an alcohol swab, thoroughly clean the earpieces as a precaution against infection.

Whether using your own instrument or one utilized by others, use another alcohol swab to thoroughly clean the diaphragm and bell. The instrument should be cleaned in this manner before and after each use to help prevent the spread of communicable diseases. Don't forget to wash your hands prior to examining your patient.

Patients in isolation will have a stethoscope in the room. Do not bring your own stethoscope into isolation. Use the one provided in the room to prevent the spread of nosocomial infections.

If you have occasion to lay down your stethoscope in a patient's room, do not place it on the bed. A preferable practice is to put it around your neck or return it to your pocket. The patient's bed and overbed table are places that may be colonized by bacteria and viruses. If you place your stethoscope on these surfaces, it may become a vehicle for transmitting nosocomial (hospital-acquired) infections.

Testing

A stethoscope may be easily and quickly tested prior to use. Place the earpieces in your auditory canals and gently tap on the diaphragm and bell. It is important not to use too much force. The stethoscope greatly amplifies sound, and too forceful a tap will cause you great discomfort. This is a good time to examine the diaphragm and bell for cracks or other signs of wear or abuse. If these parts need replacement, use only parts supplied by the manufacturer. X-ray film and other materials may be substituted in a pinch, but they rarely seal well and fail to provide good attenuation of sounds.

If your gentle tapping fails to produce any sound, verify that the diaphragm or bell is in the proper position on the chest piece. If it is not, rotate it into proper position. If the instrument still fails to perform properly, examine the chest piece carefully and make sure that all parts are assembled correctly and are tight. Examine the tubing for kinks or breaks. If any are found, free the tubing or replace it as required, using only the manufacturer's replacement parts.

Warming of the Diaphragm

It is courteous to warm the diaphragm briefly by placing it in the palm of your hand prior to applying it to your patient's chest. A cold stethoscope will prompt your patient to initiate a very deep breath, and often there is a long pause before the expiratory phase begins. The short time it takes to warm your stethoscope will make it much more comfortable for your patients and will facilitate their cooperation.

Patient Positioning

Have your patient sit in an upright position at the bedside or in a chair if possible. This position will allow for proper chest expansion and access to the chest for auscultation.

If the patient's physical condition does not permit the assumption of an upright position, modify the position as required. If your patient is too weak to sit upright, have someone assist you when you auscultate the posterior chest. In general, as long as the patient's muscle strength is the limiting factor, rather than a pathological or surgical condition, assisting your patient to assume an appropriate position is permissible.

Auscultation of the Chest
General Notes

It is always best to listen over bare skin. Don't brush against the stethoscope tubing or allow it to contact the bed rail, bed frame, or other foreign objects. Any motion or disturbance of the tubing will cause artificial sounds to be produced and confuse your examination.

Turn off radios, televisions, or other noisy appliances. Make sure the room is at a comfortable temperature, and dismiss any visitors prior to your examination.

The proper hand position is important to ensure good contact between the stethoscope and the skin surface and also to minimize motion of the chest piece. The center portion of the chest piece should be placed between your first and second digits. Place the chest piece on the chest wall and hyperextend all of your digits, making contact over a broad surface area (Figure 2-10).

Close the door or use privacy drapes or screens to preserve your patient's dignity.

Anterior Chest

Beginning on the anterior chest, listen above the clavicles between the midclavicular line and the midsternal line on each side. Progress inferiorly to just below the clavicles, listening at the same lateral position. Progress inferiorly to the third intercostal space and listen on each side between the midclavicular and midsternal lines. Move inferiorly to the fourth intercostal space and listen on each side at the same lateral positions. Moving inferiorly, listen at the sixth intercostal space at the midclavicular line below the nipples.

Progress laterally to the fourth intercostal space, listening at the anterior axillary line. Move inferiorly to the fifth intercostal space and listen at the anterior axillary line. Progress inferiorly and listen at the sixth intercostal space at the posterior axillary line. As you listen to a position on one side, be sure to compare it with the same position on the opposite side.

Posterior Chest

For auscultating the posterior chest, it is often helpful to ask the patient to shrug the shoulders forward, spreading the scapulae slightly further apart.

Begin listening at a point even with the top of the scapulae between the midscapular line and the midspinal line. Move inferiorly to the approximate midpoint of the scapulae and auscultate between the midscapular line and the midspinal line. Progress inferiorly and listen at a point

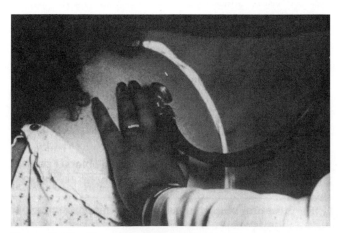

Figure 2-10 *The correct way to hold the stethoscope*

even with the bottom of the scapulae between the mid-scapular and midspinal lines. Move inferiorly and laterally to the midscapular line and listen just below the scapulae.

As with the anterior chest, be sure to compare one side with the other before you progress inferiorly.

Postauscultation

Provide assistance as required in the reapplication of the patient's gown or any clothing removed before the exami-nation. Help the patient to assume a comfortable and safe position prior to your departure. Be courteous and thank the patient for his or her cooperation and time. Wash your hands prior to leaving the room.

Clean the diaphragm or bell, or both, with an alcohol swab.

Record your findings in the patient's chart, describing the sound and its intensity, duration, phase, and location.

References

Kindig, J. R., Beeson, T. P., Campbell, R. W., Andrics, F., & Tavel, M. E. (1982). Acoustical performance of the stethoscope: A comparative analysis. *American Heart Journal, 104,* 269–275.

Additional Resources

Burton, G. G., Hodgkin, J. E., & Ward, J. (1990). *Respiratory care* (3rd ed.). Philadelphia: Lippincott.

Kozier, B., Erb, G. L., & Marcus W. (1983). *Fundamentals of nursing concepts and procedures* (2nd ed.). Reading, MA: Addison-Wesley.

Lehrer, S. (1984). *Understanding lung sounds.* Philadelphia: Saunders.

Massachusetts General Hospital, Department of Nursing. (1975). *Massachusetts General Hospital manual of nursing procedures.* Boston: Little, Brown.

Murphy, R. L. H., & Holford, S. K. (1980). Lung sounds basics of RD. *Respiratory Care, 25*(7), 763–770.Eubanks, D. H., & Bone, R. (1991). *Comprehensive respiratory care* (2nd ed.). St. Louis, MO: Mosby.

Practice Activities: Basic Patient Assessment

VITAL SIGNS

1. Using a laboratory partner, practice measuring oral body temperature. Include the following in your practice:
   a. Select appropriate equipment.
   b. Prepare the equipment for use.
   c. Shake down the thermometer (mercurial only) and clean it with alcohol or use a new probe cover (for electronic thermometer).
   d. Determine the patient's ability to breathe through the nose and determine if the patient has had anything to eat or drink or has smoked in the past 10 minutes.
   e. Correctly place the thermometer and instruct the patient.
   f. Leave the thermometer in place for 3 minutes.
   g. Correctly read the temperature and record it.

2. Using a laboratory partner, practice locating and measuring the heart rate at the following sites:
   a. Radial
   b. Brachial
   c. Femoral
   d. Carotid
   Include in your measurements:
   a. Rate
   b. Rhythm
   c. Normalcy

3. Using a laboratory partner, measure the respiratory rate, making sure the partner is unaware of your intentions.

4. Using a laboratory partner, practice measuring the blood pressure, including the following:
   a. Select the appropriate equipment.
   b. Palpate the brachial pulse.
   c. Correctly apply the cuff.
   d. Measure the blood pressure by palpation during inflation of the sphygmomanometer.
   e. Measure the blood pressure by auscultation during deflation of the sphygmomanometer.
   f. Correctly record the blood pressure.

5. Using a laboratory partner, practice sequencing the different skills together in the following way:
   a. Wash your hands.
   b. Correctly prepare and insert the thermometer for oral temperature.
   c. While waiting, measure the following:
      (1) The pulse and respirations
      (2) The blood pressure
      (3) The oral temperature (record on the chart)

BREATH SOUNDS

1. Identify all of the parts on your own stethoscope.

2. Demonstrate to your laboratory partner how to properly clean and prepare your stethoscope for use.

3. Practice auscultating the chest with a laboratory partner:
   a. Auscultate on bare skin.

b. Instruct your laboratory partner to breathe deeply and through the mouth.

c. Auscultate at each position bilaterally.

4. Following auscultation of your laboratory partner's chest, take a sheet of paper and chart your findings. Have your instructor critique your charting.

Check List: Vital Signs

_____ 1. Identify your patient.
_____ 2. Explain the procedure.
_____ 3. Wash your hands.
4. Prepare the thermometer for use:
   a. Mercury:
_____   (1) Shake it down.
_____   (2) Clean using alcohol swab.
   b. Electronic:
_____   (1) Apply new cover.
5. Determine if an oral temperature is contra-indicated:
_____ a. Determine if the patient can breathe through the nose.
_____ b. Determine if the patient has had any food or drink orally in the past 10 minutes.
_____ c. Determine if the patient has smoked in the past 10 minutes.
6. Correctly place the thermometer:
_____ a. Place it under the patient's tongue.
_____ b. Instruct the patient to close the mouth and not to bite on the thermometer.
7. Assess pulse and respirations:
   a. Pulse:

_____   (1) Locate site.
_____   (2) Measure rate.
_____   (3) Assess rhythm.
   b. Respirations:
_____   (1) Measure rate.
_____   (2) Assess depth.
_____   (3) Assess rhythm.
_____   (4) Ensure patient is unaware of assessment.
8. Measure the blood pressure:
_____ a. Locate the brachial pulse.
_____ b. Correctly apply the cuff.
_____ c. Measure the systolic blood pressure by palpation during cuff inflation.
_____ d. Measure the systolic and diastolic blood pressures by auscultation during cuff deflation.
_____ e. Correctly record the blood pressure.
_____ 9. Remove the thermometer and correctly measure the oral temperature.
_____ 10. Correctly care for the equipment following the procedure.
_____ 11. Thank the patient and wash your hands before leaving the room.

Check List: Breath Sounds

1. Collect and assemble the equipment:
_____ a. Stethoscope
_____ b. Alcohol swabs
_____ c. Pen
2. Prepare and test the equipment:
_____ a. Clean the earpieces if the stethoscope is not your own.
_____ b. Clean the diaphragm and bell.
_____ c. Test the equipment and troubleshoot.
_____ 3. Wash your hands.
4. Optimize the environment:
_____ a. Turn off the radio or television.
_____ b. Regulate the temperature as required.
_____ c. Ensure the patient's privacy.
5. Position the patient properly:
_____ a. Have the patient sit in an upright position.
_____ b. Ask for assistance if necessary or modify the position as required.
6. Auscultate the anterior chest:
_____ a. Auscultate at each position bilaterally.

_____ b. Use the stethoscope properly.
_____ c. Use a systematic method.
7. Auscultate the lateral chest:
_____ a. Auscultate at each position bilaterally.
_____ b. Use the stethoscope properly.
_____ c. Use a systematic method.
8. Auscultate the posterior chest:
_____ a. Auscultate at each position bilaterally.
_____ b. Use the stethoscope properly.
_____ c. Use a systematic method.
9. Ensure patient safety and comfort:
_____ a. Assist with clothing as required.
_____ b. Help the patient back to a comfortable position.
_____ c. Thank the patient.
_____ 10. Wash your hands.
11. Clean your equipment:
_____ a. Clean the diaphragm and bell.
_____ 12. Record the findings on the patient's chart.

Self-Evaluation Post Test: Basic Patient Assessment

1. Body temperature is regulated by the:
   a. hyperdermis.
   b. sympathetic nervous system.
   c. hypothalamus.
   d. thyroid.

2. Normal temperature for an adult is:
   a. 32°C.   c. 98°C.
   b. 35°C.   d. 37°C.

3. A child's body temperature is:
   a. the same as an adult's.
   b. lower than an adult's.
   c. higher than an adult's.
   d. more precisely regulated than an adult's.

4. A decrease in body temperature below normal is termed:
   a. hypotension.   c. hypothermia.
   b. bradypnea.   d. hypertension.

5. Hypoxemia may cause:
   a. bradypnea.   c. hyperthermia.
   b. tachycardia.   d. hypertension.

6. Sound may be conducted through:
   I.   air.
   II. fluids.
   III. solids
   a. I.   c. I, II, III
   b. I, II   d. I, III

7. Which of the following determines a sound's intensity?
   a. Frequency
   b. Amplitude
   c. Pitch
   d. Duration

8. A denser material will conduct sound:
   a. more easily than a less dense material.
   b. more slowly than a less dense material.
   c. with greater attenuation than a less dense material.
   d. only in the high-frequency ranges.

9. Vesicular breath sounds:
   I.   are normal breath sounds.
   II. are often described as quiet rustling sounds.
   III. have an expiratory phase longer than the inspiratory phase.
   IV. have no pause between inspiration and expiration.
   a. I, II, III   c. I, III, IV
   b. I, II, IV   d. II, III, IV

10. Bronchial breath sounds:
    I.   are low-pitched sounds.
    II. have an inspiratory phase shorter than the expiratory phase.
    III. have no pause between inspiration and expiration.
    IV. are often described as hollow sounding.
    a. I, III   c. II, III
    b. II, IV   d. I, IV

PERFORMANCE EVALUATION: VITAL SIGNS

Date: Lab _____ Clinical _____ Agency _____

Lab: Pass _____ Fail _____   Clinical: Pass _____ Fail _____

Student name _____ Instructor name _____

No. of times observed in clinical _____

No. of times practiced in clinical _____

PASSING CRITERIA: Obtain 90% or better on the procedure. Tasks indicated by * must receive at least 1 point, or the evaluation is terminated. Procedure must be performed within designated time, or the performance receives a failing grade.

SCORING:
2 points — Task performed satisfactorily without prompting.
1 point — Task performed satisfactorily with self-initiated correction.
0 points — Task performed incorrectly or with prompting required.
NA — Task not applicable to the patient care situation.

TASKS:

			PEER	LAB	CLINICAL
*	1.	Properly identifies the patient	☐	☐	☐
	2.	Explains the procedure to the patient	☐	☐	☐
*	3.	Observes standard precautions, including handwashing	☐	☐	☐
	4.	Prepares the thermometer for use			
*		a. Shakes down the thermometer	☐	☐	☐
*		b. Swabs off the thermometer with alcohol	☐	☐	☐
		c. Uses new disposable cover on electronic thermometer	☐	☐	☐
*	5.	Determines if an oral temperature is contraindicated	☐	☐	☐
	6.	Places the thermometer appropriately			
*		a. Places it under the tongue	☐	☐	☐
*		b. Asks the patient to close the mouth	☐	☐	☐
	7.	Correctly measures pulse and respirations			
*		a. Locates pulse	☐	☐	☐
*		b. Records rate and rhythm	☐	☐	☐
	8.	Measures respiratory rate			
*		a. Ensures patient unawareness	☐	☐	☐
*		b. Records rate, depth, and rhythm	☐	☐	☐
	9.	Measures blood pressure			
*		a. Locates brachial pulse	☐	☐	☐
*		b. Applies cuff correctly	☐	☐	☐
		c. Measures blood pressure by palpation during inflation	☐	☐	☐
*		d. Measures blood pressure by auscultation during deflation	☐	☐	☐
*		e. Correctly records blood pressure	☐	☐	☐
		f. Removes and correctly cares for equipment	☐	☐	☐

10. Removes thermometer and correctly records temperature ☐ ☐ ☐

11. Correctly cares for equipment following the procedure ☐ ☐ ☐

12. Thanks the patient and washes hands prior to leaving the room ☐ ☐ ☐

SCORE: Peer _____ points of possible 44; _____%

Lab _____ points of possible 44; _____%

Clinical _____ points of possible 44; _____%

TIME: _____ out of possible 20 minutes

STUDENT SIGNATURES   INSTRUCTOR SIGNATURES

PEER: _____   LAB: _____

STUDENT: _____   CLINICAL: _____

PERFORMANCE EVALUATION: BREATH SOUNDS

Date: Lab _____ Clinical _____ Agency _____

Lab: Pass _____ Fail _____   Clinical: Pass _____ Fail _____

Student name _____   Instructor name _____

No. of times observed in clinical _____

No. of times practiced in clinical _____

PASSING CRITERIA: Obtain 90% or better on the procedure. Tasks indicated by * must receive at least 1 point, or the evaluation is terminated. Procedure must be performed within designated time, or the performance receives a failing grade.

SCORING:
2 points — Task performed satisfactorily without prompting.
1 point — Task performed satisfactorily with self-initiated correction.
0 points — Task performed incorrectly or with prompting required.
NA — Task not applicable to the patient care situation.

TASKS:	PEER	LAB	CLINICAL
1. Obtains the required equipment			
* a. Alcohol swabs	☐	☐	☐
* b. Stethoscope	☐	☐	☐
c. Pen and paper	☐	☐	☐
2. Observes universal precautions, including handwashing	☐	☐	☐
3. Explains the procedure to the patient	☐	☐	☐
4. Optimizes the environment			
* a. Turns off the radio or television	☐	☐	☐
b. Regulates the temperature	☐	☐	☐
* c. Ensures patient privacy	☐	☐	☐
* 5. Positions the patient properly	☐	☐	☐
6. Auscultates anterior chest			
* a. Auscultates each position bilaterally	☐	☐	☐
* b. Uses the stethoscope properly	☐	☐	☐
* c. Uses a systematic method	☐	☐	☐
7. Auscultates the lateral chest			
* a. Auscultates each position bilaterally	☐	☐	☐
* b. Uses the stethoscope properly	☐	☐	☐
* c. Uses a systematic method	☐	☐	☐
8. Auscultates the posterior chest			
* a. Auscultates each position bilaterally	☐	☐	☐
* b. Uses the stethoscope properly	☐	☐	☐
* c. Uses a systematic method	☐	☐	☐
9. Ensures patient safety and comfort			

10. Thanks the patient and washes hands ☐ ☐ ☐

* 11. Cleans and cares for the equipment ☐ ☐ ☐

* 12. Records the findings on the patient's chart ☐ ☐ ☐

SCORE: Peer   _____ points of possible 44; _____%

Lab   _____ points of possible 44; _____%

Clinical   _____ points of possible 44; _____%

TIME: _____ out of possible 15 minutes

STUDENT SIGNATURES

PEER: _____

STUDENT: _____

INSTRUCTOR SIGNATURES

LAB: _____

CLINICAL: _____

CHAPTER 3

ADVANCED PATIENT ASSESSMENT: INSPECTION, PALPATION, AND PERCUSSION

INTRODUCTION

As the scope of respiratory care has broadened over the years, the respiratory care practitioner has assumed a greater responsibility for assessment of the patient and evaluation of the patient's response to therapy. Physical assessment of the chest is an important tool employed in patient care. It is a quick and easy means of clinical evaluation. It places few demands on the patient, and the only equipment required is the practitioner's hands, eyes, and ears.

Like the assessment of breath sounds, physical assessment of the chest requires that you practice to attain proficiency. It is best to learn at the side of a skilled practitioner. As your skill and confidence improve, practice will help improve your abilities.

KEY TERMS

- Barrel chest
- Biot's respiration
- Cheyne-Stokes respiration
- Collarbones
- Digital clubbing
- Eupnea
- Funnel chest
- Humpback
- Hyperpnea
- Hypopnea
- Inspection
- Kussmaul's respiration
- Kyphoscoliosis
- Kyphosis
- Lordosis
- Metabolic acidosis
- Palpation
- Pectus carinatum
- Pectus excavatum
- Percussion
- Pigeon chest
- Scoliosis
- Shoulder blades
- Sternal angle
- Swayback

OBJECTIVES

At the end of this chapter, you should be able to:

- Identify or locate the anatomical landmarks commonly used in assessing the chest:
  — Anterior Chest
    — Clavicles
    — Sternal notch
    — Sternal angle and second rib
    — Fourth rib
    — Midsternal line
    — Midclavicular line
    — Anterior axillary line
  — Lateral Chest
    — Anterior axillary line
    — Midaxillary line
    — Posterior axillary line
  — Posterior Chest
    — Scapulae
    — Seventh cervical vertebra
    — Thoracic spinal column
    — Vertebral line
    — Midscapular line
- Explain the term *inspection of the chest* and the purpose of the procedure.
- Describe the characteristics and significance of the following respiratory rates and patterns:

  — Eupnea
  — Hyperpnea
  — Kussmaul's respiration
  — Cheyne-Stokes respiration
  — Biot's respiration
  — Paradoxical breathing
- Describe how the work of breathing may be assessed by inspection.
- Differentiate among the following abnormalities of the spine and their effects on respiratory structures and their function:
  — Kyphosis
  — Scoliosis
  — Lordosis
  — Kyphoscoliosis
- Compare and contrast a normal thoracic shape with that of barrel chest.
- Describe the appearance of digital clubbing and the significance of this change.
- Differentiate between the following abnormalities of the sternum:
  — Pectus excavatum
  — Pectus carinatum

(Continued)

- Describe the purpose of palpation and how it is used in detecting the following:
  — Areas of tenderness
  — Symmetry of chest excursion
  — Tactile fremitus
  — Presence of subcutaneous emphysema
  — Deviated position of the trachea
- Describe the technique of percussion:
  — Direct percussion

— Detection of areas of tenderness
- Differentiate among the following percussion tones and the changes in air density versus tissue density that produce them:
  — Hyperresonance
  — Resonance
  — Dullness
  — Flatness

CHEST LANDMARKS FOR ASSESSMENT

Abnormal findings on physical assessment or auscultation are best described in relation to anatomical landmarks and the imaginary vertical lines that divide the chest. These two location systems serve as a coordinate system, similar to that found on most road maps. For example, assessment findings might be noted as follows: "Tenderness was reported by the patient anteriorly, on the left side, at the second rib on the midclavicular line." A skilled practitioner can use the anatomical coordinates like a map to identify or describe a specific anatomical location.

Bony Structures As Anatomical Landmarks

Anterior Chest

Figure 3-1 shows the bony landmarks on the anterior chest. These include the clavicles, suprasternal notch, sternal angle, and the fourth rib. The clavicles are the prominent horizontal bones commonly called *collarbones*.

The sternal notch is located where the clavicles join at the top of the sternum—the manubrium. The manubrium joins the body of the sternum at a horizontal ridge. This ridge is termed the *sternal angle*. Immediately lateral to the sternal angle is the second rib. The sternal angle is a landmark used to find the second rib. Other ribs may be easily palpated from this starting point. The fourth rib is located on the nipple line (imaginary horizontal line through the nipples). Like the second rib, it is easily located and serves as a starting point for locating other ribs.

Posterior Chest

The predominant bony landmarks on the posterior chest include the vertebrae and the scapulae (Figure 3-2).

An easy way to establish position on the vertebral column is to ask the patient to bend the neck forward. The prominent process at the base of the neck is the seventh cervical vertebra (C7). The process immediately below it is the first thoracic vertebra (T1). Other thoracic vertebrae may be easily determined from this point.

The scapulae are the two large triangular bones below the shoulders, often referred to as the *shoulder blades*.

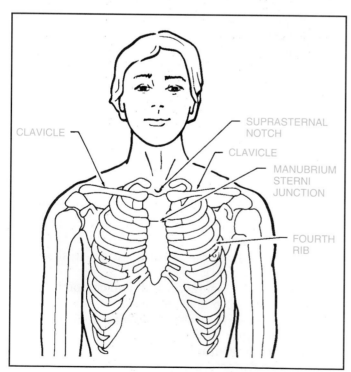

Figure 3-1   *Bony landmarks on the anterior chest*

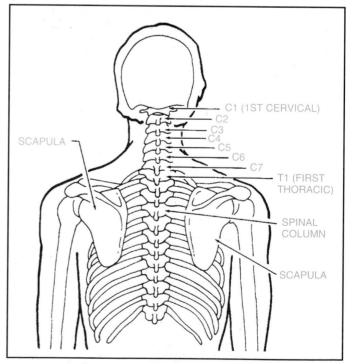

Figure 3-2   *Bony landmarks on the posterior chest*

Vertical Division Lines
Anterior Chest

Three imaginary vertical lines are used to divide the anterior chest. These lines are the midsternal line, midclavicular line, and the anterior midaxillary line (Figure 3-3). The midsternal line is an imaginary line dividing the sternum vertically in half. Imagine a line descending from the center of the sternum to the umbilicus (navel). The midclavicular lines are two vertical lines bisecting the clavicles. Each of these lines pass just medial to the nipples. The anterior axillary line is a line descending vertically from the junction of the arm and torso (at the front of the armpit).

Lateral Chest

The first division line on the lateral chest is the anterior axillary line. The two other imaginary vertical division lines are the midaxillary and posterior axillary lines (Figure 3-4). The midaxillary line is an imaginary line extending downward from the center of the armpit. The posterior axillary line is an imaginary line extending downward from the posterior junction of the arm.

Posterior Chest

There are three imaginary division lines on the posterior chest. These lines are the right and left midscapular lines and the vertebral line (Figure 3-5). The vertebral line is an imaginary line descending along the vertebral column. The left and right midscapular lines are imaginary lines bisecting the scapulae and descending vertically.

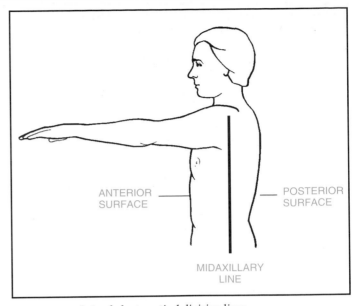

Figure 3-4   *Lateral chest vertical division lines*

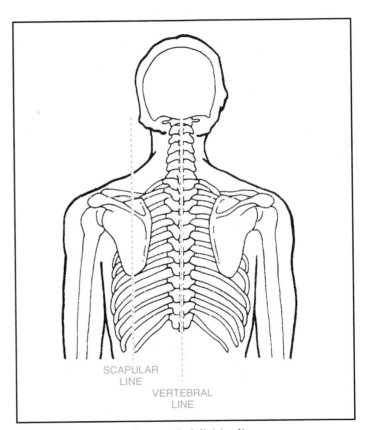

Figure 3-5   *Posterior chest vertical division lines*

ASSESSMENT TECHNIQUES AND ABNORMAL FINDINGS

Assessment of the chest includes inspection of the structure of the thorax, observation of patterns of movement during respiration, and percussion. For each component of the assessment, use of proper techniques and familiarity with the various types of abnormalities are essential for developing expertise in this area of respiratory care practice.

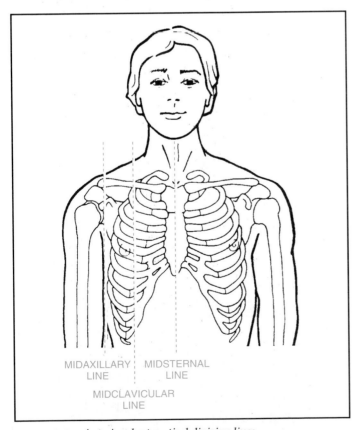

Figure 3-3   *Anterior chest vertical division lines*

Significant Aspects of Inspection of the Chest

Inspection of the chest consists of thorough observation of the chest and its motion. By careful observation of a variety of aspects including (1) the patient's skin color, (2) the work of breathing, and (3) conformation of the digits, a tremendous amount of information may be obtained.

Respiratory Rate, Rhythm, and Pattern

Observation of respiratory rate, rhythm, and pattern is an important aspect of inspection of the chest. In an adult breathing normally at rest, the respiratory rate is between 12 and 20 breaths per minute, with an inspiratory-to-expiratory ratio (I:E) of 1:2. This normal ventilatory pattern is termed *eupnea*.

An increase in the depth of respirations to greater than normal is termed *hyperpnea*. Often hyperpnea is mistakenly called hyperventilation. Hyperventilation refers to decreased carbon dioxide (CO_2) levels in the arterial blood as a result of increased ventilation, not respiratory rate or depth. Hyperpnea may exist with or without hyperventilation, or vice versa.

Hypopnea is a decrease in the depth of respirations to less than normal. When a patient is hypopneic, respirations are very shallow. There are many causes of hypopnea; one of the more serious results from a brain stem injury, which may also be accompanied by tachycardia with a weak pulse.

Variations in the respiratory pattern may be indicators of underlying conditions. Three abnormal respiratory patterns are *Kussmaul's respiration*, *Cheyne-Stokes respiration*, and *Biot's respiration*. Figure 3-6 is a graphic display comparing normal, Kussmaul's, Cheyne-Stokes, and Biot's breathing patterns. Another abnormal pattern is paradoxical breathing. It is often the result of chest wall trauma or paralysis and may significantly increase the work of breathing.

Kussmaul's respiration is an increase in rate and depth. It occurs most commonly as a result of diabetic crisis. In diabetic acidosis, excessive acid is produced and circulated in the bloodstream (condition termed *metabolic acidosis*). The brain responds by increasing the respiratory rate and depth to eliminate CO_2 from the blood, to correct the acidosis.

Cheyne-Stokes respiration is periodic in nature, with a gradual increase in depth and respiratory rate followed by a tapering of rate and depth with periods of apnea (absence of respirations). This abnormality has been described as a waxing and waning of respirations. It may be associated with congestive heart failure, damage or trauma to the central nervous system (CNS), or increased cerebrospinal fluid pressure.

Biot's respiration is irregular in rate and depth. There are variable periods of apnea between respirations. This respiratory pattern is highly variable. It is frequently associated with basal encephalitis or meningitis.

Paradoxical breathing is the result of discoordinated motion of various parts of the chest wall and/or abdomen. During normal breathing, the diaphragm descends and the ribs move up and out anteriorly and laterally. This movement increases the volume of the thoracic cavity, causing a decrease in intrathoracic pressure. Air then flows from the area of greater ambient pressure into the lungs—the area of lower pressure.

Trauma resulting in multiple rib fractures causes a loss of structural integrity of the rib cage. As the diaphragm descends, the injured section responds to the decrease in intrathoracic pressure and collapses in, rather than moving out normally. On exhalation, the increased intrathoracic pressure causes the affected area to bulge out (Figure 3-7).

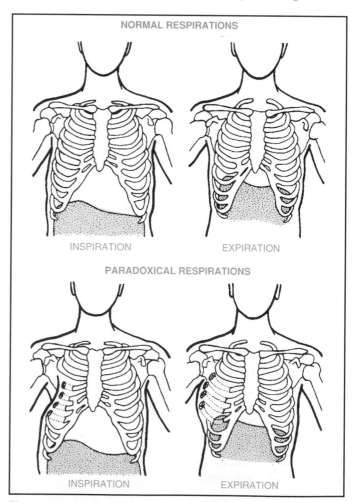

Figure 3-7 *Normal and paradoxical respirations*

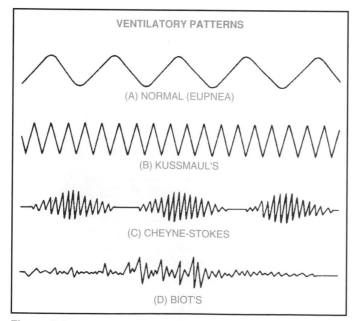

Figure 3-6 *Normal or eupnea (A), Kussmaul's (B), Cheyne-Stokes (C), and Biot's (D) respiratory patterns*

Work of Breathing

A general assessment of the work of breathing may be made by careful observation. The patient's body position gives an indication of the effort being expended. A patient assuming the position shown in Figure 3-8 is trying to transfer the effort required to sit upright to the arms instead of the abdomen. This position also shifts the abdominal contents away from the diaphragm, thus decreasing the work of breathing. This allows for less effort to be expended to sustain respiration. Observe the patient's use of accessory muscles while breathing. A patient having difficulty breathing will be unable to speak in a complete sentence. Speech will be in short bursts of words, with long pauses for breathing.

Abnormalities of the Skeleton

Abnormalities that are easily observed during inspection include abnormal thoracic diameter and shape, abnormal spinal curvature, and deformities of the sternum (Figure 3-9).

Thoracic Diameter and Shape. If you look at the chest from above, it is somewhat oval in shape. In the normal configuration of the chest, the anterior-posterior (AP) diameter (thickness) is less than the left-to-right diameter (width) (Figure 3-10).

An increase in the AP diameter to greater than normal results in a configuration termed *barrel chest*. This abnormality is commonly associated with chronic lung disease due to air trapping and a loss in lung compliance. This change in configuration is distinctive in appearance. It has the disadvantage of reducing the normal mechanical advantage of the ribs and intercostal muscles, resulting in less efficient ventilation.

Kyphosis. *Kyphosis* is an abnormal curvature of the upper spine. It is an anterior-to-posterior curvature that gives the patient a *humpback* appearance. It is frequently associated with chronic lung disease.

Scoliosis. *Scoliosis* is a lateral curvature of the spine. This lateral curvature causes the vertebrae in the affected area to rotate, flattening the rib cage anteriorly. Frequently, this abnormality can interfere with the mechanics of ventilation.

Lordosis. *Lordosis* is an inward curvature of the lumbar spine. This curvature results in a *swayback* appearance.

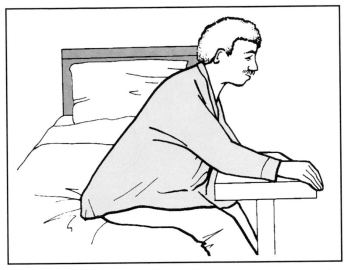

Figure 3-8 *A patient assuming a position indicating an increase in the work of breathing*

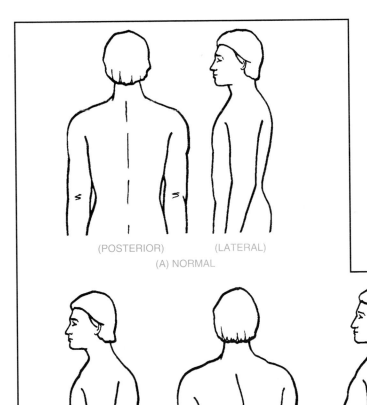

(POSTERIOR)　　(LATERAL)
(A) NORMAL

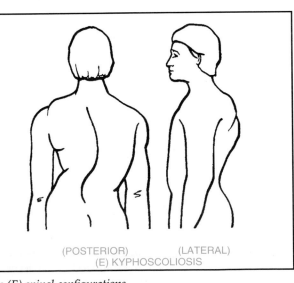

(LATERAL)　　　(POSTERIOR)　　(LATERAL)　　　(POSTERIOR)　　(LATERAL)
(B) KYPHOSIS　　(C) SCOLIOSIS　　(D) LORDOSIS　　(E) KYPHOSCOLIOSIS

Figure 3-9 *Normal (A), kyphosis (B), scoliosis (C), lordosis (D), and kyphoscoliosis (E) spinal configurations*

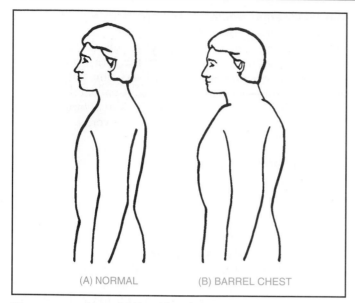

Figure 3-10 *Normal (A) and barrel chest (B) configuration*

(A) NORMAL   (B) BARREL CHEST

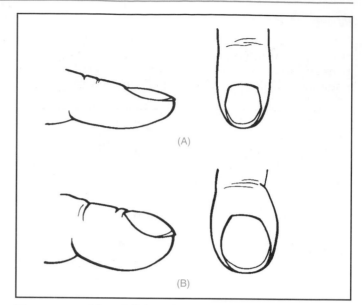

Figure 3-11 *Normal digit conformation (A) and clubbing (B)*

(A)

(B)

It is not usually associated with any pathologic respiratory condition.

Kyphoscoliosis. *Kyphoscoliosis* is a combination of kyphosis and scoliosis. Assess the lateral curvature of the spine first by comparing the heights of the scapulae. Then assess the severity of the kyphosis component. This condition can profoundly affect ventilatory volume and the mechanics of respiration. It frequently results in congestive heart failure and circulatory embarrassment as well. Many patients with severe kyphoscoliosis die at an early age of acute respiratory infection or chronic respiratory insufficiency.

Pectus Excavatum. *Pectus excavatum* is a congenital deformity of the sternum characterized by a depression in the sternum at the level of the lower body and xyphoid process. It is commonly called *funnel chest*, a term that visually describes the condition. If severe, pectus excavatum may result in decreased lung volumes.

Pectus Carinatum. *Pectus carinatum* is a congenital deformity of the sternum characterized by an outward projection of the sternum. The common term for this deformity is *pigeon chest*. This condition usually does not result in any respiratory complications.

Digital Clubbing

Chronic lung disease is one of several conditions that may cause *digital clubbing*. Hypoxemia (insufficient oxygen in the blood) results in the formation of arterial-venous anastomoses in the terminal digits. These formations are actual circulatory connections between the two sides of the circulatory system. The circulatory changes result in dramatic changes in the terminal portions of the digits (both fingers and toes) (Figure 3-11). In clubbing, the angle between the nailbed and finger becomes increased. Looking at the digits from above, the terminal portion increases in diameter as well. Often, cyanosis of the nailbeds will also be present.

Palpation of the Chest

Palpation is the physical assessment of the chest by the sense of touch. Because the hands are very sensitive, temperature differences and vibrations may be easily perceived. The hands may also be used as indicators to assess symmetry of chest movement.

Areas of Tenderness

As a practitioner palpates the chest, the patient may complain about areas that are sore or tender to the touch. This information may provide important clues to underlying conditions.

Symmetry of Excursion

Symmetry may be readily assessed by placing the hands on corresponding positions of the right and left sides of the chest and observing chest wall motion (Figures 3-12 and 3-13). As the patient inhales deeply, your hands should move apart in a symmetrical way. If one hand moves more than the other, this may indicate consolidation (airless, fluid-filled, uncollapsed lung tissue), pleural effusion (fluid in the pleural space), atelectasis (loss of air in the lung tissue), or a pneumothorax (air in the pleural space).

Tactile Fremitus

Tactile fremitus is vibration felt on the palpation of the chest during phonation, or speech. As the patient speaks, vibrations are transmitted through the bronchi and lung parenchyma to the skin surface where they can be felt. An increase in tactile fremitus indicates an increase in density of the underlying tissue. This change may be caused by pneumonia or atelectasis.

Subcutaneous Emphysema

Subcutaneous emphysema is the presence of air beneath the skin in the subcutaneous tissues. This condition may be localized or very diffuse over a large area. Subcutaneous emphysema is sometimes a complication of

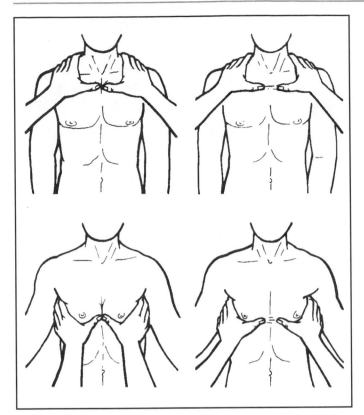

Figure 3-12 *Hand positions for assessing symmetry of the anterior chest*

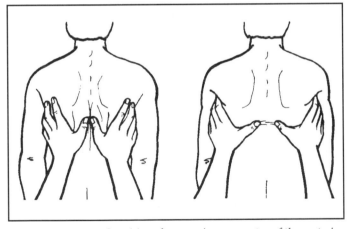

Figure 3-13 *Hand positions for assessing symmetry of the posterior chest*

TABLE 3-1: Causes of Change in Tracheal Position	
TRACHEAL SHIFT TOWARD AFFECTED SIDE	**TRACHEAL SHIFT AWAY FROM AFFECTED SIDE**
Atelectasis	Pleural effusion
Fibrosis	Pneumothorax
	Tension pneumothorax

or right—can be assessed. Table 3-1 lists the direction of tracheal shift occurring as a result of different pathological conditions.

Percussion of the Chest

Everyone has had the doctor thump on the chest as part of a routine chest or general physical examination. *Percussion* is tapping on the chest while listening for the resulting sound. There are two methods of percussing the chest, direct and indirect. The direct method involves tapping on the chest with a finger, using a short, sharp stroke. Indirect percussion involves placing a finger firmly against the chest and tapping on that finger (Figure 3-14).

Four different types of sounds may be heard during percussion of the chest: hyperresonance, resonance, dullness, and flatness.

Hyperresonance

Hyperresonance is an abnormal percussion sound heard over the chest. It occurs as a result of air trapping or from the presence of air in a closed cavity. A pneumothorax is an example of the latter category. With hyperresonance, percussion produces a loud, low-pitched sound of long duration. This percussion note is produced as sound passes through an area with a greater proportion of air in relation to tissue (high air-to-tissue ratio). This sound can also be heard over an air-filled stomach.

Resonance

Resonance is the sound heard in percussing normal lung tissue. It is a low-pitched sound of long duration. This sound is characteristic of areas that contain equal distributions of air and tissue.

Dullness

Dullness is a sound of medium intensity and pitch with a short duration. It is heard over areas containing a greater proportion of tissue or fluid than of air. This occurs in the lungs as a result of consolidation, atelectasis, or the presence of fluid in the pleural space.

Flatness

Flatness is a sound of low amplitude and pitch. It is heard over areas containing a greater proportion of tissue than of air. Frequently, flatness is an indication of pleural effusion.

tracheostomy, pneumothorax, or mechanical ventilation. The tissue changes are easily palpated; the findings are best described as feeling like a bowl of plastic beads covered with a layer of cellophane.

Tracheal Deviation

Deviation of the trachea from its normal midline position may be indicative of several underlying conditions. By depressing your index finger into the sternal notch, you can palpate the trachea. Its relative position—midline, left,

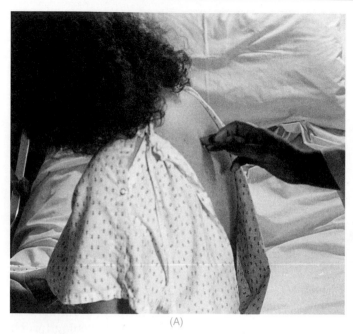
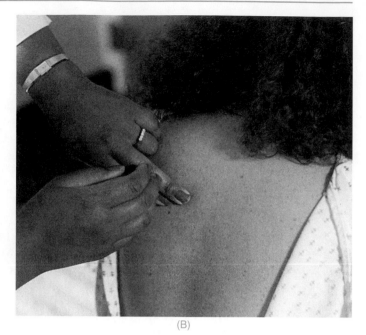

(A)   (B)

Figure 3-14   *Direct (A) and indirect (B) percussion*

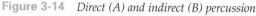

OBJECTIVES

At the end of this chapter, you should be able to:

• Describe the optimal environment for the physical assessment of the chest.

• Using a laboratory partner, properly position and prepare the partner for physical assessment of the chest.

• Using a laboratory partner, demonstrate inspection of the chest.

• Using a laboratory partner, demonstrate palpation of the chest.

• Using a laboratory partner, demonstrate percussion of the chest.

PREEXAMINATION AND OTHER CONSIDERATIONS

During physical assessment of the chest, your patient's privacy may be compromised. If possible, close the door and dismiss any visitors before beginning your examination. The temperature of the room should be comfortable and not too cold. Turn off any radios, televisions, or appliances that may be distracting to you. Explain to the patient what you will be doing and what information it may provide about his or her condition.

Male patients should disrobe to the waist for the examination. Female patients should disrobe and remove any undergarments, and then slip on a patient gown that will allow access to the chest as required.

Part of your examination will require touching the chest with your hands. This is not a breast exam. A male practitioner examining a female patient should have a female nurse or physician present in the room when conducting the exam. Failure to do so may potentially result in litigation by the patient against the practitioner. Common sense and respect for your patient's dignity will help to prevent these complications.

INSPECTION OF THE CHEST

Inspection of the chest is a detailed observation to determine the breathing pattern, assess the work of breathing, and identify skeletal abnormalities.

Observe the patient's breathing pattern. Determine if the rate and rhythm are normal. Assess the I:E ratio; it normally is 1:2.

Assess the work of breathing. Is the patient assuming an unusual posture? Listen carefully to your patient as you converse. Is the patient able to speak in complete sentences? Observe the use of accessory muscles while the patient is breathing.

Observe the chest posteriorly with the patient sitting upright. Look at the spinal column. Check to see if it is normal in appearance. Is there evidence of kyphosis, scoliosis, lordosis, or kyphoscoliosis?

Check the AP diameter. Is the AP diameter increased, suggesting evidence of barrel chest? If the patient is barrel chested, do the digits show evidence of clubbing?

Take time to carefully observe the chest. Develop a systematic approach. Initially, it is helpful to make a brief outline of all steps to be followed in assessment. Refer to this list as you practice in the laboratory. This list will help to reinforce a mental image of the tasks you will be performing.

Palpation

Methodically palpate the chest posteriorly and anteriorly. Determine if there are areas of tenderness and assess the skin temperature. Palpate for subcutaneous emphysema as you move over the surface of the chest.

To evaluate chest wall motion, place your hands as shown in Figures 3-12 and 3-13. Ask your patient to take a deep breath. Observe the motion of your hands as they move apart upon the patient's inspiration. Is the motion symmetrical? Do your hands move at all? (Patients with obstructive lung disease will exhibit little or no chest excursion on inspiration.) If one area is not symmetrical in its motion, make a mental note of it. When percussing the chest, carefully assess the side that demonstrated little motion.

To evaluate tactile fremitus, place the palmar surface of your hands on the patient's chest (Figure 3-15). Alternately, the ulnar surface of the hands may be used (Figure 3-16). Ask your patient to say "ninety-nine" repeatedly. Progressively move your hands over the chest, feeling tactile fremitus. Determine if there are areas of increased fremitus (potential consolidation).

Using your index finger, palpate at the sternal notch to assess tracheal position. Is the trachea central or deviated left or right? If it is deviated, make a mental note of which side. When percussing the chest, carefully assess the side opposite the tracheal deviation.

Percussion

Percuss the chest systematically over the entire surface. Place one finger on the chest, making sure that only the one finger is in contact with the surface of the chest. Strike that finger with the third finger on your other hand as shown in Figure 3-14. Progress from the top downward, comparing the tone generated by each side bilaterally. Position the finger in contact with the chest between the ribs. Don't percuss over the bone or a female patient's breast tissue. Note any changes in the tone, especially if it sounds dull (area of increased density).

You can easily assess diaphragmatic excursion on the posterior chest. Have your patient take a deep breath and hold it. Percuss down the posterior chest until dullness is heard. Mark this position with a felt-tip marker or grease pencil (make sure it is not a permanent marker). Now ask the patient to exhale completely and hold his or her breath. Percuss up from your mark, listening for resonance. Mark this position. The distance between the two points is the diaphragmatic excursion, which may be as much as 8 centimeters.

Recording Your Findings

It is important to make a careful record of your findings. If abnormalities are found, note their position in relation to the imaginary vertical lines and the rib number. For exam-

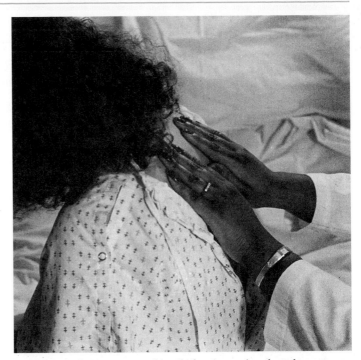

Figure 3-15 *Assessment of tactile fremitus using the palmar surface of your hands*

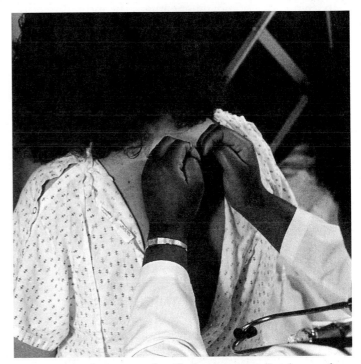

Figure 3-16 *Assessment of tactile fremitus using the ulnar surface of your hands*

ple, your charting might read: "Dullness was heard on percussion anteriorly on the right side from the second to the fourth rib on the midclavicular line." Only by recording your observations and serially comparing findings is physical assessment useful in following the course of a patient's progress.

Additional Resources

Burton, G. G., Hodgkin, J. E., & Ward, J. (1995). *Respiratory care: A guide to clinical practice* (4th ed.). Philadelphia: Lippincott.

Eubanks, D., & Bone, R. (1991). *Comprehensive respiratory care* (2nd ed.). St. Louis, MO: Mosby.

Shoup, C. A. (1988). *Laboratory exercises in respiratory therapy.* St. Louis, MO: Mosby.

Wilkins, R. L., Krider, S. J., & Sheldon, R. (1995). *Clinical assessment in respiratory care* (3rd ed.). St. Louis, MO: Mosby.

Witkowski, A. S. (1985). *Pulmonary assessment: A clinical guide.* Philadelphia: Lippincott.

Practice Activities: Advanced Patient Assessment

1. Using a laboratory partner, practice inspection of the chest. Include the following in your examination:
   a. Determination of respiratory rate and pattern
   b. Evaluation of work of breathing
   c. Examination of spine and sternum for abnormalities
   d. Comparison of AP diameter and lateral diameter
   e. Inspection of the digits for clubbing or cyanosis

2. Using a laboratory partner, practice palpation of the chest. Assess for the following in your examination:
   a. Areas of tenderness
   b. Symmetry of movement anteriorly and posteriorly:
      (1) Upper lobes
      (2) Middle and lingular lobes
      (3) Lower lobes
   c. Tactile fremitus

d. The presence of subcutaneous emphysema
e. Deviation of tracheal position

3. Using a laboratory partner, practice percussing the chest. Include the following in your examination:
   a. Correct finger position and technique
   b. Systematic approach
   c. Bilateral comparison
   d. Diaphragmatic excursion

4. Describe specifically various anatomical locations in your practice utilizing the coordinate system discussed in the theory text of this chapter.

5. Following completion of a physical examination of your laboratory partner's chest, document your findings on a piece of paper. Have your instructor critique your charting.

Check List: Advanced Patient Assessment

1. Inspect the chart:
   a. Admitting diagnosis
   b. History
   c. Laboratory tests
2. Assemble equipment:
   a. Stethoscope
   b. Paper and pen
3. Identify the patient and introduce yourself.
4. Wash your hands.
5. Optimize the environment:
   a. Turn off the radio or television.
   b. Ensure a comfortable temperature.
   c. Ensure the patient's privacy and adequate attire.
6. Explain the procedure.
7. Position the patient optimally.
8. Inspect the chest, observing the following:
   a. Respiratory rate and rhythm
   b. Work of breathing
   c. Spine and sternum for deformities

   d. AP diameter
   e. Appearance of the digits for clubbing or cyanosis
9. Palpate the chest, including the following:
   a. Identify areas of tenderness.
   b. Evaluate for symmetry.
   c. Assess for tactile fremitus.
   d. Determine if subcutaneous emphysema is present.
   e. Determine the tracheal position.
10. Percuss the chest, including the following:
    a. Proper technique
    b. Systematic method
    c. Diaphragmatic excursion
11. Solicit a cough for sputum examination.
12. Ensure the patient's safety and comfort.
13. Solicit and answer questions.
14. Wash your hands.
15. Record your findings on the patient's chart.

Self-Evaluation Post Test: Physical Assessment of the Chest

1. The second rib may be easily identified by:
   a. palpating the process of the seventh cervical vertebra.
   b. palpating the sternal angle.
   c. palpating the sternal notch.
   d. palpating the xyphoid process.

2. Which of the following is not a vertical division line on the anterior chest?
   a. Midaxillary line
   b. Midsternal line
   c. Midclavicular line
   d. Vertebral line

3. Eupnea is:
   a. rapid shallow breathing.
   b. deep and rapid breathing.
   c. deep breathing with a normal respiratory rate.
   d. normal breathing.

4. The correct term for deep rapid breathing is:
   a. eupnea.
   b. bradypnea.
   c. tachypnea.
   d. hyperpnea.

5. A lateral curvature of the spine is termed:
   a. lordosis.
   b. kyphosis.
   c. scoliosis.
   d. kyphoscoliosis.

6. A lateral curvature and humpback is termed:
   a. lordosis.
   b. kyphosis.
   c. scoliosis.
   d. kyphoscoliosis.

7. Which of the following may be assessed by palpation?
   I. Areas of tenderness
   II. Symmetry of chest excursion
   III. Resonance
   IV. Tracheal position
   a. I, III, IV
   b. II, III, IV
   c. I, IV
   d. I, II, IV

8. Which of the following percussion tones is a loud, low-pitched sound of long duration?
   a. Resonance
   b. Hyperresonance
   c. Dullness
   d. Flatness

9. Hyperresonance may be heard:
   a. over areas of increased density.
   b. over areas containing fluid.
   c. over the trachea.
   d. over areas containing trapped air.

10. A percussion tone heard over areas of roughly equal air and tissue ratio is:
    a. hyperresonance.
    b. resonance.
    c. dullness.
    d. flatness.

PERFORMANCE EVALUATION:
PHYSICAL ASSESSMENT

Date: Lab _____ Clinical _____ Agency _____

Lab: Pass _____ Fail _____   Clinical: Pass _____ Fail _____

Student name _____ Instructor name _____

No. of times observed in clinical _____

No. of times practiced in clinical _____

PASSING CRITERIA: Obtain 90% or better on the procedure. Tasks indicated by * must receive at least 1 point, or the evaluation is terminated. Procedure must be performed within designated time, or the performance receives a failing grade.

SCORING:
2 points — Task performed satisfactorily without prompting.
1 point — Task performed satisfactorily with self-initiated correction.
0 points — Task performed incorrectly or with prompting required.
NA — Task not applicable to the patient care situation.

TASKS:		PEER	LAB	CLINICAL
	1. Verifies the physician's order	☐	☐	☐
	2. Reviews the patient's chart	☐	☐	☐
	3. Identifies the patient and introduces self	☐	☐	☐
*	4. Explains the procedure	☐	☐	☐
*	5. Optimizes the environment	☐	☐	☐
*	6. Washes hands	☐	☐	☐
*	7. Positions the patient	☐	☐	☐
	8. Inspects the chest			
*	a. Respiratory rate and pattern	☐	☐	☐
	b. Work of breathing	☐	☐	☐
*	c. Spine and sternum abnormalities	☐	☐	☐
*	d. AP diameter	☐	☐	☐
*	e. Clubbing of the digits	☐	☐	☐
	9. Palpates the chest			
*	a. Identifies areas of tenderness	☐	☐	☐
*	b. Assesses symmetry of chest movements	☐	☐	☐
*	c. Assesses tactile fremitus	☐	☐	☐
*	d. Determines tracheal position	☐	☐	☐
	10. Percusses the chest			
*	a. Uses a systematic method	☐	☐	☐
*	b. Uses the proper technique	☐	☐	☐
*	c. Determines diaphragm excursion	☐	☐	☐
	11. Solicits a sputum sample	☐	☐	☐
	12. Ensures the patient's safety and comfort	☐	☐	☐

* 13. Washes hands after the procedure ☐ ☐ ☐

* 14. Records the findings on the patient's chart ☐ ☐ ☐

SCORE: Peer   _____ points of possible 46; _____%

                Lab   _____ points of possible 46; _____%

                Clinical   _____ points of possible 46; _____%

TIME: _____ out of possible 30 minutes

STUDENT SIGNATURES   **INSTRUCTOR SIGNATURES**

PEER: _____   LAB: _____

STUDENT: _____   CLINICAL: _____

CHAPTER 4
RADIOLOGIC ASSESSMENT

INTRODUCTION

The ability to interpret and review radiographic images of the chest is important to the practice of respiratory care. As a respiratory care practitioner, you will be expected to identify the presence of a pneumothorax, subcutaneous emphysema, consolidation, atelectasis, and pulmonary infiltrates. You must also be able to identify the position of endotracheal, tracheostomy, nasogastric, and chest tubes, as well as pulmonary artery and central venous catheters.

A patient's disease state is often manifested by changes in the chest radiograph. These changes may include hyperinflation, accumulation of pleural fluid, development of pulmonary edema, increase in hilar markings, and mediastinal shift. As a respiratory care practitioner, you must be able to relate changes in the chest radiograph with changes in signs and symptoms presented by the patient.

Special radiographic procedures such as ventilation-perfusion scanning and angiography are used in the diagnosis of pulmonary embolism. As a respiratory care practitioner, you must be able to recognize abnormal changes associated with ventilation-perfusion mismatching and how loss of circulation to an area or segment of the lung is manifested radiographically.

Computed tomography (CT) imaging is becoming more common in the acute care setting. As a respiratory care practitioner, you must be able to utilize CT findings to aid the diagnosis and management of your patients.

KEY TERMS

- Anterior-posterior
- Apical lordotic
- Atelectasis
- Computed tomography
- Consolidation
- Hilum
- Hyperinflation
- Infiltrate
- Exposed
- Lateral
- Left anterior oblique
- Pneumothorax
- Pneumomediastinum
- Posterior-anterior
- Pulmonary angiography
- Radiodensity
- Right anterior oblique
- Subcutaneous emphysema
- Tomogram
- Unexposed
- Ventilation-perfusion scanning

OBJECTIVES

At the end of this chapter, you should be able to:

- Describe how an x-ray film of the chest is produced.
- Describe the differences in radiodensity of the following:
  — Air
  — Water
  — Fat
  — Bone
  — Plastic
  — Metal
- Differentiate among the following x-ray views of the chest:
  — Anterior-posterior (AP)
  — Posterior-anterior (PA)
  — Lateral
  — Apical lordotic
  — Left anterior oblique
  — Right anterior oblique
  — Lateral decubitus
  — Lateral neck
- Identify the anatomical structures and landmarks observed on normal PA and lateral chest x-ray views.
- Given an abnormal chest radiograph, identify the presence of extrapulmonary air:
  — Pneumothorax
  — Subcutaneous emphysema
  — Pneumomediastinum
- Given an abnormal chest radiograph, identify the following changes in lung volume:
  — Hyperinflation
  — Atelectasis
  — Mediastinal shift
  — Consolidation
- Given an abnormal chest radiograph, identify the following fluid-related abnormalities:
  — Pleural effusion
  — Congestive heart failure
  — Pulmonary edema
  — Pulmonary infiltrates
- Given a chest radiograph of a critically ill patient, identify the following:
  — Endotracheal tube
  — Tracheostomy tube
  — Pulmonary artery catheter
  — Central venous catheter
  — Nasogastric tube
  — Feeding tube

(Continued)

— Electrocardiography (ECG) leads
— Pacemaker wires
— Surgical clips or staples
— Foreign bodies
• Describe the technique of ventilation-perfusion scanning.
• Given a ventilation-perfusion (V/Q) scan, identify the presence and location of a ventilation-perfusion mismatch.

• Describe the technique of pulmonary angiography.
• Given an abnormal pulmonary angiogram, identify circulatory occlusion.
• Describe how a computed tomography (CT) scan of the chest is made.
• Given a CT scan of the chest, locate the cut you are viewing superiorly and inferiorly with respect to the scout image.

PRODUCTION OF A CHEST RADIOGRAPH

X-rays are a form of ionizing radiation, having a very short wavelength of between 0.05 and 100 angstroms (Å). X-rays are produced by the x-ray tubes in an x-ray machine. A very high voltage (100 to 400 kilovolts) from the x-ray machine's transformer is conducted to the x-ray tube, where it bombards a positively charged tungsten target contained in the near-vacuum of the x-ray tube (Wallace, 1995). The deflected electrons undergo physical changes after striking the tungsten target and are emitted as x-radiation (Figure 4-1). Once produced, x-rays will scatter in all directions; a narrow window channels the x-ray emissions toward the desired target. The energy not emitted by the tube is absorbed and does not escape. However, because of the x-ray's tendency to scatter, the beam will spread as distance increases from the x-ray tube. This is similar to how a flashlight beam enlarges as the distance from the bulb increases.

X-ray emissions, being very-short-wavelength electromagnetic energy, tend to penetrate objects rather than to be reflected by them as happens with energy in the visible light spectrum. The degree to which x-ray energy penetrates an object is dependent on the density of the object. If the density of the object is great, penetration is low. If the density of the object is low, penetration by x-radiation is greater. When the object of interest is placed between the x-ray tube and a sheet of photographic film, shadows are cast onto the film. The density of these shadows—light or dark—will depend on the *radiodensity* of the material between the x-ray tube and the film plane. Areas of low density will appear dark, or *exposed*, whereas areas of high density will appear white, or *unexposed*, when the film is developed. For imaging of the chest using x-rays, the patient is placed between the x-ray tube and the film plane, and shadows are cast onto the film depending on the densities of the anatomical structures the x-ray energy passes through.

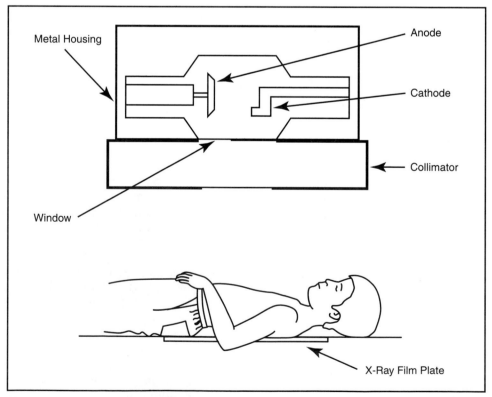

Figure 4-1 *This figure illustrates how an x-ray is produced. Note the tungsten target and the window that limits the scatter of the x-ray energy.*

RADIODENSITY OF COMMON MATERIALS

The radiodensity of anatomical structures or tissues and manmade materials is dependent on how dense the material is. An x-ray image of the chest will show many shades between black (low density) to white (high density), depending on what material the x-ray energy passes through. Common structures x-ray energy may pass through during imaging of the chest are air, water, fat, bone, plastic, and metal. All of these materials have varying radiodensities.

Air is the least radiodense of the structures x-radiation passes through during imaging of the chest. Being of low radiodensity, air is readily penetrated by the x-rays, fully exposing the x-ray film. When the film is developed, air-filled areas appear black on the x-ray image. The dark radiolucent air-filled spaces provide a good contrast to the denser tissues surrounding the air-filled alveoli and bronchi.

Water has a greater radiodensity than that of air. Some of the x-ray energy is absorbed, while the majority passes through to the x-ray film. Water, therefore, casts a gray shadow on the x-ray film when it is developed.

Fat tissue has a greater radiodensity than that of water. Fat tissue absorbs more x-ray energy than water does. The shadow produced on the developed x-ray film by fat is a lighter shade of gray than that produced by water.

Bone has the greatest density of all of the anatomical structures in the chest. The majority of x-ray energy is absorbed by bone. A bony structure, therefore, casts a white (unexposed) shadow on the developed x-ray film.

Manmade materials may also be visualized on a chest radiograph. Common materials are plastics (mostly poly vinyl chloride [PVC]) and metal. Plastics are used to make artificial airways and indwelling catheters. In its natural state, plastic has a low radiodensity, similar to that of fat. However, for easy visualization of these devices on an x-ray image, a radiopaque line is molded into the manufactured object (Figure 4-2). This feature allows for a more precise determination of the position of the object.

Metal is the most radiodense material viewed on a chest x-ray. Surgical clips, staples, and wire are common and are readily identified as small, thin white lines. These appear brighter than bony structures. Foreign objects made of metal that are nonsurgical may also appear on the chest film. Such objects may include bullets, coins, buckshot, or other items that have entered the thoracic cavity.

X-RAY VIEWS OF THE CHEST

Many different views of the chest can be obtained using x-ray techniques. Some views are named by the way the x-ray energy passes through the chest (anterior-posterior or posterior-anterior); others, by the way the patient is oriented (lordotic, oblique, lateral, lateral decubitus). You must know the common views of the chest, why specific views are used, and how they enhance the imaging of the chest.

The *posterior-anterior* (PA) view of the chest is one of the most common x-ray views (Figure 4-3). For the PA

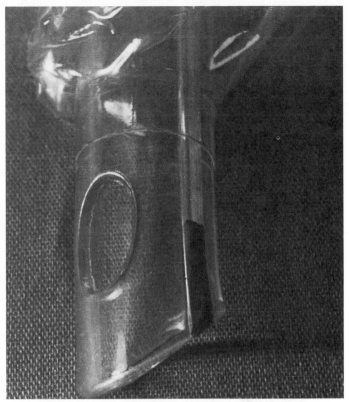

Figure 4-2 *A photograph of an endotracheal tube. Notice the radiopaque line along the length of the tube extending to the distal tip.*

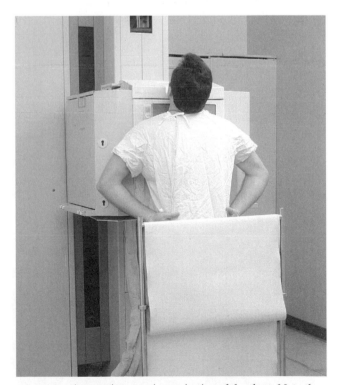

Figure 4-3 *A posterior-anterior projection of the chest. Note the position of the x-ray tube, patient, and film cassette. The x-rays pass from the posterior to the anterior surface.*

view, the film cassette rests on the anterior surface of the chest and the x-ray energy passes from the posterior surface through the chest, exposing the film on the anterior surface of the chest. Because the heart is more anterior than posterior within the chest, the heart shadow is smaller on a PA image than on the anterior-posterior view.

For the *anterior-posterior* (AP) view of the chest, the film cassette rests on the posterior surface of the chest and the x-ray energy passes from the anterior surface through the chest, exposing the film (Figure 4-4). The AP view is most commonly obtained by use of a "portable" technique. In the portable AP view, a mobile x-ray machine is brought to the patient's bedside, the film cassette is slid under the patient, and the x-ray picture is taken. Because the heart is more anterior, the heart shadow is magnified slightly in the AP view. Portable chest films are often used to verify tube placement (of an endotracheal, or chest tube, for example), to identify pneumothoraces, to locate foreign bodies, and so on.

For the *lateral* view, the film cassette rests on the left lateral surface of the chest, and the x-rays pass from the right side of the body through the chest, exposing the film (Figure 4-5). Because an x-ray image is a two-dimensional view or rendering, both the PA and the lateral films must be compared to locate precisely an anomaly or an object. By comparing the PA and the lateral films, a three-dimensional image may be created.

Sometimes it is necessary to focus attention on the upper lobes of the lungs. In a conventional PA view, the clavicles obscure part of the desired field of view. For the *apical lordotic* view (Figure 4-6), the patient leans backward at about 45°. This positioning moves the shadow of the clavicles out of the way, allowing better imaging of the upper lobes of the lungs.

For the *lateral decubitus* view of the chest, the patient is in a side-lying position, and the film cassette rests on the

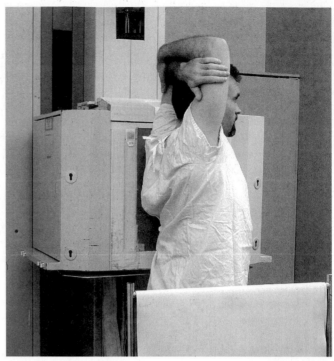

Figure 4-5 *A lateral projection of the chest. Note the position of the x-ray tube, patient, and film cassette.*

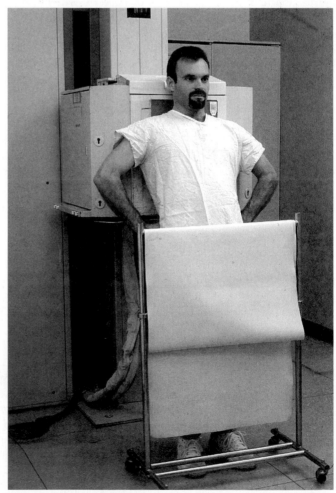

Figure 4-6 *An apical lordotic projection of the chest. Note that the patient is reclined approximately 45°, moving the clavicle's shadows.*

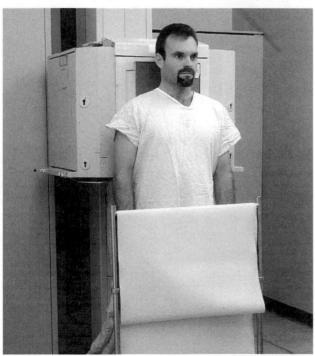

Figure 4-4 *An anterior-posterior projection of the chest. Note the position of the x-ray tube, patient, and film cassette. The x-rays pass from the anterior to the posterior surface.*

posterior surface of the chest (Figure 4-7). This view is utilized to identify and quantify the extent of pleural effusion (liquid in the pleural space). Because liquid is denser than air, it will travel to the dependent (inferior) portion of the lung, creating a shadow that lies along a plane parallel with the surface the patient is lying on (Figure 4-8).

For the *left anterior oblique* view, the patient is rotated to the right (left side more forward) with the film cassette placed against the anterior surface of the chest (Figure 4-9). For the *right anterior oblique* view, the patient is rotated to the left (right side more forward) with the film cassette placed against the anterior surface of the chest (Figure 4-10). These views are used to shift the heart shadow so that the lung (left or right) is more easily visualized. These

views are commonly used in ventilation-perfusion scanning, which is discussed later in the chapter.

The *lateral neck* view is used to image the soft tissues of the upper airway. This view is commonly used in pediatrics, to image the epiglottis and the larynx. In acute epiglottitis, the epiglottis becomes swollen, and may obstruct the airway. Figure 4-11 is a lateral neck radiograph showing an enlarged epiglottis.

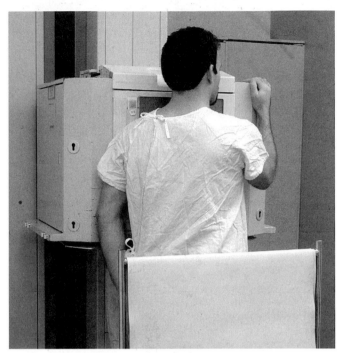

Figure 4-9 *A left anterior oblique projection of the chest. Note the position of the x-ray tube, patient, and film cassette.*

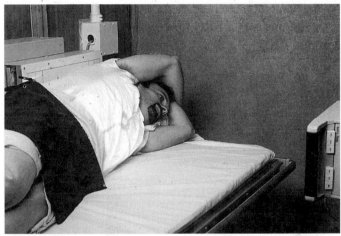

Figure 4-7 *A lateral decubitus projection. Note that the patient is in a side-lying position. Any fluid present in the pleural space will migrate dependently and appear as a layer at the most inferior point.*

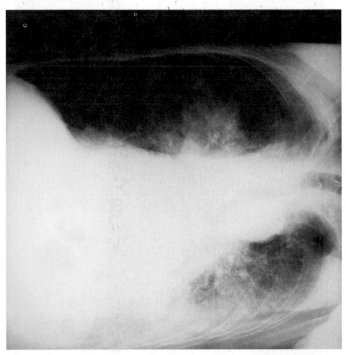

Figure 4-8 *Pleural effusion is evident on this lateral decubitus view of the chest. Note the layer along the dependent portion of the chest wall.*

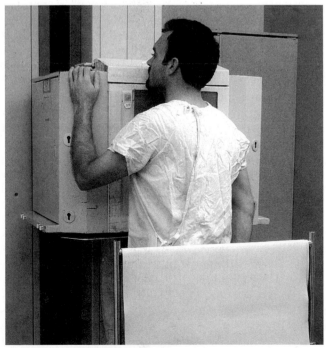

Figure 4-10 *A right anterior oblique projection of the chest. Note the position of the x-ray tube, patient, and film cassette.*

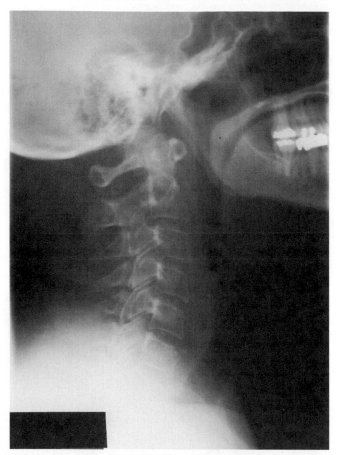

Figure 4-11 *A lateral neck x-ray for soft tissue assessment. Note the swollen epiglottis almost in the shape of a finger.*

THE NORMAL CHEST RADIOGRAPH

A normal chest radiograph contains in its image many normal anatomical structures. Reading a chest film or radiograph requires the ability to distinguish those normal structures and their normal positions from others that are abnormal. Reading chest radiographs requires repeated practice, much as in auscultating breath sounds. Your instructor may provide your initial orientation to reading chest radiographs, providing you with the basics for minimal competency in your clinical practice. However, to become more proficient, it is best to have repeated discussions with radiologists as you view and interpret films of the patients assigned to your care. Only through repeated, guided practice can you become more proficient in your abilities.

One of the most important aspects of reading chest radiographs is consistency. Often an abnormality stands out on the chest film, focusing your attention on that feature. If you are not systematic in looking at the entire film, important details may be missed. Common systematic approaches include the "outside-in" and the "inside-out" approaches. With the outside-in approach, you view the film moving from outside the chest to inside the chest. With the inside-out approach, you view the film moving from the heart to the structures lying on the outside of the chest wall. Or you may prefer to use a technique of progressing from one level of radiodensity (high density) to

the next lower density. Whatever approach you adopt, be consistent, applying it every time you view a radiograph. Remember what anatomical structures are normally present, and don't miss evaluating each one as you view the film.

Figures 4-12 and 4-13 are normal PA and lateral views of the chest. On the PA film (see Figure 4-12), first determine if the patient is rotated and how well the radiograph was penetrated (exposed).

To evaluate if the patient is rotated, find the necks of both clavicles. The spine should lie right between the clavicles (Figure 4-12). If the spine lies either to the right or to the left of center, the patient is rotated. Patient rotation can affect the way some structures appear, and therefore this finding is important to note. Penetration is evaluated by assessing the spinal processes in the center of the chest. The spinal processes should just barely be distinguishable from one another. If the spinal processes are very distinct, with dark lines separating them, the radiograph is over-

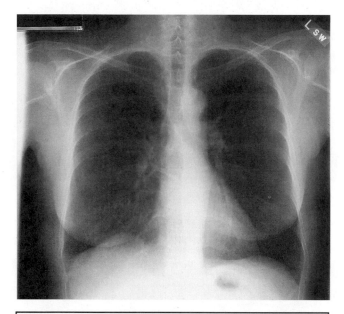

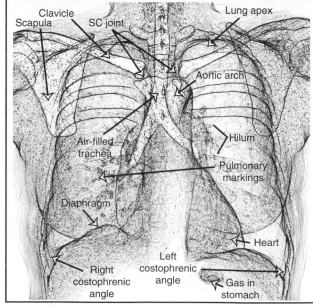

Figure 4-12 *A normal PA x-ray film of the chest.*

penetrated (overexposed) with x-ray energy. A film that is overpenetrated will appear darker and may be incorrectly interpreted as "normal" when the lung fields are evaluated. An underpenetrated film will appear lighter; this technical error may also lead to an incorrect interpretation.

The outer surface of the chest wall (light gray) is sil-

houetted against the stark dark background of air that surrounds the chest (black). Evaluate the areas outside of the chest wall, observing for dark (black) streaks against the gray tissue, indicating subcutaneous air (Figure 4-14). Air will tend to migrate upward (superiorly). Next evaluate the ribs. Trace each rib from the sternum laterally to where

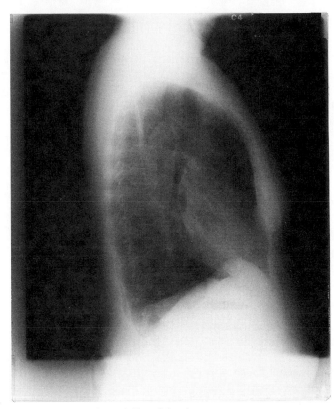

Figure 4-13   *The lateral film of the chest.*

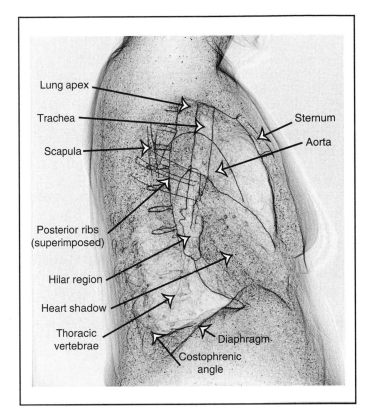

Lung apex
Trachea
Scapula
Sternum
Aorta
Posterior ribs (superimposed)
Hilar region
Heart shadow
Thoracic vertebrae
Diaphragm
Costophrenic angle

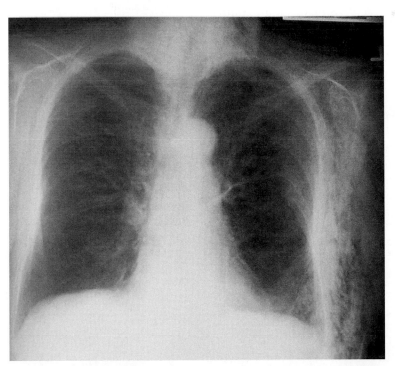

Figure 4-14   *An AP projection showing subcutaneous emphysema. Note the air markings (dark streaks) that are extrapulmonary.*

it joins the spine. Look for fractures (thin dark lines with or without separation), old healed fractures (increased radiodensity, making them whiter, and sometimes misshapen), and missing ribs or other anomalies. Evaluate the sternum, looking for any fractures or costocondral separations from the ribs (ribs separated from the sternum). Evaluate the spinal processes, observing for fractures, abnormal curvature (lordosis), or other changes. Evaluate the pleural space. Check for abnormal thickening (increased radiodensity), or air or fluid in the pleural space (as in pneumothorax, pleural effusion, or hemothorax). Next, focus your attention on the lung fields. A normal full inspiration will place the hemidiaphragms at about the level of the tenth rib. Count the ribs to the diaphragm to determine the degree of inspiration. An expiratory film will appear more dense (cloudy) and may not show the detail you are trying to evaluate. The hemidiaphragms are normally arch-shaped, domed structures, arcing superiorly. The right hemidiaphragm normally rests about 1 to 2 cm higher than the left. The lung fields should appear black (air), with vascular markings throughout (white streaks).

Occasionally you will observe round black spheres surrounded by a thin white line (a bronchus viewed end on, when viewing a lateral film). As you move toward the heart (*hilum*), the vascular markings will increase, becoming more dense. The heart is central in the chest radiograph, with the major portion of the heart lying to the left, and the aortic knob visible on the superior portion of the heart shadow. A normal heart shadow will be about one-half the diameter of the PA film at its base. The trachea can be distinguished by its dark shadow projecting downward to about the fourth vertebral body, where it bifurcates into the right and left mainstem bronchi. In most films, the carina is visible and is used as a landmark for endotracheal tube placement.

The lateral chest radiograph (Figure 4-13) may be assessed in a similar way to the PA film. Compare contrast of the tissue shadows (extrathoracic) with that of the black ambient room air. Observe for changes in the tissue density, indicating the presence of air or fluid. Evaluate the bony structures (ribs, sternum, and spine). Evaluate the radiograph for kyphosis or other abnormalities. Look at the diaphragm; there should be a slight upward curvature of the hemidiaphragms. Flattened hemidiaphragms are indicative of hyperinflation (discussed later on). Evaluate the lung fields. As on the PA view, the lung fields should appear black, with vascular markings (white streaks). Look closely at the retrosternal air space for signs of hyperinflation. The heart shadow appears narrower on the lateral film, and lies at about a 45° angle with the apex closest to the anterior chest wall. Compare the aorta shadow with that on the PA film. A calcified aorta is often very prominent on the lateral film.

COMMON ABNORMALITIES ON THE CHEST RADIOGRAPH

Extrapulmonary Air

Air is sometimes present outside of the lung parenchyma, which is not normal. Sources of extrapulmonary air

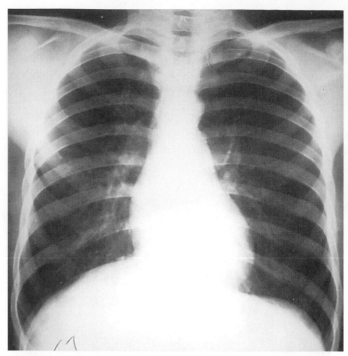

Figure 4-15 *A PA projection showing a 10% left pneumothorax. Note that the pneumothorax is more evident toward the apex of the lung in this upright patient.*

include pneumothorax (air in the pleural space), subcutaneous emphysema (air in the soft tissues surrounding the chest wall), and pneumomediastinum (air in the mediastinal space). These abnormalities all may be identified on standard PA and AP chest radiographs.

A *pneumothorax* may be observed as a dark (black) shadow along the pleural space, usually superior (Figure 4-15) because air tends to migrate upward (superiorly). A pneumothorax is distinguished from the lung fields by the absence of vascular markings. The extent of a pneumothorax is often quantified (as 5% or 10%, for example), and its location (right or left) is identified. A pneumothorax is often caused by trauma; therefore, it is important to evaluate the bony structures of the chest and the aorta for injury. Larger pneumothoraces are treated by placement of a chest tube that is connected to a vacuum source to reexpand the affected lung. Very small pneumothoraces may not be treated but may simply be watched to ensure that they don't become larger.

Subcutaneous emphysema is presence of air in the soft tissues in an extrathoracic location (Figure 4-14). Subcutaneous air is often associated with mechanical ventilation of a patient with a tracheostomy tube. Air can dissect through the stoma of the tracheostomy tube, past the tube's cuff, and migrate into the soft tissues. This extrathoracic air is not dangerous but should be noted and observed. Eventually, the air will be absorbed by the tissue, and the condition will resolve spontaneously (without treatment).

Pneumomediastinum occurs when air dissects into the mediastinal space (Figure 4-16). On an upright film, the dark, air-filled space may extend up into the neck. The air-filled space separates the visceral pleura from the parietal

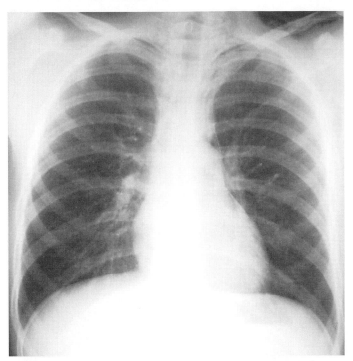

Figure 4-16   *A portable chest x-ray film showing a pneumomediastinum. Note the dark thin sliver of air along the lateral heart border.*

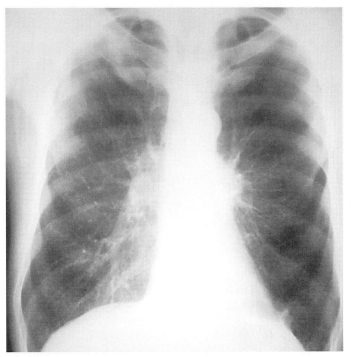

Figure 4-17   *A PA projection of the chest showing hyperinflation. Note the darker appearance of the film, the diaphragm's position (around the twelfth rib), the diaphragm's flattened shape, and the increased spacing between the ribs.*

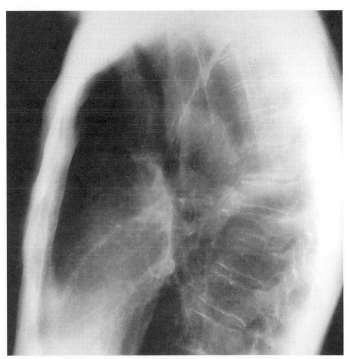

Figure 4-18   *A lateral projection illustrating hyperinflation. Note the dark appearance of the film, the flattened hemidiaphragms, and the enlarged retrosternal air space.*

pleura of the mediastinum. In adults, pneumomediastinum may be secondary to trauma, including that affecting the large airways (Pierson & Kacmarek, 1992).

Changes in Lung Volume

Changes in lung volumes may often be observed radiographically. Changes in lung volume may occur because of hyperinflation, atelectasis, or consolidation. Sometimes, as a result of unilateral lung volume changes, the mediastinum may shift to the affected side, owing to the greater expansion of the unaffected lung. This finding is termed *mediastinal shift.*

Hyperinflation is often a finding in patients with chronic obstructive pulmonary disease (COPD). In the hyperinflated chest radiograph (Figure 4-17), the hemidiaphragms extend beyond the tenth rib space and no longer maintain their characteristic domed shape. The hemidiaphragms are flatter, being displaced downward by the overdistended lung fields. In the lateral view (Figure 4-18), the retrosternal air space is enlarged, and again the hemidiaphragms are much flatter. With extreme hyperinflation, the rib spaces become larger as the ribs are forced apart by the trapped gas. Characteristically, hyperinflated chest radiographs appear darker (owing to more air space) than normal chest radiographs. In some cases, the heart shadow may also be narrower than on the normal chest film. The heart and mediastinum become compressed between the overdistended lung fields, narrowing the cardiac silhouette.

Atelectasis is manifested by a reduction in lung volume (Figure 4-19). In obstructive atelectasis, gas in the affected lung region is absorbed by the capillary blood flow, reducing the region's volume. If the atelectasis involves a lobe or segment, the diaphragm on the affected side may actually be displaced slightly upward, as the unaffected lung regions are pulled or tethered by the

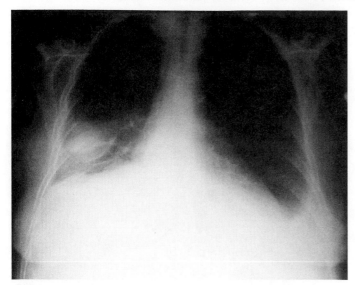

Figure 4-19 *A PA projection illustrating atelectasis in the right upper lobe. Note that the right diaphragm is elevated even more than normal; the density of the upper lobe is increased.*

affected lung. The affected area is characterized by an increase in radiodensity, appearing lighter than the surrounding regions (owing to less air density). In some cases, the fissures of the lobes and segments may be visible on the radiograph, further delineating the extent of the process (McMahon, 1999). In compressive atelectasis, pneumothorax, hemothorax, pleural effusion, or another space-occupying anomaly compresses the surrounding lung tissue, reducing its volume. The size of the anomaly will determine the extent to which the lung is compressed. In severe cases, such as in tension pneumothorax, the mediastinum is displaced toward the unaffected side and the unaffected lung is compressed (Figure 4-20). This is a life-threatening condition that requires immediate treatment (by chest tube placement).

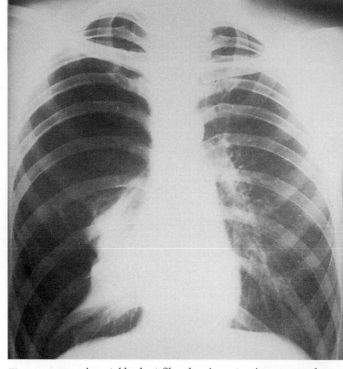

Figure 4-20 *A portable chest film showing a tension pneumothorax. Note the absence of lung markings on the right and the decreased density compared with the left. Note the mediastinal shift and that the right lung has been compressed into a very small space.*

Consolidation occurs when air-filled portions of the lung become fluid-filled, sometimes without loss of volume. Consolidation is often secondary to bacterial pneumonia. The consolidated lung region demonstrates an increased radiodensity, appearing lighter than the surrounding lung fields. Consolidation is often lobar, and when the PA projection is compared with the lateral, the lobe or segment may be easily identified (Figure 4-21).

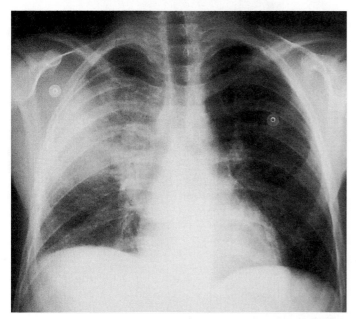
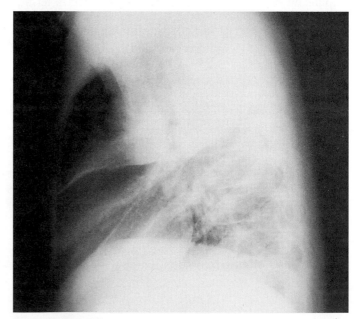

Figure 4-21 *Consolidation of the right apical posterior segment (left). Compare the lateral film (right) showing the posterior nature of the consolidation.*

Fluid Abnormalities

Fluid abnormalities manifested on chest radiographs may include pleural effusion, congestive failure, pulmonary edema, and pulmonary infiltrates. Any fluid abnormality will result in an increased opacity on the radiograph compared with that on a normal film. The type of abnormality will determine how it is characterized on the chest film.

Pleural effusion is the collection of fluid in the pleural space. The characteristic sign of pleural effusion on the PA projection is blunting of the costophrenic angles (Figure 4-22). Normally, the costophrenic angle is a sharply defined narrow angle at the lateral margin of the diaphragm (see Figure 4-12). The presence of pleural effusion will tend to obscure this angle, blunting it on the upright film. On a lateral decubitus film (see Figure 4-7), the fluid will form a uniform layer (at the most inferior portion of the lung), parallel to the surface the patient is lying on. In profound cases, pleural effusion may result in significant volume loss (compressive atelectasis). A thoracentesis may be performed to drain the fluid from the pleural space, re-expanding the lung.

Congestive heart failure (CHF) is often manifested on the chest radiograph. An early sign of CHF is an enlargement of the left ventricle of the heart (Pierson & Kacmarek, 1992). As the efficiency of the ventricle to pump blood declines, increasing pressure affects the lungs, causing fluid to migrate into the interstitial space (Kazerooni & Cascade, 1999). Pulmonary vascular consolidation occurs throughout the mediastinal area and may extend into the upper lobes (Figure 4-23). The increased fluid density results in a greater opacity of the radiograph compared with the normal film. Kerley B lines may be present along the right base of the PA film, extending horizontally from the periphery of the lung. These opaque lines represent lymphatic vessels that are engorged with fluid.

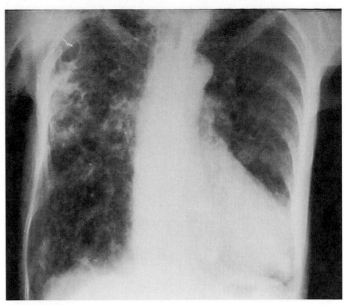

Figure 4-23 *A PA projection illustrating congestive heart failure. Note the enlarged heart shadow and the increased size and fullness of the hilum.*

Pulmonary edema may be noncardiogenic in origin, such as with the adult respiratory distress syndrome (ARDS). The chest radiograph of a patient with ARDS shows a diffuse patchy infiltrate pattern throughout the lung fields (Figure 4-24). This radiographic pattern has been referred to as a "ground glass" appearance, describing the uniform opacity the radiograph exhibits. This infiltrate pattern represents alveolar edema and interstitial edema with regions of localized atelectasis. As the disease progresses, later chest radiographs may demonstrate changes in density from fibrosis and scarring of the tissue subsequent to the disease process.

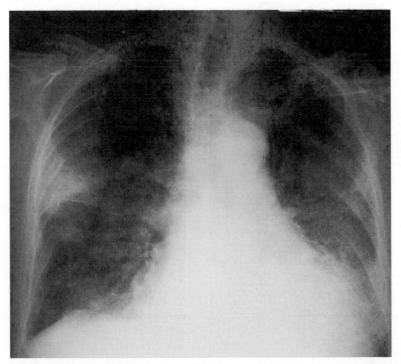

Figure 4-22 *Pleural effusion. Note that the costophrenic angle is obscured.*

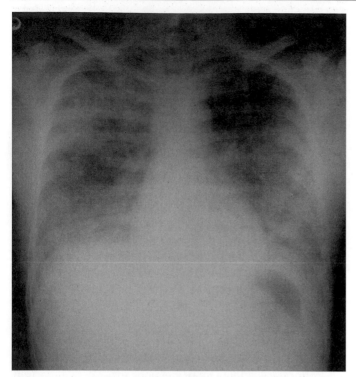

Figure 4-24 *A portable film illustrating radiographic appearance in the adult respiratory distress syndrome (ARDS). Note the almost uniform patchy infiltrate pattern throughout both lung fields.*

A *pulmonary infiltrate* is visible radiographically as an area of the lung with increased opacity, appearing lighter on the chest film (Figure 4-25). Pulmonary infiltrates are often secondary to pneumonia and involve lung tissue diffusely, often in a segmental or lobar distribution. Because of the presence of fluid in these regions, the radiodensity is greater than normal. On so-called *air bronchograms*, the bronchus is seen surrounded by fluid-filled structures, creating a distinct separation between the regions of differing densities (air versus fluid). Comparison of the lateral projection with the PA projections will help to differentiate the lobe or segment that is involved.

Foreign Objects

Besides normal anatomical structures, foreign objects may also be viewed on chest radiographs. Such objects include artificial airways, chest tubes, central catheters, feeding tubes, nasogastric tubes, and surgical clips or staples. In the critical care setting, chest radiographs are used to confirm the position and placement of these devices and to determine whether, once they have been placed, their position has changed.

Artificial airways viewed on chest radiographs include endotracheal tubes and tracheostomy tubes. The portable (AP) chest radiograph is used to confirm correct placement of the endotracheal tube following its insertion. Figure 4-26 illustrates the placement of an endotracheal tube. When the tube is placed correctly, its distal tip should be positioned 2 to 3 cm above the carina.

Tracheostomy tubes are frequently used in caring for critically ill patients and for patients requiring long-term mechanical ventilation. Figure 4-27 shows a chest radiograph of a patient with a tracheostomy tube. Occasionally, tracheostomy tubes may become displaced into the soft tissue anterior to the trachea. A lateral neck film will confirm that the tube is placed correctly in the trachea.

Chest tubes are inserted into the pleural space to evacuate air or fluid from the space to expand the lung fully. Most chest tubes are placed at about the fourth or fifth rib space laterally and are directed toward the apex of the

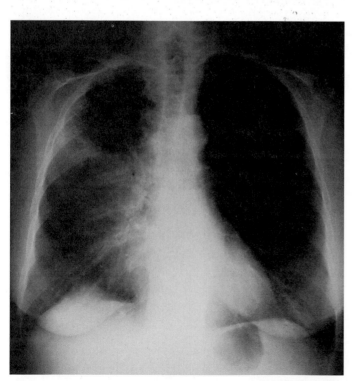

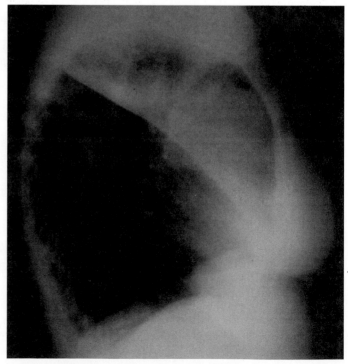

Figure 4-25 *This PA projection shows a pulmonary infiltrate in the right middle lobe. Compare the PA projection with the lateral view.*

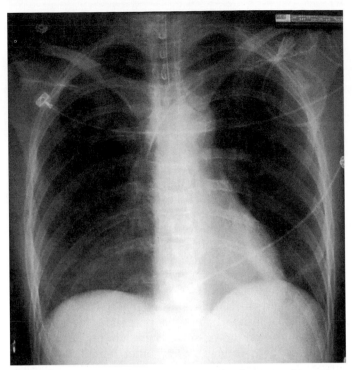

Figure 4-26 *A portable film illustrating the placement of an endotracheal tube. Note the tip of the tube resting just above the carina.*

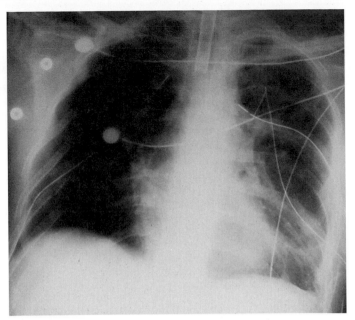

Figure 4-28 *A portable chest radiograph from a patient in the intensive care unit. Note the chest tubes that have been placed in the right chest.*

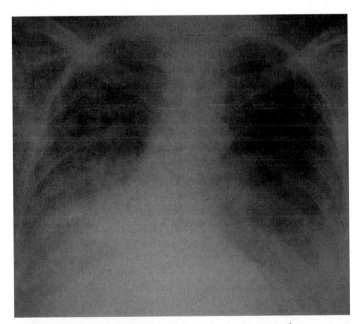

Figure 4-27 *A portable film illustrating the presence of a tracheostomy tube.*

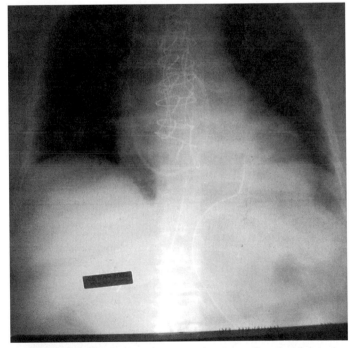

Figure 4-29 *This portable film was taken to confirm the placement of a pulmonary artery catheter.*

affected lung (Figure 4-28). The proximal end of the chest tube is connected to a vacuum source, which continuously applies subambient pressure to the pleura, maintaining its position, thereby expanding the affected lung.

Central catheters used in the critical care setting include pulmonary artery catheters, central venous catheters, and intra-aortic balloon catheters. The pulmonary artery catheter passes through the right side of the heart (right atrium and right ventricle) and rests in the pulmonary artery (Figure 4-29). The unique curve this catheter displays on the AP chest film makes it easily identifiable. The central venous catheter's tip rests in the vena cava or the right atrium. This catheter may be identified easily because it rests just inside of the cardiac silhouette. Placement of these lines may result in a pneumothorax because the venous system is accessed via the subclavian vein. Careful evaluation of the radiograph for a pneumothorax is part of the post–catheter placement assessment. The intra-aortic balloon pump is inserted through the femoral artery and advanced superiorly to the aorta.

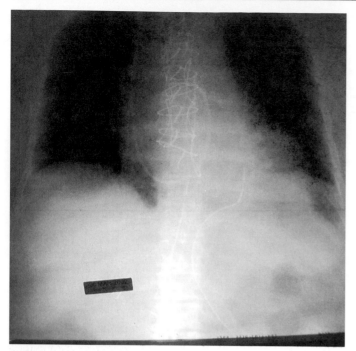

Figure 4-30 *An AP projection that was taken to confirm the position of the intra-aortic balloon.*

Figure 4-30 is a chest radiograph showing the placement of an intra-aortic balloon pump catheter.

Gastric tubes include both nasogastric tubes and feeding tubes. The nasogastric tube is passed through the esophagus and its distal tip rests in the stomach. The nasogastric tube removes the stomach contents by application of low continuous subambient (vacuum) pressure. Figure 4-31 illustrates the placement of the nasogastric tube. Sometimes the nasogastric tube is inserted following intubation, and the nasogastric tube may follow adjacent to the endotracheal tube and be inadvertently placed into the trachea. Careful evaluation of the correct placement of this tube is important. Feeding tubes are common in the intensive care environment. Feeding tubes are inserted through the esophagus and are generally placed in the small intestine. Many tubes have small weighted tips that assist in their placement and enhance radiographic visibility. Often these tubes are placed under direct radiographic visualization, using fluoroscopy.

Cardiac leads and wires include both ECG leads for monitoring purposes and cardiac pacemaker wires. The typical patient in an intensive care unit has three ECG leads placed (right and left shoulder and left axilla). Figure 4-32 illustrates the placement of these ECG leads. Cardiac pacemakers are commonly used to correct irregular heart rhythms. Figure 4-33 illustrates the placement of the pacemaker (left shoulder) and the pacemaker wire that is threaded through the venous system into the heart.

Surgical clips or staples and other foreign bodies are often seen on chest radiographs. Surgical clips and staples, used to hold bone and tissue together, are commonly used in thoracic surgery. Figure 4-34 is a chest radiograph from a patient following coronary artery bypass surgery. Note the wires holding the sternum together. Other foreign bodies may include bullets, knives, picks, nails, and other foreign objects. Figure 4-35 is a chest radiograph from a person who was shot by a shotgun. Note the numerous small pellets in the abdomen and lower thoracic cavity.

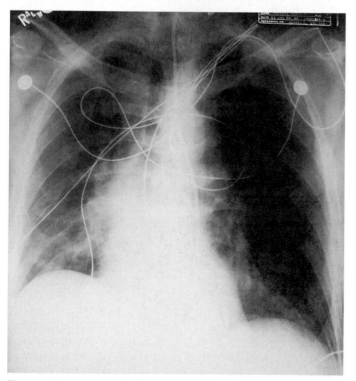

Figure 4-31 *A portable film from a patient in the intensive care unit. Note the nasogastric tube.*

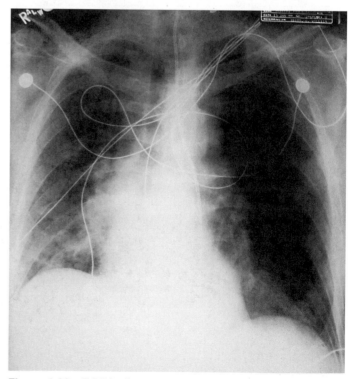

Figure 4-32 *ECG leads are evident on this portable chest film.*

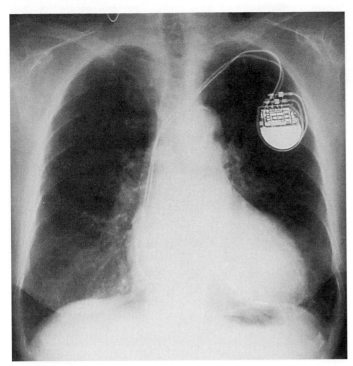

Figure 4-33 *A pacemaker has been placed subcutaneously (above the left clavicle), and the pacer wire is evident.*

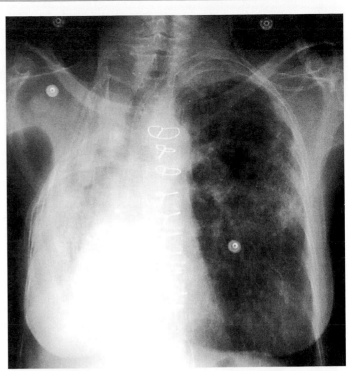

Figure 4-34 *A portable chest film from a patient who had coronary artery bypass surgery. Note the wires that hold the sternum together.*

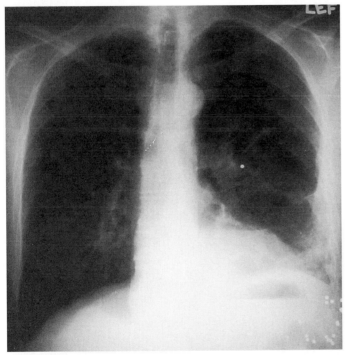

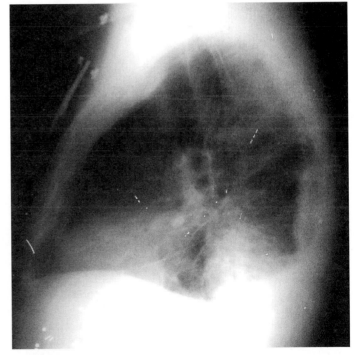

Figure 4-35 *Multiple small foreign objects are evident in the abdomen and lower chest of this gunshot victim.*

VENTILATION-PERFUSION SCANNING

Ventilation-perfusion scanning permits comparison of lung ventilation with lung perfusion. For the ventilation scan, a radioactive gas (xenon) is inhaled while the lungs are scanned radiographically. The ventilation scan can detect defects (obstruction) to ventilation to lobes or segments of the lung. Typical views include the PA, lateral, right anterior oblique, and left anterior oblique (Figure 4-36). The perfusion scan involves injection of radioisotope-tagged albumin into the venous circulation. As the tagged

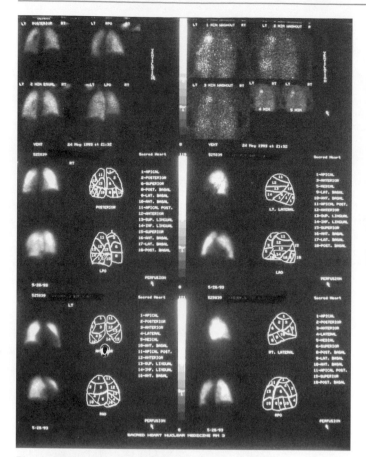

Figure 4-36 *A normal ventilation-perfusion scan.*

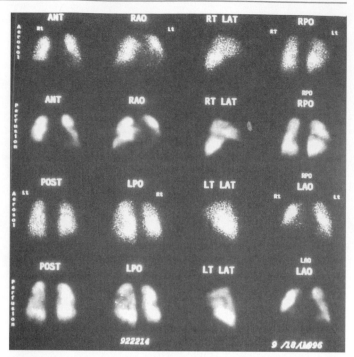

Figure 4-37 *A ventilation-perfusion scan that is positive for pulmonary embolism.*

albumin passes through the pulmonary vasculature, the lungs are scanned radiographically, using the same views as for the ventilation scan. The perfusion scan can detect obstruction in the pulmonary circulation. Ventilation-perfusion (V/Q) scans are used to diagnose or to rule out pulmonary embolism. Figure 4-37 illustrates V/Q mismatch; the scan is positive for pulmonary embolism (note the area showing absence of perfusion but the presence of ventilation).

PULMONARY ANGIOGRAPHY

Pulmonary angiography is another radiographic technique used to image the pulmonary vasculature. Pulmonary angiography is considered by some authorities to be more definitive in detecting pulmonary emboli. To perform a pulmonary angiogram, a pulmonary artery catheter is inserted through the venous system (via the subclavian vein) into the pulmonary artery, and radiopaque contrast material is injected into the pulmonary artery or into one of its branches. As the contrast medium passes through the pulmonary circulation, the chest is imaged radiographically. A positive angiogram is one in which the contrast medium fails to fill a branch or portion of the pulmonary circulation. Figure 4-38 illustrates a positive pulmonary angiogram. Note how circulation stops at one of the branches of the pulmonary artery.

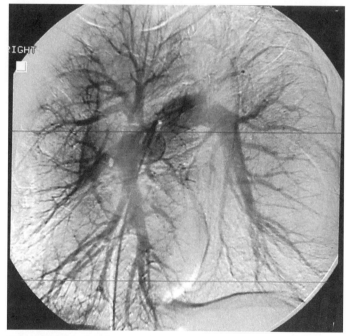

Figure 4-38 *A pulmonary angiogram that is positive for pulmonary embolism. Note the area in which perfusion ceases (arrow).*

COMPUTED TOMOGRAPHY OF THE CHEST

Computed tomography can depict many pathologic changes in greater detail than is possible with conventional chest radiography (Miller, 1999). A *tomogram* is an x-ray view in which the chest is imaged as an axial slice or cut (Figure 4-39). The image is produced by rotating the x-ray tube around the patient, focusing the x-ray energy toward a central point, making slices from superior to inferior or inferior to superior. The depth of the tomogram can vary (typically ranging from 3 to 1 cm), and as the depth becomes smaller, more detail is present. Computer systems allow much finer differentiation between shades of gray so that detection of far more subtle pathologic changes is possible (Miller, 1999). Figure 4-40 illustrates the first few cuts of a CT scan and the *scout image*. The scout image is a PA projection that indicates level and location of the slices or cuts made in the CT scan. One can relate the scout image to the desired level or cut (superior/inferior) of interest on the CT scan.

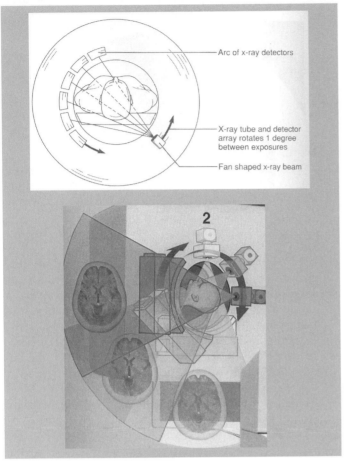

Figure 4-39 *A CT scan is produced by making narrow focused cuts, axially along the area of interest.*

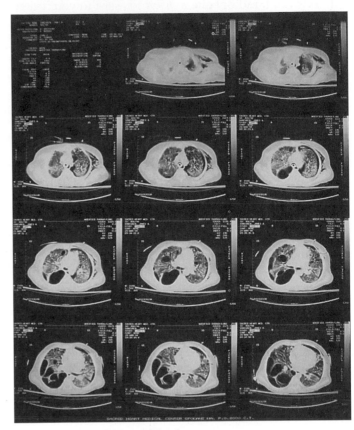

Figure 4-40 *A CT scan of the chest.*

PROFICIENCY OBJECTIVES

At the end of this chapter, you should be able to:
- Correctly orient a PA and a lateral chest radiograph on a view box for examination.
- Determine the penetration of the PA projection if the patient was rotated when the image was made.
- Demonstrate how to identify the following landmarks on the PA and lateral chest x-ray views:
  — Clavicles and scapulae
  — Spinal column
  — Ribs
  — Pleura
  — Lung fields
  — Costophrenic angle
  — Hemidiaphragms
  — Trachea
  — Carina
  — Hilum
  — Heart shadow
  — Aortic knob
  — Retrosternal air space
- View the x-ray in a systematic way:
  — Evaluate extrathoracic soft tissue
  — Evaluate the ribs tracing each
  — Evaluate the pleura
  — Evaluate the sternum and clavicles
  — Evaluate spinal processes
  — Evaluate costophrenic angle
  — Evaluate hemidiaphragms and their relative positions
  — Evaluate lung fields
  — Evaluate hilum
  — Evaluate cardiac silhouette and estimate cardiothoracic ratio
  — Identify trachea and carina
  — Identify any foreign objects or lines
  — Evaluate retrosternal air space
  — Note any spinal conformation deformities

CHEST FILM ORIENTATION

To correctly orient a PA chest film, the heart shadow should descend downward toward the right as the film is viewed on the view box. The patient's left should be aligned with your right, as if the patient were facing you. Most chest radiographs will have the right (R) and left (L) marked with a radiopaque marker to assist in your orientation of the film. The lateral film is oriented as if the patient is facing the PA film, with the lateral usually placed to the right of the PA film.

ROTATION AND PENETRATION

Patient rotation is determined by locating the neck of the clavicles and verifying that the spine lies equidistant between them. If the patient is rotated right or left, the spinal column will be closer to one side or the other or may even lie beyond the neck of one or the other clavicle.

Penetration is determined by examining the spinal column just above and extending into the cardiac silhouette. The vertebral bodies should just barely be distinguishable, without obvious dark spaces between them. If the vertebrae cannot be distinguished well, the film is underpenetrated. If the vertebrae are very pronounced, the film is overpenetrated and may appear unusually dark.

VIEWING THE CHEST RADIOGRAPH

When evaluating a chest radiograph, be sure to use a systematic approach each time. Through repeated practice, this approach will become habit, reducing the chance of your missing important details that might otherwise go unnoticed.

1. Evaluate the extrathoracic soft tissue, observing for subcutaneous air or fluid.
2. Evaluate the ribs, tracing each, looking for fractures, healed fractures, missing ribs, or other deformities.
3. Evaluate the pleura, observing for changes in thickness and presence of air or fluid.
4. Evaluate the hemidiaphragms, noting the position of each diaphragm relative to the other.
5. Evaluate the sternum and clavicles, observing for fractures or deformities.
6. Evaluate the spinal processes.
7. Evaluate the costophrenic angles, observing for blunting.
8. Evaluate the lung fields, noting any unusual lung markings, opacities, nodular densities, or other abnormalities.
9. Evaluate the hilum, noting its relative size and extent of its fullness (radiodensity).
10. Evaluate the cardiac silhouette, noting the relative ratio of cardiac size and thoracic diameter.
11. Evaluate the trachea, noting its position, and identify the carina.
12. Identify any lines, artificial airways, ECG leads or pacemaker wires, nasogastric or feeding tubes, and chest tubes.
13. Evaluate the retrosternal air space on the lateral film.
14. Evaluate the hemidiaphragms and pleura on the lateral film.
15. Note and correlate any changes in opacity or other findings with the PA projection to form a three-dimensional image.

References

Kazerooni, E. A., & Cascade, P. (1999). Chest imaging in the cardiac intensive care unit. *Respiratory Care, 44*(9), 1033–1043.

McMahon, H. (1999). Pitfalls in portable chest radiology. *Respiratory Care, 44*(9), 1018–1032.

Miller, W. T. (1999). Uses of thoracic computed tomography in the intensive care unit. *Respiratory Care, 44*(9), 1127–1136.

Pierson, D. J., & Kacmarek, R. (1992). *Foundations of respiratory care.* New York: Churchill Livingstone.

Wallace, J. E. (1995). *Radiographic exposure principles & practice.* Philadelphia: F. A. Davis.

Practice Activities: Radiographic Evaluation

1. With a lab partner, practice orienting both PA and lateral chest films for viewing.
   a. Have your partner deliberately place the film incorrectly while you are not watching, and then correct it.
2. Identify the following landmarks for your lab partner:
   a. Clavicles, scapulae, ribs, sternum, spinal processes
   b. Pleura
   c. Costophrenic angle and hemidiaphragms
   d. Trachea and carina
   e. Hilum
   f. Heart silhouette and aortic knob; estimate the cardiothoracic ratio
   g. Retrosternal air space

3. With your lab partner, identify on a radiograph the presence of these manmade objects:
   a. Artificial airways (endotracheal tube or tracheostomy tube)
   b. Chest tubes
   c. Central venous catheters
   d. Nasogastric tube or feeding tube
   e. ECG leads or cardiac pacemaker and leads
   f. Intra-aortic balloon
   g. Surgical clips or staples
4. From a set of abnormal chest radiographs, identify the following abnormalities. Have your laboratory

instructor critique your findings and offer suggestions for improving your skills.

a. Extrapulmonary air (as in pneumothorax, subcutaneous emphysema, or pneumomediastinum)

b. Changes in lung volume (as in hyperinflation, atelectasis, mediastinal shift, consolidation)

c. Fluid abnormalities (as in pleural effusion, congestive heart failure, pulmonary edema, pulmonary infiltrates)

5. With a lab partner, evaluate a lateral neck x-ray film of a pediatric patient. Identify the larynx, epiglottis, and trachea. Make a judgment about whether the epiglottis is large and if the airway is narrowed. Have your laboratory instructor confirm your findings.

6. With a lab partner, study a ventilation-perfusion scan, together assessing the scan for defects in ventilation or perfusion.

a. Identify the different x-ray views: PA, right anterior oblique, left anterior oblique, lateral.

b. Differentiate between the ventilation and perfusion scans.

7. With a lab partner, view a pulmonary angiogram. Carefully evaluate the study and try to identify where circulation is obstructed.

8. With a lab partner, evaluate a CT scan of the chest. Orient the series of images with the scout image.

a. Identify a point on the scout image and find the same point on the CT cut.

b. Identify as many landmarks as possible on each CT cut, and have your laboratory instructor critique your skills.

Check List: Chest X-Ray Evaluation

_____ 1. Review the patient's medical record.

_____ 2. Scan the patient's chart for any pertinent information.

_____ 3. Evaluate the extrathoracic soft tissue, observing for subcutaneous air or fluid.

_____ 4. Evaluate the ribs, tracing each and looking for fractures, healed fractures, missing ribs, and other deformities.

_____ 5. Evaluate the pleura, observing for changes in thickness and presence of air or fluid.

_____ 6. Evaluate the hemidiaphragms, noting the position of each diaphragm relative to the other.

_____ 7. Evaluate the sternum, clavicles, and scapulae, observing for fractures or deformities.

_____ 8. Evaluate the spinal processes.

_____ 9. Evaluate the costophrenic angles, observing for blunting (less acuity of the angle).

_____ 10. Evaluate the lung fields, noting any unusual lung markings, opacities, nodular densities, or other abnormalities.

_____ 11. Evaluate the hilum, noting its relative size and extent of its fullness (radiodensity).

_____ 12. Evaluate the cardiac silhouette, noting the relative ratio of cardiac size and thoracic diameter (should be less than half).

_____ 13. Evaluate the trachea, noting its position, and identify the carina.

_____ 14. Identify any lines, artificial airways, ECG leads or pacemaker wires, nasogastric or feeding tubes, and chest tubes.

_____ 15. Evaluate the retrosternal air space on the lateral film.

_____ 16. Evaluate the hemidiaphragms and pleura on the lateral film. Note any changes in opacity or other findings and correlate with the PA projection.

Self-Evaluation Post Test: Radiographic Imaging of the Chest

1. On a standard x-ray study of the chest, which of the following are the most common two views?
   I. Posterior-anterior
   II. Anterior-posterior
   III. Lateral
   IV. Apical lordotic

   a. I and III
   b. I and IV
   c. II and III
   d. II and IV

2. When the posterior-anterior (PA) view is compared with the anterior-posterior (AP) view:
   a. the heart shadow on the PA view is larger.
   b. the heart shadow on the AP view is larger.
   c. the apecies are more easily visualized on the AP view.
   d. the PA view is often a portable x-ray.

3. Which of the following has the greatest radiodensity?
   a. Air   c. Water
   b. Fat   d. Bone

4. A possible nodular anomaly is present in the right upper lobe on a PA film, but partially obscured by the clavicle. What view might show the anomaly better?
   a. AP projection
   b. Lateral projection
   c. Apical lordotic projection
   d. Left anterior oblique projection

5. During full inspiration, the hemidiaphragms on an adult chest film should be:
   a. at the C5 vertebra.
   b. at the level of the twelfth rib.
   c. at the L4 vertebra.
   d. at the level of the tenth rib.

6. When evaluating a PA film of the chest, you note that the right costophrenic angles are blunted. What does this suggest?
   a. A pneumothorax
   b. Presence of an infiltrate in the right lower lobe
   c. Presence of atelectasis in the right base
   d. Presence of a pleural effusion on the right

7. When evaluating a PA film of the chest, you note that in the left upper lobe there is a 1-cm-wide sliver along the lateral margin, descending from the apex, merging with the ribs at the third rib. This narrow sliver is very black and devoid of vascular markings. This could possibly be:
   a. a pneumothorax.
   b. atelectasis.
   c. pulmonary edema.
   d. hyperinflation.

8. For evaluating the position of an endotracheal tube on an AP chest film, the tip of the endotracheal tube should rest:
   a. at the carina.
   b. at the fourth rib space.
   c. at a point 2 to 3 cm above the carina.
   d. just above the clavicles.

9. When viewing a V/Q scan, you note ventilation to be even on all views. On the perfusion scan, you note absence of perfusion in the right apical posterior segment. This finding suggests:
   a. a pulmonary infiltrate.
   b. atelectasis in the right apical posterior segment.
   c. a possible pulmonary embolus.
   d. a pneumothorax in the right apical posterior segment.

10. A pulmonary angiogram is used to:
    a. image the ventilation of the lung.
    b. image the perfusion of the lung.
    c. image the lymph system of the lung.
    d. None of the above

PERFORMANCE EVALUATION:
CHEST X-RAY INTERPRETATION

Date: Lab _____ Clinical _____ Agency _____

Lab: Pass _____ Fail _____   Clinical: Pass _____ Fail _____

Student name _____ Instructor name _____

No. of times observed in clinical _____

No. of times practiced in clinical _____

PASSING CRITERIA: Obtain 90% or better on the procedure. Tasks indicated by * must receive at least 1 point, or the evaluation is terminated. Procedure must be performed within designated time, or the performance receives a failing grade.

SCORING:
2 points — Task performed satisfactorily without prompting.
1 point — Task performed satisfactorily with self-initiated correction.
0 points — Task performed incorrectly or with prompting required.
NA — Task not applicable to the patient care situation.

TASKS:

	PEER	LAB	CLINICAL
1. Reviews patient's medical record	☐	☐	☐
2. Scans the patient's chart for any pertinent information	☐	☐	☐
* 3. Evaluates the extrathoracic soft tissue			
a. Subcutaneous emphysema	☐	☐	☐
4. Evaluates the ribs			
a. Fractures	☐	☐	☐
b. Missing ribs	☐	☐	☐
c. Deformities	☐	☐	☐
5. Evaluates the pleura			
a. Thickness	☐	☐	☐
b. Pleural air	☐	☐	☐
c. Pleural fluid	☐	☐	☐
6. Evaluates the hemidiaphragms			
a. Position	☐	☐	☐
b. Elevation	☐	☐	☐
c. Conformation	☐	☐	☐
7. Evaluates the sternum and clavicles, and scapulae			
a. Fractures	☐	☐	☐
b. Deformities	☐	☐	☐
8. Evaluates the spinal processes			
a. Fractures	☐	☐	☐
b. Deformities	☐	☐	☐
9. Evaluates the costophrenic angles for blunting	☐	☐	☐

10. Evaluates the lung fields
    a. Lung markings ☐ ☐ ☐
    b. Opacities ☐ ☐ ☐
    c. Nodular densities ☐ ☐ ☐
11. Evaluates the hilum for size and fullness ☐ ☐ ☐
12. Evaluate the cardiac silhouette
    a. Estimates cardiothoracic ratio ☐ ☐ ☐
13. Evaluates the trachea
    a. Position ☐ ☐ ☐
    b. Identifies carina ☐ ☐ ☐
14. Identifies any lines
    a. Artificial airways ☐ ☐ ☐
    b. Chest tubes ☐ ☐ ☐
    c. ECG leads or pacemaker wires ☐ ☐ ☐
    d. Feeding tubes ☐ ☐ ☐
    e. Nasogastric tubes ☐ ☐ ☐
    f. Intra-aortic balloon ☐ ☐ ☐
15. Evaluates the retrosternal air space on the lateral film ☐ ☐ ☐
16. Evaluates the diaphragms and pleura on the lateral film ☐ ☐ ☐
17. Note any changes in opacity or other findings and correlates with the PA projection ☐ ☐ ☐

SCORE: Peer   _____ points of possible 66; _____%

          Lab   _____ points of possible 66; _____%

          Clinical   _____ points of possible 66; _____%

TIME: _____ out of possible 15 minutes

STUDENT SIGNATURES   INSTRUCTOR SIGNATURES

PEER: _____   LAB: _____

STUDENT: _____   CLINICAL: _____

CHAPTER 5
PULMONARY FUNCTION TESTING

INTRODUCTION

The measurement of bedside pulmonary function parameters provides important information that may be used in a variety of ways, ranging from assessing the effectiveness of bronchodilators to evaluating the adequacy of ventilation. Minimal equipment is needed, the skills are easily learned, and the procedures are noninvasive. As a respiratory care practitioner, you will also be responsible for the measurement and evaluation of a patient's lung function by performing formal pulmonary function testing. Contemporary pulmonary function testing equipment is frequently interfaced with microcomputers to eliminate the drudgery of manual calculations. Still, it is important to understand how to manually calculate pulmonary function values for assessing accuracy in the event of computer malfunction.

Basic spirometry provides volume-versus-time data. In addition, it is important to have an understanding of flow-volume loops. Flow-volume loops present the spirometry information in a way that allows easier characterization of restrictive disease and obstructive disease.

Measurement of the functional residual capacity (FRC) and residual volume (RV) is possible only through indirect methods. You must understand how gas dilution techniques allow measurement of these volumes. Additionally, body plethysmography may also be used to measure FRC and RV, as well as airway resistance.

In this chapter, you will learn how to use the portable equipment for bedside monitoring. You will also learn the techniques of routine pulmonary function testing using a water-sealed spirometer and how to calculate the results from a spirometric tracing.

KEY TERMS

- Airway resistance (R_{AW})
- Ambient temperature and pressure, saturated (ATPS)
- Anatomical dead space
- Bedside monitoring
- Body temperature and pressure, saturated (BTPS)
- Diffusion
- Expiratory reserve volume (ERV)
- $FEF_{25-75\%}$
- $FEF_{200-1200ml}$
- FEV_1
- Flow-volume loop
- Forced vital capacity (FVC)
- Frequency
- Functional residual capacity (FRC)
- Gas dilution technique
- Hyperventilation
- Inspiratory capacity
- Inspiratory reserve volume (IRV)
- Maximal inspiratory pressure (MIP)
- Maximum voluntary ventilation (MVV)
- Minute volume
- Nitrogen washout
- Peak expiratory flow rate (PEFR)
- Peak flowmeter
- Residual volume
- Respirometer
- Spirometer
- Tidal volume
- Total lung capacity
- Vital capacity

OBJECTIVES

At the end of this chapter, you should be able to:

- Discuss the rationale for monitoring bedside pulmonary function parameters.
- Compare and contrast the following spirometers and measuring devices:
  — Wright and Haloscale respirometers
  — Wright and Mini-Wright peak flowmeters
  — Boehringer inspiratory force manometer
  — Water seal spirometer
  — Fleisch Pneumotach spirometer
  Include:
  (1) Principles of operation
  (2) Accuracy ranges
  (3) Limitations
- Select an appropriate measuring device given a specific pulmonary function parameter to measure.

- Discuss the significance of and normal ranges for the following respiratory function parameters:
  — Tidal volume
  — Minute volume
  — Frequency
  — Peak expiratory flow
  — Maximal inspiratory pressure
  — Inspiratory reserve volume
  — Expiratory reserve volume
  — Residual volume
  — Total lung capacity
  — Inspiratory capacity
  — Functional residual capacity

(Continued)

- Given a normal forced vital capacity tracing, identify and explain the clinical significance of the following forced maneuvers:
  — Forced vital capacity
  — FEV_t
  — FEV_t/FVC ratio
  — $FEF_{200-1200}$
  — $FEF_{25-75\%}$
  — PEFR
- Explain how a maximum voluntary ventilation maneuver is performed and its clinical significance.
- Explain the importance of conversion from ATPS to BTPS in the reporting of pulmonary function test results.
- Given a flow-volume loop, identify the following:
  — Inspiratory portion
  — Expiratory portion

- — Vital capacity
  — Peak inspiratory flow
  — Peak expiratory flow
- Describe how a flow-volume loop changes with restrictive and obtructive disease.
- Describe how gas dilution techniques allow the measurement of FRC and RV.
- Describe how a body plethysmograph measures V_{TG}.
- Describe how gas diffusion is measured and what the single breath diffusion test (D_LCO) is.
- Discuss the hazards of pulmonary function testing, including:
  — Hyperventilation
  — Bronchodilator side effects
  — Infection

CLINICAL PRACTICE GUIDELINES

AARC Clinical Practice Guideline Spirometry, 1996 Update

S 4.0 INDICATIONS:

The indications for spirometry (4–8) include the need to

4.1 Detect the presence or absence of lung dysfunction suggested by history or physical signs and symptoms (e.g., age, smoking history, family history of lung disease, cough, dyspnea, wheezing) and/or the presence of other abnormal diagnostic tests (e.g., chest radiograph, arterial blood gas analysis);

4.2 Quantify the severity of known lung disease;

4.3 Assess the change in lung function over time or following administration of or change in therapy;

4.4 Assess the potential effects or response to environmental or occupational exposure;

4.5 Assess the risk for surgical procedures known to affect lung function;

4.6 Assess impairment and/or disability (e.g., for rehabilitation, legal reasons, military).

S 5.0 CONTRAINDICATIONS:

The requesting physician should be made aware that the circumstances listed in this section could affect the reliability of spirometry measurements. In addition, forced expiratory maneuvers may aggravate these conditions, which may make test postponement necessary until the medical condition(s) resolve(s).

Relative contraindications (9, 10) to performing spirometry are

5.1 Hemoptysis of unknown origin (forced expiratory maneuver may aggravate the underlying condition);

5.2 Pneumothorax;

5.3 Unstable cardiovascular status (forced expiratory maneuver may worsen angina or cause changes in blood pressure) or recent myocardial infarction or pulmonary embolus;

5.4 Thoracic, abdominal, or cerebral aneurysms (danger of rupture due to increased thoracic pressure);

5.5 Recent eye surgery (e.g., cataract);

5.6 Presence of an acute disease process that might interfere with test performance (e.g., nausea, vomiting);

5.7 Recent surgery of thorax or abdomen.

S 6.0 HAZARDS/COMPLICATIONS:

Although spirometry is a safe procedure, untoward reactions may occur, and the value of the information anticipated from spirometry should be weighed against potential hazards. The following have been reported anecdotally:

6.1 Pneumothorax;

6.2 Increased intracranial pressure;

6.3 Syncope, dizziness, light-headedness;

6.4 Chest pain;

6.5 Paroxysmal coughing;

6.6 Contraction of nosocomial infections;

6.7 Oxygen desaturation due to interruption of oxygen therapy;

6.8 Bronchospasm.

S 7.0 LIMITATIONS OF METHODOLOGY/ VALIDATION OF RESULTS:

7.1 Spirometry is an effort-dependent test that requires careful instruction and the cooperation of the test subject. Inability to perform acceptable maneuvers may be due to poor subject motivation or failure to understand instructions. Physical impairment and young age (e.g., <5 years of age) may also limit the subject's ability to perform spirometric maneuvers. These limitations do not preclude attempting spirometry but should be noted and taken into consideration when the results are interpreted.

7.2 The results of spirometry should meet the following criteria for number of trials, acceptability, and reproducibility. The acceptability criteria should be applied before reproducibility is checked.

7.2.1 Number of trials: A minimum of three acceptable FVC maneuvers should be performed. (3) If a subject is unable to perform a single acceptable maneuver after eight attempts, testing may be discontinued. However, after additional instruction and demonstration, more maneuvers may be performed depending on the subject's clinical condition and tolerance.

7.2.2 Acceptability: A good "start-of-test" includes:

7.2.2.1 An extrapolated volume of < or = 5% of the FVC or 150 mL, whichever is greater;

7.2.2.2 No hesitation or false start;

7.2.2.3 A rapid start to rise time.

7.2.3 Acceptability: No cough, especially during the first second of the maneuver.

7.2.4 Acceptability: No early termination of exhalation.

7.2.4.1 A minimum exhalation time of 6 seconds is recommended, unless there is an obvious plateau of reasonable duration (i.e., no volume change for at least 1 second) or the subject cannot or should not continue to exhale further. (3)

7.2.4.2 No maneuver should be eliminated solely because of early termination. The FEV_1 from such maneuvers may be valid, and the volume expired may be an estimate of the true FVC, although the FEV_1/FVC and FEF25–75% may be overestimated.

7.2.5 Reproducibility:

7.2.5.1 The two largest FVCs from acceptable maneuvers should not vary by more than 0.200 L, and the two largest FEV_1s from acceptable maneuvers should not vary by more than 0.200 L.

NOTE: The ATS has changed its recommendations from those made in the 1987 ATS guideline (2) (a reproducibility criterion of 5% or 0.100 L, whichever is larger). This change is based on evidence from Hankinson and Bang suggesting that intrasubject variability is independent of body size and that individuals of short stature are less likely to meet the older criterion than are taller subjects. (11) In addition, the 0.200 L criterion is simple to apply. However, there are two concerns with this change. The first is whether the 0.200 L criterion is too permissive in shorter individuals (e.g., children). Enright and coworkers (12) reported a failure rate of only 2.1% in 21,432 testing sessions on adults using the 5% or 100 mL criterion. In addition, they found that only 0.4% of test sessions failed to meet relaxed criteria of 5% or 200 mL. These failure rates are much lower than the 5–15% failure rates reported by Hankinson and Bang. (11) Enright and coworkers did not study children, but there was some height overlap in the two studies. Thus, we are not convinced that the 5% rule is inappropriate when applied to shorter individuals. Indeed, Hankinson and Bang stated in their report, ". . . it appears that the technician appropriately responded to the lack of a reproducible or acceptable test result by obtaining more maneuvers from these subjects." The second concern is that the 0.200 L criterion may be too rigid for very tall individuals (e.g., height >75 inches). Hankinson and Bang did not study subjects taller than 190 cm (i.e., 75 inches). In order to send a consistent message, we recommend the ATS reproducibility criterion but urge practitioners: (a) to use this criterion as a goal during data collection and not to reject a spirogram solely on the basis of its poor reproducibility; (b) to exceed the reproducibility criterion whenever possible because it will decrease interlaboratory and intralaboratory variability; and (c) to comment in the written report when reproducibility criteria cannot be met.

7.3 Maximum voluntary ventilation (MVV) is the volume of air exhaled in a specified period during rapid, forced breathing. (3) This measurement is sometimes referred to as the maximum breathing capacity (MBC).

7.3.1 The period of time for performing this maneuver should be at least 12 seconds but no more than 15 seconds, with the data reported as L/min at BTPS.

7.3.2 At least two trials should be obtained, and the two highest should agree within ±10%.

7.4 The use of a nose clip for all spirometric maneuvers is strongly encouraged.

7.5 Subjects may be studied in either the sitting or standing position. Occasionally, a subject may experience syncope or dizziness while performing the forced expiratory maneuver. Thus, the sitting position may be safer. If such a subject is standing, an appropriate chair (i.e., with arms and not on rollers) should be placed behind the subject in the event that he or she needs to be seated quickly. When the maneuver is performed from a seated position, the subject should sit erect with both feet on the floor, and be positioned correctly in relation to the equipment. Test position should be noted on the report.

(Continued)

(CPG Continued)

7.6 Spirometry is often performed before and after inhalation of a bronchodilator.

7.6.1 The drug, dose, and mode of delivery should be specifically ordered by the managing physician or determined by the laboratory and should be noted in the report.

7.6.2 The length of the interval between administration of the bronchodilator and postbronchodilator testing varies among laboratories, (13–17) but there appears to be more support for a minimum interval of 15 minutes for most short- and intermediate-acting beta-2 agonists. (14–17) This does not guarantee that peak response will be determined, and underestimation of peak bronchodilator response can occur.

7.6.3 Subjects who use inhaled short-acting bronchodilators should be tested at least four to six hours after the last use of their inhaled bronchodilator to allow proper assessment of acute bronchodilator response. Long-acting inhaled bronchodilators may need to be withheld for a more extended period. Subjects should understand that if they need to administer their bronchodilator prior to the test because of breathing problems, they should do so. Bronchodilators taken on the day of testing should be noted in the report. Table 1 lists commonly used drugs that may confound assessment of acute bronchodilator response and the recommended times for withholding.

7.6.4 Interpretation of response to a bronchodilator should take into account both magnitude and consistency of change in the pulmonary function data. The recommended criterion for response to a bronchodilator in adults for FEV_1 and FVC is a 12% improvement from baseline and an absolute change of 0.200 L. (18) However, because the peak effect of the drug may not always be determined, the inability to meet this response criterion does not exclude a response. In addition, dynamic compression of the airways during the forced expiratory maneuver may mask bronchodilator response in some subjects, and the additional measurement of airway resistance and calculation of specific conductance and resistance may provide documentation of airway responsiveness. (19)

7.7 Reporting of results:

7.7.1 The largest FVC and FEV_1 (at BTPS) should be reported even if they do not come from the same curve.

7.7.2 Other reported measures (e.g., $FEF_{25-75\%}$ and instantaneous expiratory flow rates, such as FEF_{max} and $FEF_{50\%}$) should be obtained from the single acceptable "best-test" curve (i.e., largest sum of FVC and FEV_1) and reported at BTPS.

7.7.3 All values should be recorded and stored so that comparison for reproducibility and the ability to detect spirometry-induced bronchospasm (as evidenced by a worsening in spirometric values with successive attempts — and not related to fatigue) are simplified.

7.7.4 The highest MVV trial should be reported.

7.8 Subject demographics and related information:

7.8.1 Age: The age on day of test should be used.

7.8.2 Height: The subject should stand fully erect with eyes looking straight ahead and be measured with the feet together without shoes. An accurate measuring device should be used. For subjects who cannot stand or who have a spinal deformity (e.g., kyphoscoliosis), the arm span from finger tip to finger tip with arms stretched in opposite directions can be used as an estimate of height. (20)

7.8.3 Weight: An accurate scale should be used to determine the subject's weight while wearing indoor clothes but without shoes.

7.8.4 Race: The race or ethnic background of the subject should be determined and reported to help ensure the use of appropriate reference values and appropriate interpretation of data.

7.8.5 The time of day, equipment or instrumentation used, and name of the technician administering the test should be recorded.

7.9 Open- and closed-circuit testing:

7.9.1 Open circuit: The subject takes a maximal inspiration from the room, inserts the mouthpiece into the mouth, and then blows out either slowly (SVC) or rapidly (FVC) until the end-of-test criterion is met. Although the open-circuit technique works well for some subjects, others have difficulty maintaining a maximum inspiration while trying to position the mouthpiece correctly in the mouth. These subjects may lose some of their vital capacity due to leakage prior to the expiratory maneuver. (11)

7.9.2 Closed-circuit: The subject inserts the mouthpiece into the mouth and breathes quietly for no more than five tidal breaths, takes a maximal inspiration from the reservoir, and then blows out either slowly (SVC) or rapidly (FVC) until the end-of-test criterion is met. This rebreathing technique is preferred if the spirometer system permits

TABLE 1: Recommended Times for Withholding Commonly Used Bronchodilators When Bronchodilator Response Is to Be Assessed*

DRUG	WITHHOLDING TIME (hours)
Salmeterol	12
Ipratropium	6
Terbutaline	4–8
Albuterol	4–6
Metaproterenol	4
Isoetharine	3

*Based on consensus of committee and known duration of action.

because it (1) allows the subject to obtain a tight seal with the mouthpiece prior to inspiration and (2) allows evaluation of the volume inspired.

S 8.0 ASSESSMENT OF NEED:
Need is assessed by determining that valid indications are present.

S 9.0 ASSESSMENT OF TEST QUALITY:
Spirometry performed for the listed indications is valid only if the spirometer functions acceptably and the subject is able to perform the maneuvers in an acceptable and reproducible fashion. All reports should contain a statement about the technician's assessment of test quality and specify which acceptability criteria were not met.

9.1 Quality control: (21)

9.1.1 Volume verification (i.e., calibration): at least daily prior to testing, use a calibrated known-volume syringe with a volume of at least 3 L to ascertain that the spirometer reads a known volume accurately. The known volume should be injected and/or withdrawn at least three times, at flows that vary between 2 and 12 L/s (3 L injection times of approximately 1 second, 6 seconds, and somewhere between 1 and 6 seconds). The tolerance limits for an acceptable calibration are ±3% of the known volume. Thus, for a 3 L calibration syringe, the acceptable recovered range is 2.91–3.09 L. We encourage the practitioner to exceed this guideline whenever possible (i.e., reduce the tolerance limits to <±3%).

9.1.2 Leak test: Volume-displacement spirometers must be evaluated for leaks daily. One recommendation is that any volume change of more than 10 mL/min while the spirometer is under at least 3-cm-H_2O pressure be considered excessive. (22)

9.1.3 A spirometry procedure manual should be maintained.

9.1.4 A log that documents daily instrument calibration, problems encountered, corrective action required, and system hardware and/or software changes should be maintained.

9.1.5 Computer software for measurement and computer calculations should be checked against manual calculations if possible. In addi-tion, biologic laboratory standards (i.e., healthy, nonsmoking individuals) can be tested periodically to ensure historic reproducibility, to verify software upgrades, and to evaluate new or replacement spirometers.

9.1.6 The known-volume syringe should be checked for accuracy at least quarterly using a second known-volume syringe, with the spirometer in the patient-test mode. This validates the calibration and ensures that the patient-test mode operates properly.

9.1.7 For water-seal spirometers, water level and paper tracing speed should be checked daily. The entire range of volume displacement should be checked quarterly. (21)

9.2 Quality Assurance: Each laboratory or testing site should develop, establish, and implement quality assurance indicators for equipment calibration and maintenance and patient preparation. In addition, methods should be devised and implemented to monitor technician performance (with appropriate feedback) while obtaining, recognizing, and documenting acceptability criteria.

S 11.0 MONITORING:
The following should be evaluated during the performance of spirometric measurements to ascertain the validity of the results: (3, 24)

11.1 Acceptability of maneuver and reproducibility of FVC, FEV_1 (25)

11.2 Level of effort and cooperation by the subject

11.3 Equipment function or malfunction (e.g., calibration)

11.4 The final report should contain a statement about test quality.

11.5 Spirometry results should be subject to ongoing review by a supervisor, with feedback to the technologist. (12) Quality assurance and/or quality improvement programs should be designed to monitor technician competency, both initially and on an ongoing basis.

RATIONALE FOR BEDSIDE MONITORING

Bedside monitoring is an effective tool for rapidly assessing the mechanics of ventilation. The information obtained may be useful in assessing the patient's ability to reverse atelectasis, overcome airway obstruction, mobilize secretions, and maintain ventilation, as well as to evaluate the effectiveness of bronchodilator or other therapy. Some of the bedside parameters monitored require patient cooperation. In the comatose patient, you may be able to assess only a portion of the parameters discussed in this chapter. However, those parameters that you will be able to monitor are very useful and generally provide an adequate indication of the mechanics of ventilation.

Frequently, some of these bedside parameters are monitored before and after intermittent positive-pressure breathing (IPPB) or small volume nebulizer therapy. In these instances, the patient is relatively healthy and able to sustain ventilation.

EQUIPMENT USED IN MEASURING BEDSIDE PARAMETERS

Respirometers

A *respirometer* is a device used to measure ventilatory volumes.

Wright and Haloscale Respirometers

The Wright and Haloscale respirometers are small portable respirometers (Figure 5-1).

These instruments work by rotation of a thin vane with gas flow. As the vane rotates, it turns a series of gears, rotating the hands on the dial indicating the volume. The inner workings look much like those of a watch. Slots or channels surround the vane, directing the flow of gas through it in only one direction. Figure 5-2 shows an internal schematic of the respirometers.

These respirometers are designed to operate between 3 and 300 liters per minute. Flows in excess of 300 liters per minute may cause internal damage to the delicate vane as well as affecting its accuracy. Therefore, using these devices is not recommended for forced maneuvers such as that needed to measure the forced vital capacity (FVC). Accuracy is between 5% and 10% at 60 liters per minute. These devices are susceptible to inertia. The vane can be spun up so that the measurement is taken after the flow has stopped. This can be observed by gently puffing into the respirometer and observing the dial motion.

These respirometers are very delicate and do not tolerate being dropped.

Peak Flowmeters

A *peak flowmeter* is a device that measures ventilatory flow rates.

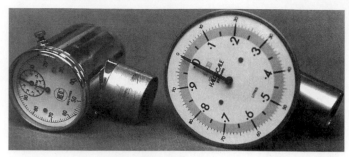

Figure 5-1   *The Wright and Haloscale respirometers*

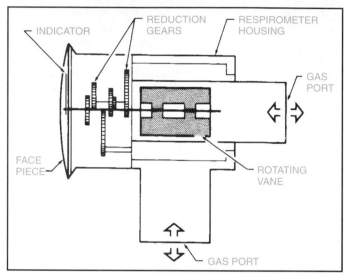

Figure 5-2   *An internal schematic of the Wright and Haloscale respirometers*

Wright and Mini-Wright Peak Flowmeters

These two devices measure expiratory flow rates. Figure 5-3 shows both the Wright and Mini-Wright peak flowmeters.

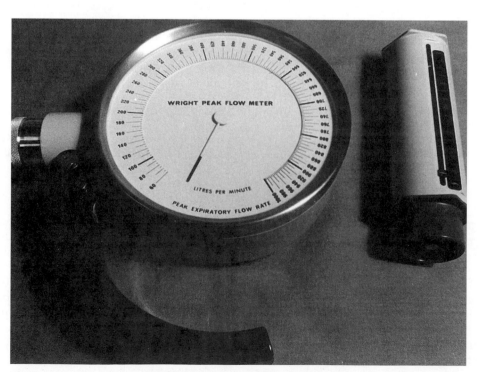

Figure 5-3   *The Wright and Mini-Wright peak flowmeters*

Expired gas pushes against a spring-loaded vane or diaphragm (as in the Mini-Wright device). As the vane or diaphragm is displaced, holes or a slot (as in the Mini-Wright) is exposed, allowing gas to escape. As more holes or more of the slot is exposed, additional flow must be generated to move the vane or diaphragm. Figure 5-4 shows a schematic of the Mini-Wright device. The scale is calibrated in liters per minute.

Both of the devices are delicate. Dropping them may result in their failure to operate properly.

The Wright peak flowmeter is calibrated from 50 to 1000 liters per minute. The Mini-Wright peak flowmeter is calibrated from 60 to 800 liters per minute.

Boehringer Inspiratory Force Manometer

This device is used to measure negative pressure generated on inspiration.

The inspiratory force manometer operates by transmittal of pressure to a sealed diaphragm and pivot assembly, as in an aneroid barometer. As more negative pressure is generated by the patient, the pivot deflects the needle further, indicating more negative pressure on the dial.

This device is delicate, and dropping or abusing it will render it inoperative.

Types of Spirometers

A *spirometer* is a device that measures ventilatory volumes and air flow.

Water Seal Spirometers

The water seal spirometer is the most common pulmonary function measuring device. As the name implies, this spirometer relies on a water seal to separate the spirometer bell from the atmosphere. The Warren E. Collins Company (Braintree, Massachusetts) manufactures several different spirometers that employ this principle. Figure 5-5 shows a cross section of this type of spirometer.

A rotating drum (kymograph) and pen is incorporated with the bell, tracing the bell's motion. This pen mechanism may be suspended by a chain and pulley or attached directly to the bell itself.

As the patient breathes from the bell, the bell rises and falls with the patient's inspired and expired volumes.

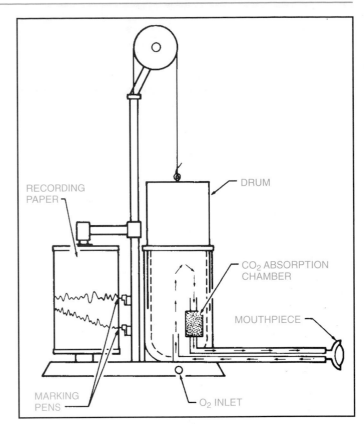

Figure 5-5   *A cross section of a Collins water seal spirometer*

These cause a corresponding motion of the pen, recording the tracing on graph paper. Different kymograph speeds allow the measurement of slow and forced maneuvers.

Fleisch Pneumotach Spirometer

This device relies on a pressure differential to measure flow. Pressure is conducted proximal and distal to a heated capillary grid and a diaphragm transducer. A pressure drop occurs distal to the capillary grid. The transducer senses and transmits the pressure differential between the two measuring points. The greater the differential, the greater the flow. This flow is then interpreted as a volume or is read directly from the device. Figure 5-6 shows a cross section of a Fleisch pneumotachometer head.

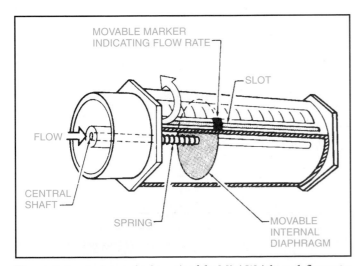

Figure 5-4   *An internal schematic of the Mini-Wright peak flowmeter*

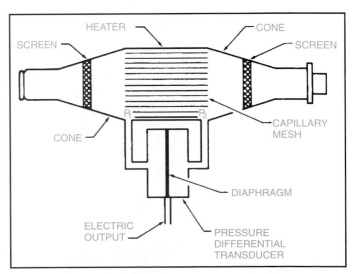

Figure 5-6   *A cross section of the Fleisch pneumotachometer*

BEDSIDE MEASUREMENTS

Minute Volume

The *minute volume* is the volume of air inhaled or exhaled during 1 minute. In the normal adult at rest, minute volume ranges between 5 and 7 liters per minute. As minute volume increases, so does the work of breathing. When minute volume decreases, hypoxemia and hypercapnia may result from less gas exchange at the alveolar level. An increase in minute ventilation may occur as a result of hypercapnia, exercise, increased dead space, or alveolar hypoventilation. A patient with sufficient muscle strength may be able to sustain an increased minute ventilation for some time without becoming severely fatigued. However, an increase in minute ventilation in excess of 10 liters per minute cannot be sustained for long and may be an indication of pending respiratory failure.

To measure the minute volume, place a pair of nose clips on your patient's nose. Instruct the patient to breathe normally into the respirometer. Observing your watch, count the respiratory rate and, after 1 minute, terminate the measurement. The exhaled volume is the minute volume.

Tidal Volume

The *tidal volume* is the amount of air moved into or out of a resting patient's lungs with each normal breath. The tidal volume can be calculated by dividing the minute volume by the respiratory rate. It is important that you measure this volume during inspiration or expiration, but not during both. Normal tidal volume may be estimated by multiplying the normal body weight (in kilograms) by 5 to 7 ml/kg. For instance, for a 75-kg man, we could estimate a tidal volume of 450 ml (75 kg × 6 ml/kg = 450 ml). Figure 5-7 shows how the tidal volume appears on a slow vital capacity tracing.

A portion of the tidal volume does not participate in respiration (actual gas exchange). This portion of the tidal volume is termed *anatomical dead space*. This volume may be estimated by multiplying the normal body weight based on height (in kilograms) by 2.2 ml/kg. For instance, a 75-kg male would have an anatomical dead space of approximately 165 ml (75 kg × 2.2 ml/kg = 165 ml).

As tidal volume decreases, the anatomical dead space does not decrease with it. Assume our 75-kg male patient's tidal volume drops to 300 ml. If you subtract the anatomical dead space (165 ml), only 135 ml is potentially participating in respiration or gas exchange. This is significant because such a small volume will not sustain a person for very long before respiratory failure occurs.

Excessive oxygenation and hyperventilation may also cause a decrease in tidal volume and respiratory rate. This is the result of an increase in the partial pressure of oxygen (PaO$_2$) and a decrease in the partial pressure of carbon dioxide (PaCO$_2$). The brain normally responds to these two conditions by decreasing ventilation.

Frequency

Respiratory *frequency* is the number of breaths per minute. Normal respiratory frequency for the adult is 12 to 20 breaths per minute. An increased respiratory rate may indicate increased hypoxemia, fear, pain, anxiety, or hypercapnia. A rate in excess of 35 breaths per minute may be an indication of pending respiratory failure.

Conversely, a low respiratory rate may result from central nervous system (CNS) depression caused by drugs, hypercapnia, or nervous system disorders. Bradypnea can lead to hypoxemia and hypercapnia.

Vital Capacity

Vital capacity is the maximum volume of air that can be exhaled after a maximal inspiration. A capacity by definition is two or more volumes. The vital capacity is made up of the *expiratory reserve volume* (ERV), tidal volume, and the *inspiratory reserve volume* (IRV). Figure 5-7 illustrates the relationship of the three volumes that in combination equal the vital capacity.

To measure the vital capacity, place a pair of nose clips on the patient's nose. Instruct the patient to inhale as deeply as possible and then exhale through the respirometer. This test requires cooperation and effort. Coach and encourage the patient as you perform this measurement.

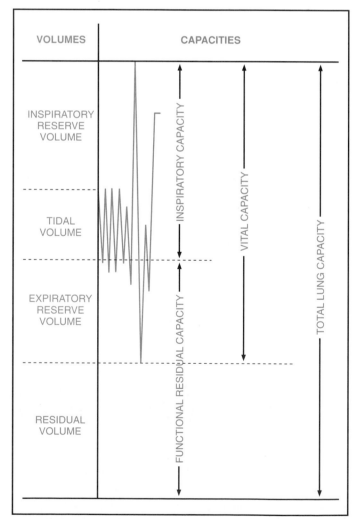

Figure 5-7 *A slow vital capacity tracing showing four volumes and four capacities*

The vital capacity is an indicator of ventilatory reserve. A patient with a large vital capacity has a large reserve and sufficient muscle strength to sustain ventilation. A patient with a low vital capacity does not have much ventilatory reserve to sustain ventilation. Normal vital capacity may be estimated by multiplying the normal body weight (in kilograms) by 65 to 75 ml/kg. Our 75-kg male patient would have an estimated vital capacity of 5.25 liters (75 kg × 70 ml/kg = 5.25 liters).

A vital capacity of less than 15 ml/kg of normal body weight may be a sign that respiratory failure is imminent. This volume/weight provides little reserve to reverse atelectasis, cough, or mobilize secretions, and to sustain ventilation. Fatigue may soon occur, resulting in a decrease in minute volume and worsening of hypoxemia and hypercapnia.

Peak Expiratory Flow Rate

The *peak expiratory flow rate* (PEFR) is the maximum flow rate attained during a forced expiration after a maximal inspiration. It requires patient cooperation to measure and is a good indicator of airway obstruction and muscle strength. This measurement is commonly used to assess the effectiveness of bronchodilators and the reversibility of an obstruction. A normal PEFR for an adult is greater than 500 L/min.

To measure the peak expiratory flow (PEF), instruct your patient to inhale as deeply as possible and then exhale as forcefully as possible through your peak flowmeter. The PEF usually occurs in the first second or two of expiration.

Maximal Inspiratory Pressure

Maximal inspiratory pressure (MIP) is the amount of negative pressure a patient is able to generate when trying to inhale. It is an indicator of muscle strength and ventilatory reserve. This relates to the patient's ability to reverse atelectasis, cough effectively, and manage airway secretions. Patient cooperation is not necessary to measure this component of pulmonary function. It can be performed on the comatose patient. MIP is measured using an inspiratory force manometer calibrated in cm H_2O. A normal patient should be able to generate a MIP of −60 cm H_2O or greater. A MIP of less than −25 cm H_2O is a sign of impending respiratory failure. A patient with a MIP value this low may not have the muscle strength to reverse atelectasis or to sustain normal ventilation before fatigue occurs, exacerbating the situation.

To measure the MIP, inform your patient that for a brief moment, inspiration of air will not be possible. Use of nose clips for the patient without an artificial airway is required. Have the patient breathe normally through the special 15-mm adapter on the inspiratory force manometer. Occlude the side port and instruct the patient to inhale as deeply as possible. The needle will deflect into the negative range, indicating the MIP generated. In the comatose patient, occlude the side port for 15 to 30 seconds and record the highest negative pressure generated along with the time interval.

BASIC SPIROMETRY

Determination of a slow vital capacity is often used to measure lung volumes and capacities. A complete inspiration slowly exhaled will often produce greater volumes than a forced maneuver, owing to airway closure causing air trapping with the latter. Figure 5-7 shows a typical slow vital capacity tracing. From this spirogram, four volumes and four capacities may be measured. A capacity by definition is two or more combined volumes.

Volumes
Tidal Volume

The tidal volume is defined as the amount of air moved into or out of a resting patient's lungs with each normal breath (see Figure 5-7).

Inspiratory Reserve Volume

The inspiratory reserve volume is defined as the maximum volume that can be inhaled after a normal inspiration (refer to Figure 5-7).

Expiratory Reserve Volume

Expiratory reserve volume is defined as the maximum amount of air that can be expired after a normal expiration (refer to Figure 5-7).

Residual Volume

The *residual volume* is the volume of gas left in the lungs following a maximal expiration. This volume cannot be measured directly but must be measured indirectly using nitrogen washout, helium dilution, or carbon monoxide methods.

CAPACITIES AND THEIR SIGNIFICANCE
Inspiratory Capacity

The *inspiratory capacity* is a combination of the tidal volume and the inspiratory reserve volume. This is the maximum volume that can be inspired from a resting expiratory level.

Normally, the inspiratory capacity approximates 75% of the vital capacity. Any increase or decrease in the inspiratory capacity will usually also be seen in the vital capacity.

Vital Capacity

The vital capacity is defined as the amount of air that can be exhaled following a maximal inspiration (see Figure 5-7). The vital capacity is a combination of the inspiratory reserve volume, tidal volume, and expiratory reserve volume.

Functional Residual Capacity

The *functional residual capacity* (FRC) is a combination of the expiratory reserve volume and the residual volume.

An increase in the FRC is considered pathologic. This change reflects hyperinflation and air trapping.

Total Lung Capacity

The *total lung capacity* is a combination of all lung volumes. An increase or decrease in total lung capacity may signify pulmonary disease. Typically, the total lung capacity is compared with the vital capacity in determining the underlying cause of the reduction or increase in volume. The total lung capacity cannot be measured at the bedside.

THE FORCED VITAL CAPACITY TRACING

Figure 5-8 illustrates a typical *forced vital capacity* (FVC) tracing. From this tracing, the FVC, timed forced expired volume (FEV_t), forced expired flow between 200 and 1200 ml ($FEF_{200-1200}$), midexpiratory forced expired flow ($FEF_{25-75\%}$), and PEFR can be measured. The FVC is measured by having the patient inhale maximally and then exhale maximally into a spirometer. This exhalation is a forced maneuver accomplished by encouraging the patient to blow the air out of the lungs as quickly as possible.

Timed Forced Expired Volume

The FEV_t is the forced expired volume over a given time interval. The common time intervals over which the volume is measured are 0.5, 1, and 3 seconds. The most common measurement is performed after 1 second. Figure 5-9 shows the FEV_1 measurement. Note the starting point of the FVC maneuver in the figure. The kymograph is rotating at 1920 mm/min or 32 mm/sec. Therefore, a 32-mm horizontal distance from the beginning of the maneuver corresponds to a 1-second time interval.

This measurement can provide an indication of obstruction. However, the test validity depends on the effort and cooperation of the patient. A decreased FEV_t may indicate obstruction and restriction. The FEV_1 is often compared to the FVC as the ratio FEV_1/FVC, or FEV%. Generally, patients with obstruction show a reduction in FVC%, whereas patients with restriction show a normal FEV_1% (Scanlan et al., 1995).

Forced Expired Flow between 200 and 1200

$FEF_{200-1200}$ is a measurement of the flow rate between 200 and 1200 ml on the FVC curve. Figure 5-10 is a measurement of this flow. Two points on the FVC curve are marked, indicating the exhalation of 200 ml and of 1200 ml. A line is drawn intersecting these points and extending over a 1-second interval. The corresponding flow may then be measured in liters per second.

The $FEF_{200-1200}$ generally indicates the air flow characteristics of the large airways. Obstructive disease processes will cause a decrease in the $FEF_{200-1200}$. A decrease in this flow rate normally occurs with aging.

Midexpiratory Forced Expired Flow

$FEF_{25-75\%}$ is the flow rate over the middle portion of the FVC maneuver. The FVC tracing is divided into four parts and

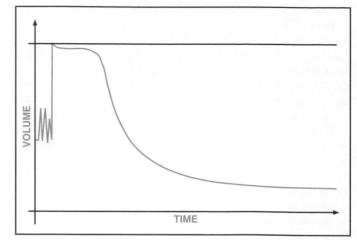

Figure 5-8 *A forced vital capacity tracing*

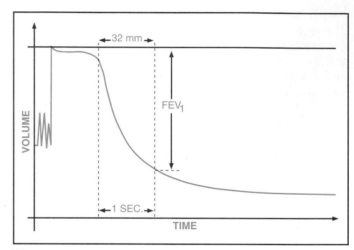

Figure 5-9 *The FEV_1 shown on the FVC tracing*

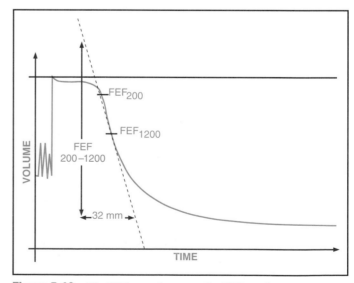

Figure 5-10 *The $FEF_{200-1200}$ shown on the FVC tracing*

the flow rate over the middle two parts (middle 50%) is calculated (Figure 5-11).

The $FEF_{25-75\%}$ is indicative of the flow characteristics of small-size airways (Scanlan et al., 1995). A decrease in the

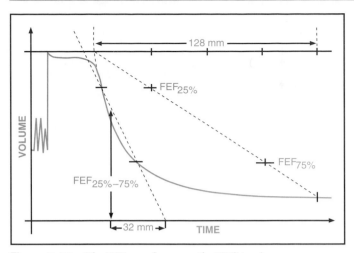

Figure 5-11 *The FEF$_{25-75\%}$ shown on the FVC tracing*

FEF$_{25-75\%}$ may signify obstruction. Since the test detects the air flow characteristics of the smaller airways, it is less dependent on effort and is often used for the early detection of obstructive disease. This flow rate decreases normally with advancing age.

Peak Expiratory Flow Rate

The PEFR may be measured by extrapolating the steepest portion of the FVC tracing over a 1-second time interval (Figure 5-12). The flow may then be calculated in liters per second.

The PEFR is of little clinical significance. A patient with obstructive disease may have an initially high PEFR that rapidly decreases over time.

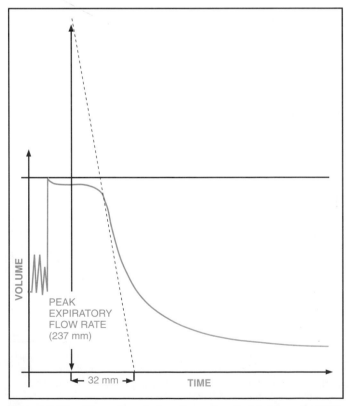

Figure 5-12 *The peak expiratory flow rate calculated from the FVC*

MAXIMUM VOLUNTARY VENTILATION

The *maximum voluntary ventilation* (MVV) is measured by having the patient stand (if possible) and breathe as deeply and rapidly as possible over a 10-, 12-, or 15-second interval. The volumes may be added individually, or if the spirometer has an accumulator pen, the volumes are added automatically. The volume is then extrapolated and measured in liters per minute.

The MVV is very effort-dependent and is therefore more of a reflection of muscle strength, airway resistance, and compliance. Patients with obstructive disease have a reduced MVV volume.

ATPS TO BTPS CONVERSION

All pulmonary function testing is performed at *ambient temperature and pressure, saturated* (ATPS). Volumes and flows must be converted to reflect conditions of *body temperature and pressure, saturated* (BTPS). This conversion is important because the volumes are larger under BTPS conditions. As the temperature of a gas increases, it expands. The difference between ambient temperature and body temperature is typically 13°C. If the measurements were not converted, the difference would represent a significant error.

FLOW-VOLUME LOOPS

Flow-volume loops present spirometry information in a way different from that used with the volume-time curves discussed so far. A flow-volume loop plots flow along the vertical axis and volume along the horizontal axis (Figure 5-13).

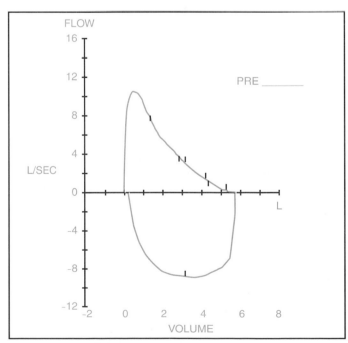

Figure 5-13 *A flow-volume loop. Note that the vertical axis is scaled in L/sec and the horizontal axis is scaled in L. Expiration is above the iso flow line, and inspiration is below it.*

The expiratory portion of the curve is above the volume axis line—the *iso flow line*. The inspiratory portion of the curve is below the iso flow line.

The FVC is determined by measuring along the horizontal axis using the volume scale provided from point *A* to point *B* on Figure 5-14. This horizontal distance (volume), as in volume-versus-time spirometry, is measured at ATPS and therefore must be converted to reflect BTPS conditions.

Flows on the flow-volume loop are determined by evaluating the tracing in relation to the vertical axis. The PEF is determined by finding the highest point the curve reaches above the iso flow line. Once this point has been determined, the flow is read directly from the flow scale (Figure 5-15). An advantage of the flow-volume loop over volume-versus-time spirometry is the capability to directly measure flow at any point on the curve. The peak inspiratory flow is determined in a similar way to the PEF. Simply identify the lowest point on the inspiratory portion of the tracing and measure the flow directly from the flow axis at that point (Figure 5-15). As with volume determination, the flows should also be converted from ATPS to BTPS and reported in BTPS.

With obstructive and restrictive pulmonary disease, the shape (morphology) of the flow-volume loop is altered. In obstructive disease, note that the expiratory portion of the curve is not as linear, as seen in Figure 5-16. Sometimes this characteristic is termed "scooping." A patient with obstructive disease is unable to generate sufficient expiratory flows; therefore, the shape of the expiratory curve changes (Fitzgerald, Speir, & Callahan, 1996). In restrictive disease, the patient is unable to inspire as fully as a normal

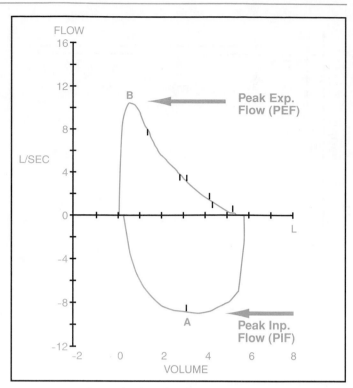

Figure 5-15 *Determination of peak inspiratory and peak expiratory flows. Peak inspiratory flow corresponds to* A *whereas peak expiratory flow corresponds to* B.

person can. Also, because of a general decrease in pulmonary compliance, there is a greater elastic recoil of the lungs. These pathophysiological changes result in a tall, skinny flow-volume loop (Figure 5-16). The volume is decreased (horizontal axis) whereas flows are normal or greater than normal (vertical axis).

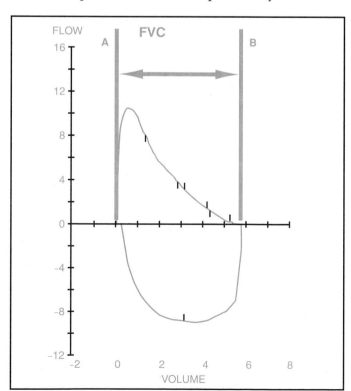

Figure 5-14 *Calculation of the FVC. Note that the FVC is the volume between points* A *and* B.

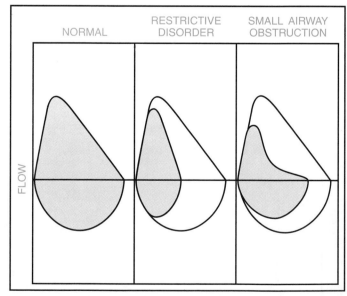

Figure 5-16 *A flow-volume loop from patients with both obstructive and restrictive components of lung disease. Note that the expiratory portion is not as linear as the normal tracing. In the restrictive tracing, note that it appears tall and "skinny."*

MEASUREMENT OF FUNCTIONAL RESIDUAL CAPACITY AND RESIDUAL VOLUME

Both the FRC and RV cannot be measured by using direct spirometry. Both volumes, however, contribute to the total lung capacity and are often helpful in the diagnosis of both obstructive and restrictive lung disease. Two common techniques are used to determine the FRC and RV: gas dilution techniques and body plethysmography.

Gas Dilution Techniques

Gas dilution techniques include nitrogen washout and helium dilution techniques. Because both techniques measure FRC and RV using a similar method, only one, *nitrogen washout*, is discussed here. Both methods are based on the following formula:

$$C_1V_1 = C_2V_2$$

where the initial concentration and volume (C_1 and V_1) and the final concentration (V_1) are known and the final volume (lung volume V_2) is unknown. For measuring FRC using the nitrogen washout technique, the patient breathes in oxygen (100%) and exhales into the spirometer system. During the test, nitrogen (from room air) in the lungs is replaced by the oxygen as it is diluted. The exhaled volume and nitrogen concentration of the exhaled gas are measured over time (Figure 5-17). After 3 to 8 minutes (typically 7), the exhaled nitrogen concentration stabilizes

and has fallen to <1.0. At that point, the test is concluded and the patient is removed from the mouthpiece. When performing this test, it is important to keep a tight seal on the mouthpiece (scuba-type mouthpieces are often used) and also to use nose clips. If a leak develops so that the patient breathes room air, a sudden spike in the exhaled nitrogen concentration will occur (Figure 5-18). Computer-based pulmonary function systems automatically measure the final nitrogen concentration and exhaled volume, calculating the FRC, RV, and TLC. This technique can only measure gas that is in communication with the mouth. Any trapped gas distal to airway obstruction will not be measured (nitrogen won't be washed out). Therefore, this technique will underestimate RV and FRC in patients with obstructive disease (Brown, 1997).

Body Plethysmography

A body plethysmograph is a closed chamber that utilizes the principle of Boyle's law to measure lung volumes (Figure 5-19). A patient is seated in the plethysmograph and the door is closed. After a minute or two, temperature stabilizes (the patient's body warms the interior of the plethysmograph). Once the temperature is stable, the patient splints the cheeks with the hands and gently pants (about 50 ml of volume at 1 pant per second [1 Hz]), as shown in Figure 5-19. A shutter closes, and mouth pressure is measured before and after shutter closure. The computer knows mouth pressure (before and after shutter closure) and plethysmograph volume. The unknown

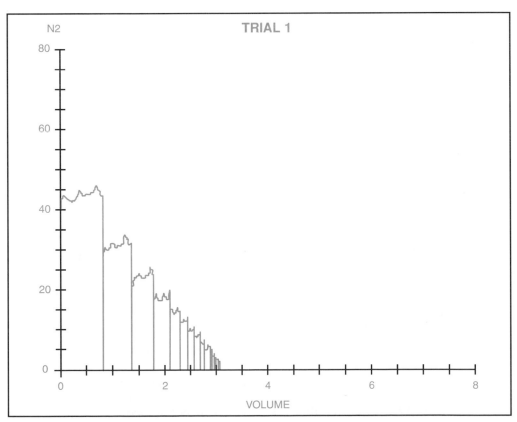

Figure 5-17 *The exhaled nitrogen tracing from a nitrogen washout determination of FRC. Note how the nitrogen concentration falls over time.*

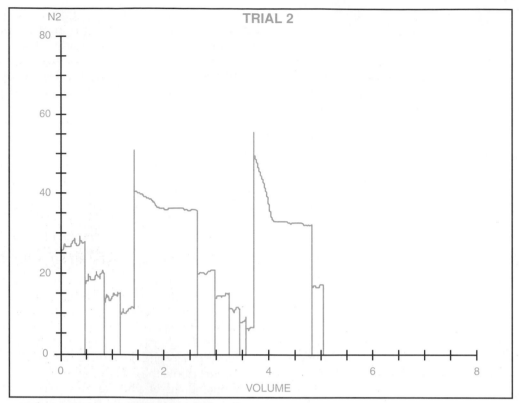

Figure 5-18 *A leak occurred during this N₂ washout study. Note the sudden spike (increase) in exhaled nitrogen concentration.*

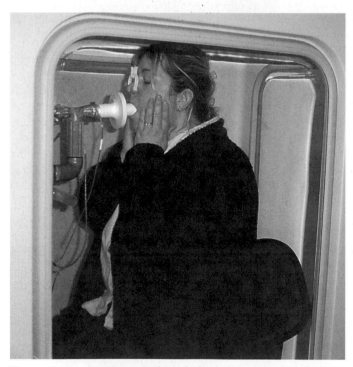

Figure 5-19 *A patient seated in a body plethysmograph ready for V_{TG} determination. Note that the hands are splinting the cheeks and the elbows are at the patient's side.*

volume (thoracic gas volume, V_{TG}) of the lungs is then calculated. This technique is more accurate for RV and TLC determination in patients who have obstructive disease (Brown, 1997).

DIFFUSION: SINGLE BREATH CARBON MONOXIDE TEST

Clinically, it would be very useful to know how well oxygen and carbon dioxide diffuse across the alveolar capillary membranes between the blood and the ambient air. However, owing to the presence of these gases both dissolved in the blood and in the air, it is not possible to measure their diffusion directly. Carbon monoxide (CO), however, is not normally present in the blood and may be present only in trace quantities in the ambient air (under normal circumstances). In addition, CO has an affinity for hemoglobin that is 210 times greater than that of oxygen (Pierson & Kacmarek, 1992). Once CO is present in the lungs, it rapidly diffuses across the alveolar-capillary membranes and binds with hemoglobin. Therefore, CO is an ideal gas to use for measuring how well *diffusion* occurs.

For the single breath CO diffusion test (single breath D_LCO test, where L refers to lung), the patient inspires CO, helium or neon, and oxygen in known concentrations. The CO is used to measure diffusion, whereas the helium or neon is used to measure alveolar volume (total lung volume) using a dilutional (washout) method. The patient inhales this mixture from RV to TLC and holds the breath at TLC for 10 seconds. Once the breath hold is met, the patient exhales back to RV. The first 750 to 1000 ml of gas is discarded. The sample volume of between 500 and 1000 ml is then collected and measured (American Thoracic Society, 1995). The computer system knows the inspired gas concentrations, measures the expired concentrations and exhaled volume, and calculates alveolar volume (V_A)

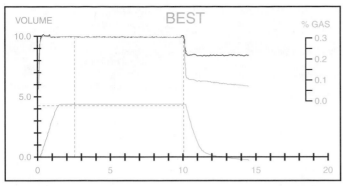

Figure 5-20 *The tracing produced from a single breath carbon monoxide diffusion test for (D$_L$CO). Note the inspiratory capacity and exhaled gas tracings.*

and D$_L$CO. Figure 5-20 illustrates the inspiration from RV to TLC, the breath hold, and the exhaled gas tracings (concentrations).

HAZARDS OF PULMONARY FUNCTION TESTING

Hyperventilation

The majority of the pulmonary function maneuvers involve greater than normal volumes and effort. Therefore, it is not uncommon for patients to become light-headed or dizzy from the corresponding decrease in PaCO$_2$. With continued effort, *hyperventilation* may result.

Careful patient monitoring is essential for the prevention of this complication. Allow frequent rest periods. The rest periods allow the patient to recover to a normal ventilatory state and also help to ensure maximal efforts for all maneuvers. Patients who are very ill may easily overextend themselves and become compromised.

Cardiac Stimulation from Bronchodilators

The most common bronchodilators are sympathomimetic agents with beta$_1$-adrenergic side effects. Bronchodilators are administered during pulmonary function testing to assess the reversibility of lung dysfunction. A potential side effect is tachycardia. Careful patient monitoring will ensure early detection of this complication.

Infection

Cross-contamination from the pulmonary function circuitry is not uncommon in patients undergoing pulmonary function testing. Patients with undiagnosed contagious pulmonary disease may be sent to your facility for testing. If permanent reusable circuitry is used, ensure that a clean, disinfected circuit is used for each patient. Disposable circuitry has recently become available, helping to minimize this potential hazard.

OBJECTIVES

At the end of this chapter, you should be able to:

- Assemble and test the equipment required for bedside monitoring and basic spirometry:
  — Respirometer
  — Peak flowmeter
  — Inspiratory force manometer
  — Flow or self-inflating manual resuscitator
  — Collins spirometer
- Using a laboratory partner, demonstrate the proper position for bedside monitoring.
- Discuss the importance of coaching and solicitation to a maximal patient effort.
- Explain the rationale for obtaining multiple tracings for pulmonary function testing.
- Using a laboratory partner, demonstrate how to measure the following bedside pulmonary function parameters:
  — Minute volume
  — Frequency
  — Tidal volume
  — Vital capacity
  — Maximal inspiratory force
  — Peak expiratory flow
- Using a laboratory partner, demonstrate how to perform the following tests using the Collins spirometer:

— Slow vital capacity
— Forced vital capacity
— Maximum minute ventilation
— From these tracings, measure and calculate the following:

Slow Vital Capacity
(1) IRV
(2) Tidal volume
(3) ERV
(4) VC

Forced Vital Capacity
(1) FVC
(2) FEV$_1$
(3) FEF$_{200-1200}$
(4) FEF$_{25-75\%}$
(5) PEFR

Maximum Voluntary Ventilation
(1) Respiratory rate
(2) Minute volume

— Using the foregoing measurements, calculate the predicted values for your laboratory partner and give each measured value as a percent of the predicted.
— Interpret the results of the tracings as normal, restricted, or obstructed.

BEDSIDE MONITORING: EQUIPMENT ASSEMBLY AND TESTING

A few pieces of specialized equipment and a watch are all that is required to measure bedside pulmonary function parameters. The equipment is generally quite simple in its design and operation; therefore, problems and trouble-shooting are minimal.

Figure 5-21 is a listing of the equipment required to measure bedside pulmonary function parameters.

These simple instruments require little in the way of preparation. Preparation and testing of the various instruments are discussed in the following paragraphs.

Respirometers

Wright and Haloscale Respirometers

These spirometers may be tested by sliding the on/off switch to the on position and gently blowing into the base of the respirometer. The dial should indicate the volume exhaled. If no reading is indicated, verify that the switch is in the on position and that the flow is directed into the spirometer through the port at the six o'clock position as the dial is read. If no recording is made, the unit is probably inoperative.

Attach a mouthpiece using a short piece of large-bore aerosol tubing and the 22-mm adapter supplied with the respirometer. This respirometer is now ready for use.

Peak Flowmeters

Wright and Mini-Wright Peak Flowmeters

Proper operation of these devices can be verified by blowing into the units and observing if flow is registered. The mouthpieces provided by the manufacturer may be used, or cardboard mouthpieces commonly used for pulmonary function testing may be substituted.

Boehringer Inspiratory Force Manometer

The operation of this device may be tested by attaching a short piece of tubing to the 15-mm adapter and inhaling, generating a negative pressure. If pressure is recorded, the unit is functional. This device has a second indication hand that may be positioned over the measuring hand on the dial. The second indication hand indicates the maximum negative pressure generated. Figure 5-22 shows the correct positioning of the two hands for inspiratory force measurement.

- Respirometer
- Inspiratory force manometer
- Peak flowmeter
- Watch (with a sweep second hand)

Figure 5–21 *Equipment required for bedside monitoring*

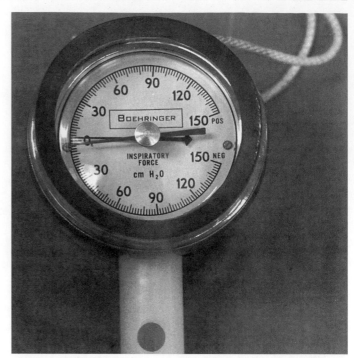

Figure 5-22 *The Boehringer inspiratory force manometer prepared for use*

PREPARATION OF THE COLLINS WATER SEAL SPIROMETER

The Collins water seal spirometer is one of the most frequently used spirometers in clinical practice today. Contemporary spirometers are often interfaced with a computer that hastens the process of calculating values for the pulmonary function measures. However, when a computer fails, a backup Collins water seal spirometer is frequently used, and all results are calculated manually.

It is very easy to learn pulmonary function testing on a computerized spirometer. However, the process and concepts are more thoroughly learned when the pulmonary function study values are manually calculated. It is important to understand the concepts and to visualize the process. Learning how to calculate pulmonary function testing values manually, without the aid of computers, will help you to understand how these values are derived.

Level the Spirometer and Fill with Water

Level the spirometer by using the leveling screws at the four corners of the spirometer. When the spirometer is level, check the water level using the glass sight gauge.

If required, fill the spirometer by raising the bell halfway and pouring water against the side of the bell. The water will run down into the reservoir surrounding the bell. Fill the spirometer with water until the water level is midway up the sight gauge.

Check for Excessive Resistance

Raise the spirometer bell and remove it. Remove the CO_2 absorber in the center of the spirometer and replace the bell. If resistance is improved, repack the CO_2 absorber with

Collins soda lime CO_2 absorbent (the indicator turns violet when it has been used), and replace the CO_2 absorber.

Adjust the Bell and Pulley System

Adjust the angle of the pulley system so that the bell is suspended without contacting the sides of the spirometer. This will ensure that the bell is free to move without excessive resistance.

Attach the Pens to the Recorder

Place fresh pens into their holders on the recorder. Black is traditionally used for the spirometry tracing, and red is used for the accumulator pen. The spirometer pen has the greater motion of the two recorders. Keep caps on the pens at all times unless you are performing a study. This precaution will help to minimize extraneous lines due to inadvertent pen contact with the paper.

Attach the Paper to the Kymograph

Turn the kymograph to its highest speed and note the direction of rotation. When attaching the paper, position it so that the overlap does not catch on rotation of the drum. Attach the paper with masking tape and ensure that it is straight and square to the kymograph drum.

Flush the Spirometer

Flush the spirometer by raising and lowering the bell several times to expel any stale air that may be in the bell. This will facilitate patient cooperation and hygiene.

Attach Clean Tubing, Valve, and Mouthpiece

When you attach clean tubing to the inlet and outlet sides of the spirometer, it is imperative to avoid accidental flow restriction; be sure to use tubing of the proper diameter. Attach clean tubing to the inlet and the outlet of the spirometer. Attach a clean valve with mouthpiece to the tubing and secure it to the support arm. You are now ready to use the spirometer for testing.

PATIENT FACTORS IN SPIROMETRY

Patient Positioning

The correct patient position for measuring these parameters is an upright position. Position the patient upright without causing undue harm. This will allow the lungs to expand freely without interference.

The Importance of Coaching

The success and validity of pulmonary function tests are largely dependent on patient response and cooperation. Therefore, it is to the practitioner's advantage to elicit the maximum patient response and cooperation. This may be facilitated in several ways. Treat the patient as a respected individual. Thoroughly explain the maneuvers to the patient, and encourage and coach the patient throughout the testing.

Patient instruction is very important. These measurements are very effort-dependent. Take time to explain in detail what is required for each test. Have the patient practice the maneuver quietly and without a great deal of effort. This rehearsal may ease any anxieties the patient has and help you to obtain good results when you measure the actual tracing.

During the testing, coach and encourage your patient. If more effort is required to obtain a good tracing, raise your voice when you coach. Pulmonary function testing is somewhat like cheerleading: it takes effort to elicit a good response.

Why Multiple Tests or Tracings?

Multiple tracings are frequently obtained from the same patient. You will often be assessing patients for disability payments. There is a monetary reward for poor performance on the tests in such cases. A patient may be deliberately malingering. If you suspect this, be very firm and insistent on obtaining the patient's best effort. Remember that your results will determine payment or nonpayment. Take more than one measurement of each tracing, preferably making three. Results for all tracings should be within 5% of each other to establish reproducibility. The best tracing is one with the greatest sum of the FVC and FEV_1.

MEASURING THE BEDSIDE PULMONARY FUNCTION PARAMETERS

Aseptic Technique

Strict adherence to aseptic technique is important to prevent the spread of nosocomial infections. A separate mouthpiece should be used for each patient. Some facilities provide a plastic bag to store mouthpieces and other equipment in a patient's room. Avoid handling the portion of the mouthpiece in contact with the patient. The possibility of acquiring and spreading bacteria by this means is obvious.

Do not lay the equipment (spirometer, peak flowmeter, MIP manometer) on the patient's bed or bedside table. These areas harbor bacteria, and the measuring devices can be the vehicle for spreading them to other areas.

Measurements

Using the appropriate equipment, measure the minute volume, frequency, tidal volume, vital capacity (VC), peak expiratory flow rate (PEFR), and maximal inspiratory pressure (MIP).

BASIC SPIROMETRY: USING THE COLLINS WATER SEAL SPIROMETER

Kymograph Speeds

There are several kymograph speeds available, depending upon the individual manufacturer. Two speeds, low and high, are fairly standard. These speeds are 32 mm/min on the low speed and 1920 mm/min on the high speed. The variation in speeds among kymographs is commonly found in the middle or medium speed. The two most common speeds are 160 mm/min and 480 mm/min, depending upon the spirometer.

The slow speed allows a better measurement of the slow vital capacity. This speed provides a complete tracing in a relatively small area of paper. All volumes are easily seen and read.

The medium speed is utilized for the MVV maneuver. At the slower speed, it becomes difficult to measure the individual volumes and count the respiratory rate. At the highest speed, the tracing would wrap itself more than once as the drum rotated. The fastest speed is used to perform the FVC tracing. This is considered to be the universally acceptable kymograph speed for FVC measurement. The tracing is relatively compact and yet easy to read.

If you are careful with your paper usage, you can obtain a slow vital capacity, FVC, and MVV tracing all on one sheet of paper.

Alignment of the Pen Mechanism to the Paper

Remove the cap from the black tracing pen and position it against the paper. Draw a vertical line by moving the bell up and down. The line will serve as a reference for measuring your values; it is a true vertical line. Recap your pen.

Measuring Testing Conditions

Note on the graph paper the conditions of the testing environment such as spirometer temperature (ambient temperature may be substituted in the absence of a spirometer thermometer) and barometric pressure in mm Hg.

Bell Factor

The *bell factor* is used to calculate the volumes and flows from your tracings. This bell factor is specific for the spirometer that you are using. The bell factor is expressed in milliliters per millimeter (ml/mm). Typical bell factors are 20.73 ml/mm and 41.27 ml/mm. Record the bell factor on the graph paper for the spirometer you are using. It is usually indicated on a plate attached to the spirometer.

PULMONARY FUNCTION TESTS

Slow Vital Capacity

Turn the valve to the off position (so that the patient is breathing room air and not into the spirometer). Remove the pen cap and position it on the paper. Explain what you want the patient to do and what to expect. Have the patient breathe quietly through the mouthpiece with the value in the off position to become accustomed to the device. Place nose clips on the patient's nose and allow a few breaths for the patient to become accustomed to this way of breathing.

Turn the kymograph to the lowest speed (32 mm/min) and check to be certain the kymograph drum is moving because it is difficult to detect motion at this speed. When you open the valve to the spirometer, the pen will begin to move, recording the patient's volumes. Have the patient breathe normally for approximately 5 breaths. Instruct the patient to inhale as deeply as possible and then to slowly blow out all the air in the lungs. Coach your patient by encouraging a maximal effort and volume. Allow the patient to relax by breathing at a "resting" tidal volume level.

Turn off the valve to the spirometer and allow your patient to rest a minute or two. Check your tracing and do a rough measurement to see if it approximates a normal value for that patient. If you suspect the patient was malingering or that the effort was not maximal, repeat the test.

Forced Vital Capacity

Remove the CO_2 absorber from the spirometer bell. The absorber creates a resistance to air as the patient's volumes move through the spirometer circuit. Leaving the absorber in place during forced maneuvers will simulate an obstructive condition.

This test requires some timing and coordination between you and your patient. Read through this section thoroughly before attempting this test.

Turn the valve to the off position (so that the patient is breathing room air and not into the spirometer). Remove the pen cap and position it on the paper.

Explain what you want the patient to do and what to expect. Have the patient breathe quietly through the mouthpiece in the off position for a few breaths to become accustomed to the device. Place nose clips on the patient's nose and allow a few breaths for the patient to become accustomed to this way of breathing.

Remove the cap from the pen and turn the kymograph on to its lowest speed (32 mm/min). Turn the valve on so that the patient is breathing through the spirometer. Have the patient inhale as deeply as possible and instruct the patient to hold up a hand when further inhaling is impossible. Be sure to coach the patient. When the patient's lungs are full, ask the patient to hold his or her breath. Immediately turn the kymograph to its fastest speed (1920 mm/min) and tell your patient to exhale as forcefully and as quickly as possible. Coach the patient to produce a maximal effort. After the patient has exhaled as much as possible, turn off the kymograph and recap the pen.

Allow your patient to rest. Take this opportunity to quickly measure the tracing to see if it is close to what you would expect. If you suspect the patient was malingering or the effort was not maximal, repeat the test. The test should be repeated a minimum of three times. Results for three tests should be within 5% of one another. The best result is defined as the one with the greatest sum of the forced vital capacity and FEV_1.

Measuring Maximal Voluntary Ventilation (MVV) with a Spirometer and Accumulator Pen

Turn the valve to the off position (so that the patient is breathing room air and not into the spirometer). Remove the pen cap and position the pen on the paper. Explain what you want the patient to do and what to expect. Have your patient breathe quietly through the mouthpiece with the value in the off position for a few breaths to become accustomed to the device. Place nose clips on the patient's nose and allow the patient a few breaths to become accustomed to this way of breathing.

Start the accumulator pen by engaging the plate/gear mechanism of the Reicher Ventilometer. Pushing the clutch plate in engages it; pulling it out disengages it. Remove the caps from the red and black recording pens and position them on the paper. Turn the kymograph to the medium speed and turn on the valve so that the patient is breathing through the spirometer. Instruct the patient to breathe as deeply and as quickly as possible. This is similar to panting. Coach your patient to obtain the best effort. Time the maneuver for 15 seconds; then turn off the kymograph and valve. Allow your patient to rest. If you suspect the patient was malingering or the effort was not maximal, repeat the test. Recap your pens. This concludes the maneuvers performed for basic spirometry.

If the spirometer you are using does not have an accumulator pen, measure the MVV using the following method. Allow the patient to become accustomed to the spirometer with the valve in the off position. Turn the kymograph to medium speed and turn the valve to the on position and have the patient breathe as deeply and quickly as possible. Time the maneuver for 15 seconds. Turn off the kymograph and allow your patient to rest.

MEASURING AND CALCULATING COMPONENTS OF A PULMONARY FUNCTION TESTING TRACING

Tidal Volume

The tidal volume is the smallest tracing on the slow vital capacity tracing (Figure 5-23). Draw horizontal lines across the top and bottom of the tracing, as shown in Figure 5–23. These lines should be at right angles to the reference line drawn by the pen before you began your testing. Perform the following steps to measure and calculate the tidal volume.

1. Measure the distance between the two lines, represented in Figure 5-23 as *A*.
2. Take this distance in millimeters and multiply it by the bell factor. This is the tidal volume.

Tidal volume = distance (mm) × bell factor (ml/mm)

Inspiratory Reserve Volume

The inspiratory reserve volume (IRV) is the maximum volume that can be inhaled after a normal inhalation. Draw a horizontal line (at a right angle to the reference line) across the point of maximal inspiration, as shown in Figure 5-22. The IRV is the distance *B* in the figure. To measure and calculate the IRV, complete the following steps:

1. Measure the distance between the point of maximum inspiration and the upper limit of a normal tidal volume (refer to Figure 5-23).
2. Multiply this distance in millimeters by the bell factor.

Inspiratory reserve volume = distance (mm) × bell factor (ml/mm)

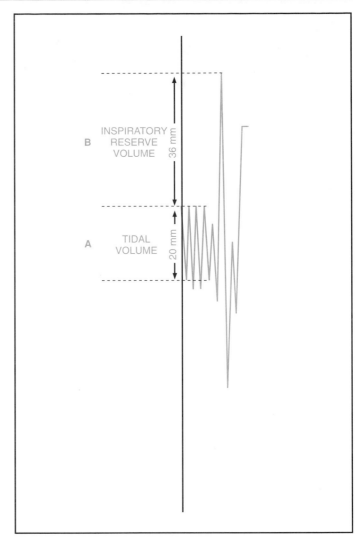

Figure 5-23   *Calculating the tidal volume and the inspiratory reserve volume*

Expiratory Reserve Volume

The expiratory reserve volume (ERV) is the maximum amount of air that can be exhaled from a resting expiratory level. Draw a horizontal line through the point of maximal exhalation (at a right angle to the reference line). Measure the distance between this line and the resting expiratory level. This is represented by distance *C* in Figure 5-24. To calculate the ERV, use the following steps:

1. Measure the distance between the point of maximal exhalation and the resting expiratory level in millimeters.
2. Multiply your measurement by the bell factor.

ERV = distance (mm) × bell factor (ml/mm)

Residual Volume

The residual volume requires a nitrogen washout test to determine the volume. It also requires special equipment to measure the nitrogen concentration. Not all schools or facilities have this equipment. If you have access to this equipment and wish to perform this test, consult the *Manual of Pulmonary Function Testing* by Gregg Ruppel (see Additional Resources at the end of the chapter) for instructions.

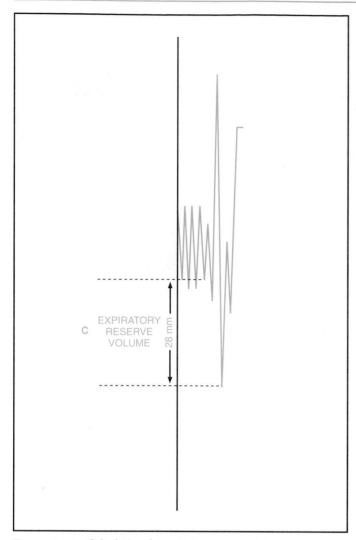

Figure 5-24   *Calculating the expiratory reserve volume*

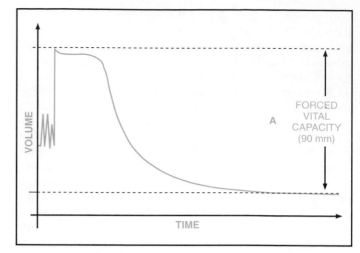

Figure 5-25   *Calculating the forced vital capacity*

To measure this you must first establish the starting point of the maneuver. On some tracings this is very clearly defined as shown in Figure 5-26, graph *A*. Note the clear, sharp transition between the point at which the patient was holding the breath (level plateau) and the FVC maneuver. This starting point is not always clear, owing to hesitation on the part of the patient. The starting point may then be extrapolated.

To extrapolate the starting point, identify the steepest portion of the FVC tracing (maximal flow). Draw a line tangent to this portion of the FVC tracing. Intersect this line with a horizontal line (at a right angle to the reference line) even with the point of maximal inspiration, as shown in Figure 5-26, graph *B*.

From this starting point, measure a 32-mm horizontal distance from the starting point. A distance of 32 mm represents 1 second (1920 mm/min for 60 seconds = 32 mm). Draw a vertical line from this point until it intersects the FVC tracing. Make certain that this line is parallel to the reference line. Measure this distance, represented by

MEASURING AND CALCULATING THE FORCED VITAL CAPACITY

Forced Vital Capacity (FVC)

The FVC is the maximum volume forcefully expired after a maximal inspiration. This can be identified as between the highest and lowest volumes on your curve. This volume is represented by distance *A* in Figure 5-25. Draw a horizontal line (at a right angle to the reference line) across the point of maximal inspiration and expiration as shown in Figure 5-25. To calculate the FVC, complete the following steps:

1. Measure the distance in millimeters from the point of maximal inspiration to maximal expiration.
2. Multiply this distance by the bell factor.

$$FVC = \text{distance (mm)} \times \text{bell factor (ml/mm)}$$

Forced Expired Volume in 1 Second (FEV$_1$)

This is the portion of the FVC that was expired in the first second of the maneuver.

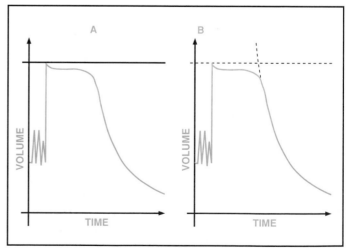

Figure 5-26   *Identifying the starting point of the forced vital capacity maneuver*

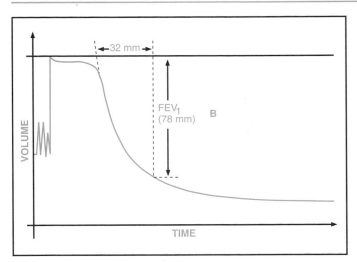

Figure 5-27   *Calculating the FEV₁*

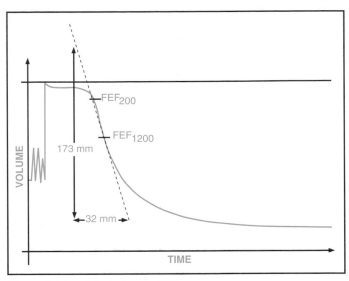

Figure 5-28   *Calculating the FEF₂₀₀₋₁₂₀₀*

distance *B* in Figure 5-27. To calculate the FEV_1, complete the following steps:

1. Measure a 32-mm horizontal distance from the start of the FVC tracing.
2. Draw a vertical line down from this point until it intersects the FVC tracing.
3. Measure the distance of this vertical line in millimeters.
4. Multiply this distance by the bell factor.

$$FEV_1 = \text{distance (mm)} \times \text{bell factor (ml/mm)}$$

Forced Expired Flow between 200 and 1200 ml

The $FEF_{200-1200}$ is the flow rate between 200 and 1200 ml on the FVC tracing. To calculate this, you must first establish the points on the FVC tracing that correspond to 200 ml and to 1200 ml.

To find these points, divide the desired volumes by the bell factor, as shown below:

$$200 \text{ ml} = 200 \text{ ml}/41.27 \text{ mm/ml}$$
$$= 4.8 \text{ mm}$$
$$1200 \text{ ml} = 1200 \text{ ml}/41.27 \text{ mm/ml}$$
$$= 29 \text{ mm}$$

Note that these distances were calculated using the bell factor for the spirometer used in the figures in this chapter. Be certain to use the bell factor for the spirometer that you are using.

Once you have calculated the distances for 200 and 1200 ml represented on your FVC tracing, measure these distances from the point of maximal inspiration, as shown in Figure 5-28. It is convenient to use the vertical line when you measure the FEV_1 to establish these points. Transfer these points onto the FVC tracing.

Draw a line intersecting these two points, and extend that line so that a 32-mm horizontal distance is covered, as shown in Figure 5-28. Measure the vertical distance *A* as shown in Figure 5-28. Multiply this distance by the bell factor. This is the $FEF_{200-1200}$ in milliliters per second.

Midexpiratory Forced Expired Flow

The $FEF_{25-75\%}$ is the flow rate over the middle portion of the FVC tracing. To calculate the $FEF_{25-75\%}$, you must first divide the FVC tracing into four parts.

To divide the tracing into four parts, measure a 128-mm horizontal distance from the beginning of the FVC tracing. Mark this horizontal line into four 32 mm-segments. Draw a horizontal line extending toward the beginning of the FVC curve even with the point of maximal expiration. Intersect this line with a vertical line from the 128-mm distance previously measured. Extend two more vertical lines extending from the 32-mm mark (25%) and the 96-mm point (75%) that intersect the FVC tracing. When you have completed this, the divisions should appear as they are in Figure 5-29. The tracing should now be divided into four equal parts.

You may also find the 25% and 75% points on the FVC tracing using the following method. Multiply the distance of the FVC in millimeters by 0.25 and 0.75.

$$25\% \text{ of FVC} = \text{FVC (mm distance)} \times 0.25$$
$$75\% \text{ of FVC} = \text{FVC (mm distance)} \times 0.75$$

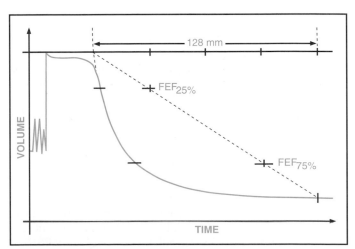

Figure 5-29   *Dividing the FVC tracing into four equal parts*

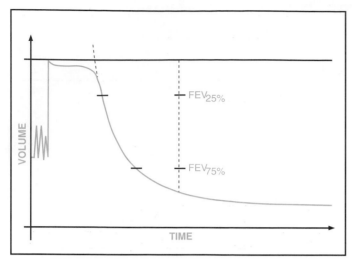

Figure 5-30 *Measuring the 25% and 75% points on the FVC tracing*

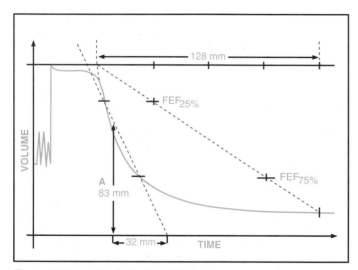

Figure 5-31 *Calculating the FEF$_{25-75\%}$*

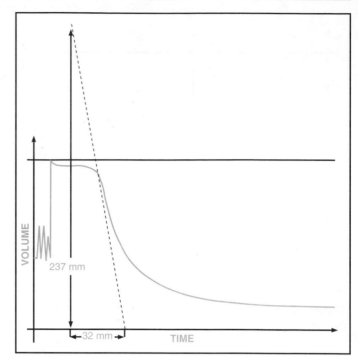

Figure 5-32 *Calculating the peak expiratory flow rate*

Once these distances have been calculated, subtract them from the beginning of the FVC tracing along a vertical line (the FEV$_1$ is convenient) and mark the corresponding points on the FVC tracing, as shown in Figure 5-30.

Once you have established the FEF$_{25\%}$ and FEF$_{75\%}$ points, draw an intersecting line through them and extend the line so that a 32-mm horizontal distance is covered. Measure the vertical distance *A* as shown in Figure 5-30. Multiply this distance by the bell factor. This is the FEF$_{25-75\%}$ in milliliters per second. Your results should correspond to what is shown in Figure 5-31.

Peak Expiratory Flow Rate

The PEFR may be calculated by identifying the steepest portion of the FVC tracing and drawing a line tangent to the tracing. Extend this line over a 32-mm horizontal distance. Measure the vertical distance in millimeters. Multiply this distance by the bell factor. This is the PEFR in milliliters per second. Your results should correspond to what is shown in Figure 5-32.

MAXIMUM VOLUNTARY VENTILATION

The MVV is the maximum amount of air that a patient can breathe in an interval of 1 minute. The test is measured over a 10-, 12-, or 15-second interval, and the measurement is extrapolated to 1 minute.

Measurement Using an Accumulator Pen (Ventilometer)

When using the accumulator pen feature, you will have two tracings for the MVV. One tracing records each breath and is sawtooth in configuration. The other tracing is a sloped line resembling a stair step pattern.

To calculate the minute volume, the stair step sloping line is used. Draw a line through the sloping line and extend this line for a distance of 32 mm. Measure the vertical rise (slope) of this line in millimeters, represented by *A* in Figure 5-33. To calculate the MVV volume, complete the following steps:

1. Measure the slope of the MVV tracing over a 32-mm distance.
2. Multiply the slope of the line by the bell factor to obtain the MVV volume.
3. Multiply the MVV volume by 25 (gear ratio of the ventilometer).
4. If the kymograph speed is 160 mm/min, multiply the foregoing result by 5 (32-mm distance = 12 sec) to determine the minute volume.

Calculating the MVV Manually

To calculate the MVV manually, mark off a 32-mm length along the sawtooth tracing. Each volume recorded on the

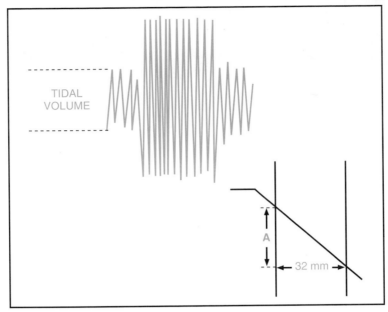

Figure 5-33 *Calculating the MVV volume from the accumulator pen tracing*

sawtooth tracing must be individually measured. Add all of the measurements together. Multiply that measurement by the bell factor. Multiply this volume by 5 (12 sec = 32 mm at a kymograph speed of 160 mm/min). This is the minute volume.

Calculating the Respiratory Rate

Using the sawtooth-shaped tracing, count the number of breaths over a 32-mm horizontal interval. Multiply this number by 5 (32-mm horizontal distance = 12 sec at a kymograph speed of 480 mm/min).

CONVERSION FROM ATPS TO BTPS

All of the measurements that were made in the pulmonary function study were recorded at ambient temperature and pressure, saturated (ATPS). These values need to be converted to reflect body temperature and pressure, saturated (BTPS) conditions to be reported accurately. To convert your values, use the following formula:

$$\text{Volume (BTPS)} = \text{volume (ATPS)} \times \frac{P_B - P_{H_2O}}{P_B - 47} \times \frac{310}{273 + T}$$

where

P_B = barometric pressure
P_{H_2O} = partial pressure of H_2O at ATPS
273 = absolute temperature conversion factor
310 = absolute body temperature
47 = partial pressure of H_2O at BTPS

The partial pressure of H_2O at ATPS may be found by consulting tables in other references (White, 1999). After completing this formula, you will have a factor enabling you to convert ATPS volume to BTPS volume by multiplying by this factor: BTPS volume = ATPS volume × factor.

CALCULATING PREDICTED VALUES

Predicted values can be determined by using nomograms. These nomograms are available in many textbooks.

A complete set of nomograms is available through the Intermountain Thoracic Society (Salt Lake City, Utah). Figure 5-34 presents two of the more common nomograms used in calculating pulmonary function tests. To use the nomograms to calculate a patient's normal values, you need to know the patient's age and height. Lay a straight-edge between the patient's height as read on the height scale and the patient's age as it appears on the age scale.

Once the normal values for your patient are known, all measured BTPS volumes should be divided by the predicted values to obtain a value reported as a percentage of predicted values.

Measured BTPS	Predicted BTPS	% Predicted
VC = 3.4 liters	VC = 4.2 liters	80.9%

INTERPRETATION OF THE RESULTS

Once the pulmonary function parameters have been measured and calculated, interpretation of the results is the last step. As a respiratory care practitioner, you must be able to recognize the significance of study findings. However, the physician is the person who reports the final results of any pulmonary function study.

Using Tables 5-1 and 5-2, determine the interpretation of the pulmonary function study results.

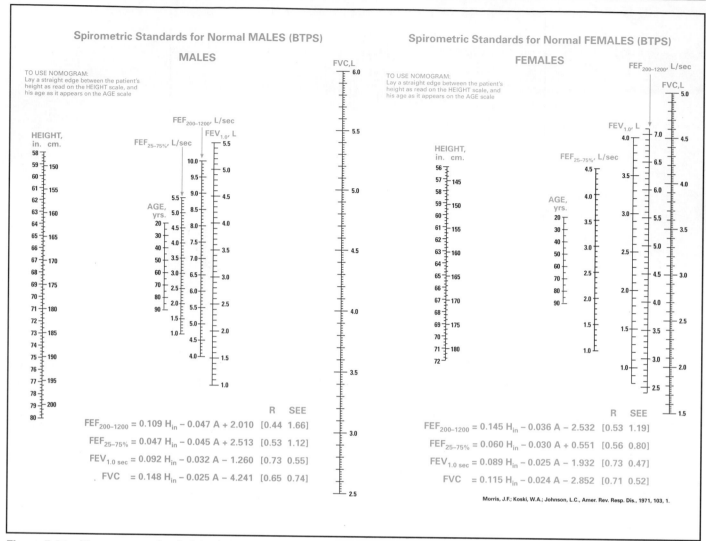

Figure 5-34 *Nomograms used to find the predicted values for male and female patients (Courtesy of* American Review of Respiratory Disease*)*

The equations shown in the nomograms:

Males:
$$FEF_{200-1200} = 0.109\ H_{in} - 0.047\ A + 2.010 \quad [0.44\ 1.66]$$
$$FEF_{25-75\%} = 0.047\ H_{in} - 0.045\ A + 2.513 \quad [0.53\ 1.12]$$
$$FEV_{1.0\ sec} = 0.092\ H_{in} - 0.032\ A - 1.260 \quad [0.73\ 0.55]$$
$$FVC = 0.148\ H_{in} - 0.025\ A - 4.241 \quad [0.65\ 0.74]$$

Females:
$$FEF_{200-1200} = 0.145\ H_{in} - 0.036\ A - 2.532 \quad [0.53\ 1.19]$$
$$FEF_{25-75\%} = 0.060\ H_{in} - 0.030\ A + 0.551 \quad [0.56\ 0.80]$$
$$FEV_{1.0\ sec} = 0.089\ H_{in} - 0.025\ A - 1.932 \quad [0.73\ 0.47]$$
$$FVC = 0.115\ H_{in} - 0.024\ A - 2.852 \quad [0.71\ 0.52]$$

Morris, J.F.; Koski, W.A.; Johnson, L.C., Amer. Rev. Resp. Dis., 1971, 103, 1.

TABLE 5-1: Restriction and Obstruction

TEST	RESTRICTION	OBSTRUCTION
Tidal volume	Decreased	Normal
IC	Decreased	Decreased
ERV	Decreased	Decreased
FVC	Decreased	Decreased
FEV_1	Normal	Decreased
$FEF_{25-75\%}$	Normal	Decreased
$FEF_{200-1200}$	Somewhat decreased	Decreased
MVV	Decreased	Decreased

TABLE 5-2: Severity of Abnormality

Normal	>80%
Mild	70–80%
Moderate	60–70%
Moderately severe	50–60%
Severe	34–50%
Very severe	<34%

References

American Association for Respiratory Care. (1996). AARC clinical practice guideline: Spirometry, 1996 update. *Respiratory Care, 41*(7), 629–636.

American Thoracic Society. (1995). Single-breath carbon monoxide diffusion capacity (transfer factor). *American Journal of Respiratory and Critical Care Medicine, 152,* 2185–2198.

Brown, R. A. (1997). Derivation, application, and utility of static lung volume measurements. *Respiratory Care Clinics of North America, 3*(2), 183–220.

Fitzgerald, D. J., Speir, W. A., & Callahan, L. A. (1996). Office evaluation of pulmonary function: Beyond the numbers. *American Family Physician, 54*(2), 525–534.

Pierson, D. J., & Kacmarek, R. (1992) *Foundations of respiratory care.* New York: Churchill Livingstone.

Scanlan, C., Spearman, C. B., & Sheldon, R. L. (1995). *Egan's fundamentals of respiratory care.* St. Louis, MO: Mosby.

White, G. C. (1999). *Equipment theory for respiratory care.* Clifton Park, NY: Delmar Learning.

Additional Resources

Burton, G. G., Hodgkin, J. E., & Ward, J. J. (1997). *Respiratory care: A guide to clinical practice* (4th ed.). Philadelphia: Lippincott.

Eubanks, D. H., & Bone, R. C. (1990). *Comprehensive respiratory care* (2nd ed.). St. Louis, MO: Mosby.

Fishman, A. P. (1980). *Assessment of pulmonary function.* New York: McGraw-Hill.

McPherson, S. P. (1995). *Respiratory therapy equipment* (5th ed.). St. Louis, MO: Mosby.

Nelson, E. J., Hunter, P. M., & Morton, E. (1983). *Critical care respiratory therapy: A laboratory and clinical manual.* Boston: Little, Brown.

Pontoppidan, H., et al. (1972). Acute respiratory failure in the adult. *New England Journal of Medicine, 287*(15), 743–752.

Ruppel, G. (1996). *Manual of Pulmonary Function Testing.* St. Louis, MO: Mosby.

Practice Activities: Pulmonary Function Testing: Bedside Monitoring and Basic Spirometry

BEDSIDE MONITORING

1. Assemble the equipment needed for monitoring bedside pulmonary function parameters:
   a. Respirometer
   b. Peak flowmeter
   c. Inspiratory force manometer
   d. Flow or self-inflating manual resuscitator
   e. Watch

2. Demonstrate the following for the listed respirometers:
   a. Assemble the spirometer.
      (1) For a spontaneously breathing patient
   b. Test the spirometer for proper operation.
      (1) Wright respirometer
      (2) Haloscale respirometer

3. Practice measuring a vital capacity on a laboratory partner, taking several determinations. Ask your laboratory instructor to confirm your measurements.
   a. Coach your laboratory partner during the procedure.
   b. Ensure flow rates are slow to avoid respirometer damage.

4. Using a laboratory partner, practice positioning for the measurement of bedside pulmonary function parameters.
   a. Place your laboratory partner in an upright position.
   b. Simulate clinical conditions that would require modification of this position.

5. Using a laboratory partner, measure all of the bedside pulmonary function parameters:
   a. Minute volume
   b. Frequency
   c. Tidal volume
   d. Vital capacity
   e. Maximal inspiratory pressure
   f. Peak expiratory flow rate
   Demonstrate the following while performing the procedure:
   (1) Instruct the patient in a clear, concise manner.
   (2) Accurately measure and record each measurement.
   (3) Use nose clips.
   (4) Allow sufficient rest periods between each measurement.

6. Following completion of your bedside pulmonary function assessment, document your findings on a blank sheet of paper. Have your instructor critique your charting.

BASIC SPIROMETRY

7. Prepare the Collins spirometer for use.

8. Turn on the kymograph to the various speeds to become accustomed to the different speeds.

9. Practice breathing through the spirometer.
   a. Note the direction of the pen motion
      (1) During inspiration
      (2) During expiration
   b. Breathe normally.
   c. Take an extra deep breath.
   d. Observe what effect different kymograph speeds have on the tracing.

10. Using a laboratory partner, practice giving instructions for the following maneuvers:
    a. Slow vital capacity
    b. Forced vital capacity
    c. Maximum voluntary ventilation

11. Using a laboratory partner, perform pulmonary function testing, including the following:
    a. Slow vital capacity
    b. FVC
    c. MVV

12. Calculate the following from the pulmonary function tracing you recorded.
    a. Slow vital capacity
       (1) IRV
       (2) Tidal volume
       (1) ERV
    b. FVC
       (1) FVC
       (2) FEV_1
       (3) $FEF_{200-1200}$
       (4) $FEF_{25-75\%}$
       (5) PEF
    c. MVV
       (1) Minute volume
       (2) Respiratory rate

13. Using a laboratory partner, simulate the following conditions:
    a. Restrictive
       (1) Use a Scultetus bandage or abdominal binder to restrict motion of the chest.
    b. Obstructive
       (2) Partially occlude the mouthpiece.
    c. Calculate the results and compare them with the results in Practice Activity 6.

Check List: Pulmonary Function Testing: Bedside Monitoring and Basic Spirometry

BEDSIDE MONITORING

1. Assemble and test all of the equipment required:
   _____ a. Respirometer
   _____ b. Peak flowmeter
   _____ c. Maximal inspiratory force manometer
   _____ d. Watch
2. Position the patient for the procedure.
3. Measure all bedside pulmonary function parameters:
   _____ a. Minute volume
   _____ b. Frequency
   _____ c. Tidal volume
   _____ d. Vital capacity
   _____ e. Maximal inspiratory force
   _____ f. Peak expiratory flow rate
4. Demonstrate the following while measuring the parameters:
   _____ a. Instruct the patient clearly and concisely.
   _____ b. Use nose clips.
   _____ c. Accurately record each measurement.
   _____ d. Allow sufficient rest periods between measurements.

_____ 5. Reposition the patient, and return to previous O_2 therapy.

_____ 6. Record the results on the patient's chart.

BASIC SPIROMETRY

_____ 1. Prepare the spirometer for use.

_____ 2. Record ambient conditions.

_____ 3. Explain the procedure to the patient.

4. Perform the testing:
   _____ a. Slow vital capacity
   _____ b. FVC
   _____ c. MVV

_____ 5. If you suspect the patient is malingering, repeat the tests. Be very firm and insistent on optimal results.

_____ 6. Thank the patient for his or her time and cooperation.

_____ 7. Calculate the results of the pulmonary function study.

_____ 8. Interpret the results.

Self-Evaluation Post Test: Pulmonary Function Testing: Bedside Monitoring and Basic Spirometry

1. Normal tidal volume may be estimated at:
   a. 2 to 3 ml/kg of body weight.
   b. 3 to 5 ml/kg of normal body weight.
   c. 3 to 7 ml/kg of normal body weight.
   d. 5 to 7 ml/kg of normal body weight.

2. Which of the following respirometers operate using a rotating vane?
   a. Collins spirometer
   b. Wright peak flowmeter
   c. Wright respirometer
   d. Boehringer inspiratory force manometer

3. It would be appropriate to use the Wright respirometer to measure which of the following parameters?
   I.   Tidal volume
   II. Vital capacity
   III. Forced vital capacity
   IV. Peak expiratory flow rate
   V.   Minute volume
   a. I, II, III
   b. I, III, IV
   c. I, II, IV
   d. I, II, V

4. Which one of the following maximal inspiratory forces indicates a reduced ventilatory reserve or possible muscle weakness?
   a. −60 cm H_2O
   b. −50 psi
   c. −30 cm H_2O
   d. −20 cm H_2O

5. Which of the following is used to assess the effectiveness of a bronchodilator?
   a. Maximal inspiratory pressure
   b. Vital capacity
   c. Tidal volume
   d. Peak expiratory flow

6. The volumes measured during a PFT are measured at:
   a. BTPS.
   b. ATPS.
   c. BTPD.
   d. STPD.

7. The vital capacity includes:
   I.   tidal volume.
   II. inspiratory reserve volume.
   III. expiratory reserve volume.
   IV. residual volume.
   a. I, II
   b. II, III
   c. I, II, III
   d. I, II, IV

8. Which of the following are derived from an FVC tracing?
   I.   Tidal volume
   II. Forced vital capacity
   III. FEV_1
   IV. $FEF_{200-1200}$
   V. $FEF_{25-75\%}$
   VI. MVV
   a. I, II, III, V
   b. I, III, IV, V
   c. II, III, IV, VI
   d. II, III, IV, V

9. A subject's MVV tracing shows 15 breaths for a 32-mm horizontal distance; the patient's actual rate in breaths per minute is (assuming a kymograph speed of 160 mm/min):
   a. 15 breaths/min.
   b. 30 breaths/min.
   c. 50 breaths/min.
   d. 75 breaths/min.

10. A subject performs an MVV maneuver for 12 seconds; the total volume expired in this interval is 32 liters. What is the MVV volume in liters per minute?
    a. 32 liters/min
    b. 64 liters/min
    c. 160 liters/min
    d. 128 liters/min

PERFORMANCE EVALUATION:
BEDSIDE PULMONARY FUNCTION TESTING

Date: Lab _____ Clinical _____ Agency _____

Lab: Pass _____ Fail _____   Clinical: Pass _____ Fail _____

Student name _____ Instructor name _____

No. of times observed in clinical _____

No. of times practiced in clinical _____

PASSING CRITERIA: Obtain 90% or better on the procedure. Tasks indicated by * must receive at least 1 point, or the evaluation is terminated. Procedure must be performed within designated time, or the performance receives a failing grade.

SCORING: 2 points — Task performed satisfactorily without prompting.
1 point — Task performed satisfactorily with self-initiated correction.
0 points — Task performed incorrectly or with prompting required.
NA — Task not applicable to the patient care situation.

TASKS:	PEER	LAB	CLINICAL
* 1. Verifies the physician's order	☐	☐	☐
2. Gathers the equipment			
* a. Respirometer	☐	☐	☐
* b. Maximal inspiratory force manometer	☐	☐	☐
* c. Peak flowmeter	☐	☐	☐
* d. Watch	☐	☐	☐
3. Assembles and tests the equipment	☐	☐	☐
* 4. Explains the procedure	☐	☐	☐
* 5. Washes hands	☐	☐	☐
* 6. Positions the patient	☐	☐	☐
* 7. Measures minute volume and frequency	☐	☐	☐
* 8. Calculates the tidal volume	☐	☐	☐
* 9. Measures the vital capacity	☐	☐	☐
* 10. Measures the maximal inspiratory pressure	☐	☐	☐
* 11. Measures the peak expiratory flow	☐	☐	☐
* 12. Allows the patient to rest as required	☐	☐	☐
* 13. Practices aseptic techniques	☐	☐	☐
* 14. Records all measurements on the patient's chart	☐	☐	☐

PERFORMANCE EVALUATION:
BASIC SPIROMETRY

Date: Lab _____ Clinical _____ Agency _____

Lab: Pass _____ Fail _____   Clinical: Pass _____ Fail _____

Student name _____   Instructor name _____

No. of times observed in clinical _____

No. of times practiced in clinical _____

PASSING CRITERIA: Obtain 90% or better on the procedure. Tasks indicated by * must receive at least 1 point, or the evaluation is terminated. Procedure must be performed within designated time, or the performance receives a failing grade.

SCORING:
2 points — Task performed satisfactorily without prompting.
1 point — Task performed satisfactorily with self-initiated correction.
0 points — Task performed incorrectly or with prompting required.
NA — Task not applicable to the patient care situation.

TASKS:		PEER	LAB	CLINICAL
*	1. Verifies the order	☐	☐	☐
	2. Scans the chart for pertinent information	☐	☐	☐
	3. Gathers the appropriate equipment	☐	☐	☐
*	4. Observes standard precautions, including washing hands	☐	☐	☐
*	5. Prepares the spirometer for use	☐	☐	☐
*	6. Introduces self and explains the procedure to the patient	☐	☐	☐
	7. Performs the following tests:			
*	a. Slow vital capacity	☐	☐	☐
*	b. FVC	☐	☐	☐
*	c. MVV	☐	☐	☐
*	8. Coaches the patient for optimal performance	☐	☐	☐
*	9. Repeats the test if the patient is malingering	☐	☐	☐
	10. Thanks the patient for cooperating	☐	☐	☐
	11. Correctly calculates:			
*	a. IRV	☐	☐	☐
*	b. Tidal volume	☐	☐	☐
*	c. ERV	☐	☐	☐
*	d. FVC and FEV_1	☐	☐	☐
*	e. $FEF_{200-1200}$ and $FEF_{25-75\%}$	☐	☐	☐
*	f. PEFR	☐	☐	☐
*	g. MVV	☐	☐	☐
*	12. Converts values to reflect BTPS conditions and reports the results as percent of the predicted result	☐	☐	☐
*	13. Interprets the results	☐	☐	☐
*	14. Reports the results to the appropriate personnel	☐	☐	☐

SCORE: Peer   _____ points of possible 44; _____%

          Lab   _____ points of possible 44; _____%

          Clinical   _____ points of possible 44; _____%

TIME: _____ out of possible 60 minutes

STUDENT SIGNATURES

PEER: _____

STUDENT: _____

INSTRUCTOR SIGNATURES

LAB: _____

CLINICAL: _____

CHAPTER 6
ELECTROCARDIOGRAPHY

INTRODUCTION

The electrocardiogram (ECG) is one of the most important diagnostic tools used in medicine. The information obtained noninvasively from the ECG tells the diagnostician about the electrical activity of the heart. From this information appropriate treatment can be prescribed to correct some of the abnormalities diagnosed using the ECG.

Because respiratory care involves the diagnosis and treatment of cardiopulmonary disorders, many respiratory care departments routinely perform electrocardiography as a part of their daily responsibilities. It is important that you, as a respiratory care practitioner, understand what an ECG is, how to recognize normal and abnormal ECG rhythms, and how to perform an ECG using an electrocardiograph machine.

In this chapter you will learn about how these ECG signals originate, and what normal and abnormal ECG tracings look like. You will also learn to recognize artifact (abnormal signal generated from sources other than the heart) and how to operate an electrocardiograph to obtain an ECG tracing.

KEY TERMS

- Atrial fibrillation
- Atrioventricular node
- Bundle of His
- Depolarization
- P wave
- Premature ventricular complexes

- Purkinje fibers
- QRS complex
- Repolarization
- Right and left bundle branches
- Sinoatrial node
- T wave

- Ventricular asystole
- Ventricular fibrillation
- Ventricular tachycardia
- Wandering baseline

OBJECTIVES

At the end of this chapter, you should be able to:

- Understand the origin of the electrical signals recorded on an ECG:
  — Describe how electrical signals are generated.
  — Describe the conduction system of the heart.
- Correlate the features of a normal ECG with the electrical activity of the heart.
- Understand why 12 leads (electrodes) are used for performing an ECG and describe the following:
  — The concept of views of the heart
  — Einthoven's triangle
  — Augmented limb leads
  — Precordial leads
- Demonstrate how to recognize the following dangerous and life-threatening arrhythmias:

  — Sinus bradycardia
  — Atrial fibrillation
  — Premature ventricular complexes
  — Ventricular tachycardia
  — Ventricular fibrillation
  — Ventricular asystole
- Demonstrate how to recognize the following artifacts on an ECG tracing:
  — Motion artifact
  — Wandering baseline
  — 60 Hz artifact
- Understand how an electrocardiograph operates and how an ECG tracing is obtained, including:
  — How the electrocardiograph makes the tracing
  — How time and voltage are read from an ECG

ELECTRICAL PHYSIOLOGY OF THE HEART

Production of Electrical Current in the Heart

The heart is a four-chambered muscle that functions as a pump to move blood through the circulatory system (Figure 6-1). This hollow muscle is composed of cardiac muscle cells. When the muscle cells are stimulated and contract, the cells undergo *depolarization* (exchanging potassium for sodium)—they become negatively charged on their outside surface (Figure 6-2). After contraction (depolarization), the muscle cells undergo *repolarization* (exchanging sodium for potassium)—they become positive on their outside surface. When this ion exchange occurs, an electrical potential (charge) of very small voltage is produced; this is conducted through the body to the surface of the skin. The resulting electrical signals (voltage changes) are what the electrocardiograph records, and the signals form an ECG tracing.

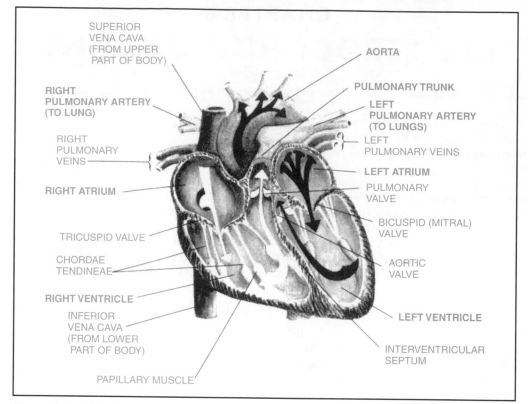

Figure 6-1 *A line drawing showing the chambers of the heart*

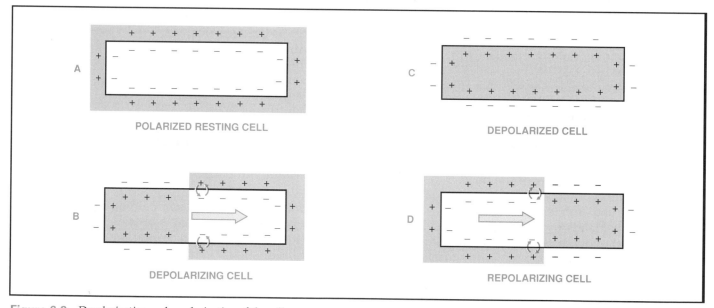

Figure 6-2 *Depolarization and repolarization of the cell*

A. *Polarized resting cell. The heart muscle is in the resting, or polarized, state; that is, the cell carries an electrical charge, with the inside negatively charged with sodium.*

B. *Depolarizing cell. When the muscle cell is stimulated, the cell begins to depolarize; that is, the positively charged ions flow into the cell, and the negatively charged ions flow out of the cell.*

C. *Depolarized cell. During the period that the cell is depolarized, all the positively charged ions are on the inside of the cell, and all the negatively charged ions are on the outside of the cell.*

D. *Repolarizing cell. After the muscle cell has depolarized, it begins to return to the resting state; that is, the negatively charged ions flow into the cell, and the positively charged ions flow out of the cell.*

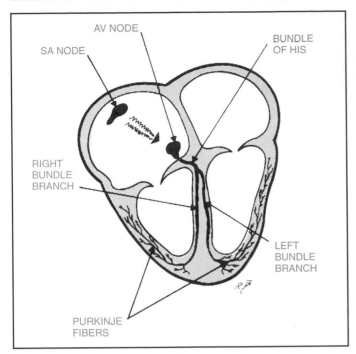

Figure 6-3   *The cardiac conduction system*

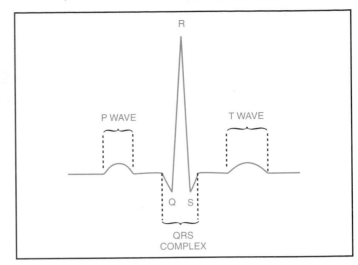

Figure 6-4   *A normal ECG tracing*

Cardiac Conduction System

The heart is really two parallel pumps—the atria and the ventricles. Therefore, an organized conduction system must exist for it to function properly. This conduction system consists of the *sinoatrial node* (SA node), *atrioventricular node* (AV node), *bundle of His*, *right and left bundle branches*, and the *Purkinje fibers* (Figure 6-3).

The SA node functions as the heart's pacemaker. It ensures that the heart will beat rhythmically without any external sources of stimulation. The cardiac conduction cycle begins at the SA node. The electrical impulse from the SA node causes the muscle cells in the atria to contract simultaneously as the impulse is conducted through the atria. When the electrical impulse from atria is conducted to the AV node, it transmits the electrical impulse to the bundle of His and the right and left bundle branches.

The right and left bundle branches conduct the electrical impulse to the apex (base) of the heart, where it is transmitted to the ventricles through the Purkinje fibers. As the impulse travels up the Purkinje fibers, the muscle cells of the ventricles contract simultaneously.

During the contraction of the ventricles, the muscle cells in the atria repolarize, bringing them to the polarized resting state. Following ventricular contraction, the ventricles repolarize, like the atria.

THE NORMAL ECG AND THE ELECTRICAL ACTIVITY OF THE HEART

Figure 6-4 represents a normal ECG tracing. The ECG tracing is divided into five waves: P, Q, R, S, T, and sometimes U. Each wave represents a portion of the heart's electrical activity.

The *P wave* is the voltage rise that occurs when the atria depolarize. As discussed earlier, depolarization results in transmission of an electrical signal to the surface of the skin.

The *QRS complex*—composed of the Q, R, and S waves—represents the depolarization of the ventricles. During ventricular depolarization, the atria repolarize. Owing to the larger number of muscle fibers in the ventricles than in the atria, the voltage generated is much larger than the voltage generated during depolarization of the atria. As a result, the repolarization of the atria is "lost" or not seen in the QRS complex. The *T wave* is a voltage that is generated as the ventricles repolarize.

The ECG tracing presents a two-dimensional view of the heart's electrical activity. You can almost think of it as an electrical "snapshot" of a cardiac cycle. The heart, however, is a three-dimensional object. To adequately describe the electrical activity of the heart, more than one view is needed.

THE TWELVE LEADS OF AN ECG

When an engineer designs a part for a ventilator, at least three views must be drawn to describe it fully (length, width, and depth). Like an engineering drawing, an ECG must contain more than one "view" to adequately describe the electrical activity of the heart. Twelve standard leads are used to obtain these views.

Einthoven's Triangle

Einthoven's triangle is named for an early pioneer of electrocardiography, Willem Einthoven. Einthoven connected positive and negative electrodes to the limbs of the body in three specific patterns—leads I through III—to generate standard ECG tracings (Stein, 1987). (More formally, "leads" are the wires connecting the patient to the electrocardiograph machine, but they also name the tracings obtained with each pattern of electrode placement.) For lead I, the left arm is positive and the right arm is negative. For lead II, the right arm is negative and the left leg is positive. For lead III, the left arm is negative and the left leg is positive (Figure 6-5). The electrical current measured

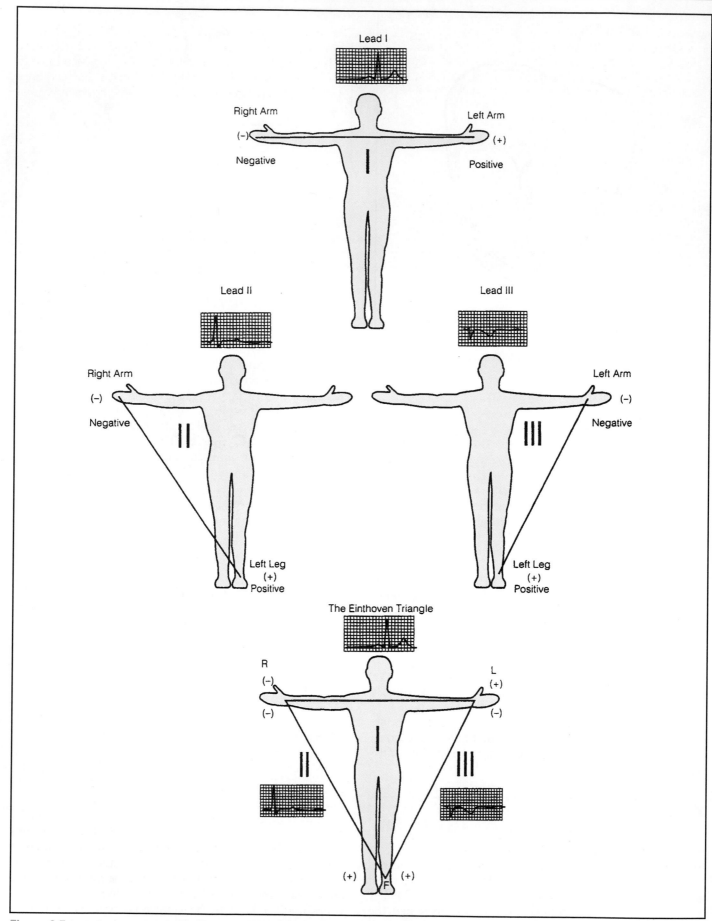

and recorded represents a vector, having a length (voltage) and a direction (orientation) (Figure 6-6). These vector orientations then represent a given view, or electrical "snapshot," of the heart. These three leads and the augmented leads are bipolar (containing both a positive and a negative electrode).

Augmented Leads

With augmented leads, the electrodes are positioned to make a single limb positive and all other limbs negative. They are termed *augmented leads* because the electrocardiograph machine must amplify or augment the weak signal more than is needed for the other leads to generate a useful tracing. Figure 6-7 shows electrode polarity for augmented leads and their associated ECG tracings. Like those for the leads in Einthoven's triangle, the tracings for augmented leads also represent vectors or views of the heart.

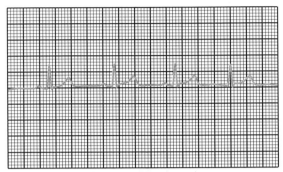

LEAD I

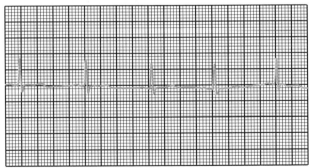

LEAD II

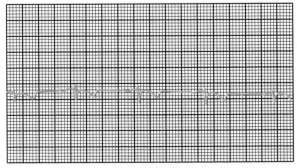

LEAD III

Figure 6-6 *The vector orientation of leads I, II, and III*

Precordial Leads

The *precordial leads* are unipolar. The tracings obtained with these leads represent horizontal views of the heart. Each tracing is recorded and then the electrode is moved to the next position (Figure 6-8). The precordial leads are helpful in the diagnosis of the location of a myocardial infarction.

DANGEROUS AND LIFE-THREATENING ARRHYTHMIAS

As a respiratory care practitioner performing ECGs, you will undoubtedly observe life-threatening conditions during the procedure. It is important for you to be able to recognize these conditions and to summon qualified help for that patient. In addition to the arrhythmias you may observe, it is also important to assess and monitor the patient during the procedure. The patient's signs, symptoms, and complaints are just as useful to a physician as the ECG tracing is during the abnormal event. Your ability to recognize these abnormalities as they occur may one day enable you to help save a patient's life.

Sinus Bradycardia

Sinus bradycardia is a normal sinus rhythm at a lower than normal heart rate (Figure 6-9). Bradycardia is defined as a heart rate of less than 60 beats per minute (Thaler, 1988; Davis, 1985). Notice that the rhythm is normal but the rate is low. Sinus bradycardia may indicate sinus node disease or increased parasympathetic tone or may be caused by drugs (digitalis).

Atrial Fibrillation

With *atrial fibrillation*, there is not an organized stimulation of the atria from the SA node. Multiple stimuli occur from many different sources. As a result, each stimulus only causes a small portion of the atria to contract. The result is an unorganized pattern with a very fast heart rate (400 to 700 beats per minute) observed on the ECG tracing (Figure 6-10). Because atrial depolarization does not occur, there is no P wave.

Because of the unorganized nature of the stimuli in atrial fibrillation, the atria never fully contract. This impedes the filling of the ventricles and reduces the cardiac output. Furthermore, because the electrical activity is disorganized, ventricular rate is also irregular.

Atrial fibrillation may be caused by underlying heart disease, hyperthyroidism, mitral valve disease, or even pulmonary emboli.

Premature Ventricular Complexes

Premature ventricular complexes (PVCs) occur when the ventricles are stimulated prematurely. This premature stimulation results in an unusually wide QRS complex (Figure 6-11). This widening occurs because one ventricle depolarizes before the other, out of sequence. PVCs are usually followed by a long pause before the next beat occurs.

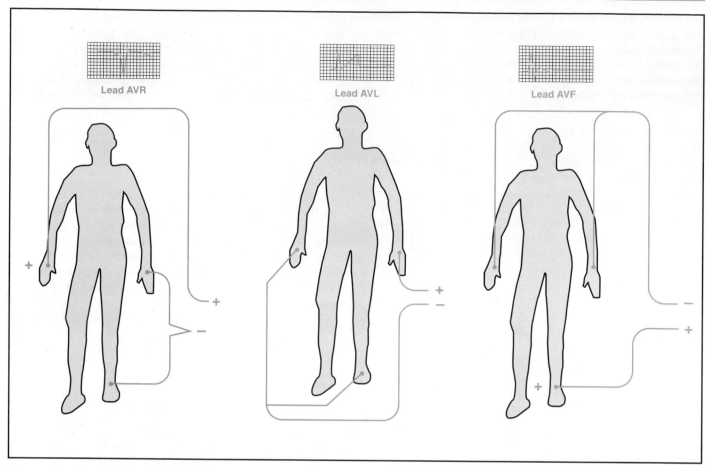

Figure 6-7 *The polarity of the augmented limb leads*

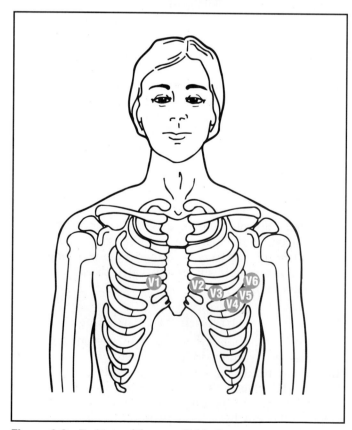

Figure 6-8 *Positions of the precordial leads*

PVCs occur randomly in normal persons; however, if they occur in runs (more than 3), or if they fall on a T wave, they are cause for concern. *Bigeminy* refers to the occurrence of PVCs every other beat (every second beat); *trigeminy* describes their occurrence every third beat (Figure 6-12).

Ventricular Tachycardia

With *ventricular tachycardia*, the ventricles are stimulated at a faster than normal rate (greater than 100 beats per minute). The ECG rhythm may be regular or irregular in appearance (Figure 6-13). Sometimes you may be able to observe P waves between the QRS complexes, and at other times you may not.

Ventricular tachycardia may represent a grave condition for the patient, especially if there is underlying heart disease. This condition should be promptly identified and appropriate treatment should be initiated.

Ventricular Fibrillation

Ventricular fibrillation, like atrial fibrillation, results from unorganized stimulation. The unorganized stimulation of the ventricles results in depolarization of only a small part of the ventricle with each stimulus. Ventricular fibrillation has a very irregular, disorganized pattern (Figure 6-14).

Ventricular fibrillation is a life-threatening condition. It requires immediate attention and treatment.

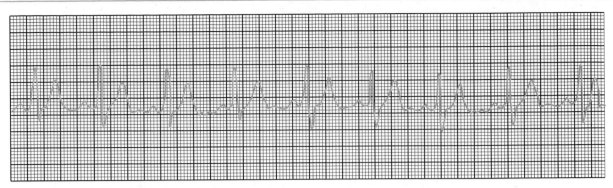

Figure 6-9   *An ECG showing sinus bradycardia*

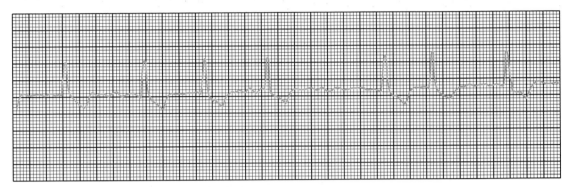

Figure 6-10   *An ECG showing atrial fibrillation*

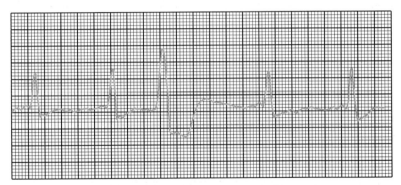

Figure 6-11   *An ECG showing a premature ventricular complex*

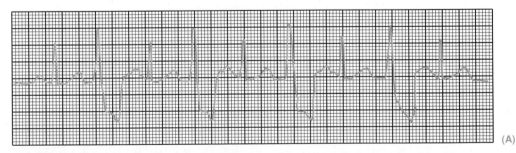

(A)

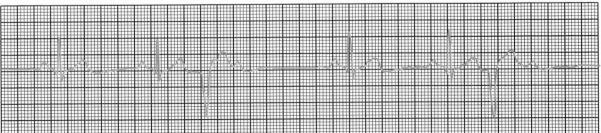

(B)

Figure 6-12   *An ECG showing bigeminy (A) and trigeminy (B)*

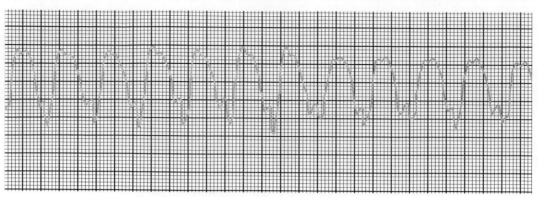

Figure 6-13   *An ECG showing ventricular tachycardia*

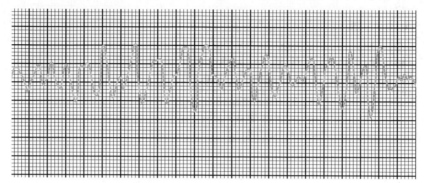

Figure 6-14   *An ECG showing ventricular fibrillation*

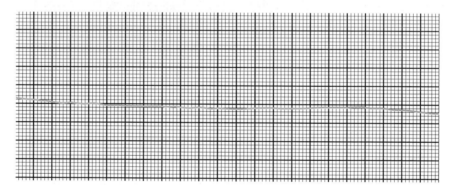

Figure 6-15   *An ECG showing ventricular asystole*

Ventricular Asystole

Ventricular asystole is the total absence of any cardiac electrical activity (Figure 6-15). It is sometimes termed *cardiac standstill*, observed as a "flat line" on the ECG tracing. Ventricular asystole is always life-threatening and requires immediate intervention.

ECG ARTIFACT

An ECG tracing represents the electrical activity of the heart. Because very small voltages (as low as 1 millivolt or less) are being amplified and recorded, artifact, or nonphysiologic (artificial) electrical current, may also be picked up. Such extraneous signal can ruin an otherwise good ECG tracing. Artifact may be patient-generated or may even be from a source external to the patient. The three most common types of artifact are patient motion artifact, wandering baseline, and 60 Hz artifact.

Patient Motion

Patient motion artifact occurs when the patient is restless or moves the limbs during the ECG. Sometimes patient motion cannot be avoided, especially if the patient is in severe distress or pain. Motion artifact usually causes an irregular appearance of the tracing. Sometimes an inexperienced respiratory care practitioner will confuse motion artifact with an atrial arrhythmia.

Wandering Baseline

A *wandering baseline* is caused by poor electrical contact between the patient and the electrodes placed on the patient to record the ECG. The baseline rises and falls as shown in Figure 6-16.

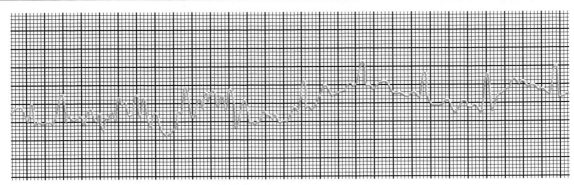

Figure 6-16 *An ECG showing a wandering baseline*

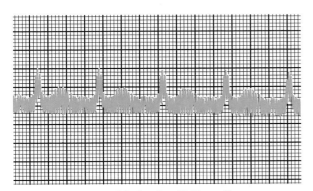

Figure 6-17 *An ECG showing 60 Hz artifact*

Electrical contact may be improved by cleaning the patient's skin with isopropyl alcohol, using more electrode cream, or cleaning the electrode contacts and connections.

60 Hz Artifact

Artifact may also occur from electrical interference external to the patient (Figure 6-17). The cause may be a faulty ground on the electrocardiograph or current leakage from adjacent equipment. This type of artifact is called 60 Hz artifact because in the United States and Canada, electricity is supplied as alternating current at 110 volts and 60 Hz.

ELECTROCARDIOGRAPH EQUIPMENT

The electrocardiograph is a very sensitive voltmeter that records the extremely small voltages generated by the heart's electrical activity. These signals are filtered and amplified and then recorded on a moving graph.

Length on the graph represents time. One small square is 0.04 second. One of the larger squares represents 0.20 second (5 small squares). If the time interval between squares is known, the heart rate may be calculated by measuring between R waves.

Height (vertical distance) on the graph paper is representative of voltage. A 1-millivolt standard is used to determine the voltages of each wave.

OBJECTIVES

At the end of this chapter, you should be able to:

- Collect and assemble the supplies necessary for an electrocardiogram.
- Demonstrate how to position the patient correctly for an electrocardiogram.
- Correctly identify anatomical landmarks and correctly place all ECG leads.
- Demonstrate how to operate the electrocardiograph machine correctly to obtain a 12-lead ECG.

- Describe how to recognize any life-threatening arrhythmias.
- Demonstrate how to recognize any artifact and correct it.
- Demonstrate what to do with the ECG tracing after it is obtained, ensuring that the appropriate personnel see the tracing.

EQUIPMENT REQUIRED FOR AN ELECTROCARDIOGRAM

Several pieces of equipment are required to perform an ECG. Many contemporary electrocardiograph machines are secured to a portable cart with wheels. Many of these carts have cupboards or pockets for storage of this equipment. Check the electrocardiograph machine's cart before searching for the following supplies.

You will need the electrical wires (leads) that will be attached to the cable providing the input to the electrocardiograph. Some machines have five wires (necessitating separate measurement of the precordial leads), whereas others have 12 wires and can record the precordial leads without moving an electrode.

You will also need suction cups and electrode jelly, or disposable adhesive electrode patches. The suction cups or patches provide the electrical contact between the patient's skin and the lead wires.

You may also need isopropyl alcohol and a clean towel or washcloth to clean the patient's skin before performing the ECG. If the patient has been brought into the emergency setting from the field and is obviously dirty, quickly clean the skin to prevent artifact before beginning the electrocardiogram.

Having a second clean towel or washcloth available is helpful for removal of any electrode jelly left by the suction cups or electrode patches after the ECG is completed.

PATIENT POSITIONING

The patient must always be placed supine for an electrocardiogram. Patient position can alter the contour of ECG tracings. The supine position is considered to be the standard ECG position.

LEAD PLACEMENT

Correct lead placement for an electrocardiogram is essential to obtain consistent results. An error of only a quarter of an inch may affect the ECG tracing (Eubanks, 1991).

The limb leads are placed on the right and left arms and on the right and left feet. The precordial leads are positioned at precise locations around the anterior chest.

The precordial leads are placed as shown in Figure 6-18. V_1 and V_2 are placed at the fourth intercostal space adjacent to the sternum. V_1 is to the right of the sternum and V_2 is at the left sternal border. Sometimes respiratory care practitioners have a difficult time identifying the

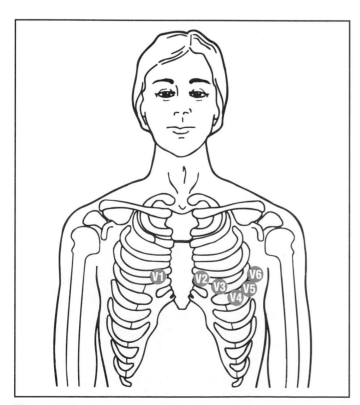

Figure 6-18 *Correct precordial lead placement*

fourth intercostal space. By palpating the manubrium sterni junction, or *sternal angle* (where the manubrium and body join), you can identify the second intercostal space. By palpating two ribs inferiorly from this point, you can identify the fourth intercostal space. V_4 is placed at the fifth intercostal space along the midclavicular line. V_3 is placed directly between V_2 and V_4. V_5 is placed at the anterior axillary line even with V_4. V_6 is placed at the midaxillary line, in line with V_4 and V_5.

ARRHYTHMIA RECOGNITION

As stated earlier, life-threatening arrhythmias may occur during an electrocardiogram. Your ability to recognize these events and obtain appropriate treatment may save a patient's life. Review the arrhythmias discussed in the theory portion of this chapter at this time. During your clinical rotation, spend some time in the coronary care unit in your assigned hospital. Ask the nursing staff to help you learn to recognize these arrhythmias on an ECG tracing. Many nurses are more than willing to run strips for you to practice with.

OPERATING THE ELECTROCARDIOGRAPH MACHINE

Many types of electrocardiographs are in use today. Some are manual, single-channel machines (requiring the operator to switch leads manually), whereas others are multichannel and automatic (recording all 12 leads automatically). Some instruments have arrhythmia recognition and interpretation built into their electronics by the manufacturers. Experienced cardiologists will agree with a machine interpretation greater than 90% of the time.

It is important for you to learn about the machine you will be using. It is not practical in this text to cover every available machine. Read the owner's manual on how to operate the machine you will be using. Observe a skilled respiratory care practitioner obtain an ECG on several patients. After observation, have the same practitioner observe you in the use of the equipment. Through practice you will become proficient.

ARTIFACT RECOGNITION

Like many other aspects of respiratory care practice, proficiency in artifact recognition requires time and exposure. Careful patient preparation (clean skin, good electrode contact, and sufficient electrode jelly) will eliminate wandering baselines. Patient motion is often difficult to control.

Your instructions to the patient to lie still and your emphasis on how important absence of motion is may help. As discussed earlier, pain, anxiety, and restlessness are difficult to control. Sometimes you must just do your best to obtain the best tracing.

In some cases, 60 Hz artifact may be eliminated by changing electrical outlets that power the electrocardiograph or by turning off unneeded electrical equipment near the patient. Fans, vacuums, or other motor-driven equipment may generate this type of artifact.

PROPER HANDLING OF AN ELECTROCARDIOGRAPHIC TRACING

Once an ECG tracing is obtained, it is usually interpreted by a physician or a cardiology specialist. In the emergency setting, the attending physician or emergency room physi-cian will want to see the ECG as soon as it is obtained. In other parts of the hospital, ECGs may be returned to the respiratory care department and placed into a file for inter-pretation or delivered to the cardiology department.

As always, it is important to record the patient's name and hospital number and the date and time of the ECG tracing. The newer machines have a computer keyboard for use in recording all pertinent information, which is automatically transferred onto the tracing.

References

Davis, D. (1985). *How to quickly and accurately master ECG interpretation.* Philadelphia: Lippincott.

Eubanks, D. H., & Bone, R. C. (1991). *Comprehensive respiratory care* (2nd ed.). St. Louis, MO: Mosby.

Stein, E. (1987). *Clinical electrocardiography: A self-study course.* Philadelphia: Lea & Febiger.

Thaler, M. S. (1988). *The only EKG book you'll ever need.* Philadelphia: Lippincott.

Practice Activities: Electrocardiography

1. Obtain a 12-lead ECG and identify tracings for the fol-lowing leads:
   a. Lead I
   b. Lead II
   c. Lead III
   d. AVR
   e. AVL
   f. AVF
   g. The six precordial leads

2. Using an arrhythmia generator, flash cards, or ECG tracings, practice arrhythmia recognition.

3. Using a laboratory partner, practice performing a 12-lead ECG.

4. With your laboratory partner, create motion artifact and a wandering baseline and then identify these com-mon artifacts.

Check List: Performing an ECG

_____ 1. Check the patient's chart for a physician's order.

_____ 2. Wash your hands. Help prevent nosocomial infections. Protect both your patient and yourself.

_____ 3. Obtain all of the appropriate equipment, as required, including:

_____ a. Electrocardiograph machine

_____ b. All leads (wires)

_____ c. Suction cups or disposable electrode pads

_____ d. Isopropyl alcohol

_____ e. Clean towels or washcloths

_____ 4. Assemble and check the equipment to ensure that it functions properly.

_____ 5. Identify the patient using the arm band.

_____ 6. Explain the procedure to the patient and emphasize the importance of being still during the procedure.

_____ 7. Place the patient in the supine position.

_____ 8. Correctly place all limb leads.

_____ 9. Identify the anatomical landmarks on the anterior chest and place the precordial leads correctly.

_____ 10. Correctly operate the electrocardiograph machine to obtain an ECG tracing.

_____ 11. Identify any life-threatening arrhythmias.

_____ 12. Recognize and, if possible, correct an artifact.

_____ 13. Clean up following the procedure by discard-ing any disposable items. Clean up the patient by wiping off any excess conductive jelly.

14. Ensure that the ECG tracing is labeled with the following information:

_____ a. Patient's name

_____ b. Patient's hospital number

_____ c. Date and time of the tracing

_____ 15. Ensure the patient's safety and comfort.

_____ 16. Wash your hands.

_____ 17. Ensure that the ECG tracing is given to the appropriate physician or is correctly filed for interpretation.

_____ 18. Document in the patient's chart the date and time of the tracing and the fact that it was performed.

Self-Evaluation Post Test: Electrocardiograms (ECGs)

1. Depolarization of the myocardium causes:
   I. ion transfer.
   II. exchange of potassium and sodium.
   III. a voltage to be produced.
   IV. the outside of the cell to become negatively charged.
   a. I
   b. I, II
   c. I, II, III
   d. I, III, IV
   e. I, II, III, IV

2. Atrial depolarization is represented on the ECG by:
   a. the P wave.
   b. the Q wave.
   c. the R wave.
   d. the S wave.
   e. the T wave.

3. Depolarization of the ventricles is represented on the ECG by:
   a. the P wave.
   b. the Q wave.
   c. the R wave.
   d. the QRS complex.
   e. the T wave.

4. Repolarization of the ventricles is represented by:
   a. the P wave.
   b. the Q wave.
   c. the R wave.
   d. the QRS complex.
   e. the T wave.

5. Which of the following are bipolar leads?
   I. Leads I, II, and III
   II. Leads AVR, AVL, and AVF
   III. The precordial leads
   a. I
   b. I, II
   c. I, III
   d. II
   e. II, III

6. Identify the following arrhythmia:

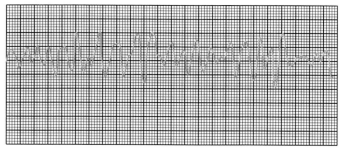

   a. Sinus bradycardia
   b. Atrial fibrillation
   c. Premature ventricular complexes (PVCs)
   d. Ventricular fibrillation
   e. Ventricular tachycardia

7. Identify the following arrhythmia:

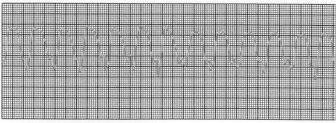

   a. Sinus bradycardia
   b. Atrial fibrillation
   c. Premature ventricular complexes (PVCs)
   d. Ventricular fibrillation
   e. Ventricular tachycardia

8. Identify the following arrhythmia:

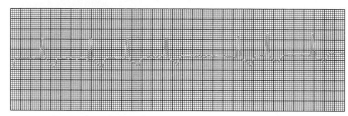

   a. Sinus bradycardia
   b. Atrial fibrillation
   c. Premature ventricular complexes (PVCs)
   d. Ventricular fibrillation
   e. Ventricular tachycardia

9. An anatomical landmark used to help identify the second intercostal space is:
   a. the xiphoid process.
   b. the manubrium.
   c. the sternal angle.
   d. the clavicle.
   e. the sternal body.

10. Common artifact on an ECG may include:
    I. motion artifact.
    II. wandering baseline.
    III. inductance interference.
    IV. 60 Hz artifact.
    a. I
    b. I, II
    c. I, II, IV
    d. II, III
    e. II, III, IV

PERFORMANCE EVALUATION: ELECTROCARDIOGRAMS (ECGs)

Date: Lab _____ Clinical _____ Agency _____

Lab: Pass _____ Fail _____   Clinical: Pass _____ Fail _____

Student name _____ Instructor name _____

No. of times observed in clinical _____

No. of times practiced in clinical _____

PASSING CRITERIA: Obtain 90% or better on the procedure. Tasks indicated by * must receive at least 1 point, or the evaluation is terminated. Procedure must be performed within designated time, or the performance receives a failing grade.

SCORING:
2 points — Task performed satisfactorily without prompting.
1 point — Task performed satisfactorily with self-initiated correction.
0 points — Task performed incorrectly or with prompting required.
NA — Task not applicable to the patient care situation.

TASKS:		PEER	LAB	CLINICAL
*	1. Verifies the physician's order	☐	☐	☐
*	2. Washes hands	☐	☐	☐
*	3. Obtains required equipment			
	a. Electrocardiograph	☐	☐	☐
	b. All leads	☐	☐	☐
	c. Suction cups or disposable pads	☐	☐	☐
	d. Isopropyl alcohol	☐	☐	☐
	e. Clean towels	☐	☐	☐
*	4. Assembles and checks all equipment for function	☐	☐	☐
	5. Identifies the patient	☐	☐	☐
	6. Explains the procedure to the patient	☐	☐	☐
*	7. Positions the patient	☐	☐	☐
*	8. Places leads correctly	☐	☐	☐
*	9. Correctly operates the electrocardiograph	☐	☐	☐
*	10. Identifies any life-threatening arrhythmias	☐	☐	☐
*	11. Recognizes and corrects artifact	☐	☐	☐
*	12. Cleans patient and cleans up the area afterward	☐	☐	☐
*	13. Ensures ECG tracing is filed or that appropriate physicians receive it	☐	☐	☐
*	14. Documents procedure in the patient's chart	☐	☐	☐

CHAPTER 7
PHLEBOTOMY
Kelly P. Jones

INTRODUCTION
INTRODUCTION

As hospitals restructure staff responsibilities to control costs, the role of respiratory care practitioners will expand to include tasks normally assigned to other staff specialists. One specialized task the respiratory therapist can perform proficiently is phlebotomy. *Phlebotomy* is the invasive puncturing of a vein for the purpose of collecting blood.

Phlebotomy is a routine task, one that can be easily learned with proper preparation and supervised practice. Respiratory care practitioners traditionally have been flexible, well-rounded clinicians who can quickly learn and absorb new skills and techniques.

This chapter presents a step-by-step procedure for drawing blood specimens. The procedure includes patient preparation, blood drawing, and follow-up actions. The chapter also discusses exposure control policies and your obligation to maintain a safe working environment.

KEY TERMS

- Butterfly needle
- Exposure control policy
- Phlebotomy
- Vacuum collection tubes

OBJECTIVES

At the end of this chapter, you should be able to:

- Identify obligations in collection of blood specimens from a patient:
  — Obligation to patient
  — Obligation to lab
  — Obligation to self
- Know how to maintain a safe environment:
  — Describe purpose of exposure control policy
  — Identify appropriate steps to take if blood exposure occurs
  — Identify steps to take if blood spill occurs
  — Identify proper waste disposal
- Demonstrate working knowledge of equipment used in venous blood collection:
  — Basic equipment

  — Needle types
  — Vacuum tubes
- Describe appropriate venipuncture technique:
  — Patient identification
  — Verification of test ordered
  — Patient preparation
  — Venipuncture site selection
  — Site decontamination
  — Needle placement
  — Blood collection
  — Removal of tourniquet
  — Needle removal and site pressure
  — Specimen labeling
  — Disposal of supplies
  — Hazards and complications
  — Delivery of samples to laboratory

OBLIGATIONS RELATED TO PERFORMANCE OF PHLEBOTOMY

As a respiratory care practitioner, you may be called upon to perform any number of tasks when a patient blood specimen is required. You may act as the support person who helps hold a combative patient in the emergency department or intensive care unit. You may be asked to transport blood samples to the laboratory. Once trained, however, you can be the person responsible for drawing blood specimens. No matter what your role, you have obligations to the patient, to the lab receiving the specimen, and to yourself.

Your first obligation is always to the patient. Make sure the patient understands the procedure to be performed. Check the blood drawing order and patient identification; make sure you are performing the proper procedure on the correct patient. Then, identify yourself to the patient and explain the procedure. Many patients are afraid of hospitals and do not like needles. Put the patient at ease; tell the patient what you are going to do. Perform the procedure quickly and safely. Protect the patient by using proper aseptic technique when preparing the skin for venipuncture. Finally, properly dress the site afterward.

The obligation to the lab is simple. Always use aseptic techniques to prevent contamination of the specimen.

Label each blood sample correctly with the patient's identification.

You are obligated to protect yourself from inadvertent exposure to blood specimens. You satisfy this obligation through knowledge, preparation, and procedure. You protect yourself by knowing what you are going to do, preparing for the procedure by assembling the correct materials, and performing the procedure step by step.

MAINTAINING A SAFE ENVIRONMENT

This last obligation is a small part of a larger objective—maintaining a safe environment. Every place in which you work will have an *exposure control policy*. This policy is the key to maintaining a safe environment.

Exposure control policy is put into place to protect health care providers as well as patients and support staff. The policy may differ slightly from workplace to workplace, so be sure to read and understand the policy instructions for each facility in which you work. Policy instructions describe what to do if you are exposed to body fluids or specimens. Exposure can come from a needle stick, a splash of secretions in the eye, or any other form of accidental exposure to patient body fluids. Along with knowing where to find this set of instructions, you should have absolute knowledge of all equipment available to treat exposure, such as eyewash stations, handwashing areas, the content of first aid kits, and the location of ointment and adhesive strips or tape.

Although exposure control policy may differ slightly from institution to institution, some general rules apply if exposure occurs. First, if an accidental needle stick occurs, notify your supervisor as soon as possible. While doing this, gently milk the area of the needle stick. You do not want to press the injured area hard enough to increase perfusion. Just gently press around the site until you get a droplet or two of blood. Next you should go to a handwashing area and perform a 2-minute scrub with antimicrobial soap. Once you have completed the scrub, apply an ointment such as polymixin-bacitracin to the area and cover the stick with an adhesive strip.

In the case of a needle stick, your supervisor will ask the patient to allow a blood draw to test for hepatitis and to screen for human immunodeficiency virus (HIV). If the patient agrees, these blood tests will be performed, and you will be notified if results are positive. If the patient denies the request for tests, then your blood will be drawn and tested immediately. Your blood will be tested again at 1, 3, 6, and 12 months after the accidental needle stick.

If a blood spill occurs, you must contain the spill by blocking off the area. Always report any blood spill or exposure to your supervisor. If the health care facility has a housekeeping or environmental service, contain the spill safely and notify the service. If the service is not available, begin by saturating the spill with an appropriate cleaning agent. Allow the saturated spill to sit for the time allotted in your exposure control policy instructions. Then clean up thoroughly with a mop or towels.

Contaminated material generated by cleaning the spill, such as towels, blankets, or mops, must be disposed of

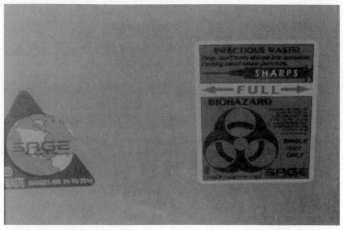

Figure 7-1 *A photograph showing a biohazard bag and the universal biohazard label*

using a red biohazard bag (Figure 7-1). Your exposure control policy instructions should tell you where the bags are stored. Put the contaminated material in the bag and tie it off. All other contaminated items that could cause injury should go into a sharps container (see Figure 7-13 later in the book).

EQUIPMENT

Blood is drawn for hundreds of different tests; some of the most common tests are emergency department panels, complete blood count (CBC), hematocrit determination (such as with Autoheme), and cardiac enzymes. If a blood test is ordered and it does not require an arterial sample or a specimen for a blood culture, then simple blood drawing equipment will suffice.

Once you have obtained an order for the blood test, gather the equipment necessary for the job. For any test, you should gather the following basic equipment (Figure 7-2):

- A set of gloves
- An alcohol and iodine swab
- Two 2 × 2-inch gauze pads
- Tourniquet
- Tape or adhesive strip

Figure 7-2 also shows one of the many types of needle and holder combinations available. The sterile packaging that contains the needle is opened, and the needle is attached to the holder. The needle size is indicated by a number on the packaging. The larger the number, the smaller the needle. For patient comfort, always use the smallest needle that will do the job.

Blood specimens are collected in "vacuum tubes" (Figure 7-3). Attach the tubes to the portion of the needle projecting through the holder after it is inserted in the patient's vein. The vacuum in the tube then draws the blood from the vein. Never attach the tube to the needle before inserting the needle in the vein; you will lose the vacuum and be unable to draw the blood. *Vacuum collection tubes* come in many different sizes and colors. Only a few are illustrated in Figure 7-3. You will need to learn the types and colors used by your medical facility. Each color indicates a different medium. You must use the correct vacuum tube, or the laboratory will not be able to perform the test on the physician's order.

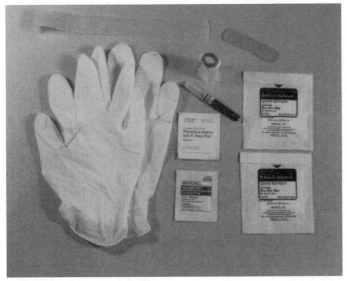

Figure 7-2 *Equipment required for phlebotomy, including gloves, alcohol and iodine swabs, 2 × 2-inch gauze pads, tourniquet, and tape or adhesive strips*

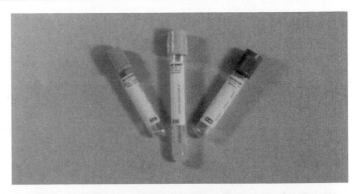

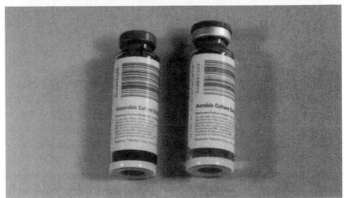

Figure 7-3 *Common vacuum tubes used to withdraw blood samples*

OBJECTIVES

At the end of this chapter, you should be able to:

- Identify roles and obligations of the phlebotomist.
- Describe how to maintain a safe environment, including institutional protocols for:
  — Exposure control policies
  — Blood exposure and spills
  — Waste disposal
- Demonstrate working knowledge of equipment used in blood drawing.
- Demonstrate how to verify properly both the test ordered and patient identification.

- Demonstrate how to prepare the patient while selecting a venipuncture site.
- Demonstrate a venipuncture, including:
  — Site decontamination
  — Needle placement
  — Blood collection
  — Specimen labeling
  — Waste disposal
- Describe possible complications and hazards of venipuncture.

VENIPUNCTURE TECHNIQUE

Once you have assembled all necessary equipment, perform the steps that follow to collect the specimen safely.

First, verify the blood drawing order and patient information. No matter where you work, always verify the written order to draw a blood specimen. Although there are exceptions for emergency treatment, and although some institutions allow telephone orders, an order to collect a specimen should normally be written in the patient's chart.

Once you have verified the order, identify the patient. The simplest and safest way to do this is to look at the patient's identification band, if available. Often patients who are confused or who cannot hear well will answer to any name. Therefore, do not address a patient by name to confirm the patient's identity. Ask the patient to state his or her name. Confirm the reply by checking the patient's identification band, if available. Compare the name with the blood drawing order. Never assume a patient's identity simply by location. Patients can be moved within the medical facility without your knowledge.

While verifying the patient's identification, look for the best venipuncture site. At the same time, assess how cooperative the patient will be, as well as the patient's fasting status and medications. If the patient seems uncooperative, get help before attempting venipuncture.

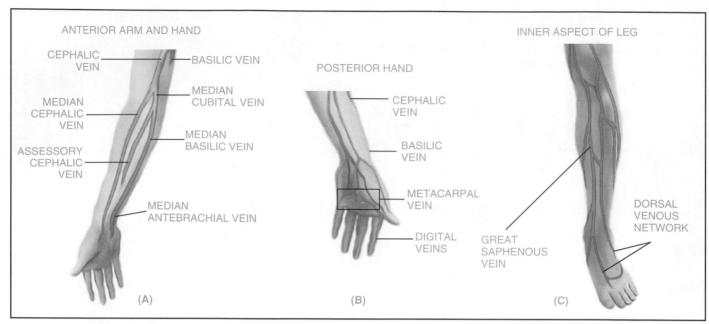

ANTERIOR ARM AND HAND

CEPHALIC VEIN — BASILIC VEIN

POSTERIOR HAND

MEDIAN CUBITAL VEIN

MEDIAN CEPHALIC VEIN — MEDIAN BASILIC VEIN

ASSESSORY CEPHALIC VEIN

MEDIAN ANTEBRACHIAL VEIN

(A)

INNER ASPECT OF LEG

CEPHALIC VEIN

BASILIC VEIN

METACARPAL VEIN

DIGITAL VEINS

GREAT SAPHENOUS VEIN

DORSAL VENOUS NETWORK

(B)

(C)

Figure 7-4 *Sites for phlebotomy on the arm (A), the hand (B), and the leg (C)*

The lab will need the patient's fasting status and medications for some tests. It is also helpful to know if the patient is taking blood-thinning medication. In patients receiving such medication, you will need to apply pressure at the venipuncture site, after removing the needle, for a longer time than is usual.

There are many veins suitable as venipuncture sites. Figure 7-4 illustrates some acceptable sites. Antecubital veins, which are found anterior to the elbow joint, are usually the largest veins and easiest to use. Often it is necessary to put the patient's extremity in a dependent position, as shown in Figure 7-5. Figure 7-5 also shows the patient's clenched fist. Holding the fist clenched will increase venous distention and make the vein easier to locate. If the patient does not have easily accessible veins, a tourniquet

can be applied 8 to 10 cm above the venipuncture site (Figure 7-6).

Once you have located a vein suitable for venipuncture, put on a pair of disposable gloves. Open the packaging on all supplies: 2 × 2-inch gauze pads, alcohol, iodine, and adhesive strip. Prepare the site by wiping the skin with alcohol, starting in the middle of the site and working outward in a circle (Figure 7-7). Never go over the same spot twice. This maintains a sterile field. Repeat this same procedure using iodine (Figure 7-8). After you have applied the alcohol and iodine to the site, wipe the area from superior to inferior with one of the 2 × 2-inch gauze pads.

Once you have finished, the site is sterile and ready for venipuncture. Warn your patient before you insert the

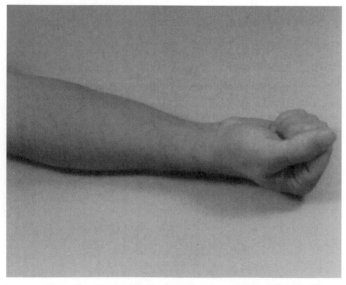

Figure 7-5 *A patient with the arm in a dependent position with a clenched fist*

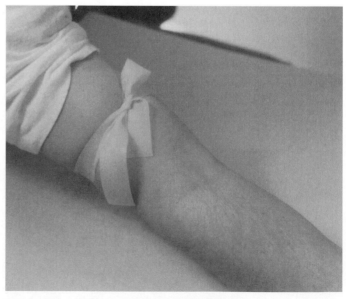

Figure 7-6 *A photograph showing the application of a tourniquet*

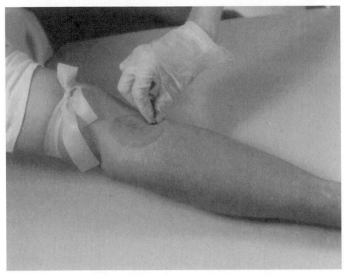

Figure 7-7   *Prepping the puncture site using an alcohol prep pad*

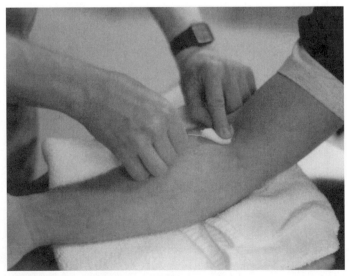

Figure 7-9   *The correct technique of puncturing the skin at a 25° to 30° angle*

needle. A reminder such as "You may feel a small stick" can prevent a reflex action that could cause pain. Take the needle and holder and position the point at a 25° to 30° angle (Figure 7-9). Place a vacuum tube loosely inside the holder but do not push it onto the needle yet. If you do, you will lose the negative pressure stored in the tube.

Insert the needle until you feel it is in the vein. Once you feel that the needle is in the vein, advance the vacuum tube onto the needle and look for blood to begin flowing into the tube. If no blood flows into the tube, advance the needle, slowly, further into the vein. If no blood flows into the tube after this second advance into the vein, remove the needle slowly. If the blood does not flow into the tube, you probably missed the vein. You need to remove the needle, obtain a new vacuum tube, and start over. It is also possible to insert the needle completely through the vein. This is characterized by a quick flash of blood into the tube; then the blood flow stops.

Besides missing the vein or advancing the needle completely through the vein, other problems can occur. The vein may collapse or the blood may clot before it can flow into the tube. If the tube begins to fill but stops halfway through, this may be an indication that the vacuum tube has caused the vein to collapse. If you remove the tube from the needle and release the tourniquet while leaving the needle in the vein, the blood flow may begin again in 30 to 40 seconds. You can then reconnect the tube and finish drawing blood. If blood does not enter the tube, you will need to start over. If the blood clots in the tube or needle, you can only start over.

Once tubes have been filled, release the tourniquet and pull the last tube off the needle and holder. Take your remaining 2 × 2-inch gauze pad and apply gentle pressure to the venipuncture site as you withdraw the needle (Figure 7-10). Apply pressure for 1 minute if the patient has no history of bleeding or is not taking blood-thinning

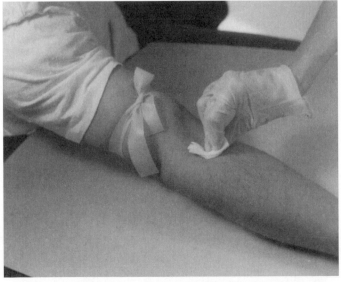

Figure 7-8   *Prepping the puncture site using an iodine prep pad*

Figure 7-10   *Application of pressure with a 2 × 2-inch gauze pad on withdrawal of the needle*

medication. If the patient has a history of bleeding or is taking blood-thinning medication, apply pressure for 2 to 5 minutes, or until bleeding stops (Figure 7-11). Once bleeding has stopped, cover the venipuncture site with an adhesive strip or tape (Figure 7-12). Dispose of the needle by placing it in a sharps container with the appropriate biohazard markings (Figure 7-13).

When using a *butterfly needle* for blood cultures or difficult blood draws, you will need the same equipment, minus the needle and holder. You will need a butterfly needle and syringes to draw the specimen (Figure 7-14).

Follow the same steps, starting with the alcohol swab followed by the povidone-iodine swab. Wipe the area dry with one sterile 2 × 2-inch gauze pad. Insert the butterfly needle at a 25° to 30° angle (Figure 7-15). Once the needle is in place and blood enters the line, place a piece of tape on the butterfly (Figure 7-16). Attach either a 5-ml or a 10-ml syringe to the line. Gently pull the syringe plunger back to draw blood into the syringe (see Figure 7-16). If blood is in the line but does not enter the syringe, reposition the butterfly. If no blood enters the syringe after

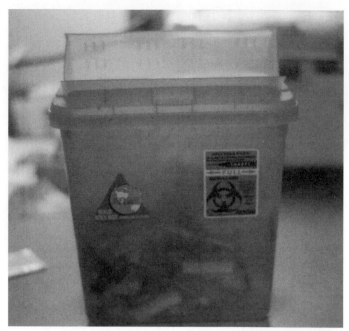

Figure 7-13 *A photograph of a sharps container for disposal of the needle used for venous access*

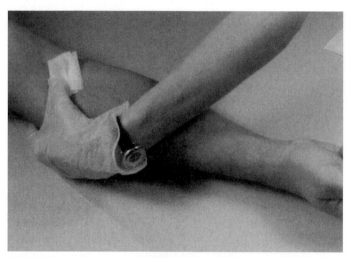

Figure 7-11 *Application of firm pressure using a 2 × 2-inch gauze pad following venous access*

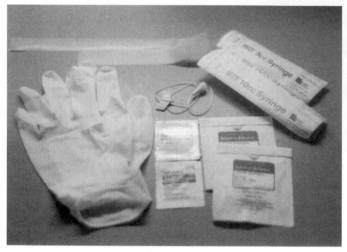

Figure 7-14 *A photograph of the equipment required for venipuncture using a butterfly needle: gloves, alcohol and iodine prep pads, 5-ml and 10-ml syringes, tourniquet, adhesive strip, and a butterfly needle*

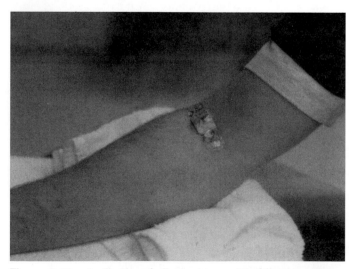

Figure 7-12 *Application of adhesive tape or strip following venous puncture*

moving the butterfly, change syringes and try again. If this fails, remove the butterfly and restart. When the syringe is full, remove it from the line and attach a sterile needle to the end of the syringe. Then break the seal on top of the blood culture bottles. Clean the top of the blood culture bottles to prevent contamination. Insert the needle on the syringe into the blood culture bottle (Figure 7-17). The vacuum in the bottles will automatically draw an exact amount of blood out of the syringe.

When you have completed drawing blood cultures, use gentle pressure to apply a 2 × 2-inch gauze pad at the venipuncture site while slowly removing the needle. Apply pressure to the site for 1 minute, or until bleeding has stopped. Place a piece of tape or an adhesive strip over the site.

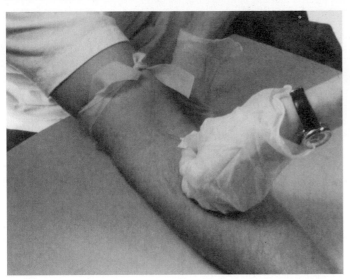

Figure 7-15   *Insertion of a butterfly needle at a shallow (25°–30°) angle*

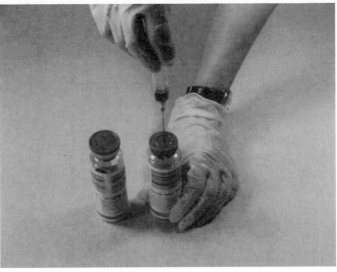

Figure 7-17   *A photograph showing injection of the blood sample into the vacuum (blood culture) bottle*

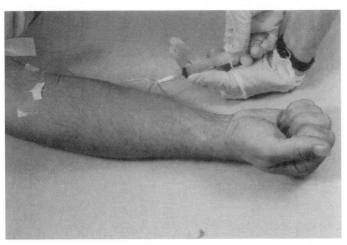

Figure 7-16   *A photograph showing the butterfly needle taped in position and a syringe being used to withdraw the blood from the vein*

There are several complications and hazards associated with venipuncture. Complications can range from slight bruising to large hematomas at the venipuncture site. The extent of bruising or bleeding can be aggravated by blood thinners. Always apply pressure at the site after needle removal. If you insert the needle too deeply or move it from side to side while under the skin, nerve damage is possible, though extremely rare. Carefully inserting the needle and completely removing the needle to reposition it will avoid nerve damage. Infection is a technique-dependent complication. Venipuncture invades the patient's body, breaking down the defense system by puncturing the skin. Good aseptic technique before venipuncture and proper cover over the site afterward will greatly reduce the probability of infection.

After you complete the blood draw, label the tubes. After you have completed all blood draws, transport them to the laboratory. Most institutions require the label to include the patient's identification number and name. The label may also include the patient's date of birth, the time and date the sample was drawn, the name of the person who drew the sample, and that person's initials. This is all that is usually required, but check your employer's policy requirements.

Transporting is accomplished through several ways. You may carry the blood to the lab yourself, or the lab may pick up the samples at some collection point. Some institutions use pneumatic tubes that run throughout the facility. Pneumatic tubes can sometimes be unreliable and samples may be lost. Keep this possibility in mind for code situations or difficult patients. Also, transport through these tubes is rough going, so for very fragile samples, like blood culture specimens, walk them to the lab yourself.

The skills needed for you to become proficient at venipuncture are not demanding. If you study the procedure outlined here and practice under supervision, you can add phlebotomy to your list of skills as a respiratory care practitioner.

Additional Resources

Black, J. M. (1997). *Medical surgical nursing* (5th ed.). Philadelphia: Saunders.

Dantzker, D. R., MacIntyre, N. R., & Bakow, E. D. (1995). *Comprehensive respiratory care.* Philadelphia: Saunders.

DeLaune, S. C., & Ladner, P. K. (2002). *Fundamentals of nursing: Standards & practice* (2nd ed.). Clifton Park, NY: Delmar Learning.

Delmar's nursing image library [Computer software]. (1999). Clifton Park, NY: Delmar Learning.

Holy family hospital policy and procedure manuals. (1995). Spokane, WA.

Practice Activities: Phlebotomy

1. Collect, identify, and describe the function of all materials needed for venipuncture:
   a. Gloves
   b. Alcohol and iodine swabs
   c. Two 2 × 2-inch gauze pads
   d. Tourniquet
   e. Tape or bandage
   f. Needle and vacuum tubes

2. Apply tourniquet 8 to 10 cm above the site and practice palpating for veins.

3. Practice removing tourniquet and applying gentle pressure to site.

4. Describe what information should be included on all labels of specimens.

Check List: Venipuncture

_____ 1. Review obligations to patient, lab, and self.
_____ 2. Review exposure control policy.
_____ 3. Identify steps to take if accidental needle stick occurs.
_____ 4. Identify and locate proper waste disposal.
5. Obtain all equipment necessary for venipuncture:
_____ a. Pair of gloves
_____ b. Alcohol and iodine swabs
_____ c. Two 2 × 2-inch gauze pads
_____ d. Tourniquet
_____ e. Tape or bandage
_____ f. Needle or butterfly
6. Verify physician orders:
_____ a. Refer to physician order sheet.
7. Verify patient identification:
_____ a. Check identification band.
_____ b. Ask patient's name.
8. Prepare patient:
_____ a. Assess patient attitude.
_____ b. Check fasting status/medications.
_____ c. Apply one pair of gloves.
9. Select venipuncture site and instruct patient:
_____ a. Place extremity in dependent position.
_____ b. Have patient clench fist and hold.
_____ c. Use tourniquet if needed.

10. Decontaminate site:
_____ a. Alcohol
_____ b. Povidone-iodine
_____ c. 2 × 2-inch gauze pad
11. Use correct needle placement:
_____ a. 25° to 30° angle
12. Draw the blood specimen, using the following as indicated:
_____ a. Vacuum tubes
_____ b. Blood culture bottles
_____ 13. Remove tourniquet.
_____ 14. Pull vacuum tube off needle and holder.
15. Remove needle and attend to puncture site:
_____ a. Apply pressure to site.
_____ b. Apply bandage or tape.
_____ 16. Properly dispose of materials.
17. Label specimen:
_____ a. Patient identification
_____ b. Time
_____ c. Date
_____ d. Your initials
_____ 18. Transport specimen.

Self-Evaluation Post Test: Phlebotomy

1. In which role might you find a respiratory therapist?
   a. Support staff
   b. Transport staff
   c. Staff responsible for actual blood draw
   d. All of the above

2. Why is the exposure control policy put into place?
   a. To protect patients and staff
   b. To maintain a safe environment
   c. To give employees something to read during slow times
   d. Both a and b

3. If an accidental needle stick occurs, what should you do?
   a. Squeeze your finger and hold it.
   b. Gently milk the area.
   c. Apply a tourniquet to your arm.

4. Which of these materials will _not_ be needed for a blood draw?
   a. Gloves
   b. Syringe and needle
   c. Alcohol and iodine
   d. Tourniquet and bandages
   e. Antibiotic ointment

5. It is acceptable _not_ to check the patient's identification band if the patient can state his or her name.
   a. True
   b. False

6. It is acceptable to move the needle side to side once under the skin.
   a. True
   b. False

7. What are some hazards and complications of venipuncture?
   a. Slight bruising
   b. Hematomas at the site
   c. Infection
   d. Nerve damage
   e. All of the above

8. At which angle do you insert the needle for blood draws?
   a. 10° to 20° angle
   b. 25° to 30° angle
   c. 45° to 50° angle
   d. 90° angle

9. If a patient has a bleeding history or is taking blood thinners, how long must pressure be applied to the venipuncture site?
   a. For 2 to 5 minutes
   b. For 1 minute
   c. For 30 seconds
   d. For 10 minutes

10. Gloves are not required if you believe that the patient does not have HIV infection.
    a. True
    b. False

PERFORMANCE EVALUATION: VENIPUNCTURE

Date: Lab _____ Clinical _____ Agency _____

Lab: Pass _____ Fail _____   Clinical: Pass _____ Fail _____

Student name _____   Instructor name _____

No. of times observed in clinical _____

No. of times practiced in clinical _____

PASSING CRITERIA: Obtain 90% or better on the procedure. Tasks indicated by * must receive at least 1 point, or the evaluation is terminated. Procedure must be performed within designated time, or the performance receives a failing grade.

SCORING:
2 points — Task performed satisfactorily without prompting.
1 point — Task performed satisfactorily with self-initiated correction.
0 points — Task performed incorrectly or with prompting required.
NA — Task not applicable to the patient care situation.

TASKS:		PEER	LAB	CLINICAL
*	1. Reviews obligation to patient, self, and lab	☐	☐	☐
*	2. Reviews exposure control policy	☐	☐	☐
*	3. Identifies steps to be taken if accidental needle stick occurs	☐	☐	☐
*	4. Identifies and locates proper waste disposal	☐	☐	☐
*	5. Obtains all necessary equipment:			
	a. Pair of gloves	☐	☐	☐
	b. Alcohol and iodine swabs	☐	☐	☐
	c. Two 2 × 2-inch gauze pads	☐	☐	☐
	d. Tape or bandage	☐	☐	☐
	e. Tourniquet	☐	☐	☐
	f. Needle or butterfly	☐	☐	☐
*	6. Verifies physician orders	☐	☐	☐
*	7. Verifies patient's identification band	☐	☐	☐
*	8. Prepares patient for venipuncture:			
	a. Assesses patient's cooperativeness	☐	☐	☐
	b. Explains procedure to patient	☐	☐	☐
	c. Checks patient's fasting status and medications	☐	☐	☐
*	9. Applies gloves	☐	☐	☐
*	10. Selects a venipuncture site:			
	a. Extremity in dependent position	☐	☐	☐
	b. Fist clenched and held	☐	☐	☐
	c. Applies tourniquet 8 to 10 cm above site	☐	☐	☐

* 11. Properly decontaminates site:

     a. Alcohol swab in circular motion   ☐ ☐ ☐

     b. Iodine swab in circular motion   ☐ ☐ ☐

     c. Swipes area with a 2 × 2-inch gauze pad one time   ☐ ☐ ☐

* 12. Places needle at 25° to 30° angle   ☐ ☐ ☐

* 13. Applies proper blood collection tubes   ☐ ☐ ☐

* 14. Removes collection tubes from needle   ☐ ☐ ☐

* 15. Removes tourniquet   ☐ ☐ ☐

* 16. Removes needle and applies pressure and bandage   ☐ ☐ ☐

* 17. Disposes of all sharps and biohazard material in proper waste disposal container   ☐ ☐ ☐

* 18. Properly labels blood samples:

     a. Patient identification number   ☐ ☐ ☐

     b. Date and time blood was drawn   ☐ ☐ ☐

     c. Initials of person who drew blood   ☐ ☐ ☐

  19. Transports blood tubes to lab via appropriate means   ☐ ☐ ☐

SCORE: Peer   _____ points of possible 64; _____%

           Lab   _____ points of possible 64; _____%

           Clinical   _____ points of possible 64; _____%

TIME: _____ out of possible 20 minutes

STUDENT SIGNATURES

PEER: _____

STUDENT: _____

INSTRUCTOR SIGNATURES

LAB: _____

CLINICAL: _____

CHAPTER 8
ARTERIAL BLOOD GAS SAMPLING

INTRODUCTION

Arterial blood gas (ABG) analysis is an extremely useful diagnostic test used for the clinical assessment of ventilation, acid-base status, and oxygenation. The collection of an arterial sample may be done quickly, and it provides important information for decision making in the management of the patient requiring oxygen or ventilatory assistance.

The collection of an arterial blood sample is commonly done by arterial puncture or, in the intensive care unit, by drawing a sample from an indwelling arterial catheter. In an infant weighing less than 30 pounds, arterialized blood may be obtained from a capillary stick, or in a newborn, from an umbilical artery catheter.

Arterial puncture is a skill that is easily learned. However, it is not without hazards and potential complications because it disrupts the integrity of a large high-pressure vessel of the arterial system. Possible complications of arterial puncture at any site are vessel trauma and occlusion, embolization, infection, and vessel spasm. If properly done by a skilled practitioner, arterial puncture provides safe, reliable information for patient management.

In this chapter you will learn the three common sites for arterial puncture, how to perform an arterial puncture, and the advantages and disadvantages of each site. You will also learn how to perform arterial line sampling and the hazards and complications of this procedure.

KEY TERMS

- Arterialization
- Arterial sampling
- Capillary blood gas sampling
- Flash
- Modified Allen's test

OBJECTIVES

At the end of this chapter, you should be able to:

- Identify the three common anatomical locations for arterial puncture:
  — Radial
  — Brachial
  — Femoral
  State the advantages and disadvantages of each site.
- Explain the complications associated with arterial puncture.
- Explain the rationale for the modified Allen's test for evaluation of collateral circulation.
- Discuss the use of a glass syringe versus a specialized plastic syringe for arterial sampling.
- Describe the six most common technical causes of blood gas sampling errors and their prevention:

  — Room air mixed with the sample
  — Delay in analyzing the sample
  — Drawing a venous sample by mistake
  — Heparin contamination
  — Patient anxiety causing hyperventilation
  — Plastic syringes
- State the appropriate anticoagulant to use when drawing an arterial sample for blood gas analysis.
- Explain the advantages, disadvantages, and hazards of drawing blood from an arterial line.
- Describe the rationale for capillary blood sampling in infants.
- Describe the three most common errors in capillary blood sampling:
  — Poor blood flow during sampling
  — Introduction of air into the capillary sample
  — Inadequate mixing of heparin in the sample

CLINICAL PRACTICE GUIDELINES

AARC Clinical Practice Guideline
Sampling for Arterial Blood Gas Analysis

ABGA 4.0 INDICATIONS:

4.1 The need to evaluate the adequacy of ventilatory ($PaCO_2$) acid-base (pH and $PaCO_2$), and oxygenation (PaO_2 and SaO_2) status, and the oxygen-carrying capacity of blood (PaO_2, HbO_2, Hb_{total}, and dyshemoglobins) (1,2,7,8)

4.2 The need to quantitate the patient's response to therapeutic intervention (1,2,5) and/or diagnostic evaluation (e.g., oxygen therapy, exercise testing) (2)

4.3 The need to monitor severity and progression of a documented disease process (1,2)

(Continued)

(CPG *Continued*)

ABGA 5.0 CONTRAINDICATIONS:

Contraindications are absolute unless specified otherwise.

5.1 Negative results of a modified Allen's test (collateral circulation test) are indicative of inadequate blood supply to the hand and suggest the need to select another extremity as the site for puncture.

5.2 Arterial puncture should not be performed through a lesion or through or distal to a surgical shunt (e.g., as in a dialysis patient). If there is evidence of infection or peripheral vascular disease involving the selected limb, an alternate site should be selected.

5.3 Agreement is lacking regarding the puncture sites associated with a lesser likelihood of complications; however, because of the need for monitoring the femoral puncture site for an extended period, femoral punctures should not be performed outside the hospital.

5.4 A coagulopathy or medium-to-high-dose anticoagulation therapy (e.g., heparin or Coumadin, streptokinase, and tissue plasminogen activator but not necessarily aspirin) may be a relative contraindication for arterial puncture.

ABGA 6.0 HAZARDS/COMPLICATIONS:

6.1 Hematoma (1,2,7,8)
6.2 Arteriospasm (1,7,8)
6.3 Air or clotted-blood emboli (1–3,7,8)
6.4 Anaphylaxis from local anesthetic (7,8)
6.5 Introduction of contagion at sampling site and consequent infection in patient; introduction of contagion to sampler by inadvertent needle "stick" (1–3,7,8)
6.6 Hemorrhage (2,3)
6.7 Trauma to the vessel (1,3)
6.8 Arterial occlusion (2)
6.9 Vasovagal response
6.10 Pain

ABGA 8.0 ASSESSMENT OF NEED:

The following findings may assist the clinician in deciding whether arterial blood sampling is indicated:

8.1 History and physical indicators (e.g., positive smoking history, recent onset of difficulty in breathing independent of activity level, trauma) (2)

8.2 Presence of other abnormal diagnostic tests or indices (e.g., abnormal pulse oximetry reading, chest x-ray) (2)

8.3 Initiation of, administration of, or change in therapeutic modalities (e.g., initiation, titration, or discontinuance of supplemental oxygen or initiation of, changes in, or discontinuance of mechanical ventilation) (1,2,4,5)

8.4 Projected surgical interventions for patients at risk (5,17)

8.5 Projected enrollment in a pulmonary rehabilitation program

ABGA 11.0 MONITORING:

The following should be monitored as part of arterial blood sampling:

11.1 FiO_2 (analyzed) or prescribed flow rate (1,2,7,8)

11.2 Proper application of patient device (e.g., mask or cannula) (1,2,7,8)

11.3 Mode of supported ventilation and relevant ventilator settings (7,8)

11.4 Pulsatile blood return (1,6,8)

11.5 Presence or absence of air bubbles or clots in syringe or sample (1,2,6–8)

11.6 Patient's respiratory rate (7,8)

11.7 Patient's temperature (7,8)

11.8 Position and/or level of activity (if other than resting)

11.9 Patient's clinical appearance

11.10 Ease of (or difficulty with) blood sampling (1,7,8)

11.11 Appearance of puncture site after direct pressure has been applied and before application of pressure dressing for potential hematoma formation (1,6–8) (a detailed protocol for postsampling management should be in place)

Reprinted with permission from *Respiratory Care* 1992; 37: 913–917. The complete AARC Clinical Practice Guidelines are available from the AARC Web site (http://www.aarc.org), from the AARC Executive Office, or from *Respiratory Care* journal.

AARC Clinical Practice Guideline
Capillary Blood Gas Sampling for Neonatal and Pediatric Patients

CBGS 4.0 INDICATIONS:

Capillary blood gas sampling is indicated when:

4.1 Arterial blood gas analysis is indicated but arterial access is not available.

4.2 Noninvasive monitor readings are abnormal: transcutaneous values, end-tidal CO_2, pulse oximetry.

4.3 Assessment of initiation, administration, or change in therapeutic modalities (i.e., mechanical ventilation) is indicated.

4.4 A change in patient status is detected by history or physical assessment.

4.5 Monitoring the severity and progression of a documented disease process is desirable.

CBGS 5.0 CONTRAINDICATIONS:

5.1 Capillary punctures should not be performed:

5.1.1 At or through the following sites (10):

5.1.1.1 Posterior curvature of the heel, as the device may puncture the bone (11)

5.1.1.2 The heel of a patient who has begun walking and has callus development (12)

5.1.1.3 The fingers of neonates (to avoid nerve damage) (13)

5.1.1.4 Previous puncture sites (14,15)

5.1.1.5 Inflamed, swollen, or edematous tissues (14,15)

5.1.1.6 Cyanotic or poorly perfused tissues (14,15)

5.1.1.7 Localized areas of infection (14,15)

5.1.1.8 Peripheral arteries

5.1.2 On patients less than 24 hours old, due to poor peripheral perfusion (1)

5.1.3 When there is need for direct analysis of oxygenation (1–3)

5.1.4 When there is need for direct analysis of arterial blood

5.2 Relative contraindications include:

5.2.1 Peripheral vasoconstriction (1)

5.2.2 Polycythemia (due to shorter clotting times) (1)

5.2.3 Hypotension may be a relative contraindication (1)

CBGS 6.0 HAZARDS/COMPLICATIONS:

6.1 Infection

6.1.1 Introduction of contagion at sampling site and consequent infection in patient, including calcaneus osteomyelitis (9,16) and cellulitis

6.1.2 Inadvertent puncture or incision and consequent infection in sampler

6.2 Burns

6.3 Hematoma

6.4 Bone calcification (14)

6.5 Nerve damage (9)

6.6 Bruising

6.7 Scarring (12)

6.8 Puncture of posterior medial aspect of heel may result in tibial artery laceration (11)

6.9 Pain

6.10 Bleeding

6.11 Inappropriate patient management may result from reliance on capillary PO_2 values (17,18)

CBGS 8.0 ASSESSMENT OF NEED:

Capillary blood gas sampling is an intermittent procedure and should be performed when a documented need exists. Routine or standing orders for capillary puncture are not recommended. The following may assist the clinician in assessing the need for capillary blood gas sampling:

8.1 History and physical assessment (23)

8.2 Noninvasive respiratory monitoring values

8.2.1 Pulse oximetry (23)

8.2.2 Transcutaneous values

8.2.3 End-tidal CO_2 values

8.3 Patient response to initiation, administration, or change in therapeutic modalities (23–25)

8.4 Lack of arterial access for blood gas sampling (1–3)

CBGS 11.0 MONITORING:

11.1 FIO_2 or prescribed oxygen flow (10,23, 28,29)

11.2 Oxygen administration device or ventilator settings (10,23,27,28)

11.3 Free flow of blood without the necessity for "milking" the foot or finger to obtain a sample (10,14)

11.4 Presence/absence of air or clot in sample (10,26,27)

11.5 Patient temperature, respiratory rate, position or level of activity, and clinical appearance (10,27)

11.6 Ease or difficulty of obtaining sample (10,27,28)

11.7 Appearance of puncture site (14,15)

11.8 Complications or adverse reactions to the procedure

11.9 Date, time, and sampling site (10)

11.10 Noninvasive monitoring values: transcutaneous O_2 & CO_2, end-tidal CO_2, and/or pulse oximetry (23)

11.11 Results of the blood gas analysis

Reprinted with permission from *Respiratory Care* 1994; 39: 1180–1183. The complete AARC Clinical Practice Guidelines are available from the AARC Web site (http://www.aarc.org), from the AARC Executive Office, or from *Respiratory Care* journal.

ANATOMICAL LOCATIONS FOR ARTERIAL PUNCTURE

Radial Artery

The radial artery's location makes it easily accessible. It is located in the wrist on the radial side (thumb side), close to the surface of the skin. It is the site most commonly used for taking a patient's pulse. Figure 8-1 shows the location of the radial artery where it is most accessible for puncture.

A big advantage of performing arterial puncture at the radial site is the safety afforded by the presence of collateral circulation. The hand is supplied with blood by both the radial and ulnar arteries. Because repeated punctures may result in vessel damage, swelling with partial or complete occlusion of the vessel may occur. If circulation is inadvertently interrupted resulting from radial artery puncture, the ulnar artery will continue to supply the circulatory needs of the hand. There are no veins or nerves immediately adjacent to the radial artery; consequently, arterial sampling at this site is facilitated by a reduced chance of inadvertent venous puncture or nerve damage.

The disadvantage of radial artery puncture is the small size of this artery. The radial artery is a small target. But through careful observation, palpation, and considerable

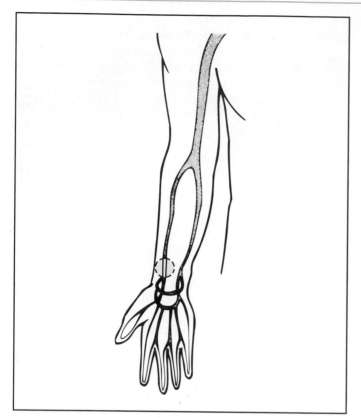

Figure 8-1   *The radial puncture site*

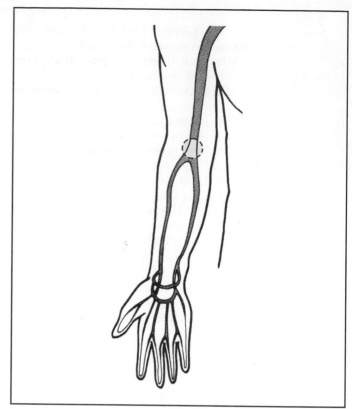

Figure 8-2   *The brachial puncture site*

practice, the radial artery can be punctured easily. However, in case of hypotensive and hypovolemic states or low cardiac output, puncture at this site may be particularly difficult.

Brachial Artery

The site where the brachial artery is commonly punctured is at the elbow in the antecubital fossa. Figure 8-2 shows its location. It is located on the medial side of the fossa near the insertion of the biceps muscle at the radial tuberosity.

An advantage of the brachial artery puncture site is its size. It is large and easily palpated.

There are several disadvantages to using the brachial artery. It is close to both a large vein and a nerve. Inadvertent venous sampling is common at this site. Accidental contact with the nerves at this site may cause extreme discomfort. Also, this site does not have the advantage of collateral circulation. Inadvertent injury leading to stoppage of circulation may result in the loss of the limb.

Femoral Artery

The femoral artery is accessible for arterial sampling in the groin. It may be palpated laterally from the pubis bone. Figure 8-3 shows the location for arterial puncture at this site.

The femoral artery is very large. It is easily palpated and presents a large target. The femoral artery may be the only site where arterial sampling is possible in cases of hypovolemia or hypotension, during cardiopulmonary resuscitation (CPR), or with low cardiac output.

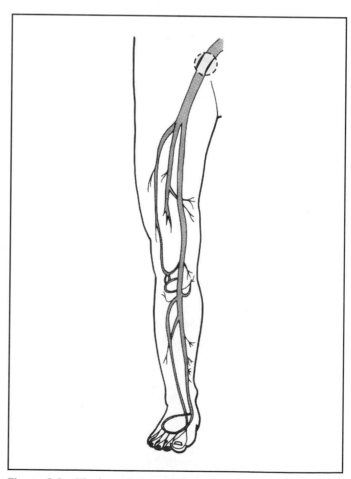

Figure 8-3   *The femoral puncture site*

There are several disadvantages to arterial puncture at this site, including the proximity of a major vein and a lack of collateral circulation. The artery may also be deep and difficult to locate. Atherosclerotic plaques commonly form in the femoral artery. If a plaque is dislodged as a result of arterial puncture, circulation to the entire leg may be compromised by formation of emboli. In addition, the close proximity of the femoral vein makes the certainty of arterial sampling questionable. It is often difficult to tell by inspection of the sample whether you have punctured the femoral artery or a vein.

COMPLICATIONS OF ARTERIAL PUNCTURE

There are several potential complications and hazards of arterial puncture, including vessel spasm and formation of thrombi or emboli, infection, and loss of blood flow and circulation. When an artery is punctured, arteriospasm may result. The artery is surrounded by a layer of muscle. The irritation caused by the penetration of the hypodermic needle may induce the muscle to spasm. There is a possibility of dislodging an atherosclerotic plaque or thrombus as a result of arterial puncture. If this happens, circulation to that limb or area may be seriously compromised. It could be severe enough that the circulation would be totally interrupted. Air emboli may also be inadvertently introduced into the vessel by improper technique. These emboli may result in serious consequences. Repeated punctures may compromise the vessel's integrity and circulation.

The Modified Allen's Test for Collateral Circulation

An advantage of performing an arterial puncture at the radial site is that the vascular anatomy allows testing for collateral circulation. The *modified Allen's test* should be done before arterial puncture to determine the adequacy of circulation supplied by the ulnar artery.

To perform the modified Allen's test, occlude both the radial and ulnar arteries with a firm grip, using your index fingers. Hold the patient's hand higher than the level of the heart and have the patient open and close the hand rapidly several times. Release the pressure on the ulnar artery. The hand should flush pink within 15 seconds. If it does, the test is positive, and the ulnar artery is supplying sufficient blood flow. Figure 8-4 shows the correct hand position for the Allen's test.

If the hand does not flush pink, it is likely that blood flow through the ulnar artery is insufficient to provide circulation if the radial artery loses patency. If this happens, try the other hand. If this also fails, choose the brachial site for puncture.

This test may be done on an unconscious patient by holding the hand above the heart for 30 to 60 seconds to 1 minute before releasing pressure on the ulnar artery.

Sampling Syringes

Recent advances in plastics technology have eliminated accuracy errors that result from diffusion of gases through

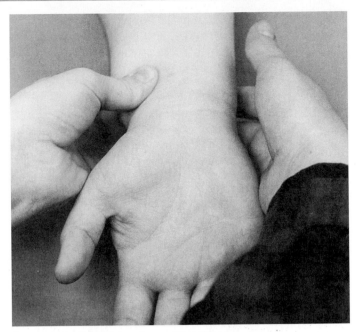

Figure 8-4 *Performing the modified Allen's test*

the plastic of the syringe. Many specialized plastic syringes are commercially available for arterial sampling. If these syringes are used according to the manufacturer's directions, little or no error will be introduced.

ABG sampling kits are commonly available. These kits contain a syringe, needle, alcohol and/or iodine-based prep pads, label, cork or stopper, and a bag or container for transport of the specimen.

BLOOD GAS SAMPLING ERRORS

The reliability of blood gas analysis is very technique-dependent. Every step of the process, from preparation of equipment through reporting the data, has potential problems that affect data reliability. That is, your knowledge and skill as a respiratory care practitioner will often determine the accuracy of the procedure. Knowledge of the factors that contribute to sampling errors will help to prevent their occurrence in clinical practice. If a sample is questionable, the relevant facts should be noted with the results of analysis. Clinical decisions are frequently based on data assumed to be entirely accurate.

Bubbles

Particularly if the sample is aspirated, air bubbles are often present in the collected blood sample. These bubbles must be expelled immediately upon collection. Room air contains enough oxygen that it can diffuse into the sample, increasing the arterial oxygen tension (PaO_2), or if the PaO_2 is greater than 160 mm Hg, it can decrease the PaO_2. This diffusion problem is especially true in hypoxemic patients. Carbon dioxide is present in the atmosphere in a concentration of only 0.003%, or around 2 mm Hg at sea level. Because arterial blood normally has a carbon dioxide tension ($PaCO_2$) ranging from 35 to 45 mm Hg, CO_2 dissolved in blood will tend to diffuse into the bubbles in the sample, lowering the measured value.

Ideally, if a large quantity of bubbles is present in the sample, it is best to discard it and draw another sample, being more attentive with your technique. However, this may not be practical in the clinical setting.

Delay in Sample Analysis

Blood contains living cells with their own metabolism and metabolic needs. These cells will continue to consume oxygen and nutrients and to produce acids and CO_2 even after being withdrawn from the body. Thus, if 15 minutes elapses before the sample is analyzed, the results can change dramatically (Shapiro, 1994).

Immediately after collection, cool the sample in a slush of ice and water. Ice slows the cells' metabolism, and even a delay of 30 minutes will not significantly affect the analysis results. It is best, however, to analyze the sample as soon after collection as you can. Ten minutes is optimal. Samples held longer than this may show lower PaO_2, higher $PaCO_2$, or a pH less than the patient's actual pH.

Use of the Proper Anticoagulant

Oxalates, ethylenediaminetetra-acetic acid (EDTA), and the citrate anticoagulants available for use will alter the pH of the arterial sample (Shapiro, 1994). Sodium heparin is the best anticoagulant to use in arterial blood sampling. Even sodium heparin, if too much is used (more than 0.1 ml of heparin per 1 ml of whole blood), will cause acidosis in the blood sample. If you are preparing a glass syringe for use, a safe general rule to follow is to expel all excess heparin. Heparin will be left in the needle and needle hub, occupying a minimal volume.

The syringes in blood gas sampling kits often contain crystalline heparin or lithium heparin. No aspiration of additional anticoagulant is necessary. Simply draw the sample, and the anticoagulant will dissolve. However, it is important to mix the sample by gently rolling or shaking the syringe after collection.

Venous Sampling

In a sample drawn from a hypoxemic patient, it is difficult to distinguish arterial blood from venous blood by color. When an arterial sample is drawn, the plunger of the syringe tends to pulsate as the sample fills the barrel. If the syringe does not fill without assistance, be suspicious of the sample site.

Patients in cardiopulmonary arrest, hypovolemia, hypotension, or low cardiac output often have low blood pressure. Samples from these patients must usually be aspirated. Drawing from the brachial or femoral site will help to ensure obtaining an arterial sample.

In the event of collection of a venous sample, draw another sample for analysis. If this is not possible, note with the sample results that it may be a venous sample.

Under some circumstances, a venous sample may be intentionally drawn, as well as an arterial sample. The technique for venipuncture is different from that for arterial puncture and is discussed in Chapter 7.

Patient Anxiety

It is a rare person who enjoys having blood drawn. It is natural to be a little apprehensive before the skin is punctured by a needle. However, if extreme, this anxiety may lead to hyperventilation and consequent altering of the $PaCO_2$.

Anxiety can be minimized by doing the procedure quickly and being prepared before reaching the bedside. Do not stress the pain and discomfort a patient may experience with arterial puncture. There is a difference between informed consent and scaring the patient. A statement such as "You will feel a little poke" is sufficient. If an arterial puncture is performed properly by a skilled practitioner, the blood sample can be drawn with minimal pain and discomfort.

CAPILLARY BLOOD GAS SAMPLING

In infants, *capillary blood gas sampling* is frequently performed in lieu of arterial puncture. Performing arterial puncture in an infant requires a large degree of skill and good technique for best results. The infant's vessels are very small and are difficult to palpate and puncture.

Technique

Capillary samples are usually obtained from the infant's heel but may also be obtained from the finger. When capillary blood is drawn from the heel, this sampling technique is sometimes referred to as a *heel stick*. *Arterialization* (warming to maximize blood flow) of the infant's heel is done before sampling, and then a lancet is used to puncture the skin surface. A sample from an adequately arterialized limb will yield reliable pH and $PaCO_2$ values, whereas PaO_2 values will vary from those determined using blood drawn by arterial puncture.

Capillary Sampling Errors

Poor Blood Flow

In performing capillary blood sampling, it is important to obtain a free-flowing sample. Do not squeeze the infant's foot when drawing the sample into a capillary tube. Squeezing the foot excessively could result in injury to the foot, leading to altered blood gas values. If blood at the puncture site does not flow freely, repeat the puncture to obtain a freely flowing blood sample.

Introduction of Air into the Sample

As with arterial puncture techniques, it is important to minimize the blood sample's exposure to air. Air may be introduced when it is drawn into the capillary tube, causing bubbles. The presence of air bubbles will alter the blood gas results; therefore, introduction of air should be avoided. If your sample contains visible bubbles, discard it and draw another (or remove the air bubbles as they enter the capillary tube).

Inadequate Mixing of Heparin

Once the sample has been drawn into the capillary tube, one end may be sealed with clay or a rubber stopper. A small metal rod is inserted into the capillary tube and a magnet is passed back and forth along the length of the tube to mix the heparin in the capillary tube with the blood sample. It is important to mix the heparin well to avoid clotting prior to sampling.

OBJECTIVES

At the end of this chapter, you should be able to:

ARTERIAL PUNCTURE

- Collect and properly assemble the supplies needed for arterial puncture.
- Demonstrate how to prepare a syringe properly for arterial puncture.
- Locate the three sites for arterial puncture:
  — Radial
  — Brachial
  — Femoral
- Using a laboratory partner, demonstrate the modified Allen's test for collateral circulation.
- Using an arterial arm simulator or the arm of a laboratory partner, demonstrate:
  — Radial artery puncture
  — Brachial artery puncture
- Demonstrate how to properly label and prepare the sample for transport.

- Demonstrate how to draw an arterial sample from an indwelling radial artery catheter.

CAPILLARY SAMPLING

- Collect and properly assemble the supplies needed for capillary blood sampling.
- Using a resuscitation mannequin or an infant, correctly demonstrate how to arterialize an infant's heel prior to puncture.
- Using a resuscitation mannequin or an infant, demonstrate correct techniques for obtaining a capillary blood sample:
  — Site preparation
  — Use of the lancet
  — Drawing the capillary sample
  — Mixing the heparin
  — Care of the puncture site following the procedure

SUPPLIES NEEDED FOR ARTERIAL PUNCTURE

The supplies needed for arterial puncture are usually contained in an ABG kit. If you need to assemble your supplies separately, the supplies needed are listed in Figure 8-5.

PUNCTURE TECHNIQUES

General Considerations

Standard Precautions

As discussed in Chapter 1, blood and blood products are body fluids that come under the classification of biohazards. As such, it is important that you adhere to the guidelines provided by the Centers for Disease Control and Prevention (CDC) and comply with all standard precautions.

To perform arterial puncture, arterial line sampling, or capillary blood sampling (heel sticks), you should

5-ml preheparinized disposable sampling syringe
Needles (20 to 25 gauge, in various lengths)
Rubber stopper or rubber syringe cap
Adhesive strip or Elastoplast tape
Iodine and alcohol prep pads
Plastic bag or other container to transport sample
Ice slush
Lidocaine anesthetic 2% solution (if ordered)
Personal protective equipment
—Disposable latex gloves
—Eye protection (goggles or face shield)

Figure 8-5 Supplies needed for arterial puncture

wear personal protective equipment. As a minimum, you should wear disposable latex gloves and eye protection (either goggles or a face shield). You should always exercise caution when using sharps (needles or lancet) to prevent sticks or punctures of your own skin. Always handle sharps carefully, and properly dispose of them into an approved biohazard sharps container.

Patient-Related Considerations

A physician's order is required before performing this or any other procedure. It is important to check the patient's chart for a physician's order for anticoagulant therapy or oxygen therapy before arterial sampling.

Anticoagulant therapy may necessitate your putting pressure on the site for up to 15 minutes to stop the bleeding following arterial puncture.

It is important to assess if the patient is receiving the proper oxygen therapy (or to identify the lack of therapy) before doing the puncture. ABG analysis is a useful tool for judging the adequacy of oxygen therapy. If blood is drawn while the patient is receiving the wrong oxygen regimen, however, a repeat arterial puncture is necessary. Mistakes can be avoided by checking the chart and the patient first. Usually, 10 to 30 minutes is needed before arterial puncture after any oxygen concentration change.

The patient should be reassessed 20 to 30 minutes following arterial puncture. Check the circulation distal to the puncture site and for any bleeding at the site.

Use of an Anesthetic

The use of an anesthetic prior to arterial puncture requires a physician's order and a specific protocol. The puncture site should be prepared as though you were doing an arterial puncture. Draw up 0.1 to 0.2 ml of 2% lidocaine into a tuberculin syringe with a 25-gauge needle. Puncture the skin near the artery and draw back on the plunger. If blood appears in the syringe, it is in a vessel. Withdraw the syringe and redirect the needle. Repeat the aspiration step. If there is no blood return, make a small wheal by injecting part of the anesthetic. Try to surround the artery with anesthetic. Allow 2 to 3 minutes to lapse before performing the arterial puncture.

Puncture Preparation

Prepare your syringe as outlined in the previous section. If you are using a preheparinized syringe, follow the manufacturer's instructions for preparation. It is best to arrange all of the supplies you will need within easy reach. The rubber stopper, 2×2-inch gauze pads, container with ice slush, and adhesive strip should be arranged so that immediate retrieval is possible.

If you are doing a radial puncture, perform the modified Allen's test. Carefully palpate the puncture site. Try to form a mental image of the course and direction of the artery. Note the strength of the pulse and try to estimate the depth of the artery below the skin.

Using an iodine-based prep pad, cleanse the site. Use firm pressure, scribing a circle from the puncture site out. Use what is left of the pad to cleanse the thumb and forefinger with which you will palpate. Follow the iodine-based preparation with an alcohol prep pad, using the same technique.

Obtaining the Specimen
Radial and Brachial Sites

Hold the syringe like a pencil. Palpate the pulse and visualize the artery location.

For sampling at the radial site, with the needle bevel up, puncture the skin at a 45° angle. Once the needle is below the skin surface, visualize the artery location and slowly advance the needle toward the artery. Observe the hub of the needle. When the artery is punctured, blood will quickly appear in the needle hub. This is termed a *flash*. When you see the flash, do not move. Allow the syringe to fill.

For sampling at the brachial site, with the needle bevel up, puncture the skin at a 45° to 90° angle. Advance the needle slowly toward the artery, watching for the flash. When the flash is observed, do not move. Allow the syringe to fill.

Femoral Site

The femoral artery is deep and may require a longer needle for successful puncture. With the bevel of the needle facing the patient's head and perpendicular to the skin's surface, puncture the skin. Watch for the flash and allow the syringe to fill.

POSTPUNCTURE CARE

After the sample is collected, withdraw the needle and apply firm pressure with a 2×2-inch gauze pad. Expel any air and insert the needle into a rubber stopper to seal it. Continue to apply firm pressure to the puncture site for a minimum of 5 minutes.

While you are holding firm pressure to the puncture site, mix the sample in the syringe. The sample may be mixed by gently rolling the syringe between your thumb and forefinger. Rolling the syringe will mix the heparin with the blood and prevent clotting.

Ice the sample after mixing by placing it into the container of ice slush.

Check the puncture site after 5 minutes have passed. Observe the color of the skin distal to the puncture. Check for circulation by palpating the artery distal to the puncture site. The skin should be warm to the touch, and when the tissue is firmly pressed and released, capillary refill should be evident. An adhesive strip may be applied now.

Label the sample with the patient's name and room number, time of collection, and the fraction of inspired oxygen (FiO_2) inhaled by the patient, respiratory rate, or ventilator settings as appropriate. Transport the sample to the laboratory for analysis.

After 20 minutes, check the puncture site again, using the same criteria described earlier.

INDWELLING ARTERIAL CATHETER SAMPLING

The placement of an indwelling arterial catheter is common in critically ill patients. The catheter supplies moment-by-moment pressure monitoring and allows repeated arterial sampling with minimal trauma to the patient. However, *arterial line sampling* poses certain hazards, including the introduction of air emboli, infection, and inadvertent loss of the line by decannulation.

To prevent the catheter from clotting, a continuous drip of sodium heparin at a pressure greater than arterial pressure is maintained. If a sample is drawn without first flushing the line, the sample would be severely diluted with heparin.

To flush the line, remove the cap from the sampling port. Clean the port with an alcohol prep pad. Attach a sterile 3-ml syringe, and rotate the stopcock so that blood flows to the sampling port. Withdraw 3 to 5 ml of blood so that undiluted blood flows freely into the syringe. Close the stopcock and discard the syringe.

Attach a new 5-ml syringe, properly prepared, for arterial sampling and draw 3 to 5 ml of undiluted arterial blood. Close the stopcock at the sampling port. Cap the syringe to maintain anaerobic conditions and ice the sample.

Flush the catheter by opening the stopcock to the heparin reservoir bag and allowing heparin to flow through the catheter. Continue flushing the line until it is clear. Figure 8-6 shows the sequence of arterial sampling from an indwelling arterial catheter.

SUPPLIES FOR CAPILLARY SAMPLING

The supplies needed for capillary sampling are listed in Figure 8-7. It is important to have all of the supplies required for this procedure on hand and ready to use. Infants are very active, and it is difficult to obtain equipment when you need it under the best of circumstances.

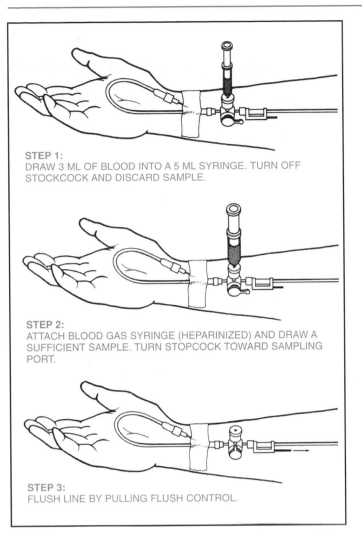

STEP 1:
DRAW 3 ML OF BLOOD INTO A 5 ML SYRINGE. TURN OFF STOCKCOCK AND DISCARD SAMPLE.

STEP 2:
ATTACH BLOOD GAS SYRINGE (HEPARINIZED) AND DRAW A SUFFICIENT SAMPLE. TURN STOPCOCK TOWARD SAMPLING PORT.

STEP 3:
FLUSH LINE BY PULLING FLUSH CONTROL.

Figure 8-6 *The sequence for obtaining a sample from an arterial line*

STANDARD PRECAUTIONS

As discussed in Chapter 1, blood and blood products are body fluids that come under the classification of biohazards. As such, it is important that you adhere to the CDC guidelines and comply with all standard precautions.

Latex gloves
Eye protection
Heparinized capillary tubes
Metal rod
Hot packs or towels soaked in hot water
Clay or rubber caps for capillary sample tubes
Lancets
Povidone-iodine, alcohol prep pads, and 2 × 2-inch gauze pads
Adhesive strip
Paper cup filled with an ice slush

Figure 8-7 *Supplies needed for capillary sampling*

To perform arterial puncture, arterial line sampling, or capillary blood sampling (heel sticks), you should wear personal protective equipment. As a minimum you should wear disposable latex gloves and eye protection (either goggles or a face shield). You should always exercise caution when using sharps (needles or lancet) to prevent sticks or punctures of your own skin. Always handle sharps carefully, and properly dispose of them into an approved biohazard sharps container.

ARTERIALIZATION OF THE PUNCTURE SITE

It is important to arterialize the puncture site before obtaining the sample, to increase blood flow to the area. A hot (45°C) pack or towels soaked in warm water should be applied to the heel for at least 5 minutes prior to performing the puncture. The site should be very pink or red following the application of heat, indicating an increase in capillary circulation.

SITE PREPARATION

The site should be cleansed with an alcohol prep pad followed by a povidone/iodine prep pad. It is important to use aseptic technique to avoid exposing your patient to the risks of infection.

OBTAINING THE SAMPLE

Using the lancet, quickly puncture the skin on the lateral surface of the heel. The lancet should penetrate approximately 3 mm to ensure adequate blood flow. The blood should flow freely from the puncture site without having to squeeze the infant's heel to augment blood flow.

The initial blood should be discarded and not obtained as part of the sample. Once the blood is flowing freely, use the heparinized capillary tube to draw your sample. Be careful not to introduce air or bubbles into the sample.

CARE OF THE SAMPLE

Once the capillary sample has been obtained, seal one end of the tube with clay or a rubber stopper. Introduce a metal rod into the open end, and using a magnet, move the rod back and forth through the tube, mixing the heparin.

Ice the sample and analyze it as quickly as possible. An ice slush promotes good heat transfer and will cool the sample more quickly than ice alone.

CARE OF THE PUNCTURE SITE

Using a sterile 2 × 2-inch gauze pad, apply pressure to the site if blood is continuing to flow. Once blood flow has stopped, apply an adhesive strip or another dry dressing to protect the site.

References

American Association for Respiratory Care. (1992). AARC clinical practice guideline: Sampling for arterial blood gas analysis. *Respiratory Care, 37*(8), 913–917.

American Association for Respiratory Care. (1994). AARC clinical practice guideline: Capillary blood gas sampling for neonatal and pediatric patients. *Respiratory Care, 39*(12), 1180–1183.

Shapiro, B. A., (1994). *Clinical application of blood gases* (5th ed.). Chicago: Mosby–Year Book.

Additional Resources

Burton, G. G., Hodgkin, J., & Ward, J. (1991). *Respiratory care* (3rd ed.). Philadelphia: Lippincott.

Garner, J. S., & the Hospital Infection Control Practices Advisory Committee. (1996). Guideline for isolation precautions in hospitals. *American Journal of Infection Control, 24*(2), 24–52.

Nelson, E. J., Hunter, P., & Morton, E. (1983). *Critical care respiratory therapy: A laboratory and clinical manual*. Boston: Little, Brown.

Practice Activities: Arterial Blood Gas Sampling

1. Using a laboratory partner, perform the following for the listed arterial puncture sites:
   a. Properly position the patient.
   b. Locate the site.
   c. Palpate the site.
      (1) Radial site
      (2) Brachial site
      (3) Femoral site
2. Properly prepare a glass syringe or ABG kit for arterial puncture.
   a. Use aseptic technique.
   b. Lubricate the barrel with sodium heparin or prepare a disposable syringe.
   c. Expel excess heparin.
   d. Handle syringe without introducing room air.

3. Using a laboratory partner, perform the modified Allen's test for collateral circulation.

4. Using an arterial arm simulator:
   a. Practice correct technique for radial artery puncture.
   b. Practice correct technique for brachial artery puncture.
   Incorporate the following:
      (1) Practice using standard precautions.
      (2) Practice aseptic technique.
      (3) Practice puncture skills.
      (4) Practice correct sample-handling skills.

5. Using an arterial arm simulator, draw an arterial sample from an indwelling radial artery catheter.

Check List: Arterial Blood Gas Sampling

_____ 1. Verify physician's order.
2. Check the patient's chart:
_____ a. Anticoagulant therapy
_____ b. Oxygen therapy
3. Gather required supplies.
_____ a. Latex gloves
_____ b. Eye protection
_____ c. 5-ml syringe
_____ d. 20- to 25-gauge needle
_____ e. Sodium heparin
_____ f. Syringe cap and rubber stopper
_____ g. Adhesive strip
_____ h. Elastoplast tape
_____ i. Iodine-based prep pad
_____ j. Alcohol-based prep pad
_____ k. Lidocaine anesthetic, if ordered
_____ l. Ice
_____ 4. Wash your hands.
_____ 5. Don latex gloves prior to patient contact.
_____ 6. Explain the procedure to the patient.

7. Position the patient:
   a. Radial site
_____ (1) Hyperextend the wrist and support it slightly with a towel or washcloth.
   b. Brachial site
_____ (1) Lay the arm flat, palm side up.
   c. Femoral site
_____ (1) Lay the patient in a supine position with access to the groin.
8. Palpate the puncture site:
_____ a. Visualize course of the artery.
_____ b. Estimate the depth.
_____ 9. For a radial artery puncture, perform the modified Allen's test for collateral circulation.
10. Prepare the site:
_____ a. Use iodine first.
_____ b. Cleanse with alcohol.
_____ c. Clean the fingers you will use to palpate the site.

11. If one has been ordered, administer the anesthetic:
_____ a. Do not use more than 0.2 ml.
_____ b. Use a small-gauge needle (25 gauge recommended).
_____ c. Surround the puncture site and artery.

12. Properly perform the puncture:
_____ a. Use the correct angle and bevel position.
_____ b. Penetrate the skin quickly.
_____ c. Advance the needle, watching for the flash in the hub of the needle.

13. Collect the sample:
_____ a. 3 to 5 ml

_____ 14. Withdraw the needle and apply firm pressure to the area.

15. Insert the needle into the stopper or safety cap and ice the sample:

_____ a. Expel any air bubbles.
_____ b. Insert the needle into stopper or safety cap.
_____ c. Ice the sample.
_____ d. Label the sample.

16. Check for circulation distal to the puncture site.
_____ a. Color
_____ b. Pulse

17. Make the patient comfortable:
_____ a. Apply an adhesive strip.
_____ b. Help the patient to a comfortable position.

18. Transport the sample to the laboratory:
_____ a. Label the sample.
_____ b. Prepare the required laboratory slips and paperwork.

19. Check the puncture site after 20 minutes:
_____ a. Check the circulation.
_____ b. Check for bleeding.

_____ 20. Correctly record the procedure on the chart.

Check List: Arterial Line Sampling

_____ 1. Verify the physician's order for therapy.
_____ 2. Verify the oxygen concentration.
3. Gather the appropriate equipment:
_____ a. Latex gloves
_____ b. Eye protection
_____ c. 5-ml syringe
_____ d. Blood gas syringe
_____ e. Sodium heparin
_____ f. Syringe cap or stopper
_____ g. Ice slush
_____ 4. Wash your hands.
_____ 5. Don latex gloves prior to patient contact.
_____ 6. Explain the procedure and position the patient.
_____ 7. Assemble and prepare the equipment.
_____ 8. Turn off monitoring alarms.
_____ 9. Open the sampling port, removing the cap aseptically.
_____ 10. Attach a disposable syringe.

_____ 11. Turn the stopcock to fill the syringe and draw 3 ml of blood.
_____ 12. Turn off the stopcock and remove the syringe.
_____ 13. Attach the heparinized blood gas syringe.
_____ 14. Open the stopcock and draw a sufficient sample.
_____ 15. Close the stopcock and remove the syringe.
_____ 16. Expel any air from the sample.
_____ 17. Cap and ice the sample.
_____ 18. Flush the sampling port with heparin, using the flush control.
_____ 19. Clean up the area and dispose of the 3-ml blood sample collected before the blood gas.
_____ 20. Reset the alarm and observe the monitor for the correct wave form.
_____ 21. Label and transport the sample.
_____ 22. Record the procedure on the chart.

Check List: Capillary Sampling

_____ 1. Verify the physician's order for therapy.
_____ 2. Wash your hands.
3. Obtain the required supplies for the procedure:
_____ a. Latex gloves
_____ b. Eye protection
_____ c. Heparinized capillary tubes
_____ d. Clay or rubber stopper
_____ e. Povidone-iodine and alcohol prep pads
_____ f. Hot pack or hot towels
_____ g. Metal rod and magnet
_____ h. 2 × 2-inch gauze pads and adhesive strips
_____ i. Cup filled with an ice slush

_____ 4. Wash your hands before the procedure.
_____ 5. Apply latex gloves prior to patient contact.
_____ 6. Position the patient and interact with the patient and the patient's family appropriately.
_____ 7. Apply the hot pack or hot towels for 5 minutes to arterialize the sample site.
_____ 8. Prepare the puncture site using alcohol and a povidone-iodine prep pad.
_____ 9. Using the lancet, quickly puncture the lateral surface of the heel. Pierce the skin to a depth of 3 mm to ensure adequate blood flow.
_____ 10. Obtain a blood sample using the capillary tubes.

_____ 11. Correctly care for the sample:

_____ a. Cap one end of the capillary tube with clay or a rubber stopper.

_____ b. Insert the metal rod, and using the magnet, mix the heparin with the blood sample.

_____ c. Ice the sample.

_____ 12. Using a 2 × 2-inch gauze pad, apply pressure to the puncture site until bleeding has stopped.

_____ 13. Apply another 2 × 2-inch gauze pad as a dressing or use an adhesive strip to protect the puncture site.

_____ 14. Clean up the area following the procedure.

_____ 15. Label and transport the sample to the laboratory for analysis.

_____ 16. Record the procedure in the patient's chart.

Self-Evaluation Post Test: Arterial Blood Gas Sampling

1. The modified Allen's test is a test for:
   a. adequate blood pressure.
   b. collateral circulation.
   c. ulnar pulse.
   d. muscle tone of the hand.
   e. nervous reflexes in the extremities.

2. The radial artery is a preferred arterial site because:
   a. it is near the surface.
   b. the ulnar artery can provide collateral circulation to the hand.
   c. no major veins are nearby.
   d. it is the largest vessel accessible.
   e. it has the greatest blood pressure.

3. Air bubbles, that are present in an arterial blood sample after collection:
   a. have no significant effect.
   b. will be compensated for by the blood gas analyzer.
   c. should be expelled immediately.
   d. should be forced into solution immediately.
   e. enhance the results of the test.

4. If an arterial blood sample contains large amounts of air bubbles after collection:
   a. it should be iced immediately.
   b. discard it and draw another sample.
   c. the bubbles should be forced into solution.
   d. they will have no effect on the sample.
   e. the syringe should be mixed until they dissolve.

5. Air bubbles, if present in an arterial blood sample, will:
   I. increase PaO_2.   IV. decrease $PaCO_2$.
   II. decrease PaO_2.   V. increase pH.
   III. increase $PaCO_2$.
   a. I, IV   d. II, IV
   b. I, III   e. II, IV, V
   c. II, III

6. If the patient is on oxygen therapy, you should do the following before collecting ABG samples:
   a. Verify the physician's order.
   b. Verify that the patient is receiving the correct oxygen therapy.
   c. Remove the oxygen because it adversely affects results.
   d. Both a and b
   e. None of the above

7. If the patient is very hypotensive, the best site(s) for arterial blood sampling is (are):
   a. the radial site.   d. a and b
   b. the brachial site.   e. a and c
   c. the femoral site.

8. The site for arterial blood sampling that is associated with the highest likelihood of obtaining a venous sample is:
   a. the radial site.   d. the carotid.
   b. the brachial site.   e. a and d
   c. the femoral site.

9. If the modified Allen's test is negative, you should:
   a. go ahead and use the radial artery.
   b. call the doctor.
   c. perform an Allen's test on the other arm.
   d. use the brachial site.
   e. use the femoral site.

10. The site for arterial blood sampling with the greatest risk of complications resulting from arterial puncture is:
    a. the radial site.   d. the saphenous vein.
    b. the femoral site.   e. a and d
    c. the brachial site.

PERFORMANCE EVALUATION:
ARTERIAL PUNCTURE

Date: Lab _____   Clinical _____   Agency _____

Lab: Pass _____ Fail _____   Clinical: Pass _____ Fail _____

Student name _____   Instructor name _____

No. of times observed in clinical _____

No. of times practiced in clinical _____

PASSING CRITERIA: Obtain 90% or better on the procedure. Tasks indicated by * must receive at least 1 point, or the evaluation is terminated. Procedure must be performed within designated time, or the performance receives a failing grade.

SCORING: 2 points — Task performed satisfactorily without prompting.
                1 point — Task performed satisfactorily with self-initiated correction.
                0 points — Task performed incorrectly or with prompting required.
                NA — Task not applicable to the patient care situation.

TASKS:		PEER	LAB	CLINICAL
*	1. Verifies the physician's order	☐	☐	☐
	2. Scans the chart	☐	☐	☐
*	3. Verifies the oxygen concentration	☐	☐	☐
	4. Gathers the required equipment			
*	a. Latex gloves	☐	☐	☐
*	b. Eye protection	☐	☐	☐
*	c. 5-ml syringe and needles	☐	☐	☐
*	d. Rubber stopper or cap	☐	☐	☐
*	e. Adhesive strip	☐	☐	☐
*	f. Iodine and alcohol prep pads	☐	☐	☐
	g. Lidocaine anesthetic	☐	☐	☐
*	h. Ice	☐	☐	☐
*	5. Washes hands	☐	☐	☐
	6. Dons protective equipment before patient contact	☐	☐	☐
	7. Explains the procedure and positions the patient	☐	☐	☐
*	8. Assembles and prepares the equipment	☐	☐	☐
*	9. Palpates the puncture site	☐	☐	☐
*	10. Performs the modified Allen's test	☐	☐	☐
*	11. Prepares the site before puncture	☐	☐	☐
	12. Administers an anesthetic, if ordered	☐	☐	☐
*	13. Palpates the puncture site	☐	☐	☐
*	14. Correctly performs the puncture	☐	☐	☐
*	15. Applies firm pressure to the site	☐	☐	☐
*	16. Expels any air from the sample	☐	☐	☐

*	17.	Caps and ices the sample	☐	☐	☐
*	18.	Checks the circulation distal to the site	☐	☐	☐
	19.	Ensures patient safety and comfort	☐	☐	☐
	20.	Cleans up	☐	☐	☐
*	21.	Labels and transports the sample	☐	☐	☐
*	22.	Checks the site after 20 minutes	☐	☐	☐
*	23.	Records the procedure in the chart	☐	☐	☐

SCORE: Peer   _____ points of possible 62; _____%

             Lab   _____ points of possible 62; _____%

             Clinical   _____ points of possible 62; _____%

TIME: _____ out of possible 20 minutes

STUDENT SIGNATURES   **INSTRUCTOR SIGNATURES**

PEER: _____   LAB: _____

STUDENT: _____   CLINICAL: _____

PERFORMANCE EVALUATION: ARTERIAL LINE SAMPLING

Date: Lab _____ Clinical _____ Agency _____

Lab: Pass _____ Fail _____   Clinical: Pass _____ Fail _____

Student name _____ Instructor name _____

No. of times observed in clinical _____

No. of times practiced in clinical _____

PASSING CRITERIA: Obtain 90% or better on the procedure. Tasks indicated by * must receive at least 1 point, or the evaluation is terminated. Procedure must be performed within designated time, or the performance receives a failing grade.

SCORING:
2 points — Task performed satisfactorily without prompting.
1 point — Task performed satisfactorily with self-initiated correction.
0 points — Task performed incorrectly or with prompting required.
NA — Task not applicable to the patient care situation.

TASKS:		PEER	LAB	CLINICAL
*	1. Verifies the physician's order	☐	☐	☐
	2. Scans the chart	☐	☐	☐
*	3. Verifies the oxygen concentration	☐	☐	☐
	4. Gathers the required equipment			
*	a. Latex gloves	☐	☐	☐
*	b. Eye protection	☐	☐	☐
*	c. 5-ml syringe	☐	☐	☐
*	d. Blood gas syringe	☐	☐	☐
*	e. Syringe cap or rubber stopper	☐	☐	☐
*	f. Ice	☐	☐	☐
*	5. Washes hands	☐	☐	☐
	6. Dons protective equipment before patient contact	☐	☐	☐
	7. Explains the procedure and positions the patient	☐	☐	☐
*	8. Assembles and prepares the equipment	☐	☐	☐
	9. Turns off monitor alarms	☐	☐	☐
	10. Opens the sampling port			
*	a. Removes the cap and sets it on sterile gauze	☐	☐	☐
*	11. Attaches a disposable syringe	☐	☐	☐
*	12. Turns the stopcock to fill the syringe and draws 3 ml of blood	☐	☐	☐
*	13. Turns off the stopcock and removes the syringe	☐	☐	☐
*	14. Attaches the heparinized blood gas syringe	☐	☐	☐
*	15. Opens the stopcock and draws a sufficient sample	☐	☐	☐
*	16. Closes the stopcock and removes the syringe	☐	☐	☐
*	17. Expels any air from the sample	☐	☐	☐

* 18. Caps and ices the sample ☐ ☐ ☐

* 19. Flushes the sampling port with heparin, using the flush control ☐ ☐ ☐

20. Ensures the patient's safety and comfort ☐ ☐ ☐

* 21. Cleans up the area and disposes of the
3-ml blood sample properly ☐ ☐ ☐

* 22. Resets the alarm and observes the monitor for the
correct wave form ☐ ☐ ☐

* 23. Labels and transports the sample ☐ ☐ ☐

* 24. Records the procedure in the chart ☐ ☐ ☐

SCORE: Peer   _____ points of possible 60; _____%

Lab   _____ points of possible 60; _____%

Clinical   _____ points of possible 60; _____%

TIME: _____ out of possible 20 minutes

STUDENT SIGNATURES   INSTRUCTOR SIGNATURES

PEER: _____   LAB: _____

STUDENT: _____   CLINICAL: _____

PERFORMANCE EVALUATION:
CAPILLARY SAMPLING

Date: Lab _____ Clinical _____ Agency _____

Lab: Pass _____ Fail _____   Clinical: Pass _____ Fail _____

Student name _____ Instructor name _____

No. of times observed in clinical _____

No. of times practiced in clinical _____

PASSING CRITERIA: Obtain 90% or better on the procedure. Tasks indicated by * must receive at least 1 point, or the evaluation is terminated. Procedure must be performed within designated time, or the performance receives a failing grade.

SCORING:
2 points — Task performed satisfactorily without prompting.
1 point — Task performed satisfactorily with self-initiated correction.
0 points — Task performed incorrectly or with prompting required.
NA — Task not applicable to the patient care situation.

TASKS:		PEER	LAB	CLINICAL
*	1. Verifies the physician's order	☐	☐	☐
*	2. Washes hands	☐	☐	☐
*	3. Obtains required supplies			
	a. Latex gloves	☐	☐	☐
	b. Eye protection	☐	☐	☐
	c. Heparinized capillary collection tubes	☐	☐	☐
	d. Clay or rubber stopper	☐	☐	☐
	e. Prep pads	☐	☐	☐
	f. Hot pack or hot towels	☐	☐	☐
	g. Metal rod and magnet	☐	☐	☐
	h. 2 × 2-inch gauze pads and adhesive strip	☐	☐	☐
	i. Cup filled with ice slush	☐	☐	☐
*	4. Dons protective equipment before patient contact	☐	☐	☐
	5. Positions and interacts with the patient appropriately	☐	☐	☐
*	6. Applies hot packs for correct time before sampling	☐	☐	☐
*	7. Prepares site before sampling	☐	☐	☐
*	8. Correctly obtains blood sample	☐	☐	☐
*	9. Correctly cares for sample			
	a. Mixes heparin	☐	☐	☐
	b. Ices sample	☐	☐	☐
*	10. Correctly cares for puncture site	☐	☐	☐
*	11. Cleans up after the procedure	☐	☐	☐
*	12. Labels and transports sample	☐	☐	☐
*	13. Records procedure in the patient's chart	☐	☐	☐

SCORE: Peer   _____ points of possible 48; _____%

             Lab   _____ points of possible 48; _____%

             Clinical   _____ points of possible 48; _____%

TIME: _____ out of possible 30 minutes

STUDENT SIGNATURES   INSTRUCTOR SIGNATURES

PEER: _____   LAB: _____

STUDENT: _____   CLINICAL: _____

CHAPTER 9
HEMODYNAMIC MONITORING

INTRODUCTION

Hemodynamic monitoring provides important clinical information regarding blood pressure, fluid volume, cardiac preload and afterload, cardiac output, and the pulmonary and systemic vascular resistance. Hemodynamic monitoring in its simplest terms is the measurement of pressures within the vascular system, utilizing invasive, indwelling catheters. Besides simply measuring pressures, these catheters provide a convenient route for fluid and drug administration and access for blood sampling (venous and arterial). Not all acutely ill patients will have invasive catheters placed to provide this information; however, the need for such monitoring will be greatest in the most acutely ill patients. It is important that as a respiratory care practitioner, you understand where these catheters are placed anatomically, how the data provided by these catheters relate to cardiac function and fluid balance, how to utilize these catheters, and the hazards and complications associated with their placement and usage.

KEY TERMS

- Central venous pressure catheter
- Damping
- Distal lumen
- Inflation lumen and balloon
- Pascal's law

- Phlebostatic axis
- Proximal lumen
- Pulmonary artery
- Pulmonary artery catheter
- Pulmonary artery wedge pressure (PAWP)

- Swan-Ganz catheter
- Thermistor
- Thermistor lumen
- Transducer
- Vena cava

OBJECTIVES

At the end of this chapter, you should be able to:

- Describe Pascal's law and how it applies to hemodynamic monitoring.
- Describe what a transducer is and how it is utilized in hemodynamic monitoring.
- For central venous pressure (CVP) catheters:
  — Describe the preferred routes of vessel access.
  — Describe the correct anatomical placement of the catheter.
  — Identify the parts of a CVP wave form.
  — List the normal values for the CVP.
  — Discuss how a CVP catheter can provide data to help determine:
    — Fluid volume
    — Adequacy of venous return
    — Right ventricular preload
  — Describe what other functions a CVP catheter may serve besides pressure monitoring.
- For pulmonary artery catheters or Swan-Ganz catheters:
  — Identify the parts of a pulmonary artery catheter.
  — Describe the preferred routes of vessel access.
  — Describe the correct anatomical placement of the catheter.
  — Identify the wave form morphology as the catheter is placed.
  — Identify the parts of the pulmonary artery and pulmonary artery wedge pressure tracing.
  — List the normal ranges for:
    — Right atrial pressure

  — Right ventricular pressure
  — Pulmonary artery pressure
  — Pulmonary artery wedge pressure
- Discuss how a pulmonary artery catheter can provide data to help determine:
  — Fluid volume
  — Adequacy of venous return
  — Right ventricular preload
  — Right ventricular afterload
  — Left ventricular preload
  — Cardiac output
  — Mixed venous oxygen saturation
  — Pulmonary vascular resistance
  — Systemic vascular resistance
- Given a set of hemodynamic data, determine which of the following may be occurring:
  — Hypovolemia
  — Hypervolemia
  — Right ventricular failure
  — Left ventricular failure
  — Effects of positive-pressure ventilation
- For an arterial line:
  — Describe the preferred routes of vessel access.
  — Identify the parts of an arterial pressure wave form.
  — List the normal values for the arterial pressure.
- Discuss the hazards and complications associated with indwelling vascular catheters, their placement, and usage.

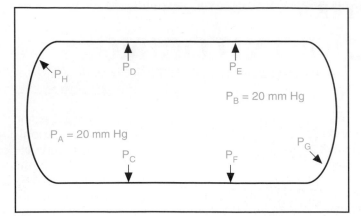

Figure 9-1 *A diagram illustrating Pascal's law. Note that the pressure at point A is equal to the pressure at point B and that the forces act perpendicular to the walls of the container.*

PASCAL'S LAW

Blaise Pascal was a seventeenth-century investigator. Quite inadvertently, Pascal discovered an important principle in fluid mechanics. He discovered that when the base of a full champagne bottle lying on its side was struck smartly with a mallet, the neck of the bottle would break off and not the base that was struck. Pascal concluded two important concepts from his early experimentation: (1) the pressure of a fluid in a closed container is equal at all points within the container and (2) the pressure acts perpendicularly against the walls of the container (Figure 9-1).

Pascal's law also applies to the vascular system as well as to champagne bottles. For example, for a catheter inserted into the radial artery of a patient, the pressure monitored at the point of insertion is equal to the pressure within the arterial system. We apply Pascal's law to determine arterial, right atrial, and left ventricular end-diastolic pressures using indwelling catheters, as you will learn later in this chapter. Pascal's law holds true as long as the vascular system at the point of interest does not have valves or any other anatomical structures that would alter the reflected pressure being measured.

TRANSDUCERS

A *transducer* is a device that converts one form of energy into another. Hemodynamic monitoring depends heavily on transducers to convert pressures into analog electrical signals, which can then be used to display pressures or graphical wave forms. A typical transducer used in hemodynamic monitoring consists of a diaphragm with a strain gauge embedded into it or attached to it (Figure 9-2). As the pressure applied to the diaphragm increases, the diaphragm distorts, causing the strain gauge to lengthen. The longer the strain gauge becomes, the more resistance it creates to electrical current passed through it. Therefore, a change in electrical current is proportional to a change in pressure (Figure 9-3). These small changes in current are utilized by the microprocessors in the monitoring systems to provide both the graphical and the digital information used in patient management.

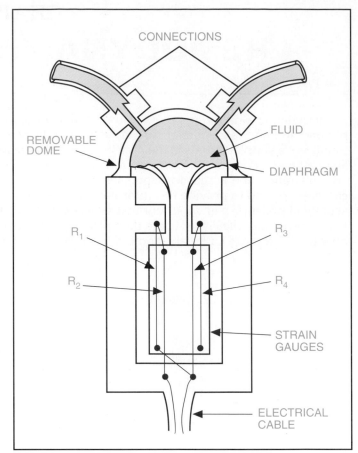

Figure 9-2 *A figure illustrating a strain gauge pressure transducer*

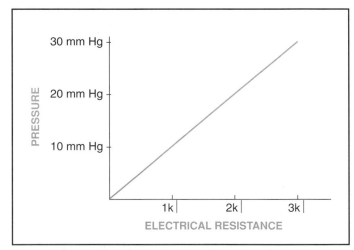

Figure 9-3 *A graph illustrating that a change in pressure is proportional to a change in electrical resistance*

CENTRAL VENOUS PRESSURE CATHETERS

A *central venous pressure catheter* (CVP catheter) is placed in the venous system so that the distal tip of the catheter rests in the *vena cava* or right atrium (Figure 9-4). The outflow from the vena cava empties into the right atrium. Because there are no heart valves between the vena cava

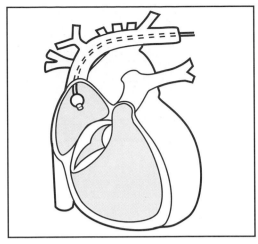

Figure 9-4   *The anatomical location of a central venous catheter. Note that the tip rests in the right atrium.*

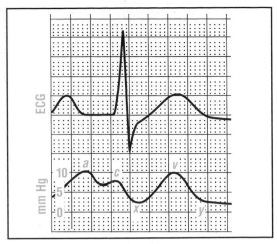

Figure 9-5   *The CVP tracing and its component parts—the* a, c, x, v, *and* y *waves—and the relationship of the wave form to the electrocardiogram.*

and the right atrium, the pressure in the vena cava is the same as the pressure in the right atrium.

Preferred Routes of Access

Several sites are used for the insertion of CVP catheters. These include the antecubital fossa and the basilic, internal jugular, and subclavian veins. The most commonly used sites are the internal jugular and subclavian sites. A large-bore needle is used percutaneously to puncture the vessel wall and is inserted into the vein. The catheter is advanced while the needle is held steady and then is threaded through the venous system until the distal tip rests in the vena cava or right atrium.

Central Venous Pressure Wave Form and Pressures

Figure 9-5 illustrates a typical CVP tracing, including the *a* wave, *x* wave descent, *c* and *v* waves, and the *y* wave descent. The *a* wave reflects the atrial contraction and follows the P wave on the electrocardiogram (ECG). The height of the *a* wave is dependent on how much pressure is generated by the atrium as it ejects blood into the ventricle at the end of diastole.

The *x* wave descent represents the fall in atrial pressure and CVP as the atrium relaxes. As the muscle fibers relax, fluid pressure diminishes as the muscle fibers elongate to their normal resting potential length. Another factor contributing to the fall in pressure is the downward pull on the atrioventricular (AV) junction during ventricular contraction.

The *c* wave reflects the closure of the tricuspid valve at the beginning of ventricular systole. As the tricuspid valve closes, pressure plateaus as it equalizes against the closed valve.

The *v* wave reflects the filling of the atrium during ventricular systole. As the atrium fills, pressure increases as the muscle fibers become stretched, peaking at a point when the atrium has filled completely with blood prior to contraction.

The *y* wave descent reflects the fall in pressure as the tricuspid valve opens, allowing the right ventricles to fill. As blood is emptied from the atria, CVP falls proportionately as the ventricles fill.

Normal CVP values range from 0 to 7 mm Hg (0 to 10 cm of H_2O). CVP varies with inspiration and expiration. As intrathoracic pressure decreases during a normal inspiratory effort, CVP falls (Figure 9-6). Therefore, CVP is always measured during resting exhalation. Positive intrathoracic pressure—as with mechanical ventilation, positive end-expiratory pressure (PEEP), continuous positive airway pressure (CPAP), or bilevel positive airway pressure (bi-PAP)—will elevate CVP pressures.

Clinical Applications of the Central Venous Pressure Catheter

The CVP catheter provides useful clinical information that may be applied to determine hypervolemia, hypovolemia, and right ventricular preload, and it is a convenient site for mixed venous blood sampling and for fluid administration. The CVP pressure is a direct reflection of vascular volume and venous return. As vascular volume increases, CVP values will also increase. It is important to correlate increased CVP with fluid intake and output data, daily weights, and blood pressures. An increase in the difference between the CVP and the mean systemic blood pressure (constant blood pressure) reflects an increase in systemic fluid volume (Kiess Daily, & Schroeder, 1994). An increased volume causes the atrium to be distended (stretched), increasing the reflected pressure into the vena cava owing to the increased pressures within the chamber.

A decrease in fluid volume causes the difference between the CVP and the mean systemic blood pressure (constant blood pressure) to fall until the pressure reaches zero, at which point the central veins begin to collapse (Kiess Daily, & Schroeder, 1994). Again, correlation with fluid intake and output helps to confirm the relevance of the CVP and mean arterial pressure as being truly reflective of changes in fluid volume.

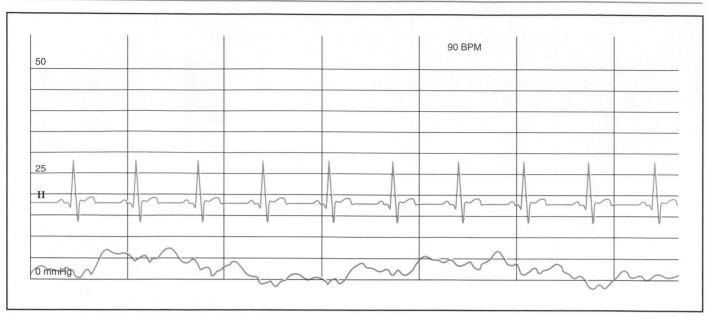

Figure 9-6 *Variation of the CVP with the ventilatory cycle, falling during inspiration*

The CVP (right atrial pressure) is reflective of right ventricular preload. During diastole when the ventricles are filling, the tricuspid valve is open, allowing the pressure in the right ventricle to be reflected back to the vena cava (Pascal's law). As CVP values increase, the preload of the right ventricle also increases. Clinically, it is important to optimize preload to obtain the greatest efficiency from the myocardial contraction. If preload is increased too much, the myocardium loses efficiency (Starling's law); therefore, optimization of preload is clinically important.

The CVP catheter also provides an important route for mixed venous blood sampling. The blood in the right atrium is a mixture of all of the venous blood returning to the heart from all parts of the body. Therefore, a blood sample from the right atrium represents a mixed sample and does not reflect any regional differences in oxygen consumption, as would a sample obtained from a more peripheral vein. Mixed venous samples are important clinically in that they are used to determine oxygen consumption and to determine the clinical shunt fraction.

Fluid administration is also enhanced by the placement of a CVP catheter. The CVP catheter is a large-bore catheter compared with most intravenous catheters. Therefore, when large volumes of fluid administration are required (fluid resuscitation), the CVP catheter can facilitate delivery of fluid.

PULMONARY ARTERY CATHETERS OR SWAN-GANZ CATHETERS

The *pulmonary artery catheter* or *Swan-Ganz catheter* is inserted percutaneously and threaded through the right heart with its distal tip resting in the *pulmonary artery* (Figure 9-7). The pulmonary artery catheter provides CVP or right atrial pressures, as does the CVP catheter, but it also provides measurement of the pulmonary artery pressure and *pulmonary artery wedge pressure (PAWP)*. Today, most Swan-Ganz catheters also have the capability to provide cardiac output data when coupled to an appropriate monitor. In addition to pressure monitoring and cardiac output monitoring, the Swan-Ganz catheter also provides a route for mixed venous sampling and fluid administration, just like the CVP catheter. Clinically, the Swan-Ganz catheter truly represents a leap forward in terms of its capabilities; however, hazards and complications increase proportionately with the length of time the catheter remains indwelling in the right side of the heart.

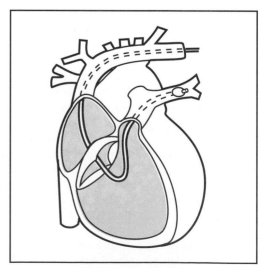

Figure 9-7 *Position of a pulmonary artery catheter within the heart*

Parts of a Pulmonary Artery Catheter

The pulmonary artery catheter is a multilumen catheter, with each lumen or port having a specific function. These ports include the proximal lumen, the distal lumen, the thermistor lumen, and the inflation lumen (Figure 9-8). The *proximal lumen*, when the catheter is correctly placed, rests either in the vena cava or in the right atrium. In this position, the pressure information provided by this port or lumen has the same clinical application of the CVP catheter discussed earlier in this chapter.

The *distal lumen* rests in the pulmonary artery when the catheter is correctly placed. The open distal end reflects the pressure in the pulmonary artery (when the balloon is deflated) and is a direct reflection of the right ventricular afterload, or the resistance that the right ventricle must overcome to eject blood.

The *thermistor lumen* is a lumen that contains the electrical conductors emanating from the *thermistor* located near the distal tip of the catheter. The thermistor is a temperature-sensitive resistor (electrical resistance changes proportionally to changes in temperature) that is used to measure cardiac output using the thermal dilution technique, which is discussed later in this chapter.

The *inflation lumen and balloon* are analogous to the pilot line and cuff of an endotracheal or tracheostomy tube. When air (approximately 1 to 2 ml) is injected into the inflation lumen, the balloon inflates. Balloon inflation is used to float the catheter through the right heart.

The pulmonary artery catheter is sometimes called a flow-directed catheter because of the use of the inflated balloon. Blood flow carries the catheter forward into the pulmonary artery until the diameter of the artery diminishes to the point that it becomes stuck, or "wedged." Once the catheter is wedged, the pressure measured at the distal tip (PAWP) reflects the pressure distal to it all the way to the left ventricle (when the mitral valve is opened), in accordance with Pascal's law.

Preferred Routes of Access

Several sites are used for the insertion of pulmonary artery catheters. These include the antecubital fossa and the basilic, internal jugular, and subclavian veins. The most commonly used sites are the internal jugular and subclavian sites. A large-bore needle is used percutaneously to puncture the vessel wall and is inserted into the vein. The catheter is advanced while the needle is held steady. Once the balloon is inflated, the catheter can be advanced through the venous system until the distal tip rests in the pulmonary artery.

Pulmonary Artery Catheter Wave Form Morphology

The morphology of the pressure tracing or wave form obtained from a pulmonary artery catheter varies with its position or location. Wave form characteristics are particularly important to observe and recognize as the catheter is advanced (Figure 9-9). The wave form undergoes distinct morphologic changes as the catheter passes from the right atrium to the right ventricle to the pulmonary artery and

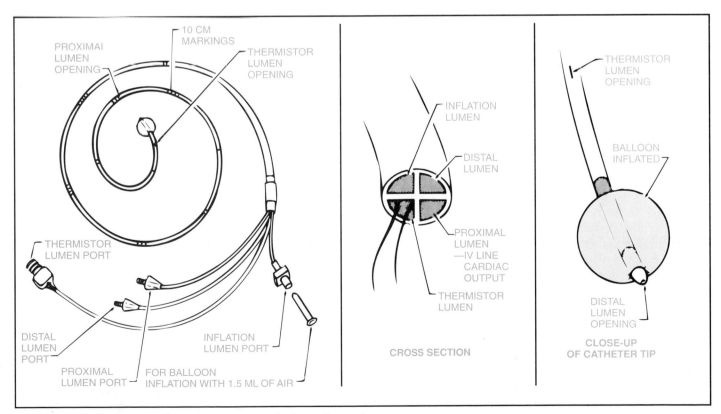

Figure 9-8 *A diagram identifying the components of a Swan-Ganz catheter*

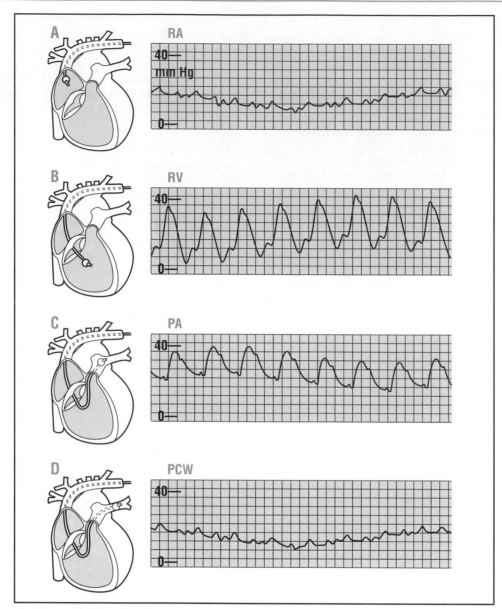

Figure 9-9 *Wave form characteristics during advancement of the pulmonary artery catheter: (A) right atrium (RA) and right atrial (central venous) wave form; (B) right ventricle (RV) and right ventricular wave form; (C) pulmonary artery (PA) and pulmonary arterial wave form; and (D) pulmonary capillary wedge (PCW) and pulmonary capillary wedge pressure wave form.*

finally to its wedged position. The ability to recognize these wave form characteristics is important in the identification of the correct placement of the catheter and in determining whether the catheter has become dislodged from its original placement position. Once the pulmonary artery catheter has been floated into position, the balloon is deflated. The balloon is subsequently inflated only when it is necessary to measure the pulmonary artery wedge pressure.

Pulmonary Artery Pressure and Pulmonary Artery Wedge Pressure Wave Form Morphology

It is important to recognize the morphology of the pulmonary artery pressure and pulmonary artery wedge pressure tracings. The morphology of the pressure tracings

is a direct result of the underlying physiologic, pathophysiologic, and cardiac cyclic events. Pressure changes are a direct reflection of changes in fluid volume (myocardial preload and afterload), changes in ventricular compliance, or vascular resistance to blood flow.

Pulmonary Artery Pressure Morphology

The pulmonary artery pressure tracing reflects pressure gradients caused by the systolic and diastolic events of the right ventricle. During systole, the ventricle contracts and the pulmonic valve opens, causing a rapid ejection of blood into the pulmonary artery. There is a subsequent rise in pressure as the blood fills the pulmonary artery (Figure 9-10). As the volume of blood decreases, the pressure values also decrease. Once the pressure in the pulmonary artery equals the pressure in the right ventricle,

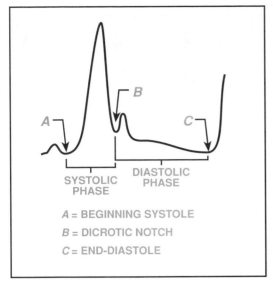

Figure 9-10 *Pulmonary arterial pressure (PAP) wave form: beginning systole (A), dicrotic notch (closure of semilunar valves) (B), and end-diastole (C).*

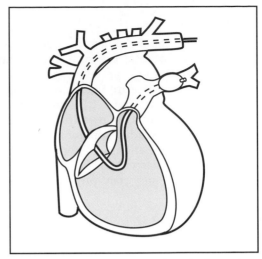

Figure 9-11 *The pulmonary artery catheter in the wedge position*

the pulmonic valve closes, causing a small dip in the pressure tracing (dicrotic notch) (see Figure 9-10).

During diastole, the right ventricle is filling. Because no additional blood is ejected into the pulmonary artery (pulmonic valve has closed), the pressure slowly decreases until just before the next systolic event (end-diastole).

The pulmonary artery pressure should be measured at end-diastole.

The respiratory cycle will affect the pulmonary artery pressure tracing. During inspiration (reduced intrathoracic pressure), the pulmonary artery pressure baseline falls. During exhalation (increased intrathoracic pressure), the baseline pressure increases. The pulmonary artery pressure should always be read at end-expiration.

Positive-pressure ventilation will also cause changes in the pulmonary artery pressure tracing. Positive intrathoracic pressures reduce venous return and therefore reduce the preload to the right ventricle, decreasing its output. Therefore, pulmonary artery pressures are typically lower during positive-pressure ventilation because less blood is ejected into the vessels (decreased cardiac output).

Pulmonary Artery Wedge Pressure Morphology

Once the balloon of the pulmonary artery catheter is inflated, blood flow carries the catheter forward until it wedges or becomes stuck, occluding blood flow as the vessel narrows. Once the catheter is wedged, the distal tip of the catheter reflects pressures distal to the point at which it has become wedged (Figure 9-11). This pressure reflects events occurring in the left atrium and left ventricle (when the mitral valve is opened during diastole). This is so because the pulmonary vasculature lacks the valves present in the systemic vasculature, and Pascal's law applies. The morphology of the PAWP is similar to that of the right atrial or central venous pressure tracing.

The pulmonary artery wedge pressure tracing consists of the *a* wave, the *x* descent, the *v* wave, and the *y* descent (Figure 9-12). These pressure changes are caused by the cardiac cycle of the left atrium and ventricle. The *a* wave is produced as a result of left atrial contraction, the pressure wave building with myocardial fiber contraction. The *x* descent reflects the fall in pressure that occurs following left atrial systole. The *v* wave pressure increase is a result of filling of the left atrium during diastole. The *y* descent occurs after the mitral valve opens, when blood passively fills the left ventricle.

Like the pulmonary artery pressure tracing, the pulmonary artery wedge pressure tracing is also affected by spontaneous respiration and positive-pressure ventilation. During inspiration (reduced intrathoracic pressure), the pulmonary artery pressure baseline falls. During exhalation (increased intrathoracic pressure), the baseline pressure increases. The pulmonary artery wedge pressure should always be read at end-expiration.

Positive-pressure ventilation will also cause changes in the pulmonary artery pressure tracing. Positive intrathoracic pressures reduce venous return and therefore reduce the preload to the right ventricle, decreasing its output. Therefore, pulmonary artery pressures are typically lower during positive-pressure ventilation because less blood is ejected into the vessels (decreased cardiac output).

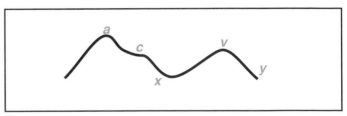

Figure 9-12 *Pulmonary capillary wedge pressure (PCWP) wave form: a wave: left atrial contraction; c wave (may be absent): closure of mitral valve; x downslope (descent): decrease of left atrial pressure following atrial contraction; v wave: left ventricular contraction and passive atrial filling; y downslope (descent): decrease of blood volume (pressure) following the opening of mitral valve*

NORMAL PRESSURE RANGES

It is important to recognize what the normal pressure ranges are for the right atrial pressure, right ventricular pressure, pulmonary artery pressure, and pulmonary artery wedge pressure. Pressure values reflect right ventricular preload, afterload, and left ventricular preload. Once you commit the normal ranges to memory, abnormal values will become more readily apparent, enhancing your grasp of the clinical applications of the pulmonary artery catheter in patient management. Table 9-1 summarizes the normal ranges for these important pressure values.

CLINICAL APPLICATIONS OF THE PULMONARY ARTERY CATHETER

The pulmonary artery catheter provides very important clinical information regarding fluid volume, right and left heart preloads and function, cardiac output, mixed venous saturation and sampling, and the vascular resistance of the pulmonary and systemic systems. As a respiratory care practitioner, you must know the normal values and how abnormal values relate to fluid balance and cardiac function.

Fluid Volume and Venous Return

When the pulmonary artery catheter is positioned correctly, its proximal port rests in the right atrium or vena cava. In the previous discussion of central venous pressure, you learned that an increase in CVP or right atrial pressures with a constant systolic blood pressure reflects an increase in fluid volume, and that the converse is also true. As stated previously, it is important to correlate the right atrial pressure or CVP with fluid intake and output, systemic blood pressure, and daily weights because the pressures measured reflect only a small part of the data necessary for correct decision making.

Assessment of Right Ventricular Function

The pulmonary artery catheter provides a means to assess right ventricular function, including preload and afterload. As discussed previously, the right atrial pressure (CVP) reflects the preload or stretch of the right ventricle. Increasing right atrial pressures indicate ejection of greater volumes of blood into the right ventricle, and the converse is also true.

The pulmonary artery pressure reflects the pressure that the right ventricle must work against to eject blood. Increased pulmonary artery pressure increases the afterload of the right ventricle, increasing the work required to pump blood. Common causes of increased pulmonary artery pressures include increased pulmonary vascular resistance, mitral stenosis, left ventricular failure (decreased compliance), increased fluid volume, and positive-pressure ventilation.

A decrease in pulmonary artery pressure results in a decreased afterload of the right ventricle. A decrease in afterload results in less work that the right ventricle must overcome. Decreased pulmonary artery pressure may be caused by hypovolemia or reduced venous return.

TABLE 9-1: Normal Pressure Ranges

	MEAN	SYSTOLIC	DIASTOLIC
Right atrium	0–8 mm Hg 0–11 cm H_2O		
Right ventricle	10–22 mm Hg 13–30 cm H_2O	15–28 mm Hg 20–36 cm H_2O	0–8 mm Hg 0–11 cm H_2O
Pulmonary artery	10–22 mm Hg 13–18 cm H_2O	15–28 mm Hg 20–36 cm H_2O	5–16 mm Hg 7–22 cm H_2O
Pulmonary artery wedge	6–12 mm Hg 8–16 cm H_2O		

Assessment of Left Ventricular Preload

Measurement of the pulmonary artery wedge pressure (with balloon inflated and wedged) reflects the preload of the left ventricle. The pulmonary artery wedge pressure at end-diastole (while the mitral valve is still open) reflects the filling pressure or preload of the left ventricle. This is so because there is an absence of valves in the pulmonary vascular system, and Pascal's law applies.

It is important to note that the pulmonary artery wedge pressure is independent of pulmonary vascular resistance. This is true because once the catheter is wedged, blood flow distal to the inflated balloon has ceased. *Resistance* by definition is a change in pressure divided by a flow; because blood flow has stopped, resistance must be zero. Therefore, the pressure measured from the distal port of the catheter is the reflected pressure of the left atrium and left ventricle (when the mitral valve is open) during diastole.

A decreased pulmonary artery wedge pressure may be caused by hypovolemia or increased intrathoracic pressures (as with PEEP or CPAP), resulting in reduced venous return. Hypovolemia results in circulation of a lower volume of blood, causing a reduction in left ventricular filling pressure (Starling's law). Positive intrathoracic pressures result in decreased venous return and in reduced right ventricular output and PA pressures and, consequently, a lower filling pressure in the left ventricle.

An increased pulmonary artery wedge pressure may be caused by hypervolemia, left ventricular failure, or mitral stenosis. Hypervolemia causes increased left ventricular diastolic pressures because increased blood volume results in the distention of the ventricle (Starling's law). Left ventricular failure may manifest itself as an increased pulmonary artery wedge pressure because a decreased left ventricular compliance causes a concomitant increase in ventricular filling pressure. Mitral stenosis causes an increased resistance as the left ventricle fills, resulting in a higher reflected pressure to the pulmonary artery catheter.

Assessment of Cardiac Output

The pulmonary artery catheter uses a technique called *thermal dilution*, which allows the clinician to assess a patient's cardiac output. Cardiac output is what generates blood pressure and is the "engine" that drives the circulatory system. *Cardiac output* is a product of stroke volume multiplied by heart rate. The thermal dilution technique utilizes the cardiac output computer monitor and a cold solution to measure cardiac output.

A cold solution, usually 5% dextrose in water (D_5W) or normal (physiologic) saline, is injected through the proximal lumen of the pulmonary artery catheter into the right atrium. The temperature of the solution must be at least 4°C less than the patient's body temperature. If the cardiac output is less than 3 liters per minute or greater than 10 liters per minute, iced (0°C) injectate must be used. Blood flow carries the cold solution downstream to the thermistor lumen, where a temperature drop is detected. The cardiac output computer monitor measures the temperature change using the thermistor located near the distal tip of the catheter. The cardiac output computer monitor factors in the distance (proximal port to thermistor, usually 30 cm), amount of injectate (typically 10 ml), and the temperature change to determine the cardiac output. Thermal dilution cardiac output determination is very technique-dependent.

Several factors may alter the results of thermal dilution cardiac output measurements. These include patient position, the time required for injection of cold solution, respiratory phase when injection occurs (inspiration versus expiration), and whether the clinician injects solution unevenly (variance of pressures). Cardiac output should always be determined with the patient in the same position. It is not necessary to position the patient supine. However, the patient should always be in the same position (supine or semi-Fowler's, for example) every time cardiac output is determined. When you inject the cold solution, injection of 10 ml should take no longer than 4 seconds. It will take a strong, quick, and steady push on the syringe to move 10 ml of fluid through the narrow proximal lumen in the required time. Focus on the task at hand and concentrate on maintaining a firm, quick, and even force on the plunger of the syringe. The cold solution should always be injected during the expiratory phase of ventilation. Timing can be tricky, especially at higher ventilatory rates. Because variability exists in the technique, it is important to take several measurements.

When measuring cardiac output using thermal dilution technique, you should make at least three cardiac output determinations (more will be required if there is a high degree of variability). You should strive for all determinations to be within 10% of one another. When three values are plus or minus 10%, calculate the average for those three values.

Determination of Mixed Venous Oxygen Saturation

A pulmonary artery catheter provides a convenient route for mixed venous blood sampling through the proximal port, located in the right atrium. In addition, a specialized catheter is manufactured that incorporates fiberoptic technology into its design, allowing it to continuously monitor mixed venous oxygen saturation. Mixed venous oxygen saturation is normally 68% to 75%. The continuous monitoring of mixed venous saturation allows determination of

the patient's oxygen consumption ($CaO_2 - CvO_2$), and the oxygen supply ($10 (CaO_2 \times C.O.)$) and metabolic demand made by the body.

Determination of Pulmonary Vascular Resistance

As stated earlier, the pulmonary artery wedge pressure (with the balloon inflated) is independent of the pulmonary vascular resistance because blood flow has been halted. Therefore, the difference between the pulmonary artery pressure and the pulmonary artery wedge pressure is reflective of the pulmonary vascular resistance. The pulmonary vascular resistance may be calculated using the following formula:

$$PVR = \frac{PAWP - PA}{\text{cardiac output}} \times 80$$

Pulmonary vascular resistance may be increased by alveolar hypoxemia, acidemia, hypercapnia, positive intrathoracic pressures (as with PEEP or CPAP), vascular blockage, vascular compression, or vascular wall disease. Pulmonary vascular resistance may be decreased owing to pharmacologic agents (oxygen, isoproterenol, aminophylline, or calcium channel blockers) and humoral substances.

Determination of Systemic Vascular Resistance

The pulmonary artery catheter provides a convenient way to determine the systemic vascular resistance, which is the resistance the left ventricle must overcome to pump blood. Systemic vascular resistance may be calculated using the following formula:

$$SVR = \frac{\text{mean arterial pressure} - \text{central venous pressure}}{\text{cardiac output}} \times 80$$

Systemic vascular resistance may be increased owing to hypertension or vasopressor drugs (such as dopamine or norepinephrine). Decreased systemic vascular resistance may be the result of vasodilators (such as nitroglycerin, nitroprusside, or morphine) or hypovolemic or septic shock.

CASE STUDIES ILLUSTRATING THE APPLICATION OF A PULMONARY ARTERY CATHETER

In the previous section, you learned how central venous, pulmonary artery, and wedge pressures change in various disease states. You also learned how the pulmonary artery catheter enables you to measure cardiac output and pulmonary and systemic vascular resistances. In this section, these specific applications of the pulmonary artery catheter are applied to specific case studies or scenarios.

Determination of Hypovolemia

A 23-year-old female patient is admitted to your intensive care unit (ICU) following surgery. She was involved in a motor vehicle accident and suffered a fractured right femur, pelvis, and humerus. Her femoral fracture was a compound fracture requiring open reduction, and she suffered considerable blood loss in the field.

Her admitting blood pressure is 85/60 mm Hg and her heart rate is 125 beats per minute. Because of concerns about her hemodynamic status, a pulmonary artery catheter is inserted. On catheter insertion you obtain the following data:

RA   = 1 mm Hg
PA   = 18/3 mm Hg
PAWP = 6 mm Hg
$C(a-v)O_2$ = 8 vol %

where RA is right atrial pressure, PA is pulmonary artery pressure, PAWP is pulmonary artery wedge pressure, and $C(a-v)O_2$ is the arteriovenous oxygen content difference.

Interpretation of the Data

The data in combination with the patient's history suggest hypovolemia. The right atrial pressure reflects a low blood volume return to the right heart (right ventricular preload). The low pulmonary artery pressure and increased $C(a-v)O_2$ value suggest a low cardiac output, while the decreased pulmonary artery wedge pressure suggests a low left ventricular preload. The patient was treated by the administration of several units of blood.

Determination of Hypervolemia

You are assessing the hemodynamic status of a 43-year-old postoperative patient. Over the course of the past 12 hours, the resident in charge has been treating a low blood pressure with fluid administration. You obtain the following hemodynamic data following your first patient/ventilator system assessment:

BP   = 95/70 mm Hg
RA   = 10 mm Hg
PA   = 48/25 mm Hg
PAWP = 23 mm Hg
CO   = 7.4 L/min
$C(a-v)O_2$ = 3 vol %

Interpretation of the Data

The data suggest that the patient is experiencing fluid overload. The right atrial pressure reflects a high preload to the right ventricle from excessive fluid return to the right heart. Elevated pulmonary artery and pulmonary artery wedge pressures also reflect excessive fluid volumes. The elevated cardiac output is a result of the high fluid return and operation of the cardiac muscle at the upper limits of Starling's curve. The patient was treated with vasopressors and aggressive diuresis.

Assessment of Right Ventricular Failure

You are caring for an acutely ill 74-year-old patient with chronic obstructive pulmonary disease (COPD) admitted to your ICU. He is currently on 50% oxygen delivered by a Venturi mask. Because of concerns about his hemodynamic status and the possibility of impending respiratory failure, a pulmonary artery catheter is placed. You obtain the following set of data:

RA   = 8 mm Hg
PA   = 42/23 mm Hg
PAWP = 10 mm Hg
CO   = 3.4 L/min

Interpretation of the Data

The elevated right atrial pressure suggests an increased preload on the right ventricle. This could be caused by increased fluid return or by a decreased right ventricular compliance (infarction or failure). The elevated pulmonary artery pressure reflects an increased afterload to the right ventricle. The normal pulmonary artery wedge pressure, however, suggests normal preload to the left ventricle and normal left heart function. The cardiac output is diminished. If you calculate the pulmonary vascular resistance, it is substantially elevated. This set of data suggests right heart failure secondary to pulmonary hypertension (history of COPD).

Determination of Left Ventricular Failure

You are assessing the hemodynamic status of a patient in the cardiac care unit (CCU). She is 58 years of age and was admitted with an acute myocardial infarction 2 days ago through your Emergency Department. Her cardiac catheterization last night suggests obstruction in three of her coronary arteries. You obtain the following set of hemodynamic data before she is transferred for surgery:

RA   = 4 mm Hg
PA   = 32/26 mm Hg
PAWP = 23 mm Hg
CO   = 3.1 L/min
$C(a-v)O_2$ = 3 vol %

Interpretation of the Data

The normal right atrial pressure reflects a normal return to the right heart and normal preload. The elevated pulmonary artery pressure may be caused by increased pulmonary vascular resistance, mitral stenosis, or decreased left ventricular compliance. The elevated pulmonary artery wedge pressure confirms that left ventricular compliance is decreased. If you calculate the pulmonary vascular resistance, it is within normal limits. The decreased cardiac output is also suggestive of ventricular failure.

Assessment of the Effects Caused by Positive-Pressure Ventilation

You are assessing the hemodynamic data from a 58-year-old male patient who underwent coronary artery bypass grafting 7 hours earlier. He is on synchronized intermittent mandatory ventilation (SIMV) with a rate of 7 breaths per minute and a PEEP setting of 10 cm H_2O. You obtain the following hemodynamic data:

RA   = 2 mm Hg
PA   = 23/15 mm Hg
PAWP = 12 mm Hg
BP   = 100/70 mm Hg
CO   = 4.3 L/min

Interpretation of the Data

The right atrial pressure is on the low side of normal, reflecting a decrease in blood volume returning to the heart. Although this could be caused by hypovolemia, in this case it is due to increased intrathoracic pressure. The pulmonary artery and pulmonary artery wedge pressures are normal, reflecting a normal pulmonary vascular resistance and left heart function. The reduction in cardiac output would also match the suggestion of diminished venous return to the heart from elevated intrapleural pressures.

ARTERIAL LINES

An arterial line provides several types of data helpful in the management of critically ill patients. It is a convenient site for arterial blood sampling and real-time measurement of the systemic blood pressure. Besides real-time digital data, an analog graphic display can be used to reflect the systolic and diastolic characteristics of the blood pressure tracing.

Preferred Routes of Vessel Access

The two preferred routes for the insertion of arterial lines are the radial and femoral arteries. Generally, the radial site is preferred owing to presence of collateral circulation (ulnar artery) and ease of vessel access. The femoral site carries with it increased risk of complications, which include loss of the limb with venal injury (because there is no collateral circulation) and the likelihood of arterial plaque that may become dislodged with catheter placement.

When the catheter has been correctly placed, an introducer needle is used to puncture the desired artery. The catheter is advanced while holding the introducer needle steady. After successful placement of the catheter, the introducer needle is removed. The arterial catheter is then secured, resting inside the vessel.

Parts of an Arterial Pressure Wave Form

Figure 9-13 illustrates a typical arterial pressure wave form. The rapid upstroke between C and A reflects the rapid change in pressure that occurs as the ventricles contract. As they contract, blood is rapidly ejected into the arterial system, causing a rapid rise in pressure. The downward slope from A to C reflects the fall in pressure that occurs during diastole. During diastole, the ventricles are passively filling as the ventricles relax. The dicrotic notch B reflects the closure of the semilunar valves. The lowest point on the pressure tracing reflects the end-diastolic pressure, whereas the highest point of the tracing is the systolic pressure. Normal values for arterial pressures are 100 to 140 mm Hg systolic and 60 to 90 mm Hg diastolic.

HAZARDS WITH INDWELLING VASCULAR CATHETERS

Hazards with indwelling vascular catheters include ischemia, infection, and hemorrhage. The pulmonary artery catheter also carries with it the additional risk of cardiac arrhythmias and, in rare instances, pulmonary artery rupture with inflation of the balloon.

Ischemic complications of indwelling vascular catheters are usually secondary to thrombus or embolus formation. The thrombus or embolus then is carried distal to the catheter, where it becomes lodged, resulting in ischemic injury. The arterial catheter is always maintained with a constant drip of heparin to prevent thrombus formation.

Hemorrhage can occur if the vascular catheter becomes accidentally dislodged or if the sampling port is inadvertently left open. Proper securing of the catheter and care with its use in sampling blood are important in the prevention of this complication.

Infection is always a hazard when any invasive procedure is performed. Therefore, strict use of aseptic techniques is essential; in addition, adherence to standard precautions is required in work with vascular catheters.

The pulmonary artery catheter has its unique hazards and complications. Presence of this catheter may lead to cardiac arrhythmias. Because the catheter passes through the heart, myocardial irritation may result, causing arrhythmias. In rare instances, when the balloon is inflated to measure the pulmonary artery wedge pressure, pulmonary artery rupture may occur (Kiess Daily, & Schroeder, 1994). This complication is usually associated with patients of advanced age with hypertension.

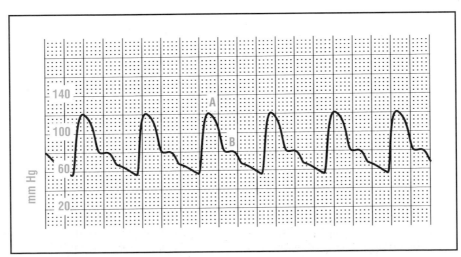

Figure 9-13 *Normal arterial pressure wave form. The systolic and diastolic pressures are about 120 mm Hg and 60 mm Hg, respectively: systolic peak (A); dicrotic notch (B)*

OBJECTIVES

At the end of this chapter, you should be able to:

- Assemble the equipment required for hemodynamic pressure monitoring.
- Demonstrate how to set up the equipment needed for hemodynamic pressure monitoring.
- Demonstrate how to zero the pressure-monitoring system.
- Demonstrate how to correctly locate the phlebostatic axis and level the transducer to that point.
- Recognize and describe four causes of a damped wave form.

- Demonstrate how to correctly wedge a pulmonary artery catheter.
- Recognize overwedging and describe what may cause it.
- Demonstrate how to measure cardiac output using the thermodilution technique.
- Demonstrate how to maintain an arterial line.
- Demonstrate how to zero an arterial line transducer.

EQUIPMENT REQUIRED FOR HEMODYNAMIC MONITORING

The equipment required for hemodynamic monitoring is similar for CVP, pulmonary artery, and arterial catheters. Table 9-2 lists the equipment required for hemodynamic pressure monitoring.

Infection is one of the hazards of placement and use of indwelling vascular catheters. Therefore, in assembling and preparing the equipment, it is important to maintain aseptic technique.

EQUIPMENT SETUP AND PREPARATION

It is important to prepare your equipment carefully, using aseptic technique as described earlier. Also, embolism is one of the hazards of invasive vascular catheters. Therefore, you must always remove any air bubbles from the tubing, transducer, and connections. Air bubbles will also cause damping of the wave form (discussed later) because they become compressed and the fluid does not.

Medication Preparation

When preparing equipment to monitor hemodynamic pressures, mix the heparin to the correct concentration. Add 500 units of heparin to the 500-ml normal saline bag. Note the medication and dosage on the medication label and affix it to the solution bag. For heparinizing an arterial solution bag, up to 1000 units may be added to the 500-ml solution bag.

Spiking the Bag and Priming the Tubing

Using the pressurized intravenous (IV) tubing, aseptically spike (pierce) the solution bag. Ensure that the air is removed from the bag. Prime the tubing by allowing solution to flow through it and ensure that all bubbles have been removed; then close the stopcock. Insert the solution bag into the pressure bag. Increase the pressure in the pressure bag to 300 mm Hg by pumping up the hand bulb.

TABLE 9-2: Equipment Required for Hemodynamic Monitoring

	CVP CATHETER	PA CATHETER	ARTERIAL CATHETER
500-ml bag of 0.9% saline	X	X	X
500 units of heparin	X	X	X
Medication label	X	X	X
Pressure bag	X	X	X
Disposable transducer	X	X	X
Transducer holder	X	X	X
Pressure monitoring cable	X	X	X
IV pressure tubing	X	X	X
Pressure monitor	X	X	X

Transducer Preparation

Insert the disposable transducer into its holder. Attach the monitoring cable to its connection on the transducer and the other end to the pressure monitor or patient monitoring system. Attach the infusion IV line to the transducer, locking it into place. Place a three-way stopcock on the other port of the transducer and connect the patient catheter to it.

ZEROING THE TRANSDUCER

All physiologic hemodynamic monitoring is referenced to atmospheric pressure, which by convention is zero. Therefore, it is important to "zero" the transducer before making measurements so that the pressure is always referenced to the same value. You must zero the transducer on initial setup and preparation and at the beginning of each shift. By doing so, you know all measurements made will have the same reference point.

When you zero the transducer for CVP or pulmonary artery pressure measurements, the transducer should be at the same level as the patient's *phlebostatic axis*. Identification of the phlebostatic axis is described in the next section. Once this reference point has been identified, the transducer should be located at the same height. A carpenter's level is a helpful tool to ensure that the transducer and the phlebostatic axis are on the same plane.

Zero the transducer by first turning off the system to the patient (closing the stopcock) and then opening the reference stopcock to air. This sequence will allow the system to equilibrate to atmospheric pressure. Allow a few seconds for equilibration and then depress the zero button or switch on the monitor.

IDENTIFICATION OF THE PHLEBOSTATIC AXIS

It is assumed that the CVP and pulmonary artery catheters are located in the middle of the chest. When making mea-

surements, ensure that the patient is positioned supine and level. Once the patient has been positioned, identify the phlebostatic axis on the patient's axilla. This reference point is identified by the midaxillary line at the junction of the fourth rib.

Once the axis has been identified, as described, position the transducer in the same plane by using a carpenter's level. If the transducer is higher than the phlebostatic axis, pressure readings will be lower. Conversely, if the transducer is located lower than the phlebostatic axis, pressures will be higher. These pressure variations are caused by the gravitational effect on the fluid in the lines.

WAVE FORM DAMPING

A damped (suppressed) wave form is important to recognize. Figures 9-14 and 9-15 illustrate a normal arterial wave form and a damped arterial wave form. Wave form

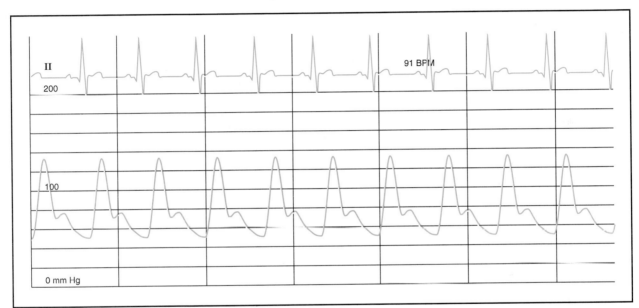

Figure 9-14 *A damped arterial pressure wave form*

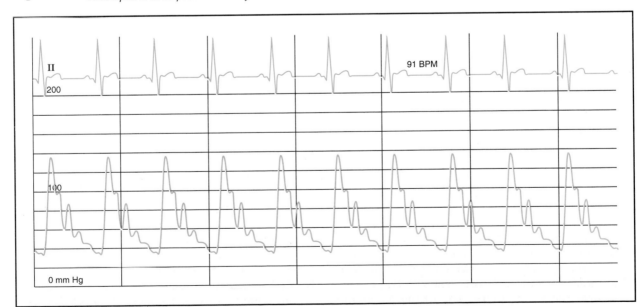

Figure 9-15 *A normal arterial pressure wave form*

damping may occur during monitoring of any hemodynamic data. Damping may be caused by several factors, including air in the system, improper zeroing of the transducer, blood clots in the system, catheter occlusion (clots, balloon, tip touching the vessel wall), leaks in the system, inadequate pressure in the pressure bag, and kinks in the tubing.

OBTAINING A PULMONARY ARTERY WEDGE PRESSURE

As described in previous sections, the pulmonary artery wedge pressure is measured when the balloon on the pulmonary artery catheter is inflated and wedged in the pulmonary artery. Correct wedging is important to obtain accurate data but also for patient safety.

Check to ensure that the transducer is located at the phlebostatic axis and that it is zeroed with the patient in a supine level position. Observe the pressure monitor and verify that the wave form displayed is the pulmonary artery wave form and that pressures correspond as such. Draw air into a tuberculin syringe and attach it to the inflation lumen of the catheter. Run a continuous strip on your monitor. Inject approximately 0.8 cc of air into the inflation lumen while observing the pressure monitor. Inject only enough air to obtain the desired wedged wave form. Observe for the wave form to change from the pulmonary artery pressure morphology to the wedge pressure morphology. Once the catheter is wedged, keep it wedged until pressures stabilize and the patient has breathed for several ventilatory cycles. Evacuate air from the balloon by withdrawing the syringe and observe for the monitor to return to the pulmonary artery wave form characteristics. Last, stop the continuous strip recording.

OVERWEDGING OF THE BALLOON

If too much air is injected, a damped pulmonary artery wedge wave form will result. Do not inject more than 1 to 1.5 cc of air into the inflation lumen of the catheter. If you suspect you have overwedged the catheter, withdraw all air from the inflation lumen. Next, verify that you have the correct pulmonary artery wave form morphology. Then inject only enough air to obtain the desired pulmonary artery wedge wave form morphology.

CARDIAC OUTPUT DETERMINATION

It is not imperative that the patient always be positioned supine for cardiac output determination; however, the patient should be in the same position (supine or semi-Fowler's, for example) each time these measurements are performed. Change the monitor's function to cardiac output determination and ensure that you have a supply of cold injectate (D_5W or normal saline). Draw up 10 ml of injectate and attach the syringe to the proximal port. Trigger the monitor to prompt you when to begin your injection. Once instructed to do so, firmly push the syringe's contents into the proximal port's lumen. You

have approximately 4 seconds to complete the injection. Observe your data and obtain three values within 10% of one another. Take the average of these results for the cardiac output value.

ARTERIAL LINE MAINTENANCE

Maintenance of an arterial line is facilitated by using heparinized solution in the pressure bag. Also, the catheter should be flushed periodically using a syringe and heparinized solution. The catheter should be checked frequently for loose connections because a leak could result in severe hemorrhage. Pulses should also be checked proximal and distal to the catheter to verify that circulation has not been impaired.

ZEROING AN ARTERIAL LINE

The transducer assembly for an arterial line is usually taped to the patient's limb, proximal to the insertion point of the catheter (Figure 9-16). Therefore, the phlebostatic axis or leveling of the transducer is not required. However, the transducer must be zeroed just as for the pulmonary artery and CVP catheters. Turn off the system to the patient by rotating the stopcock. Open the reference stopcock to atmospheric pressure, allow for equilibration, and zero the monitor.

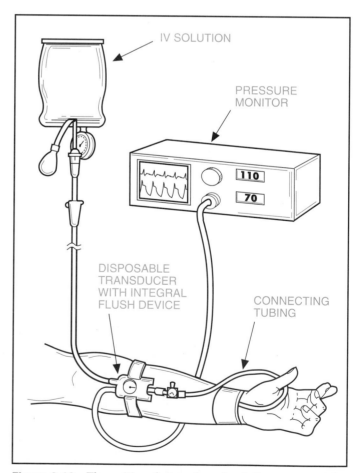

Figure 9-16 *The position of a transducer in relation to an arterial catheter*

References

Kiess Daily, E., & Schroeder, J. S. (1994). *Techniques in bedside hemodynamic monitoring* (5th ed.). St. Louis, MO: Mosby–Year Book.

Additional Resources

Chang, D. W. (1997). *Clinical application of mechanical ventilation.* Clifton Park, NY: Delmar Learning.

Des Jardins, T. R. (1993). *Cardiopulmonary anatomy and physiology* (2nd ed.). Clifton Park, NY: Delmar Learning.

Mowreader, M. (1995). *Hemodynamics learning module.* Unpublished manuscript. Sacred Heart Medical Center, Spokane, WA.

Wilkins, R. L. (1995). *Clinical assessment in respiratory care* (3rd ed.). St. Louis, MO: Mosby–Year Book.

Practice Activities: CVP and Pulmonary Artery Catheter Monitoring

1. In the laboratory, assemble all of the equipment required to monitor the CVP and pulmonary artery pressures:
   a. 500-ml normal saline solution bag
   b. 500 units of sodium heparin
   c. Medication label
   d. IV tubing
   e. Disposable transducer and holder
   f. Stopcocks
   g. Pressure bag
   h. Transducer cable
   i. Monitor

2. Using your laboratory setup, prime the tubing and purge it of all air.

3. Close the distal port and practice zeroing the transducer in the laboratory.

4. Using a laboratory partner, correctly position him/her and identify the phlebostatic axis.

5. Level the transducer to the same plane as for the phlebostatic axis using your laboratory partner.

6. In the laboratory, insert a pulmonary artery catheter into a basin of water. Practice inflating the balloon with air and injecting 10 ml of saline.

Practice Activities: Arterial Line Monitoring

1. In the laboratory, assemble all of the equipment required to monitor arterial pressures:
   a. 500-ml normal saline solution bag
   b. 500 units of sodium heparin
   c. Medication label
   d. IV tubing
   e. Disposable transducer and holder
   f. Stopcocks
   g. Pressure bag
   h. Transducer cable
   i. Monitor

2. Using your laboratory setup, prime the tubing and purge it of all air.

3. Close the distal port and practice zeroing the transducer in the laboratory.

4. Practice flushing an arterial catheter set up in the laboratory using 3 to 5 ml of saline.

Check List: CVP and Pulmonary Artery Catheter Monitoring

1. Assemble and prepare the required equipment:
   ___ a. 500-ml normal saline solution bag
   ___ b. 500 units of sodium heparin
   ___ c. Medication label
   ___ d. IV tubing
   ___ e. Disposable transducer and holder
   ___ f. Stopcocks
   ___ g. Pressure bag
   ___ h. Transducer cable
   ___ i. Monitor
   ___ 2. Purge all air and prime the system with flush solution.

___ 3. Identify the phlebostatic axis and level the transducer.

___ 4. Zero the transducer.

___ 5. Obtain the pulmonary artery pressure measurement.

___ 6. Wedge the catheter and obtain the pulmonary artery wedge pressure measurement.

___ 7. Measure the cardiac output.

___ 8. Document all findings and affix the strip chart recording to the appropriate location in the patient's chart.

___ 9. Maintain aseptic technique at all times.

Check List: Arterial Line Monitoring

1. Assemble and prepare the required equipment:
   _____ a. 500-ml normal saline solution bag
   _____ b. 500 units of sodium heparin
   _____ c. Medication label
   _____ d. IV tubing
   _____ e. Disposable transducer and holder
   _____ f. Stopcocks
   _____ g. Pressure bag

   _____ h. Transducer cable
   _____ i. Monitor
   _____ 2. Purge all air and prime the system with flush solution.
   _____ 3. Zero the transducer.
   _____ 4. Obtain a tracing and record your values.
   _____ 5. Maintain aseptic technique at all times.
   _____ 6. Document your results in the patient's chart.

Self-Evaluation Post Test: Hemodynamic Monitoring

1. Which of the following best describes Pascal's law?
   a. Volume changes proportionally with the pressure at the same temperature.
   b. The pressure in a closed system is the same at different points in the system.
   c. Pressure varies inversely with the temperature at the same volume.
   d. Volume varies inversely with temperature at the same pressure.

2. What is the purpose of a transducer in a hemodynamic monitoring system?
   a. It measures pressures.
   b. It converts a physical parameter into an electrical signal.
   c. It separates the blood from the infusion fluid.
   d. It converts cm H_2O to mm Hg.

3. Which of the following can a central venous catheter (CVP) determine?
   I.   Right ventricular preload
   II. Right ventricular afterload
   III. Left ventricular preload
   IV. Cardiac output
   a. I   c. I, II, III
   b. I, II   d. I, II, III, IV

4. Which of the following can a pulmonary artery catheter determine?
   I.   Right ventricular preload
   II. Right ventricular afterload
   III. Left ventricular preload
   IV. Cardiac output
   a. I   c. I, II, III
   b. I, II   d. I, II, III, IV

5. Which of the following pressures is a measure of right ventricular afterload?
   a. CVP   c. PA
   b. RA   d. PAWP

6. Which of the following pressures is a measure of left ventricular preload?
   a. CVP   c. PA
   b. RA   d. PAWP

7. You are assigned to the ICU and are caring for a patient who experienced traumatic injury. Owing to blood loss, the patient was aggressively fluid resuscitated 24 hours ago. You obtain the following hemodynamic data:

   RA   = 7 mm Hg
   PA   = 48/30 mm Hg
   PAWP = 24 mm Hg
   CO   = 7.3 L/min
   BP   = 110/74 mm Hg

   Which of the following assessments best matches your data?
   a. The patient is hypovolemic.
   b. The patient is experiencing right heart failure.
   c. The patient is experiencing left heart failure.
   d. The patient is experiencing fluid overload.

8. You are assigned to the CCU and are assessing a patient who was admitted yesterday for chest pain. His heart rate is 125 beats per minute. You obtain the following hemodynamic data:

   RA   = 4 mm Hg
   PA   = 40/28 mm Hg
   PAWP = 24 mm Hg
   CO   = 3.2 L/min

   Which of the following assessments best matches your data?
   a. The patient is hypovolemic.
   b. The patient is experiencing right heart failure.
   c. The patient is experiencing left heart failure.
   d. The patient is experiencing fluid overload.

9. Given the following set of data:
   CO   = 4.3 L/min
   PAWP = 15 mm Hg
   PA   = 45/30 mm Hg
   RA   = 8 mm Hg

   calculate the pulmonary vascular resistance:
   a. 419 dynes•sec•cm^{-5}
   b. 130 dynes•sec•cm^{-5}
   c. 279 dynes•sec•cm^{-5}
   d. 539 dynes•sec•cm^{-5}

10. Which of the following is a hazard/are hazards of indwelling vascular catheters?
    I.   Infection
    II. Emboli
    III. Hemorrhage
    IV. Arrhythmias
    a. I
    b. I, II
    c. I, II, III
    d. I, II, III, IV

PERFORMANCE EVALUATION:
CVP AND PULMONARY ARTERY CATHETER MONITORING

Date: Lab _____ Clinical _____ Agency _____

Lab: Pass _____ Fail _____   Clinical: Pass _____ Fail _____

Student name _____   Instructor name _____

No. of times observed in clinical _____

No. of times practiced in clinical _____

PASSING CRITERIA: Obtain 90% or better on the procedure. Tasks indicated by * must receive at least 1 point, or the evaluation is terminated. Procedure must be performed within designated time, or the performance receives a failing grade.

SCORING:
2 points — Task performed satisfactorily without prompting.
1 point — Task performed satisfactorily with self-initiated correction.
0 points — Task performed incorrectly or with prompting required.
NA — Task not applicable to the patient care situation.

TASKS:		PEER	LAB	CLINICAL
*	1. Practices standard precautions, including washing hands	☐	☐	☐
*	2. Assembles and prepares the required equipment			
	a. 500-ml normal saline solution bag	☐	☐	☐
	b. 500 units of sodium heparin	☐	☐	☐
	c. Medication label	☐	☐	☐
	d. IV tubing	☐	☐	☐
	e. Disposable transducer and holder	☐	☐	☐
	f. Stopcocks	☐	☐	☐
	g. Pressure bag	☐	☐	☐
	h. Transducer cable	☐	☐	☐
	i. Monitor	☐	☐	☐
*	3. Sets up and primes the tubing, purging it of air	☐	☐	☐
*	4. Positions the patient, identifying the phlebostatic axis	☐	☐	☐
*	5. Zeroes the transducer	☐	☐	☐
*	6. Levels the transducer at the phlebostatic axis	☐	☐	☐
*	7. Obtains the pulmonary artery pressure measurement	☐	☐	☐
*	8. Wedges the catheter, obtaining the pulmonary artery wedge pressure	☐	☐	☐
*	9. Measures the cardiac output	☐	☐	☐
*	10. Documents all findings and affixes a strip to the chart	☐	☐	☐
*	11. Maintains aseptic technique at all times	☐	☐	☐

PERFORMANCE EVALUATION: ARTERIAL LINE MONITORING

Date: Lab _____ Clinical _____ Agency _____

Lab: Pass _____ Fail _____   Clinical: Pass _____ Fail _____

Student name _____   Instructor name _____

No. of times observed in clinical _____

No. of times practiced in clinical _____

PASSING CRITERIA: Obtain 90% or better on the procedure. Tasks indicated by * must receive at least 1 point, or the evaluation is terminated. Procedure must be performed within designated time, or the performance receives a failing grade.

SCORING:
2 points — Task performed satisfactorily without prompting.
1 point — Task performed satisfactorily with self-initiated correction.
0 points — Task performed incorrectly or with prompting required.
NA — Task not applicable to the patient care situation.

TASKS:

			PEER	LAB	CLINICAL
*	1.	Practices standard precautions, including washing hands	☐	☐	☐
*	2.	Assembles and prepares the required equipment	☐	☐	☐
		a. 500-ml normal saline solution bag	☐	☐	☐
		b. 500 units of sodium heparin	☐	☐	☐
		c. Medication label	☐	☐	☐
		d. IV tubing	☐	☐	☐
		e. Disposable transducer and holder	☐	☐	☐
		f. Stopcocks	☐	☐	☐
		g. Pressure bag	☐	☐	☐
		h. Transducer cable	☐	☐	☐
		i. Monitor	☐	☐	☐
*	3.	Sets up and primes the tubing, purging it of air	☐	☐	☐
*	4.	Zeroes the transducer	☐	☐	☐
*	5.	Obtains a tracing and records values	☐	☐	☐
*	6.	Documents all findings and affixes a strip to the chart	☐	☐	☐
*	7.	Maintains aseptic technique at all times	☐	☐	☐

SCORE:
Peer _____ points of possible 30; _____%
Lab _____ points of possible 30; _____%
Clinical _____ points of possible 30; _____%

TIME: _____ out of possible 20 minutes

STUDENT SIGNATURES

PEER: _____

STUDENT: _____

INSTRUCTOR SIGNATURES

LAB: _____

CLINICAL: _____

CHAPTER 10
NONINVASIVE MONITORING

INTRODUCTION

Noninvasive patient monitoring has become routine in the acute care setting. Advances in microcomputer and microchip technology with advancements in photospectrometry have allowed the development of small, reliable instruments. Being microprocessor-controlled, these instruments display data in real time—as events happen. Clinically, knowing immediately how your patient is responding is a tremendous advantage over having to wait for lab results to return.

Noninvasive monitoring, by definition, is ongoing assessment of the patient's condition without entry into the body (through body orifices or via puncture of the skin or vessels). Current noninvasive monitoring allows measurement of transcutaneous (through the skin) oxygen tension ($PtcO_2$), transcutaneous carbon dioxide tension ($PtcCO_2$), arterial oxygen saturation obtained by pulse oximetry (SpO_2), and end-tidal carbon dioxide ($PetCO_2$).

In this chapter you will learn about the purpose and clinical applications of noninvasive monitoring. You will also learn how the equipment operates and how to apply it correctly to your patients. As with all procedures, there are hazards and limitations associated with noninvasive monitoring techniques. An appreciation of these risks and limitations is important so that you can apply these techniques optimally in the acute care setting.

KEY TERMS

- End-tidal CO_2 monitor
- Heating element
- Mainstream monitor
- Pulse oximeter
- Sidestream monitor
- Thermocouple
- Transcutaneous CO_2 monitor
- Transcutaneous PO_2 electrode

OBJECTIVES

At the end of this chapter, you should be able to:

- Discuss the purpose and clinical applications of noninvasive monitoring.
- Describe the principles of operation for the following noninvasive monitors:

  — Pulse oximeter
  — Transcutaneous CO_2 monitor
  — Transcutaneous O_2 monitor
  — End-tidal CO_2 monitor
- Describe the limitations of noninvasive monitoring.
- Discuss the hazards of noninvasive monitoring.

CLINICAL PRACTICE GUIDELINES

AARC Clinical Practice Guideline
Pulse Oximetry

PO 4.0 INDICATIONS:
4.1 The need to monitor the adequacy of arterial oxyhemoglobin saturation (1,4,6,9)
4.2 The need to quantitate the response of arterial oxyhemoglobin saturation to therapeutic intervention (4,9,10) or to a diagnostic procedure (e.g., bronchoscopy)
4.3 The need to comply with mandated regulations (11,12) or recommendations by authoritative groups (13,14)

PO 5.0 CONTRAINDICATIONS:
The presence of an ongoing need for measurement of pH, $PaCO_2$, total hemoglobin, and abnormal hemoglobins may be a relative contraindication to pulse oximetry.

PO 6.0 HAZARDS/COMPLICATIONS:
Pulse oximetry is considered a safe procedure, but because of device limitations, false-negative results for hypoxemia (4) and/or false-positive results for normoxemia (15,16) or hyperoxemia (17,18) may lead to inappropriate treatment of the patient. In addition, tissue injury may occur at the measuring site as a result of probe misuse (e.g., pressure sores from prolonged application of electrical shock and burns from the substitution of incompatible probes between instruments). (19)

PO 8.0 ASSESSMENT OF NEED:
8.1 When direct measurement of SaO_2 is not available or accessible in a timely fashion, an SpO_2 measurement may temporarily suffice if the limitations of the data are appreciated. (9,10)
8.2 SpO_2 is appropriate for continuous and prolonged monitoring (e.g., during sleep, exercise, bronchoscopy). (1,6,7,9,10,14,31)
8.3 SpO_2 may be adequate when assessment of acid-base status and/or PaO_2 is not required. (1,4,9,10)

(Continued)

(CPG Continued)

PO 9.0 ASSESSMENT OF OUTCOME:

The following should be utilized to evaluate the benefit of pulse oximetry:

9.1 SpO_2 results should reflect the patient's clinical condition (i.e., validate the basis for ordering the test).

9.2 Documentation of results, therapeutic intervention (or lack of), and/or clinical decisions based on the SpO_2 measurement should be noted in the medical record.

PO 11.0 MONITORING:

The clinician is referred to Section 7.0 Validation of Results. The monitoring schedule of patient and equipment during continuous oximetry should be tied to bedside assessment and vital signs determinations.

Reprinted with permission from *Respiratory Care* 1991; 36: 1406–1409. The complete AARC Clinical Practice Guidelines are available from the AARC Web site (http://www.aarc.org), from the AARC Executive Office, or from *Respiratory Care Journal*.

AARC Clinical Practice Guideline Transcutaneous Blood Gas Monitoring for Neonatal & Pediatric Patients

TCM 4.0 INDICATIONS:

4.1 The need to monitor the adequacy of arterial oxygenation and/or ventilation (9,10)

4.2 The need to quantitate the response to diagnostic and therapeutic interventions as evidenced by $PtcO_2$ and/or $PtcCO_2$ values (9–11)

TCM 5.0 CONTRAINDICATIONS:

In patients with poor skin integrity and/or adhesive allergy, transcutaneous monitoring may be relatively contraindicated. (9)

TCM 6.0 HAZARDS/COMPLICATIONS:

$PtcO_2$ and/or $PtcCO_2$ monitoring is considered a safe procedure, but because of device limitations, false-negative and false-positive results may lead to inappropriate treatment of the patient. (10,12,13) In addition, tissue injury may occur at the measuring site (e.g., erythema, blisters, burns, skin tears). (1,8,10)

TCM 8.0 ASSESSMENT OF NEED:

8.1 When direct measurement of arterial blood is not available or accessible in a timely fashion, $PtcO_2$ and/or $PtcCO_2$ measurements may temporarily suffice if the limitations of the data are appreciated. (9)

8.2 Transcutaneous blood gas monitoring is appropriate for continuous and prolonged monitoring (e.g., during mechanical ventilation, CPAP, and supplemental oxygen administration). (9,10)

8.3 $PtcO_2$ values can be used for diagnostic purposes as in the assessment of functional shunts (e.g., persistent pulmonary hypertension of the newborn, PPHN, or persistent fetal circulation (21–23) or to determine the response to oxygen challenge in the assessment of congenital heart disease. (21–23)

TCM 9.0 ASSESSMENT OF OUTCOME:

9.1 Results should reflect the patient's clinical condition (i.e., validate the basis for ordering the monitoring). (3,5,7)

9.2 Documentation of results, therapeutic intervention (or lack of), and/or clinical decisions based on the transcutaneous measurements should be noted in the medical record.

TCM 11.0 MONITORING:

The monitoring schedule of patient and equipment during transcutaneous monitoring should be integrated into patient assessment and vital signs determinations. Results should be documented in the patient's medical record and should detail the conditions under which the readings were obtained:

11.1 The date and time of measurement, transcutaneous reading, patient's position, respiratory rate, and activity level;

11.2 Inspired oxygen concentration or supplemental oxygen flow, specifying the type of oxygen delivery device;

11.3 Mode of ventilatory support, ventilator, or CPAP settings;

11.4 Electrode placement site, electrode temperature, and time of placement;

11.5 Results of simultaneously obtained PaO_2, $PaCO_2$, and pH when available;

11.6 Clinical appearance of patient, subjective assessment of perfusion, pallor, and skin temperature.

Reprinted with permission from *Respiratory Care* 1994; 39: 1176–1179. The complete AARC Clinical Practice Guidelines are available from the AARC Web site (http://www.aarc.org), from the AARC Executive Office, or from *Respiratory Care* journal.

AARC Clinical Practice Guideline Capnography/Capnometry during Mechanical Ventilation

CO_2 MV 4.0 INDICATIONS:

On the basis of available evidence, capnography should not be mandated for all patients receiving mechanical ventilatory support, but it may be indicated for:

4.1 Evaluation of the exhaled $[CO_2]$, especially end-tidal CO_2, which is the maximum partial pressure of CO_2 exhaled during a tidal breath (just prior to the beginning of inspiration) and is designated PetCO$_2$; (5,6)

4.2 Monitoring severity of pulmonary disease (5) and evaluating response to therapy, especially therapy intended to improve the ratio of dead space to tidal volume (VD/VT) (7,8) and the matching of ventilation to perfusion (V/Q), (9) and, possibly, to therapy intended to increase coronary blood flow; (5,10,11)

4.3 Determining that tracheal rather than esophageal intubation has taken place (low or absent cardiac output may negate its use for this indication); (12–16)

4.4 Continued monitoring of the integrity of the ventilatory circuit, including the artificial airway; (12,15)

4.5 Evaluation of the efficiency of mechanical ventilatory support by determination of the difference between the arterial partial pressure for CO$_2$ (PaCO$_2$) and the PetCO$_2$; (17,18)

4.6 Reflecting CO$_2$ elimination; (19)

4.7 Monitoring adequacy of pulmonary and coronary blood flow; (10,11,20–22)

4.8 Monitoring inspired CO$_2$ when CO$_2$ gas is being therapeutically administered; (23)

4.9 Graphic evaluation of the ventilator-patient interface. Evaluation of the capnogram may be useful in detecting rebreathing of CO$_2$, obstructive pulmonary disease, waning neuromuscular blockade ("curare cleft"), cardiogenic oscillations, esophageal intubation, cardiac arrest, and contamination of the monitor or sampling line with secretions or mucus. (24)

CO$_2$ MV 5.0 CONTRAINDICATIONS:

There are no absolute contraindications to capnography in mechanically ventilated adults, provided that the data obtained are evaluated with consideration given to the patient's clinical condition.

CO$_2$ MV 6.0 HAZARDS/COMPLICATIONS:

Capnography with a clinically approved device is a safe, noninvasive test, associated with few hazards. With mainstream analyzers, the use of too large a sampling window may introduce an excessive amount of dead space into the ventilator circuit. (2,25) Care must be taken to minimize the amount of additional weight placed on the artificial airway by the addition of the sampling window or, in the case of a sidestream analyzer, the sampling line.

CO$_2$ MV 8.0 ASSESSMENT OF NEED:

Capnography is considered a standard of care during anesthesia. (12) The Society of Critical Care Medicine has suggested that capnography be available in every ICU. (39) Assessment of the need to use capnography with a specific patient should be guided by the clinical situation. The patient's primary cause of respiratory failure and the acuteness of his or her condition should be considered. Patients with severe dynamic disease, such as ARDS, should be considered candidates for capnography. (5,6)

CO$_2$ MV 9.0 ASSESSMENT OF OUTCOME:

Results should reflect the patient's condition and should validate the basis for ordering the monitoring. Documentation of results (along with all ventilatory and hemodynamic variables available), therapeutic interventions, and/or clinical decisions made based on the capnogram should be included in the patient's chart.

CO$_2$ MV 11.0 MONITORING:

During capnography the following should be considered and monitored:

11.1 Ventilatory variables: tidal volume, respiratory rate, positive end-expiratory pressure, inspiratory-to-expiratory time ratio (I:E), peak airway pressure, and concentrations of respiratory gas mixture (24,26)

11.2 Hemodynamic variables: systemic and pulmonary blood pressures, cardiac output, shunt, and ventilation-perfusion imbalances (24,26)

Reprinted with permission from *Respiratory Care* 1995; 40: 1321–1324. The complete AARC Clinical Practice Guidelines are available from the AARC Web site (http://www.aarc.org), from the AARC Executive Office, or from *Respiratory Care* journal..

RATIONALE FOR NONINVASIVE MONITORING

Noninvasive monitoring allows you to monitor in real time (immediately) a patient's oxygen saturation, partial pressure of oxygen, or partial pressure of carbon dioxide. Historically, this information was available only through blood gas analysis. Blood gas analysis is still the standard by which noninvasive monitors are compared, and by which monitoring data are related to the patient's condition. However, noninvasive monitoring has greatly reduced the number of arterial blood gas (ABG) samples drawn in the acute care setting.

By its very nature, noninvasive monitoring is more comfortable for the patient. There is less risk from infection or other complications associated with invasive techniques. Noninvasive monitoring also provides a continuous form of monitoring and tending, which is clinically very useful.

NONINVASIVE MONITORING EQUIPMENT

Pulse Oximeters

Pulse oximeters allow you to monitor the oxygen saturation in the arterial blood. Rather than directly measuring the saturation of the blood as a co-oximeter does (SaO_2), the pulse oximeter uses photospectrometry to measure the oxygen saturation of a capillary bed (SpO_2).

Pulse oximeters use two light-emitting diodes (LEDs) and a photodetector (Figure 10-1). One LED emits light that is red at a wavelength of approximately 660 nm, and the other emits infrared light at approximately 900 nm

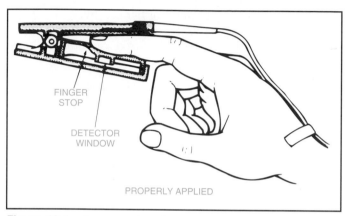

FINGER STOP

DETECTOR WINDOW

PROPERLY APPLIED

Figure 10-1   *A cross section of a pulse oximeter probe (Courtesy of Ohmeda Critical Care, a Division of the BOC Group, Inc., Columbia, MD)*

(Craig, 1990). The light passes through the capillary bed, and depending on the amount of saturated hemoglobin, the color of the vascular bed varies (desaturated hemoglobin being darker). Because oxygenated blood is more permeable to red light, the oximeter is able to relate this color change to oxygen saturation.

Common sites of measurement are the fingers, toes, and the ears. Different probes are designed for use at specific sites. Newborn and pediatric probes usually wrap around the foot (Figure 10-2).

Transcutaneous Monitors

Transcutaneous CO_2 Monitor

The *transcutaneous CO_2 monitor* is a modified PCO_2 electrode (Severinghaus electrode) with a heater incorporated into its design (Figure 10-3). The pH glass membrane is molded into a flat surface that is perpendicular to the surface of the skin. The pH glass membrane separates the measuring and reference electrodes. The heating element and thermocouple maintain skin temperatures at 44°C. The increased temperature arterializes the vascular bed under the electrode, increasing circulation to that area.

CO_2 diffuses across the skin and through the membrane (permeable only to CO_2) and is measured by the electrode. An airtight seal around the electrode prevents ambient air from entering the sample site.

Transcutaneous O_2 Monitor

The *transcutaneous PO_2 electrode* is a modified Clark electrode, incorporating the addition of a heating element and

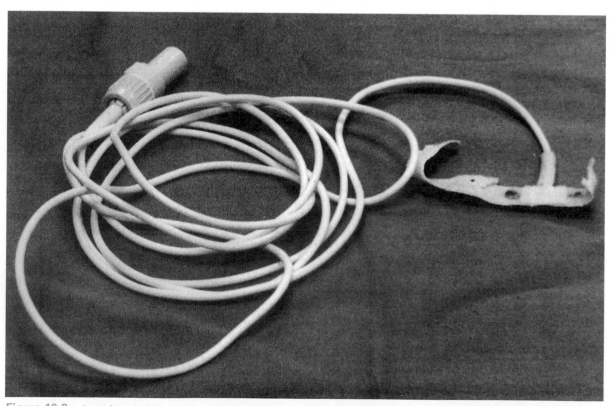

Figure 10-2   *A newborn/pediatric pulse oximeter probe*

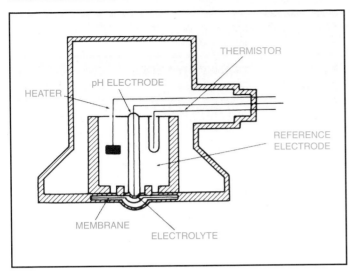

Figure 10-3 *A cross section of a transcutaneous CO_2 electrode (Courtesy of Novametrix Medical Systems, Wallingford, CT)*

a thermocouple. As in the transcutaneous PCO_2 electrode, the PO_2 electrode's heating element arterializes the sample site by increasing the skin temperature to 44°C. Oxygen diffuses through the skin and is measured by the electrode.

Combination PO_2 and PCO_2 Monitors

Some manufacturers make a combination PO_2 and PCO_2 transcutaneous electrode. In these designs both types of transcutaneous electrodes are incorporated into one sensor assembly. This combination allows the monitoring of the transcutaneous partial pressures of both gases with one instrument.

The principles of operation are identical to those of the individual instruments; only the design differs.

End-Tidal CO_2 Monitors

End-tidal CO_2 monitors are used to monitor the partial pressure of CO_2 in exhaled gas ($PetCO_2$). End-tidal CO_2 monitors are used in the anesthesia setting and the critical care setting to monitor the adequacy of ventilation.

End-tidal CO_2 monitors use infrared light absorption to measure the $PetCO_2$. CO_2 will absorb infrared light. The end-tidal CO_2 monitor compares CO_2 absorption between a reference chamber (no CO_2 present) and a sampling chamber (exhaled gas). The difference in absorption is proportional to the $PetCO_2$.

There are two types of end-tidal CO_2 monitors: *mainstream* and *sidestream*. The mainstream monitors use a sensor that is attached directly to the airway. The sidestream monitors draw the exhaled gas sample from the airway through a capillary tube to an analyzer that is located near the patient.

LIMITATIONS OF NONINVASIVE MONITORING

Although noninvasive monitoring has provided real-time data that facilitates good patient care, the values observed on the monitors do not always reflect the patient's true condition. Noninvasive monitors may provide inaccurate readings owing to the patient's physiological condition or other environmental influences. Therefore, it is important that as a respiratory care practitioner you understand the limitations of noninvasive monitors and use each type on patients who will benefit the most from the application of that particular monitor.

Limitations of Pulse Oximetry

Pulse oximetry is widely used in the acute care setting (Welch & DeCesare, 1990). Many respiratory care practitioners and other health care workers blindly accept the data obtained with these instruments as correct and accurate, when in fact the results obtained may be inaccurate for a variety of reasons. It is important to understand the limitations of these instruments so that they may be applied and utilized correctly. The factors that can influence their accuracy are listed in Table 10-1 (Craig, 1990; Welch & DeCesare, 1990).

As you can see from Table 10-1, many factors may influence the accuracy of these instruments. Therefore, it is important to correlate the readings from these instruments with ABG values and co-oximetry results. From this comparison you may recognize discrepancies and trend the data accordingly.

Limitations of Transcutaneous Monitoring

Transcutaneous monitoring, like pulse oximetry and other technologies, has its limitations. Understanding these limitations and knowing when to draw blood for ABG analysis is part of applying these instruments correctly in the acute care setting. The limitations of transcutaneous monitoring are summarized in Table 10-2 (Aloan, 1987; Martin, 1990).

TABLE 10-1: Factors Influencing Pulse Oximeter Accuracy
Motion
Sensor misalignment
Dysfunctional hemoglobin
Low perfusion states (patient hemodynamics)
Ambient light interference
Vascular dyes
Skin pigmentation and nail polish

TABLE 10-2: Limitations of Transcutaneous Monitoring
Edema of the skin
Insufficient heat applied to the skin from the electrode
Blistering from skin burns
Use of vasopressive drugs
Poor perfusion to the skin

TABLE 10-3: Limitations of End-Tidal CO_2 Monitoring

Shunt producing pulmonary disease

Pulmonary emboli

Tubing obstructions (sidestream devices)

As with pulse oximeters, readings from transcutaneous monitors should be correlated with ABG values and co-oximetry results. Frequent membrane changes, site changes, and calibrations help to minimize some of this technology's limitations.

Limitations of End-Tidal CO_2 Monitoring

End-tidal CO_2 monitoring also has its limitations. These limitations must be recognized, and appropriate tending with blood gas analysis initiated when appropriate. The limitations of end-tidal CO_2 monitoring are summarized in Table 10-3 (Hess, 1990).

TABLE 10-4: Hazards and Complications of Noninvasive Monitoring

PULSE OXIMETRY	TRANSCUTANEOUS MONITORING	END-TIDAL CO_2 MONITORING
Skin burns Pressure necrosis	Skin burns	Airway occlusion

HAZARDS OF NONINVASIVE MONITORING

As with most medical procedures and techniques, noninvasive monitoring has its risks as well as its benefits. Understanding the hazards and potential complications is important in the effective clinical application of these techniques. The hazards and complications are summarized in Table 10-4.

PROFICIENCY OBJECTIVES

At the end of this chapter, you should be able to:

- Assemble, test for function, and if required, calibrate the equipment required for noninvasive monitoring:
  — Pulse oximeter
  — Transcutaneous monitor
  — End-tidal CO_2 monitor
- Demonstrate how to correctly apply the noninvasive monitor to the patient:
  — Pulse oximeter
  — Transcutaneous monitor
  — End-tidal CO_2 monitor
- Observe the preliminary readings from the instrument and determine if the monitor has been applied correctly and is working normally.
- As required, correlate the data from the non-invasive monitor with ABG values.

ASSEMBLY, TROUBLESHOOTING, AND CALIBRATION

Pulse Oximeter

Assembly

Little assembly is required for most pulse oximeters. Many different manufacturers and models of pulse oximeters are used in the acute care setting. A general assembly guide, which should be generic enough for most models, is provided in Table 10-5.

Troubleshooting

Troubleshooting a pulse oximeter is not difficult but may take some sleuthing on your part to correct the problem. Table 10-6 is a summary of the most common problems that may require troubleshooting.

TABLE 10-5: Pulse Oximeter Assembly

1. Connect the power cord to a 110 V 60 Hz electrical outlet.
2. Connect the oximeter probe to the monitor:
   a. Finger probe
   b. Ear probe
   c. Pediatric probe
3. Turn on the power switch.
4. Wipe the probe clean using an alcohol prep pad before applying it to the patient.
5. Apply the probe to the patient:
   a. Finger
   b. Toe
   c. Ear
   d. Foot (infant or pediatric patient)
6. Observe for adequate wave forms (pulse signal) and reading.
7. Set alarm limits as required.

TABLE 10-6: Pulse Oximeter Troubleshooting

1. Patient site may be dirty. Clean the site with an alcohol prep pad.
2. Probe may be dirty. Clean the probe with an alcohol prep pad.
3. Probe may be misaligned. Check the probe placement and adjust it, or move it to a different site.
4. If the patient is wearing fingernail polish, remove it and reapply the probe.
5. If steps 1 through 4 have been checked and the oximeter is still not functioning, replace the probe.
6. If the room appears unusually bright (strong ambient light), shield the probe from the light using a towel or other covering.

Transcutaneous O_2 and CO_2 Monitors
Assembly

Many different types of transcutaneous monitors are employed in the acute care setting. When assembling the transcutaneous monitor in your clinical site, consult the owner's manual for specific information about your monitor. The information in Table 10-7 is a summary of assembly instructions that should apply to most monitors.

Troubleshooting

The common problems in transcutaneous monitors that may require troubleshooting are summarized in Table 10-8.

TABLE 10-7: Transcutaneous Monitor Assembly

1. Connect the monitor to a 110 V 60 Hz electrical outlet.
2. Calibrate the monitor to known gas levels of O_2 (using sodium sulfite and room air), CO_2 (usually 5% and 10% CO_2) as recommended by the manufacturer.
3. Attach a membrane to the electrode following the manufacturer's guidelines.
4. Adjust the temperature setting to the desired range.
5. Select an appropriate site and prep the site with a clean alcohol prep pad.
6. Apply a ring of double-sided tape to the electrode.
7. Place a drop of contact solution or distilled water onto the electrode and apply the electrode to the skin.
8. Allow the reading to stabilize and correlate the reading to blood gas values.

End-Tidal CO_2 Monitors
Assembly

Assembly instructions for end-tidal CO_2 monitors are summarized in Table 10-9.

Troubleshooting

Common sources of problems to look for in troubleshooting are summarized in Table 10-10.

TABLE 10-8: Transcutaneous Monitor Troubleshooting

1. If readings fluctuate or differ greatly from arterial blood gases:
   a. The membrane may need to be changed.
   b. The site may need to be changed.
   c. The site may be too edematous.
   d. The patient may be receiving vasoactive drugs.
   e. An air leak may be present. Change the site and reapply the electrode to the patient.

TABLE 10-9: End-Tidal CO_2 Monitor Assembly Instructions

1. Connect the monitor to a 110 V 60 Hz electrical outlet.
2. Calibrate the monitor to known CO_2 levels according to the manufacturer's instructions.
3. Connect the monitor to the patient's airway:
   a. Using the special adapter if using a sidestream monitor:
      (1) Adjust the sample flow until a plateau is seen on the capnograph.
   b. Directly to the airway if using a mainstream monitor.
4. Correlate the monitor's readings with ABG values.

TABLE 10-10: End-Tidal CO_2 Monitor Troubleshooting

1. If the readings vary significantly from blood gas values:
   a. Recalibrate the monitor.
   b. Clear the sampling tubing of moisture or secretions if using a sidestream monitor.
   c. Check the patient's history for indications of chronic obstructive lung disease, pulmonary embolism, left ventricular failure, or low perfusion (shock).

References

Aloan, C. A. (1987). *Respiratory care of the newborn*. Philadelphia: Lippincott.

American Association for Respiratory Care. (1991). AARC clinical practice guideline: Pulse oximetry. *Respiratory Care*, 36(12), 1406–1409.

American Association for Respiratory Care. (1994). AARC clinical practice guideline: Transcutaneous blood gas monitoring for neonatal & pediatric patients. *Respiratory Care*, 39(12), 1176–1179.

American Association for Respiratory Care. (1995). AARC clinical practice guideline: Capnography/capnometry during mechanical ventilation. *Respiratory Care*, 40(12), 1321–1324.

Craig, K. (1990, Summer). *Clinical performance limitations of pulse oximetry*. (Progress Notes). Carlsbad, CA: Puritan Bennett Corporation.

Hess, D. (1990). Capnometry and capnography: Technical aspects, physiologic aspects, and clinical applications. *Respiratory Care*, 35(6), 557–576.

Martin, R. J. (1990). Transcutaneous monitoring: Instrumentation and clinical applications. *Respiratory Care*, 35(6), 577–583.

Welch, J. P., & DeCesare, R. (1990). Pulse oximetry: Instrumentation and clinical applications. *Respiratory Care*, 35(6), 584–601.

Practice Activities: Noninvasive Monitoring

1. Practice setting up and calibrating (if required) the following noninvasive monitors:
   a. Pulse oximeter
   b. Transcutaneous CO_2 or O_2 monitor
   c. End-tidal CO_2 monitor:
      (1) Mainstream
      (2) Sidestream

2. Practice applying noninvasive monitors to your laboratory partner:
   a. Pulse oximeter
   b. Transcutaneous CO_2 or O_2 monitor
   c. End-tidal CO_2 monitor:
      (1) Mainstream
      (2) Sidestream

3. Troubleshoot the monitors if they fail to function properly.

4. With your laboratory partner, deliberately attempt to make the noninvasive monitor give erroneous readings:

   Pulse oximeter:
   a. Apply nail polish to your partner.
   b. Make the site dirty and apply the probe.
   c. Misalign the emitter and detector when applying the probe.
   d. Shine a strong light source on the probe when it is applied.

   Transcutaneous monitor:
   a. Create a small leak around the electrode's membrane.
   b. Fail to calibrate the monitor before applying it.
   c. Apply the electrode to a poorly perfused site.

   End-tidal CO_2 monitor:
   a. Fail to calibrate the monitor before applying it.
   b. Adjust the sample chamber flow so it is too low.
   c. Disconnect the probe to simulate an airway disconnection.

Check List: Pulse Oximeter Monitor

_____ 1. Verify the physician's order for a monitor.
_____ 2. Wash your hands.
3. Obtain the appropriate equipment as required:
_____ a. Pulse oximeter
_____ b. Probe(s)
_____ c. Alcohol prep pads
_____ 4. Explain the procedure to the patient.
_____ 5. Connect the power cord to a 110 V 60 Hz electrical outlet.
6. Connect the oximeter probe to the monitor:
_____ a. Finger probe
_____ b. Ear probe
_____ c. Pediatric probe
_____ 7. Turn on the power switch.

_____ 8. Wipe the probe clean using an alcohol prep pad before applying it to the patient.
9. Apply the probe to the patient:
_____ a. Finger
_____ b. Toe
_____ c. Ear
_____ d. Foot (infant or pediatric patient)
_____ 10. Observe for adequate wave forms (pulse signal) and reading.
_____ 11. Set alarm limits as required.
_____ 12. Remove any supplies from the patient's room and clean up the area.
_____ 13. Document the procedure and initial readings in the patient's chart.

Check List: Transcutaneous CO₂ and O₂ Monitoring

_____ 1. Verify the physician's order for transcutaneous monitoring.

_____ 2. Wash your hands.

_____ 3. Explain the procedure to the patient or the patient's family (infants).

_____ 4. Connect the monitor to a 110 V 60 Hz electrical outlet.

_____ 5. Calibrate the monitor to known gas levels of O_2 (using sodium sulfite and room air) and of CO_2 (usually 5% and 10% CO_2) as recommended by the manufacturer.

_____ 6. Attach a membrane to the electrode following the manufacturer's guidelines.

_____ 7. Adjust the temperature setting to the desired range.

_____ 8. Select an appropriate site and prep the site with a clean alcohol prep pad.

_____ 9. Apply a ring of double-sided tape to the electrode.

_____ 10. Place a drop of contact solution or distilled water onto the electrode and apply the electrode to the skin.

_____ 11. Allow the reading to stabilize and correlate the reading with blood gas values.

_____ 12. Clean up the patient's area, removing all disposable supplies.

_____ 13. Document the procedure in the patient's chart, including initial readings.

Check List: End-Tidal CO₂ Monitoring

_____ 1. Verify the physician's order for an end-tidal CO_2 monitor.

_____ 2. Wash your hands.

_____ 3. Assemble the appropriate equipment required:

_____ a. End-tidal CO_2 monitor

_____ b. Mainstream or sidestream probe

_____ c. Calibration gases

_____ 4. Explain the procedure to the patient.

_____ 5. Connect the monitor to a 100 V 60 Hz electrical outlet.

_____ 6. Calibrate the monitor to known CO_2 levels according to the manufacturer's instructions.

_____ 7. Connect the monitor to the patient's airway:

_____ a. Use the special adapter if using a sidestream monitor.

_____ (1) Adjust the sample flow until a plateau is seen on the capnograph.

_____ b. Connect directly to the airway if using a mainstream monitor.

_____ 8. Correlate the monitor's readings with ABG values.

_____ 9. Clean up the patient's area, removing all supplies.

_____ 10. Document the procedure in the patient's chart, including the initial readings.

Self-Evaluation Post Test: Noninvasive Monitoring

1. Which of the following instruments is able to measure hemoglobin saturation?
   a. Pulse oximeter
   b. Transcutaneous monitor
   c. Oxygen analyzer
   d. Arterial blood gas analyzer

2. Which of the following instruments measures the partial pressures of oxygen and carbon dioxide noninvasively?
   a. Pulse oximeter
   b. Transcutaneous monitor
   c. Oxygen analyzer
   d. Arterial blood gas analyzer

3. What is the purpose of the heater on the transcutaneous electrode?

   a. It warms the blood before sampling.
   b. It increases perfusion by arterializing the capillary bed.
   c. It improves patient comfort.
   d. It is needed to correct the readings to body temperature.

4. You are setting up an end-tidal CO_2 monitor on a pediatric patient who is intubated and on a ventilator. You are concerned regarding the security of the endotracheal tube and the traction the monitor might place on it. What end-tidal CO_2 monitor might be best in this situation?
   a. Mainstream
   b. Sidestream

5. You are evaluating a patient in the emergency room who was admitted following a motor vehicle accident. The patient's extremities are very cold and the patient is demonstrating signs and symptoms of shock. The pulse oximeter shows an SpO_2 of 78% and a heart rate of 52 beats per minute, yet the cardiac monitor shows a heart rate of 125 beats per minute. Why is there such a discrepancy between the two heart rates?
   a. The cardiac monitor always reads higher than the pulse oximeter.
   b. They are different because they are measured differently.
   c. The pulse oximeter is not reading accurately because of poor perfusion.
   d. The pulse oximeter is accurate and the cardiac monitor is not.

6. You are called to assess a pediatric patient who is being monitored via pulse oximetry. The nurse is concerned that the patient's saturation is low with activation of the oximeter alarm. When you initially observe the patient, you observe a very active 18-month-old boy who is squirming about his crib and mist tent (room air) with abandon. Which of the following would account for the low reading and alarm condition?
   a. The saturation is low because of the increased patient activity.
   b. The saturation is low because activity increases perfusion.
   c. The saturation is low because the mist tent is powered by room air.
   d. Patient motion is causing artifact.

7. How does an end-tidal CO_2 monitor measure the tension of the exhaled CO_2?
   a. It uses infrared light absorption.
   b. It uses photospectrometry.
   c. It uses a CO_2 electrode similar to that of a blood gas analyzer.
   d. It relies on a chemical change to occur.

8. Which of the following is a hazard/are hazards of pulse oximetry?
   I. Skin burns
   II. Pressure necrosis
   III. Airway occlusion
   a. I
   b. I, II
   c. II, III
   d. I, II, III

9. Which of the following is a hazard/are hazards of transcutaneous monitoring?
   I. Skin burns
   II. Pressure necrosis
   III. Airway occlusion
   a. I
   b. I, II
   c. II, III
   d. I, II, III

10. Which of the following is a hazard/are hazards of end-tidal CO_2 monitoring?
   I. Skin burns
   II. Pressure necrosis
   III. Airway occlusion
   a. I
   b. II
   c. III
   d. II, III

PERFORMANCE EVALUATION:
PULSE OXIMETER MONITORING

Date: Lab _____ Clinical _____ Agency _____

Lab: Pass _____ Fail _____   Clinical: Pass _____ Fail _____

Student name _____ Instructor name _____

No. of times observed in clinical _____

No. of times practiced in clinical _____

PASSING CRITERIA: Obtain 90% or better on the procedure. Tasks indicated by * must receive at least 1 point, or the evaluation is terminated. Procedure must be performed within designated time, or the performance receives a failing grade.

SCORING:
2 points — Task performed satisfactorily without prompting.
1 point — Task performed satisfactorily with self-initiated correction.
0 points — Task performed incorrectly or with prompting required.
NA — Task not applicable to the patient care situation.

TASKS:		PEER	LAB	CLINICAL
*	1. Verifies the physician's order for a monitor	☐	☐	☐
*	2. Washes hands	☐	☐	☐
*	3. Obtains the appropriate equipment as required			
	a. Pulse oximeter	☐	☐	☐
	b. Probe(s)	☐	☐	☐
	c. Alcohol prep pads	☐	☐	☐
	4. Explains the procedure to the patient	☐	☐	☐
*	5. Connects the power cord to a 110 V 60 Hz electrical outlet	☐	☐	☐
*	6. Connects the oximeter probe to the monitor			
	a. Finger probe	☐	☐	☐
	b. Ear probe	☐	☐	☐
	c. Pediatric probe	☐	☐	☐
*	7. Turns on the power switch	☐	☐	☐
*	8. Wipes the probe clean using an alcohol prep pad prior to applying it to the patient	☐	☐	☐
*	9. Applies the probe			
	a. Finger	☐	☐	☐
	b. Toe	☐	☐	☐
	c. Ear	☐	☐	☐
	d. Foot (infant or pediatric patient)	☐	☐	☐
*	10. Observes for adequate wave forms (pulse signal) and reading	☐	☐	☐
*	11. Sets alarm limits as required	☐	☐	☐
	12. Removes any supplies from the patient room and cleans up the area	☐	☐	☐

*   13. Documents the procedure and initial readings in the patient's chart   ☐   ☐   ☐

SCORE: Peer   _____ points of possible 40; _____%

             Lab   _____ points of possible 40; _____%

             Clinical   _____ points of possible 40; _____%

TIME: _____ out of possible 30 minutes

STUDENT SIGNATURES   INSTRUCTOR SIGNATURES

PEER: _____   LAB: _____

STUDENT: _____   CLINICAL: _____

PERFORMANCE EVALUATION:
TRANSCUTANEOUS MONITORING

Date: Lab _____ Clinical _____ Agency _____

Lab: Pass _____ Fail _____   Clinical: Pass _____ Fail _____

Student name _____   Instructor name _____

No. of times observed in clinical _____

No. of times practiced in clinical _____

PASSING CRITERIA: Obtain 90% or better on the procedure. Tasks indicated by * must receive at least 1 point, or the evaluation is terminated. Procedure must be performed within designated time, or the performance receives a failing grade.

SCORING:

2 points — Task performed satisfactorily without prompting.
1 point — Task performed satisfactorily with self-initiated correction.
0 points — Task performed incorrectly or with prompting required.
NA — Task not applicable to the patient care situation.

TASKS:

			PEER	LAB	CLINICAL
*	1.	Verifies the physician's order	☐	☐	☐
*	2.	Washes hands	☐	☐	☐
	3.	Explains the procedure to the patient or family members	☐	☐	☐
*	4.	Connects the monitor to a 110 V 60 Hz electrical outlet	☐	☐	☐
*	5.	Calibrates the monitor	☐	☐	☐
*	6.	Attaches a membrane to the electrode	☐	☐	☐
*	7.	Adjusts the temperature setting to the desired range	☐	☐	☐
*	8.	Selects an appropriate site and prepares it	☐	☐	☐
*	9.	Applies a ring of double-sided tape to the electrode	☐	☐	☐
*	10.	Places a drop of contact solution or distilled water onto the electrode and applies it	☐	☐	☐
*	11.	Allows the reading to stabilize and correlates it with ABG values	☐	☐	☐
	12.	Cleans up the patient's area, removing all supplies	☐	☐	☐
*	13.	Documents the procedure in the patient's chart	☐	☐	☐

SCORE: Peer   _____ points of possible 26; _____%

Lab   _____ points of possible 26; _____%

Clinical   _____ points of possible 26; _____%

TIME: _____ out of possible 30 minutes

STUDENT SIGNATURES   **INSTRUCTOR SIGNATURES**

PEER: _____   LAB: _____

STUDENT: _____   CLINICAL: _____

PERFORMANCE EVALUATION:
END-TIDAL MONITORING

Date: Lab _____ Clinical _____ Agency _____

Lab: Pass _____ Fail _____   Clinical: Pass _____ Fail _____

Student name _____ Instructor name _____

No. of times observed in clinical _____

No. of times practiced in clinical _____

PASSING CRITERIA: Obtain 90% or better on the procedure. Tasks indicated by * must receive at least 1 point, or the evaluation is terminated. Procedure must be performed within designated time, or the performance receives a failing grade.

SCORING:
2 points — Task performed satisfactorily without prompting.
1 point — Task performed satisfactorily with self-initiated correction.
0 points — Task performed incorrectly or with prompting required.
NA — Task not applicable to the patient care situation.

TASKS:	PEER	LAB	CLINICAL
* 1. Verifies the physician's order for an end-tidal monitor	☐	☐	☐
* 2. Washes hands	☐	☐	☐
* 3. Obtains the appropriate equipment as required			
a. End tidal monitor	☐	☐	☐
b. Probes or adapters	☐	☐	☐
c. Calibration gases	☐	☐	☐
4. Introduces self and explains the procedure to the patient	☐	☐	☐
* 5. Connects the monitor to a 100 V 60 Hz electrical outlet	☐	☐	☐
* 6. Calibrates the monitor to known CO_2 levels according to the manufacturer's instructions	☐	☐	☐
* 7. Connects the monitor to the patient's airway			
a. Using the special adapter (sidestream monitor)	☐	☐	☐
(1) Adjusts the sample flow until a plateau is seen on the capnograph	☐	☐	☐
b. Directly to the airway (mainstream monitor)	☐	☐	☐
* 8. Correlates the monitor's readings with ABG values	☐	☐	☐
9. Cleans up the patient's area	☐	☐	☐
* 10. Documents the procedure and the initial readings in the patient's chart	☐	☐	☐

CHAPTER 11

DOCUMENTATION AND GOALS ASSESSMENT

INTRODUCTION

Documentation is an important part of patient care. Documentation is synonymous with care itself (Castonguay, 2001). Legally, if an event is not documented in the patient's medical record, it was not done. The medical record provides an exact sequential record of the patient's condition, illness, and treatment. The medical record is the common source on a given patient referred to by all health care professionals, including physicians, respiratory care practitioners, nurses, physical and occupational therapists, and other allied health practitioners. This record is the one place where nearly all pertinent medical information on a patient is recorded and accessible to all health care professionals caring for that patient.

Assessment(s), treatment(s), procedure(s), and test(s) are all recorded in the patient's medical record. This documentation must be timely, factual, and complete. The medical record serves as legal proof of the nature of care, quality of care, and timeliness of care. The hospital may use the medical record for risk management, reimbursement purposes, continuous quality improvement, case management, or research purposes. Documentation is an important part of patient care. Therefore, the accuracy and completeness of your entries are important in the total care of the patient.

Goals assessment is another important part of patient care. Goals are measurable, demonstrated outcomes that can be assessed following patient treatment or intervention. The purpose of the respiratory care practitioner's working with a patient is to improve the patient's cardiopulmonary health and quality of life. Specific goals in reference to oxygenation, ventilation, bronchial hygiene, or other interventions may be determined and assessed before and following treatment. The Joint Commission on Accreditation of Healthcare Organizations (JCAHO) stresses the integration of interdisciplinary teams in the care of the patient (JCAHO, 2001). As such, goals assessment and determination are shared among the health care team members collaboratively, mutually benefiting the patient's care. As such, goals and their attainment for each discipline must be documented in the patient's medical record (JCAHO, 2001).

KEY TERMS

- Charting by exception
- Clinical goal
- Graphic record

- HEENT
- Objective data
- Physician's orders

- Progress notes
- Subjective data

OBJECTIVES

At the end of this chapter, you should be able to:

- Describe the purpose of the medical record.
- Describe the components of the medical record.
- Discuss the importance of the medical record for legal and reimbursement purposes.
- Describe the contents of a complete medical record entry.

- Discuss the procedure of charting by exception.
- Define a goal or outcome in reference to:
  — Oxygenation
  — Ventilation
  — Bronchial hygiene
  — Hyperinflation
- Discuss medical record documentation using computer technology.

THE MEDICAL RECORD

The medical record is a compilation of pertinent facts of a patient's life and health history, illness(es), and treatment(s) written by health care professionals who have contributed to the care of that patient (Huffman, 1994). The purpose of the medical record is to provide a written source of information regarding that patient's health, conditions, and treatments, providing a common source of information for all caregivers. The medical record is the one definitive source referenced by all caregivers about a patient. Because the medical record is such an important source of information, all entries must be clear, concise, and factual.

The medical record is also a legal document. Evidence from the medical record may be entered into a court of law as evidence or as supporting evidence. The entries in a patient's medical record may determine if care was appropriate, timely, and delivered in a competent manner. Therefore, falsification of deletion of information in a patient's medical record can result in legal action against the person or institution altering or destroying the record.

Entries in the patient's medical record are chronological. Entries begin from the first time the patient is seen or hospitalized and progress from there. Each entry has a date and time, indicating what was assessed, given (medications), or performed (tests or therapies). Because the medical record is chronological, you need to make entries as soon as practicable after working with the patient or giving medications. Timeliness is important because many other health care providers may depend on your entry to provide them with information regarding the patient's status.

Components of the Medical Record

The medical record is organized into several broad content areas. Each area is identified using tabs, color dividers, or other face sheets so that each section may be readily identified and located. Typically, in the acute care (hospital) setting, the medical record is divided into the admission record, physician's orders, progress notes, medical history and physical examination and consultation records, nursing data, graphic record, laboratory reports, imaging reports, operative data, medication administration record, ancillary services, and discharge plan.

Admission Record

The admission record states the date and time the patient was admitted to the acute care facility. The patient's name, birth date, address, Social Security number, telephone number(s), and next of kin are recorded on this form. Insurance information and policy numbers are also recorded on the admission record. The patient's diagnosis must be written out in full without abbreviations. The patient's attending physician is responsible for authenticating the admission diagnosis (Huffman, 1994).

Physician's Orders

Typically, *physician's orders* follow the admission record, proceeding from the front to the back of the medical record. All orders must contain the date and time, the order(s), and the physician's signature. Verbal or telephone orders on hospital admission are typically accepted and countersigned at a later time (JCAHO standards specify within 24 hours) when the attending physician first visits the patient in the acute care setting. Each subsequent order follows the initial one, in chronological order. All orders must be signed and dated by the attending or consulting physician(s), including all verbal and telephone orders. New standards may require the time the order was written to also be indicated.

Progress Notes

Every time the patient is visited by a physician, *progress notes* are made in the medical record. Most physicians follow the SOAP (subjective, objective, assessment, plan) format when charting progress notes.

Information provided to the physician by the patient constitutes *subjective data*. When asked specific questions, the patient responds indicating discomfort, dysfunction, pain, and so on. Sometimes patient responses are quite specific and helpful, whereas at other times only vague responses are possible.

Information that is obtained directly constitutes *objective data*. For example, vital signs, breath sounds, jugular venous distention, heart tones, SpO_2, bowel sounds, and edema can all be directly assessed and noted.

Assessment is the physician's interpretation of the subjective and objective information. Additional diagnoses or progress may be indicated in this section. For example, "SpO_2 85% on room air," "lung fields remain consolidated," and "temperature within normal limits" all are assessments of the data obtained.

The planning section denotes how the patient will be treated to help resolve some of the continuing problems. Documented plans might include the following: "continue low-flow oxygen for SpO_2 >90%," "continue hyperinflation therapy," and "discontinue IV antibiotics and switch to oral meds."

Physiology and pathophysiology are both dynamic processes. Rarely does a patient go from one moment to the next without a change in some physiologic process. The progress record allows the physician to assess the patient's response to treatment over time and to track the patient's general progress toward wellness.

History and Physical Examination and Consultation Examinations

The patient's history and physical examination are dictated by the attending physician. If the patient is able to communicate, the history may take up to 30 or 40 minutes to obtain. If the patient is unable to communicate, family members or others who are able to relate the facts accurately are solicited for the information.

The initial physical examination is performed by the attending physician. The physical exam includes a head-to-toe assessment of all major organ systems. Included are head, eyes, ears, nose, and throat (HEENT), respiratory, neurological, musculoskeletal, cardiovascular, gastrointestinal, genitourinary, endocrine, hematological and psychosocial assessments. A thorough physical exam may require an additional 20 to 30 minutes to complete.

Any consultations are recorded by the consulting physician (such as a cardiologist or pulmonologist) reporting the patient's history and findings on physical examination. These consultation notes follow chronologically the admission history and physical findings.

Included at the conclusion of each history and physical section is usually a section for assessment—listing diagnosis(es)—and planning. Each potential diagnosis is determined and an initial plan for treatment is specified.

Nursing Data

Nursing data include nursing notes (similar to physician progress notes), nursing assessment records, and nursing teaching records. Usually included in this section are the multidisciplinary plan forms.

The multidisciplinary plan forms are goals or outcomes determined by nursing and other ancillary services (respiratory care, physical therapy, occupational therapy, speech therapy, and so on) for that patient. Each outcome must be measurable, and for each outcome, a treatment or plan to attain it must be specified. Once the outcome or goal is achieved, the date and measured assessment are recorded.

Graphic Record

The graphic record contains temperature, pulse, respiration, blood pressure, urine output, oral intake (fluids), and daily weights. The graphic record may be updated as frequently as hourly or as infrequently as every 8 hours in the acute care setting, depending on the patient's acuity level (how ill the patient is).

Laboratory Reports

The laboratory report section includes hematology, chemistry, microbiology, histology, and endocrinology reports. Results of arterial blood gas (ABG) analyses are also typically included in this section.

Imaging Reports

The imaging reports section includes x-ray studies, computed tomography (CT) scans, magnetic resonance imaging (MRI) scans, ultrasound, and other imaging reports. As a respiratory care practitioner, you will find that the imaging report (dictated by a radiologist) as well as viewing the actual films (scans) is an important part of patient assessment.

Operative Data

The operative data section includes operative consent(s), operative reports, and anesthesia and postanesthesia records. The operative consent form(s) are signed by the patient or the patient's legal representative and witnessed by a member of the acute care organization's staff (physician or nurse). The operative report is dictated by the surgeon, describing the procedure, what was found, and what surgical therapy was performed. The anesthesia/postanesthesia record indicates the anesthetic agent(s) used and the patient's vital signs during and following surgery. In this section some forms are for the physician's use, others for nursing staff, and others may be utilized by allied health professionals.

Medication Administration Record

The medication administration record provides a chronology of the medications given to the patient, quantity, dosage, route, and date and time of administration. This information is important in the assessment of the patient's response to medical therapy and any adverse reactions that may occur as a result.

Ancillary Services

The ancillary services section is reserved for services such as respiratory care, physical therapy, speech therapy, occupational therapy, and other ancillary services. Various forms (charting by exception), narratives (progress notes), and goal/outcome measure sheets are used by the various ancillary services to denote medical treatments, therapies or other interventions. Specific respiratory care documentation is discussed in a later section of this chapter.

Discharge Plan

The discharge plan denotes the patient's condition and date and time of discharge. Any prescribed medication(s) and patient teaching for medication administration are documented on this form. The person receiving or accompanying the patient on discharge may also be indicated. If a discharge record is not complete, the patient may have signed out of the facility against medical advice (AMA).

The Medical Record: Legal and Reimbursement Issues

Legal

As stated previously, the medical record is considered a legal document. A patient's medical record may be submitted in court as evidence. Based on the entries in the medical record, the care provided for that patient, including medication, therapies, timeliness of treatment, appropriateness of care, and quality of care, are determined in the court of law. The medical record is the single best source of information regarding the care and treatment of a patient—even though it may have been years since the patient was last admitted or discharged. When making entries in the medical record as a respiratory care practitioner, you should imagine trying to reconstruct what was performed based on your documentation.

Because of the legal nature of the medical record, falsification of its contents may result in legal action. Concealment of an incident, attempting to protect oneself or the acute care institution, falsifying data (such as vital signs, ventilator settings, or oxygen concentrations), intentional deceit (charting something that wasn't performed) all are forms of falsification. What is documented must be concise, accurate, and truthful. Documentation in any other way is not acceptable and may be punishable in a court of law.

Reimbursement

The medical record is used by third-party payers (such as Medicare, Medicaid, or insurance companies) for purposes of reimbursement. Patients' medical records are periodically audited, verifying that what the acute care institution billed corresponds to what is documented in the medical record. Failure to document your activities accurately may result in loss of significant reimbursement. Remember that if it isn't documented, it wasn't performed and therefore may not be billable or reimbursed for payment.

The Medical Record Entry

Accuracy, timeliness, and truthfulness all are important when you are documenting in the patient's medical record. However, for optimal charting, you need to ask the following question: "Of everything I just performed, what is important to chart?" The medical record entry should include the date and time the event occurred, your assessment of the patient, what you did, what technique you employed (including medications administered and dosages when applicable), the length of time you spent, the patient's response (results of what you did), and any special circumstances (unique to the interaction).

The date and time you interacted with the patient and provided respiratory care services should be documented in the entry. You should never document anything merely in anticipation of doing it; what happens if you are called away and are unable to return? Document only what *has* been performed, not what you intend to do in the future. Time can be important in administering medications. Some medications may not be given too frequently; therefore, the time of administration of the last dosage is important.

Your assessment of the patient is important. You should document vital signs (heart rate, respiratory rate, blood pressure), patient appearance or inspection, breath sounds, oxygen saturation (SpO_2), and specifics of oxygen administration, including the device and flow rate or concentration (if the patient is on supplemental oxygen). Often other health care professionals make determinations based on the respiratory care practitioner's assessment (home oxygen, supplemental oxygen for exercise or ambulation, and so on).

What you did with the patient includes any therapies (aerosol, oxygen, chest physiotherapy [CPT], and so on) and medications administered including dosage (in mg or other units as appropriate) and diluents (normal saline, sterile water, etc.). Besides the therapy performed, include what techniques or methods were employed (manual or mechanical percussion, for example). The amount of time spent with the patient should also be documented in the patient's medical record.

The patient's response to your efforts may be documented both subjectively and objectively. Subjectively, the patient may state that breathing is easier (less work of breathing), or that his or her chest doesn't feel as tight. Objectively, you can assess changes in breath sounds, vital signs (heart rate, respiratory rate, blood pressure), SpO_2 changes, or bedside pulmonary function testing (changes in forced vital capacity [FVC] or in forced expiratory volume in 1 second [FEV_1]). The patient's response is important to document. If you can't prove that you have accomplished the desired goal, why are you there?

Unique or special circumstances may include adverse reactions, complaints by the patient about the taste of medications, incorrect oxygen settings, and so on. Document how you found that patient (e.g., on oxygen therapy or SpO_2 assessment) and document the patient's state when you left.

One important part of your medical record entry is both your initials (first and last) and your signature followed by your professional credentials (such as CRT or RRT). Most medical records have a signature log at the front of the chart (Figure 11-1) or at the bottom of that particular form. Each day when entries are made in the medical record, the person making the entry records his or her initials and signature in full, department or service area, and then printed name and credentials. The signature sheet clearly identifies each person making entries into the medical record.

Charting by Exception

Charting by exception is a method of charting, usually employing fill-in-the-blank forms where only data that change are documented (Figure 11-2). Charting by exception can save considerable time in documentation in the medical record (Short, 1997). Often arrows or other symbols are used to denote that nothing for that data point has changed (Figure 11-2). Most charting by exception forms allow space for brief narratives, supplied if something significant or unusual occurs. Spaces for the date and time of the occurrence are provided.

GOALS ASSESSMENT AND DOCUMENTATION

Clinical goals are measurable outcomes the patient is expected to achieve following the intervention of a health care practitioner. Every procedure performed should have a desired outcome in which the patient's condition or quality of life can show demonstrated improvement. Clinical goals should be objective measures, rather than subjective as provided by the patient. Documentation of objective clinical improvements is one way in which the allied health discipline of respiratory care can demonstrate the clinical benefit by being at the bedside, working with patients.

Oxygenation Goals

Oxygen therapy is indicated for patients with an SpO_2 of less than 90% or a PaO_2 of less than 60 mm Hg (American Association for Respiratory Care [AARC], 1991). Therefore, the clinical goal of oxygen therapy is to increase the SpO_2 to 90% or greater or to increase the PaO_2 to 60 mm Hg or greater. The method and delivery device will be dependent on the patient's response to therapy. The desired outcome (ideally) is to reach an end point where the patient may achieve the clinical goal (SpO_2, PaO_2) without supplemental oxygen (depending on the patient's pathophysiology). In many cases, the desired outcome may not be achieved (long-standing COPD or pulmonary disease), and the patient may be discharged from the facility on supplemental oxygen.

Ventilation Goals

The best indicator of ventilation is the patient's arterial $PaCO_2$ and secondarily the patient's pH. Ventilation goals are often expressed as maintenance of both $PaCO_2$ and pH levels within a specific range. For example, a goal may be to decrease the pressure support but maintain $PaCO_2$ at less than 60 mm Hg and pH at greater than 7.35. The ideal goal or outcome is to achieve the desired $PaCO_2$ and pH without ventilatory assistance (so that the patient is breathing spontaneously). In most patients, this outcome can be successfully met. Those patients in whom this clinical goal cannot be met may be discharged on ventilatory support, using home mechanical ventilators.

STAFF SIGNATURE SHEET
★PERMANENT CHART FORM. DO NOT DISCARD★

Staff responsible for documentation in this patient's record must record their Initials, Signature, Title, their **PRINTED NAME** and the Date on this form when the first entry is made anywhere in the chart. Entries on individual chart forms may be identified with initials unless form directs otherwise.

DATE	INI	SIGNATURE, TITLE	DEPT.	PRINT NAME
(Addressograph)				**STAFF SIGNATURE SHEET**

Figure 11-1 *An example of a signature sheet, identifying by date all people who have made entries into the medical record.*

#	ASSESSMENT/ORDER/ TREATMENT	✔ = NORMAL *SIGNIFICANT FINDINGS/COMMENTS → = NO CHANGE FROM PREVIOUS*											
1	INHALED MED. PROTOCOL: *Assessment/Reassessment (See Resp. Therapy Assessment Record)												
2	THERAPY MODE: I = IPPB S = SVN M = MDI R = return demonstration from patient with reinforcement/cues Other: _____												
3	MED.:												
4	MED.:												
5	MED.:												
6	HEART RATE PRE: POST:												
7	RESP RATE PRE: POST												
8	BREATH SOUNDS												
9	VISCOSITY: AMOUNT/COLOR CL = clear; WH = white; GY = grey; B = brown; R = red; Y = yellow; GR = green												
10	O₂ MODE/LITER FLOW*												
11	OXIMETRY %												
12	PATIENT EDUCATION: (See purple Multidisciplinary Care Plan—Part 2)												
	DATE												
	TIME												
	INITIALS												

#	DATE	TIME	*SIGNIFICANT FINDINGS/COMMENTS	INI

HM = Heat Mist;   HF = High Flow;   NC = nasal cannula;   T = Tent;   USN = ultrasonic nebulizer;   VM = ventimask;   NRB = non-rebreather

INI	NAME/TITLE	INI	NAME/TITLE	INI	NAME/TITLE	INI	NAME/TITLE

Figure 11-2   An example of a form used for charting by exception. Note that only the data that have changed are documented using this type of form.

Another ventilation goal that is objective and measurable is reversal of atelectasis. Serial chest x-ray films may be obtained to evaluate the effectiveness of hyperinflation therapy or chest physiotherapy (CPT). With resolution of atelectasis, ventilation also improves. Patients not receiving ventilatory support (mechanical ventilation) can benefit from adjunctive techniques with the goal of improving ventilation.

Bronchial Hygiene

The goals of bronchial hygiene include production of sputum following coughing, assessment of clinical improvement, improved subjective response, and stabilization of pulmonary hygiene with chronic pulmonary disease and a history of secretion retention (AARC, 1993). Bronchial hygiene techniques may include directed cough, airway aspiration (suctioning), CPT, positive expiratory pressure (PEP) mask therapy, high-frequency chest wall oscillation (HFCWO), and incentive spirometry. Documentation of sputum production and of the amount, color, consistency, and odor is important. Changes in sputum may indicate the presence of a pulmonary infection, warranting culture and sensitivity testing. The desired clinical goal is for the patient to be able to maintain adequate bronchial hygiene (sputum production and expectoration) without intervention or assistance.

Hyperinflation Goals

Goals of hyperinflation therapy include improvement or reversal of atelectasis, improved vital signs, improved breath sounds, resolution of abnormalities on the chest radiograph, improved PaO_2, and increased vital capacity (VC) and FVC (AARC, 1991). Hyperinflation techniques may include breathing retraining, incentive spirometry, intermittent positive-pressure breathing (IPPB), intrapulmonary percussive ventilation (IPV), and intermittent continuous positive airway pressure (CPAP). Documentation of objective improvement such as improvement in breath sounds, PaO_2, VC, FVC, and so on is preferable to subjective assessments. Reversal or lessening of atelectasis may be documented through serial chest x-ray films and also by improvement in breath sounds heard over affected areas. As with other interventions, the ultimate goal is for the patient to maintain spontaneous ventilation without the need for adjunctive medications or intervention.

Computer-Aided Documentation

Computer-aided documentation and medical record keeping are currently in use throughout the world. Eventually, the majority of medical record documentation will be performed using computer technology. Many documentation programs are the fill-in-the-blank variety, requiring the user to fill in data into specific fields before the program will allow progression to the next section.

Computer documentation has several advantages (Castonguay, 2001). Computer-aided documentation may improve quality and accuracy, keep the information more up to date, provide prompting for important (required) fields, promote legibility, and improve the availability of information. Once the practitioner becomes accustomed to the computer program, documentation may progress at a much faster pace, conserving time.

OBJECTIVES

At the end of this chapter, you should be able to:

- Document a procedure in the medical record using concise, accurate, and descriptive language.
- Demonstrate the ability to use common abbreviations when documenting in the medical record.
- When documenting a procedure, include the following:
  — Date and time
  — Procedures/interventions performed and techniques utilized
  — The length of time spent with the patient
  — The patient's response
  — Any unusual circumstances or occurrences
  — Your initials, signature, and credentials
- Demonstrate the ability to chart by exception.
- Given a therapeutic modality, identify two desirable measurable clinical outcomes.

DOCUMENTATION GUIDELINES AND ABBREVIATIONS

Documentation of your activities in the patient's medical record must be accurate, clear, and concise. The objective is not to write a novel but rather to provide enough information to the reader so that your activities may be accurately reconstructed. Remember that the medical record is a legal document. There always is a potential that at a later time, you may be on the witness stand, attempting to justify and or defend your actions based on what you have documented in the medical record!

Accuracy in documentation does not mean that it must be lengthy. Accepted abbreviations may be used to conserve space and reduce time. The operative words in documentation are *brevity* and *accuracy*. Common abbreviations are included in Table 11-1.

Remembering all that occurs at the bedside is often a challenge. The patient, family members, physicians, and other health care professionals may provide distractions at the bedside. Carrying a small spiral notebook (3 × 5 inches) for recording pertinent data will facilitate remembering the patient's vital signs, saturations, breath sounds, and so on. If you are called away, you will have a record of what

TABLE 11-1: Accepted Abbreviations for Medical Records

$\bar{a}$	before
bid	twice a day
BS	breath sounds, blood sugar, bowel sounds
$\bar{c}$	with
cc	cubic centimeters (same as milliliters)
C	Celsius
cm	centimeter
F	Fahrenheit
f	frequency
Fr, F	French
gt	drop
HR	heart rate
hs	hour of sleep (i.e., at bedtime)
Hx	kistory
kg	kilogram
L/min	liters per minute
mg	milligram
mcg, μg	microgram
$\bar{p}$	after
prn	as needed
qh	every hour
q4h	every four hours (also q4 may be used)
qid	four times daily
RR	respiratory rate
Rx	prescription
$\bar{S}$	without
stat	at once or immediately
tid	three times daily
Tx	treatment

you did and what you saw that will assist you in correct documentation later.

Every facility should have in its procedures manual a list of accepted abbreviations that may be used for documentation. What is accepted may vary depending on the facility and the region in which it is located. Therefore, it is important that as a respiratory care practitioner you become familiar with all abbreviations utilized by the facility that employs you.

Identification of the Medical Record

Before beginning documentation, you must correctly identify the patient's medical record. On the front cover or spine of the record is the patient's name (first and last), room number, and attending physician's name. By checking the cover sheet, you can verify the patient's full name and medical record number or hospital number, along with the patient's age and gender. Once the correct medical record has been identified, documentation may begin.

Documentation

Documentation in the patient's medical record needs to include date and time; what was performed; the length of time spent; the patient's response; any unusual circumstances; and your initials, signature, and credentials. The format this documentation takes will be largely dependent on the type of charting used in the facility (narrative versus tabular versus charting by exception). Clear, concise, and accurate should be descriptors of your documentation.

Date and Time

The date and time of the event are important parts of the medical record entry. The date may be abbreviated (01/22/02 or Jan 22, 2002). Military time (based on a 24-hour clock) is used in most facilities for periods following twelve o'clock noon until midnight. If you are not familiar with military time, inexpensive watches may be purchased that have both notations on the face of the watch, which may aid you until you become accustomed to it. The time should be documented in hours and minutes. For example, 9:32 PM is documented as 21:32.

What You Performed

This section should accurately describe what you did. This includes your assessment of the patient (for heart rate, respiratory rate, breath sounds, SpO_2, inspection, and so on); any procedures or tests performed; and any medications given, including dosage (in mg or appropriate units), diluents used, and quantity (in ml). Be brief and concise in your narrative, describing precisely what was done using as few words as possible.

Length of Time

The length of time spent with the patient is also important. This documentation may be used for reimbursement purposes, for determination of patient acuity, or to determine the workload for the facility's respiratory care practitioners. This documentation should be accurate to the nearest minute.

Patient's Response

The patient's response to the procedure should reflect both subjective and objective information. Subjective information provided by the patient may be prefaced by the words "The patient states . . . " or "The patient states she feels . . . " to indicate the subjective nature of the information.

Objective data are measurable information that may provide evidence that clinical objectives are being met. This can include breath sounds, heart and respiratory rates, SpO_2, and other data. Documentation of objective criteria is important to validate the benefits of the time and effort spent with the patient. Reimbursement will be closely linked to achievement of objective criteria.

Unusual Circumstances

Documentation of unusual circumstances is also important. These might include adverse reactions or other occurrences that normally may not occur.

Initials and Signature

Each person making the entry in the patient record must be able to be clearly identified. Therefore, your initials, full signature, and credentials must be indicated for each entry. Many medical record forms have fill-in-the-blank spaces for initials, with spaces at the lower margin for initials followed by the full signature (see Figure 11-2). In addition to the requirement for signing and/or initialing each entry, a signature form may also be included as part of the medical record (see Figure 11-1).

Charting By Exception

Charting by exception is documentation of only items that change from what has been previously documented earlier in time. If the event or item has not changed, arrows, ditto marks, or other shorthand nomenclature may be used to indicate that the data are the same. Only when changes occur is information documented by indicating what changed and what time it changed. Figure 11-2 is an example of a form using charting by exception.

Clinical Goals

Clinical goals were described in the previous section. It is important that you understand the indications and outcomes for each procedure you are performing. The AARC has published numerous research-based clinical practice guidelines for the majority of respiratory care modalities. These guidelines are available for purchase or on the AARC's Web site (http://www.aarc.org); many are included in this text. As a respiratory care practitioner, you will find these clinical practice guidelines to be useful resources as you learn the desired clinical outcomes and what you must assess to determine if they have been met.

References

American Association for Respiratory Care. (1991). AARC clinical practice guideline: Incentive spirometry. *Respiratory Care, 36*(12), 1402–1405.

American Association for Respiratory Care. (1991). AARC clinical practice guideline: Oxygen therapy in the acute care hospital. *Respiratory Care, 36*(12), 1410–1413.

American Association for Respiratory Care (1993). AARC clinical practice guideline: Directed cough. *Respiratory Care, 38*(5), 495–499.

Castonguay, D. (2001). Nursing documentation—how important is it? *Nursing News* (New Hampshire), 25(1).

Huffman, F. K. (1994). *Health information management*. Berwyn, IL: Physicians' Record Company.

Joint Commission on Accreditation of Healthcare Organizations. (2001). *Hospital accreditation standards*. Oakbrook Terrace, IL: Author.

Short, M. (1997). Charting by exception on a clinical pathway. *Nurse Manager, 28*(8), 45–46.

Practice Activities: Documentation

1. Practice the following skills using a laboratory partner:
   a. Auscultation of breath sounds
   b. Physical assessment of the chest
   c. Determination of vital signs
   Once you have completed the skills, document the procedure using a SOAP format.

2. Working together with your laboratory partner, teach the following skills:
   a. Incentive spirometry
   b. Use of a metered dose inhaler (with and without a spacer)
   Once you have completed the instruction, document the procedure.

3. Write three sentences using the following abbreviations:
   a. $\bar{a}$
   b. $\bar{p}$
   c. qid

   Ask your laboratory instructor to check your documentation for correct use of the abbreviations, clarity, and brevity.

4. Using Figure 11-2 as an example, practice charting by exception the information you charted in Practice Activity 1.

5. With a laboratory partner, identify two measurable clinical outcomes for the following modalities and discuss how you could assess whether they are met.
   a. Incentive spirometry
   b. Oxygen delivery via nasal cannula
   c. Chest physiotherapy
   d. IPPB therapy

Check List: Documentation and Goals Assessment

1. Records pertinent information in a small note-book:
   - _____ a. Vital signs
   - _____ b. Breath sounds
   - _____ c. Oxygen saturation
   - _____ d. Type of therapy/test
   - _____ e. Medications administered
   - _____ f. Patient's response
   - _____ g. Any unusual circumstances
2. Identifies the patient's medical record:
   - _____ a. Matches name
   - _____ b. Matches attending physician's name
   - _____ c. Matches room number

3. _____ Identifies the correct section for documentation.
4. Appropriately documents in the medical record:
   - _____ a. Date/time
   - _____ b. Patient assessment data
   - _____ c. Procedures/interventions performed, including technique
   - _____ d. Medications administered (dose and diluents)
   - _____ e. The patient's response
   - _____ f. Any unusual occurrences
   - _____ g. Signature and credentials
5. _____ Returns the medical record to its proper location.

Self-Evaluation Post Test: Documentation and Goals Assessment

1. Which of the following best describes the patient's medical record?
   a. A document containing subjective information
   b. The one best source of medical information about the patient
   c. A legal document
   d. b and c

2. Which of the following are components of the medical record?
   I.   History and physical
   II. Laboratory reports
   III. Discharge summary
   IV. Progress notes
   a. I   c. I, II, III
   b. I, II   d. I, II, III, IV

3. Which of the following sections of the medical record are utilized most by physicians for documentation purposes?
   I.   History and physical
   II. Laboratory reports
   III. Medication administration record
   IV. Progress notes
   a. I, II   c. II, III
   b. I, III   d. I, IV

4. Which of the following is/are important in documenting in a patient's medical record?
   I.   Document only facts.
   II. Be brief.
   III. Use medical terminology.
   IV. Describe precisely what has occurred.
   a. I   c. I, II, III
   b. I, II   d. I, II, III, IV

5. The patient's medical record may:
   a. Be taken home when the patient is discharged.
   b. Be used as evidence in a court of law.
   c. Falsified to protect the institution caring for the patient.
   d. Be destroyed on the patient's discharge.

6. Which of the following constitute objective data?
   I.   Heart rate
   II. A patient's complaint of dyspnea
   III. Breath sounds
   IV. The patient's statement "I feel crummy"
   a. I, II   c. II, III
   b. I, III   d. II, IV

7. Which of the following constitute subjective data?
   I.   Heart rate
   II. A patient's complaint of dyspnea
   III. Breath sounds
   IV. The patient's statement "I feel crummy"
   a. I, II   c. II, III
   b. I, III   d. II, IV

8. Charting by exception is best described as:
   a. documenting everything that occurs using a narrative style.
   b. documenting only what remains the same.
   c. documenting that data that changes.
   d. using computer-aided charting methods.

9. You are administering oxygen via nasal cannula at 3 L/min. What are appropriate clinical goals?
   I.   Oxygen saturation of >90%
   II. A normal $PaCO_2$
   III. A PaO_2 of >60 mm Hg
   IV. An increased vital capacity
   a. I, II   c. I, IV
   b. I, III   d. II, III

10. The physician requests that you begin a bronchial hygiene protocol. What are the expected clinical outcomes of this protocol?
   I.   Evidence of sputum production
   II. Patient's subjective improvement
   III. Stabilization of pulmonary hygiene in chronic pulmonary disease
   IV. Clinical observation of improvement
   a. I   c. I, II, III
   b. I, II   d. I, II, III, IV

PERFORMANCE EVALUATION:
DOCUMENTATION AND GOALS ASSESSMENT

Date: Lab _____ Clinical _____ Agency _____

Lab: Pass _____ Fail _____   Clinical: Pass _____ Fail _____

Student name _____   Instructor name _____

No. of times observed in clinical _____

No. of times practiced in clinical _____

PASSING CRITERIA: Obtain 90% or better on the procedure. Tasks indicated by * must receive at least 1 point, or the evaluation is terminated. Procedure must be performed within designated time, or the performance receives a failing grade.

SCORING: 2 points — Task performed satisfactorily without prompting.
1 point — Task performed satisfactorily with self-initiated correction.
0 points — Task performed incorrectly or with prompting required.
NA — Task not applicable to the patient care situation.

TASKS:	PEER	LAB	CLINICAL
* 1. Records pertinent information in a small notebook:			
a. Vital signs	☐	☐	☐
b. Breath sounds	☐	☐	☐
c. Oxygen saturation	☐	☐	☐
d. Type of therapy/test	☐	☐	☐
e. Medications administered	☐	☐	☐
f. Patient's response	☐	☐	☐
g. Any unusual circumstances	☐	☐	☐
* 2. Identifies the patient's medical record			
a. Matches name	☐	☐	☐
b. Matches attending physician's name	☐	☐	☐
c. Matches room number	☐	☐	☐
* 3. Identifies the correct section for documentation	☐	☐	☐
* 4. Appropriately documents in the medical record			
a. Date/time	☐	☐	☐
b. Patient assessment data	☐	☐	☐
c. Procedures/interventions performed, including technique	☐	☐	☐
d. Medications administered (dose and diluents)	☐	☐	☐
e. The patient's response	☐	☐	☐
f. Any unusual occurrences	☐	☐	☐
g. Signature and credentials	☐	☐	☐
* 5. Returns the medical record to its proper place	☐	☐	☐

SCORE: Peer   _____ points of possible 40; _____%

          Lab   _____ points of possible 40; _____%

          Clinical   _____ points of possible 40; _____%

TIME: _____ out of possible 15 minutes

STUDENT SIGNATURES   INSTRUCTOR SIGNATURES

PEER: _____   LAB: _____

STUDENT: _____   CLINICAL: _____

CHAPTER 12

OXYGEN SUPPLY SYSTEMS

INTRODUCTION

As a respiratory care practitioner, you will be expected to know how to utilize safely the various medical gas supply systems available in your institution. These supply systems include medical gas cylinders, medical gas piping systems, liquid systems, and oxygen concentrators.

When used appropriately, these systems are safe and effective. If mishandled, they can be potentially lethal.

In this chapter, the theory of how the systems are constructed, principles of operation, and safety features are discussed. Following this is a section covering the procedure for using the supply systems.

KEY TERMS

- Air/oxygen blender
- ASSS
- Cracking
- DISS
- Downstream
- Flowmeter
- Hydrostatic testing
- Oxygen concentrator
- PISS
- Preset reducing valve
- Reducing valve
- Riser
- Spontaneous combustion
- Station outlet
- Tank factor
- Upstream
- Zone valve

OBJECTIVES

At the end of this chapter, you should be able to:

MEDICAL GAS CYLINDERS

- Identify the contents of a medical gas cylinder using the United States and International color code system, and the label for the following gases or gas mixtures:
  — Air
  — Oxygen
  — Nitrogen
  — Nitrous oxide
  — Helium
  — Helium/oxygen mixtures
  — Carbon dioxide
  — Carbon dioxide/oxygen mixtures
- Interpret the following data for a full "E" and "H" oxygen cylinder:
  — Gauge pressure when full
  — Contents in liters
  — Contents in cubic feet
- Describe the two main types of valves found on "E" and "H" medical gas cylinders. Identify and describe the function of the following parts:
  — Stem
  — Outlet
  — Safety features
  — Valve plunger
  — Valve seat
  — Gas entrance channel
- Interpret the markings found on a medical gas cylinder shoulder including:
  — DOT specification number
  — Cylinder composition code
  — Serial number and purchaser/user identification mark
  — Inspector's mark and testing date

  — Manufacturer's mark
  — The mark indicating that a cylinder has successfully passed a hydrostatic test
  — The mark indicating that a cylinder may be filled in excess of a service pressure by 10%
- List fifteen rules for the safe storage and handling of compressed medical gas cylinders.
- Given a gauge pressure, cylinder size ("E" or "H"), and liter flow rate, calculate the duration of gas flow remaining for an oxygen cylinder.
- Describe the appropriate actions to be taken if the contents of a medical gas cylinder are in doubt.
- Describe the appropriate actions to be taken when one is requested to transfill a medical gas cylinder.

OXYGEN PIPING SYSTEMS

- Describe the safety features associated with an oxygen piping system.
- Describe the purpose of a zone valve.
- Describe a station outlet and the different types of connections available for the attachment of equipment.

LIQUID OXYGEN SYSTEMS

- Describe the physical characteristics of a small liquid oxygen reservoir.
- Describe the advantages and disadvantages of a liquid oxygen system for home use.

OXYGEN CONCENTRATORS

- Differentiate between the two types of oxygen concentrators available.
- Describe the principles of operation for each type.
- Describe how liter flow affects the output of an oxygen concentrator.

(Continued)

MEDICAL GAS CYLINDERS

Cylinders manufactured for the transport of medical gases are constructed in accordance with regulations specifically established by the U.S. Department of Transportation (DOT). The DOT specifies the materials and methods by which medical gas cylinders may be constructed.

In accordance with regulations, medical gas cylinders are generally constructed from seamless steel meeting chemical and physical requirements. Cylinders are formed by either spinning or stamping a flat sheet into the proper shape. Following construction, cylinders are heat-treated to retain the steel's tensile strength.

Cylinder Markings

Medical gas cylinders, in compliance with DOT regulations, are required to have specific markings permanently stamped onto the shoulder (Figures 12-1 and 12-2). The first marking stamped on the shoulder of a medical gas cylinder is "DOT 3AA." This indicates that the cylinder meets the DOT standards for 3AA-type compressed gas cylinders. These standards require that the cylinder be of seamless construction and made from high-strength, heat-treated alloy steels with specific chemical compositions. These metals can withstand high stress. Because of the high-tensile-strength alloy construction, this cylinder has a wall thickness less than that of other cylinder types and

therefore weighs less than cylinders of comparable size and service pressure.

The next stamp following the cylinder type is the service pressure. This is the pressure, given in *pounds per square inch* (psi), under which the cylinder was designed to operate. The most common service pressure for cylinders in medical use is 2015 psi for oxygen.

The number stamped immediately below the specification number is the serial number for that cylinder. This number is unique and assigned by the manufacturer to that cylinder.

Next, the manufacturer's mark appears below the serial number. The manufacturer's mark may be represented by initials or an abbreviation of the manufacturer's name.

The ownership mark appears on the next line. Like the manufacturer's mark, it may be represented by initials or an abbreviation.

If hydrostatic testing has been performed on the cylinder, the date of the hydrostatic test and the inspector's mark will also be stamped on the cylinder shoulder. The inspector's mark may appear between the month and day of the test, or it may appear after the month and day. If a plus sign (+) follows the testing date, this indicates that the cylinder may be charged up to 10% greater than the service pressure. In the case of the cylinder under discussion, the cylinder may be filled to 2200 psi (see Figure 12-2).

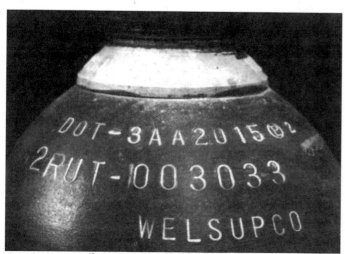

Figure 12-1 *Cylinder markings stamped on the cylinder shoulder*

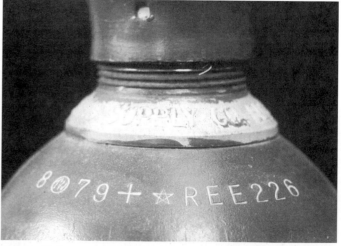

Figure 12-2 *Cylinder markings stamped on the cylinder shoulder, indicating month and year of hydrostatic testing and results*

Hydrostatic testing every 5 or 10 years is required for all cylinders in service. The test is conducted by placing a cylinder in a vessel filled with water and filling the cylinder to 5/3 the service pressure (for 3A and 3AA cylinders). The expansion of the cylinder is measured while it is under pressure. If the expansion is within acceptable limits, the test date and expansion data are recorded. The cylinder is then stamped with the date of the test and the inspector's mark. If a cylinder fails a hydrostatic test, it is destroyed.

Common Medical Gas Cylinder Sizes

The two most common medical gas cylinder sizes encountered in the clinical setting are "E" and "H." Other cylinder sizes are shown in Figure 12-3.

The E cylinder is used for brief intervals owing to its relatively small capacity. Its most common use is for the transport of a patient from one area of the hospital to another, or in ambulance vehicles and short-term therapy where piped gases are not available. The cylinder's small size makes it ideal for use in transport situations. Small mobile cylinder carts make transporting a patient in a wheelchair or gurney much easier.

The H cylinder is much larger than the E cylinder and contains a little more than 10 times as much gas. Owing to its size and construction, it is quite heavy, usually weighing approximately 135 pounds. Special cylinder carts have been designed to facilitate the transport of these cylinders from one area to another.

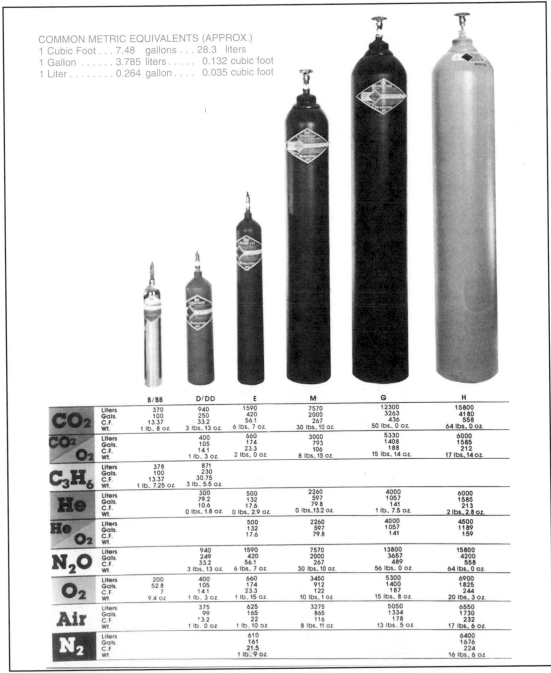

COMMON METRIC EQUIVALENTS (APPROX.)
1 Cubic Foot . . . 7.48   gallons . . . 28.3   liters
1 Gallon . . . . . . 3.785 liters . . . . . 0.132 cubic foot
1 Liter . . . . 0.264 gallon . . . . 0.035 cubic foot

Gas		B/BB	D/DD	E	M	G	H
CO_2	Liters	370	940	1590	7570	12300	15800
	Gals.	100	250	420	2000	3263	4180
	C.F.	13.37	33.2	56.1	267	436	558
	Wt.	1 lb. 8 oz.	3 lbs. 13 oz.	6 lbs. 7 oz.	30 lbs. 10 oz.	50 lbs. 0 oz.	64 lbs. 0 oz.
$\frac{CO_2}{O_2}$	Liters		400	660	3000	5330	6000
	Gals.		105	174	793	1408	1585
	C.F.		14.1	23.3	106	188	212
	Wt.		1 lb. 3 oz.	2 lbs. 0 oz.	8 lbs. 15 oz.	15 lbs. 14 oz.	17 lbs. 14 oz.
C_3H_6	Liters	378	871				
	Gals.	100	230				
	C.F.	13.37	30.75				
	Wt.	1 lb. 7.25 oz.	3 lb. 5.5 oz.				
He	Liters		300	500	2260	4000	6000
	Gals.		79.2	132	597	1057	1585
	C.F.		10.6	17.6	79.8	141	213
	Wt.		0 lbs. 1.8 oz.	0 lbs. 2.9 oz.	0 lbs. 13.2 oz.	1 lb. 7.5 oz.	2 lbs. 2.8 oz.
$\frac{He}{O_2}$	Liters			500	2260	4000	4500
	Gals.			132	597	1057	1189
	C.F.			17.6	79.8	141	159
	Wt.						
N_2O	Liters		940	1590	7570	13800	15800
	Gals.		249	420	2000	3657	4200
	C.F.		33.2	56.1	267	489	558
	Wt.		3 lbs. 13 oz.	6 lbs. 7 oz.	30 lbs. 10 oz.	56 lbs. 0 oz.	64 lbs. 0 oz.
O_2	Liters	200	400	660	3450	5300	6900
	Gals.	52.8	105	174	912	1400	1825
	C.F.	7	14.1	23.3	122	187	244
	Wt.	9.4 oz.	1 lb. 3 oz.	1 lb. 15 oz.	10 lbs. 1 oz.	15 lbs. 8 oz.	20 lbs. 3 oz.
Air	Liters		375	625	3275	5050	6550
	Gals.		99	165	865	1334	1730
	C.F.		13.2	22	116	178	232
	Wt.		1 lb. 0 oz.	1 lb. 10 oz.	8 lbs. 11 oz.	13 lbs. 5 oz.	17 lbs. 6 oz.
N_2	Liters		610				6400
	Gals.		161				1676
	C.F.		21.5				224
	Wt.		1 lb. 9 oz.				16 lbs. 6 oz.

Figure 12-3 *Various cylinder sizes (Courtesy of* BOC Gases, formerly Airco, Murray Hill, NJ)

TABLE 12-1: Cylinder Color Coding

GAS	COLOR CODE	
	United States	International
Oxygen	Green	White
Carbon dioxide	Gray	Gray
Nitrous oxide	Light blue	Light blue
Cyclopropane	Orange	Orange
Helium	Brown	Brown
Carbon dioxide and oxygen	Gray and green	Gray and white
Helium and oxygen	Brown and green	Brown and white
Air	Yellow	White and black

Color Coding

The Compressed Gas Association (CGA) has developed a color code for the different gases and gas mixtures. Each gas or gas mixture has its own unique color code. This code is published by the U.S. Department of Commerce under recommendation from the Bureau of Standards. Table 12-1 illustrates the United States (U.S.) color code system and the International color code system. The only difference between the U.S. and International systems is the color code for oxygen.

Besides the color code, all medical gas cylinders are required to have a label affixed to the cylinder identifying its contents. The label's color code and the cylinder's color code should match.

If you are in doubt about the contents of a medical gas cylinder (for example, if a label is missing or if the label and the color code of the cylinder do not match), do not administer gas from that cylinder. Tag the cylinder as being mislabeled and return it to the medical gas supplier.

Only by verifying the color code of the cylinder and matching the label to the color code can you be certain of the cylinder's contents.

Cylinder Valves and Cylinder Valve Safety Systems

Because of the high pressure contained in a medical gas cylinder, a device is needed to contain the gas and to provide a point of attachment for equipment. These devices are termed *cylinder valves*. The cylinder valves are located at the top of the cylinder and are of two types: direct-acting and diaphragm.

The *direct-acting* cylinder valve is in essence a needle valve. To prevent leakage of the high-pressure gas through the threaded portion of the needle valve, washers and polytetrafluoroethylene (Teflon) gasket material are provided. As the stem of the valve is rotated counterclockwise, the plunger is raised from its seat and gas flows from the cylinder. Figure 12-4 shows the component parts of a direct-acting cylinder valve. This type of cylinder valve is able to withstand high pressure and is found on cylinders containing gas at 1500 psi pressure and greater.

The *diaphragm* cylinder valve contains a diaphragm that rests on the seat of the valve. As the valve stem is

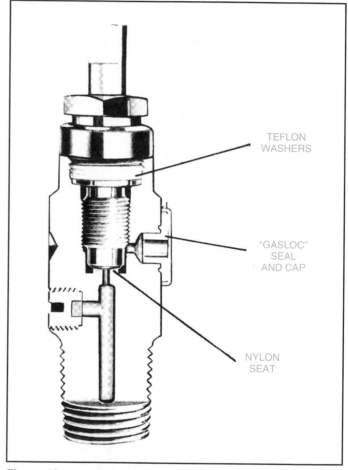

Figure 12-4 *A direct-acting cylinder valve (Courtesy of* BOC Gases, formerly Airco, Murray Hill, NJ)

TEFLON WASHERS

"GASLOC" SEAL AND CAP

NYLON SEAT

turned counterclockwise, the pressure in the cylinder displaces the diaphragm and gas flows from the cylinder. In this type of valve, the valve plunger does not act directly on the valve seat. The diaphragm cylinder valve is not prone to leakage but cannot withstand high pressure. It is generally found on cylinders containing less than 1500 psi of pressure. Figure 12-5 depicts a typical diaphragm cylinder valve.

There are two safety systems incorporated into cylinder valves: one recommended by the Bureau of Explosives

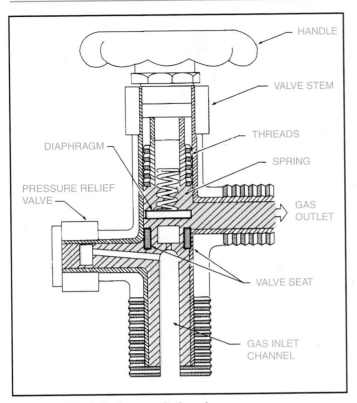

Figure 12-5 *A diaphragm cylinder valve*

and the other recommended by the CGA. For use in the event that excessive pressure builds up within the cylinder, a safety pressure relief is provided on the cylinder valve. The system recommended by the Bureau of Explosives consists of a frangible disk or a fusible plug. When the frangible disk is exposed to excessive pressure, the disk fragments into small pieces, releasing the pressure in the cylinder. The fusible plug is made from a metal with a low

melting point. If the temperature rises beyond the melting point of the metal plug, the plug melts and releases the pressure in the cylinder. A cylinder valve may contain one or both types of safety relief devices (Figure 12-6).

Because medical gas cylinders may contain a variety of gases besides oxygen, a safety system was designed by the CGA to prevent the interchange of cylinders containing dissimilar gases. This system was formally adopted by the American Standards Association and called the American Standard Index system, or the American Standard Safety System (*ASSS*).

There are two safety systems designed to prevent the interchange of cylinders containing different gases: one for large cylinders and one for E cylinders and other small cylinder sizes.

The large cylinder safety system consists of different thread sizes and pitches and both internal and external threading. Because of variations in threading, a cylinder containing one gas may not be connected to equipment indexed for a different gas.

In addition to the safety system just described, large medical gas cylinders have a protective cap that covers the cylinder valve. This cap is threaded and matches threads on the cylinder shoulder just below the valve. Whenever the cylinder is transported, safe practice dictates that the protective cylinder valve cap must be kept in place.

Small cylinder (D and E) valves utilize a yoke connection rather than a threaded connection for equipment attachment. The face of the cylinder valve has two holes drilled in two of six specific positions. The yoke that attaches to the cylinder valve has pins indexed in corresponding positions. If the pin and hole positions do not match, the cylinder and yoke cannot be mated. This indexing is designed to prevent the interchange of equipment or cylinders containing dissimilar gases. This system is commonly known as the pin index safety system (*PISS*).

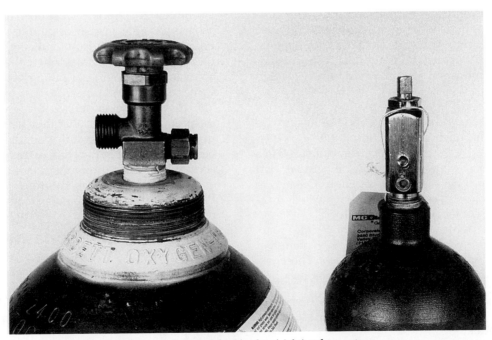

Figure 12-6 *The frangible disk (left) and fusible plug (right) safety systems*

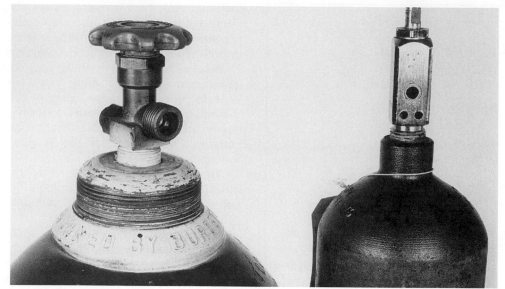

Figure 12-7 *The American Standard Safety System (ASSS) and the pin index safety system (PISS)*

Figure 12-7 shows the threaded safety system and the PISS for large and small cylinder sizes.

Safety Precautions with Use of Medical Gas Cylinders

As a respiratory care practitioner, you must use common sense and care when handling compressed gas cylinders. When handled properly and with care, medical gas cylinders are completely safe. However, there are numerous documented instances of damage to personnel, buildings, and vehicles resulting from improper handling of cylinders (Grenard, 1973).

The most common gas you will administer from a medical gas cylinder is oxygen. Knowledge of the physical characteristics of oxygen will help in your handling of these medical gas cylinders. Oxygen is colorless, odorless, and tasteless. It supports life and is a requirement for combustion of any material. Although oxygen is not flammable, it does support combustion. If anything is burning in close proximity, combustion will occur at a greatly accelerated rate.

Certain substances, when exposed to oxygen, may ignite with great force without the addition of heat to initiate the process. This phenomenon is termed *spontaneous combustion*. Such substances that may be encountered in a hospital or transport situation include oil, grease, and petroleum-based products such as Vaseline. Great care must be exercised to prevent the cylinder valves and fittings from making contact with these products.

The CGA has published recommended safe practices for handling medical gases in its 1971 pamphlet *Characteristics and Safe Handling of Medical Gases*. These recommendations are summarized in the following lists.

MOVING CYLINDERS

1. Always leave protective valve caps in place when moving a cylinder.
2. Do not lift a cylinder by its cap.
3. Do not drop a cylinder or strike two cylinders against one another, or strike other surfaces.
4. Do not drag or slide cylinders; use a cart.
5. Use a cart whenever loading or unloading cylinders.

STORING CYLINDERS

1. Comply with local and state regulations for cylinder storage as well as those established by the National Fire Protection Association (NFPA).
2. Post the names of the gases stored.
3. Keep full and empty cylinders separate. Place the full cylinders in a convenient spot to minimize handling of cylinders.
4. Keep storage areas dry, cool, and well ventilated. Storage rooms should be fire resistant.
5. Do not store cylinders close to flammable substances such as gasoline, grease, or petroleum products.
6. Protect the cylinders from damage by cuts or abrasion. Do not store them in areas where they may be subject to damage from moving or falling objects. Keep cylinder valve caps on at all times.
7. You may store cylinders in the open; however, keep them on a platform so that they are above the ground. In some parts of the country, shading may be required because of high temperature extremes. If ice and snow accumulate, thaw at room temperature or use water not exceeding 125°F in temperature.
8. Protect cylinders from potential tampering by untrained, unauthorized persons.

WITHDRAWING CYLINDER CONTENTS

1. Allow cylinders to be handled only by experienced, trained persons.
2. The user of the cylinder is responsible for verifying the cylinder contents before use. If the contents are in doubt, do not use that cylinder. Return it to the supplier.

3. Leave the protective valve cap in place until you are ready to attach a regulator or other equipment.
4. Use safe practices, making sure the cylinder is well supported and protected from falling over.
5. Use appropriate reducing valves or regulators when attaching equipment designed for lower operating pressures than those contained in the cylinder.
6. Do not force any threaded connections. Verify that the threads you are using are designed for the same gas or gas mixture in accordance with the American Standard Index system.
7. Connect a cylinder only to a manifold designed for high-pressure cylinders.
8. Use equipment only with cylinders containing the gases for which the equipment was designed.
9. Open cylinder valves slowly. Never use a wrench or hammer to force a cylinder valve open. Treat cylinders and cylinder valves with care.
10. Do not use compressed gases to dust off yourself or your clothing.
11. Keep all connections tight to prevent leakage.
12. Before removing a regulator, turn off the valve and bleed it to depressurize the connection.
13. Never use a flame to detect leaks with flammable gases.
14. Do not store flammable gases with oxygen. Keep all flammable anesthetic gases stored in a separate area.

Calculation of Cylinder Contents

It is important to determine the duration of time a cylinder will last at a given flow rate in using medical gas cylinders. The ability to perform this task quickly and accurately is essential when patients are being transported.

When full, the most common sizes of oxygen cylinders —H and E—contain 244 cubic feet and 22 cubic feet of oxygen, respectively. As discussed earlier, the gauge pressure of a full cylinder is also 2200 psi. These are constants for full cylinders.

A special constant termed a *tank factor* is used in the calculation for each cylinder size. The following calculations show how these constants are derived:

Tank factor for an H cylinder:

$$\frac{\text{Tank size in cu ft} \times 28.3 \text{ liters/cu ft}}{\text{Full tank pressure}} = \text{tank factor}$$

$$\frac{244 \text{ cu ft} \times 28.3 \text{ liters/cu ft}}{2200 \text{ psi}} = 3.14 \text{ liters/psi}$$

Tank factor for an E cylinder:

$$\frac{\text{Tank size in cu ft} \times 28.3 \text{ liters/cu ft}}{\text{Full tank pressure}} = \text{tank factor}$$

$$\frac{22 \text{ cu ft} \times 28.3 \text{ liters/cu ft}}{2200 \text{ psi}} = 0.28 \text{ liters/psi}$$

To utilize these new tank factors or constants to determine cylinder contents, multiply the constant by the pressure indicated on the gauge.

Problem

You are using an E cylinder to transport a patient 60 miles by ambulance. You are using oxygen at a flow rate of 3 liters per minute. The gauge indicates a pressure of 1500 psi. Will the tank last for the duration of the 1 hour and 15 minute trip?

a. Multiply the gauge pressure by the tank factor for an E cylinder.

$$1500 \text{ psi} \times 0.28 \text{ L/psi} = 420 \text{ L}$$

b. Now, divide the liters remaining by the flow rate of 3 liters per minute to determine the time in minutes remaining in the cylinder.

$$\frac{420 \text{ L}}{3 \text{ L/min}} = 140 \text{ minutes}$$

c. Convert the time remaining in minutes to hours and minutes.

$$\frac{140 \text{ min}}{60 \text{ min/h}} = 2.3 \text{ hours or 2 hours 18 minutes}$$

Following this method, it is possible to calculate the amount of time a cylinder of oxygen will last at a given flow rate. However, at the end of the calculated time period, the cylinder will be completely empty.

It is common practice to change an oxygen cylinder in use when the gauge pressure reads 500 psi. The pressure at which cylinders are changed may vary with hospital policy. This leaves a slight reserve of oxygen for the patient. Also, by leaving a little pressure in the cylinder, air, water, or other undesirable contaminants cannot enter the cylinder.

Transfilling of Medical Gas Cylinders

The process of transfilling medical gas cylinders involves the connection of an empty cylinder to one that contains gas under pressure. Usually the practice involves the filling of a small portable cylinder from a large H cylinder.

Transfilling of medical gas cylinders remains a controversial topic in respiratory care. As with all controversies, there are two schools of thought.

There are definite hazards involved in the transfilling of medical gas cylinders. If transfilling is performed improperly, excessive heat can be generated, posing a potential fire hazard. If the pressure limits of a small cylinder are accidentally exceeded, the result may be a disastrous rupture of the cylinder. There is also the possibility of mixing two dissimilar gases by accident. Serious hazards are associated with the transfilling of gas from one cylinder to another; therefore, it is recommended that the practice be discontinued (Compressed Gas Association, 1981).

Some authors and practitioners maintain that transfilling is a safe, routinely practiced activity. They maintain that if common sense is exercised, cylinders may be transfilled safely.

It is my opinion, however, that the benefits of transfilling cylinders are not worth the risk. Requests for transfilling a cylinder should be referred to an appropriate medical gas supply company.

MEDICAL GAS PIPING SYSTEMS

Because of increased convenience, safety, and cost savings, medical gas piping systems have grown in popularity over the years. Like medical gas cylinders, medical gas piping systems are regulated and must conform to specific standards of design and construction. The National Fire Protection Association (NFPA) is the organization that recommends the standards for construction of medical gas piping systems.

These piping systems may be supplied by a bulk liquid supply of gas or a manifold composed of two or more large medical gas cylinders, or both. Should the bulk supply system run out, a safety system is provided. A piping system is required to have a reserve or backup supply of oxygen. As the pressure in the supply line drops after the main oxygen supply is exhausted, the reserve system is automatically switched on. This reserve system may consist of a liquid bulk supply, a manifold of two or more cylinders, or a combination of the two. The reserve system must be able to meet a facility's oxygen needs for a minimum of 24 hours, according to NFPA regulations.

The bulk gas supply pressure must be reduced to a working pressure of 50 psi by a regulator. From the regulator, oxygen is conducted into the building through a pipe. In a multistoried building, each floor is provided with oxygen by a pipe termed a *riser*. Each riser is required to have a safety shutoff valve in the event of a fire.

Each floor of a building is divided into several zones. Each zone has a safety shutoff valve, termed a *zone valve*. In the event of a fire in one zone or wing of a floor, that zone's oxygen supply can be shut off without affecting other areas on the same floor.

In the facilities where you are working, it is important to know where the riser and zone valves are located. In the event of a fire, you may be asked to terminate the oxygen supply to an area to help contain the fire. Figure 12-8 shows a typical zone valve.

The connection for attaching equipment for patient use is termed a *station outlet*. These outlets may have a diameter-indexed safety system (*DISS*) or quick-connect fittings. Both of these fittings have check valves to prevent oxygen loss when they are not in use (Figure 12-9).

The DISS safety system is designed for pressures of 200 psi and lower. It was designed by the CGA. This system prevents the interchange of equipment designed for dissimilar gases or gas mixtures.

Reducing Valves

Medical gas cylinders, as discussed earlier, contain gas under high pressure. This high pressure must be reduced to a working pressure of 50 psi. Respiratory care equipment is designed to function at this lower working pressure. Operating equipment at the lower pressure has obvious safety advantages. A device that reduces the pressure in the medical gas cylinder from 2200 psi to 50 psi is termed a *reducing valve*. There are many types of reducing valves: single-stage, modified single-stage, and multistage valves.

Single-Stage Reducing Valve

A single-stage reducing valve has one chamber for the reduction of cylinder pressure to 50 psi. The single-stage reducing valve operates as a result of two opposing forces (Figure 12-10). The two opposing forces allowing this device to operate are spring tension and gas pressure. The diaphragm allows these two forces to work in opposition. High pressure forces gas into the chamber. As the gas enters the chamber through the nozzle, the valve seat is displaced. If gas flow at the outlet were to remain unobstructed, the valve seat would remain open. Resistance at the outlet causes pressure to build within the chamber. As pressure builds, the diaphragm is forced up against the tension of the spring. When gas pressure in the chamber equals the tension of the spring, the valve seat closes. A pressure drop or decrease in resistance at the outlet allows the cycle to begin again.

Also, note that the portion of the reducing valve housing the spring has openings for atmospheric pressure. This is by design so that movement of the diaphragm does not cause pressure to increase in this portion of the reducing

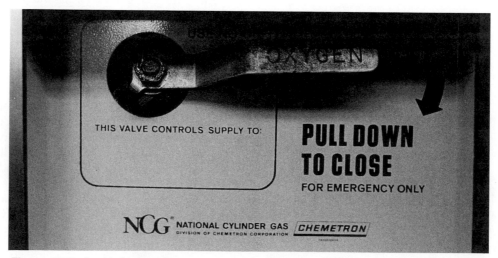

Figure 12-8 *A typical zone valve*

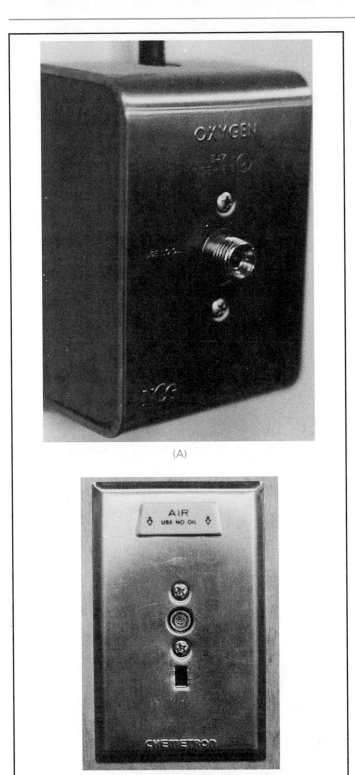

(A)

(B)

Figure 12-9 *DISS (A) and quick-connect (B) fittings*

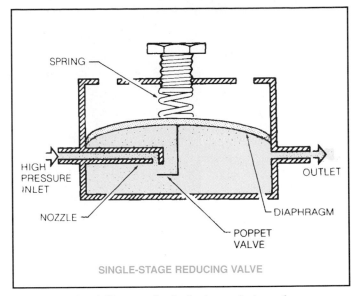

SINGLE-STAGE REDUCING VALVE

Figure 12-10 *A diagram of a single-stage reducing valve*

Modified Single-Stage Reducing Valve

A modified single-stage reducing valve is very similar in design to a single-stage reducing valve. The only difference is the addition of a poppet-closing spring (Figure 12-11).

The poppet-closing spring provides a force in addition to gas pressure to oppose the force of the spring tension. The additional force provided by the poppet-closing spring allows the valve to open and close at a faster rate. The faster rate enables this reducing valve to provide higher flow rates than those possible with a standard single-stage reducing valve. Also, because of the faster action of the valve, pressure is more accurately regulated.

The outlet pressure on some of these reducing valves may be adjusted. By adjusting the tension of the spring using a screw adjustment, pressure may be increased or decreased.

Multistage Reducing Valves

A multistage reducing valve consists of two or more single-stage reducing valves working in series. The gas

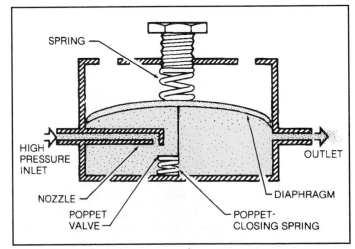

Figure 12-11 *A diagram of a modified single-stage reducing valve*

valve. If pressure builds in this section of the reducing valve, there is then an additional force to be overcome as the gas is compressed.

The outlet pressure on some of these reducing valves may be adjusted. By adjusting the tension of the spring using a screw adjustment, pressure may be increased or decreased. If no adjustment is provided, the reducing valve is termed a *preset reducing valve*.

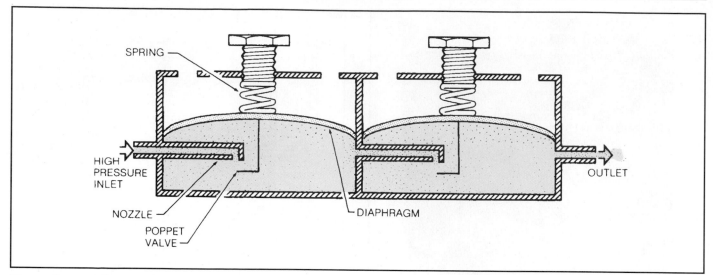

Figure 12-12 *A diagram of a two-stage reducing valve*

entering the first stage is reduced to an intermediate pressure. This first stage of the reducing valve is usually preset by the factory to a pressure of approximately 200 psi. The gas then enters the second stage and is reduced to the correct working pressure of 50 psi. The second stage spring tension is less than the spring tension of the first stage—hence the lower pressure (Figure 12-12).

Three or more stages may be connected in series. In clinical practice, two-stage and, on rare occasions, three-stage reducing valves may be encountered.

The advantages of a multistage reducing valve are more accurate regulation of pressure, smoother operation, and consistently higher flow rates.

Safety Features

In the event of the build-up of excessive pressure within the reducing valve, there are several safety features incorporated into the design. These safety features are listed in Figure 12-13.

Flowmeters
Bourdon Gauge Flowmeters

A Bourdon gauge *flowmeter* may also be referred to as a *fixed orifice flowmeter*. This flowmeter is really not a flowmeter at all but rather a pressure gauge calibrated to measure flow.

A Bourdon tube flowmeter has a thin tube formed into a portion of a circle. The lower end of the tube is exposed

to the pressure released from the reducing valve. The upper end is sealed. Distal to the placement of the Bourdon tube is a restricted orifice (Figure 12-14).

As gas flows past the Bourdon tube and encounters the restricted orifice, pressure builds proximal to the orifice. As the pressure builds, the thin Bourdon tube straightens slightly. As the tube straightens, this motion is translated to rotary motion by a gear mechanism that changes the dial indication on the face of the gauge.

These flowmeters are small and quite compact. They have an advantage in that they will operate in any position. This capability has definite advantages in a transport situation.

Certain precautions must be observed with use of this type of flowmeter. The accuracy of the flowmeter is dependent on the size of the orifice of the flowmeter outlet. Therefore, restriction or back pressure at the outlet will render the reading inaccurate. It is possible to occlude the

---

- Safety popoff valve for each stage
- Beveled glass face on all gauges
- Thin, unsealed metal back on the pressure gauge
- American Standard, pin index, and diameter-indexed safety systems as appropriate

---

Figure 12-13 *Oxygen reducing valve safety features*

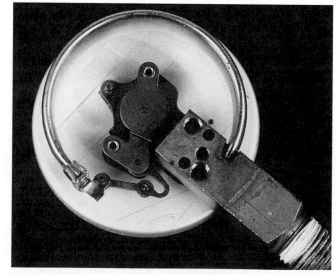

Figure 12-14 *A Bourdon gauge flowmeter*

opening of the flowmeter totally so that no flow exists and the gauge will show a flow rate higher than the original setting. Care must be exercised to prevent any restriction to flow with use of this type of flowmeter. When accurate flow rates are required, it is best to use another type of flowmeter.

Thorpe Tube Flowmeters

Thorpe tube flowmeters employ a Thorpe tube in their design. A Thorpe tube is a tapered tube with a small end at the bottom and a large end at the top. This V-shaped tube provides a variable orifice. The internal diameter of the tube varies from the bottom to the top, increasing in area toward the top.

A float device is suspended in the tube by the flow of gas. In oxygen and air flowmeters, the float is typically a small-diameter steel ball. The ball or float remains suspended as a result of a pressure differential between the top and the bottom of the float. The higher the flow rate, the higher the pressure is below the float, causing the float to be suspended at a higher level. Of course, the higher the float is suspended, the larger the opening around the float. Thus, more gas is allowed to exit around the float. The opposing forces at work are the weight of the ball and the pressure differential that is related to the flow of gas.

Thorpe tube flowmeters can be classified into two general categories: uncompensated and back pressure–compensated. The placement of the needle valve in the flowmeter design determines whether it is uncompensated or back pressure–compensated (Figure 12-15).

Uncompensated Thorpe Tube Flowmeters

The uncompensated Thorpe tube flowmeter has the needle valve placed proximal to the Thorpe tube or *upstream*. With the flowmeter operating normally, the pressure proximal to the needle valve is equal to the line pressure or 50 psi. The pressure distal to the needle valve is equal to the atmospheric pressure.

With partial obstruction of the outlet of the flowmeter, the pressure inside the Thorpe tube would increase owing to the increased resistance. As the pressure within the tube increases, the pressure differential between the top and bottom of the float decreases and the float is suspended at a lower position. This would indicate a lower flow than originally set. In reality, the actual flow rate may not change at all. It is possible, in the face of back pressure distal to the needle valve, to deliver flows higher than indicated by the suspension of the float.

Back Pressure–Compensated Flowmeter

The back pressure–compensated flowmeter has the needle valve placed distal or *downstream* from the Thorpe tube. By placing the needle valve in this position, the pressure within the Thorpe tube proximal to the needle valve remains at the line pressure of 50 psi. The pressure distal to (downstream from) the needle valve is ambient or atmospheric pressure.

If the outlet of a back pressure–compensated flowmeter is partially occluded, the flow rate will still be indicated accurately. As long as there is flow, the pressure distal to the needle valve will not exceed the line pressure of 50 psi.

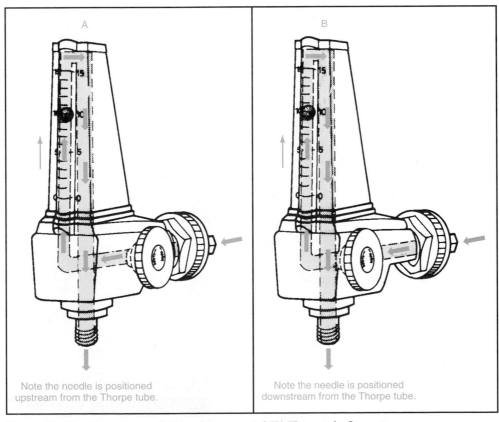

Note the needle is positioned upstream from the Thorpe tube.

Note the needle is positioned downstream from the Thorpe tube.

Figure 12-15 *Uncompensated (A) and compensated (B) Thorpe tube flowmeters*

The restriction is simply serving as another needle valve restricting the flow. With total occlusion of the outlet, the pressure distal to the needle valve would be equal to the line pressure of 50 psi and the float would not be suspended, indicating zero flow.

Liquid Oxygen Systems

Liquid oxygen systems have become very popular in home care primarily for economic reasons. A large reservoir is the primary system the patient uses. The reservoir contains as much oxygen as in several H cylinders and is less expensive to fill. The large reservoir can power a humidifier, a nebulizer, or positive-pressure breathing devices from its 50 psi outlet. The construction of the liquid reservoir is similar to that of a large thermos bottle. Liquid oxygen is contained in the reservoir at −297°F. When demand causes gas to flow from the reservoir, the liquid moves through condensing coils that vaporize the liquid into a gas.

For portable use, a smaller reservoir can be filled from the large one. The smaller reservoir is similar in design and construction to the larger unit. At a low flow rate, the smaller reservoir can last several hours. It is small and compact, weighing approximately 11 pounds when full. Figure 12-16 shows a smaller reservoir mated to the larger one for refilling.

Oxygen Concentrators

Within the past 10 years, oxygen concentrators have been developed primarily for low-flow oxygen therapy in the home. An *oxygen concentrator* takes air from the atmosphere and separates the oxygen from the other gases in the air. These units provide an adequate oxygen concentration of between 40% to 90%, depending on the type of unit.

There are currently two types of oxygen concentrators on the market. The two types are membrane (oxygen enricher) and molecular sieve oxygen concentrators.

The membrane type of oxygen enricher uses a thin membrane made out of a polymer. This membrane is only 1 micrometer thick. A compressor provides a pressure gradient across the membrane. Oxygen and water vapor pass through the membrane at a faster rate than is the case with nitrogen. This type of concentrator can provide a humidified oxygen concentration of approximately 40%.

The molecular sieve concentrator utilizes a chemical (sodium–aluminum silicate) to scrub the nitrogen from the air. A compressor forces the ambient air through the sieve. The gas, after passing through the sieve, has a concentration of oxygen between 50% and 90%. At low flow rates (2 L/min or less) the concentration of oxygen is 90%. At a flow rate of 10 L/min, the oxygen concentration drops to 50%. At the lower flow rate, the ambient air has a greater exposure time in the sieve and therefore more nitrogen is separated. Figure 12-17 shows a typical oxygen concentrator.

Air/Oxygen Blenders

An *air/oxygen blender* is a device that provides a precise oxygen concentration by mixing air and oxygen. The concentration may be adjusted to any value from room air to

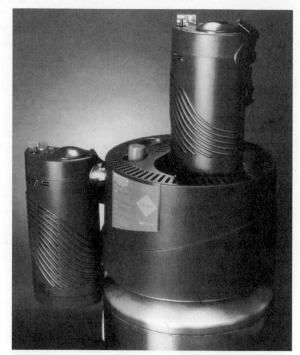

Figure 12-16 *A large liquid oxygen reservoir and a portable liquid reservoir for home use (Courtesy of* CAIRE, Inc., Bloomington, MN)

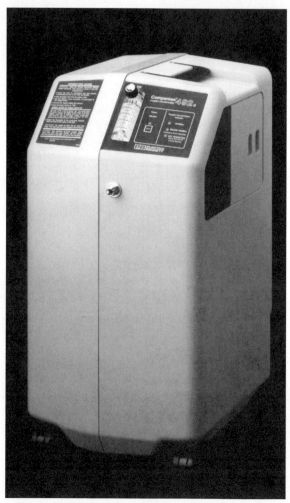

Figure 12-17 *An oxygen concentrator (Courtesy of* Puritan Bennett Corporation, Lenexa, KS)

100% oxygen. All air/oxygen blenders have a 50 psi outlet and some have a Thorpe tube flowmeter attached, in addition to the outlet.

Air/oxygen blenders have a 50 psi inlet for both air and oxygen. Internally, a proportioning valve mixes the incoming air and oxygen as the oxygen percentage dial is adjusted. Variations in line pressure or in flow or pressure requirements for any attached device will not affect the oxygen concentration. Air/oxygen blenders are ideally suited for use with ventilators or other devices with high flow and pressure demands because oxygen delivery is not affected.

OBJECTIVES

At the end of this chapter, you should be able to:

- Correctly select an E or an H cylinder for use.
- Correctly maneuver a medical gas cylinder onto and off a cylinder cart.
- Demonstrate the correct handling of a cylinder and cart on level ground.

- Properly prepare a cylinder for attachment of a reducing valve or gas delivery device.
- Correctly demonstrate the process of bleeding a reducing valve before removal.
- Demonstrate how to prepare an air/oxygen blender for use.

USING MEDICAL GAS CYLINDERS

Obtaining the Cylinder from Storage

Large medical gas cylinders are stored along a wall where, for optimal safety, chains or straps are provided to secure the cylinders to the wall. The safety chains will prevent the cylinders from accidentally falling from the upright position.

The first step in obtaining a medical gas cylinder for use is cylinder identification. Color code and the adhesive label affixed to the cylinder should match. If they do not match, do not use that cylinder. Mark the cylinder and return it to the medical gas supplier.

Once the correct cylinder has been identified, you may maneuver it onto the cart designed to facilitate the safe transport of large cylinders.

Maneuvering Large Medical Gas Cylinders

An oxygen H cylinder weighs approximately 135 pounds when full. Care must be exercised when handling this much weight concentrated in a relatively small package. Besides the weight factor, the pressure in a full cylinder, if it is mistreated, could cause serious injury.

To maneuver a cylinder onto the cart, unchain the cylinder or bank of cylinders from the wall. Grasp the cylinder of choice by placing one hand on the protective cap over the cylinder valve and the other hand on the cylinder shoulder. Tilt the cylinder toward your body slightly. With the cylinder in a tilted position, it is easy to roll the cylinder on its base in the desired direction. The hand placed on the safety cap provides stability, while the other hand provides the locomotion (Figure 12-18).

The cylinder cart should be placed in a convenient location close to the bank of cylinders, allowing sufficient room to maneuver. The cart should be in an upright position with the third wheel in the retracted position.

To maneuver the cylinder onto the cart, block one of the main wheels with a chock or your foot to prevent the cart from tipping over when the cylinder is rolled onto it (Figure 12-19). After the cylinder is on the cart, securely chain it with the chain provided. After the cylinder is secured, lock the third wheel into position and, by placing your foot on one of the main wheels, rotate the cart onto the third wheel. The cylinder and cart should now be resting on all three wheels. Return to the main bank of cylinders where you obtained your cylinder and reattach the chain securing the other cylinders as required.

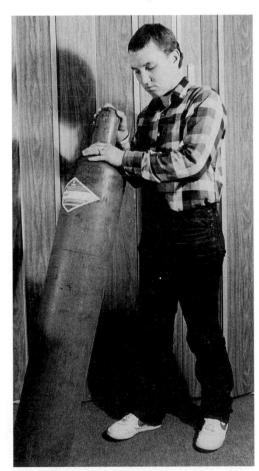

Figure 12-18 *Rolling an H cylinder*

Transporting the Cylinder and Cart

You are now ready to transport the cylinder and cart to the desired location. To transport the cylinder and cart, place one hand on the safety cap over the cylinder valve and the other hand on the handle of the cart. Figure 12-19 illustrates the process of moving a cylinder on a cylinder cart. This hand position will provide you with the best control of the cylinder and cart. Push the cylinder and cart in front of you while keeping a sharp eye out for other personnel, objects, or hazards. When approaching a corner or busy area, slow down. It is often difficult to see other personnel when approaching these areas.

Cracking the Cylinder

Before attachment of any equipment to a cylinder, the cylinder valve must be cracked. *Cracking* the cylinder removes any dust, or particulate matter, from the outlet of the cylinder valve. This prevents contaminants from entering your equipment. If the materials are flammable, fire hazard is minimized because they are removed before the application of high-pressure oxygen.

To crack a cylinder, place the cart in an upright position and release the third wheel into the retracted position. Remove the safety cap from the cylinder valve. Ideally, this should be done in an area away from patient rooms. Point the outlet of the cylinder valve away from you and other personnel. Remove the protective cover from the cylinder valve outlet, if one is provided. Announce to any personnel around you that you are going to crack the tank and that it will make a loud noise. Place your hand around the rim of the cylinder valve handle and quickly rotate the handle one-quarter turn counterclockwise; then quickly rotate it clockwise back to the closed position. When a cylinder is cracked, gas at 2200 psi pressure exiting through the narrow opening of the cylinder valve makes a very loud hissing noise. The sudden noise is enough to startle anyone. The cylinder is now ready for attachment of a reducing valve or other equipment.

Attaching a Reducing Valve

A reducing valve for an H cylinder has the American Standard Index thread safety system. You will need a wrench to attach the reducing valve to the cylinder.

Place the female end of the American Standard Index fitting of the reducing valve onto the male portion of the cylinder valve. Attach the nut "finger tight" by rotating the nut clockwise. Now, using the wrench, tighten the nut by rotating it farther in the clockwise direction.

After the reducing valve is secure, slowly open the cylinder valve by turning the handle counterclockwise. Keep your hand on the outside of the handle's rim. Never place the palm of your hand so that it covers the entire handle. Listen and feel for leaks at the cylinder valve connection. If you are in doubt about the presence of a leak, a solution of soapy water may be used to detect it. Open the cylinder valve completely; then rotate it clockwise one-quarter turn. You are now ready to attach any further equipment requiring a 50 psi oxygen source.

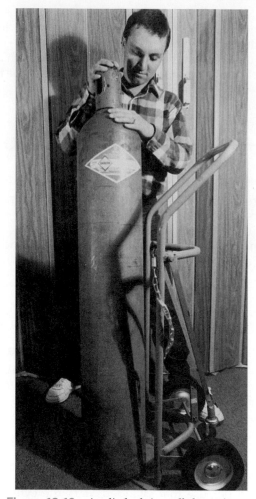

Figure 12-19 *A cylinder being rolled onto its cart*

Using an H Cylinder in a Patient Area

For use of cylinders at the patient's bedside, there should be safety chains on the wall to secure the cylinder. If chains are not available, a cylinder base may be used to secure the cylinder. For short-term use, the cylinder cart can be tilted in the upright position and the third wheel placed in the retracted position.

It is imperative to place the cylinder in a spot where it will not be disturbed by traffic into or out of the room. Keep it away from heat registers and electrical outlets. Placard the room with signs inside and outside stating "No smoking—oxygen in use." If the patient has a history of smoking and is not coherent, remove any smoking materials.

Do not leave a cylinder standing on its base, unsecured by a chain, cart, or cylinder base.

Maneuvering an E Cylinder

E cylinders are often found in the same storage area as for the larger H cylinders. Owing to their smaller size, they are often kept in a divided box, somewhat like an egg crate. This divided box keeps the cylinders upright and separated from one another. Just like H cylinders, E cylinders have a special cart to facilitate their transport.

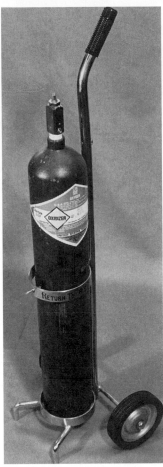

Figure 12-20 *An E cylinder secured to its cart*

To place an E cylinder onto its cart, lift the cylinder and gently lower it into its cart. Secure the cylinder with one or more wing nuts provided for the purpose (Figure 12-20).

The best way to maneuver an E cylinder cart is to pull it behind you. If you maneuver the cart in front of you, your feet will become tangled with the wheels on the cart.

Cracking an E Cylinder

Cracking an E cylinder is quite similar to cracking an H cylinder. The same rules apply. Point the cylinder valve outlet in a safe direction and issue a verbal warning before cracking the tank. Be sure to use the correct end of the cylinder wrench provided for an E cylinder. Use the small slot that fits the stem of the cylinder valve. The large hexagonal opening fits the upper end of the cylinder valve. If this nut were to be removed, 2200 psi would propel the valve stem with potentially lethal force. Some hospitals cut off the hexagonal end of the wrench to prevent the inadvertent use of the wrong end.

Attaching a Reducing Valve to an E Cylinder

After cracking the cylinder, you are now ready to attach a reducing valve or other equipment. Unlike an H cylinder, an E cylinder utilizes a doughnut-shaped Teflon washer between the flat face of the cylinder valve and the yoke.

Place the washer onto the male inlet on the yoke, match the PISS safety pins, and tighten the yoke in place using the large wing nut provided. Do not use a wrench. When you change an E cylinder, always change the Teflon washer, putting a new one on with the new cylinder. This precaution will help prevent leaks. After the reducing valve or equipment is secure, slowly turn on the cylinder valve and check your attachments for leaks. Open the cylinder valve completely; then rotate it clockwise one-quarter of a turn.

Bleeding a Reducing Valve

The process of bleeding a reducing valve relieves the pressure contained in the reducing valve and attachment fittings before removal. The reducing valve should also be bled when the attached device is not in use. To bleed a reducing valve, turn off the cylinder valve. Turn on the flowmeter or the pneumatically powered equipment attached to the reducing valve, allowing the pressure to bleed off. Next, turn off the flowmeter or equipment and remove it from the cylinder.

USE OF PORTABLE LIQUID OXYGEN SYSTEMS

Portable liquid oxygen systems have become popular for home and ambulatory use (see Figure 12-16). The primary liquid systems are relatively small (12 to 15 inches in diameter and 27 to 38 inches tall, weighing between 84 and 160 pounds), whereas the ambulatory systems weigh between 5.3 and 9.0 pounds and are very compact. These portable systems can contain between 20 and 43 liquid liters of oxygen whereas the ambulatory systems may contain between 0.6 and 1.2 liquid liters of oxygen. Because each liter of liquid oxygen is equivalent to 861 liters of gaseous oxygen, capacities will vary, ranging between 16,000 and 35,000 liters for the primary systems and 500 and 1025 liters for the ambulatory systems.

Transfilling the Ambulatory System

Before transfilling a portable system from a primary liquid reservoir, it is important to review some important safety considerations. Liquid oxygen is stored at −280°F, and contact with the liquid will result in cryogenic burns. Like gaseous oxygen, liquid oxygen will support and accelerate combustion. Transfilling should never be done in the vicinity of anyone smoking or around any open flames. During the transfilling process and afterward, the couplings are extremely cold and may cause cryogenic burns. Always store both the primary liquid reservoir and the portable system upright; tipping them on their side will cause them to vent liquid oxygen.

Attach the ambulatory system to the primary system by coupling them together by connecting the male fill port of the portable system to the female fitting on the primary reservoir. Rotate the portable system until it is locked into place on the primary reservoir. Once the two systems are connected to one another, open the vent port on the portable system to allow liquid to flow from the primary reservoir into the portable system. The vent must be opened for oxygen to flow. Continue filling the portable system until you can observe liquid oxygen being expelled from the vent on the portable system. Closing the vent valve terminates the flow of oxygen into the portable system. Disconnect the portable system from the primary reservoir by rotating the portable system until it detaches from the primary liquid reservoir.

Primary Liquid Reservoir Use

Connect an oxygen flowmeter to the DISS threaded outlet fitting. Adjust the liter flow to the desired setting and connect an appropriate oxygen delivery device. Some liquid primary reservoirs have a built-in flow control valve: adjust the flow control valve to the desired setting and connect an appropriate oxygen delivery device to the threaded DISS outlet.

Portable System Use

Once the portable system has been transfilled and is full, connect an appropriate oxygen delivery device to the nipple outlet of the portable system. Adjust the flow control valve to the desired setting.

Determining Liquid Oxygen Duration

The duration of liquid oxygen systems is determined by the weight of the reservoir (primary or portable). Each pound of liquid oxygen contains 342.8 liters of gaseous oxygen. To determine the duration of the reservoir, complete the following steps:

1. Weigh the reservoir.
2. Subtract the empty weight of the reservoir from its current weight to determine the weight of the liquid oxygen in the reservoir.
3. Multiply the liquid oxygen weight by 342.8 L/lb and multiply that product by 0.8 (a factor used to allow for variations in spring scales).
4. Divide the result obtained in step 3 by the liter flow rate being used.

Example

Mrs. Jones has filled her portable system. It weighs 9.5 lb following filling and has an empty weight of 6.5 lb. At a liter flow of 3 L/min, how long will her portable system last?

1. 9.5 lb − 6.5 lb = 3.0 lb liquid oxygen weight
2. (3.0 lb × 342.8 L/lb)0.8 = 824 L
3. 824 L ÷ 3 L/min = 274 minutes or 4.5 hours

USE OF AN OXYGEN CONCENTRATOR

Oxygen concentrators provide a convenient method for the delivery of oxygen for home or subacute use that is less expensive than use of cylinders or liquid systems. The only expense of these systems, once purchased, is the electricity used to run the unit's compressor, because oxygen is separated from atmospheric air.

Place the concentrator in the room in which your patient plans to spend the majority of his or her time. Locate the concentrator away from radiators, heaters, or any hot air registers. Be certain that the back and sides of the unit are at least 6 inches away from any walls, draperies, or surfaces that may interfere with air movement or flow into or out of the concentrator.

When selecting the electrical outlet to power the concentrator, try to select a circuit that has very little additional electrical load on it. Do not choose a circuit that also powers larger, high electrical current–drawing appliances or devices. When plugging the concentrator into the electrical outlet, verify that the power switch is first turned off before connecting the power cord to the outlet.

It is important to check the gross particle filter at the concentrator inlet for cleanliness or obstructions. If the filter is dirty, clean it in a mild solution of water and household dishwashing detergent. Rinse it thoroughly in tap water and use a towel to blot it dry. Reinstall the filter after it has been cleaned. A dirty or obstructed filter will greatly hamper the performance of an oxygen concentrator.

Attach a humidifier or appropriate oxygen delivery device to the outlet of the oxygen concentrator. Additional oxygen extension tubing may be added to facilitate patient mobility and relative freedom for movement about the home. Do not use more than 50 feet of extension tubing. Turn on the power switch and adjust the oxygen flowmeter to the desired setting.

USE OF AIR/OXYGEN BLENDERS

Preparation of an air/oxygen blender generally consists of the attachment of 50 psi air and oxygen sources to the device. High-pressure hoses are usually the most convenient way to attach the two source gases to the air/oxygen blender. Once the source gases are attached, inlet pressures may be checked on some blenders by checking the attached pressure gauge.

In the event of line pressure failure (less than 30 psi pressure), an audible alarm will sound. This alarm is strictly a pressure alarm and not an oxygen percentage alarm. This safety feature may be tested by disconnecting either the air or the oxygen source.

Once the inlet gases are attached and the air/oxygen blender is well secured to a stand or wall mount, it is ready for use. Attach the device to be operated to the 50 psi outlet or a flowmeter attached to the outlet. Adjust the desired oxygen concentration and confirm the delivered oxygen concentration with an oxygen analyzer.

References

Compressed Gas Association. (1981). *Handbook of compressed gases*. New York: Reinhold Publishing.

Grenard, S. (1973). *The hazards of respiratory therapy*. Monsey, NJ: Glenn Educational Medical Services.

Additional Resources

Cryogenics Associates Liberator 20, 30, 45, and Stroller, Sprint service manual. (1992). Bloomington, MN: Cryogenics Associates.

DeVilbiss DeVO/MC 44–90 oxygen concentrator service manual. (1987). Somerset, PA: DeVilbiss Health Care.

Garrett, D., & Donaldson, W. P. (1978). *Physical principles of respiratory therapy equipment.* Madison, WI: Ohio Medical Products.

Hunsinger, D., Lisnerski, K. J., Maurizi, J. J., & Phillips, M. L. (1980). *Respiratory technology: A procedure manual.* Reston, VA: Reston Publishing.

McPherson, S. (1995). *Respiratory therapy equipment* (5th ed.). St. Louis, MO: Mosby.

Nellcor-Puritan Bennett Companion 492a oxygen concentrator service manual. (1990). Lenexa, KS: Nellcor-Puritan Bennett.

Scanlan, C., Spearman, C. B., & Sheldon, R. L. (1995). *Egan's fundamentals of respiratory therapy* (6th ed.). St. Louis, MO: Mosby.

Practice Activities: Oxygen Supply Systems

1. Practice maneuvering an H cylinder and an E cylinder onto and off a transport cart:
   a. Use good body mechanics.
   b. Utilize safety chains.
   c. Maintain contact with cylinder at the valve cap and shoulder.

2. Practice maneuvering a cylinder and cart around the laboratory.

3. Practice cracking both cylinder types.
   a. Observe all safety rules.

4. Practice selecting and attaching the appropriate reducing valves:
   a. Identify and describe all safety features.
   b. Determine by inspection whether the reducing valve is single-stage or multistage.
   c. Observe all safety rules.

5. Practice bleeding a reducing valve following use.
   a. Observe good safety practices.

6. Practice returning cylinders to the storage area.
   a. Observe cylinder storage safety rules:
      (1) Empty and full cylinders are separate.
      (2) Flammable anesthetics are not stored with oxygen.
      (3) Cylinders are chained.
      (4) Door is kept closed.

7. Practice preparing an air/oxygen blender for use:
   a. Attach 50 psi air and oxygen sources.
   b. Secure the air/oxygen blender to a stand or wall mount.
   c. Attach a delivery device to the air/oxygen blender.
   d. Adjust the percentage control to the desired concentration.
   e. Confirm the concentration with an oxygen analyzer.

Check List: Oxygen Supply Systems

_____ 1. Obtain an E or H cylinder from storage.
_____ 2. Release the safety chain.
_____   a. Ensure that other cylinders will not fall or be disturbed.
     3. Maneuver the cylinder onto the cart.
_____   a. Roll or spin the cylinder but do not try to carry it.
_____   b. Observe principles of good body mechanics.
     4. Secure the cylinder to the cart with the safety chain.
_____   a. Secure the safety chain on the cylinders in storage.
     5. Tilt the cart upright and release the third wheel.
_____   a. The cart should rest on three wheels for transport.
     6. Transport the cylinder to the desired area.
_____   a. Use caution around the other foot or vehicular traffic.

     7. Remove cylinder valve safety cap.
_____   a. Remove the cap outside the patient's room.
     8. Crack the cylinder.
_____   a. Use good hand position.
_____   b. Give an audible warning.
     9. Select and attach the correct reducing valve for use.
_____   a. Secure tightly with a wrench.
    10. Check and correct for leaks.
_____   a. Look, listen, and feel.
_____   b. Correct for leaks by tightening connections.
_____ 11. Calculate the time remaining using the gauge pressure and a given flow rate.
_____ 12. After use, push the cart back to storage.
_____ 13. Return all equipment to its proper location.

Check List: Portable Liquid Oxygen Systems

_____ 1. Weigh the portable system to determine its need for transfilling or utilize the electronic indicator gauge to determine the contents of the portable unit if one is provided.

_____ 2. Connect the portable system to the stationary reservoir by mating the male fill port fitting to the female fill port on the stationary reservoir, rotating the portable system until it locks into place.

_____ 3. Open the vent valve to begin the filling process.

4. Observe all safety rules regarding use of liquid oxygen:

_____ a. No smoking or open flame is permitted in the area.

_____ b. Avoid contact with the liquid contents.

_____ c. Avoid contact with fill port or filling fittings.

_____ d. Always store the portable and stationary reservoirs in an upright position.

_____ 5. Once liquid oxygen can be observed exiting the vent fitting, close the vent valve to stop the filling process.

_____ 6. Disconnect the portable system from the stationary reservoir.

_____ 7. Verify by weight or the unit's electronic gauge that the portable system is full.

_____ 8. Calculate the duration of time the portable system will last at the desired liter flow rate.

_____ 9. Connect the oxygen delivery device to the nipple outlet of the portable system.

_____ 10. Set the liter flow to the desired rate using the flowmeter on the portable system.

_____ 11. Document the liter flow rate and delivery device in the patient's record.

Check List: Oxygen Concentrator

1. Place the concentrator correctly at the point of use:

_____ a. Back and sides must be at least 6 inches away from walls, draperies, or potential obstructions to air flow.

_____ b. Locate the concentrator away from heaters, heat registers, or radiators.

_____ 2. Verify that the power switch is in the off position.

3. Connect the power cord to an electrical outlet.

_____ a. Check to ensure that a minimal load is shared on that particular circuit.

_____ 4. Check the gross particle filter at the air inlet for cleanliness or obstructions, and clean it as required.

_____ 5. Connect a humidifier to the outlet (if required or prescribed), or connect the oxygen delivery device directly to the outlet of the concentrator.

_____ 6. If required for patient mobility, connect up to 50 feet of oxygen extension tubing between the concentrator and the delivery device.

_____ 7. Turn on the power switch.

_____ 8. Adjust the liter flow to the desired setting.

_____ 9. Document the liter flow rate and delivery device in the patient's record.

Self-Evaluation Post Test: Oxygen Supply Systems

1. A molecular sieve oxygen concentrator is delivering oxygen at a flow of 10 L/min. The delivered oxygen percentage is approximately:
   a. 100%.
   b. 80%.
   c. 60%.
   d. 50%.

2. Which of the following safety systems is utilized for equipment operating at less than 200 psi?
   a. Diameter-indexed safety system
   b. American Standard Safety System
   c. Pin index safety system
   d. Frangible disc and fusible plug combination
   e. American index system

3. With use of a compensated Thorpe tube flowmeter in the face of resistance distal to the flowmeter, the reading on the flowmeter will be:
   a. less than the delivered flow.
   b. greater than the delivered flow.
   c. equal to the delivered flow.
   d. dependent on temperature and pressure.

4. How many liters are there in 1 cubic foot of gaseous oxygen?
   a. 32.8 L
   b. 23.8 L
   c. 3.14 L
   d. 0.28 L

5. If the outlet of a Bourdon gauge became partially obstructed, the indicated flow would:
   a. be higher than you set.
   b. be lower than you set.
   c. indicate no flow (zero).
   d. not change.

6. An H cylinder contains how many cubic feet of oxygen when full?
   a. 22 cu ft
   b. 38 cu ft
   c. 220 cu ft
   d. 244 cu ft

7. Stamped on the shoulder of an H cylinder are the markings "3AA 2015." These markings indicate the:
   a. DOT code number and filling pressure.
   b. ICC code number.
   c. serial number of the cylinder.
   d. USP purity number.

8. In a compressed gas storage area, oxygen should not be stored with:
   a. carbon dioxide.
   b. helium.
   c. nitrogen.
   d. flammable anesthetics.

9. The difference between a single-stage and a modified single-stage reducing valve is:
   a. an additional pressure relief valve.
   b. a poppet-closing spring.
   c. the presence of two diaphragms.
   d. a second reducing stage.

10. Mr. Brown is a patient with COPD who is on home oxygen. He wants to go out for dinner. If he takes a full E cylinder and uses 4 L/min, leaving at 6:00 PM, by what time must he return to avoid running out of oxygen?
    a. 6:30 PM   c. 8:20 PM
    b. 7:15 PM   d. 9:00 PM

PERFORMANCE EVALUATION: OXYGEN SUPPLY SYSTEMS

Date: Lab _____ Clinical _____ Agency _____

Lab: Pass _____ Fail _____   Clinical: Pass _____ Fail _____

Student name _____   Instructor name _____

No. of times observed in clinical _____

No. of times practiced in clinical _____

PASSING CRITERIA: Obtain 90% or better on the procedure. Tasks indicated by * must receive at least 1 point, or the evaluation is terminated. Procedure must be performed within designated time, or the performance receives a failing grade.

SCORING:
2 points — Task performed satisfactorily without prompting.
1 point — Task performed satisfactorily with self-initiated correction.
0 points — Task performed incorrectly or with prompting required.
NA — Task not applicable to the patient care situation.

TASKS:

		PEER	LAB	CLINICAL
*	1. Obtains an H and an E cylinder and appropriate regulators from storage areas	☐	☐	☐
	2. Releases the safety chain	☐	☐	☐
	3. Maneuvers the cylinder onto cart	☐	☐	☐
*	4. Secures the cylinder to the cart with the safety chain	☐	☐	☐
*	5. Tilts the cart upright	☐	☐	☐
*	6. Releases the third wheel	☐	☐	☐
*	7. Removes the cylinder valve cap and gives an audible warning of the impending noise	☐	☐	☐
*	8. Cracks the cylinder with safe hand and valve positions	☐	☐	☐
*	9. Selects the correct reducing valve for intended use	☐	☐	☐
*	10. Secures the reducing valve to the cylinder	☐	☐	☐
x	11. Checks for and corrects any leaks	☐	☐	☐
*	12. Calculates the amount of time before the cylinder must be changed at a liter flow designated by the instructor	☐	☐	☐
*	13. Pushes the cart correctly to the patient area and back to storage	☐	☐	☐
*	14. Returns all the equipment to storage and properly secures it	☐	☐	☐

SCORE:
Peer _____ points of possible 28; _____%
Lab _____ points of possible 28; _____%
Clinical _____ points of possible 28; _____%

TIME: _____ out of possible 15 minutes

STUDENT SIGNATURES   **INSTRUCTOR SIGNATURES**

PEER: _____   LAB: _____

STUDENT: _____   CLINICAL: _____

PERFORMANCE EVALUATION:
LIQUID OXYGEN SYSTEMS

Date: Lab _____ Clinical _____ Agency _____

Lab: Pass _____ Fail _____ Clinical: Pass _____ Fail _____

Student name _____ Instructor name _____

No. of times observed in clinical _____

No. of times practiced in clinical _____

PASSING CRITERIA: Obtain 90% or better on the procedure. Tasks indicated by * must receive at least 1 point, or the evaluation is terminated. Procedure must be performed within designated time, or the performance receives a failing grade.

SCORING: 2 points — Task performed satisfactorily without prompting.
1 point — Task performed satisfactorily with self-initiated correction.
0 points — Task performed incorrectly or with prompting required.
NA — Task not applicable to the patient care situation.

TASKS:		PEER	LAB	CLINICAL
	1. Weighs the portable system or reads the gauge to determine if filling is required	☐	☐	☐
*	2. Follows all safety rules:			
	a. No smoking or open flame is permitted	☐	☐	☐
	b. Avoid contact with fill port fittings	☐	☐	☐
	c. Liquid reservoirs are stored upright	☐	☐	☐
*	3. Connects the portable system to the stationary one	☐	☐	☐
*	4. Opens the vent valve	☐	☐	☐
*	5. Closes the vent valve when liquid oxygen can be observed venting through the vent port	☐	☐	☐
*	6. Disconnects the two systems from one another	☐	☐	☐
*	7. Verifies that the portable system is full	☐	☐	☐
*	8. Calculates the time that the portable system will last	☐	☐	☐
*	9. Connects the oxygen delivery device	☐	☐	☐
*	10. Sets the liter flow	☐	☐	☐
*	11. Documents procedure in the patient's record	☐	☐	☐

SCORE: Peer _____ points of possible 26; _____%

Lab _____ points of possible 26; _____%

Clinical _____ points of possible 26; _____%

TIME: _____ out of possible 30 minutes

STUDENT SIGNATURES   INSTRUCTOR SIGNATURES

PEER: _____   LAB: _____

STUDENT: _____   CLINICAL: _____

PERFORMANCE EVALUATION: OXYGEN CONCENTRATORS

Date: Lab _____ Clinical _____ Agency _____

Lab: Pass _____ Fail _____   Clinical: Pass _____ Fail _____

Student name _____   Instructor name _____

No. of times observed in clinical _____

No. of times practiced in clinical _____

PASSING CRITERIA: Obtain 90% or better on the procedure. Tasks indicated by * must receive at least 1 point, or the evaluation is terminated. Procedure must be performed within designated time, or the performance receives a failing grade.

SCORING:
2 points — Task performed satisfactorily without prompting.
1 point — Task performed satisfactorily with self-initiated correction.
0 points — Task performed incorrectly or with prompting required.
NA — Task not applicable to the patient care situation.

TASKS: PEER   LAB   CLINICAL

		TASK	PEER	LAB	CLINICAL
	1.	Places the concentrator correctly at the point of use			
*	a.	Away from walls or draperies	☐	☐	☐
*	b.	Away from heaters, heat registers, or radiators	☐	☐	☐
*	2.	Connects the power cord, ensuring that the circuit has minimal electrical load	☐	☐	☐
*	3.	Checks the gross particle filter and cleans as needed	☐	☐	☐
*	4.	Connects a humidifier as required	☐	☐	☐
*	5.	Connects the oxygen delivery device	☐	☐	☐
*	6.	Adds up to 50 feet of extension tubing as needed	☐	☐	☐
*	7.	Turns on the power switch	☐	☐	☐
*	8.	Sets the liter flow rate	☐	☐	☐
*	9.	Documents procedure in the patient record	☐	☐	☐

SCORE: Peer   _____ points of possible 20; _____%

            Lab   _____ points of possible 20; _____%

            Clinical _____ points of possible 20; _____%

TIME: _____ out of possible 30 minutes

STUDENT SIGNATURES   INSTRUCTOR SIGNATURES

PEER: _____   LAB: _____

STUDENT: _____   CLINICAL: _____

CHAPTER 13
OXYGEN ADMINISTRATION

INTRODUCTION

Oxygen therapy, when indicated and when administered by a knowledgeable respiratory care practitioner, may have a dramatic effect on the condition of a patient suffering from hypoxemia. However, under certain circumstances, overadministration of oxygen may be harmful and even fatal.

Oxygen is listed in the *United States Pharmacopoeia* (USP) as a drug. Therefore, it may be administered only upon an order from a physician. Oxygen therapy is frequently abused and misused. It is important that you become knowledgeable about the various oxygen delivery devices. Acquaint yourself with the advantages of each, as well as the associated hazards and complications.

Because the initiation of oxygen administration calls for relatively simple skills, it is easy to overlook the hazards and potential complications associated with this modality. Your knowledge of these factors may prevent injury or even death resulting from the inappropriate administration of oxygen.

KEY TERMS

- Absorption atelectasis
- Anatomic reservoir
- Croupette
- FiO_2
- Head box
- High-flow oxygen delivery system

- Hypoxemia
- Isolette
- Low-flow oxygen delivery system
- Nasal cannula
- Nonrebreathing mask

- Oxygen analyzer
- Partial rebreathing mask
- Retinopathy of prematurity
- Simple oxygen mask
- Transtracheal catheter

OBJECTIVES

At the end of this chapter, you should be able to:

- State the indications for oxygen therapy.
- Define *high-flow* and *low-flow oxygen delivery systems*, and categorize six administration devices.
- Explain the role of the nasopharynx and the oropharynx, and effect of tidal volume and respiratory rate, on the delivered FiO_2 by low-flow oxygen systems.
- Explain the principle of operation for the majority of high-flow oxygen delivery systems.
- Diagram the flow of oxygen and air through a multivent mask.
- Given an oxygen flow rate and entrainment ratio, calculate the total flow.
- Differentiate between the indications for the use of a low-flow or high-flow oxygen system.

- Explain the rationale for the use of a humidifier with oxygen delivery devices.
- List the oxygen delivery devices that can be categorized as enclosures, and their advantages and disadvantages and FiO_2 ranges.
- Describe the oxygen percentages that can be delivered by the different enclosures.
- Describe the proper use of an oxygen analyzer.
- Describe the two most common types of oxygen analyzers.
- Explain the following conditions associated with oxygen administration:
  — Absorption atelectasis
  — Interruption of hypoxic drive
  — Oxygen toxicity
  — Retinopathy of Prematurity
- Discuss the role of arterial blood gas analysis in the administration of oxygen.

CLINICAL PRACTICE GUIDELINES

AARC Clinical Practice Guideline
Oxygen Therapy in the Acute Care Hospital

OT-AC 4.0 INDICATIONS:

  4.1 Documented hypoxemia

   4.1.1 In adults, children, and infants older than 28 days, arterial oxygen tension (PaO_2) of <60 torr or arterial oxygen satu-

ration (SaO_2) of <90% in subject's breathing room air or with PaO_2 and/or SaO_2 below desirable range for specific clinical situation (1,2)

   4.1.2 In neonates, PaO_2 <50 torr and/or SaO_2 <88% or capillary oxygen tension (PcO_2) <40 torr (1,3,4)

(Continued)

219

(CPG *Continued*)

4.2 An acute care situation in which hypoxemia is suspected (1,5,6–8) — substantiation of hypoxemia is required within an appropriate period of time following initiation of therapy.
4.3 Severe trauma (7,8)
4.4 Acute myocardial infarction (1,9)
4.5 Short-term therapy (e.g., postanesthesia recovery) (7,10)

OT-AC 5.0 CONTRAINDICATIONS:
No specific contraindications to oxygen therapy exist when indications are judged to be present.

OT-AC 6.0 PRECAUTIONS AND/OR POSSIBLE COMPLICATIONS:
6.1 With PaO_2 > or = 60 torr, ventilatory depression may occur in spontaneously breathing patients with elevated $PaCO_2$. (8,11,12)
6.2 With FIO_2 > or = 0.5, absorption atelectasis, oxygen toxicity, and/or depression of ciliary and/or leukocytic function may occur. (12,13)
6.3 In newborns
    6.3.1 In premature infants, PaO_2 of >80 torr should be avoided because of the possibility of retinopathy of prematurity. (2,14)
    6.3.2 Increased PaO_2 can contribute to closure or constriction of the ductus arteriosus — a possible concern in infants with ductus-dependent heart lesions. (15)
6.4 Supplemental oxygen should be administered with caution to patients suffering from paraquat poisoning (16) and to patients receiving bleomycin. (17)
6.5 During laser bronchoscopy, minimal levels of supplemental oxygen should be used to avoid intratracheal ignition. (18)
6.6 Fire hazard is increased in the presence of increased oxygen concentrations.
6.7 Bacterial contamination associated with certain nebulization and humidification systems is a possible hazard. (19–21)

OT-AC 7.0 LIMITATIONS OF PROCEDURE:
Oxygen therapy has only limited benefit for the treatment of hypoxia due to anemia, and benefit may be limited with circulatory disturbances.

Oxygen therapy should not be used in lieu of but in addition to mechanical ventilation when ventilatory support is indicated.

OT-AC 8.0 ASSESSMENT OF NEED:
Need is determined by measurement of inadequate oxygen tensions and/or saturations, by invasive or noninvasive methods, and/or the presence of clinical indicators as previously described.

OT-AC 9.0 ASSESSMENT OF OUTCOME:
Outcome is determined by clinical and physiologic assessment to establish adequacy of patient response to therapy.

OT-AC 11.0 MONITORING:
11.1 Patient
    11.1.1 Clinical assessment including, but not limited to, cardiac, pulmonary, and neurologic status
    11.1.2 Assessment of physiologic parameters: measurement of oxygen tensions or saturation in any patient treated with oxygen
        11.1.2.1 In conjunction with the initiation of therapy; or
        11.1.2.2 Within 12 hours of initiation with FIO_2 <0.40
        11.1.2.3 Within 8 hours, with FIO_2 > or = 0.40 (including postanesthesia recovery)
        11.1.2.4 Within 72 hours in acute myocardial infarction (9)
        11.1.2.5 Within 2 hours for any patient with the principal diagnosis of COPD
        11.1.2.6 Within 1 hour for the neonate (2)
11.2 Equipment
    11.2.1 All oxygen delivery systems should be checked at least once per day.
    11.2.2 More frequent checks by calibrated analyzer are necessary in systems.
        11.2.2.1 Susceptible to variation in oxygen concentration (e.g., hoods, high-flow blending systems)
        11.2.2.2 Applied to patients with artificial airways
        11.2.2.3 Delivering a heated gas mixture
        11.2.2.4 Applied to patients who are clinically unstable or who require an FIO_2 of 0.50 or higher
    11.2.3 The standard of practice for newborns appears to be continuous analysis of F_DO_2 with a system check at least every 4 hours, but data to support this practice may not be available.

Reprinted with permission from *Respiratory Care* 1991; 36: 1410–1413. The complete AARC Clinical Practice Guidelines are available from the AARC Web site (http://www.aarc.org), from the AARC Executive Office, or from *Respiratory Care* journal.

AARC Clinical Practice Guideline
Oxygen Therapy in the Home or
Extended Care Facility

OT-CC 4.0 INDICATIONS:
Documented hypoxemia: In adults, children, and infants older than 28 days: (1) PaO_2 < or = 55 torr or SaO_2 < or = 88% in subject's breathing room air, (1,2) or (2) PaO_2 of

$56–59$ torr or SaO_2 or $SpO_2 <$ or $= 89\%$ in association with specific clinical conditions (e.g., cor pulmonale, congestive heart failure, or erythrocythemia with hematocrit >56). (3,4)Π

Some patients may not qualify for oxygen therapy at rest but will qualify for oxygen during ambulation, sleep, or exercise. Oxygen therapy is indicated during these specific activities when SaO_2 is demonstrated to fall to < or $= 88\%$. (5)

OT-CC 5.0 CONTRAINDICATIONS:

No absolute contraindications to oxygen therapy exist when indications are present.

OT-CC 6.0 PRECAUTIONS AND/OR POSSIBLE COMPLICATIONS:

6.1 In spontaneously breathing hypoxemic patients with chronic obstructive pulmonary disease, oxygen administration may lead to an increase in $PaCO_2$. (6–8)

6.2 Undesirable results or events may result from noncompliance with physician's orders or inadequate instruction in home oxygen therapy.

6.3 Complications may result from use of nasal cannulae (9) or transtracheal catheters. (10)

6.4 Fire hazard is increased in the presence of increased oxygen concentrations.

6.5 Bacterial contamination associated with certain nebulizers and humidification systems is a possible hazard. (11–13)

6.6 Possible physical hazards can be posed by unsecured cylinders, ungrounded equipment, or mishandling of liquid oxygen (resulting in burns). Power or equipment failure can lead to an inadequate oxygen supply.

OT-CC 7.0 LIMITATIONS OF PROCEDURE:

Oxygen therapy has only limited benefit for the treatment of hypoxia due to anemia and benefit may be limited when circulatory disturbances are present.

OT-CC 8.0 ASSESSMENT OF NEED:

8.1 Initial assessment: Need is determined by the presence of clinical indicators as previously described and the presence of inadequate oxygen tension and/or saturation as demonstrated by the analysis of arterial blood. Concurrent pulse oximetry values must be documented and reconciled with the results of the baseline blood gas analysis if future assessment is to involve pulse oximetry.

8.2 Ongoing evaluation or reassessment: Additional arterial blood gas analysis is indicated whenever there is a major change in clinical status that may be cardiopulmonary-related. Arterial blood gas measurements should be repeated in 1–3 months when oxygen therapy is begun in the hospital in a clinically unstable patient to determine the need for long-term oxygen therapy (LTOT). (14) Once the need for LTOT has been documented, repeat arterial blood gas analysis or oxygen saturation measurements are unnecessary other than to follow the course of the disease, to assess changes in clinical status, or to facilitate changes in the oxygen prescription. (14,15)

OT-CC 9.0 ASSESSMENT OF OUTCOME:

Outcome is determined by clinical and physiologic assessment to establish adequacy of patient response to therapy.

OT-CC 11.0 MONITORING:

11.1 Patient

11.1.1 Clinical assessment should routinely be performed by the patient and/or the caregiver to determine changes in clinical status (e.g., use of dyspnea scales and diary cards). Patients should be visited/monitored at least once a month by credentialed personnel unless conditions warrant more frequent visits.

11.1.2 Measurement of baseline oxygen tension and saturation is essential before oxygen therapy is begun. (5,15) These measurements should be repeated when clinically indicated or to follow the course of the disease. Measurements of SO_2 also may be made to determine appropriate oxygen flow for ambulation, exercise, or sleep.

11.2 Equipment Maintenance and Supervision: All oxygen delivery equipment should be checked at least once daily by the patient or caregiver. Facets to be assessed include proper function of the equipment, prescribed flow rates, FDO_2, remaining liquid or compressed gas content, and backup supply. A respiratory care practitioner or equivalent should during monthly visits reinforce appropriate practices and performance by the patient and caregivers and ensure that the oxygen equipment is being maintained in accordance with manufacturers' recommendations. Liquid systems need to be checked to ensure adequate delivery. (25) Oxygen concentrators should be checked regularly to ensure that they are delivering 85% oxygen or greater at 4 L/min. (24)

Reprinted with permission from *Respiratory Care* 1992; 37: 918–922. The complete AARC Clinical Practice Guidelines are available from the AARC Web site (http://www.aarc.org), from the AARC Executive Office, or from *Respiratory Care* journal.

INDICATIONS FOR OXYGEN THERAPY

The primary indication for oxygen therapy is hypoxemia. *Hypoxemia* is defined as an oxygen tension in arterial blood (PaO_2) that is below normal. You can estimate PaO_2 for a patient breathing room air by using the following formula: $103.5 - (0.42 \times age) \pm 4$ (Sabrini et al., 1968). As a respiratory care practitioner, you keep in mind the effects that altitude has on what is considered normal.

The amount of oxygen required to correct the hypoxemia will vary depending on the patient's clinical condition. The best way to assess the effects of oxygen therapy is by arterial blood gas analysis or monitoring by oximetry. Sampling arterial blood allows the oxygen therapy to be tailored to meet the patient's specific needs.

There are other therapeutic goals for oxygen administration in addition to correction of hypoxemia (Shapiro, Kacmarek, Cane, & Hauptman, 1991). These goals are listed in Figure 13-1.

Hypoxemia may cause an increase in ventilation and cardiac output as the body compensates (the hypoxic drive). By increasing the oxygen content of the arterial blood, the muscle (energy) requirements of the pulmonary and cardiovascular systems are reduced.

Low-Flow Oxygen Delivery Systems

A *low-flow oxygen delivery system* is defined as a system that supplies oxygen-enriched gas as part of a patient's inspiratory flow needs. The patient must be able to inhale sufficiently to meet ventilatory needs, but may require the administration of a limited amount of 100% oxygen, which is then mixed with room air as the patient inhales.

Low-flow devices rely on the nasopharynx and oropharynx to serve as a reservoir, enhancing FiO_2 by temporarily holding a small amount of 100% oxygen. This reservoir is referred to as the *anatomic reservoir*. In an average adult, it is estimated that this reservoir has a volume of about 50 cc (Shapiro et al., 1991).

Because the low-flow devices provide only part of the inspiratory needs, the delivered fraction of inspired oxygen (FiO_2, usually expressed as a decimal fraction) may vary depending on several factors. One factor that may alter FiO_2 is the flow of oxygen through the device. Generally, the higher the flow, the higher the FiO_2. The patient's respiratory rate and tidal volume may also affect the FiO_2.

A patient with shallower than normal tidal volumes will receive proportionately more oxygen than that delivered to the patient with a normal tidal volume. The 100% oxygen inhaled from the anatomic reservoir (approximately 50 cc) is proportionately greater in a patient with a 250-cc tidal volume than in a patient with a 500-cc tidal volume. Therefore, the FiO_2 is higher. Keep in mind that the oxygen flow through the device also influences the delivered FiO_2, as noted.

A respiratory rate higher than normal may also dilute the oxygen concentration by not allowing time for the anatomic reservoir to fill sufficiently with oxygen. Under these circumstances, more room air is inspired, diluting the oxygen concentration.

Owing to these variables, the best way to assess the adequacy of oxygen therapy with these devices is by arterial blood gas analysis and careful patient observation.

LOW-FLOW OXYGEN DEVICES

Nasal Cannula

The *nasal cannula* is designed to rest on the upper lip with the two prongs directed into each naris (nostril) of the nose. Oxygen is directed into the nasal passage, where it is warmed and humidified as the gas passes over the turbinates. This device utilizes the anatomic reservoir to deliver increased FiO_2. In a short period of time, most patients become quite comfortable with this device and hardly notice its presence.

When the cannula is correctly applied, the cannula tubing is looped over each ear and the slide is adjusted so that it is barely snug under the chin. Application of a cannula in this manner provides for safety. Without the loops, if the patient turns suddenly and stretches the connecting tubing to its limit, the cannula will pull off the face. A cannula applied incorrectly by looping the free tubing around the head may serve as a noose on a confused, combative patient. Figures 13-2 and 13-3 illustrate a nasal cannula and its correct application, respectively. Figure 13-4 is a diagram of the anatomic reservoir.

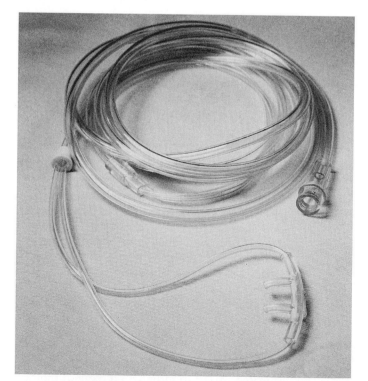

- To correct hypoxemia
- To decrease myocardial work
- To decrease the work of breathing

Figure 13-1 *Goals of oxygen therapy*

Figure 13-2 *A nasal cannula*

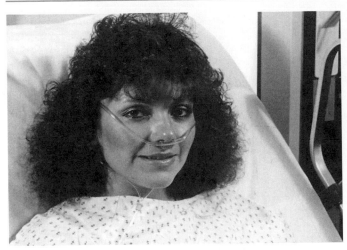

Figure 13-3   *A nasal cannula correctly applied on a patient*

TABLE 13-1:   Nasal Cannula Oxygen Concentrations

100% O_2 FLOW	OXYGEN CONCENTRATION
1 L/min	24%
2 L/min	28%
3 L/min	32%
4 L/min	36%
5 L/min	40%
6 L/min	44%

Reprinted, by permission, from Barry A. Shapiro, Clinical applications of respiratory care (3rd ed.), Table 12-2. © 1985 by Year Book Medical Publishers.

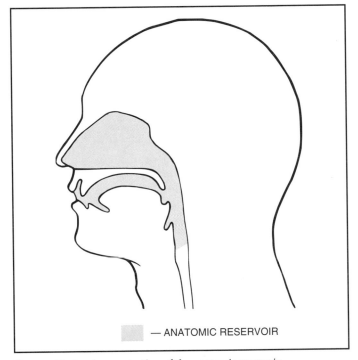

— ANATOMIC RESERVOIR

Figure 13-4   *A cross section of the anatomic reservoir*

Oxygen Concentration

The FiO$_2$ delivered by a nasal cannula will vary with the liter flow and the patient's ventilatory patterns, as discussed earlier. Table 13-1 shows approximate oxygen concentrations at various oxygen flows.

Transtracheal Catheter

A *transtracheal catheter* is a small catheter that is inserted into the trachea surgically at the second cartilaginous ring of the trachea (Figure 13-5). Because this device delivers the oxygen directly into the trachea, lower liter flows may be used than are required with a simple nasal cannula to maintain a desired PaO$_2$ or SpO$_2$ (pulse oximeter–determined arterial blood oxygen saturation). These devices are used for patients who require continuous low-flow oxygen delivery. Substantial cost savings may be realized by these patients because often an oxygen flow of 0.25 to 0.50 L/min is all that is required by these patients.

These devices are not without their hazards and complications. Because surgical intervention is required to place them, the risk of infection is always present. Therefore, these catheters must be routinely cleaned and maintained by the patient or the patient's caregiver. Also, the cost advantages must be carefully weighed against the risk of infection and the patient's cosmetic appearance.

Simple Oxygen Mask

The *simple oxygen mask* delivers a low flow of oxygen, meeting only part of a patient's inspiratory flow needs. The underlying principle in use of a mask is to add an oxygen reservoir external to the patient. The volume of the mask serves as this reservoir. Typically, the volume of this reservoir is greater than that of the anatomic reservoir.

The mask is filled with 100% oxygen at the end of inspiration. As the patient inhales, the first portion of the inspired air is the 100% oxygen contained in the mask, followed by a mixture of air and oxygen for the remainder of the inspiratory phase. The room air is allowed to enter the mask through the ports on the side of the mask. Because of the greater volume of oxygen being delivered, the FiO$_2$ provided by this device is higher than what can be administered using a nasal cannula or catheter.

The FiO$_2$ delivered by a simple mask ranges between 35% and 55% (Scanlan, Spearman & Sheldon, 1995). The FiO$_2$ will vary depending on oxygen flow rate and the patient's breathing pattern. Figures 13-6 and 13-7 show a disposable simple oxygen mask and its correct application, respectively.

Partial Rebreathing Mask

A *partial rebreathing mask* takes the reservoir concept of a simple mask one step further by the addition of a reservoir bag. Now, in addition to the mask, a large bag also serves as a reservoir. The oxygen enters the device between the bag and the reservoir. Figures 13-8 and 13-9 show a typical disposable partial rebreathing mask and its application, respectively.

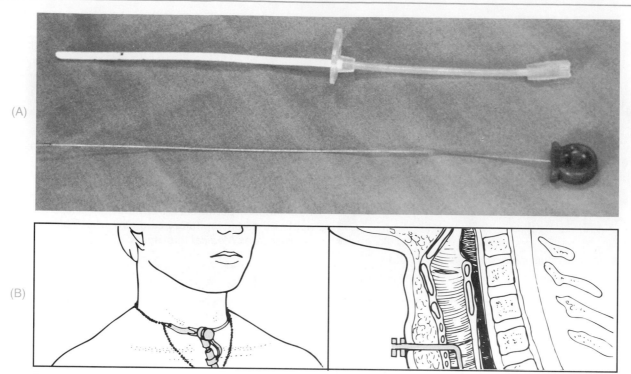

Figure 13-5 *A transtracheal catheter (A) and its correct placement (B)*

Oxygen enters the mask, filling the reservoir bag. As the patient inhales, part of the breath is inhaled from the bag and mask. The remainder of the breath is air drawn in through the ports on the side of the mask, mixing with the incoming oxygen. As the patient exhales, approximately the first third of exhaled gas fills the reservoir bag. This first part of expiratory volume is predominantly dead space and has not participated in gas exchange in the lungs. Therefore, it is relatively high in oxygen concentration. The remainder of the exhaled gas exits the mask through the ports on the side.

Because the partial rebreathing mask has a larger reservoir volume, it is capable of delivering a higher FIO_2. This mask is capable of delivering up to 60% oxygen (Scanlan et al., 1995).

When this mask is fitted properly, the flow rate should be adjusted so that the bag is not allowed to collapse completely on inspiration (Scanlan et al., 1995).

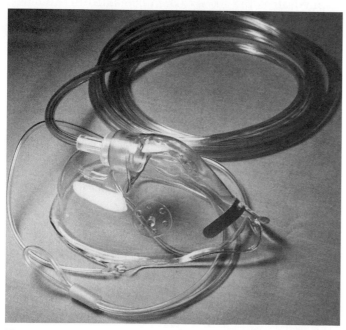

Figure 13-6 *A simple oxygen mask*

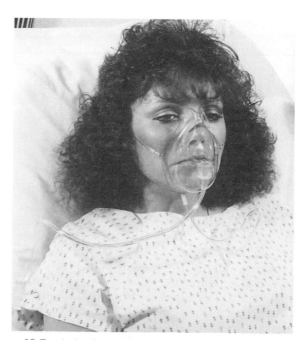

Figure 13-7 *A simple oxygen mask correctly applied on a patient*

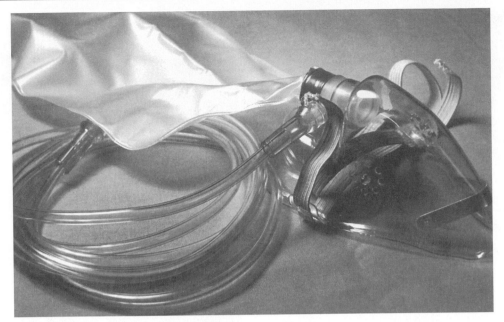

Figure 13-8 *A partial rebreathing mask*

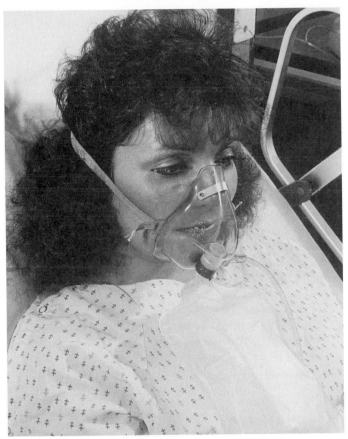

Figure 13-9 *A partial rebreathing mask correctly applied on a patient*

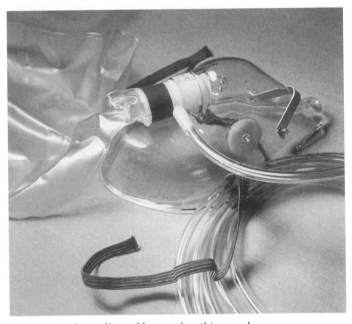

Figure 13-10 *A disposable nonrebreathing mask*

Figures 13-10 and 13-11 show a typical nonrebreathing mask and its application, respectively.

The one-way valve between the mask and bag serves to prevent the exhaled gas from entering the bag. This valve may consist of a disk and spring or may be a simple diaphragm valve. Valves over the side ports prevent the entrainment of ambient air on inspiration.

If the fit of the mask is good, both side ports have one-way valves, and if all one-way valves are functional, then it is possible to deliver up to 100% oxygen. However, with some disposable masks, only one side port is fitted with a one-way valve, and it is rarely possible to obtain a good tight fit. Under these conditions, this type of mask becomes a low-flow device because not all of

Nonrebreathing Mask

The disposable *nonrebreathing mask* is similar in design to a partial rebreathing mask. The differences lie in the addition of a one-way valve between the bag and the mask and the addition of valves on the side ports of the mask.

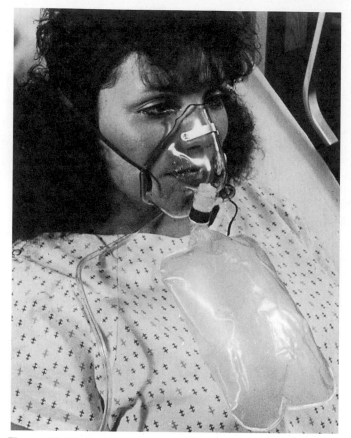

Figure 13-11 *A disposable nonrebreathing mask applied on a patient*

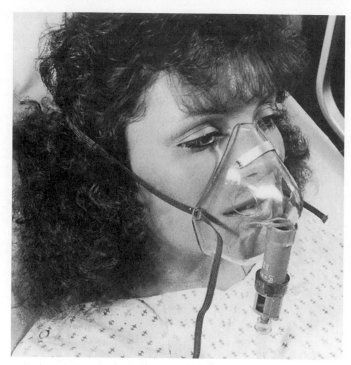

Figure 13-13 *A Venturi mask applied on a patient*

the inspiratory needs of the patient are met. The oxygen delivery would fall considerably below 100% (Scanlan et al., 1995).

As with the partial rebreathing mask, it is important to adjust the flow rate so that the reservoir bag is not allowed to completely collapse on inspiration.

HIGH-FLOW OXYGEN DELIVERY SYSTEMS

A *high-flow oxygen delivery system* provides all of the total inspiratory flow required by the patient. Any inspired gas is provided solely by the device. Respiratory pattern and rate will not affect the FIO_2 delivered by these devices.

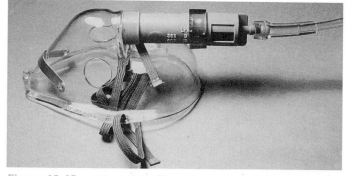

Figure 13-12 *A Venturi mask*

The majority of high-flow oxygen systems utilize jet mixing and precisely mix oxygen and ambient air to deliver a specific FIO_2. Figures 13-12 and 13-13 show a typical Venturi mask and its application, respectively.

The way in which these devices function is based on the principles of viscous shearing and vorticity (Scacci, 1979). The high-velocity gas (oxygen) exiting the nozzle (jet) causes shear forces to develop distal to the nozzle orifice and along the axis of the gas flow. These shear forces accelerate the relatively stationary ambient air, forming vortices. The ambient air is entrained by (drawn into) the oxygen flow by these vortices (Figure 13-14). By varying the size of the nozzle (jet) and entrainment ports, air and oxygen may be mixed in precise ratios to achieve known oxygen percentages. These masks are sometimes called Venturi, Venti, or multivent masks. This principle is also employed in many nebulizers to adjust the oxygen concentration.

Entrainment ratios of oxygen to room air used in establishing various FIO_2 concentrations are listed in Table 13-2.

Let us examine the significance of these entrainment ratios and see how the high-flow devices using this principle satisfy total inspiratory needs. Let's assume you have set the entrainment device to deliver 35% oxygen with a corresponding entrainment ratio of 5:1. The oxygen flowmeter is set at 6 L/min. According to the entrainment ratio, each liter of oxygen will entrain 5 liters of ambient air. With the oxygen flow at 6 L/min, the device will entrain 30 liters of ambient air per minute. The entrained ambient air is added to the flow from the oxygen flowmeter for a total flow of 36 L/min. This device, when set at an oxygen flow rate of 6 L/min, provides a total flow of 36 L/min.

Assuming an average adult has a tidal volume of 500 cc and is breathing at a rate of 14 breaths per minute with an

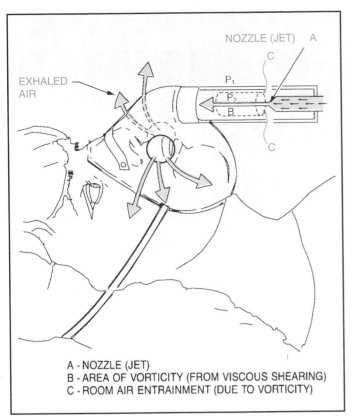

A - NOZZLE (JET)
B - AREA OF VORTICITY (FROM VISCOUS SHEARING)
C - ROOM AIR ENTRAINMENT (DUE TO VORTICITY)

Figure 13-14 *Application of viscous shearing and vorticity to entrain room air into a mask to provide a precise concentration of oxygen*

inspiratory to expiratory ratio (I:E) of 1:2, the patient would require approximately 22 L/min to meet inspiratory needs. This device floods the patient with oxygen at 35%. It is important to note that the oxygen percentage is changed by adjusting the amount of entrained ambient air, not by adjusting the flowmeter. Increasing the liter flow from 6 L/min to 10 L/min will not affect the delivered FIO_2.

Assume again that the device is adjusted for 35% oxygen, at an entrainment ratio of 5:1. As you can see by the example, increasing the oxygen flow rate simply increases ambient air entrainment at the same ratio as before.

TABLE 13-2: Air to Oxygen Entrainment Ratios	
ROOM AIR TO OXYGEN RATIO	**OXYGEN CONCENTRATION**
25:1	24%
10:1	28%
8:1	30%
5:1	35%
3:1	40%
1.7:1	50%
1:1	60%
0:1	100%

Although there is an increase in oxygen flow, this does not affect the delivered FIO_2. The total flow to the patient increases, however. In this example, the total flow increases from 36 L/min to 60 L/min, but the ratio remains the same, as does the FIO_2. To prevent dilution of entrained gas by the room air being drawn in around the mask, it is important that the total gas flow exceed the patient minute ventilation (total volume of gas inspired in 1 minute).

Effects of Back Pressure Distal to the Point of Entrainment

Back pressure applied distal to the point of entrainment causes an increase in the delivered FIO_2. This back pressure may occur as a result of a kink in the delivery tubing, water build-up, humidification, secretions in the delivery tubing, or any of a number of other factors.

An obstruction distal to the nozzle (jet) causes pressure to increase upstream to the point of entrainment. If the pressure at the entrainment ports becomes greater than ambient (atmospheric) pressure, ambient air is no longer mixed by vorticity because no air can enter (Scacci, 1979); therefore, the FIO_2 will increase.

CLINICAL APPLICATIONS OF LOW-FLOW AND HIGH-FLOW OXYGEN SYSTEMS

The low-flow oxygen devices are adequate for administering oxygen to the majority of patients. As discussed earlier, the FIO_2 cannot be accurately measured. Therefore, if the patient must receive a precise oxygen concentration, these devices would not be indicated. Also, unusual respiratory rates and depths can significantly alter the FIO_2.

High-flow oxygen systems are indicated for patients who require a constant, precise FIO_2 (Table 13-3). With use of these devices, FIO_2 will not vary from what has been set. If for physiological reasons a specific or consistent FIO_2 is desired, the high-flow device would be indicated.

HUMIDIFICATION

Oxygen from a cylinder or piping system is anhydrous. In the manufacture of medical gases, all water and water vapor are removed. The administration of dry gas is very irritating to the mucosa of the upper airway and may lead to thickened secretions, impaired ciliary activity, and retained secretions (Chalon, 1980). These adverse effects can be prevented by proper humidification with administration of oxygen.

TABLE 13-3: Effect of Increasing Oxygen Flow through High-Flow Device			
ENTRAIN-MENT RATIO	**AMBIENT AIR ENTRAIN-MENT**	**OXYGEN FLOW RATE**	**OXYGEN CONCEN-TRATION**
5:1	30 L/min	6 L/min	35%
5:1	50 L/min	10 L/min	35%

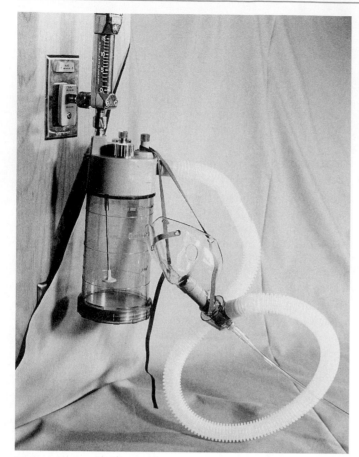

Figure 13-15 *Use of a large-volume nebulizer to humidify a Venturi mask*

All oxygen administration devices should be used with a separate humidifier. If a humidifier or nebulizer is an integral part of the design, it should be utilized.

With a Venturi mask, it is more efficient to provide humidification externally by using a collar to attach a nebulizer to the air entrainment port. By the attachment of a nebulizer, the entrained ambient air is humidified before reaching the patient. Figure 13-15 shows the attachment of a large-volume nebulizer to a Venturi mask. Note that the external nebulizer, if it is pneumatically driven, should be operated by compressed air so that the FiO_2 is not affected.

ENCLOSURES

Oxygen enclosures are devices designed to contain all or part of the patient's body in an oxygen-enriched atmosphere. The most common applications of these devices are for newborns and infants. The use of adult enclosures is on the decline, owing to the more efficient oxygen administration devices available.

Croupette

A *Croupette* is a small tent designed to provide an oxygen-enriched, humidified environment for infants and small children. Its most common application is in the treatment of croup.

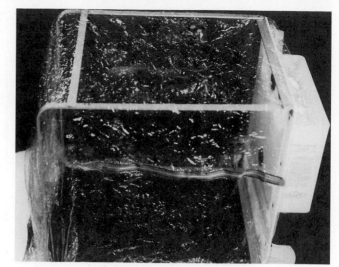

Figure 13-16 *A Croupette*

The device consists of a framework that supports a clear plastic canopy, a back piece housing a container for ice, and a jet nebulizer. When the device is connected to an oxygen flowmeter running at 12 to 15 L/min, oxygen percentages in the tent can be maintained at around 40%. Figure 13-16 shows a typical Croupette.

The use of an oxygen analyzer is important with a Croupette. The FiO_2 should be carefully maintained and monitored. Note, however, that FiO_2 will be higher at the bottom of the enclosure owing to the greater density of oxygen.

To ensure consistent FiO_2 and humidification, it is important to keep the child in the tent and to keep the edges sealed as tightly as possible. Access to the child should be through the zippers provided in the sides of the canopy.

Isolette

An *isolette* is a chamber designed to provide a thermally controlled, oxygen-enriched, humid environment for a newborn. The chamber is constructed of clear Plexiglas, with access to the newborn provided by ports on the sides of the isolette.

To maintain a consistent environment, it is important in caring for the newborn to gain access through the ports provided for delivery of care. When the ports are not in use, they should remain closed.

Most isolette models have safety features that prevent administration of high FiO_2 concentrations. Careful monitoring of blood gases (to maintain the PaO_2 between 50 and 80 mm Hg) is important to prevent *retinopathy of prematurity* (ROP). Figure 13-17 shows an older-model isolette.

Head Box

A *head box* is an enclosure designed for use on a newborn infant. It encloses only the head, leaving good access to the rest of the infant's body for nursing care. The head box is typically made from Plexiglas. Some models have removable tops to provide access to the head if needed. Figure 13-18 depicts a typical head box.

Warmed, humidified oxygen is supplied to the box by means of large-bore aerosol tubing. A fitting is provided at

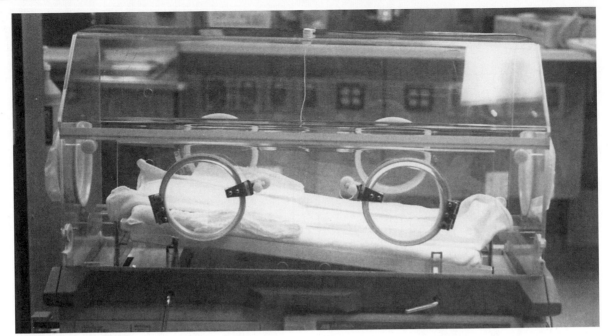

Figure 13-17 *An isolette*

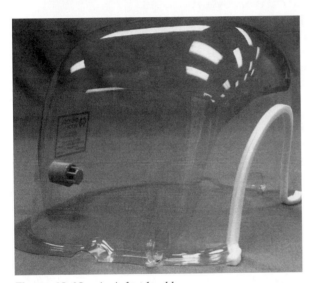

Figure 13-18 *An infant head box*

the end of the box for the attachment of the tubing. Precautions similar to those taken with the isolette should be employed with head boxes. Careful monitoring of blood gases and FiO_2 is important in the prevention of ROP.

Hazards Associated with Enclosures

Oxygen enclosures having large volumes of oxygen-enriched air can pose a considerable fire hazard if not treated properly.

Children in enclosures should not be allowed to have battery-powered electric toys, radios, or other electrically powered appliances. If possible, limit the child's playthings to stuffed animals or other nonmetallic objects incapable of generating sparks.

All visitors should be prohibited from smoking in the room, and *No smoking* signs should be placed in several conspicuous locations inside and outside the room.

Types of Oxygen Analyzers

Four types of *oxygen analyzer* devices have been produced commercially. These are the physical (based on the principle of paramagnetism), electrical (Wheatstone bridge), and electrochemical, both galvanic and polarographic. Of the four types, the galvanic and polarographic analyzers are the most commonly used types.

Galvanic Oxygen Analyzer

The galvanic oxygen analyzer uses a chemical reaction of oxygen combining with water and electrons to form hydroxyl ions (OH^-). This reaction is a type of *oxidation-reduction reaction*. The hydroxyl ions migrate to a positive electrode (anode), which reduces the lead, forming more free electrons (Figure 13-19). Formation of these electrons is measured as current flow, and the current is proportional to the oxygen concentration.

Galvanic oxygen analyzers rely strictly on the chemical reaction to produce the electrical current flow that is measured. The response time may be somewhat slower than that with use of a polarographic oxygen analyzer.

Polarographic Oxygen Analyzers

Polarographic oxygen analyzers are similar to galvanic oxygen analyzers, with the addition of a battery to polarize the electrodes (Figure 13-20). The polarographic oxygen analyzer uses a similar oxidation-reduction reaction to form free electrons at the anode.

Polarographic analyzers generally have a more rapid response time than galvanic analyzers. The polarization of the electrodes speeds the reaction, reducing the response time.

Use of an Oxygen Analyzer

Various types of oxygen analyzers using different physical principles of operation are available for the measurement

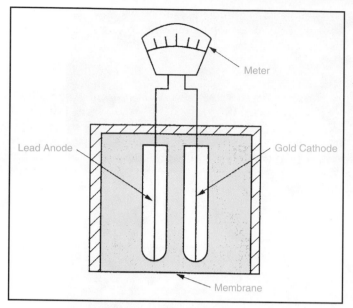

Figure 13-19 *A diagram of a galvanic oxygen analyzer*

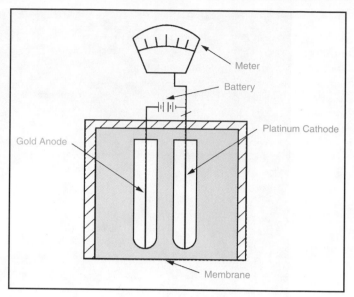

Figure 13-20 *A diagram of a polarographic oxygen analyzer*

of oxygen concentrations. Whenever possible, oxygen concentrations should be measured and documented in the patient's chart at least once each shift, or every 8 hours.

Before measurement of the oxygen concentration, the oxygen analyzer should be calibrated. Calibration is performed at room air (21%) and at 100% (pure oxygen). Calibrate the analyzer at 21% or room air, then calibrate it at 100% by immersing the probe in a reservoir of 100% oxygen.

To measure the FiO$_2$, sample the gas as close to the patient as possible. The oxygen concentration may be documented either as a percentage (40% oxygen) or as a fraction of the inspired oxygen (FiO$_2$ 0.40). Do not mix the two methods of documentation.

In some cases, it is very difficult to analyze the oxygen concentration. For example, with a low-flow oxygen delivery system for a patient on a nasal cannula receiving oxygen at 2 L/min, a specific oxygen concentration cannot be measured. In this instance, the oxygen concentration may be documented by the liter flow rate; for example, you may chart as follows: "Patient on a nasal cannula at an oxygen flow rate of 2 L/min." If oxygen concentration cannot be measured, at least document the oxygen flow rate.

HAZARDS OF OXYGEN THERAPY

There are several hazards and complications associated with oxygen therapy. This section briefly discusses the more common hazards and complications you may encounter in clinical practice. It is important to note that the majority may be avoided entirely by the proper administration and monitoring of oxygen therapy. The common hazards and complications discussed here are absorption atelectasis, oxygen-induced hypoventilation, oxygen toxicity, and retinopathy of prematurity (ROP). For a more in-depth study, consult one of the references listed at the end of this chapter.

Absorption Atelectasis

Prolonged exposure to high concentrations of oxygen causes the gradual washout of nitrogen from the lungs. The atmosphere is composed of approximately 78% nitrogen. The nitrogen in the atmosphere is inert and does not participate significantly in the normal gas exchange across the alveolar-capillary membrane. Because the majority of nitrogen remains in the alveoli, this gas helps to keep the alveoli open at the end of expiration.

As the nitrogen is washed out and replaced by oxygen, the oxygen is absorbed into the blood. As more and more volume is absorbed, the alveolar volume decreases, resulting in a diffuse microatelectasis. In the patient who is compromised and breathing very shallowly, this effect, termed *absorption atelectasis*, can be quite pronounced.

Oxygen-Induced Hypoventilation

Some patients who have a history of chronic obstructive pulmonary disease (COPD) tend to retain higher than normal levels of carbon dioxide in the blood (hypercapnia). As a result of CO$_2$ retention, the body's normal stimulus to breathe in response to high levels of CO$_2$ is not as responsive. The patient with chronic obstructive lung disease is breathing primarily on an oxygen stimulus rather than a carbon dioxide stimulus.

When these patients are given moderate to high concentrations of oxygen, the body's chemoreceptors slow respiratory rate and depth as a result of the now adequate levels of PaO$_2$ (Robinson, 2000; American Association for Respiratory Care, 1991). As a result of the induced hypoventilation, arterial carbon dioxide levels may rapidly increase, with resulting rapid shifts in pH. Oxygen therapy for these patients should be carefully controlled by observation and by arterial blood gas measurements to ensure that hypercapnia is not made worse by oxygen therapy.

Patients using oxygen at home should be cautioned about the potentially lethal effects of increasing the oxygen flow rate beyond the level prescribed by their physician.

Oxygen Toxicity

Prolonged exposures to high concentrations of oxygen at ambient pressures have been shown to produce detrimental changes in the pulmonary system. Progressive changes that occur as a result of this exposure may include consolidation, thickening of the capillary beds, formation of hyaline membranes and fibrosis, edema, and atelectasis (Scanlan et al., 1995; Shapiro, et al., 1991).

It is generally accepted that exposure to 100% oxygen for 24 hours is not severely detrimental to the patient. However, the response to oxygen toxicity varies from one person to the next. Exposure to 100% oxygen for longer periods of time should be viewed with great caution. Serial measurements of the vital capacity have been shown to be helpful in monitoring the effects of oxygen toxicity (Clark, 1974).

If adequate PaO_2 levels cannot be maintained by 100% oxygen administration, continuous mechanical ventilation or continuous positive airway pressure (CPAP) in the spontaneously breathing patient may allow the administration of lower levels of oxygen with subsequent improvement in arterial oxygen tension.

Retinopathy of Prematurity

Retinopathy of prematurity (ROP) is a potential complication of oxygen therapy in the newborn. Administration of a high concentration of oxygen causes vasoconstriction in the retina. The vessels become obliterated, and normal growth ceases in the periphery of the retina. Eventually, these changes may lead to partial retinal detachment and blindness. ROP may be prevented by careful monitoring of arterial blood gases. PaO_2 should be maintained between 50 and 80 mm Hg.

It may be difficult to maintain newborns in distress who require high oxygen concentrations. CPAP has helped many newborns by the maintenance of adequate arterial oxygen concentrations on lower FIO_2 levels.

OBJECTIVES

At the end of this chapter, you should be able to:

- Correctly assemble, test for function, safely apply, and troubleshoot the following:
  — Nasal cannula
  — Simple oxygen mask
  — Partial rebreathing oxygen mask
  — Nonrebreathing oxygen mask
  — Venturi oxygen mask
  — Oxygen enclosure
  — Croupette
  — Isolette
- Demonstrate how to analyze FIO_2:
  — Calibrate the oxygen analyzer.
  — Analyze at an appropriate position.
  — Adjust delivery device as appropriate.
  — Document the oxygen concentration.

Review the Patient's Chart

Before proceeding with any prescribed respiratory therapy, take time to review the patient's chart. Check for indications and hazards. In an emergency situation, you may not have the time to perform this procedure. Obviously, if life is in danger and you are ordered directly to proceed, do so.

When reviewing the chart, check for a physician's order. If the order is not written, check with the charge nurse on duty. Ascertain whether the nurse received a verbal or telephone order, verify it, and make sure the order is documented in the patient's chart. It is also important to check the order for completeness (device ordered, liter flow or FIO_2, duration and goal of therapy).

Next, check the laboratory report section of the chart and look for an arterial blood gas analysis report. If an arterial blood gas sample has been drawn, it will indicate the severity of the hypoxemia and the patient's acid-base status. A blood gas analysis report will also help you to document the goal of therapy, which is required more frequently as health care providers come under more stringent government regulation.

Gather the Appropriate Equipment

The order for O_2 should specify a delivery device, as well as FIO_2. Specified FIO_2 will dictate which equipment is essential or required. Figure 13-21 lists the equipment required for the majority of clinical situations requiring oxygen administration.

Assemble Your Equipment

After washing your hands, assemble the equipment needed to administer the oxygen therapy ordered by the physician. Most disposable oxygen cannulas and masks are packaged with everything needed except the flowmeter, humidifier, *No smoking* sign, and oxygen analyzer. Assembly consists of opening the package, connecting the device to the humidifier or flowmeter, and then applying it to the patient.

- Oxygen flowmeter
- Humidifier (if required)
- Sterile water (if required)
- Oxygen connecting tubing (if required)
- Oxygen administration device
- *No smoking* sign
- Oxygen analyzer (if appropriate)

Figure 13-21 *Equipment required for oxygen administration*

Simple oxygen masks, partial rebreathing masks, and nonrebreathing masks generally should not be operated at a flow rate of less than 5 L/min. This higher flow rate will ensure that the exhaled carbon dioxide is adequately flushed from the mask. The head straps should be adjusted to prevent the mask from slipping off the face, but should not be so tight as to cause pressure sores to develop.

Enclosures require more assembly. The canopy frame must be set up (if required), nebulizer jar filled (if provided), oxygen connecting tubing attached, ice reservoir filled (if required), and the canopy attached (if required). It is important that you practice assembling, testing for function, and troubleshooting the various enclosures commonly used in your geographic region. Only through repeated practice can you become truly familiar with the equipment you will be required to use.

Explain the Procedure to the Patient

Before actually applying the device to the patient, take a minute to explain who you are, what department you are from, what you will be doing, and why you are doing it. Ask the patient's permission. Patients have the right to know what is being done to their bodies and why.

A little salesmanship on your part will help to promote the patient's cooperation and understanding. It takes only a moment. A smile, a polite and concise presentation, and a show of genuine concern for the patient make a great difference to the patient's acceptance of you and your therapy.

Nasal Cannula

Practice applying a nasal cannula with a laboratory partner. Apply the cannula so that the curve of the prongs points down (the airway through the nose progresses posteriorly and then down, not up). Adjust the ear loops or lariat around the back of the ears and then down under the chin. Move the cinch adjustment up so that it is snug enough to keep the prongs in the nose but not so snug as to be uncomfortable.

Turn on the oxygen flow and check it before applying the cannula to the patient. Set the flow rate between 1 and 6 L/min as ordered by the physician.

Oxygen Masks

Oxygen masks are applied to the bridge of the nose first and then positioned over the chin. The strap should be adjusted snugly around the head to keep the mask in place, but not so tight as to cause discomfort or pressure sores.

TABLE 13-4: Oxygen Mask Application

MASK	FLOW RATE	OXYGEN PERCENTAGE
Simple	6 to 10 L/min	35–55%
Partial rebreathing	Enough to keep bag from collapsing	Up to 60%
Nonrebreathing	Enough to keep bag from collapsing	Up to 100%

Liter flows should be adjusted between 6 and 10 L/min. Table 13-4 shows the different liter flows and approximate FIO_2 ranges for the different masks.

Entrainment Masks

The assembly and oxygen flow rate adjustment will vary depending on the manufacturer of the mask. It is imperative that you familiarize yourself with the various directions supplied by the mask manufacturers because they vary from company to company. Some manufacturers have a separate oxygen dilutor for each desired oxygen percentage (usually color coded). Other manufacturers provide for the oxygen percentage adjustment by adjusting the size of the air entrainment ports. Become familiar with the types of Venturi masks used in your geographic region.

Adjust the liter flow as specified by the manufacturer. Analyze the FIO_2 at the gas entrance port in the mask. Adjust the flow or air entrainment as required to establish the desired FIO_2.

Apply the mask to the bridge of the nose first and then apply it to the chin. Adjust the head strap to keep the mask on the face but not too snugly, as pressure sores may result.

Croupette

First attach the frame to the head of the bed using the adjustable clamp provided. If the Croupette is a smaller version, set the frame of the Croupette at the head of the bed, and make sure it is supported in the vertical position.

Open the canopy and attach it to the supporting frame of the Croupette. The canopy may be attached by sliding rubber rings onto the frame or by snaps provided on the canopy. Tuck the edges securely under the mattress and roll the loose end of the canopy in a bath blanket to help to seal it tightly.

Add ice to the ice reservoir.

Fill the nebulizer jar with sterile distilled water. Attach the nebulizer to a flowmeter using oxygen-connecting tubing. Adjust the oxygen flowmeter to 12 to 15 L/min. Verify the function of the nebulizer.

Open the canopy using the zippers provided. Place the infant into the canopy and close the zipper. Analyze the FIO_2 after approximately 10 to 20 minutes have elapsed since closing the canopy. This time period will allow for the equilibration of the FIO_2.

Isolette

To prepare the isolette for use, fill the water reservoir chamber with sterile distilled water.

Using oxygen connecting tubing, attach the isolette to an oxygen flowmeter. Adjust the flow to 12 to 15 L/min.

Adjust the temperature and humidity controls to the desired ranges.

Analyze the FIO_2 after 10 to 20 minutes has elapsed to allow for equilibration.

Head Box

It is very difficult to maintain a consistent FIO_2 and humidity for an infant in an isolette because of the constant opening and closing of the enclosure for nursing care.

By using a head box to deliver the desired FIO_2 and humidity, adequate access is provided for the rest of the infant's body.

A head box is usually operated from a large-volume nebulizer or a humidifier capable of delivering 100% body humidity. The FIO_2 adjustments provided on the nebulizer/humidifier may be used, or the nebulizer/humidifier may be operated from an oxygen blender to adjust the FIO_2. Supplemental heat must be provided by a stick heater or a wraparound heater.

Using large-bore aerosol tubing, attach the large-volume nebulizer to the head box. Monitor temperature (35 to 37°C is the desired range) and the FIO_2 using an oxygen analyzer. Analyze the FIO_2 proximal to the infant's face. Routinely and carefully monitor both the temperature and the FIO_2 as long as the infant requires therapy.

Use of an Oxygen Analyzer

The most common type of oxygen analyzer used in clinical practice is the polarographic oxygen analyzer. It has become popular owing to its small size, its ability to analyze gas in motion, and its rapid response time.

Testing and Calibration

The polarographic analyzers utilize a battery in their operation. Most manufacturers provide some means to test the battery prior to the use of the analyzer.

Calibrate the oxygen analyzer at 21% or room air. Following this, calibrate the analyzer at 100% by immersing the sensor into a reservoir of 100% oxygen. After calibrating the analyzer at 100%, return the sensor to room air. The reading should stabilize back to 21% within 1 minute.

Analysis

It is important to analyze the oxygen concentration as close to the patient as possible. You want to know what the patient is receiving. If you analyze distal to the patient, there may be the possibility of room air entrainment between the point of analysis and the patient.

Humidity can shorten the life of some oxygen analyzer sensors. At today's hospital supply prices, one sensor is almost a day's pay for the average respiratory therapist. If an oxygen analyzer is to be used continuously, make sure that humidity will not adversely affect the sensor.

Dispose of Excess Equipment Properly

After initiating therapy, remove any unneeded equipment. The patient rooms are small and quite cramped for space. Removal of unnecessary equipment will keep the patient area less cluttered and, more important, safer. Extra supplies and plastic are a particular hazard in pediatric units.

Document the Procedure in the Patient Chart

It is helpful to know the liter flow and the FIO_2 on some devices. The oxygen concentration may be documented as a percentage, or as a fraction of inspired oxygen concentration (FIO_2). Use one method or the other, but do not mix the two systems.

Document on the patient's chart the date and time, the equipment used when you initiated therapy on the patient, and the oxygen concentration or flow rate—for example: "12/20/2001, 09:00, Mr. J. Smith, room 214, was set up on a simple oxygen mask at a flow rate of 8 L/min. Respiratory rate is steady at 13 breaths per minute and SpO_2 is 93%."

References

American Association for Respiratory Care. (1991). AARC clinical practice guideline: Oxygen therapy in the acute care hospital. *Respiratory Care, 36*(12), 1410–1413.

American Association for Respiratory Care. (1992). AARC clinical practice guideline: Oxygen therapy in the home or extended care facility. *Respiratory Care, 37*(8), 918–922.

Chalon, J. (1980). Low humidity damage to the tracheal mucosa. *Bulletin of the New York Academy of Medicine, 56*, 314–332.

Clark, J. M. (1974). The toxicity of oxygen. *American Review of Respiratory Diseases, 110*(2), 40.

Robinson, T. D. (2000). The role of hypoventilation and ventilation-perfusion redistribution in oxygen-induced hypercapnia during acute exacerbations of chronic obstructive pulmonary disease. *American Journal of Respiratory and Critical Care Medicine, 161*(5), 1524-1529.

Sabrini, C. A., et al. (1968). Arterial oxygen tension in relation to age in healthy subjects. *Respiration, 25*(3).

Scacci, R. (1979). Air entrainment masks: Jet mixing is how they work; the Bernoulli and Venturi principles are how they don't. *Respiratory Care, 24*(10), 928–931.

Scanlan, C., Spearman, C. B., & Sheldon, R. L. (1995). *Egan's fundamentals of respiratory therapy* (6th ed.). St. Louis, MO: Mosby.

Shapiro, B. A., Kacmarek, R. M., Cane, R. D., & Hauptman, D. (1991). *Clinical application of respiratory care* (4th ed.). Chicago: Year Book.

Practice Activities: Oxygen Administration

1. Practice setting up the following equipment using an intubation mannequin or infant resuscitation mannequin as appropriate. Practice with each device until you are familiar with its correct application and operation:
   a. nasal cannula
   b. simple oxygen mask
   c. partial rebreathing mask
   d. nonrebreathing mask
   e. Venturi mask
   f. Croupette
   g. isolette
   h. head box

2. Practice applying the following devices to a laboratory partner:
   a. nasal cannula at 4 L/min
   b. simple oxygen mask at 8 L/min
   c. partial rebreathing mask at 10 L/min
   d. nonrebreathing mask at 10 L/min
   e. Venturi mask

3. Practice troubleshooting any of the devices by deliberately sabotaging them and then attempting to restore them to normal operation.

4. Practice the calibration of an oxygen analyzer to room air and 100% oxygen settings. Analyze the FIO_2 of a Venturi mask operating at 28%, 35%, and 50%.

5. Set up a Croupette or an isolette at an oxygen flow rate of 12 L/min. Establish a stable FIO_2 reading. Open the Croupette canopy using the zippered sides or by opening the hinge of the isolette for 45 seconds. Note what happens to the FIO_2 and how long it takes to return to the previous level.

Check List: Oxygen Administration

_____ 1. Wash your hands. Help prevent nosocomial infections. Protect both your patient and yourself.
2. Obtain the appropriate equipment as required, including:
_____ a. Oxygen flowmeter
_____ b. Humidifier or nebulizer
_____ c. Sterile water (if humidifier or nebulizer is not prefilled)
_____ d. Oxygen connecting tubing (if required)
_____ e. Oxygen administration device:
_____ (1) nasal cannula
_____ (2) simple oxygen mask
_____ (3) partial rebreathing mask
_____ (4) nonrebreathing mask
_____ (5) Venturi mask
_____ (6) head box
_____ (7) Croupette
_____ (8) isolette
_____ (9) _No smoking_ sign
_____ 3. Assemble the equipment. Assembly will be determined by what oxygen therapy has been ordered.

_____ 4. Identify the patient using the arm band.
_____ 5. Explain the procedure to the patient. Give a brief explanation of the benefits of therapy and do your best to elicit the patient's cooperation.
_____ 6. Apply the device to the patient. As appropriate, adjust the device to an acceptable comfort level for the patient.
_____ 7. Adjust the oxygen concentration or flow rate as ordered by the physician.
_____ 8. Confirm the delivered oxygen concentration with an oxygen analyzer as appropriate.
_____ 9. Clean up the patient's area. Dispose of any plastic wrappers, excess tubing, or other unused items.
_____ 10. Ensure the patient's comfort and safety.
_____ 11. Wash your hands.
_____ 12. Document in the patient's chart the date, time, oxygen device applied, flow rate or oxygen concentration, and the patient's condition.

Self-Evaluation Post Test: Oxygen Administration

1. A nasal cannula with a liter flow rate of 2 L/min applied to a patient with a normal ventilatory pattern delivers an oxygen concentration of approximately:
   a. 24%.   d. 36%.
   b. 28%.   e. 40%.
   c. 32%.

2. Which of these is/are (a) high-flow device(s)?
   I.   Partial rebreathing mask   a. I, IV, V
   II. Nasal cannula   b. III
   III. Venturi mask   c. I, III, IV
   IV. Simple oxygen mask   d. I, II, III, IV
   V.   Oxygen tent   e. II, III, IV

3. Factors that affect the delivered oxygen concentration from a simple mask are:
   I. patient's tidal volume.
   II. patient's respiratory rate.
   III. liter flow of oxygen.
   IV. fit of the mask.
   a. I, II
   b. II, III
   c. I, III, IV
   d. I, IV
   e. I, II, III, IV

4. All of the following are enclosures except:
   a. head box.
   b. oxygen tent.
   c. Croupette.
   d. isolette.
   e. nasal cannula.

5. If the oxygen cannot be analyzed, it is best to record the concentration delivered in the chart using:
   a. arterial blood gases.
   b. an oxygen analyzer.
   c. liter flows.
   d. duration of therapy.
   e. minute volume and respiratory rate.

6. A Croupette with a minimum oxygen flow rate of 10 to 12 L/min will deliver an FIO_2 of approximately:
   a. 30%.
   b. 40%.
   c. 50%.
   d. up to 60%.
   e. up to 80%.

7. An isolette is an example of a(n):
   a. Venturi device.
   b. tent.
   c. low-flow device.
   d. enclosure.
   e. high-flow device.

8. An oxygen analyzer should be calibrated at:
   a. room air.
   b. 50% oxygen.
   c. 70% oxygen.
   d. 100% oxygen.
   e. a and d

9. A low-flow oxygen administration device meets all of a patient's inspiratory needs.
   a. True
   b. False

10. With use of a nonrebreathing mask, the liter flow should be:
    a. at least 2 L/min.
    b. at least 5 L/min.
    c. at least 10 L/min.
    d. high enough to prevent the bag from deflating completely on inspiration.
    e. high enough to prevent the bag from deflating completely on expiration.

PERFORMANCE EVALUATION:
OXYGEN ADMINISTRATION

Date: Lab _____ Clinical _____ Agency _____

Lab: Pass _____ Fail _____   Clinical: Pass _____ Fail _____

Student name _____   Instructor name _____

No. of times observed in clinical _____

No. of times practiced in clinical _____

PASSING CRITERIA: Obtain 90% or better on the procedure. Tasks indicated by * must receive at least 1 point, or the evaluation is terminated. Procedure must be performed within designated time, or the performance receives a failing grade.

SCORING:
2 points — Task performed satisfactorily without prompting.
1 point — Task performed satisfactorily with self-initiated correction.
0 points — Task performed incorrectly or with prompting required.
NA — Task not applicable to the patient care situation.

TASKS:

		PEER	LAB	CLINICAL
*	1. Verifies the physician's order	☐	☐	☐
*	2. Observes universal precautions, including washing hands	☐	☐	☐
	3. Obtains the required equipment			
*	a. Oxygen flowmeter	☐	☐	☐
*	b. Humidifier	☐	☐	☐
*	c. Sterile water	☐	☐	☐
*	d. Oxygen connecting tubing	☐	☐	☐
*	e. Oxygen administration device	☐	☐	☐
*	f. *No smoking* sign(s)	☐	☐	☐
	4. Identifies the patient	☐	☐	☐
	5. Explains the procedure to the patient	☐	☐	☐
*	6. Adjusts the device to the ordered level	☐	☐	☐
*	7. Applies the device to the patient	☐	☐	☐
*	8. Confirms FiO_2 as appropriate	☐	☐	☐
	9. Disposes of excess equipment	☐	☐	☐
	10. Leaves the patient area clean and safe	☐	☐	☐
*	11. Washes hands before leaving room	☐	☐	☐
*	12. Documents equipment, concentration, or liter flow rate in the patient's chart	☐	☐	☐

CHAPTER 14

INTRODUCTION TO RESPIRATORY CARE PHARMACOLOGY

INTRODUCTION

The administration of specific drugs that act on the respiratory system is one of many tasks performed by respiratory care practitioners. To administer pharmacologic agents safely and effectively, you must understand the indications and contraindications for these drugs, how they act on the body, their side effects and associated hazards, and common dosages.

In this chapter you will learn about the common drugs administered by respiratory care practitioners. You will also learn about how these drugs work, when they are indicated, and their side effects and hazards.

KEY TERMS

- Alpha receptors
- Anticholinergic drugs
- Antigen
- Antimicrobial agents
- Beta-1 receptors
- Beta-2 receptors
- Cholinergic receptors
- Corticosteroids
- Degranulation
- Dry powder inhaler
- Histamine
- IgE
- Leukotrienes
- Mast cells
- Metered dose inhaler
- Mucokinetic drugs
- Muscarinic effect
- Nicotinic effect
- Phosphodiesterase inhibitors
- Prophylactic
- Prostaglandins
- Receptor sites
- Spacer
- Sympathomimetic drugs

OBJECTIVES

At the end of this chapter, you should be able to:

- Discuss the autonomic receptor site theory for the pharmacologic action of the following types of drugs:
  — Adrenergic receptors
    — Alpha receptors
    — Beta-1 receptors
    — Beta-2 receptors
  — Cholinergic receptors
- Describe the mechanisms of bronchospasm:
  — Mast cell degranulation
    — Leukotrienes
    — Histamines
    — Prostaglandins
  — Release of acetylcholine
- Explain how sympathomimetic agents work and state their indications and hazards:
  — Salmeterol xinafoate
  — Pirbuterol acetate
  — Bitolterol mesylate
  — Albuterol sulfate
  — Metaproterenol sulfate
  — Isoetharine HCl
  — Isoproterenol
  — Epinephrine
  — Terbutaline sulfate
  — Racemic epinephrine
- Explain how phosphodiesterase inhibitors work and state their indications and hazards:
  — Aminophylline
  — Theophylline
- Explain how anticholinergic agents work and state their indications and hazards:
  — Atropine sulfate
  — Ipratropium bromide
- Describe the role of corticosteroids in the management of reactive airways disease:
  — Prednisone
  — Dexamethasone
  — Triamcinolone
  — Beclomethasone
  — Flunisolide
- Describe the role of cromolyn sodium and nedocromil sodium in the management of reactive airways disease.
- Describe the role of mucokinetic agents in respiratory care:
  — Acetylcysteine
  — Sodium bicarbonate
  — Deoxyribonuclease
- Describe the role of bland aerosols in humidity therapy.
- Describe the role of antimicrobial agents in respiratory care:
  — Antibiotics
  — Antiviral agents
  — Antiprotozoal agents
- Explain the advantages and disadvantages of metered dose inhalers (MDIs) in the administration of pharmacologic agents.
- Describe a dry powder inhaler (DPI) and its potential advantages over an MDI.

RECEPTOR SITE THEORY

Throughout the body are *receptor sites*. Receptor sites are specialized cells that will respond predictably to an outside (external to the cell) stimulus. The airways of the lung contain a multitude of receptor sites. Stimulation of some of these sites results in profound bronchospasm, whereas stimulation of others results in bronchodilation. Therefore, it is important that as a respiratory care practitioner you understand these receptor sites and their activity.

Adrenergic Receptor Sites

Alpha Receptors

Alpha receptors are located in the peripheral vasculature, the heart, bronchial muscle, and bronchial blood vessels (Ziment, 1978). Stimulation of these receptors causes peripheral vasoconstriction and mild bronchoconstriction in the lungs. Relatively few of these receptor sites are found in the lungs. This accounts for the mild bronchoconstrictive response when these sites are stimulated.

Beta-1 Receptors

Beta-1 receptors are found in the bronchial blood vessels and the heart (Ziment, 1978). Stimulation of the beta-1 receptors results in tachycardia, an increased potential for arrhythmias, and an increased cardiac output. In administering drugs to the pulmonary system, stimulation of the beta-1 sites is not desired. However, most respiratory pharmacologic agents have some beta-1 stimulatory effect.

Beta-2 Receptors

Beta-2 receptors are located in the bronchial smooth muscle, the bronchial blood vessels, the systemic blood vessels, and the skeletal muscles. Stimulation of the beta-2 receptors in the lungs causes bronchodilation. A constant goal in the development of new adrenergic drugs for the pulmonary system is to maximize the beta-2 effect while minimizing the beta-1 effect.

Cholinergic Receptors

Cholinergic receptors are cells that respond when stimulated by acetylcholine. Cholinergic receptors cause profound bronchospasm in the lungs when stimulated. As you may remember from studying anatomy and physiology, acetylcholine is a chemical unique to the parasympathetic nervous system. Vagal stimulation causes the release of acetylcholine, known as the *muscarinic effect*. The muscarinic system consists of those organs innervated by the tenth cranial nerve (vagus nerve). The other cholinergic effect is the *nicotinic effect*. The nicotinic system consists of the motor nerves of the skeletal muscles.

MECHANISMS OF BRONCHOSPASM

As you have learned from the previous discussion, bronchospasm can result from adrenergic and cholinergic stimulation. Bronchospasm, however, may also result from other mechanisms. As a respiratory care practitioner, it is important that you understand the mechanisms of bronchospasm so that appropriate drugs can be given to reverse it.

Mast Cell Degranulation

Mast cells are specialized cells in the lungs that are located in the smooth muscle of the bronchi, the intra-alveolar septa, and the submucosal glands (Des Jardins, 2002). The humoral immunity response (allergic response) causes *degranulation* of these cells, releasing chemical mediators such as histamine, heparin, and leukotrienes. The humoral response is caused by an *antigen* (e.g., pollen, animal proteins, feathers) causing the peripheral lymphoid tissue to release immunoglobulin E (*IgE*) antibodies. The IgE (reagin) antibodies sensitize the mast cell. Repeated exposure to the antigen causes the degranulation of the mast cell (Figure 14-1). When the mast cell degranulates, chemical mediators are released, causing bronchospasm and other adverse effects.

Leukotrienes

Leukotrienes are one of many chemical mediators released by the mast cells. Leukotrienes cause a direct, strong bronchoconstriction (Ziment, 1978). Leukotrienes also increase vascular permeability, causing edema to occur.

Histamine

Histamine is also a potent bronchoconstrictor. In addition to its bronchoconstrictive activity, histamine increases bronchial gland secretion, causing an increase in the amount of mucus present in the airways (Ziment, 1978). Histamine may also have an effect on vascular permeability similar to the effect of SRS-A.

Prostaglandins

Prostaglandins cause a strong bronchospasm, especially in asthmatic patients (Ziment, 1978). Prostaglandins are produced in the lung and other organs in the body. Prostaglandins have also been implicated in the acute (adult) respiratory distress syndrome (ARDS) (Bonner, 1985; Bone, 1984).

Acetylcholine

As you learned earlier, release of acetylcholine causes bronchospasm. The muscarinic effect is the one primarily responsible for bronchospasm in the lungs. The bronchospasm from this mechanism is very strong and long-lasting.

SYMPATHOMIMETIC DRUGS

Action of Sympathomimetic Drugs

As their name implies, *sympathomimetic drugs* mimic the actions of the sympathetic nervous system. There are many different drugs that fall under this classification. Sympathomimetic agents are the drugs most commonly used to reverse bronchospasm.

Sympathomimetics stimulate the beta-1 and beta-2 receptor sites. The desired site of stimulation is the beta-2

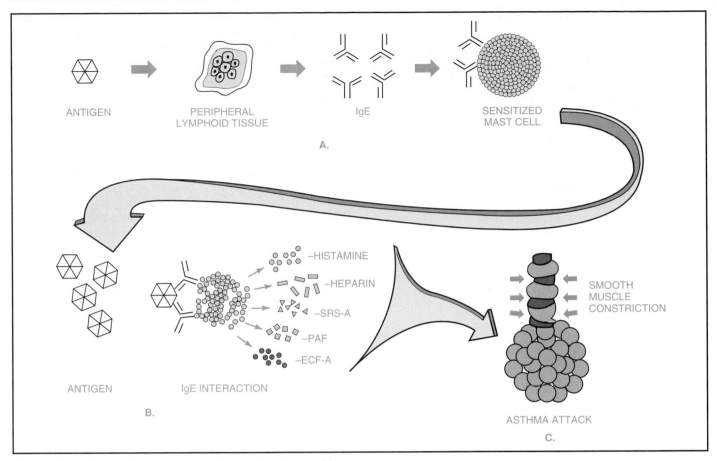

Figure 14-1 *Immunologic response causing mast cell degranulation*

site, which causes bronchodilation. However, few drugs are purely beta-2 stimulants.

Beta-2 stimulation causes the formation of adenylate cyclase (Figure 14-2). Adenylate cyclase combines with magnesium and ATP (adenosine triphosphate) to form cyclic 3′,5′-AMP (adenosine monophosphate). Cyclic 3′,5′-AMP results in bronchial smooth muscle relaxation and hence bronchodilation. Cyclic 3′,5′-AMP is not a long-lived agent. It is readily broken down by another enzyme present in the lungs called phosphodiesterase. Phosphodiesterase breaks 3′,5′-AMP down into 5′-AMP, which no longer causes bronchodilation.

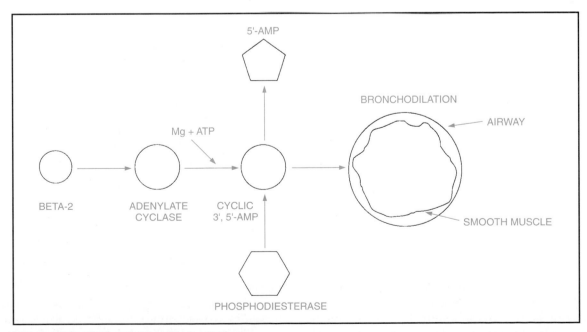

Figure 14-2 *Action of sympathomimetic drugs*

Indications for Sympathomimetic Agents

The primary indication for the administration of sympathomimetic drugs is to reverse bronchospasm. These drugs are very effective and, when given by aerosol route, have few side effects (compared with systemic administration). The different drugs, however, have differing beta-1 and beta-2 effects; therefore, it is important to understand each one so that they can be administered for optimal pharmacological effect.

Specific Sympathomimetic Drugs

Salmeterol Xinafoate

Salmeterol xinafoate (Serevent) is a long-acting beta agonist that has beta-2 effects stronger than its beta-1 effects. It is longer-acting than many other beta agonist drugs, with a 12-hour duration of action and a 60-minute time to onset of action. It is available only as a metered dose inhaler (MDI) preparation that delivers 50 micrograms (mcg or μg) per puff. Most patients require two puffs every 12 hours.

Salmeterol is intended for maintenance therapy (typically administered twice per day, morning and night). It is not intended as a rescue drug because its time to onset is at least 60 minutes. Patients using salmeterol usually require a fast-acting beta agonist (such as albuterol or metaproterenol) for periods of dyspnea between doses of salmeterol.

Side effects include tachycardia, nausea, palpitations, hypertension, headaches, and tremors. Side effects may be additive if this drug is used in conjunction with other, shorter-acting beta agonists.

Pirbuterol Acetate

Pirbuterol acetate (Maxair) is another beta agonist available as an MDI preparation (200 mcg/puff). It is also long-acting, with a time to onset of action of 5 minutes and a duration of action of 5 hours. Most patients require two puffs every 4 to 6 hours.

Side effects include tachycardia, nausea, palpitations, hypertension, headaches, and tremors. These side effects are related to beta-1 stimulation. However, this drug has more beta-2 effects than beta-1 effects.

Bitolterol Mesylate

Bitolterol mesylate (Tornalate) is a beta agonist available as an MDI preparation (200 mcg/puff). It is a long-acting drug with a time to onset of 3 to 4 minutes and a duration of action of 5 to 8 hours. Most patients require two puffs every 8 hours.

Side effects include tachycardia, nausea, palpitations, hypertension, headaches, and tremors. These side effects are related to beta-1 stimulation. However, this drug has more beta-2 effects than beta-1 effects.

Albuterol Sulfate

Albuterol sulfate (Ventolin, Proventil) is a drug with primarily a beta-2 effect. There is some beta-1 effect, but when compared with other sympathomimetics in use in the United States, it has the least beta-1 effect. Albuterol is supplied as a solution for inhalation (0.5% or 5 mg/ml), and as an MDI preparation, and also in oral form and in solution for intravenous injection. Recommended dosage is 1.25 to 2.5 mg mixed in normal saline or other diluent.

Side effects of albuterol include tachycardia, nausea, palpitations, hypertension, headaches, and tremors. These side effects are related to beta-1 stimulation. Administration via aerosol route can minimize these effects by administration directly to the target organ (the lungs).

Metaproterenol Sulfate

Metaproterenol sulfate (Alupent) is another sympathomimetic drug. It acts primarily on the beta-2 sites, although it does have some beta-1 activity. It is provided as a solution for inhalation (5% solution or 50 mg/ml) and as an oral preparation, and in MDI inhalers. Recommended dosage via aerosol is 5, 10, or 15 mg mixed in normal saline or other diluent.

Metaproterenol has more beta-1 effects than does albuterol. The side effects are similar and include tachycardia, nausea, palpitations, hypertension, headaches, and tremors. Systemic administration results in greater side effects than when it is administered by the aerosol route.

Isoetharine

Isoetharine HCl (Bronkosol), like albuterol and metaproterenol, is a beta-2 stimulant. However, it has greater beta-1 effects than do the other two sympathomimetics. Therefore, the side effects are greater with this drug than with albuterol or metaproterenol. Isoetharine is available as a solution for inhalation (1% or 10 mg/ml) and as an oral preparation. Recommended dosage via aerosol is 2.5 to 5 mg mixed 1:3 with normal saline or other diluent.

The side effects are similar to those of the other sympathomimetics and include the same symptoms. These symptoms are caused by the beta-1 stimulation that occurs in concert with the beta-2 stimulation.

Isoproterenol

Isoproterenol (Isuprel) is a powerful bronchodilator. Along with its strong beta-2 effects, it has an almost equally strong beta-1 effect. Isoproterenol is available in solution for aerosol administration (1:200 and 1:100 stock solutions) and is also available for injection. Recommended dosage via aerosol route is 1:1000 final concentration in normal saline or other diluent.

With isoproterenol's strong beta-1 effects, careful monitoring of heart rate, blood pressure, and other symptoms is indicated before, during, and after administration.

Epinephrine

Epinephrine is one of the strongest bronchodilators available. However, it also has the strongest beta-1 side effects and alpha effects. It can be administered by injection or via aerosol. It is most commonly used in the management of acute asthma attacks and is administered intramuscularly.

If epinephrine is given via aerosol, recommended dosage is two deep inhalations spaced about 1 minute apart in a dilution of 1:100 (Scanlan, Spearman, & Sheldon, 1995).

Patients receiving epinephrine should be monitored closely for beta-1 side effects. Be especially alert for adverse effects when it is given to elderly patients. The side effects are similar to those of the other drugs and include tachycardia, nausea, palpitations, hypertension, headaches, and tremors.

Terbutaline Sulfate

Terbutaline sulfate (Brethine) is a sympathomimetic that is available as an oral preparation, in solution for injection or inhalation, and also as an MDI preparation. It has strong beta-2 effects and a lesser beta-1 effect. Recommended aerosol dosage is 0.25 to 0.5 mg diluted in normal saline or other diluent.

Terbutaline has some beta-1 effects although not as strong as those of metaproterenol. The patient should be monitored for the typical symptoms associated with beta-1 stimulation.

Racemic Epinephrine

Racemic epinephrine (Vaponephrine) is a sympathomimetic like the other drugs previously discussed. However, its alpha effects are strong and it is commonly used to relieve croup and epiglottitis symptoms in children. It may also be used for adults following extubation to relieve subglottic edema and its associated airway obstruction. It is supplied in a solution of 2.25% or 22.5 mg/ml. Recommended dosage via aerosol is 7 mg to 14 mg mixed in normal saline or other diluent.

Racemic epinephrine has beta-1 effects as well as beta-2 and alpha effects. Monitoring of the patient for adverse reactions due to beta-1 effects is indicated with use of this drug.

PHOSPHODIESTERASE INHIBITORS

As you learned earlier, cyclic 3',5'-AMP is broken down into 5'-AMP by the enzyme phosphodiesterase. If the action of phosphodiesterase can be blocked or inhibited, more 3',5'-AMP will remain in the lungs, resulting in better bronchodilation. *Phosphodiesterase inhibitors* act in this way. Common phosphodiesterase drugs are found in the *methylxanthine group*, which are sometimes called just "xanthines." Caffeine and theophylline are two examples of drugs in the xanthine group.

Aminophylline

Aminophylline is a phosphodiesterase inhibitor that is commonly given intravenously for the management of asthma. It is also available for oral administration in tablet form. Aminophylline dosage intravenously is 5 to 10 mg/kg of normal body weight. Serum concentrations should be monitored, and dosage adjusted to maintain a therapeutic level (serum theophylline) of 10 to 20 mcg/100 ml. Aminophylline exerts its bronchodilating effect by a pathway other than the sympathomimetic pathway. This difference can be useful clinically.

Aminophylline has several side effects, including nausea, vomiting, nervousness, agitation, and tachycardia. Aminophylline may also cause tachypnea and hyperventilation.

Theophylline

Like aminophylline, theophylline is another methylxanthine. It acts by blocking phosphodiesterase. Theophylline is available in tablet and elixir form. Like aminophylline, it should be titrated until a therapeutic blood level (serum theophylline) of 10 to 20 mcg/100 ml is attained.

Side effects of theophylline and aminophylline are similar and include gastrointestinal discomfort, tachycardia, restlessness, tachypnea, and hyperventilation.

ANTICHOLINERGIC DRUGS

Anticholinergic drugs block the cholinergic receptor sites, preventing that route of bronchospasm. Anticholinergics provide a third pathway for bronchodilation in addition to those described for the sympathomimetics and phosphodiesterase inhibitors.

Atropine Sulfate

Atropine sulfate (Atropine) is available in tablet and liquid form. Dosage for aerosol administration is 1 mg diluted in normal saline or other diluent.

Side effects of atropine include dryness of the nose and mouth, bradycardia, palpitations, and flushing of the skin.

Ipratropium Bromide

Ipratropium bromide (Atrovent) is another agent that, like atropine, blocks the cholinergic receptor site. It is available as an MDI preparation and in solution. Recommended aerosol dosage is two puffs up to 4 times per day or 0.5 mg every 4 hours. The side effects of this drug are similar to atropine's side effects.

CORTICOSTEROIDS IN RESPIRATORY CARE

Corticosteroids are widely used in the management of the inflammatory process associated with asthma, reactive airways disease, and other pulmonary disorders. Corticosteroids may be administered systemically (orally or via the intravenous route) or via aerosol. Most corticosteroids that are administered via the aerosol route are given using MDI inhalers. It is important that you understand the actions of these drugs and how they are applied in the management of inflammatory disorders.

Prednisone

Prednisone is an oral preparation (tablet) of a glucocorticoid drug. Its action is twofold: (1) inflammation is reduced and (2) the action of sympathomimetic agents is potentiated (enhanced) (Ziment, 1978). Depending on the patient's disease state and need for therapy, prednisone may be given for a 2- to 3-week period followed by a rapid tapering of the dosage, or it may be administered for a longer term to manage the patient's condition more adequately. A typical dosage would be a loading dose of 4 mg per kg of body weight; then a maintenance dose of 1 mg/kg is used until a therapeutic level is reached. Therapeutic serum levels are 100 to 150 mcg/100 ml.

Side effects include cushingoid effects, impairment of the immune system, and steroid dependency. The side effects of steroids can be severe, and they are used only when the patient can significantly benefit from their pharmacological action.

Dexamethasone

Dexamethasone (Decadron) is available as an MDI preparation. The use of this drug in aerosol form allows the physician to target the lungs specifically in its administration. Fewer side effects may be noticed because systemic administration is avoided. Recommended dosage is three puffs 3 or 4 times per day.

The side effects of dexamethasone are similar to those of other steroids and include cushingoid effects, impaired immunity, and steroid dependency. In addition, patients may experience throat irritation or hoarseness from the MDI form of delivery.

Beclomethasone Dipropionate

Beclomethasone dipropionate (Beclovent, Vanceril) are two corticosteroids available as an MDI preparation (42 mcg/puff). Most patients require two puffs 3 or 4 times per day. Like other corticosteroids, these drugs act as anti-inflammatory agents. However, because they are inhaled, systemic side effects are fewer than if they were taken orally or intravenously.

Side effects include coughing, oral candidiasis, and dysphonia (difficulty speaking). Side effects may be minimized by thoroughly rinsing the mouth and oropharynx following use of the MDI.

Triamcinolone Acetonide

Triamcinolone acetonide (Azmacort, Pulmicort) is another corticosteroid available as an MDI preparation (100 mcg/puff). Most patients require two to four puffs 4 times per day. Azmacort is another anti-inflammatory agent that when given by inhalation has fewer side effects.

Side effects include coughing, oral candidiasis, and dysphonia. Side effects may be minimized by thoroughly rinsing the mouth and oropharynx following use of the MDI.

Flunisolide

Flunisolide (AeroBid) is another MDI corticosteroid preparation (250 mcg/puff). Most patients take two puffs twice each day. Because it is an inhaled corticosteroid, systemic side effects are fewer than with other steroids given parenterally or orally.

Side effects include coughing, oral candidiasis, and dysphonia. Side effects may be minimized by thoroughly rinsing the mouth and oropharynx following use of the MDI.

Fluticasone Propionate

Fluticasone propionate (Flowvent) is a synthetic glucocorticoid with good anti-inflammatory properties. It is available in an MDI preparation (44, 110, and 220 mcg/puff) and as a DPI. Most patients use two puffs twice daily for maintenance. As with other inhaled corticosteroids, systemic side effects are fewer than with systemic administration.

Side effects include coughing, oral candidiasis, and dysphonia. Side effects can be minimized by rinsing the mouth following drug administration.

Fluticasone Propionate—Salmeterol

Fluticasone propionate (Flowvent) and salmeterol (Serevent) have been combined into a DPI preparation containing 100 mcg of fluticasone propionate and 50 mcg of salmeterol. By taking both drugs together, the long-term effects of both (anti-inflammatory and long-acting bronchodilation) can be achieved. Most patients use two puffs twice each day. Side effects of each have been previously described.

CROMOLYN SODIUM AND ASTHMA MANAGEMENT

Cromolyn sodium is an agent that inhibits the degranulation of sensitized mast cells. The drug is very useful in the management of extrinsic (allergic) asthma. It is available in powdered form (capsules used with a Spinhaler to form an aerosol), in a liquid form for nebulization, and as an MDI preparation. Recommended dosage is 20 to 40 mg per day (of aerosolized solution) or two puffs 4 times per day using the MDI preparation.

Cromolyn sodium is a *prophylactic agent*. That is, it prevents mast cell degranulation. Administration of cromolyn sodium during an acute attack is not indicated. The drug does not have any bronchodilatory action or effect. A patient must use the drug on a regular basis to prevent acute bronchospastic episodes.

Most side effects of the drug are related to the MDI device and include hoarseness and dry mouth. Patients sometimes experience periods of coughing with both the MDI preparation and the aerosolized liquid form of the drug.

Nedocromil Sodium

Nedocromil sodium (Tilade) is a disodium salt of a pyranoquinolone dicarboxylic acid, which is a drug used in asthma management. Nedocromil sodium blocks both the early and late asthmatic responses to a variety of allergic and nonallergic asthma triggers. Like cromolyn sodium, it is most effective when used as a prophylactic agent. Nedocromil sodium is available as an MDI preparation (1.75 mcg/puff), with most patients requiring two puffs between 2 and 4 times per day.

MUCOKINETIC AGENTS

Mucokinetic drugs are agents that decrease the viscosity of pulmonary secretions, increase mucus production, hydrate retained secretions, or affect the composition of mucus proteins. The goal of all mucokinetic therapy is to increase pulmonary clearance through the normal mechanism and to promote coughing.

Acetylcysteine

Acetylcysteine (Mucomyst) is a drug that acts on the disulfide bond of mucus proteins. The action of the drug is to break down the disulfide bonds, weakening the mucus molecule (Ziment, 1978). The net effect is to reduce the viscosity of mucus, thinning it so that it is easier to expectorate. The recommended dosage is 1 to 10 ml of the 20% solution every 2 to 6 hours.

Side effects of acetylcysteine include nausea, bronchospasm in asthmatic patients, and rhinorrhea. Usually, acetylcysteine is given with a bronchodilator to prevent the bronchospastic side effect.

Sodium Bicarbonate

Sodium bicarbonate increases the pH of sputum, making it more alkaline (Ziment, 1978). The viscosity of sputum decreases in an alkaline environment. When the viscosity is reduced, sputum is easier to expectorate. Also, sodium bicarbonate is hypertonic and may increase the water content of sputum through its oncotic action. Recommended dosage is 2 to 5 ml of 2% solution, aerosolized, 3 or 4 times per day.

Side effects are primarily related to irritation of the respiratory tract. These symptoms include hoarseness and a sore throat.

Deoxyribonuclease

Deoxyribonuclease (Dornavac) is an enzyme preparation that is used to break down purulent sputum. It is a proteolytic enzyme that breaks the DNA bonds of purulent sputum. The net effect is to reduce the viscosity of the sputum, making it easier to expectorate. Recommended dosage is 50,000 to 100,000 units aerosolized up to 4 times per day.

Side effects are pharyngeal and tracheal irritation. Some patients may complain of a burning sensation in the mouth during administration.

USE OF BLAND AEROSOLS IN RESPIRATORY CARE

Bland aerosols are commonly administered in respiratory care. The goals of bland aerosol therapy include humidification of medical gases, mobilization of pulmonary secretions, and sputum induction. Bland aerosols include distilled water, saline solutions, and propylene glycol.

The use of distilled water and saline solutions is discussed in Chapter 15. Propylene glycol is used primarily as a stabilizing agent for other drugs administered via the aerosol route. It stabilizes solutions because of its detergent-like property that reduces surface tension.

AEROSOLIZED ANTIMICROBIAL AGENTS

Antimicrobial agents such as antibiotics have been aerosolized for the treatment of pulmonary infections. The aerosol route targets the lungs specifically, while in some cases avoiding systemic side effects (pentamidine administration). It is important to understand these drugs, what they are, and why they are administered.

Antibiotics

The aerosol administration of antibiotics is frequently performed in conjunction with systemic administration of other antibiotics (Scanlan et al., 1995). Tobramycin and gentamicin are sometimes aerosolized for use in patients with cystic fibrosis and have shown some efficacy in treatment of the recurrent infections these patients experience. One disadvantage of aerosolized antibiotics is the difficulty in controlling dosage.

Antiviral Agents

The primary aerosolized antiviral agent is ribavirin, used in the treatment of respiratory syncytial virus (RSV) infection in pediatric patients. Ribavirin is administered using a special small-particle aerosol generator (SPAG) nebulizer. Ribavirin has been shown to be effective in conjunction with other therapies in the treatment of RSV infection.

Antiprotozoal Agents

Pentamidine is often administered to patients with *Pneumocystis carinii* infections, a secondary complication of human immunodeficiency virus (HIV) infection. Aerosolized pentamidine is more effective and has fewer side effects than are seen with systemic administration of the same drug. When aerosolized, this drug targets the lungs specifically with few systemic effects. Furthermore, a lower aerosolized dosage may be given while achieving higher therapeutic serum levels.

METERED DOSE INHALERS

A *metered dose inhaler* (MDI) is a small, portable aerosol-dispensing device (Figure 14-3). These devices are hand-operated and are powered by a Freon propellant, much like an aerosol spray can.

Each activation of the trigger dispenses a known dose of medication. The patient squeezes the MDI trigger during a deep inhalation, depositing the aerosol into the respiratory tract. These devices are convenient to use and with proper technique can be very effective.

The greatest difficulty in MDI application is patient instruction. The patient must understand completely how to use this device. Clear, concise instructions must be given, and a placebo MDI should be used for instructional purposes and demonstration. Ideally, written directions should also be given to the patient for future reference. The medication will be administered as prescribed only when the patient uses the MDI correctly.

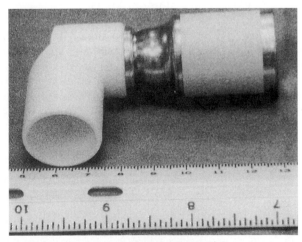

Figure 14-3 *A metered dose inhaler (MDI)*

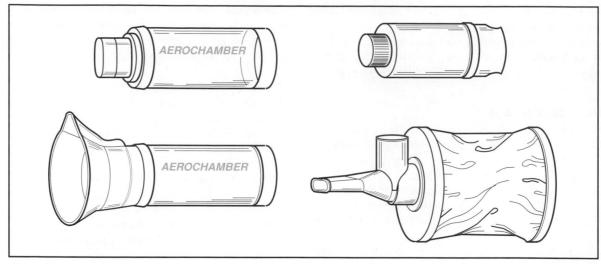

Figure 14-4 *A drawing showing several different spacer devices*

MDI Spacer Devices

MDI *spacer* devices are used in conjunction with MDIs and enhance the effectiveness of aerosol deposition and improve medication delivery (Figure 14-4). The spacer serves as a baffle, removing larger particles from suspension, and as a reservoir that helps to increase the evaporation of the MDI propellant. The use of a spacer ensures that a smaller particle size is delivered to the patient. Patients who have difficulty coordinating their breathing (inspiration) with hand coordination (squeezing) will achieve better results by using a spacer.

DRY POWDER INHALERS (DPI)

A *dry powder inhaler* (DPI) is another type of device for delivering drugs by the pulmonary route. A DPI creates an aerosol by drawing air through a small dose of dry powder. If the powder is fine enough (small particles), and sufficient air flow is generated by the patient, an aerosol of dry particles will be produced.

Unlike MDIs, DPIs do not require a propellant to expel the medication through the device. Most MDIs use chlorofluorocarbons (CFCs) as a propellant, and soon the use of CFCs will be banned from use in MDIs.

DPIs require less patient coordination than is needed for use of MDIs, do not require a breath hold, and are breath-activated (Fink, 2000). However, DPIs require a greater inspiratory flow for adequate aerosolization of the dry powdered medication. Figure 14-5 shows an example of a DPI. Table 14-1 is a summary of the drugs available in DPI form.

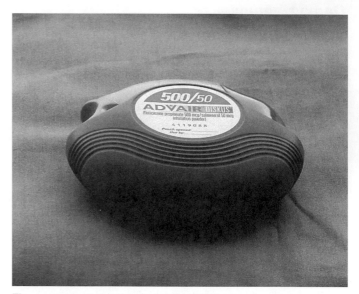

Figure 14-5 *A dry powder inhaler (DPI)*

TABLE 14-1 Drugs Available in DPI Form

DRUG	DEVICE
Albuterol sulfate	Rotahaler
Salmeterol	Diskus
Budesonide	Turbuhaler
Fluticasone propionate–salmeterol	Diskhaler

OBJECTIVES

At the end of this chapter, you should be able to:

- Demonstrate how to use a metered dose inhaler (MDI) to deliver a medication.

- Demonstrate how to use a spacer device in conjunction with an MDI to deliver a medication.

- Demonstrate the use of a dry powder inhaler (DPI)

METERED DOSE INHALER

It is important to know how to administer a medication using an MDI. The convenience and popularity of this type of aerosol administration have increased in recent years. However, as discussed previously, this method of aerosol administration is very technique-dependent; therefore, it is important to understand how to use these devices properly.

Position the Patient

It is important to position the patient properly for optimal administration of medication delivered via MDI. The optimal position is sitting erect or in high Fowler's position. This position allows for good chest expansion. Ensure that the patient is not wearing any clothing that may interfere with chest wall excursion.

Monitor the Patient

Auscultate the chest and note any abnormal breath sounds or other findings. Measure the heart rate and respiratory rate prior to medication administration. Measure the peak expiratory flow as indicated to measure the effectiveness of bronchodilator therapy.

Instruct the Patient

As discussed previously, it is important to instruct the patient thoroughly to obtain the best results with this type of aerosol administration. Allow the patient opportunity to ask questions about any aspect of the technique he or she doesn't understand. Ideally, use an MDI containing a placebo and demonstrate the technique yourself.

Assemble the Equipment

Thoroughly shake the MDI prior to use. Attach the mouthpiece to the canister and remove the cap from the mouthpiece.

Administer the Medication

Have the patient hold the MDI a few centimeters from the open mouth. Instruct the patient to inhale slowly and deeply while activating the MDI by squeezing it. Instruct the patient to continue to inhale and to hold the breath at the end of inhalation for 5 to 7 seconds. Have the patient slowly exhale following the medication administration. Repeat the procedure as many times as ordered by the patient's physician, waiting between puffs.

Monitor the Patient following Therapy

Monitor the patient's heart and respiratory rates following medication administration. Auscultate the chest and note any changes in breath sounds. If administering a bronchodilator, measure the peak expiratory flow following aerosol administration.

Clean the Patient's Room and Chart Procedure

Remove any unneeded supplies from the patient's room and ensure that the patient is safe and comfortable. Chart the procedure in the patient's record, noting heart and respiratory rates, breath sounds, peak flows (if measured), and what medication and the number of puffs that were given.

USE OF A SPACER WITH A METERED DOSE INHALER

Spacers are small chambers that are designed to be used in conjunction with MDI aerosol administration. Spacer devices help to slow the velocity of aerosol particles, enhance the vaporization of the propellant, and reduce the amount of coordination required to obtain optimal results.

Position the Patient

It is important to position the patient properly for optimal administration of medication via metered dose inhaler. The optimal position is sitting erect or in high Fowler's position. This position allows for good chest expansion. Ensure that the patient is not wearing any clothing that may interfere with chest wall excursion.

Monitor the Patient

Auscultate the chest and note any abnormal breath sounds or other findings. Measure the heart rate and respiratory rate prior to medication administration. Measure the peak expiratory flow as indicated to measure the effectiveness of bronchodilator therapy.

Instruct the Patient

As discussed previously, it is important to instruct the patient thoroughly to obtain the best results with this type of aerosol administration. Allow the patient opportunity to ask questions about any aspect of the technique he or she doesn't understand. Ideally, use an MDI containing a placebo and demonstrate the technique yourself.

Assemble the Equipment

Thoroughly shake the MDI prior to use. Attach the mouthpiece to the canister and remove the cap from the mouthpiece. Attach the spacer device to the MDI. Ensure that the aerosol can pass through the spacer without obstruction.

Administer the Medication

Have the patient hold the MDI and spacer in the mouth. Instruct the patient to inhale slowly and deeply while activating the MDI by squeezing it. Instruct the patient to continue to inhale and to hold the breath at the end of inhalation for 5 to 7 seconds. Have the patient slowly exhale following the medication administration. Repeat the procedure as many times as ordered by the patient's physician, waiting between puffs.

Monitor the Patient following Therapy

Monitor the patient's heart and respiratory rates following medication administration. Auscultate the chest and note any changes in breath sounds. If administering a bronchodilator, measure the peak expiratory flow following aerosol administration.

Clean the Patient's Room and Chart Procedure

Remove any unneeded supplies from the patient's room and ensure that the patient is safe and comfortable. Chart the procedure in the patient's record, noting heart and respiratory rates, breath sounds, peak flows (if measured), and what medication and the number of puffs that were given. It is also important to note in the record that a spacer was used.

DRY POWDER INHALERS

The correct use of a DPI is dependent on what type of DPI is to be used (Diskhaler, Diskus, or Turbuhaler). Each type requires a slightly different technique, as described in this section. However, it is strongly recommended that as a practitioner, you read the package insert provided by the manufacturer including the directions for use for each DPI prior to teaching your patient how to use the device.

Practice using a DPI containing placebo. Familiarity with the experience of using these devices will enhance your ability to instruct your patient in correct technique.

Diskhaler

Figure 14-6 is a photograph of the Diskhaler. Begin by removing the mouthpiece cover by sliding it off. Pull the tray out from the device (holds the disk), and place the disk on the center wheel of the Diskhaler with the num-

bers facing up. Rotate the disk by sliding the tray in and out of the Diskhaler. Lift the back of the lid fully upright; this punctures the small blister on the disk, allowing the drug to be released. Keeping the Diskhaler level, insert the open mouthpiece into your mouth. Take a slow deep breath, inhaling the medication. Remove the device from your mouth to exhale.

Diskus

Figure 14-7 is a photograph of the Diskus DPI. Open the device by rotating the inner and outer portions in opposite directions. This exposes the mouthpiece opening. Slide the lever on the side of the device; this advances the foil strip containing medication doses and exposes the contents for inhalation. Keeping the Diskhaler level, insert the open mouthpiece into your mouth. Take a slow deep breath, inhaling the medication. Remove the device from your mouth to exhale.

Turbuhaler

Like the majority of DPIs, the Turbuhaler contains both the delivery device (DPI) and the medication in one unit (Figure 14-8). To use the device, remove the cover from the mouthpiece. Holding the Turbuhaler upright (mouthpiece

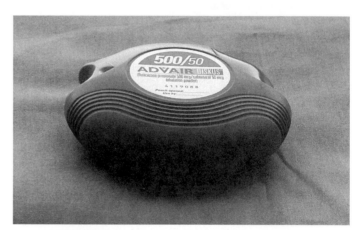

Figure 14-7   *A photograph of the Diskus DPI*

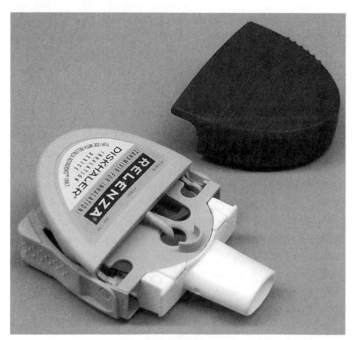

Figure 14-6   *A photograph of the Diskhaler*

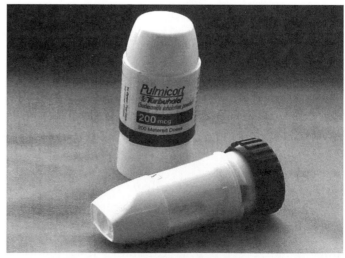

Figure 14-8 *A photograph of the Turbuhaler DPI*

up), rotate the lower grip first right and then left while holding the upper portion (mouthpiece) stationary. When this manuever is performed correctly, a "click" can be heard. Place the mouthpiece into your mouth. Keeping the Turbuhaler level, insert the open mouthpiece into your mouth. Take a slow, deep breath, inhaling the medication. Remove the device from your mouth to exhale. Replace the mouthpiece cover, and store the device in a cool, dry place.

References

Bone, R. C. (1984). The adult respiratory distress syndrome: Treatment in the next decade. *Respiratory Care, 29*(3), 249.

Bonner, J. T. (1985). *Respiratory intensive care of the adult patient.* St. Louis, MO: Mosby.

Des Jardins, T. R. (2002). *Cardiopulmonary anatomy & physiology: Essentials for respiratory care* (4th ed.). Clifton Park, NY: Delmar Learning.

Fink, J. B. (2000). Metered-dose inhalers, dry powder inhalers, and transistions. *Respiratory Care, 45*(6), 623–635.

Scanlan, C., Spearman, C. B., & Sheldon, R. L. (1995). *Egan's fundamentals of respiratory therapy* (6th ed.). St. Louis, MO: Mosby.

Ziment, I. (1978). *Respiratory pharmacology and therapeutics.* Philadelphia: Saunders.

Practice Activities: Introduction to Respiratory Care Pharmacology

1. Using a laboratory partner, practice instructing each other on how to use an MDI. Carefully critique each other's instructions.

2. Using a laboratory partner, practice using an MDI containing a placebo:

   a. With a spacer
   b. Without a spacer

3. Practice charting what you would record in a patient's record following MDI administration.

Check List: Metered Dose Inhaler

_____ 1. Properly identify and position the patient for MDI administration.
_____ 2. Wash your hands.
3. Give complete and thorough instructions on how to use an MDI:
_____ a. Without a spacer
_____ b. With a spacer
4. Monitor the patient:
_____ a. Heart rate
_____ b. Respiratory rate
_____ c. Breath sounds
_____ d. Peak expiratory flows (if giving a bronchodilator)

5. Administer the medication using an MDI:
_____ a. Without a spacer
_____ b. With a spacer
6. Monitor the patient following MDI administration.
_____ a. Heart rate
_____ b. Respiratory rate
_____ c. Breath sounds
_____ d. Peak expiratory flows (if giving a bronchodilator)
_____ 7. Ensure the patient's safety and comfort.
_____ 8. Clean the patient's room.
_____ 9. Chart the procedure in the patient's record.

Self-Evaluation Post Test: Introduction to Respiratory Care Pharmacology

1. Adrenergic receptor sites include which of the following?

   I. Alpha
   II. Beta-1
   III. Beta-2
   IV. Cholinergic

   a. I
   b. I, II
   c. I, II, III
   d. II, III

2. Which of the following mediators is/are released during bronchospasm following mast cell degranulation?

   I. Leukotrienes
   II. Histamine
   III. Prostaglandins
   IV. Acetylcholine

   a. I
   b. I, II
   c. I, II, III
   d. II, III, IV

3. Sympathomimetic agents work by:
   a. releasing acetylcholine.
   b. increasing production of adenylate cyclase.
   c. increasing production of phosphodiesterase.
   d. blocking phosphodiesterase.

4. Examples of sympathomimetic agents are:
   I. albuterol.   a. I, II
   II. atropine.   b. I, III
   III. isoproterenol.   c. II, III
   IV. theophylline.   d. II, IV

5. Metaproterenol comes in a stock solution of 5%. To draw up 10 mg of metaproterenol, you would withdraw how many ml from the bottle?
   a. 0.1 ml   c. 0.3 ml
   b. 0.2 ml   d. 0.4 ml

6. Advantages of aerosol administration of respiratory drugs include which of the following?
   I. The lungs are specifically targeted.
   II. There are fewer systemic side effects.
   III. Dosing is always precise.
   IV. It is less expensive than other routes.
   a. I   c. II, III
   b. I, II   d. II, IV

7. An example of an anticholinergic drug is:
   a. albuterol.   c. acetylcysteine.
   b. atropine.   d. prednisone.

8. Advantages of MDIs include:
   I. ease of use.
   II. portability.
   III. the lungs are specifically targeted.
   IV. fewer systemic side effects.
   a. I   c. I, II, III
   b. I, II   d. I, II, III, IV

9. The following mucokinetic agents break chemical bonds in the mucus protein:
   I. Acetylcysteine
   II. Sodium bicarbonate
   III. Deoxyribonuclease
   IV. Prednisone
   a. I, II   c. II, III
   b. I, III   d. II, IV

10. Which of the following drugs is routinely administered prophylactically to prevent asthma?
    a. Albuterol   c. Cromolyn sodium
    b. Atropine   d. Acetylcysteine

PERFORMANCE EVALUATION:
MDI ADMINISTRATION

Date: Lab _____ Clinical _____ Agency _____

Lab: Pass _____ Fail _____   Clinical: Pass _____ Fail _____

Student name _____   Instructor name _____

No. of times observed in clinical _____

No. of times practiced in clinical _____

PASSING CRITERIA: Obtain 90% or better on the procedure. Tasks indicated by * must receive at least 1 point, or the evaluation is terminated. Procedure must be performed within designated time, or the performance receives a failing grade.

SCORING:
2 points — Task performed satisfactorily without prompting.
1 point — Task performed satisfactorily with self-initiated correction.
0 points — Task performed incorrectly or with prompting required.
NA — Task not applicable to the patient care situation.

TASKS:		PEER	LAB	CLINICAL
*	1. Verifies the physician's order	☐	☐	☐
*	2. Washes hands	☐	☐	☐
*	3. Obtains required supplies			
	a. MDI	☐	☐	☐
	b. Spacer	☐	☐	☐
*	4. Gives thorough and complete instructions	☐	☐	☐
*	5. Monitors the patient			
	a. Heart rate	☐	☐	☐
	b. Respiratory rate	☐	☐	☐
	c. Breath sounds	☐	☐	☐
	d. Peak expiratory flow	☐	☐	☐
*	6. Administers aerosol using the MDI			
	a. Without a spacer	☐	☐	☐
	b. With a spacer	☐	☐	☐
*	7. Monitors the patient following aerosol administration			
	a. Heart rate	☐	☐	☐
	b. Respiratory rate	☐	☐	☐
	c. Breath sounds	☐	☐	☐
	d. Peak expiratory flow	☐	☐	☐
	8. Cleans up after the procedure	☐	☐	☐
*	9. Records procedure in the patient's chart	☐	☐	☐

SCORE: Peer _____ points of possible 34; _____%

Lab _____ points of possible 34; _____%

Clinical _____ points of possible 34; _____%

TIME: _____ out of possible 30 minutes

STUDENT SIGNATURES

PEER: _____

STUDENT: _____

INSTRUCTOR SIGNATURES

LAB: _____

CLINICAL: _____

PERFORMANCE EVALUATION:
DPI ADMINISTRATION

Date: Lab _____ Clinical _____ Agency _____

Lab: Pass _____ Fail _____   Clinical: Pass _____ Fail _____

Student name _____ Instructor name _____

No. of times observed in clinical _____

No. of times practiced in clinical _____

PASSING CRITERIA: Obtain 90% or better on the procedure. Tasks indicated by * must receive at least 1 point, or the evaluation is terminated. Procedure must be performed within designated time, or the performance receives a failing grade.

SCORING:
2 points — Task performed satisfactorily without prompting.
1 point — Task performed satisfactorily with self-initiated correction.
0 points — Task performed incorrectly or with prompting required.
NA — Task not applicable to the patient care situation.

TASKS:		PEER	LAB	CLINICAL
*	1. Verifies the physician's order	☐	☐	☐
*	2. Observes universal precautions, including washing hands.	☐	☐	☐
*	3. Obtains DPI	☐	☐	☐
*	4. Gives thorough and complete instructions	☐	☐	☐
*	5. Monitors the patient			
	a. Heart rate	☐	☐	☐
	b. Respiratory rate	☐	☐	☐
	c. Breath sounds	☐	☐	☐
	d. Peak expiratory flow	☐	☐	☐
*	6. Administers DPI	☐	☐	☐
*	7. Monitors the patient following aerosol administration			
	a. Heart rate	☐	☐	☐
	b. Respiratory rate	☐	☐	☐
	c. Breath sounds	☐	☐	☐
	d. Peak expiratory flow	☐	☐	☐
	8. Cleans up after the procedure	☐	☐	☐
*	9. Records procedure in the patient's chart	☐	☐	☐

SCORE: Peer   _____ points of possible 30; _____%

           Lab   _____ points of possible 30; _____%

           Clinical   _____ points of possible 30; _____%

TIME: _____ out of possible 30 minutes

CHAPTER 15

HUMIDITY AND AEROSOL THERAPY

─── **INTRODUCTION** ───

Humidity and aerosol therapy is a frequently used modality in clinical practice. A great deal of your time in respiratory care practice will be spent setting up, monitoring, and troubleshooting humidity and aerosol therapy equipment. It is important that you understand the components and theory of operation of the various types of humidity and aerosol equipment. This knowledge base will allow you to select and set up appropriate devices to meet clinical goals. You will also be expected to know how to troubleshoot the equipment, rendering it operational.

This chapter discusses the various types of equipment used to administer humidity and aerosol therapy, their principles of operation, clinical applications, and hazards and complications.

KEY TERMS

- Absolute humidity
- Aerosol
- Amplitude
- Body humidity
- Capacity
- Frequency
- Humidifier
- Humidity
- Maximum humidity
- Nebulizer
- Relative humidity
- Steamer

OBJECTIVES

At the end of this chapter, you should be able to:

- Define *humidity* and *aerosol*.
- Explain the difference between a humidifier and a nebulizer.
- State the three factors that can affect humidity output.
- For the following humidifiers, describe the principles of operation, efficiency, and application in the clinical setting:
  — Bubble humidifier
  — Cascade humidifier
  — Bird Wick humidifier
- For the following large-volume nebulizers, describe the principles of operation, efficiency, and application in the clinical setting:

- — Puritan All-Purpose nebulizer
- — Ohio Deluxe nebulizer
- — MistyOx nebulizers
- — McGaw Solo Sphere
- Discuss the following features of an ultrasonic nebulizer:
  — Principles of operation
    — Energy generation
    — Function of piezoelectric crystal
    — Significance of amplitude and frequency
  — Clinical application
  — Hazards of use
- Compare and contrast the types of small-volume nebulizers and their clinical applications.

CLINICAL PRACTICE GUIDELINES

AARC Clinical Practice Guideline:
Bland Aerosol Administration

BAA 4.0 INDICATIONS:
    4.1 The presence of upper airway edema — cool bland aerosol (1,2)
        4.1.1 Laryngeotracheobronchitis (LTB) (1,2)
        4.1.2 Subglottic edema (1,2)
        4.1.3 Postextubation edema (1,2)
        4.1.4 Postoperative management of the upper airway
    4.2 The presence of a bypassed upper airway (3)
    4.3 The need for sputum specimens (3,4)

BAA 5.0 CONTRAINDICATIONS:
    5.1 Bronchoconstriction (1,3,5,6)

    5.2 History of airway hyperresponsiveness (1,2, 5,6)

BAA 6.0 HAZARDS/COMPLICATIONS:
    6.1 Wheezing or bronchospasm (1,3,5,6)
    6.2 Bronchoconstriction when artificial airway is employed (7–11)
    6.3 Infection (12)
    6.4 Overhydration (12)
    6.5 Patient discomfort
    6.6 Caregiver exposure to droplet nuclei of *Mycobacterium tuberculosis* or other airborne contagion produced as a consequence of coughing, particularly during sputum induction.

(Continued)

(CPG Continued)

BAA 8.0 ASSESSMENT OF NEED:

8.1 The presence of one or more of the following may be an indication for administration of a water or isotonic or hypotonic saline aerosol:

8.1.1 Stridor

8.1.2 Brassy, crouplike cough

8.1.3 Hoarseness following extubation

8.1.4 Diagnosis of LTB or croup

8.1.5 Clinical history suggesting upper airway irritation and increased work of breathing (e.g., smoke inhalation)

8.1.6 Patient discomfort associated with airway instrumentation or insult

8.2 The presence of the need for sputum induction (e.g., for diagnosis of *Pneumocystis carinii* pneumonia [14–16] tuberculosis) is an indication for administration of hypertonic saline aerosol.

BAA 9.0 ASSESSMENT OF OUTCOME:

9.1 With administration of water or hypotonic or isotonic saline, the desired outcome is the presence of one or more of the following:

9.1.1 Decreased work of breathing

9.1.2 Improved vital signs

9.1.3 Decreased stridor

9.1.4 Decreased dyspnea

9.1.5 Improved arterial blood gas values

9.1.6 Improved oxygen saturation as indicated by pulse oximetry (SpO_2)

9.2 With administration of hypertonic saline, the desired outcome is a sputum sample adequate for analysis.

BAA 11.0 MONITORING:

The extent of patient monitoring should be determined on the basis of the stability and severity of the patient's condition:

11.1 Patient subjective response—pain, discomfort, dyspnea, restlessness

11.2 Heart rate and rhythm, blood pressure

11.3 Respiratory rate, pattern, mechanics, accessory muscle use

11.4 Sputum production quantity, color, consistency, odor

11.5 Skin color

11.6 Breath sounds

11.7 Pulse oximetry (if hypoxemia is suspected)

Reprinted with permission from *Respiratory Care* 1993; 38: 1196–1200. The complete AARC Clinical Practice Guidelines are available from the AARC Web site (http://www.aarc.org), from the AARC Executive Office, or from *Respiratory Care* journal.

AARC Clinical Practice Guideline: Selection of Aerosol Delivery Device

AD 4.0 INDICATIONS:

The need to deliver — as an aerosol to the lower airways — a medication from one of the following drug classifications:

Beta adrenergic agents

Anticholinergic agents (antimuscarinics)

Anti-inflammatory agents (e.g., corticosteroids)

Mediator-modifying compounds (e.g., cromolyn sodium)

Mucokinetics

The selection of a device for delivery of aerosol for parenchymal deposition (e.g., antibiotics) will be addressed in another Guideline.

AD 5.0 CONTRAINDICATIONS:

5.1 No contraindications exist for the administration of aerosols by inhalation.

5.2 Contraindications related to the substances being delivered may exist. Consult the package insert for product-specific contraindications.

AD 6.0 HAZARDS/COMPLICATIONS:

6.1 Malfunction of device (3–5) and/or improper technique (6–12) may result in underdosing.

6.2 The potential exists for malfunction of device and/or improper technique (inappropriate patient use) to result in overdosing.

6.3 Complications of specific pharmacologic agent may occur.

6.4 Cardiotoxic effects of Freon have been reported as an idiosyncratic response that may be a problem with excessive use of MDI. (13–18)

6.5 Freon may affect the environment by its effect on the ozone layer. (19–21)

6.6 Repeated exposure to aerosols has been reported to produce asthmatic symptoms in some caregivers. (22)

AD 8.0 ASSESSMENT OF NEED:

8.1 Based on proven therapeutic efficacy, (25, 51–60) variety of available medications, and cost-effectiveness, (51,61–64) the MDI with accessory device should be the first method to consider for administration of aerosol to the airway.

8.2 Lack of availability of prescribed drug in MDI, dry powder, or solution form

8.3 Inability of the patient to use device properly with coaching and instruction should lead to consideration of other devices.

8.4 Patient preference for a given device that meets therapeutic objectives should be honored.

8.5 When there is need for large doses, MDI, SVN, or LVN may be used. Clear superiority of any one method has not been established. Convenience and patient tolerance of procedure should be considered.

8.6 When spontaneous ventilation is inadequate (e.g., as in kyphoscoliosis or neuromuscular disorders, exacerbation of severe bronchospasm with impending respiratory failure that does not respond to other forms of therapy), delivery by a positive-pressure breathing device (IPPB) should be considered. (65–67)

AD 9.0 ASSESSMENT OF OUTCOME:
9.1 Proper technique applying device
9.2 Patient response to or compliance with procedure
9.3 Objectively measured improvement (e.g., increased FEV_1 or peak flow)

AD 11.0 MONITORING:
11.1 Performance of the device
11.2 Technique of device application
11.3 Assessment of patient response including changes in vital signs

---

Reprinted with permission from *Respiratory Care* 1992; 37: 891–897. The complete AARC Clinical Practice Guidelines are available from the AARC Web site (http://www.aarc.org), from the AARC Executive Office, or from *Respiratory Care* journal.

AARC Clinical Practice Guideline:
Delivery of Aerosols to the Upper Airway

AUA 4.0 INDICATIONS:
4.1 Upper airway inflammation (e.g., to relieve inflammation due to laryngeotracheobronchitis (2))
4.2 Anesthesia (e.g., to control pain and gagging during endoscopic procedures (3–7))
4.3 Rhinitis (e.g., to relieve inflammation and vascular congestion (8,9))
4.4 Systemic disease (e.g., to deliver peptides such as insulin (10))

AUA 5.0 CONTRAINDICATIONS:
Known hypersensitivity to the medication being delivered

AUA 6.0 HAZARDS/COMPLICATIONS:
6.1 Administration of medications for upper airway inflammation may result in:
 6.1.1 Bronchospasm (11,12)
 6.1.2 Rebound of symptoms
 6.1.3 Systemic side effects
6.2 Administration of medications for anesthesia (3–7) may result in:
 6.2.1 Inhibition of gag reflex
 6.2.2 Choking
 6.2.3 Dehydration of epithelium
 6.2.4 Allergic reactions
 6.2.5 Excessive systemic effect
 6.2.6 Bronchospasm
 6.2.7 Nosocomial infection from contaminated delivery device or medication (See

AARC CPG on Selection of Aerosol Delivery Device (13)) (14)
6.3 Administration of medications for rhinitis (15–21) may result in:
 6.3.1 Nasal rebound (including rhinitis medicamentosa) after extended use of alpha adrenergic decongestants
 6.3.2 Delayed effect (e.g., effects of steroids are not immediate)
 6.3.3 Sensation of irritation and burning in the nose
 6.3.4 Sneezing attacks (immediately following administration)
 6.3.5 Mucosal ulceration and bleeding
 6.3.6 Postnasal drip
6.4 Systemic disease — medication may cause nasal irritation or toxic effects (9,10)

AUA 8.0 ASSESSMENT OF NEED:
The presence of one or more of the following may suggest the need for aerosol application.
 8.1 In upper airway inflammation:
  8.1.1 Stridor
  8.1.2 Brassy crouplike cough
  8.1.3 Hoarseness following extubation
  8.1.4 Diagnosis of laryngeotracheobronchitis or croup
  8.1.5 Recent extubation
  8.1.6 Evidence of inflamed upper airway
  8.1.7 Soft-tissue radiograph suggesting edema
  8.1.8 Increased work of breathing
 8.2 For anesthesia:
  8.2.1 Severe localized pain in upper airway
  8.2.2 Impending invasive instrumentation of the upper airway
 8.3 In rhinitis:
  8.3.1 Diagnosis of allergic, nonallergic, or infectious rhinitis
  8.3.2 Symptomatic need:
   8.3.2.1 Nasal congestion
   8.3.2.2 Rhinorrhea
   8.3.2.3 Sneezing
   8.3.2.4 Itching of nose, eyes, or palate
 8.4 In systemic disease — presence of a systemic disease that warrants intranasal delivery of a therapeutic agent

AUA 9.0 ASSESSMENT OF OUTCOME:
9.1 In upper airway inflammation, effectiveness of administration may be indicated by:
 9.1.1 Reduced stridor
 9.1.2 Reduced hoarseness
 9.1.3 Improvement in soft-tissue radiograph
 9.1.4 Decreased work of breathing, as evidenced by decreased use of accessory muscles

(Continued)

(CPG Continued)

9.2 For anesthesia, effectiveness of administration is marked by reduced discomfort in the patient.

9.3 In rhinitis, effectiveness of administration may be indicated by:

9.3.1 Reduced nasal congestion

9.3.2 Improved air flow through nose

9.3.3 Reduced rhinorrhea

9.3.4 Reduced sneezing

9.3.5 Reduced itching of nose, eyes, or palate

9.4 Systemic disease — effectiveness of administration of agent is marked by the presence of the appropriate systemic therapeutic response.

AUA 11.0 MONITORING:

The extent of patient monitoring should be determined on the basis of the stability and severity of the patient's condition:

11.1 Patient compliance and increase or decrease in symptoms, signs, and patient subjective response as specified in Section 8

11.2 Heart rate and rhythm, blood pressure

11.3 Change in indicators of therapeutic effect (e.g., blood-glucose level with insulin)

Reprinted with permission from *Respiratory Care* 1994; 39(8): 803–807. The complete AARC Clinical Practice Guidelines are available from the AARC Web site (http://www.aarc.org), from the AARC Executive Office, or from *Respiratory Care* journal.

AARC Clinical Practice Guideline: Selection of a Device for Delivery of Aerosol to the Lung Parenchyma

DALP 4.0 INDICATIONS:

The indication for selecting a suitable device is the need to deliver a topical medication (in aerosol form) that has its site of action in the lung parenchyma or is intended for systemic absorption. Such medications may possibly include antibiotics, antivirals, antifungals, surfactants, and enzymes.

DALP 5.0 CONTRAINDICATIONS:

5.1 No contraindications exist for choosing an appropriate device for parenchymal deposition.

5.2 Contraindications related to the substances being delivered may exist. Consult the package insert for product-specific contraindications to medication delivery.

DALP 6.0 HAZARDS/COMPLICATIONS:

6.1 Malfunction of device and/or improper technique may result in underdosing or overdosing.

6.2 In mechanically ventilated patients, the nebulizer design and characteristics of the medication may affect ventilator function (e.g., filter obstruction, altered tidal volume, decreased trigger sensitivity) and medication deposition. (10,11)

6.3 Complications related to specific pharmacologic agents can occur.

6.4 Aerosols may cause bronchospasm or irritation of the airway.

6.5 Exposure to medications (12–23) and patient-generated droplet nuclei may be hazardous to clinicians. (24)

6.5.1 Exposure to medication should be limited to the patient for whom it has been ordered. Nebulized medication that is released into the atmosphere from the nebulizer or exhaled by the patient becomes a form of "secondhand" exposure that may affect health care providers and others in the vicinity of the treatment.

There has been increased awareness of possible health effects of aerosols, such as ribavirin and pentamidine. Anecdotal reports associate symptoms such as conjunctivitis, decreased tolerance to presence of contact lenses, headaches, bronchospasm, shortness of breath, and rashes in health care workers exposed to secondhand aerosols. Similar concerns have been expressed concerning health care workers who are pregnant or are planning to be pregnant within eight weeks of administration. Less often discussed are the potential exposure effects of aerosolized antibiotics (which may contribute to the development of resistant organisms), steroids, and bronchodilators. (25)

Because the data regarding adverse health effects on the health care worker and on those casually exposed are incomplete, the prudent course is to minimize exposure in all situations. (26)

6.5.2 The Centers for Disease Control and Prevention recommends addressing exposure control issues by (1) administrative policy, (2) engineering controls, and (3) personal protective equipment, in that order. (27,28)

6.5.2.1 Administrative controls: Should include warning signs to apprise all who enter a treatment area of potential hazards of exposure. Accidental exposures should be documented and reported according to accepted standards.

Measures to reduce aerosol contamination of room air include:

6.5.2.1.1 Discontinuing nebulization of medication while patient is not breathing the aerosol

6.5.2.1.2 Ensuring that staff who administer medications understand risks inherent with the medication and procedures for safely disposing of hazardous wastes

6.5.2.1.3 Screening of staff for adverse effects of exposure to aerosol medication

6.5.2.1.4 Providing alternative assignments for those staff who are at high risk of adverse effects from exposure (e.g., pregnant women or those with demonstrated sensitivity to the specific agent)

6.5.2.2 Engineering controls:

6.5.2.2.1 Filters or filtered scavenger systems to remove aerosols that cannot be contained

6.5.2.2.2 Frequent air exchanges to dilute concentration of aerosol in room to eliminate 99% of aerosol before the next patient enters and receives treatment in the area

6.5.2.2.3 Booths or stalls for sputum induction and aerosolized medication administration in areas in which multiple patients are treated. Booths or stalls should be designed to provide adequate air flow to draw aerosol and droplet nuclei from the patient and into an appropriate filtration system, with exhaust directed to an appropriate outside vent.

6.5.2.2.4 Handling of filters, nebulizers, and other contaminated components of the aerosol delivery system used with suspect agents (such as pentamidine and ribavirin) as hazardous waste

6.5.2.3 Personal protection devices:

6.5.2.3.1 Personal protection devices should be used to reduce exposure when engineering alternatives are not in place or are not adequate. Use properly fitted respirators with adequate filtration when exhaust flow cannot adequately remove aerosol particles. (28)

6.5.2.3.2 Goggles, gloves, and gowns should be used as splatter shields and to reduce exposure to medication residues and body substances.

DALP 8.0 ASSESSMENT OF NEED (Selection Criteria for Device):

8.1 Availability of prescribed drug in solution or MDI formulation

8.2 Availability of appropriate scavenging or filtration equipment

8.3 Patient preference for a given device that meets therapeutic objectives

8.4 Although specific devices may give known ranges of particle size and output, clear superiority of any one method or device for achieving specific clinical outcomes has not been established. Cost, convenience, effectiveness, and patient tolerance of procedure should be considered. (26,53)

8.5 When spontaneous ventilation is inadequate (e.g., kyphoscoliosis, neuromuscular disorders, or respiratory failure) consider augmentation with mechanical ventilation.

DALP 9.0 ASSESSMENT OF OUTCOME:

Appropriate device selection is reflected by evidence of:

9.1 Use of proper technique in applying device

9.2 Patient compliance with procedure

9.3 A positive clinical outcome (However, appropriate device selection and application does not guarantee a positive outcome.)

DALP 11.0 MONITORING:

11.1 Performance of the device and scavenging system

11.2 Technique of device application

11.3 Assessment of patient response

Reprinted with permission from *Respiratory Care* 1996; 41(7): 647–653. The complete AARC Clinical Practice Guidelines are available from the AARC Web site (http://www.aarc.org), from the AARC Executive Office, or from *Respiratory Care* journal.

(Continued)

(CPG Continued)

AARC Clinical Practice Guideline:
Humidification during Mechanical Ventilation

HMV 4.0 INDICATIONS:

Humidification of inspired gas during mechanical ventilation is mandatory when an endotracheal or tracheostomy tube is present. (1–7)

HMV 5.0 CONTRAINDICATIONS:

There are no contraindications [to] providing physiologic conditioning of inspired gas during mechanical ventilation. An HME is contraindicated under some circumstances.

5.1 Use of an HME is contraindicated for patients with thick, copious, or bloody secretions. (8,26–28)

5.2 Use of an HME is contraindicated for patients with an expired tidal volume less than 70% of the delivered tidal volume (e.g., those with large bronchopleurocutaneous fistulas or incompetent or absent endotracheal tube cuffs). (5–25)

5.3 Use of an HME is contraindicated for patients with body temperatures less than 32°C. (8,29)

5.4 Use of an HME may be contraindicated for patients with high spontaneous minute volumes (> 10 L/min). (8,26,29)

5.5 An HME must be removed from the patient circuit during aerosol treatments when the nebulizer is placed in the patient circuit. (8–29)

HMV 6.0 HAZARDS/COMPLICATIONS:

Hazards and complications associated with the use of humidification devices include:

6.1 Potential for electrical shock — heated humidifiers (11–14)

6.2 Hypothermia — HME or heated humidifiers; hyperthermia — heated humidifiers (11–14)

6.3 Thermal injury to the airway from heated humidifiers; (30) burns to the patient and tubing meltdown if heated-wire circuits are covered or circuits and humidifiers are incompatible

6.4 Underhydration and impaction of mucus secretions — HME or heated humidifiers (1–7)

6.5 Hypoventilation and/or alveolar gas trapping due to mucous plugging of airways — HME or heated humidifier (1–7)

6.6 Possible increased resistive work of breathing due to mucous plugging of airways — HME or heated humidifiers (1–7)

6.7 Possible increased resistive work of breathing through the humidifier — HME or heated humidifiers (31–34)

6.8 Possible hypoventilation due to increased dead space — HME (8,15–25,26–30)

6.9 Inadvertent overfilling resulting in unintentional tracheal lavage — heated reservoir humidifiers (35)

6.10 The fact that when disconnected from the patient, some ventilators generate a high flow through the patient circuit that may aerosolize contaminated condensate, putting both the patient and clinician at risk for nosocomial infection — heated humidifiers (35)

6.11 Potential for burns to caregivers from hot metal — heated humidifiers

6.12 Inadvertent tracheal lavage from pooled condensate in patient circuit — heated humidifiers (35)

6.13 Elevated airway pressures due to pooled condensation — heated humidifiers

6.14 Patient-ventilator dysynchrony and improper ventilator performance due to pooled condensation in the circuit — heated humidifiers

6.15 Ineffective low-pressure alarm during disconnection due to resistance through HME (36)

HMV 8.0 ASSESSMENT OF NEED:

Humidification is needed by all patients requiring mechanical ventilation via an artificial airway. Conditioning of inspired gases should be instituted using either an HME or a heated humidifier.

8.1 HMEs are better suited for short-term use (< or = 96 hours) and during transport. (8,29)

8.2 Heated humidifiers should be used for patients requiring long-term mechanical ventilation (>96 hours) or for patients who exhibit contraindications [to] HME use. (8,29)

HMV 9.0 ASSESSMENT OF OUTCOME:

Humidification is assumed to be appropriate if, on regular careful inspection, the patient exhibits none of the hazards or complications listed in HMV 6.0.

HMV 11.0 MONITORING:

The humidification device should be inspected visually during the patient-ventilator system check and condensate should be removed from the patient circuit as necessary. HMEs should be inspected and replaced if secretions have contaminated the insert or filter. The following variables should be recorded during equipment inspection:

11.1 Humidifier setting (temperature setting or numeric dial setting or both). During routine use on an intubated patient, a heated humidifier should be set to deliver an inspired gas temperature of 33 ± 2°C and should provide a minimum of 30 mg/L of water vapor. (8–10)

11.2 Inspired gas temperature. Temperature should be monitored as near the patient's airway opening as possible, if a heated humidifier is used.

11.2.1 Specific temperatures may vary with patient condition, but the inspiratory gas should not exceed 37°C at the airway threshold.

11.2.2 When a heated-wire patient circuit is used (to prevent condensation) on an infant, the temperature probe should be located outside of the incubator or away from the direct heat of the radiant warmer. (12)

11.3 Alarm settings (if applicable). High temperature alarm should be set no higher than 37°C, and the low temperature alarm should be set no lower than 30°C. (8,10)

11.4 Water level and function of automatic feed system (if applicable)

11.5 Quantity and consistency of secretions. Characteristics should be noted and recorded. When using an HME, if secretions become copious or appear increasingly tenacious, a heated humidifier should replace the HME.

Reprinted with permission from *Respiratory Care* 1992; 37: 887–890. The complete AARC Clinical Practice Guidelines are available from the AARC Web site (http://www.aarc.org), from the AARC Executive Office, or from *Respiratory Care* journal.

WHAT IS HUMIDITY AND WHAT IS AEROSOL?

Humidity is water in gaseous form, or vapor. As such, water vapor or humidity cannot be seen. Humidification is used to add water vapor to an anhydrous gas during oxygen administration and to raise the relative humidity of a room to prevent or loosen thick retained secretions. It is also used to provide humidity to the lower airways when the upper airway is bypassed by intubation or tracheostomy.

An *aerosol* is the suspension of particulate water in a gas. Technically, we can generate an aerosol of any matter if there is sufficient energy to suspend it. In the practice of respiratory care, aerosol generation generally serves two purposes: bland aerosol therapy and the aerosolization of medication. A bland aerosol is usually nebulized water or saline and is used to increase the water content of secretions, thereby thinning them. Medications such as bronchodilators may be aerosolized to reverse bronchoconstriction. Mucokinetics may be aerosolized to break down mucus. Decongestants may be aerosolized to shrink swollen mucous membranes by vasoconstriction. Racemic epinephrine is an example and is commonly used to treat epiglottitis.

Humidifiers and Nebulizers

A *humidifier* is a device that produces water in gaseous form (vapor) through the process of evaporation. There are many types of humidifiers that range in efficiency from poor to excellent. An ideal humidifier is capable of completely saturating a gas (100% humidity) at body temperature and pressure (termed *body humidity*: 37°C, 47 mm Hg partial press [H_2O], and 100% saturation).

A *nebulizer* is a device used to aerosolize liquids. Efficiency and particle sizes vary depending on the device and its principle of operation.

Heating a humidifier or nebulizer increases the content of water in the aerosol output, closely matching that of the body. Some people may be sensitive to the nature of the aerosol itself—the water may be irritating as well as the increased temperature. The temperature should be closely regulated to prevent adverse affects on the patient such as fever or burns.

Factors Affecting Humidity Output

Three factors that influence humidity output are temperature, surface area, and gas-liquid contact time. From a design or engineering standpoint, these factors can be manipulated to increase or decrease the output of a device. Temperature is the most easily controlled method of regulating humidity output. The warmer gas is, the more water vapor it can hold. When a gas is fully saturated with water vapor, the amount of water in grams per liter is termed *absolute humidity*. If a gas is fully saturated with water vapor (100% saturated), it is said to have *maximum humidity* or *capacity*. When the temperature of a gas is increased, its capacity will also increase. A gas heated to body temperature can therefore reach a humidity approaching that of the gas contained in the lungs.

Surface area and exposure time are other ways to control humidity output. By increasing the surface area for the gas-water interface, more gas is exposed to the water and more water vapor is picked up. Surface areas can be increased to only a limited degree; otherwise, the device would be too large and awkward. The time during which a gas is exposed to the water can also influence humidity output by providing time for evaporation to occur. Time of gas exposure, however, is difficult to influence.

EQUIPMENT FOR HUMIDITY AND AEROSOL THERAPY

Room Humidifier

The simplest room humidifier is an open pan of water. This is not very efficient, so other means are used to increase room humidity. As discussed here, a *room humidifier* is a device that generates an aerosol. When the aerosol is exposed to the ambient air, it evaporates, thereby increasing the *relative humidity* of the room:

$$\text{Relative humidity} = \frac{\text{actual humidity}}{\text{absolute humidity}} \times 100$$

Some common room humidifiers operate by means of centrifugal force. A disk and hollow shaft are driven at high speed by an electric motor. Water is drawn up the shaft by capillary action. When the water reaches the top of the shaft, centrifugal force propels the water from the

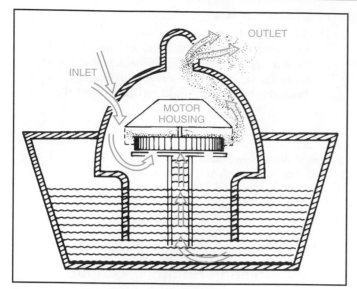

Figure 15-1 *A schematic of a centrifugal room humidifier*

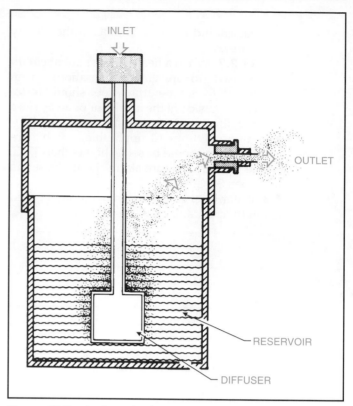

Figure 15-2 *A schematic of a typical bubble humidifier*

disk. Surrounding the spinning disk are *breaker combs*. These combs break the water particles into smaller sizes. The aerosol then flows out of the unit. Hankscraft and Devilbiss both make room humidifiers that utilize this principle of operation. Figure 15-1 is a schematic of a centrifugal room humidifier.

Another type of room humidifier is a *steamer*. These devices heat the water to the boiling point, producing water vapor. The vapor is then discharged into the room, where it evaporates. Many home steamer-humidifiers bought from pharmacies use this principle.

These devices were quite popular for home use in the late 1950s and early 1960s. They are not frequently found in clinical practice, primarily owing to the hazards associated with a reservoir of hot water, poor efficiency, and their potential as a source for nosocomial infections.

Bubble Humidifier

The bubble humidifier is the most commonly used humidifier in clinical practice. These devices are not very efficient in terms of humidity output. Their primary application is in the humidification of oxygen delivered by nasal cannula or by mask.

Bubble humidifiers work by conducting gas down a small tube that is submerged in water. The gas passes through a diffuser, which breaks the released gas into small bubbles, increasing the surface area. The bubbles float passively to the surface, absorbing water vapor. The humidified gas then flows through the outlet, out of the unit. Figure 15-2 is a schematic of a typical bubble humidifier.

Bubble humidifiers may be permanent, nondisposable units that are cleaned and sterilized between patient applications. Bubble humidifiers may also be purchased as disposable units designed for single-patient use. The disposable units are also available prefilled with sterile distilled water.

The outlets of bubble humidifiers have a tapered nipple, designed to fit small-diameter oxygen connecting tubing.

The oxygen delivery devices used with a bubble humidifier include the nasal cannula, simple oxygen mask, partial rebreathing mask, and the nonrebreathing mask.

These devices produce water vapor, or water in gaseous form. You cannot see the humidity output of these devices. Occasionally, water may be seen in the oxygen connecting tubing if temperature conditions promote condensation.

Cascade Humidifier

The cascade or diffuser type humidifier is one of the most efficient humidifiers available. These devices are capable of producing 100% body humidity.

The heart of the cascade humidifier is the tower. Gas entering the unit is conducted down the tower, below the surface of the water, and is forced through a one-way valve. This one-way valve prevents the gas from following the path of least resistance, back up the tower. As the gas enters a chamber below the level of the one-way valve, water is displaced by the gas. This displacement raises the water level in the unit and allows water to enter through a small port above the diffusion grid in the tower, where it forms a thin layer. Simultaneously, gas rises up through the grid, mixing with the water to form a fine foam. The cascade humidifier also contains a heating element, and an adjustable control is provided for thermostatic maintenance of a specific temperature. In addition, a small hole near the top of the cascade tower permits pressure changes (from the patient's spontaneous respiratory effort) to be conducted to whatever device is attached to the inlet. Figure 15-3 is a schematic of a cascade humidifier. The

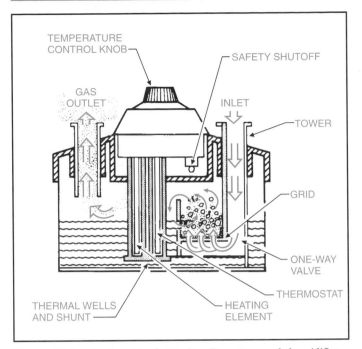

Figure 15-3 *A schematic of a Puritan-Bennett cascade humidifier*

cascade humidifier is capable of producing body humidity (100% saturation at 37°C).

The efficiency of the cascade humidifier makes it ideal for use with mechanical ventilation and artificial airways. Inlets and outlets on the humidifier are designed for large-bore aerosol tubing, which assists in the conduction of humidified gas at a high volume and flow. These put out such a large volume of vapor that as gas is conducted through large-bore tubing, the temperature drops, filling the tubing with condensed water.

Wick Humidifiers

Wick humidifiers are also very efficient humidifiers. By increasing the temperature and surface area, efficiency is enhanced. The wicks are typically made from a relatively thick blotter-type paper. This paper is very absorbent and quickly conducts water by capillary action.

The Bird Wick humidifier has a wick surrounded by a heating element. The bottom of the wick is submerged below the water level at the bottom of the chamber. Gas is conducted down close to the base of the unit and then

allowed to flow up adjacent to the wick. As the gas passes the wick, water is absorbed by evaporation.

The Bird Wick humidifier is ideal for use with mechanical ventilation and artificial airways. Inlets and outlets on the humidifier are designed for large-bore aerosol tubing, which assists in the conduction of humidified gas at a high volume and flow.

Water level is maintained automatically by a float system. As the water level reaches the upper fill limit, a float rises and shuts off any further flow of water. When the water level drops as a result of evaporation, the float also drops and allows water to enter the chamber. Figure 15-4 is a schematic of a Bird Wick humidifier.

Heat and Moisture Exchanger

A *heat and moisture exchanger* (HME) is a small hygroscopic device placed proximal to a patient's artificial airway, where it absorbs water vapor from the patient's exhaled gas (Figure 15-5). When the patient breathes or the

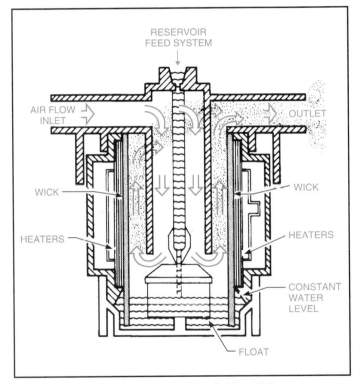

Figure 15-4 *A cross section of a Bird Wick humidifier*

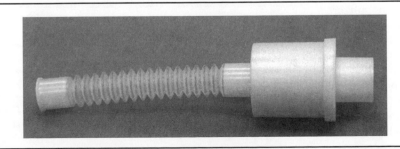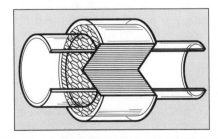

Figure 15-5 *A photograph and a cross section of a heat and moisture exchanger (HME)*

mechanical ventilator delivers the next breath, moisture trapped in the HME evaporates, humidifying the airway. The efficiency of these devices varies, ranging from around 70% to 90% at temperatures of 30 to 31°C. These devices are best used for shorter durations (less than 96 hours). The patient should be carefully monitored for increases in airway resistance and increased work of breathing.

Large-Volume Nebulizers

Use of large-volume nebulizers is very common in respiratory care practice. These devices deliver cool or heated aerosol, and they precisely regulate oxygen concentration using an oxygen diluter.

Jet mixing occurs by viscous shearing and vorticity as described in Chapter 13 to dilute oxygen with room air. These devices provide a range of inspired oxygen levels, operating in a manner similar to that of entrainment masks. Adjustment of the entrainment port size varies the amount of room air added to the oxygen flow. As with other entrainment devices, back pressure distal to the entrainment ports can cause an increase in the fraction of inspired oxygen delivered (FIO_2). The large-volume nebulizers are especially susceptible to this effect because of their high aerosol output, which may "rain out" and partially obstruct the delivery tubing. Therefore, the tubing should be checked and drained on a routine basis. A drainage bag or 3-L anesthesia bag may be positioned in line with the delivery tubing to serve both as a gas reservoir and as a collection bag for rain-out.

The high-velocity gas exiting from the nozzle (jet) is directed perpendicular to a small capillary tube whose base is immersed in water (Figure 15-6). Shear forces cause water to be removed from the capillary tube into the flow of gas. Because mass has been removed from the capillary tube (water), a void forms because the gas flow across the top of the tube effectively caps it (Scacci, 1979). This void forms a small area of reduced (subambient) pressure within the capillary tube itself. Capillary action draws water up the tube to fill the void (conservation of mass). Once the water level reaches the top, it is removed again by shear forces. This is a continuous process, and the water removed forms a dense aerosol.

Downstream a short distance from the jet is a baffle that serves to stabilize particle size. When the aerosolized particles meet the baffle, larger particles, having greater inertia, are rained out.

Ports for an immersion heater are commonly provided. A cap closes one of the ports with a 2 psi safety popoff feature, releasing pressure if the outlet is occluded.

Two common permanent, nondisposable nebulizers in this category are the Puritan All-Purpose and the Ohio Deluxe nebulizers. Several manufacturers also produce disposable nebulizers that operate using similar principles.

The outlet of the nebulizer has a connector for large-bore aerosol tubing. The common applications for the unit are in bland aerosol therapy via aerosol mask or face tent and in humidification of artificial airways via a Briggs adapter or tracheostomy mask.

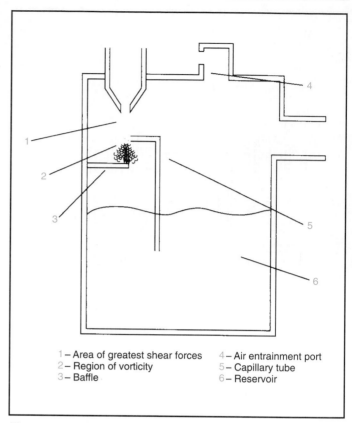

1 – Area of greatest shear forces
2 – Region of vorticity
3 – Baffle
4 – Air entrainment port
5 – Capillary tube
6 – Reservoir

Figure 15-6 *A schematic diagram of a large-volume jet nebulizer: 1, area of greatest shear forces; 2, region of vorticity; 3, baffle to stabilize particle size; 4, air entrainment port; 5, capillary tube; 6, liquid reservoir*

Total gas flow from these nebulizers will vary depending on the FIO_2 setting and entrained room air. Vorticity is utilized to dilute the source gas with room air entrained by the device. The total flow depends on the entrainment ratio. Tables 15-1 and 15-2 show the various entrainment ratios for the three FIO_2 settings for the Puritan All-Purpose and Ohio Deluxe nebulizers.

TABLE 15-1: Puritan All-Purpose Nebulizer Flow Output

SETTING	RATIO	OUTPUT
40%	3:1	60 L/min
70%	0.6:1	24 L/min
100%	0:1	15 L/min

TABLE 15-2: Ohio Deluxe Nebulizer Output

SETTING	RATIO	OUTPUT
40%	3:1	60 L/min
60%	1:1	30 L/min
100%	0:1	15 L/min

It becomes evident that flow decreases at the higher FIO_2 settings. It is not uncommon to simultaneously use more than one nebulizer to meet the flow needs of the patient.

MistyOx Nebulizers

The MistyOx Hi-Fi nebulizer and the MistyOx Gas Injection Nebulizer (GIN), Costa Mesa, CA, are two nebulizers that are designed to provide high-density aerosol delivery at high total flow rates (Figure 15-7). The Hi-Fi nebulizer can provide a flow of 43 L/min at an FIO_2 of 0.96 and of 77 L/min at an FIO_2 of 0.60 from a single oxygen source. The GIN device is capable of providing flows of more than 100 L/min when powered by two gas sources. Tables 15-3 and 15-4 summarize the GIN device oxygen concentrations and flow deliveries.

Both nebulizers have a standard 38-mm threaded fitting that allows connection of the nebulizer to most disposable sterile solution bottles. This capability is advantageous in that significant cost savings can be realized in comparison with other prefilled nebulizer brands. Heated aerosol may be provided by the attachment of the optional TurboHeater.

Babbington Nebulizers

The Babbington principle is a unique method of aerosol generation. A Babbington nebulizer consists of a small glass sphere or ball pressurized with source gas. On the sphere at the midpoint of its circumference is a tiny hole. High-pressure gas exits this hole at a very high flow rate. Liquid is drawn up a small capillary tube to a small reservoir situated above the sphere. The liquid is propelled up

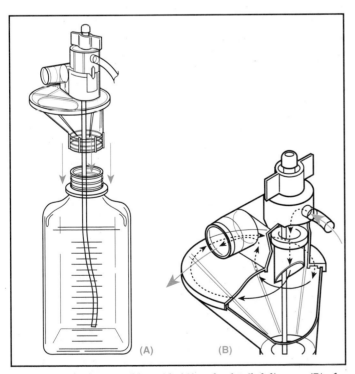

Figure 15-7 *An assembly guide (A) and a detailed diagram (B) of the MistyOx Gas Injection Nebulizer (GIN)*

TABLE 15-3: Concentration of Oxygen As Primary Gas and Total Flow for MistyOx GIN Nebulizer

PRIMARY GAS: OXYGEN (L/min)	SECONDARY GAS: AIR (L/min)	TOTAL FLOW	CONCEN-TRATION
40	0	40	100%
40	10	50	84.2%
40	20	60	73.6%
40	30	70	66.1%
40	40	80	60.5%
40	50	90	56.1%
40	60	100	52.6%
40	70	110	49.7%

TABLE 15-4: Concentration of Oxygen As Secondary Gas and Total Flow for MistyOx GIN Nebulizer

PRIMARY GAS: AIR (L/min)	SECONDARY GAS: OXYGEN (L/min)	TOTAL FLOW	CONCEN-TRATION
40	0	40	20.9%
40	10	50	36.8%
40	20	60	47.3%
40	30	70	54.9%
40	40	80	60.5%
40	50	90	64.9%
40	60	100	68.4%
40	70	110	71.3%

the tube by bubble action. Part of the flow to the sphere is directed to a chamber below the water level in the main reservoir.

The incoming gas forms bubbles that rise up the tube. Each bubble carries a small amount of water that eventually fills the small reservoir above the sphere. Water is allowed to drip over the sphere, forming a very thin film. When the film of water encounters the supersonic-velocity gas exiting the sphere, a very fine aerosol results. A ball positioned at the outlet of the sphere helps to stabilize the particle size by impaction. Particles are quite small, about the same size and stability as particles produced by an ultrasonic nebulizer (discussed next). Figure 15-8 is a schematic of a Babbington nebulizer.

McGaw Laboratories (Irvine, CA) produce several nebulizers using the Babbington principle, including the Hydrosphere and Solo Sphere.

The outlet of the nebulizer has a connector for large-bore aerosol tubing. The common application for ultrasonic nebulizers is in bland aerosol therapy delivered via aerosol mask or face tent.

The Babbington nebulizers do not provide an attachment for a heater, so their use is limited to the application of a cold mist.

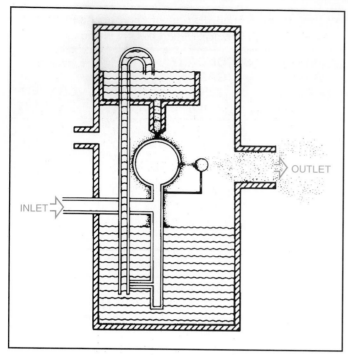

Figure 15-8 *A cross section illustrating the operation of a Babbington nebulizer*

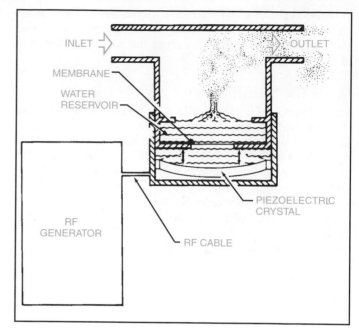

Figure 15-9 *A schematic of an ultrasonic nebulizer*

Ultrasonic Nebulizers

Ultrasonic nebulizers rely on electrical and mechanical energy to generate an aerosol. Because of their greater level of sophistication, they are more expensive and generally more costly to repair than pneumatically powered devices.

The generation of the energy required to produce an aerosol begins with a radio frequency generator (rf generator). You can draw an analogy by comparing the rf generator with a radio transmitter. However, the frequencies generated are generally higher, in the range of 1.3 to 1.4 megahertz (MHz) (the AM commercial broadcast band is 54 to 160 kilohertz [KHz] and the FM broadcast band is 88 to 108 MHz). The frequencies generated are conducted to a special crystal with a shielded cable.

The special crystal, called a *piezoelectric crystal*, has the ability to change shape in resonance with the rf energy. For each wavelength or impulse of energy, the crystal will oscillate back and forth, creating mechanical energy. These waves are conducted through the water in the reservoir to the surface, breaking the water surface into fine aerosol particles having a mean diameter of 3 to 5 micrometers. The piezoelectric crystal has the ability to convert electrical energy into mechanical energy. Figure 15-9 is a schematic of an ultrasonic nebulizer.

Output from an ultrasonic nebulizer may be altered in one of two ways: either by changing the frequency or by changing the amplitude. *Amplitude* refers to the depth of the wave form from the upper to the lower crest of the wave. Amplitude can vary from a large amplitude to a small amplitude. By increasing the amplitude, the amount of aerosol output increases. *Frequency* refers to the number of wave forms per second. The rf energy in an ultrasonic nebulizer may range from 1.3 million cycles per second to 1.4 million cycles per second. Figure 15-10 shows schemat-

ically two different amplitudes and frequencies. By increasing the frequency, more wave forms strike the water surface each second. Because of the greater number of impacts per second, the result is a smaller particle size. The frequency is usually not adjustable on the majority of ultrasonic nebulizers.

Ultrasonic nebulizers are utilized in the clinical setting to administer bland aerosol therapy. Due to the small particle size, pulmonary deposition is greater than with other nebulizers that have outputs of larger particle size. This therapy is very effective in thinning retained, inspissated secretions.

The hazards of therapy with an ultrasonic nebulizer are related to its output in cubic centimeters of water per minute. An ultrasonic nebulizer is capable of producing 6 cc of aerosol per minute. There is a potential hazard of overhydrating a patient if they are exposed to long-term administration. This overhydration may lead to an

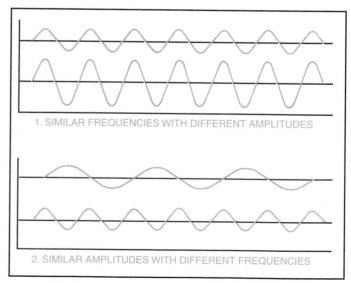

Figure 15-10 *A comparison of frequency and amplitude*

increased volume of secretions and a narrowing of the airway lumen. These changes will result in increased resistance, wheezing, and dyspnea. Bronchospasm may also be a hazard associated with the use of an ultrasonic nebulizer.

Small-Volume Nebulizers

Small-volume nebulizer therapy has become a very popular means of administering medication in the clinical setting. This is so because of its effectiveness, simplicity, and relatively low cost. Small-volume nebulizers provide a convenient, inexpensive way to aerosolize liquid medications.

Mainstream and sidestream devices are the two general types of small-volume nebulizers. The two are differentiated by the placement of the nebulizer in relation to the main flow of gas through the device. The nebulizer in a mainstream device is positioned directly in the path of the gas flow. A sidestream device has the nebulizer positioned adjacent to and connected to the main flow of gas, usually with a Briggs adapter or aerosol T piece. A sidestream nebulizer will generally produce smaller particles owing to the longer pathway the aerosol must travel to reach the main gas flow. Figure 15-11 is a schematic showing both types of nebulizers.

The delivery devices compatible with small-volume nebulizers include a mouthpiece, a Briggs adapter, an aerosol mask, a tracheostomy mask, and a face tent. The outlet on most nebulizers is designed with an inside diameter that will fit a mouthpiece and an outside diameter to fit larger-bore aerosol tubing.

Commonly Administered Medications

For a more detailed discussion of medications delivered by aerosol, refer to Chapter 14, "Introduction to Respiratory Care Pharmacology," or consult any of a number of excellent books on the topic.

Monitoring Therapy for Effectiveness

Small-volume nebulizer therapy may be monitored for effectiveness by measuring the vital capacity and peak flow rate before and after therapy when administering a bronchodilator. Peak flow rate is generally a more sensitive indicator of bronchodilation than the vital capacity; however, both are easily monitored and documented. Besides the parameters mentioned above, breath sounds and sputum should also be monitored. Pretherapy and posttherapy breath sounds should be compared. The patient should be encouraged to cough after therapy, and sputum color, amount, and odor (if present) should be noted.

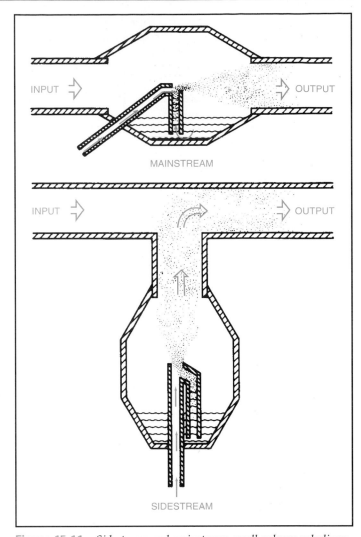

Figure 15-11 *Sidestream and mainstream small-volume nebulizers*

Heart rate and blood pressure should be monitored before, during, and after therapy. An increase in the heart rate greater than 20 beats per minute over the baseline rate should be the criteria for discontinuing the therapy. The patient should be monitored for other medication side effects, which should be noted on the medical record.

Hazards and Complications

Hazards and complications of small-volume nebulizer therapy are primarily associated with the side effects from the medications administered. Loosening of secretions may also precipitate obstruction if not cleared by coughing.

OBJECTIVES

At the end of this chapter, you should be able to:

• Correctly assemble, test for function, safely apply, and troubleshoot the following humidifiers:
  — Bubble humidifier
  — Cascade humidifier
  — Bird Wick humidifier

— Demonstrate use of the humidifiers with appropriate delivery devices.
— Correctly monitor the following as appropriate:
  — Oxygen concentration
  — Temperature

(Continued)

- Correctly assemble, test for function, safely apply, and troubleshoot the following nebulizers:
  — Puritan All-Purpose nebulizer
  — Ohio Deluxe nebulizer
  — MistyOx nebulizers
  — McGaw Solo Sphere
  — Ultrasonic nebulizer
  — Demonstrate use of the nebulizers with appropriate delivery devices.
  — Correctly monitor the following as appropriate:
    — Oxygen concentration

  — Temperature
- Correctly assemble, test for function, safely apply, and troubleshoot a small-volume nebulizer:
  — Demonstrate the use of a small-volume nebulizer with the following delivery devices:
    — Aerosol mask
    — Briggs adapter/aerosol T piece
    — Mouthpiece
  — Correctly monitor a patient while delivering a small-volume nebulizer treatment with a bronchodilator.

HUMIDITY AND AEROSOL THERAPY

Operation of humidification equipment, including assembly, testing, application, and troubleshooting, is quite simple and consists primarily of the filling of reservoirs with sterile, distilled water and the attachment of delivery devices. Refer to the operation manual for the specific device you are using.

Room Humidifiers

Room humidifiers require the filling of the reservoir with sterile, distilled water and the connection of the device to an appropriate electrical power source (usually 115 V alternating current [AC]).

To test for function, observe for aerosol output. After operation of the device for an hour or so, a sling psychrometer may be employed to establish whether the relative humidity of the room has been increased.

Troubleshooting consists of checking electrical connections and verifying the proper assembly of components. Bacterial contamination is common in home units. This problem may be minimized by nebulizing a vinegar solution each day and then thoroughly rinsing the unit. Make the solution by combining equal parts of white vinegar and boiled water. Parts that can be disassembled and removed should be soaked in the solution for 20 minutes and then rinsed. Damage to breaker combs, if excessive, may necessitate replacement of the unit.

Bubble Humidifier

Preparation consists of filling the reservoir with sterile, distilled water (unless unit is prefilled) and attaching the device to an oxygen flowmeter. Adjust the flow to the ordered level and attach the ordered delivery device.

Testing can be accomplished by observing for bubbling and checking for flow at the outlet. The outlet should also be occluded to test the safety popoff for function.

Loose fittings or connections cause the most frequent problems during troubleshooting. If the device is a prefilled disposable unit, make sure all seals have been appropriately broken on assembly.

Cascade Humidifier

The reservoir should be filled with sterile, distilled water to the *full* line inscribed on the jar. It is preferable to fill the unit through the outlet fitting rather than opening the jar

and exposing it to potential bacterial contamination from the room. Insert the cascade onto the heater and adjust the heater to an appropriate temperature. Attach the inlet and outlet to the appropriate devices.

Leaks constitute the majority of troubleshooting problems with the cascade. Check the O rings at the heater wells (exercise extreme caution if the unit is in use; they will be very hot), the cascade tower stud, and the gasket around the rim of the lid. Sometimes the heater fails to function because the safety shut-off switch has not been depressed. Tighten the studs holding the blue tabs on the lid by lightly tapping them with a small hammer.

Bird Wick Humidifier

The Bird Wick humidifier is readied for use by attaching a continuous feed system to the water inlet located on the top. Snap the humidifier onto its heater and adjust the thermostat as appropriate. Attach the delivery devices to the inlet and outlet of the unit.

Troubleshooting consists of checking for leaks around the O rings at the top and bottom of the device. The temperature probe may also develop electrical shorts over time, causing the temperature alarm to trigger inappropriately.

Large-Volume Nebulizers

A large-volume nebulizer is prepared for use by filling the reservoir with sterile, distilled water. It is then attached to a flowmeter with the DISS fitting at the top of the unit. Adjust the oxygen flow rate to between 8 and 12 L/min. Observe the nebulizer for aerosol output. Insert an immersion or base heater if heated aerosol is ordered. A 115 V AC outlet must be nearby. Adjust the diluter to the desired oxygen percentage and analyze the FIO_2 with an oxygen analyzer. Do not obstruct the outlet when determining the FIO_2 because the back pressure will cause the FIO_2 to increase. Attach a sufficient length of large-bore aerosol tubing to the outlet and position a drainage bag at the lowest point of the tubing. Attach an aerosol mask, tracheostomy mask, Briggs adapter, or face tent as appropriate.

The majority of problems encountered with this type of nebulizer occur at the diluter jet. The jet often becomes obstructed. Some nebulizers are provided with a thin wire on a lever arm to clean the orifice of the jet. To clean the jet, push the button adjacent to the oxygen inlet several times. If this fails to clear the jet, disassembly and cleaning may be required.

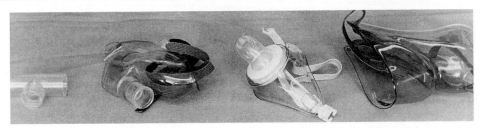

Figure 15-12   *Aerosol delivery devices (left to right: Briggs adapter, aerosol mask, tracheostomy mask, face tent)*

MistyOx Hi-Fi and GIN Nebulizers

Remove the cap from the sterile solution distilled water bottle, aseptically remove the nebulizer from its packaging, insert the capillary tube into the bottle, and screw the bottle onto the 38-mm fitting on the nebulizer (for both the Hi-Fi and the GIN nebulizers). Make certain that the nebulizer is attached tightly and not cross threaded.

Connect the nebulizer to an oxygen flowmeter or two flowmeters and set the desired oxygen concentration or adjust the flow rates (for the GIN nebulizer; refer to Tables 15-3 and 15-4). If heated aerosol is desired, connect the TurboHeater between the nebulizer and the reservoir bottle and connect it to an electrical outlet. Monitor inspired gas temperature using a thermometer placed close to the patient. Monitor the oxygen concentrations using an oxygen analyzer and adjust the nebulizer to achieve the desired concentration and total flow rate.

Babbington Nebulizers

Fill the reservoir with sterile, distilled water. Connect the nebulizer to a flowmeter; if it is a Hydrosphere, a gas source of 50 psi is required. Observe the unit for aerosol output. Adjust the diluter to the desired oxygen percentage and analyze the FIO_2 with an oxygen analyzer. Attach large-bore aerosol tubing to the outlet and position a drainage bag at the low point of the tubing. If you are using a Hydrosphere, use the extra-large tubing provided, owing to the high aerosol output.

These nebulizers are relatively trouble-free. Leaks can occur at the O rings below the glass spheres. Check them periodically for integrity. The glass spheres may also be damaged easily, so handle the unit with care.

Ultrasonic Nebulizers

If the ultrasonic nebulizer you are using has a coupling chamber, fill it with tap water; then fill the nebulizer compartment with sterile, distilled water. For an ultrasonic nebulizer without a coupling chamber, simply fill the nebulizer compartment. Attach large-bore aerosol tubing from the fan to the inlet of the nebulizer compartment. Connect the power cord(s) to an appropriate electrical outlet. Turn on the nebulizer and adjust the output control to the desired aerosol output. Attach large-bore aerosol tubing to the outlet and attach an appropriate aerosol delivery device to the distal end of the tubing.

Troubleshooting these devices is often a frustrating experience. Water level in the coupling chamber is critical; too much or too little will decrease the output. Adjust the

level for optimal output. The piezoelectric crystal may become contaminated with mineral deposits. Use an ultrasonic nebulizer cleaner and operate the unit for several minutes; then rinse the crystal and chamber with water and try again. Check the electrical connections. Check the tubing for obstruction from rain-out. If all of these efforts fail to restore the nebulizer to an operational condition, send it to your facility's biomedical engineering department for testing and repair or to an authorized service center.

AEROSOL/OXYGEN DELIVERY DEVICES

There are four commonly used aerosol administration delivery devices. These are the Briggs adapter, aerosol mask, tracheostomy mask, and the face tent. These devices are shown in Figure 15-12. The aerosol mask and tracheostomy mask are used by connecting the large male fitting on the device to the large-bore aerosol tubing.

The Briggs adapter or aerosol T is attached directly to the distal end of the aerosol delivery tubing. In addition, a short, 6-inch piece of aerosol tubing is attached to the opposite end of the Briggs adapter. This serves as a 50-ml oxygen/aerosol reservoir, preventing room air entrainment when the patient first begins inspiration.

The face tent is designed to be positioned under the chin, as shown in Figure 15-13. This device is commonly used in the recovery room following surgery.

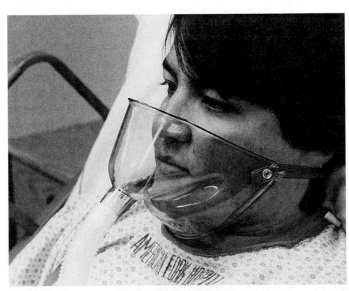

Figure 15-13   *Application of a face tent*

Small-Volume Nebulizer Therapy

The assembly of small-volume nebulizers will vary depending on the manufacturer. Some disposable units pull apart into two halves; others have threads that join the two parts. Some are equipped with a soft rubber fitting for the injection of a medication with a syringe. These different designs all provide for the introduction of medication into the reservoir in the proper amount and dilution as ordered by the physician.

Attach an appropriate delivery device to the outlet. An aerosol mask, mouthpiece, Briggs adapter, tracheostomy mask, or face tent may be appropriate.

Small-diameter oxygen connecting tubing joins the nebulizer to a flowmeter equipped with a nipple adapter or Christmas tree adapter. Oxygen flow is adjusted to between 4 and 8 L/min, depending on the unit. Adjust the flow until a dense aerosol can be observed.

If the nebulizer fails to function properly, check the jet for obstruction and the supply tubing for kinks. If this does not fix the problem, discard the nebulizer and obtain another.

Give the nebulizer to the patient and instruct the patient to take slow, deep breaths with a slight pause before exhaling. This end-inspiratory pause will help the aerosol to deposit in the lungs. If the patient becomes lightheaded because of the deep breathing, turn off the flowmeter, and allow the patient to rest for a short period.

Monitor the patient carefully for any side effects caused by the medication you are using. If administering a bronchodilator, measure a pretreatment and posttreatment vital capacity and a peak expiratory flow rate.

References

American Association for Respiratory Care. (1992). AARC clinical practice guideline: Selection of aerosol delivery device. *Respiratory Care, 37*(8), 891–897.

American Association for Respiratory Care. (1993). AARC clinical practice guideline: Bland aerosol administration. *Respiratory Care, 38*(11), 1196–1200.

American Association for Respiratory Care. (1994). AARC clinical practice guideline: Delivery of aerosols to the upper airway. *Respiratory Care, 39*(8), 803–807.

American Association for Respiratory Care. (1996). AARC clinical practice guideline: Selection of a device for delivery of aerosol to the lung parenchyma. *Respiratory Care, 41*(7), 647–653.

Scacci, R. (1979). Air entrainment masks: Jet mixing is how they work; the Bernoulli and Venturi principles are how they don't. *Respiratory Care, 24*(10), 928–931.

Additional Resources

Bagwell, T. (1986). U.S. Patent Number: 4,767,576. Costa Mesa, CA: Medical Molding Corporation of America.

Garrett, D., & Donaldson, W. P. (1978). *Physical principles of respiratory therapy equipment.* Madison, WI: Ohio Medical Products.

Hunsinger, D., Lisnerski, K. J., Mauriz, J. J., & Phillips, M. L. (1980). *Respiratory technology: A procedure manual.* Reston, VA: Reston Publishing.

Lehnert, B. E. (1980). *The pharmacology of respiratory care.* St. Louis, MO: Mosby.

McPherson, S. (1995). *Respiratory therapy equipment* (5th ed.). St. Louis, MO: Mosby.

Scanlan, C., Spearman, C. B., & Sheldon, R. L. (1999). *Egan's fundamentals of respiratory therapy* (7th ed.). St. Louis, MO: Mosby.

Practice Activities: Humidity and Aerosol Therapy

1. Practice setting up the following humidifiers to the indicated delivery devices when appropriate.
   a. Room humidifier
   b. Bubble humidifier
   c. Bubble jet humidifier
   Delivery Devices
   (1) Nasal cannula
   (2) Simple oxygen mask
   (3) Partial rebreathing mask
   (4) Nonrebreathing mask

2. Practice setting up the following humidifiers to the indicated delivery devices. Use large-bore tubing, including a drainage bag and a thermometer, to monitor the inspiratory temperature.
   a. Cascade humidifier
   b. Bird Wick humidifier
   Delivery Devices
   (1) Aerosol mask
   (2) Tracheostomy mask
   (3) Face tent
   (4) Briggs adapter

3. Practice setting up the following nebulizers to the indicated delivery devices. Use large-bore tubing, including a drainage bag. When a nebulizer has provisions for a heater, apply a heated aerosol and use a thermometer to monitor the inspiratory temperature.
   a. Puritan All-Purpose nebulizer
   b. Ohio Deluxe nebulizer

c. McGaw Solo Sphere
d. Ultrasonic nebulizer
Delivery Devices
(1) Aerosol mask
(2) Tracheostomy mask
(3) Face tent
(4) Briggs adapter

4. Practice troubleshooting any of the foregoing humidity or aerosol devices by deliberately sabotaging them and restoring them to an operational condition.

5. Adjust the Puritan All-Purpose nebulizer to 40% oxygen or the Ohio Deluxe nebulizer to 60% oxygen. Remove the drainage bag and make a large loop in the aerosol tubing below the level of the humidifier and raise the distal end to an appropriate level.
a. Measure the FIO_2.
b. Add 100 ml of water into the distal end of the tubing, causing a partial obstruction at the dependent loop.
c. Measure the FIO_2 with the water partially obstructing the flow.
(1) How can you explain the difference?

6. Practice applying any of the foregoing humidity or aerosol devices to a laboratory partner. Note how cold and heated humidity/aerosol delivery feels.

7. Practice setting up both a sidestream and a mainstream small-volume nebulizer. Note if there is a perceivable difference in output between the two devices running at the same flow rate.

8. Practice troubleshooting the small-volume nebulizers by deliberately sabotaging them and restoring them to proper operation.

9. Deliver a small-volume nebulizer treatment to a laboratory partner using normal saline. *Note:* Do not use a bronchodilator without a physician's order. Monitor the following parameters:
Before treatment
a. Pulse and respiratory rate
b. Breath sounds
c. Vital capacity
d. Peak expiratory flow
During treatment
a. Pulse and respiratory rate
b. Breath sounds
c. Vital capacity
d. Peak expiratory flow

10. Using a blank sheet of paper, document the humidity or aerosol device used and how the "treatment" was administered to your laboratory partner. Have your instructor critique your documentation.

Check List: Humidity and Aerosol Therapy

_____ 1. Verify the physician's order for therapy.
_____ 2. Follow standard precautions, including washing hands.
3. Obtain the appropriate equipment as required:
_____ a. Oxygen flowmeter
_____ b. Sterile water
_____ c. Large-bore aerosol tubing
_____ d. Drainage bag
_____ e. Thermometer (if heated therapy is required)
_____ f. Humidifier or nebulizer
_____ g. *No smoking* sign
_____ h. Oxygen analyzer, if required

_____ 4. Assemble the equipment.
_____ 5. Confirm operation of equipment and troubleshoot, as required.
_____ 6. Apply the device to the patient.
_____ 7. Reassure the patient.
_____ 8. Monitor temperature and FIO_2, as required.
_____ 9. Clean up any plastic wrappers or unneeded equipment before leaving the room.
_____ 10. Wash your hands.
_____ 11. Document the procedure on the patient's chart.

Check List: Small-Volume Nebulizer Therapy

_____ 1. Verify the order in the chart. Check for medication, amount, dilution, and frequency of therapy.
_____ 2. Follow standard precautions, including handwashing.
3. Obtain and assemble your equipment, which may include:
_____ a. Oxygen flowmeter
_____ b. Small-volume nebulizer
_____ c. Medication
_____ d. Peak expiratory flowmeter
_____ e. Respirometer or vital capacity bag
_____ 4. Prepare the medication as ordered by the physician.
_____ 5. Introduce yourself.

_____ 6. Assemble your equipment.
_____ 7. Explain the procedure, including respiratory pattern.
8. Obtain the following parameters before therapy:
_____ a. Breath sounds
_____ b. Heart and respiratory rate
_____ c. Peak expiratory flow
_____ d. Vital capacity
_____ 9. Administer the small-volume nebulizer treatment, encouraging your patient as you progress.
_____ 10. Monitor your patient closely for side effects.
_____ 11. Encourage your patient to cough following therapy. If the cough is productive, note color, amount, and odor of sputum.

12. Measure the following parameters after therapy:
_____ a. Breath sounds
_____ b. Heart and respiratory rate
_____ c. Peak expiratory flow rate
_____ d. Vital capacity
_____ 13. Clean up the area.

_____ 14. Reassure your patient and check to see if he or she is comfortable.
_____ 15. In the patient's chart, record the date, time, medication (amount and dilution), pretherapy and posttherapy parameters, any sputum production, and the patient's tolerance of the therapy.

Self-Evaluation Post Test: Humidity and Aerosol Therapy

1. Humidity is referred to as:
   a. particulate water.
   b. liquid water.
   c. vaporized water.
   d. nebulized water.

2. Why should large-bore tubing used during aerosol therapy have a loop and drainage bag below the patient and the nebulizer?
   a. To prevent condensate from entering the inspiratory site
   b. To prevent back pressure from affecting the Venturi
   c. To prevent condensate from entering the nebulizer
   d. All of the above

3. A patient who received a bronchodilator via a small-volume nebulizer now demonstrates signs of tachycardia and nervousness. The reason is that:
   a. the patient was hyperventilating.
   b. the patient received too much bronchodilator.
   c. the patient probably received the wrong drug by mistake.
   d. the patient received too much oxygen.

4. The piezoelectric crystal of an ultrasonic nebulizer has the ability to:
   a. convert electrical energy to mechanical energy.
   b. convert the couplant fluid to a gas.
   c. cause the particles to form new compounds.
   d. cause variations in the current generated by the rf module.

5. One method to increase the delivered humidity is to:
   a. decrease the temperature.
   b. increase the temperature.
   c. add more tubing between the device and the patient.
   d. increase the line pressure powering the device.

6. A cascade humidifier:
   I. is not efficient.
   II. supplies 100% body humidity.
   III. is heated.
   IV. is not heated.
   a. I, II
   b. I, III
   c. II, III
   d. II, IV

7. An example of a nebulizer that works on the viscous shearing principle and also uses the principle to adjust the oxygen concentration is the:
   a. Bennett cascade nebulizer.
   b. Ohio bubble jet nebulizer.
   c. Devilbiss ultrasonic nebulizer.
   d. Puritan All-Purpose nebulizer.

8. Body humidity is:
   a. 50% saturated at body temperature and pressure.
   b. 100% saturated at room temperature and pressure.
   c. 50% saturated at room temperature and pressure.
   d. 100% saturated at body temperature and pressure.

9. The use of a baffle in a nebulizer causes:
   a. a mist of larger droplets to be delivered.
   b. no change in the size of the particles.
   c. the mist to be less irritating.
   d. a more uniform-size droplet to be produced.

10. The ideal breathing pattern for maximal aerosol deposition and retention is:
    a. rapid, shallow respirations.
    b. a slow, deep inspiration and a fast, forced exhalation.
    c. a pause of several seconds' duration at the peak of every other breath.
    d. a slow, deep inspiration with an end-inspiratory hold followed by a passive exhalation.

PERFORMANCE EVALUATION: HUMIDITY AND AEROSOL THERAPY

Date: Lab _____ Clinical _____ Agency _____

Lab: Pass _____ Fail _____   Clinical: Pass _____ Fail _____

Student name _____   Instructor name _____

No. of times observed in clinical _____

No. of times practiced in clinical _____

PASSING CRITERIA: Obtain 90% or better on the procedure. Tasks indicated by * must receive at least 1 point, or the evaluation is terminated. Procedure must be performed within designated time, or the performance receives a failing grade.

SCORING:
2 points — Task performed satisfactorily without prompting.
1 point — Task performed satisfactorily with self-initiated correction.
0 points — Task performed incorrectly or with prompting required.
NA — Task not applicable to the patient care situation.

TASKS:		PEER	LAB	CLINICAL
*	1. Verifies the physician's order	☐	☐	☐
*	2. Follows standard precautions, including handwashing	☐	☐	☐
	3. Obtains the required equipment			
*	a. Oxygen flowmeter	☐	☐	☐
*	b. Humidifier/nebulizer	☐	☐	☐
*	c. Sterile water	☐	☐	☐
*	d. Large-bore tubing or O_2 connecting tubing	☐	☐	☐
*	e. Administration device	☐	☐	☐
*	f. Heater (if required)	☐	☐	☐
*	g. Drainage bag and T piece	☐	☐	☐
*	h. Thermometer (if required)	☐	☐	☐
*	i. *No smoking* sign(s)	☐	☐	☐
	4. Explains the procedure to the patient	☐	☐	☐
*	5. Confirms the operation of the device	☐	☐	☐
*	6. Applies the device to the patient	☐	☐	☐
	7. Reassures the patient	☐	☐	☐
*	8. Confirms FiO_2 as appropriate	☐	☐	☐
*	9. Monitors the gas temperature	☐	☐	☐
	10. Disposes of excess equipment	☐	☐	☐
	11. Leaves the patient's area clean and safe	☐	☐	☐
*	12. Washes hands before leaving the room	☐	☐	☐
*	13. Documents equipment, concentration, or liter flow on the patient's chart	☐	☐	☐

SCORE: Peer   _____ points of possible 42; _____%

           Lab   _____ points of possible 42; _____%

           Clinical   _____ points of possible 42; _____%

TIME: _____ out of possible 20 minutes

PEER: _____   LAB: _____

STUDENT: _____   CLINICAL: _____

Date: Lab _____ Clinical _____ Agency _____

Lab: Pass _____ Fail _____   Clinical: Pass _____ Fail _____

Student name _____ Instructor name _____

No. of times observed in clinical _____

No. of times practiced in clinical _____

PASSING CRITERIA: Obtain 90% or better on the procedure. Tasks indicated by * must receive at least 1 point, or the evaluation is terminated. Procedure must be performed within designated time, or the performance receives a failing grade.

SCORING:
2 points — Task performed satisfactorily without prompting.
1 point — Task performed satisfactorily with self-initiated correction.
0 points — Task performed incorrectly or with prompting required.
NA — Task not applicable to the patient care situation.

TASKS:		PEER	LAB	CLINICAL
*	1. Verifies the physician's order	☐	☐	☐
	2. Scans the chart	☐	☐	☐
*	3. Follow standard precautions, including handwashing	☐	☐	☐
	4. Obtains the required equipment			
*	a. Oxygen flowmeter	☐	☐	☐
*	b. Small-volume nebulizer	☐	☐	☐
*	c. Peak flowmeter	☐	☐	☐
*	d. Respirometer	☐	☐	☐
*	5. Prepares the medication in accordance with the physician's order	☐	☐	☐
	6. Monitors the patient before therapy			
*	a. Pulse and respiratory rate	☐	☐	☐
*	b. Peak flow rate	☐	☐	☐
*	c. Vital capacity	☐	☐	☐
*	d. Breath sounds	☐	☐	☐
*	7. Uses the appropriate gas for a propellant	☐	☐	☐
	8. Coaches and encourages the patient	☐	☐	☐
	9. Monitors the patient			
*	a. Pulse	☐	☐	☐
*	b. Respiratory rate	☐	☐	☐
	10. Encourages and assists the patient to cough	☐	☐	☐
	11. Monitors therapy effectiveness			
*	a. Peak expiratory flow rate	☐	☐	☐
*	b. Vital capacity	☐	☐	☐
*	12. Uses aseptic technique	☐	☐	☐

13. Removes unneeded equipment   ☐   ☐   ☐

14. Leaves the patient area safe and clean   ☐   ☐   ☐

*   15. Charts the therapy appropriately   ☐   ☐   ☐

SCORE: Peer   _____ points of possible 46; _____%

            Lab   _____ points of possible 46; _____%

            Clinical   _____ points of possible 46; _____%

TIME: _____ out of possible 20 minutes

STUDENT SIGNATURES   **INSTRUCTOR SIGNATURES**

PEER: _____   LAB: _____

STUDENT: _____   CLINICAL: _____

CHAPTER 16

BRONCHIAL HYGIENE THERAPY

INTRODUCTION

Bronchial hygiene therapy is an important aspect of respiratory care. Many patients have increased secretion production, impairment of cough, or other pathologic conditions that prevent effective removal of pulmonary secretions. Retained secretions and poor pulmonary hygiene may lead to atelectasis and pulmonary infections. Therefore, it is important for you to know the techniques that will assist the patient in the removal of pulmonary secretions.

Postural drainage and chest percussion are indicated for patients who have difficulty mobilizing thick or copious pulmonary secretions. They are simple techniques that can be easily learned and may be performed at home. Like other therapeutic modalities, postural drainage and chest percussion may be performed only when ordered by a physician.

To position a patient safely and properly for postural drainage, an understanding of patient positioning, body mechanics, and the hazards associated with changes in position is required.

Positive expiratory pressure (PEP) mask therapy is the application of positive end-expiratory pressure during active exhalation to functional residual capacity (FRC) following a larger than normal tidal breath. The equipment required is simple and relatively inexpensive. PEP therapy has been shown to be effective in helping to remove secretions in patients with chronic lung diseases such as cystic fibrosis, bronchiectasis, and chronic bronchitis (Mahlmeister, Fink, Hoffman, & Fifer, 1991).

Flutter valve therapy is similar to PEP therapy in that an expiratory resistance device is employed. However, unlike in PEP therapy, the expiratory resistance created by the Flutter device varies; as the valve opens and closes, it creates pressure pulses within the chest. Like PEP therapy, Flutter valve therapy has been successfully employed in the treatment of cystic fibrosis.

Adjunctive breathing techniques include unilateral chest expansion, diaphragmatic breathing, pursed-lip breathing, and controlled cough techniques. All of these techniques are indicated to help the patient improve the ability to clear pulmonary secretions. Through demonstration and patient instruction these techniques are easily learned and may be self-administered by the patient.

In this chapter you will learn about body mechanics and how to correctly position a patient in the common positions utilized in the hospital setting. Additionally, you will learn 12 positions utilized to drain the bronchopulmonary segments and how to percuss and vibrate the chest properly to facilitate the removal of secretions from the lungs. You will also learn how to apply PEP and Flutter valve therapy, and you will learn how to demonstrate and teach adjunctive breathing techniques to the patient.

KEY TERMS

- Chest percussion
- Diaphragmatic breathing
- Directed cough
- Flutter valve therapy
- High-frequency chest wall oscillation (HFCWO) therapy

- Mechanical percussor
- Patient positions
- Positive expiratory pressure (PEP) therapy
- Postural drainage
- Pursed-lip breathing

- Turning
- Unilateral chest expansion
- Vibration

OBJECTIVES

At the end of this chapter, you should be able to:

- Describe the role of stance, balance, and body alignment in safe movement by the practitioner.
- Explain why body alignment and the use of good body mechanics are important in the positioning of the patient.
- Describe the following patient positions:
  — Fowler's and semi-Fowler's
  — Supine
  — Prone
  — Side-lying

  — Sims'
  — Trendelenburg
  — Reverse Trendelenburg
- Explain the use and purpose of these safety devices:
  — Bed rails
  — Restraints
    — Chest
    — Waist
    — Wrist and ankle
  — Nurse call button
  — Code switch

(Continued)

- Explain how chest percussion, postural drainage, and vibration can facilitate the removal of pulmonary secretions.
- Explain how to use mechanical percussors, noting:
  — Hazards
  — Limitations
- List the components of a complete physician's order for postural drainage and chest percussion.
- Describe the contraindications to and hazards of postural drainage and chest percussion.
- In the absence of a complete physician's order, describe how a patient may be assessed to determine the segments requiring postural drainage and chest percussion.

PEP THERAPY

- Define *PEP therapy*.
- Describe the circuit used for PEP therapy.
- Describe the indications for PEP therapy.
- List the hazards of PEP therapy.

FLUTTER VALVE THERAPY

- Define *Flutter valve therapy*.
- Describe the circuit used for Flutter valve therapy.
- Describe the indications for Flutter valve therapy.
- List the hazards of Flutter valve therapy.

HIGH-FREQUENCY CHEST WALL OSCILLATION (HFCWO) THERAPY

- Define *HFCWO therapy* and describe the equipment used for HFCWO therapy.
- Describe the indications for HFCWO therapy.
- Discuss the hazards associated with HFCWO therapy.
- Describe how to perform the following the following adjunctive breathing techniques:
  — Diaphragmatic breathing
  — Unilateral chest expansion
  — Pursed-lip breathing
  — Directed cough
- Discuss the indications for adjunctive breathing techniques and the hazards associated with those techniques.

CLINICAL PRACTICE GUIDELINES

AARC Clinical Practice Guideline
Postural Drainage Therapy

PDT 4.0 INDICATIONS:

    4.1 Turning
        4.1.1 Inability or reluctance of patient to change body position (e.g., mechanical ventilation, neuromuscular disease, drug-induced paralysis)
        4.1.2 Poor oxygenation associated with position (20,22,48–50) (e.g., unilateral lung disease)
        4.1.3 Potential for or presence of atelectasis (24,26,30)
        4.1.4 Presence of artificial airway
    4.2 Postural drainage
        4.2.1 Evidence or suggestion of difficulty with secretion clearance
            4.2.1.1 Difficulty clearing secretions with expectorated sputum production greater than 25–30 ml/day (adult) (3,7,9,11,12,27,38,40,46,51–53)
            4.2.1.2 Evidence or suggestion of retained secretions in the presence of an artificial airway
        4.2.2 Presence of atelectasis caused by or suspected of being caused by mucous plugging (24,26,29,30,54)
        4.2.3 Diagnosis of diseases such as cystic fibrosis, (1,5,6,13–15,18,36,55) bronchiectasis, (4,5,14) or cavitating lung disease

        4.2.4 Presence of foreign body in airway (56–58)
    4.3 External manipulation of the thorax
        4.3.1 Sputum volume or consistency suggesting a need for additional manipulation (e.g., percussion and/or vibration) to assist movement of secretions by gravity in a patient receiving postural drainage

PDT 5.0 CONTRAINDICATIONS:

The decision to use postural drainage therapy requires assessment of potential benefits versus potential risks. Therapy should be provided for no longer than necessary to obtain the desired therapeutic results. Listed contraindications are relative unless marked as absolute (A).

    5.1 Positioning
        5.1.1 All positions are contraindicated for:
            5.1.1.1 Intracranial pressure (ICP) > 20 mm Hg (59,60)
            5.1.1.2 Head and neck injury until stabilized (A)
            5.1.1.3 Active hemorrhage with hemodynamic instability (A)
            5.1.1.4 Recent spinal surgery (e.g., laminectomy) or acute spinal injury
            5.1.1.5 Acute spinal injury or active hemoptysis
            5.1.1.6 Empyema
            5.1.1.7 Bronchopleural fistula
            5.1.1.8 Pulmonary edema associated with congestive heart failure

5.1.1.9 Large pleural effusions
5.1.1.10 Pulmonary embolism
5.1.1.11 Aged, confused, or anxious patients who do not tolerate position changes
5.1.1.12 Rib fracture, with or without flail chest
5.1.1.13 Surgical wound or healing tissue
5.1.2 Trendelenburg position is contraindicated for:
5.1.2.1 Intracranial pressure (ICP) > 20 mm Hg (59,60)
5.1.2.2 Patients in whom increased intracranial pressure is to be avoided (e.g., neurosurgery, aneurysms, eye surgery)
5.1.2.3 Uncontrolled hypertension
5.1.2.4 Distended abdomen
5.1.2.5 Esophageal surgery
5.1.2.6 Recent gross hemoptysis related to recent lung carcinoma treated surgically or with radiation therapy (59)
5.1.2.7 Uncontrolled airway at risk for aspiration (tube feeding or recent meal)
5.1.3 Reverse Trendelenburg is contraindicated in the presence of hypotension or vasoactive medication.
5.2 External manipulation of the thorax
In addition to contraindications previously listed:
5.2.1 Subcutaneous emphysema
5.2.2 Recent epidural spinal infusion or spinal anesthesia
5.2.3 Recent skin grafts, or flaps, on the thorax
5.2.4 Burns, open wounds, and skin infections of the thorax
5.2.5 Recently placed transvenous pacemaker or subcutaneous pacemaker (particularly if mechanical devices are to be used)
5.2.6 Suspected pulmonary tuberculosis
5.2.7 Lung contusion
5.2.8 Bronchospasm
5.2.9 Osteomyelitis of the ribs
5.2.10 Osteoporosis
5.2.11 Coagulopathy
5.2.12 Complaint of chest-wall pain

PDT 6.0 HAZARDS/COMPLICATIONS:

6.1 Hypoxemia
Action to Be Taken/Possible Intervention: Administer higher oxygen concentrations during procedure if potential for or observed hypoxemia exists. If patient becomes hypoxemic during treatment, administer 100% oxygen, stop therapy immediately, return patient to original resting position, and consult physician. Ensure adequate ventilation. Hypoxemia during postural drainage may be avoided in unilateral lung disease by placing the involved lung uppermost with patient on his or her side. (20,22,48–50)

6.2 Increased intracranial pressure
Action to Be Taken/Possible Intervention: Stop therapy, return patient to original resting position, and consult physician.

6.3 Acute hypotension during procedure
Action to Be Taken/Possible Intervention: Stop therapy, return patient to original resting position, and consult physician.

6.4 Pulmonary hemorrhage
Action to Be Taken/Possible Intervention: Stop therapy, return patient to original resting position, call physician immediately. Administer oxygen and maintain an airway until physician responds.

6.5 Pain or injury to muscles, ribs, or spine
Action to Be Taken/Possible Intervention: Stop therapy that appears directly associated with pain or problem, exercise care in moving patient, and consult physician.

6.6 Vomiting and aspiration
Action to Be Taken/Possible Intervention: Stop therapy, clear airway and suction as needed, administer oxygen, maintain airway, return patient to previous resting position, and contact physician immediately.

6.7 Bronchospasm
Action to Be Taken/Possible Intervention: Stop therapy, return patient to original resting position, administer or increase oxygen delivery while contacting physician. Administer physician-ordered bronchodilators.

6.8 Dysrhythmias
Action to Be Taken/Possible Intervention: Stop therapy, return patient to previous resting position, administer or increase oxygen delivery while contacting physician.

PDT 8.0 ASSESSMENT OF NEED:
The following should be assessed together to establish a need for postural drainage therapy:
8.1 Excessive sputum production
8.2 Effectiveness of cough
8.3 History of pulmonary problems treated successfully with PDT (e.g., bronchiectasis, cystic fibrosis, lung abscess)
8.4 Decreased breath sounds or crackles or rhonchi suggesting secretions in the airway
8.5 Change in vital signs
8.6 Abnormal chest x-ray consistent with atelectasis, mucous plugging, or infiltrates
8.7 Deterioration in arterial blood gas values or oxygen saturation

(Continued)

(CPG Continued)

PDT 9.0 ASSESSMENT OF OUTCOME:

These represent individual criteria that indicate a positive response to therapy (and support continuation of therapy). Not all criteria are required to justify continuation of therapy (e.g., a ventilated patient may not have sputum production >30 ml/day, but may have improvement in breath sounds, chest x-ray, or increased compliance or decreased resistance).

9.1 Change in sputum production

If sputum production in an optimally hydrated patient is less than 25 ml/day with PDT, the procedure is not justified. (3,5,7,9,11,12,38, 40,46,51–53) Some patients have productive coughs with sputum production from 15 to 30 ml/day (occasionally as high as 70 or 100 ml/day) without postural drainage. If postural drainage does not increase sputum in a patient who produces >30 ml/day of sputum without postural drainage, the continuation of the therapy is not indicated. Because sputum production is affected by systemic hydration, apparently ineffective PDT probably should be continued for at least 24 hours after optimal hydration has been judged to be present.

9.2 Change in breath sounds of lung fields being drained

With effective therapy, breath sounds may "worsen" following the therapy as secretions move into the larger airways and increase rhonchi. An increase in adventitious breath sounds can be a marked improvement over absent or diminished breath sounds. Note any effect that coughing may have on breath sounds. One of the favorable effects of coughing is clearing of adventitious breath sounds.

9.3 Patient subjective response to therapy

The caregiver should ask patient how he or she feels before, during, and after therapy. Feelings of pain, discomfort, shortness of breath, dizziness, and nausea should be considered in decisions to modify or stop therapy. Easier clearance of secretions and increased volume of secretions during and after treatments support continuation.

9.4 Change in vital signs

Moderate changes in respiratory rate and/or pulse rate are expected. Bradycardia, tachycardia, or an increase in irregularity of pulse, or fall or dramatic increase in blood pressure are indications for stopping therapy.

9.5 Change in chest x-ray

Resolution or improvement of atelectasis may be slow or dramatic.

9.6 Change in arterial blood gas values or oxygen saturation

Oxygenation should improve as atelectasis resolves.

9.7 Change in ventilator variables

Resolution of atelectasis and plugging reduces resistance and increases compliance.

PDT 11.0 MONITORING:

The following should be chosen as appropriate for monitoring a patient's response to postural drainage therapy, before, during, and after therapy.

11.1 Subjective response — pain, discomfort, dyspnea, response to therapy

11.2 Pulse rate, dysrhythmia, and ECG if available

11.3 Breathing pattern and rate, symmetrical chest expansion, synchronous thoracico-abdominal movement, flail chest

11.4 Sputum production (quantity, color, consistency, odor) and cough effectiveness

11.5 Mental function

11.6 Skin color

11.7 Breath sounds

11.8 Blood pressure

11.9 Oxygen saturation by pulse oximetry (if hypoxemia is suspected)

11.10 Intracranial pressure (ICP)

Reprinted with permission from *Respiratory Care* 1991; 36: 1418–1426. The complete AARC Clinical Practice Guidelines are available from the AARC Web site (http://www.aarc.org), from the AARC Executive Office, or from *Respiratory Care* journal.

AARC Clinical Practice Guideline: Directed Cough

DC 4.0 INDICATIONS:

4.1 The need to aid in the removal of retained secretions from central airways (3–6)—(the suggestion that FET at lower lung volumes may be effective in preferentially mobilizing secretions in the peripheral airways while larger volumes facilitate movement in the central airways lacks validation).

4.2 The presence of atelectasis (3,7,8)

4.3 As prophylaxis against postoperative pulmonary complications (7)

4.4 As a routine part of bronchial hygiene in patients with cystic fibrosis, (2,4,6,9) bronchiectasis, chronic bronchitis, (3,10,11) narcotizing pulmonary infection, or spinal cord injury (12)

4.5 As an integral part of other bronchial hygiene therapies such as postural drainage therapy (PDT), (2,13) positive expiratory pressure therapy (PEP), and incentive spirometry (IS)

4.6 To obtain sputum specimens for diagnostic analysis

DC 5.0 CONTRAINDICATIONS:

Directed cough is rarely contraindicated. The contraindications listed must be weighed against potential benefit in deciding to eliminate cough from the care of the patient. Listed contraindications are relative.

5.1 Inability to control possible transmission of infection from patients suspected or known to have pathogens transmittable by droplet nuclei (e.g., *M. tuberculosis*)

5.2 Presence of an elevated intracranial pressure or known intracranial aneurysm

5.3 Presence of reduced coronary artery perfusion, such as in acute myocardial infarction (14)

5.4 Acute unstable head, neck, or spine injury

Manually assisted directed cough with pressure to the epigastrium may be contraindicated in presence of:

5.5 increased potential for regurgitation/aspiration (e.g., unconscious patient with unprotected airway)

5.6 acute abdominal pathology, abdominal aortic aneurysm, hiatal hernia, or pregnancy

5.7 a bleeding diathesis

5.8 untreated pneumothorax

Manually assisted directed cough with pressure to the thoracic cage may be contraindicated in presence of:

5.9 osteoporosis, flail chest

DC 6.0 HAZARDS/COMPLICATIONS:

6.1 Reduced coronary artery perfusion (14)

6.2 Reduced cerebral perfusion leading to syncope or alterations in consciousness, such as lightheadedness or confusion, (15) vertebral artery dissection

6.3 Incontinence

6.4 Fatigue

6.5 Headaches

6.6 Paresthesia or numbness (15)

6.7 Bronchospasm (11)

6.8 Muscular damage or discomfort

6.9 Spontaneous pneumothorax, pneumomediastinum, subcutaneous emphysema

6.10 Cough paroxysms

6.11 Chest pain

6.12 Rib or costochondral junction fracture

6.13 Incisional pain, evisceration

6.14 Anorexia, vomiting, and retching

6.15 Visual disturbances including retinal hemorrhage (15)

6.16 Central line displacement

6.17 Gastroesophageal reflux (17)

DC 8.0 ASSESSMENT OF NEED

8.1 Spontaneous cough that fails to clear secretions from the airway

8.2 Ineffective spontaneous cough as judged by:

    8.2.1 Clinical observation

    8.2.2 Evidence of atelectasis

    8.2.3 Results of pulmonary function testing

8.3 Postoperative upper abdominal or thoracic surgery patient (7)

8.4 Long-term care of patients with tendency to retain airway secretions

8.5 Presence of endotracheal or tracheostomy tube

DC 9.0 ASSESSMENT OF OUTCOME:

9.1 The presence of sputum specimen following a cough (4)

9.2 Clinical observation of improvement

9.3 Patient's subjective response to therapy

9.4 Stabilization of pulmonary hygiene in patients with chronic pulmonary disease and a history of secretion retention

DC 11.0 MONITORING:

Items from the following list should be chosen as appropriate for monitoring a patient's response to cough technique.

11.1 Patient response: pain, discomfort, dyspnea

11.2 Sputum expectorated following cough to note color, consistency, odor, volume of sputum produced

11.3 Breath sounds

11.4 Presence of any adverse neurologic signs or symptoms following cough (15)

11.5 Presence of any cardiac dysrhythmias or alterations in hemodynamics following coughing

11.6 Measures of pulmonary mechanics, when indicated, may include vital capacity, peak inspiratory pressure, peak expiratory pressure, peak expiratory flow, and airway resistance

---

Reprinted with permission from *Respiratory Care* 1993; 38: 495–499. The complete AARC Clinical Practice Guidelines are available from the AARC Web site (http://www.aarc.org), from the AARC Executive Office, or from *Respiratory Care* journal.

AARC Clinical Practice Guideline:
Use of Positive Airway Pressure Adjuncts to Bronchial Hygiene Therapy

PAP 4.0 INDICATIONS:

4.1 To reduce air trapping in asthma and COPD (16,29–31)

4.2 To aid in mobilization of retained secretions (in cystic fibrosis and chronic bronchitis) (14,15,17–24,32,33)

4.3 To prevent or reverse atelectasis (6–13,34–36)

4.4 To optimize delivery of bronchodilators in patients receiving bronchial hygiene therapy (37,38)

(Continued)

(CPG *Continued)*

PAP 5.0 CONTRAINDICATIONS:

Although no absolute contraindications [to] the use of PEP, CPAP, or EPAP mask therapy have been reported (4,39), the following should be carefully evaluated before a decision is made to initiate PAP mask therapy:

5.1 Patients unable to tolerate the increased work of breathing (acute asthma, COPD)

5.2 Intracranial pressure (ICP) >20 mm Hg

5.3 Hemodynamic instability (4)

5.4 Recent facial, oral, or skull surgery or trauma (4)

5.5 Acute sinusitis (39)

5.6 Epistaxis

5.7 Esophageal surgery

5.8 Active hemoptysis (39)

5.9 Nausea

5.10 Known or suspected tympanic membrane rupture or other middle ear pathology

5.11 Untreated pneumothorax

PAP 6.0 HAZARDS/COMPLICATIONS:

6.1 Increased work of breathing (4) that may lead to hypoventilation and hypercarbia

6.2 Increased intracranial pressure

6.3 Cardiovascular compromise

    6.3.1 Myocardial ischemia

    6.3.2 Decreased venous return (4)

6.4 Air swallowing, (4) with increased likelihood of vomiting and aspiration

6.5 Claustrophobia (4)

6.6 Skin breakdown and discomfort from mask (4)

6.7 Pulmonary barotrauma (4)

PAP 8.0 ASSESSMENT OF NEED:

The following should be assessed together to establish a need for PAP therapy:

8.1 Sputum retention not responsive to spontaneous or directed coughing

8.2 History of pulmonary problems treated successfully with postural drainage therapy

8.3 Decreased breath sounds or adventitious sounds suggesting secretions in the airway

8.4 Change in vital signs — increase in breathing frequency, tachycardia

8.5 Abnormal chest radiograph consistent with atelectasis, mucous plugging, or infiltrates

8.6 Deterioration in arterial blood gas values or oxygen saturation

PAP 9.0 ASSESSMENT OF OUTCOME:

9.1 Change in sputum production — if PEP does not increase sputum production in a patient who produces >30 ml/day of sputum without PEP, the continued use of PEP may not be indicated.

9.2 Change in breath sounds — with effective therapy, breath sounds may clear or the movement of secretions into the larger airways may cause an increase in adventitious breath sounds. The increase in adventitious breath sounds is often a marked improvement over no (or diminished) breath sounds. Note any effect that coughing may have had on the breath sounds.

9.3 Patient subjective response to therapy — the caregiver should ask the patient how he or she feels before, during, and after therapy. Feelings of pain, discomfort, shortness of breath, dizziness, and nausea should be considered in modifying and stopping therapy. Improved ease of clearing secretions and increased volume of secretions during and after treatments support continuation.

9.4 Change in vital signs — moderate changes in respiratory rate and/or pulse rate are expected. Bradycardia, tachycardia, increasingly irregular pulse, or a drop or dramatic increase in blood pressure are indications for stopping therapy.

9.5 Change in chest radiograph — resolution or improvement of atelectasis and localized infiltrates may be slow or dramatic.

9.6 Change in arterial blood gas values or oxygen saturation — normal oxygenation should return as atelectasis resolves.

PAP 11.0 MONITORING:

Items from the following list should be chosen as is appropriate for monitoring a specific patient's response to PAP:

11.1 Patient subjective response — pain, discomfort, dyspnea, response to therapy

11.2 Pulse rate and cardiac rhythm (if ECG is available)

11.3 Breathing pattern and rate, symmetrical lateral costal expansion, synchronous thoracico-abdominal movement

11.4 Sputum production (quantity, color, consistency, and odor)

11.5 Mental function

11.6 Skin color

11.7 Breath sounds

11.8 Blood pressure

11.9 Pulse oximetry (if hypoxemia with procedure has been previously demonstrated or is suspected); blood gas analysis (if indicated)

11.10 Intracranial pressure (ICP) in patients for whom ICP is of critical importance

Reprinted with permission from *Respiratory Care* 1993; 38: 516–521. The complete AARC Clinical Practice Guidelines are available from the AARC Web site (http://www.aarc.org), from the AARC Executive Office, or from *Respiratory Care* journal.

BODY ALIGNMENT AND STANCE

Body alignment and stance are crucial to safe movement in helping patients. A patient who is unable to move is very heavy. When your body is aligned properly, you are able to move smoothly. Minimal strain is placed on your muscles, tendons, bones, and joints. The muscles assume a state of slight tension or tone.

Injuries are more common when the body is not in alignment. These injuries commonly include muscles of the back, legs, tendons, and joints. Hernias may also result from improper alignment and undue muscle strain. Furthermore, improper alignment adversely affects balance. Balance is critical when you are assisting a patient to move.

Erect, the body should assume a position as shown in Figure 16-1. The upright body is aligned along an axis with the center of gravity. The feet should be slightly spread to provide a larger base of support. The closer together your feet are, the less stability you have in your balance.

When lifting heavy objects, you should always assume a squatting position, as shown in Figure 16-2. Lifting should be performed with your legs, not your back. Keep the object close to your body, minimizing muscle strain. The squatting position should also be assumed for adjusting beds or performing other tasks that are near the floor. This position minimizes the back strain experienced in bending from the waist. In the figure, notice how the feet are spread slightly, facilitating balance.

Patient comfort and prevention of disability from contractures are facilitated with correct body alignment. When the patient's body is properly aligned, the muscles, tendons, and joints are at rest. Pillows aid in providing

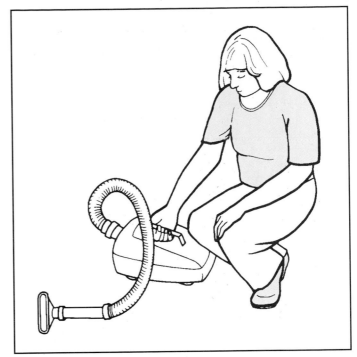

Figure 16-2   *Correct lifting stance*

additional support and removing pressure at contact points in the maintenance of correct alignment.

GENERAL GUIDELINES FOR MOVING PATIENTS

Common sense is required in moving patients. If you follow a few simple rules, you will prevent injury to yourself and the task will require less effort. Figure 16-3 is a summary of these rules.

Before attempting to move a patient, you should check on the patient's general condition and ascertain if a change of position is contraindicated. Some types of surgical procedures limit patient position. A patient who has undergone back surgery may be required to remain supine postoperatively. A patient with a head injury or who has undergone eye surgery may also have limits on positioning. Patients with cardiovascular problems may experience postural hypotension when raised to a sitting or standing position.

Figure 16-4 illustrates the common therapeutic patient positions that are utilized in the hospital setting. Note the use of pillows for additional comfort and support.

- Adjust the working surface to waist level if possible
- Use major muscle groups (legs and arms), not your back
- Use your body weight to your advantage
- Allow gravity to assist in your movements
- Allow the patient to assist if possible
- Seek help if needed

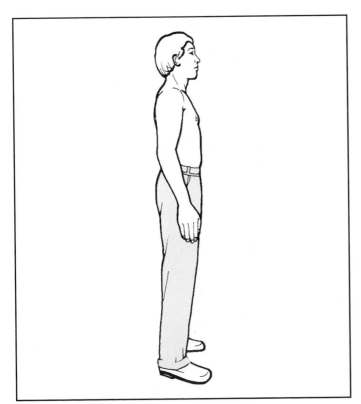

Figure 16-1   *Correct body alignment and stance*

Figure 16-3   *Rules for patient positioning*

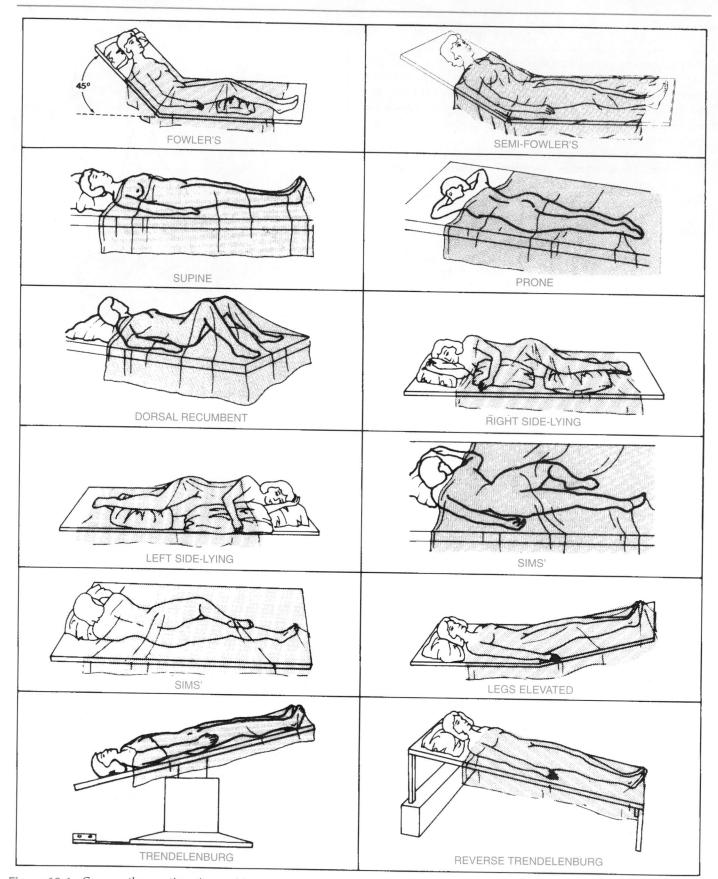

Figure 16-4 *Common therapeutic patient positions*

SAFETY DEVICES

Bed Rails

Bed rails are provided on hospital beds for the patient's protection. Under certain circumstances, the patient may become disoriented as to time and place. Bed rails help to minimize the likelihood of a patient's falling out of bed. Bed rails should always be used with confused or elderly patients. Side rails on a crib must always be up unless you are standing with your hands on the child. If the patient emphatically refuses to use bed rails, explain their purpose and try to convince the patient of their benefit. If the patient still refuses to use them, note the refusal on the patient's chart. If a patient is allowed out of bed without assistance during the day, the bed rail should be left down on one side and the bed should be lowered to its lowest level so that the patient does not fall in trying to crawl over the rail.

Restraints

Many patients who are awake, alert, and oriented during the day may become confused at night, especially elderly patients who are medicated. A patient may become confused, combative, or disoriented because of medication, anesthesia, or psychological conditions. Restraints are utilized to prevent the patient from removing life support equipment or to prevent self-injury or injury of hospital personnel.

Chest restraints and waist restraints prevent patients from extracting themselves from bed. The restraints should be snug, but not tight. Restraints should never impair circulation. It should be easy to insert a finger between the restraint and the patient's skin or gown. The restraint should always be tied to the bed frame, not the side rail.

Wrist and leg restraints reduce the mobility of the limb they are tied to. They are commonly used to prevent the patient from removing endotracheal tubes and intravenous and arterial lines.

Nurse Call Button

The nurse call button is the patient's lifeline. It frequently is the only way a patient can summon help in an emergency situation. Without access to the button, the patient is, in effect, unable to communicate. It is important to leave this device within reach of the patient at all times. If the patient watches television, leave the remote control within reach. Check with the patient before you leave to see if other things need to be within reach. Patients have fallen out of bed trying to reach items placed too far away.

Code Switch

In many intensive care units, a "code" switch is provided to notify appropriate personnel that a life-threatening emergency such as cardiac or respiratory arrest has occurred. The use of the code switch should be limited to appropriate circumstances. False alarms are frowned on.

CHEST PERCUSSION AND POSTURAL DRAINAGE

Manual techniques for bronchial hygiene therapy include postural drainage, chest percussion, and vibration. Chest percussion can also be performed using mechanical percussion devices.

Postural drainage is a technique wherein the patient is positioned in specific ways that allow gravity to facilitate the removal of pulmonary secretions. The rationale for specific positioning is the principle that water runs downhill. The bronchopulmonary tree is complex, with the various segments of the lung branching out from the larger airways at unique angles. A thorough knowledge of the pulmonary anatomy is essential for proper performance of this procedure.

Chest percussion is a technique of clapping on the chest wall with cupped hands. The small amount of air trapped under the hand induces vibration in the lung parenchyma that literally shakes the pulmonary secretions loose.

Vibration is an isometric maneuver performed with the arm and hand. The practitioner's hands are in contact with the patient's chest wall, and the induced vibrations are transmitted to the lung parenchyma, shaking the pulmonary secretions free. This technique is employed only on exhalation.

Postural Drainage

Postural drainage may be employed as a single modality or in combination with chest percussion. This technique involves placing the patient in specific positions that ensure that the desired pulmonary segment drains straight down.

The human body is, by nature, bilateral. If an imaginary line were drawn between the eyes and the end of the pelvis, the left and right sides would mirror each other. This is also generally true with the structure of the lungs. However, owing to the position of the heart, the left lung has two lobes while the right lung has three. There are 18 bronchopulmonary segments. All 18 segments may be drained using only 12 positions. In some positions, both segments on the left and right sides may be drained.

An outline of the segments being drained with the 12 positions is listed below and includes the landmarks for percussion. Figure 16-5 is a pictorial schematic of the 12 positions and their segments.

1. Anterior apical segments of the right and left upper lobes
   a. Position the patient sitting and leaning back at about a 45° angle.
   b. Area to percuss is just below the clavicle.
2. Posterior apical segments of the right and left upper lobes
   a. Position the patient sitting and leaning forward at about a 45° angle.
   b. Area to percuss is just above the scapula with the fingers extending up onto the shoulders.

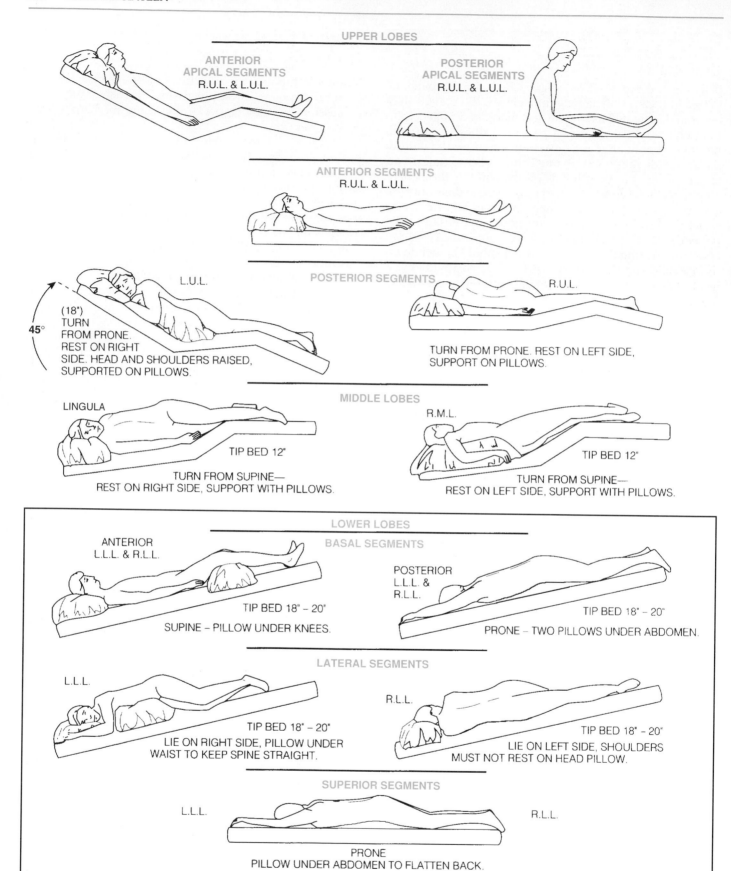

UPPER LOBES

ANTERIOR APICAL SEGMENTS
R.U.L. & L.U.L.

POSTERIOR APICAL SEGMENTS
R.U.L. & L.U.L.

ANTERIOR SEGMENTS
R.U.L. & L.U.L.

POSTERIOR SEGMENTS

L.U.L.

45° (18")
TURN FROM PRONE. REST ON RIGHT SIDE. HEAD AND SHOULDERS RAISED, SUPPORTED ON PILLOWS.

R.U.L.

TURN FROM PRONE. REST ON LEFT SIDE, SUPPORT ON PILLOWS.

MIDDLE LOBES

LINGULA

TIP BED 12"
TURN FROM SUPINE—REST ON RIGHT SIDE, SUPPORT WITH PILLOWS.

R.M.L.

TIP BED 12"
TURN FROM SUPINE—REST ON LEFT SIDE, SUPPORT WITH PILLOWS.

LOWER LOBES

BASAL SEGMENTS

ANTERIOR
L.L.L. & R.L.L.

TIP BED 18" – 20"
SUPINE – PILLOW UNDER KNEES.

POSTERIOR
L.L.L. & R.L.L.

TIP BED 18" – 20"
PRONE – TWO PILLOWS UNDER ABDOMEN.

LATERAL SEGMENTS

L.L.L.

TIP BED 18" – 20"
LIE ON RIGHT SIDE, PILLOW UNDER WAIST TO KEEP SPINE STRAIGHT.

R.L.L.

TIP BED 18" – 20"
LIE ON LEFT SIDE, SHOULDERS MUST NOT REST ON HEAD PILLOW.

SUPERIOR SEGMENTS

L.L.L.

R.L.L.

PRONE
PILLOW UNDER ABDOMEN TO FLATTEN BACK.

Figure 16-5 *The 12 postural drainage positions*

3. Anterior segments of the right and left upper lobes
   a. Position the patient supine with the bed flat.
   b. Area to percuss is just above the nipple.
4. Posterior segment of the left upper lobe
   a. Position the patient one-quarter turn from prone and resting on the right side with the head of the bed elevated 18 inches.
   b. Area to percuss is over the left scapula.
5. Posterior segment of the right upper lobe
   a. Position the patient one-quarter turn from prone and resting on the left side with the bed flat.
   b. Area to percuss is just above the right scapula.
6. Left lingula
   a. Position the patient one-quarter turn from supine and resting on the right side with the foot of the bed elevated 12 inches.
   b. Area to percuss is just above the left nipple and under the armpit.
7. Right middle lobe
   a. Position the patient one-quarter turn from supine with the foot of the bed elevated 12 inches.
   b. Area to percuss is just above the right nipple and under the armpit.
8. Anterior basal segments of the right and left lung
   a. Position the patient supine with the foot of the bed elevated 18 to 20 inches.
   b. Area to percuss is over the lower ribs.
9. Posterior basal segments of the right and left lung
   a. Position the patient prone with the foot of the bed elevated 18 to 20 inches.
   b. Area to percuss is over the lower ribs.
10. Left lateral segment of the lower lobes
    a. Position the patient on the right side with the foot of the bed elevated 18 to 20 inches.
    b. Area to percuss is over the lower ribs.
11. Right lateral segment of the lower lobes
    a. Position the patient on the left side with the foot of the bed elevated 18 to 20 inches.
    b. Area to percuss is over the lower ribs.
12. Superior segments of the right and left lower lobes
    a. Position the patient prone with the bed flat.
    b. Area to percuss is just below the lower margin of the scapula.

Equipment Requirements

An electric hospital bed is not a requirement for postural drainage. Use of several pillows will suffice very nicely. Usually, a minimum of four is required to position the patient to drain the lower lobes. In the home setting, an ironing board propped appropriately will work. Even dangling head down from a coach or sofa has served some patients very well.

Position Modifications

Postural drainage may have effects on the cardiovascular system, intracranial pressure, and the arterial partial pressure of oxygen (PaO_2). If your patients have problems in any of these areas, modification of the positions may be necessary.

Cardiac output may decrease as a result of postural drainage, especially in the head-down position. Those patients with cardiac insufficiency may be especially susceptible in this position. In the critical care unit, patients with an arterial line may have blood pressure conveniently monitored during this procedure. If any adverse changes occur, the therapy may be discontinued. Those patients without sophisticated monitoring devices will need to be carefully observed for any adverse effects of the positioning.

Intracranial pressure will increase when a patient is positioned head down. Blood will tend to pool in the dependent portion of the body because of gravity. Venous return will decrease, owing to the fact that the blood must now flow uphill. Those patients who have known intracranial disease or have undergone neurological surgery may need to have their positions modified to prevent complications.

PaO_2 may decrease with postural drainage owing to changes in the relationship between ventilation and perfusion in the lung. Patients positioned so that blood is pooled in an area of atelectasis or consolidation may experience a significant shunt. Patients with chronic obstructive lung disease may also be quite orthopneic. In these patients, changes in position may cause shortness of breath. Some patients simply cannot tolerate the head-down position, so positioning for postural drainage will need to be modified. Using the increasingly popular technique of pulse oximetry, patients at risk may be monitored for a decrease in SpO_2 so that therapy can be discontinued before complications result.

The judgment of the patient's physician and your own experience as a clinician will help determine the modification of the various positions. You must weigh the benefits against any potential complications.

Percussion

Percussion is a technique of clapping on the patient's chest wall with cupped hands. To position your hands properly, rest your arms and hands comfortably at your side while standing. Approximate your fingers together with your hands in the resting configuration. On inspection, your hands should have a slight curve and be cupped in shape.

By striking the chest wall alternately with each hand, a small air pocket is trapped, inducing a vibration through the lung parenchyma. The ideal frequency is between 50 and 60 percussions per minute. When the technique is performed properly, a hollow popping sound will result, and no red marks will be visible on the surface of the skin. The sound is low in pitch and hollow in timbre. If the sound becomes higher in pitch, you are probably slapping the patient. On inspection of the skin, you will probably observe some reddening. Percussion is ideally performed over a light covering such as a hospital gown or bedsheet.

Areas to Avoid

Avoid bony structures, the spine, the abdomen, and breast tissue in a female patient. Percussion over bony structures is painful and may result in injury. Percussion over the spine is not indicated because of the severe neurological injury that may result in the event of a fracture. Patients with osteoporosis are especially susceptible to fractures. The abdominal organs, especially the kidneys, may be damaged by percussing over the abdomen. Finally, a woman's breast tissue is extremely sensitive. Percussion over this area is very painful and definitely not indicated. If access is difficult, politely ask your patient to hold the breast away from the area of percussion. If the patient is unable to cooperate, you may be required to move the breast yourself while preserving your patient's dignity.

Mechanical Percussors

Mechanical percussor devices have been developed to facilitate chest percussion. Prolonged chest percussion requires energy and well-trained muscles. Manually completing eight or nine treatments of 20 to 30 minutes each is tiring. Use of a mechanical percussor can ensure that the last patient receives the same quality of therapy as the first. Figure 16-6 is a sample of the variety of mechanical percussors available for use in clinical practice.

There is a great variety of mechanical percussors available. Some are well-designed electric and pneumatic devices. Others are not as well designed or effective. Because there are many different percussors available, the one you select determines the mode of application.

There are, however, some general guidelines for the use of mechanical percussors. Use the same anatomical landmarks as if you were manually percussing a patient. Do not apply excessive force, but rather allow the unit to operate at its own speed and frequency. Avoid bony structures, the spine, the abdomen, and a breast tissue in female patients. Move the device around in a moderately sized area about 10 to 20 cm in diameter. Constant application of the device to one area may irritate the skin and cause sores to develop.

You should begin percussion at a lower frequency and gradually increase the frequency to a higher rate as you progress. This practice helps to alleviate any fear the patient may experience initially.

Do not exert excessive force with the device. Let gravity apply a downward force vector. Use your hands to guide the percussor — not to apply additional force. Some percussors will operate at a lower frequency if pressure is exerted on them.

Hazards. Some mechanical devices have a pad or cup attached to a narrow rod about ¼ inch in diameter and 3 to 4 inches long. The cup or pad oscillates back and forth over a range of about 5 cm. Often, the pad is held in place by one or two set screws. If the set screws came loose, the pad could easily fall off and the rod could then injure the patient. Always check and tighten the set screws as required before using these percussors.

Limitations. The limitations of these devices are primarily dependent on the patient's ability to tolerate their use. Some patients will be able to tolerate them without difficulty and others will not. It is not unusual for a patient to express a fear of mechanical devices, especially in the unfamiliar hospital setting. The therapy of touch as used in manual percussion may be more effective for some patients than the use of mechanical percussors.

Physician's Order

A complete order for postural drainage and chest percussion includes the frequency and duration of therapy and the location or target area. If an order is not complete, it may be up to the respiratory therapist to determine what is required for optimal treatment of the patient. Check the policy and procedures manual.

In the absence of a complete order, contact the physician in person or by telephone to ascertain the frequency, duration, or location of therapy. If the physician requests that the therapy be performed as indicated, you will need to rely on your diagnostic skills and chest x-ray appearance to determine the areas requiring therapy.

If you are requested to assess the patient and determine what areas of the chest require therapy, begin with the patient's chart. Check the patient's history for any indications of cardiovascular insufficiency, past surgery on the thorax or spine, or any other abnormalities of the chest or spine that may limit the patient's tolerance to positioning. Look in the chart for any chest x-ray reports. Areas of consolidation or atelectasis constitute areas to drain and percuss. If it is possible, view the chest radiograph yourself to form a mental picture of the areas you will be treating. When you first see the patient, auscultate and percuss the chest to help clarify areas of consolidation and hypoaeration. By using these findings, you are reasonably assured of selecting the correct areas for therapy.

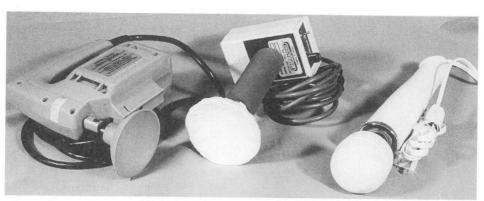

Figure 16-6 *A variety of mechanical percussors*

Duration of the therapy should be a minimum of 5 to 10 minutes for a lobe or segment. If all segments are to be drained, the total duration of therapy should not exceed 40 to 45 minutes. Often in this situation, upper lobes are treated in the morning, middle lobes in the afternoon, and lower lobes in the evening.

Contraindications and Hazards

The contraindications to postural drainage and chest percussion are primarily limited to presence of cardiovascular instability and other specific diseases of the pulmonary system. The performance of postural drainage and chest percussion on the patient whose cardiovascular status is unstable may have potentially serious consequences. As discussed previously, decrease in cardiac output and ventilation-perfusion mismatches may be severe enough for the patient to go into shock. Any patient who has a history of cardiovascular instability should be carefully monitored and the drainage positions modified as required.

Pathologic conditions of the lung that may be worsened by postural drainage and chest percussion include an undrained empyema, or lung abscess, and large-volume hemoptysis of unknown cause. In such cases, it is entirely possible for the maneuver of physiotherapy to release suddenly a large amount of loculated fluid or to induce excessive bleeding. Patients may literally drown in their own fluids. The best practice is to have the loculated fluid surgically drained by a physician before proceeding with further therapy.

The safety of your patients rests on your judgment as a clinician. If you have doubts about a patient's ability to tolerate an ordered procedure, document your reasoning and discuss it with the patient's attending physician. Perhaps with some slight modifications, adequate therapy may be administered without jeopardizing the patient's safety.

OTHER THERAPIES FOR BRONCHIAL HYGIENE

Positive Expiratory Pressure Therapy
Definition and Equipment

Positive expiratory pressure (PEP) therapy is the application of positive pressure (10 to 15 cm H_2O) during active exhalation to increase functional residual capacity (FRC) following a larger than normal tidal breath. The equipment (Figure 16–7) consists of a soft-seal mask, T assembly, one-way valve, pressure manometer, threshold resistor or fixed orifice (2.5 to 4.0 mm diameter), and a nebulizer (optional for aerosol administration). The patient holds the mask tightly against the face using both hands and then is instructed to take a deeper than normal breath and to exhale actively, against the resistance, to FRC level. The purpose of PEP therapy is to mechanically (pressure) splint the airways open during exhalation. PEP therapy promotes better distribution of ventilation and improved mucus clearance.

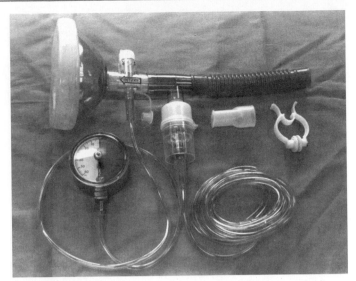

Figure 16–7 *A photograph of a PEP mask therapy device with a small-volume nebulizer for aerosol delivery attached*

Indications

Indications for PEP therapy include the need to aid in removal of retained secretions, atelectasis, and prophylaxis of pulmonary infections and as routine therapy in the treatment of cystic fibrosis. By splinting the airway open mechanically using positive pressure, PEP therapy allows gas to move distally to obstructed areas. When the patient coughs forcefully, the removal of these secretions is facilitated.

Hazards

The risk of barotrauma and hemodynamic compromise exists with PEP therapy owing to the application of positive intrathoracic pressure (Mahlmeister et al., 1991). However, with the low pressures involved (10 to 15 cm H_2O), the risk is minimal. As with incentive spirometry, patients may complain of light-headedness or confusion, headaches, fatigue, or other symptoms relating to taking deeper than normal breaths.

Flutter Valve Therapy
Definition and Equipment

Flutter valve therapy is similar to PEP therapy in that an expiratory resistance device is employed during exhalation. The difference, however, is that the Flutter valve has a weighted ball resting on a conical seat (Figure 16-8). The ball rises, then falls, blocking the outlet, and then rises again during exhalation. This happens repeatedly, causing the Flutter device to "chatter" during exhalation. The alternating opening and closing of the valve causes pressure pulses to be transmitted throughout the lung parenchyma. The pulsing in conjunction with mechanical splinting of the airways (like PEP therapy) helps to facilitate secretion mobilization.

Indications

The indications for Flutter valve therapy are similar to those for PEP therapy. Flutter valve therapy is indicated

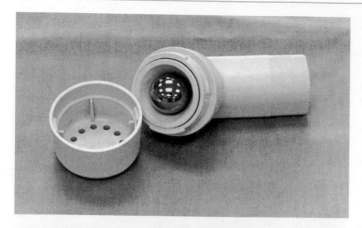

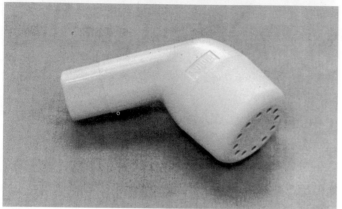

Figure 16-8 *An illustration of the Flutter valve. Note the conical seat and the ball that is displaced by exhaling into the seat.*

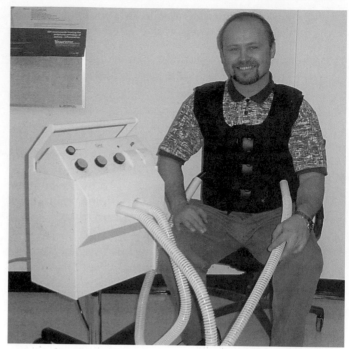

Figure 16-9 *A photograph of the Vest™ airway clearance system made by Advanced Respiratory, St. Paul, MN.*

for the need to aid in removal of retained secretions, atelectasis, and prophylaxis of pulmonary infections and as routine therapy in the treatment of cystic fibrosis. When the patient coughs forcefully, the removal of these secretions is facilitated.

Hazards

The hazards of Flutter valve therapy are similar to those of PEP therapy. These hazards are related to the application of positive pressure (barotrauma, cardiovascular compromise) and hyperinflation (light-headedness, headaches).

High-Frequency Chest Wall Oscillation Therapy

High-frequency chest wall oscillation (HFCWO) therapy is the application of pressure pulses to the thoracic cage via a pneumatic inflatable vest (Figure 16-9). The patient applies the vest and connects it to the air-pulse generator, which rapidly inflates and deflates the vest. The alternating inflation and deflation causes oscillatory pressure pulses (5 to 25 times per second) to be transmitted throughout the thorax. This pulsing facilitates the removal of retained secretions and facilitates home self-application of therapy for airway clearance.

Indications

HFCWO therapy is indicated for mucous plugging, retained secretions, and treatment of chronic diseases such as cystic fibrosis. HFCWO facilitates the patient's self-care in the administration of therapy.

Hazards

Patients using HFCWO therapy should follow the physician's and manufacturer's recommendations for the application of the device. Use of HFCWO therapy in patients with fractures of the thoracic cage dictates extreme caution. Disruption of unstable fractures in such cases could result in pneumothorax or other complications.

Adjunctive Breathing Techniques

Adjunctive breathing techniques are breathing exercises that are taught to the patient for self-administration. These exercises include diaphragmatic breathing, unilateral chest expansion, pursed-lip breathing, and directed cough techniques. The goal of these techniques is hyperinflation of the lungs, which will facilitate secretion removal by coughing.

Indications

Indications for adjunctive breathing techniques include removal of retained secretions, atelectasis, and prophylaxis of pulmonary infections and as routine care for patients with cystic fibrosis. These techniques facilitate mobilization of secretions and may be performed independently by the patient in the absence of a caregiver.

Hazards

Hazards of these adjunct breathing techniques are related to the hazards of hyperinflation. Potential symptoms include light-headedness, dizziness, and headaches. Proper patient instruction on awareness of these symptoms and what to do when they occur is important when you teach these adjunctive breathing techniques.

OBJECTIVES

At the end of this chapter, you should be able to:

- Demonstrate proper body alignment and stance when performing patient care skills.
- Demonstrate the use of good body alignment and body mechanics when positioning or assisting a laboratory partner.
- Demonstrate how to properly position a patient in the following positions:
  — Fowler's and semi-Fowler's positions
  — Supine position
  — Prone position
  — Side-lying position
  — Sims' position
  — Trendelenburg position
- Demonstrate how to assist a patient from the bed into a chair and back into bed.
- Demonstrate how to properly secure the following restraints:
  — Chest restraint
  — Waist restraint
  — Wrist and ankle restraints
- Demonstrate the correct use of bed rails and other safety devices while performing patient care.
- Using a laboratory partner as a patient substitute, properly perform postural drainage and chest percussion on any specified segment(s) of the lung, including:
  — Proper positioning
  — Identification of anatomical landmarks
  — Proper manual percussion and vibration techniques
  — Proper use of a mechanical percussor
- Demonstrate use of a PEP mask device:
  — Demonstrate how to assemble a PEP mask device with and without a nebulizer.
  — Correctly instruct a patient on how to use a PEP device.
- Demonstrate use of a Flutter valve:
  — Correctly assemble the Flutter valve for use.
  — Correctly instruct the patient on how to use the Flutter valve.
- Demonstrate use of the The Vest airway clearance system
  — Correctly assemble The Vest airway clearance system
  — Correctly teach the patient how to use The Vest airway clearance system
- Demonstrate the following adjunctive breathing exercises:
  — Diaphragmatic breathing
  — Unilateral chest expansion
  — Pursed-lip breathing
  — Controlled cough, including splinting
  — Acute chest compression coughing

GENERAL GUIDELINES

Bed Rails

Bed rails should always be in the up position except when you are working on that side of the bed.

Positioning Yourself

You should always position yourself as close to the patient and the side of the bed as possible. It is easier to maintain good body alignment when you are close to the bed and less strain is placed on your muscles. Additionally, to keep the patient from inadvertently rolling out of bed, you may use your body as a bed rail to prevent a fall.

PATIENT POSITIONING

There are a number of standardized *patient positions*.

Fowler's and Semi-Fowler's Positions

Electric beds have simplified the positioning of patients in the two Fowler's positions. You may need to pull the patient up in bed so that the bend of the bed is located where the patient bends at the waist. Simply raising or lowering the head of the bed is all that is required. Elevating the knees slightly will help to prevent the patient from sliding to the foot of the bed and relieve pressure on the back and buttocks.

Supine Position

To place the patient in the supine position, lower the bed until it is flat. Position a blanket that has been formed into a roll or small pillow under the knees to slightly flex them and under the small of the back to support the spine. Use of a foot board is helpful to prevent adverse flexing of the feet. Footdrop from the continual pressure of the bedding on the feet can result in permanent disability. Avoid leaving the comatose or helpless patient supine, as there is a danger of vomiting and aspiration.

Prone Position

Positioning the patient in the prone position requires *turning* the patient. You must roll the patient first into a side-lying and then into the prone position. Care must be exercised to ensure that enough room is provided to complete the maneuver without rolling the patient out of bed.

Begin by positioning the patient to one side of the bed in the supine position. If the patient is unable to assist you, use the following technique: Imagine that the patient is divided into thirds: feet and legs, waist and buttocks, and chest and head. Each third may be easily moved by placing your hands under that portion and then shifting your weight. This is illustrated in Figure 16-10. Slide the patient's feet over first (this is the lightest part). Slide the waist and buttocks over and, finally, the chest and head.

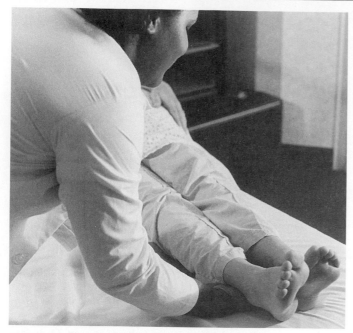

Figure 16-10 *Moving a patient by thirds*

shown in Figure 16-11. Raise the bed rail and move to the other side of the bed.

Roll the patient into a side-lying position by pulling the patient toward yourself. You again may accomplish this with a simple weight shift. Continue rolling the patient to the prone position. Realign the patient so that the patient is centered in the bed and the spinal column is in alignment. A small pillow should be placed under the abdomen to maintain proper spinal alignment. Another, larger pillow may be placed under the ankles and lower legs to prevent adverse flexing of the feet, as shown in Figure 16-12.

Side-Lying Position

To position a patient in the side-lying position, turn the patient onto the patient's side, centered in the bed. Position pillows as shown in Figure 16-13 for support. Slightly flex the patient's knees and arms to relieve strain on muscles and tendons.

Sims' Position

Sims' position (Figure 16-14) is similar to the side-lying position, and some patients find it more comfortable. When rolling a patient to the side, care must be taken not to position the lower arm in a location where the patient can roll over onto it.

Preserve the patient's spinal alignment as much as possible during the procedure.

Once the patient is on one side of the bed, cross the patient's legs and move the patient's arm to the position

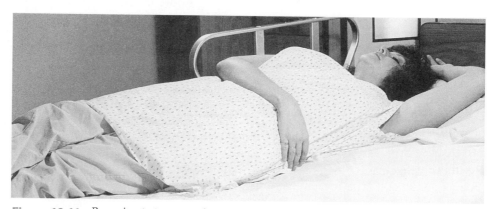

Figure 16-11 *Preparing to turn a patient*

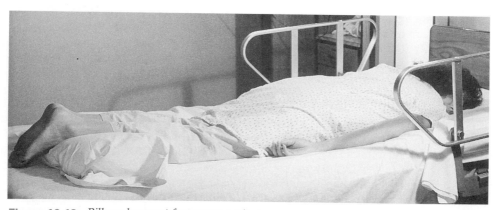

Figure 16-12 *Pillow placement for a prone patient*

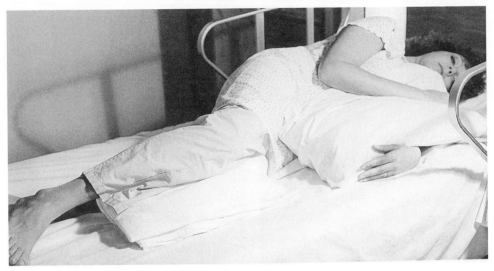

Figure 16-13   *A patient in side-lying position*

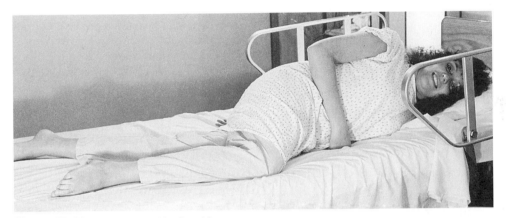

Figure 16-14   *A patient in Sims' position*

Trendelenburg Position

Electric beds have simplified the positioning of patients into the Trendelenburg position. Beds vary, so read the printed directions on the bed and follow them to position your patient. If you do not understand how to work the bed, obtain assistance.

Once the patient is in Trendelenburg position, monitor the patient closely. Check heart rate, skin color, and respiratory rate for any significant changes. The Trendelenburg position is not a natural position, and complications occasionally arise. Avoid leaving the patient unattended and do not allow the patient to cough spasmodically in this head-down position, as it may increase intracranial pressure to dangerous levels.

Reverse Trendelenburg Position

Using the electric bed, follow the directions and position the patient in the reverse Trendelenburg position. Your patient will have a tendency to slide toward the foot of the bed. Use of a foot board will help to prevent this.

Assisting a Patient into a Chair

Begin by lowering the bed as low as its design permits. Raise the head of the bed to full Fowler's position (as far up as it will go). When you raise the bed, be certain that the patient is high enough toward the head of the bed so that the patient will bend at the waist and not the chest. These maneuvers accomplish two things. First, the patient is low enough to make an exit easy. Second, raising the head of the bed reduces the work you need to do to assist the patient to a sitting position. You may wish to allow the patient to sit in this position for a moment to avoid dizziness.

Assist the patient into a dangling position at the side of the bed, as shown in Figure 16-15.

Spread the patient's feet slightly and position your foot closer to the patient between the patient's feet. Grasp the patient under the arms and assist the patient to a standing position as shown in Figure 16-16. Pivot the patient 90° and lower him or her into the chair.

If this is the patient's first time in a chair after a prolonged period of bed rest, two people should assist. If the patient becomes shaky, two people may be required to prevent a fall.

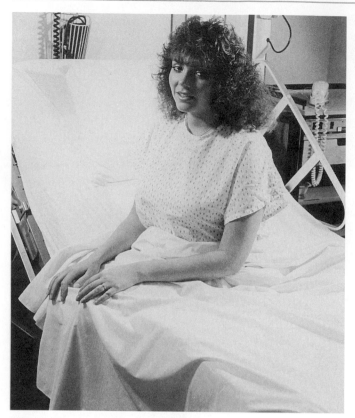

Figure 16-15 *A patient in the dangling position, ready to be assisted into a chair*

USE OF RESTRAINTS

Chest and Waist Restraints

Chest restraints are used to prevent the patient from falling or climbing out of bed. They are also used to help a patient who is sitting in a chair or wheelchair. When these devices are used, they should completely encircle the body. Restraints should be snug but not tight, so a finger can be easily slipped underneath.

Tie the restraint to the bed frame, not the bed rail. The knot should be out of the reach of the patient. Use a square knot to secure the restraint. This knot is easily untied by personnel but cannot be easily undone by the patient. Do not use a knot that cannot be quickly untied in an emergency situation. The patient's movement should be only slightly restricted.

Wrist and Ankle Restraints

Wrist and ankle restraints are used to reduce the mobility of the limb they are attached to. Frequently one hand may be restrained to maintain an intravenous line. The restraint should completely encircle the limb. With soft or Posey restraints, a clove hitch is commonly used to secure the restraint to the limb. Figure 16-17 illustrates how to tie a clove hitch. The two free ends are then tied to the bed frame. Like the chest and waist restraints, these should be snug but not tight.

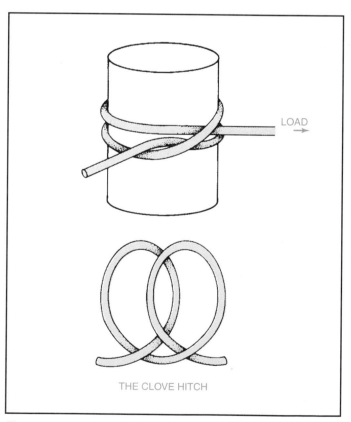

LOAD

THE CLOVE HITCH

Figure 16-16 *Correct foot placement to assist a patient into a chair*

Figure 16-17 *How to tie a clove hitch*

MANUAL BEDS

Some facilities may have manual beds instead of electric beds. These beds operate using hand cranks at the foot of the bed. Usually the center crank raises or lowers the bed. The crank on the left side raises the head and the one on the right raises the feet. A manual bed is shown in Figure 16-18. Trendelenburg and reverse Trendelenburg positions are accomplished by releasing or raising supports between the mattress frame and the bed frame.

When the handles are not in use, it is important to store them in the retracted position under the bed. Handles left in the out position are very hazardous.

PERCUSSION TECHNIQUE

Applying the knowledge you gained in the theory portion of this chapter, practice postural drainage and percussion on a laboratory partner.

Position your hands by letting your arms fall to a resting position at your side while standing. The palmar surface of your hand should face toward your thighs. Keep your fingers together and your hands in the resting configuration. If you look at the shape of your hands, they should be slightly cupped as shown in Figure 16-19.

Practice chest percussion initially by percussing your own thigh. Try to achieve a hollow, popping sound. Notice the difference in sound and tactile stimulation between correct and incorrect technique. When you have mastered the hand positioning, practice percussion on a laboratory partner. Figure 16-20 illustrates correct percussion technique. Using both hands, work toward a frequency of 50 to 60 percussions per minute. The muscle action is predominantly in the wrist and forearm, with the wrist acting as a pivot. Observe for red marks on the surface of the skin. Position your laboratory partner into the 12 drainage positions, identify the landmarks for percussion, and properly perform the technique, observing your partner for any adverse effects from the procedure.

POSITIVE EXPIRATORY PRESSURE THERAPY

Verify the Physician's Order

Before initiating PEP therapy, verify the physician's order for PEP therapy. Determine whether or not aerosolized medication delivery is desired along with PEP therapy, the desired pressure level, and the frequency of therapy. If any of these is not clearly stated, contact the patient's physician for clarification.

Scan the Chart

Scan the patient's history documented in the patient's medical record. Verify that the patient does not have acute sinusitis or a history of ear infections or epistaxis. Confirm that facial, oral, or skull surgery has not recently been performed. Also verify that the patient does not have active

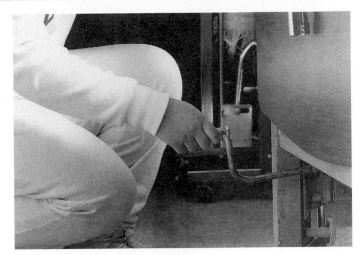

Figure 16-18   *A manual hospital bed*

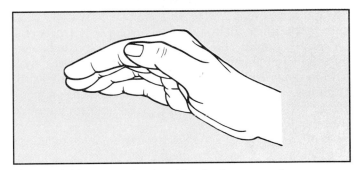

Figure 16-19   *Correct hand position for chest percussion*

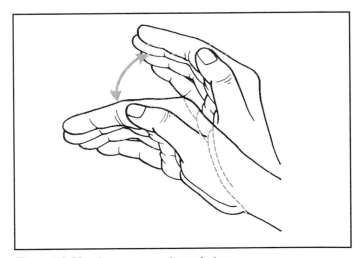

Figure 16-20   *Correct percussion technique*

hemoptysis or an untreated pneumothorax. All of these conditions are contraindications to PEP therapy.

Check the patient's chart, looking for recent blood gas analysis reports, chest x-ray films and report, laboratory data, orders for oxygen administration, and any other items that will help you to assess the patient's current pulmonary status. Review the physician's progress notes, which may help you to determine the goals of PEP therapy. Note the current vital signs, which will provide you with a frame of reference when you first see the patient.

Administration of Therapy

Patient Positioning

The ideal patient position for PEP therapy is sitting comfortably with the elbows resting on a table. This position allows good chest expansion while freeing both hands to provide a good seal for the mask around the nose and mouth. If the patient is unable to sit upright, a full Fowler's or high semi-Fowler's position may be adequate. If you modify the patient's position, use good clinical judgment, monitor for any adverse effects, and assess whether the goals and objectives of PEP therapy are being met.

Appropriate Monitoring before Therapy

Prior to beginning PEP therapy, you should auscultate the patient's chest, measure heart rate and respiratory rate, and observe the patient's ventilatory pattern and symmetry of chest wall motion (by inspection). The goals of PEP therapy are to mobilize secretions, to reverse atelectasis, and to optimize delivery of aerosolized medications. Therefore, quantification of sputum production and determination of pretherapy and posttherapy vital capacity will help to document the effectiveness of therapy. If you are administering a bronchodilator, measurement of peak expiratory flow or forced expired volume in 1 minute (FEV_1) will be appropriate.

If the patient's oxygen therapy is being interrupted for PEP therapy, monitor the patient's arterial oxygen concentration (SpO_2) with the pulse oximeter before and during therapy. To perform PEP therapy, the patient may need to remove the oxygen delivery device to obtain an adequate seal. If this is the case, it is important to monitor the patient's oxygenation status.

Ideal Breathing Pattern

The ideal breathing pattern for PEP therapy is as follows: Instruct the patient to take a larger than normal tidal breath (but not to total lung capacity), and then to exhale actively, but not forcefully, against the resistance to functional residual capacity (FRC). The patient should be relaxed, and diaphragmatic breathing should be emphasized. The patient should be instructed to take between 10 and 20 PEP breaths and then to cough. This cycle should be repeated four to six times. Most PEP therapy sessions take approximately 10 to 20 minutes.

Monitoring the Patient during Therapy

The patient's subjective response (e.g., pain, discomfort, dyspnea) should be monitored and noted. Any dyspnea, tachycardia, or tachypnea should be carefully monitored. If oxygen therapy is being interrupted for PEP therapy, monitor the SpO_2; you may need to discontinue PEP therapy and place the patient on oxygen therapy if levels drop too low.

Monitor the patient's sputum production. PEP therapy should assist the patient in increasing the quantity of sputum produced. Note the color, consistency, and quantity of the sputum, and the presence or absence of odor.

If a bronchodilator is being given, it is important to monitor the heart rate during therapy. Because most sympathomimetic bronchodilators have some cardiac side effects, any significant increase in heart rate warrants stopping therapy and monitoring the patient closely.

FLUTTER VALVE THERAPY

Verify the Physician's Order

Prior to initiating Flutter valve therapy, verify the physician's order for Flutter valve therapy. If the order is not clearly stated, contact the patient's physician for clarification.

Scan the Chart

Scan the patient's history documented in the medical record. Verify that the patient does not have contraindications to Flutter valve therapy. Verify that the patient does not have active hemoptysis or an untreated pneumothorax. Both of these conditions are contraindications to therapy.

Check the patient's chart, looking for recent reports of blood gas analysis, chest x-ray films and report, laboratory data, orders for oxygen administration, and any other items that will help you to assess the patient's current pulmonary status. Review the physician's progress notes, which may help you to determine the goals of Flutter valve therapy. Note the current vital signs, which will provide you with a frame of reference when you first see the patient.

Administration of Therapy

Patient Positioning

The ideal patient position for Flutter valve therapy is sitting comfortably with his/her elbows resting on a table. This position allows good chest expansion while freeing both hands to provide a good seal for the mask around the nose and mouth. If the patient is unable to sit upright, a full Fowler's or high semi-Fowler's position may be adequate. If you modify the patient's position, use good clinical judgment, monitor for any adverse side effects, and assess whether the goals and objectives of Flutter valve therapy are being met.

Appropriate Monitoring before Therapy

Prior to beginning Flutter valve therapy, you should auscultate the patient's chest, measure heart rate and respiratory rate, and observe the patient's ventilatory pattern and symmetry of chest wall motion (inspection). The goals of Flutter valve therapy are to mobilize secretions and reverse atelectasis. Therefore, quantification of sputum production and determination of pretherapy and posttherapy vital capacity will help to document the effectiveness of therapy.

If the patient's oxygen therapy is being interrupted for Flutter valve therapy, monitor the patient's SpO_2 before and during therapy. To perform Flutter valve therapy, the patient may need to remove the oxygen delivery device to obtain an adequate seal. If this is the case, it is important to monitor the patient's oxygenation status.

Ideal Breathing Pattern

The ideal breathing pattern for Flutter valve therapy is as follows: Instruct the patient to take a larger than normal tidal breath (but not to total lung capacity), and then to exhale actively, but not forcefully, against the resistance to FRC. The patient should be relaxed, and diaphragmatic breathing should be emphasized. The patient should be instructed to take between 10 and 20 Flutter valve breaths and then to cough. This cycle should be repeated four to six times. Most Flutter valve therapy sessions take approximately 10 to 20 minutes.

Monitoring the Patient during Therapy

The patient's subjective response (e.g., pain, discomfort, dyspnea) should be monitored and noted. Any dyspnea, tachycardia, or tachypnea should be carefully monitored. If oxygen therapy must be interrupted for Flutter valve therapy, monitor the SpO_2, discontinue therapy, and place the patient on oxygen therapy as required.

Monitor the patient's sputum production. Flutter valve therapy should assist the patient in increasing the quantity of sputum produced. Note the color, consistency, and quantity of sputum and the presence or absence of odor.

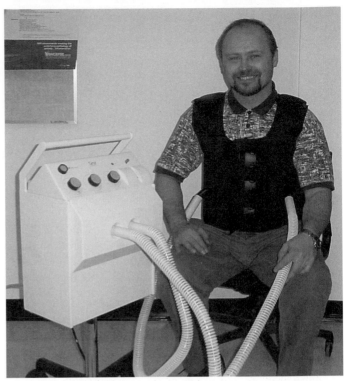

Figure 16-21 *Application of The Vest™ airway clearance system vest to the patient's chest*

HIGH-FREQUENCY CHEST WALL OSCILLATION THERAPY ADMINISTRATION

The Vest™ Airway Clearance System Assembly

Assist and instruct the patient in applying the vest to the chest. Ensure that the vest is properly secured using the self-fastening straps, with the head and arms free to move (Figure 16-21). It is important to secure the vest so that it doesn't ride too high or too low on the chest.

Connect both large-diameter hoses to the air-pulse generator unit, matching left and right sides with the labeled outlets. Connect the power cord to a standard wall electrical outlet, verifying that the voltage is set correctly for your facility. Set the controls (frequency and pressure) to the correct settings.

Verify the Physician's Order

Prior to initiating HFCWO therapy, verify the physician's order for therapy. If the order is not clearly stated, contact the patient's physician for clarification.

Scan the Chart

Scan the patient's history documented in the patient's medical record. Verify that the patient does not have contraindications to HFCWO therapy. Verify that the patient does not have active hemoptysis, an untreated pneumothorax, or unstable chest wall fractures. All of these conditions are contraindications to therapy.

Check the patient's chart, looking for recent results of blood gas analysis, chest x-ray films and report, laboratory data, orders for oxygen administration, and any other items that will help you to assess the patient's current pulmonary status. Review the physician's progress notes, which may help you to determine the goals of HFCWO therapy. Note the current vital signs, which will provide you with a frame of reference when you first see the patient.

Administration of Therapy
Patient Positioning

The ideal patient position for HFCWO therapy is sitting comfortably erect with the chest in a good position for expansion. If you modify the patient's position, use good clinical judgment, monitor for any adverse effects, and assess whether the goals and objectives of HFCWO therapy are being met.

Technique

Turn the unit on. Have the patient relax and take slow, deep breaths during therapy. If the patient needs to cough, the unit may be turned off if coughing is easier without HFCWO. A typical session takes about 20 minutes.

Monitoring the Patient during Therapy

The patient's subjective response (e.g., pain, discomfort, dyspnea) should be monitored and noted. Any dyspnea, tachycardia, or tachypnea should be carefully monitored. Monitor the patient's SpO_2; place the patient on oxygen therapy as required if oxygen desaturation occurs.

Monitor the patient's sputum production. HFCWO therapy should assist the patient in increasing the quantity of sputum produced. Note the color, consistency, and quantity of sputum and the presence or absence of odor.

ADJUNCTIVE BREATHING TECHNIQUES

Adjunctive breathing techniques such as controlled coughing and splinting may be used postoperatively to improve secretion mobilization. Because of pain, a patient may expend considerable energy with weak, ineffective coughs, desperately trying to clear secretions. A low volume combined with a weak effort is insufficient to generate the flow rates necessary to clear any retained secretions.

Diaphragmatic Breathing

Diaphragmatic breathing may be accomplished on both inspiration and expiration. For this technique, the patient is encouraged to distend the abdomen with the inspiratory effort. Use of the abdominal muscles in this way helps to lower the diaphragm, expanding the lungs further. A patient may also be coached to observe the intercostal margin and encouraged to expand it outward. This maneuver takes considerable effort and is the reverse of the breathing pattern most people use (stomach in, chest out).

On expiration, the patient is encouraged to flatten the abdomen, thus pushing the diaphragm up and thereby improving the strength of exhalation. With time, the contractile force of the abdominal muscles will be increased. The patient may feel the effects on the diaphragm by placing the hands over the rib cage at the level of the xiphoid process.

Unilateral Chest Expansion

By placing a hand along the midaxillary line (Figure 16-22), expanding one side of the chest preferentially (unilateral) is facilitated. This position results in a slight kyphosis, compressing the opposite chest. Therefore, when the patient performs deep breathing, the side where the hand is placed preferentially expands. This technique of *unilateral chest expansion* may be helpful in reversing middle or lower lobe atelectasis.

Pursed-Lip Breathing

For *pursed-lip breathing*, the patient is instructed to take a deep breath and exhale through pursed lips. The narrowing of the airway generates a resistance to exhalation, causing pressure to be maintained throughout the bronchial tree. This sustained pressure prevents air trapping and keeps the alveoli inflated for a longer time period on exhalation. This is a natural phenomenon that may be observed when a patient is short of breath.

Controlled Coughing

For controlled coughing, or *directed cough*, the patient is instructed to take three breaths as deep as possible. This maneuver will help to reverse atelectasis and to increase the volume available for the cough effort. At the end of the third breath, the patient is encouraged to

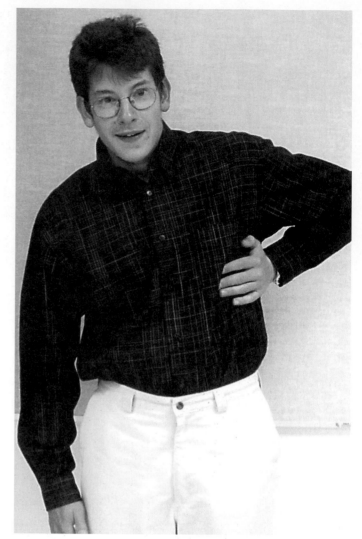

Figure 16-22 *A photo showing unilateral chest expansion*

cough twice very firmly. With the larger volume behind the cough, flow can be improved and the cough becomes more effective.

Splinting is a technique wherein the surgical incision or injured area is supported with your hands, a pillow, or a bath blanket. By applying pressure across the incision and minimizing its movement, pain during coughing is reduced. Splinting may be accomplished by either the therapist or the patient, if able. Any time pain can be reduced, cooperation is generally better.

Acute Chest Compression

Acute chest compression is effective for those patients with a poor cough effort, which is often due to weak musculature. The patient is instructed to take as deep a breath as possible. Then place your hands on the patient's lateral costal margins. When the patient exhales, apply firm but gentle pressure. This helps to generate the flows and pressures necessary to move secretions into the larger airways from where they may be expelled. Figure 16-23 illustrates the technique of acute chest compression.

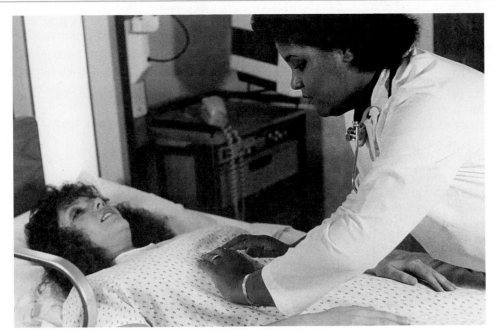

Figure 16-23   *A respiratory care practitioner performing acute chest compression*

References

American Association for Respiratory Care. (1991). AARC clinical practice guideline: Postural drainage therapy. *Respiratory Care, 36*(12), 1418–1426.

American Association for Respiratory Care. (1993). AARC clinical practice guideline: Directed cough. *Respiratory Care, 38*(5), 495–499.

American Association for Respiratory Care. (1993). AARC clinical practice guideline: Use of positive airway pressure adjuncts to bronchial hygiene therapy. *Respiratory Care, 38*(5), 516–521.

Mahlmeister, M., Fink, J. B., Hoffman, G. L., & Fifer, L. F. (1991). Positive-expiratory-pressure mask therapy: Theoretical and practical considerations and a review of the literature. *Respiratory Care, 36*(11).

Additional Resources

Allsop, K. (1976). *Body mechanics and patient transfer techniques.* Ogden, UT: Weber State College.

Burton, G. C., Hodgkin, J., & Ward, J. (1997). *Respiratory care: A guide to clinical practice.* (4th ed.). Philadelphia: Lippincott.

DeLaune, S. C., & Ladner, P. K. (2002). *Fundamentals of nursing concepts and procedures* (2nd ed.). Reading, MA: Addison-Wesley.

Eubanks, D. H., & Bone, R. C. (1991). *Comprehensive respiratory care* (2nd ed.). St. Louis, MO: Mosby.

Scanlan, C., Spearman, C. B., & Sheldon, R. L. (1999). *Egan's fundamentals of respiratory therapy* (7th ed.). St. Louis, MO: Mosby.

Tyler, M. (1982). Complications of positioning and chest physiotherapy. *Respiratory Care, 27*(4), 458–466.

Practice Activities: Patient Positioning and Chest Physiotherapy

1. With a laboratory partner, demonstrate how to position the patient into the following positions:
   a. Fowler's and semi-Fowler's
   b. Dangling
   c. Prone
   d. Side-lying
   e. Sims'
   f. Trendelenburg
   g. Reverse Trendelenburg

2. With a laboratory partner, demonstrate how to use the following restraints:
   a. Chest
   b. Waist
   c. Wrist
   d. Ankle

3. Position a laboratory partner for postural drainage:
   a. Position your partner into the 12 positions, verbally stating what region or structure each position drains.
   b. Ask your partner to test your abilities by specifying a lobe or segment to be drained; then position your partner as appropriate. Observe the following:
      (1) Pulse
      (2) Respiratory rate and depth
      (3) Color

4. With a laboratory partner, practice manual chest percussion. During your practice, observe the following:
   a. Properly identify all anatomical landmarks.
   b. Use correct hand positioning.
   c. Percussion should produce a hollow popping sound.
   d. The skin should not have any evidence of red marks.
   e. Do not percuss bony structures, the spine, the abdomen, or breast tissue in a female patient.

5. With a laboratory partner, practice manual vibration. During your practice, observe the following:
   a. Properly identify all anatomical landmarks.
   b. Use correct hand positioning.
   c. Vibration is performed only on exhalation.

6. With a laboratory partner, practice use of a mechanical percussor. During your practice, observe the following:
   a. Do not use excessive force.
   b. Properly identify all anatomical landmarks.
   c. Do not percuss over bony structures, the spine, the abdomen, or breast tissue in a female patient.
   d. Move the percussor over an area of about 10 to 20 cm.

7. Using a blank sheet of paper, document the positioning used, the technique (manual or mechanical) of chest percussion, and the lobe and segment treated. Have your laboratory instructor critique your charting.

Practice Activities: PEP Mask Therapy

CIRCUIT ASSEMBLY

Connect a soft seal mask of the correct size to the outlet T assembly with the one-way valves and threshold resistor. Connect a pressure manometer to the opposite side of the T assembly from the threshold resistor for pressure monitoring. If a nebulized medication is desired, connect the nebulizer to the inlet of the T assembly and connect a 6-inch length of aerosol tubing (reservoir) to the opposite end of the nebulizer (Figure 16-24), and connect the nebulizer to a compressed gas source (air or oxygen).

Alternatively, a mouthpiece and nose clips may be substituted for the soft-seal mask. Some patients may find the mask confining and feel claustrophobic. It is important to use nose clips when a mouthpiece is used, in that pressure may be lost through the nose without them.

PRESSURE ADJUSTMENT

Adjust the threshold resistor until the desired expiratory pressure is achieved. Most often pressures between 10 to 20 cm H_2O are applied during PEP mask therapy.

ACTIVITIES

1. Correctly assemble the circuit for PEP mask therapy.
2. With a laboratory partner acting as your patient:
   a. Correctly assess your patient prior to therapy.
   b. Correctly instruct your patient on the use of the PEP mask device.
   c. Correctly monitor your patient during therapy.

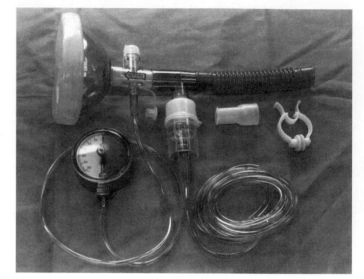

Figure 16-24 *The correct assembly of the PEP therapy device*

   d. Correctly monitor your patient following PEP mask therapy.
   e. Using a blank sheet of paper, document the procedure as if you were charting in a medical record and have your laboratory instructor critique your charting.
3. Assemble a PEP mask device for aerosol delivery.

Practice Activities: Flutter Valve Therapy

---

1. Correctly assemble the Flutter valve for use.
2. With a laboratory partner acting as your patient:
   a. Correctly assess your patient prior to therapy.
   b. Correctly instruct your patient on the use of the Flutter valve.
   c. Correctly monitor your patient during therapy.

   d. Correctly monitor your patient following Flutter valve therapy.
   e. Using a blank sheet of paper, document the procedure as if you were charting in a medical record and have your laboratory instructor critique your charting.

Practice Activities: The Vest Airway Clearance System

1. Assemble the required equipment:
   a. The vest
   b. Two large-bore tubes
   c. The air-pulse generator
2. Using a laboratory partner as your patient, assist in correctly applying the vest.
3. Set the control (frequency) to 15 Hz at a medium pressure.
4. Connect the hoses to the air-pulse generator and plug the unit into an AC electrical outlet.
5. Correctly assess your patient prior to therapy.
6. Instruct the patient on the use of the device.
7. Monitor the patient during therapy:
   a. Shortness of breath
   b. Coughing
   c. Oximetry
8. Using a blank sheet of paper, document the procedure as if you were charting in a medical record and have your laboratory instructor critique your charting.

Practice Activities: Adjunctive Breathing Techniques

1. With a laboratory partner, practice giving each other directions on how to perform the following techniques:
   a. Diaphragmatic breathing
   b. Unilateral chest expansion
   c. Pursed-lip breathing
   d. Directed cough
   Note: When a patient does not seem to do well, it usually may be attributed to poor instruction.
2. Complete the following steps as if you were going to perform these techniques with a patient:
   a. Wash your hands.
   b. Assess the patient:
      (1) Auscultation of breath sounds
      (2) Oximetry
      (3) Determination of heart and respiratory rates
      (4) Assess the work of breathing
   c. Instruct the patient on these techniques:
      (1) Diaphragmatic breathing
      (2) Unilateral chest expansion
      (3) Pursed-lip breathing
      (4) Directed cough
   d. Assist the patient with coughing following the adjunctive exercises.
   e. Wash your hands.
   f. Using a blank sheet of paper, chart the procedure and have your laboratory instructor critique it.

Check List: Patient Positioning

_____ 1. Properly identify the patient.
_____ 2. Wash your hands.
_____ 3. Explain the procedure to the patient.
4. Use the following guidelines in moving your patient:
_____ a. Stand with correct alignment and balance.
_____ b. Adjust the working surface to waist height.
_____ c. Use the major muscle groups.
_____ d. Use a wide stance for a good base of support.
_____ e. Use your body weight to your advantage.
_____ f. Allow gravity to assist.
_____ 5. Operate the electric bed correctly.
6. Position the patient to the desired position:
_____ a. Allow the patient to assist.
_____ b. Allow the patient to move at his or her own speed.
_____ c. Maintain patient safety at all times.
_____ d. Maintain good body alignment.
7. Use safety devices properly:
_____ a. Use bed rails correctly.
   b. Use restraints properly as required:
_____ (1) Chest and waist
_____ (2) Wrist and ankle
_____ c. Position the nurse call button within reach.
_____ d. Observe the position of the code switch.
_____ 8. Check for hazards before leaving the room.

Check List: Postural Drainage and Chest Percussion

_____ 1. Review the patient's chart.
2. Gather the appropriate equipment:
_____ a. Tissues for the patient (if there are none at the bedside)
_____ b. Stethoscope
_____ c. Sputum cup or container
_____ d. Mechanical percussors if required
3. Introduce yourself and explain the procedure.
_____ a. Use simple, easily understood terms.
_____ 4. Follow standard precautions, including handwashing.
5. Assess your patient as follows:
_____ a. Take the pulse.
_____ b. Inspect skin color.

_____   c. Determine respiratory rate.
_____   d. Auscultate the chest.
_____   e. Percuss the chest.
_____   6. Position the patient to drain the correct segments or lobes.
     7. Following drainage, perform chest percussion or clapping:
_____   a. Identify landmarks.
_____   b. Do not redden the skin.
_____   c. Avoid bony structures, the spine, the abdomen, and breast tissue in a female patient.
     8. Perform vibration following percussion.
_____   a. Use proper technique.
_____   b. Vibrate only on exhalation.

_____   9. Leave the patient in each position for the proper duration.
   10. Monitor the following:
_____   a. Pulse
_____   b. Skin color
_____   c. Respiratory rate
_____   d. Redness of the skin
_____   11. Assist the patient with coughing after treating an area.
   12. Leave the patient safe and comfortable.
_____   a. Clean up the area and dispose of materials as appropriate
_____   13. Reassess breath sounds.
_____   14. Record the procedure in the patient's chart.

Check List: PEP Mask Therapy

_____   1. Verify the physician's order.
_____   2. Scan the chart for relevant information.
_____   3. Follow standard precautions, including handwashing.
_____   4. Obtain and assemble your equipment.
_____   5. Introduce yourself and explain the procedure.
_____   6. Position the patient properly.
_____   7. Assess the patient prior to therapy.

_____   8. Instruct the patient on PEP mask therapy.
_____   9. Assist and coach the patient during therapy.
_____   10. Periodically, have the patient cough.
_____   11. Monitor the patient during therapy.
_____   12. Assess the patient following therapy.
_____   13. Clean up after yourself.
_____   14. Ensure that the patient is safe and comfortable.
_____   15. Document the procedure in the patient's chart.

Check List: Flutter Valve Therapy

_____   1. Verify the physician's order.
_____   2. Scan the chart for relevant information.
_____   3. Follow standard precautions, including handwashing.
_____   4. Obtain and assemble your equipment.
_____   5. Introduce yourself and explain the procedure.
_____   6. Position the patient properly.
_____   7. Assess the patient prior to therapy.

_____   8. Instruct the patient on Flutter valve therapy.
_____   9. Assist and coach the patient during therapy.
_____   10. Periodically, have the patient cough.
_____   11. Monitor the patient during therapy.
_____   12. Assess the patient following therapy.
_____   13. Clean up after yourself.
_____   14. Ensure that the patient is safe and comfortable.
_____   15. Document the procedure in the patient's chart.

Check List: HFCWO Therapy—(The Vest Airway Clearance System)

_____   1. Verify the physician's order.
_____   2. Scan the chart for relevant information.
_____   3. Follow standard precautions, including handwashing.
     4. Obtain and assemble the equipment:
_____   a. The vest
_____   b. Two large-diameter tubes
_____   c. The air-pulse generator
_____   5. Introduce yourself and explain the procedure.
_____   6. Position the patient properly.

_____   7. Assess the patient prior to therapy.
_____   8. Instruct the patient on applying the vest.
_____   9. Set the controls correctly.
_____   10. Assist and coach the patient during therapy.
_____   11. Periodically, have the patient cough.
_____   12. Monitor the patient during therapy.
_____   13. Assess the patient following therapy.
_____   14. Clean up after yourself.
_____   15. Ensure that the patient is safe and comfortable.
_____   16. Document the procedure in the patient's chart.

Check List: Adjunctive Breathing Exercises

_____ 1. Verify the physician's order.
_____ 2. Scan the chart for relevant information.
_____ 3. Follow standard precautions, including hand-washing.
_____ 4. Introduce yourself and explain the procedure.
_____ 5. Position the patient properly.
_____ 6. Assess the patient prior to therapy.
   7. Instruct the patient on the adjunctive techniques:
_____   a. Diaphragmatic breathing
_____   b. Unilateral chest expansion
_____   c. Pursed-lip breathing
_____   d. Directed cough
_____ 8. Assist and coach the patient during technique performance.
_____ 9. Periodically, have the patient cough.
_____ 10. Monitor the patient during therapy.
_____ 11. Assess the patient following therapy.
_____ 12. Clean up after yourself.
_____ 13. Ensure that the patient is safe and comfortable.
_____ 14. Document the procedure in the patient's chart.

Self-Evaluation Post Test: Bronchial Hygiene Therapy

1. The practice of good body mechanics is necessary to:
   a. prevent damage to hospital equipment.
   b. aid in patient rehabilitation.
   c. prevent strain, fatigue, and injuries.
   d. aid in equipment maintenance.

2. To lift a heavy object, you should:
   I. bend at the waist.
   II. use your back.
   III. squat.
   IV. use your legs.
   a. I, IV
   b. I, II
   c. III, IV
   d. II, III

3. Injuries are more frequent when:
   a. the body is in poor alignment.
   b. the body is balanced.
   c. a wide base of support is used.
   d. large muscle groups are utilized.

4. The position that facilitates the greatest chest expansion is:
   a. dangling.
   b. Fowler's.
   c. prone.
   d. supine.

5. The contraindications to PEP therapy may include:
   a. acute sinusitis.
   b. atelectasis.
   c. pneumonia.
   d. cystic fibrosis.

6. You should never percuss:
   I. the sternum.
   II. breast tissue in an adult female patient.
   III. the spinal column.
   IV. the abdomen.
   a. I
   b. I, II
   c. I, II, III
   d. I, II, III, IV

7. Which of the following is/are (an) indication(s) for Flutter valve therapy?
   a. Retained secretions
   b. Atelectasis
   c. Routine therapy for cystic fibrosis
   d. All of the above

8. A patient in position for draining the posterior basal segments of both lungs complains of a headache when coughing. The most likely cause is:
   a. increased abdominal pressure.
   b. neck vein engorgement.
   c. increased intrapleural pressure.
   d. increased intracranial pressure.

9. A patient positioned one-quarter turn from prone, resting on the left side and supported against pillows, will experience drainage of:
   a. the superior segment of the right lower lobe.
   b. the apical segment of the right upper lobe.
   c. the posterior segment of the right upper lobe.
   d. the superior segment of the left lower lobe.

10. Vibration is an isometric type of maneuver performed:
   a. only on inspiration.
   b. during exhalation only.
   c. to facilitate removal of secretions.
   d. b and c

PERFORMANCE EVALUATION:
PATIENT POSITIONING

Date: Lab _____ Clinical _____ Agency _____

Lab: Pass _____ Fail _____   Clinical: Pass _____ Fail _____

Student name _____   Instructor name _____

No. of times observed in clinical _____

No. of times practiced in clinical _____

PASSING CRITERIA: Obtain 90% or better on the procedure. Tasks indicated by * must receive at least 1 point, or the evaluation is terminated. Procedure must be performed within designated time, or the performance receives a failing grade.

SCORING:
2 points — Task performed satisfactorily without prompting.
1 point — Task performed satisfactorily with self-initiated correction.
0 points — Task performed incorrectly or with prompting required.
NA — Task not applicable to the patient care situation.

TASKS:		PEER	LAB	CLINICAL
*	1. Properly identifies the patient	☐	☐	☐
	2. Explains the procedure to the patient	☐	☐	☐
*	3. Follows standard precautions, including handwashing	☐	☐	☐
	4. Uses the following during procedure:			
*	a. Stands with correct alignment	☐	☐	☐
*	b. Adjusts working surface level	☐	☐	☐
*	c. Uses major muscle groups	☐	☐	☐
*	d. Uses a wide base of support	☐	☐	☐
*	e. Uses body weight to advantage	☐	☐	☐
*	f. Utilizes gravity when possible	☐	☐	☐
*	5. Operates electric bed correctly	☐	☐	☐
*	6. Places patient in desired position			
*	a. Allows the patient to assist	☐	☐	☐
*	b. Allows the patient to move at the his or her own speed	☐	☐	☐
*	c. Maintains patient safety	☐	☐	☐
*	d. Maintains good alignment	☐	☐	☐
	7. Uses safety devices properly			
*	a. Restraints secured correctly	☐	☐	☐
*	b. Nurse call button within reach	☐	☐	☐
*	c. Identifies code switch	☐	☐	☐
	d. Ensures bed rails are up	☐	☐	☐
*	8. Checks room for safety hazards	☐	☐	☐

Score: Peer   _____ points of possible 38; _____%

          Lab   _____ points of possible 38; _____%

          Clinical   _____ points of possible 38; _____%

TIME: _____ out of possible 20 minutes

STUDENT SIGNATURES   INSTRUCTOR SIGNATURES

PEER: _____   LAB: _____

STUDENT: _____   CLINICAL: _____

PERFORMANCE EVALUATION:
CHEST PERCUSSION AND POSTURAL DRAINAGE

Date: Lab _____ Clinical _____ Agency _____

Lab: Pass _____ Fail _____   Clinical: Pass _____ Fail _____

Student name _____   Instructor name _____

No. of times observed in clinical _____

No. of times practiced in clinical _____

PASSING CRITERIA: Obtain 90% or better on the procedure. Tasks indicated by * must receive at least 1 point, or the evaluation is terminated. Procedure must be performed within designated time, or the performance receives a failing grade.

SCORING:
2 points — Task performed satisfactorily without prompting.
1 point — Task performed satisfactorily with self-initiated correction.
0 points — Task performed incorrectly or with prompting required.
NA — Task not applicable to the patient care situation.

TASKS:			PEER	LAB	CLINICAL
*	1.	Verifies the physician's order	☐	☐	☐
*	2.	Follows standard precautions, including handwashing	☐	☐	☐
	3.	Introduces self and explains procedure	☐	☐	☐
*	4.	Places patient into proper position	☐	☐	☐
	5.	Percusses patient's chest			
*		a. Does not redden skin	☐	☐	☐
*		b. Makes a loud popping sound	☐	☐	☐
*		c. Percusses over segments being drained	☐	☐	☐
*	6.	Vibration does not exert excessive pressure	☐	☐	☐
*	7.	Vibrates only on exhalation	☐	☐	☐
	8.	Percusses and vibrates over light cover	☐	☐	☐
*	9.	Leaves patient in position for proper length of time	☐	☐	☐
	10.	Monitors patient's condition			
*		a. Pulse	☐	☐	☐
*		b. Color	☐	☐	☐
*		c. Respiratory rate	☐	☐	☐
*	11.	Assists patient to cough	☐	☐	☐
*	12.	Has expectoration supplies nearby	☐	☐	☐
	13.	Leaves patient safe and comfortable	☐	☐	☐
*	14.	Records the procedure on the chart	☐	☐	☐

Score: Peer   _____ points of possible 36; _____%

            Lab   _____ points of possible 36; _____%

            Clinical   _____ points of possible 36; _____%

TIME: _____ out of possible 20 minutes

STUDENT SIGNATURES   INSTRUCTOR SIGNATURES

PEER: _____   LAB: _____

STUDENT: _____   CLINICAL: _____

PERFORMANCE EVALUATION:
PEP MASK THERAPY

Date: Lab _____ Clinical _____ Agency _____

Lab: Pass _____ Fail _____   Clinical: Pass _____ Fail _____

Student name _____   Instructor name _____

No. of times observed in clinical _____

No. of times practiced in clinical _____

PASSING CRITERIA: Obtain 90% or better on the procedure. Tasks indicated by * must receive at least 1 point, or the evaluation is terminated. Procedure must be performed within designated time, or the performance receives a failing grade.

SCORING:
2 points — Task performed satisfactorily without prompting.
1 point — Task performed satisfactorily with self-initiated correction.
0 points — Task performed incorrectly or with prompting required.
NA — Task not applicable to the patient care situation.

TASKS:

		PEER	LAB	CLINICAL
*	1. Verifies the physician's order	☐	☐	☐
*	2. Scans the chart for relevant information	☐	☐	☐
*	3. Follows standard precautions, including handwashing	☐	☐	☐
	4. Obtains and assembles the equipment	☐	☐	☐
	5. Introduces self and explains procedure	☐	☐	☐
	6. Positions the patient properly	☐	☐	☐
*	7. Assesses the patient prior to therapy	☐	☐	☐
*	8. Instructs the patient on PEP mask therapy	☐	☐	☐
*	9. Assists and coaches the patient during therapy	☐	☐	☐
	10. Periodically has the patient cough	☐	☐	☐
	11. Monitors the patient during therapy	☐	☐	☐
	12. Assesses the patient following therapy	☐	☐	☐
	13. Cleans up	☐	☐	☐
	14. Ensures that the patient is safe and comfortable	☐	☐	☐
	15. Documents the procedure in the patient's chart	☐	☐	☐

SCORE:
Peer _____ points of possible 30; _____%
Lab _____ points of possible 30; _____%
Clinical _____ points of possible 30; _____%

TIME: _____ out of possible 30 minutes

STUDENT SIGNATURES   **INSTRUCTOR SIGNATURES**

PEER: _____   LAB: _____

STUDENT: _____   CLINICAL: _____

PERFORMANCE EVALUATION: FLUTTER VALVE THERAPY

Date: Lab _____ Clinical _____ Agency _____

Lab: Pass _____ Fail _____   Clinical: Pass _____ Fail _____

Student name _____   Instructor name _____

No. of times observed in clinical _____

No. of times practiced in clinical _____

PASSING CRITERIA: Obtain 90% or better on the procedure. Tasks indicated by * must receive at least 1 point, or the evaluation is terminated. Procedure must be performed within designated time, or the performance receives a failing grade.

SCORING:
2 points — Task performed satisfactorily without prompting.
1 point — Task performed satisfactorily with self-initiated correction.
0 points — Task performed incorrectly or with prompting required.
NA — Task not applicable to the patient care situation.

TASKS:

		PEER	LAB	CLINICAL
*	1. Verifies the physician's order	☐	☐	☐
*	2. Scans the chart for relevant information	☐	☐	☐
*	3. Follows standard precautions, including handwashing	☐	☐	☐
	4. Obtains and assembles the equipment	☐	☐	☐
	5. Introduces self and explains procedure	☐	☐	☐
	6. Positions the patient properly	☐	☐	☐
*	7. Assesses the patient prior to therapy	☐	☐	☐
*	8. Instructs the patient on Flutter valve therapy	☐	☐	☐
*	9. Assists and coaches the patient during therapy	☐	☐	☐
	10. Periodically has the patient cough	☐	☐	☐
	11. Monitors the patient during therapy	☐	☐	☐
	12. Assesses the patient following therapy	☐	☐	☐
	13. Cleans up	☐	☐	☐
	14. Ensures that the patient is safe and comfortable	☐	☐	☐
	15. Documents the procedure in the patient's chart	☐	☐	☐

SCORE: Peer _____ points of possible 30; _____ %

Lab _____ points of possible 30; _____ %

Clinical _____ points of possible 30; _____ %

TIME: _____ out of possible 30 minutes

STUDENT SIGNATURES   INSTRUCTOR SIGNATURES

PEER: _____   LAB: _____

STUDENT: _____   CLINICAL: _____

311

PERFORMANCE EVALUATION:
HFCWO (THE VEST AIRWAY CLEARANCE SYSTEM)

Date: Lab _____ Clinical _____ Agency _____

Lab: Pass _____ Fail _____   Clinical: Pass _____ Fail _____

Student name _____ Instructor name _____

No. of times observed in clinical _____

No. of times practiced in clinical _____

PASSING CRITERIA: Obtain 90% or better on the procedure. Tasks indicated by * must receive at least 1 point, or the evaluation is terminated. Procedure must be performed within designated time, or the performance receives a failing grade.

SCORING:
2 points — Task performed satisfactorily without prompting.
1 point — Task performed satisfactorily with self-initiated correction.
0 points — Task performed incorrectly or with prompting required.
NA — Task not applicable to the patient care situation.

TASKS:

			PEER	LAB	CLINICAL
*	1.	Verifies the physician's order	☐	☐	☐
*	2.	Scans the chart for relevant information	☐	☐	☐
*	3.	Follows standard precautions, including handwashing	☐	☐	☐
	4.	Obtains and assembles the equipment			
		a. The vest	☐	☐	☐
		b. Two large-diameter tubes	☐	☐	☐
		c. The air-pulse generator	☐	☐	☐
	5.	Introduces self and explains procedure	☐	☐	☐
	6.	Positions the patient properly	☐	☐	☐
*	7.	Assesses the patient prior to therapy	☐	☐	☐
*	8.	Instructs the patient on applying vest	☐	☐	☐
*	9.	Sets the controls correctly	☐	☐	☐
*	10.	Assists and coaches the patient during therapy	☐	☐	☐
	11.	Periodically, has the patient cough	☐	☐	☐
	12.	Monitors the patient during therapy	☐	☐	☐
	13.	Assesses the patient following therapy	☐	☐	☐
	14.	Cleans up	☐	☐	☐
	15.	Ensures that the patient is safe and comfortable	☐	☐	☐
	16.	Documents the procedure in the patient's chart	☐	☐	☐

PERFORMANCE EVALUATION:
ADJUNCTIVE BREATHING TECHNIQUES

Date: Lab _____ Clinical _____ Agency _____

Lab: Pass _____ Fail _____   Clinical: Pass _____ Fail _____

Student name _____   Instructor name _____

No. of times observed in clinical _____

No. of times practiced in clinical _____

PASSING CRITERIA: Obtain 90% or better on the procedure. Tasks indicated by * must receive at least 1 point, or the evaluation is terminated. Procedure must be performed within designated time, or the performance receives a failing grade.

SCORING:
2 points — Task performed satisfactorily without prompting.
1 point — Task performed satisfactorily with self-initiated correction.
0 points — Task performed incorrectly or with prompting required.
NA — Task not applicable to the patient care situation.

TASKS:		PEER	LAB	CLINICAL
*	1. Verifies the physician's order	☐	☐	☐
*	2. Scans the chart for relevant information	☐	☐	☐
*	3. Follows standard precautions, including handwashing	☐	☐	☐
	4. Introduces self and explains the procedure	☐	☐	☐
*	5. Positions the patient properly	☐	☐	☐
*	6. Assesses the patient prior to therapy	☐	☐	☐
	7. Instructs the patient on the adjunctive techniques			
*	a. Diaphragmatic breathing	☐	☐	☐
*	b. Unilateral chest expansion	☐	☐	☐
*	c. Pursed-lip breathing	☐	☐	☐
*	d. Directed cough	☐	☐	☐
*	8. Assists and coaches the patient during technique performance	☐	☐	☐
	9. Periodically, has the patient cough	☐	☐	☐
	10. Monitors the patient during therapy	☐	☐	☐
	11. Assesses the patient following therapy	☐	☐	☐
	12. Cleans up after procedure	☐	☐	☐
	13. Ensures that patient is safe and comfortable	☐	☐	☐
	14. Documents the procedure in the patient's chart	☐	☐	☐

CHAPTER 17
HYPERINFLATION THERAPY

INTRODUCTION

The goal of hyperinflation therapy is to facilitate hyperinflation of the lungs, thereby preventing or reversing atelectasis, facilitating mobilization of secretions, and promoting effective coughing. Incentive spirometry, intermittent positive-pressure breathing (IPPB) therapy, and intrapulmonary percussive ventilation (IPV) therapy all are common modalities used to accomplish these goals.

Incentive spirometry relies on patient effort and muscular strength to accomplish its therapeutic goal. The incentive spirometer is used primarily to monitor and reinforce a patient's effort. It is a relatively inexpensive device that is effective in reducing postoperative complications (Indihar, Forsberg, & Adams, 1982).

IPPB therapy utilizes a mechanical ventilator to deliver positive pressure during inspiration. The extra pressure assists the patient to take deeper breaths.

IPV therapy is a combination of high-frequency phased pulse gas delivery and the administration of a dense aerosol. IPV therapy is administered using a special high-frequency ventilator. The high-frequency pulsed inspiratory gas flow increases mean airway pressure, while the percussive effect of the pulses assists in mobilization and clearance of secretions.

As a respiratory care practitioner, you must be familiar with the procedures and equipment used. The potential hazards, complications, and the desired therapeutic goals and objectives should be thoroughly understood.

KEY TERMS

- Incentive spirometer
- Incentive spirometry
- Intermittent positive-pressure breathing (IPPB)
- Intrapulmonary percussive ventilation (IPV)

OBJECTIVES

At the end of this chapter, you should be able to:

- Define the following:
  — Incentive spirometry
  — Intermittent positive-pressure breathing (IPPB) therapy
  — Intrapulmonary percussive ventilation (IPV) therapy
- Compare and contrast the clinical goals and indications of the following hyperinflation modalities:
  — Incentive spirometry
  — IPPB therapy
  — IPV therapy
- State the hazards, contraindications, and complications associated with the following hyperinflation modalities:
  — Incentive spirometry
  — IPPB therapy
  — IPV therapy
- Compare and contrast the following incentive spirometers:
  — Monaghan Spirocare
  — Voldyne

BIRD MARK 7 OR 8 VENTILATOR:

- Identify the following component parts:
  — Ambient chamber
  — Pressure chamber
  — Center body

- Identify and explain the function of the following controls:
  — Sensitivity
  — Flow rate
  — Air mix
  — Expiratory timer
  — Pressure
  Describe the effect each of the controls has on the following:
  — Tidal volume
  — FIO_2
  — I:E ratio
- Trace the flow of gas through the Bird Mark 7 breathing circuit.

BENNETT PR-2 VENTILATOR:

- Identify and explain the function of the following controls:
  — Pressure
  — Air dilution
  — Rate
  — Expiration time
  — Nebulizer controls (inspiratory and expiratory)
  — Negative pressure
  — Sensitivity
  — Terminal flow
  — Peak flow
  — System and control pressure manometers

(Continued)

- Identify the Bennett valve and describe the gas flow through it.
  — Explain how the Bennett valve terminates inspiration.
- Describe the effect of each control on the following:
  — Tidal volume
  — FiO_2
  — I:E ratio

BENNETT AP-5 VENTILATOR:

- Identify and explain the function of the following controls:
  — On/off
  — Pressure
  — Nebulizer

- Describe how the pressure control affects tidal volume delivery.
- Trace the flow of gas through a Bennett breathing circuit.

IPV THERAPY:

- Describe the controls of the IPV-1 ventilator:
  — Source pressure
  — Impact control
  — Manual inspiration
- Identify the components of the Phasitron and how it works.
- Describe how to increase tidal delivery and how to increase or decrease the percussive frequency.

CLINICAL PRACTICE GUIDELINES

AARC Clinical Practice Guideline
Incentive Spirometry

IS 4.0 INDICATIONS:

4.1 Presence of conditions predisposing to the development of pulmonary atelectasis
  4.1.1 Upper-abdominal surgery (2,4,9–14)
  4.1.2 Thoracic surgery (9,10,13–15)
  4.1.3 Surgery in patients with chronic obstructive pulmonary disease (COPD) (7,13–15)
4.2 Presence of pulmonary atelectasis (16)
4.3 Presence of a restrictive lung defect associated with quadraplegia and/or dysfunctional diaphragm (6,8,14,17,18)

IS 5.0 CONTRAINDICATIONS:

5.1 Patient cannot be instructed or supervised to assure appropriate use of the device.
5.2 Patient cooperation is absent (2,16) or patient is unable to understand or demonstrate proper use of the device. (16)
5.3 Is contraindicated in patients unable to deep breathe effectively (e.g., with vital capacity [VC] less than about 10 ml/kg or inspiratory capacity [IC] less than about one third of predicted).
5.4 The presence of an open tracheal stoma is not a contraindication but requires adaptation of the spirometer.

IS 6.0 HAZARDS AND COMPLICATIONS:

6.1 Ineffective unless closely supervised or performed as ordered (6)
6.2 Inappropriate as sole treatment for major lung collapse or consolidation
6.3 Hyperventilation
6.4 Barotrauma (emphysematous lungs) (19)
6.5 Discomfort secondary to inadequate pain control (15,18)
6.6 Hypoxia secondary to interruption of prescribed oxygen therapy if face mask or shield is being used

6.7 Exacerbation of bronchospasm
6.8 Fatigue (20,21)

IS 8.0 ASSESSMENT OF NEED:

8.1 Surgical procedure involving upper abdomen or thorax (4,5)
8.2 Conditions predisposing to development of atelectasis including immobility, poor pain control, and abdominal binders
8.3 Presence of neuromuscular disease involving respiratory musculature (8)

IS 9.0 ASSESSMENT OF OUTCOME:

9.1 Absence of or improvement in signs of atelectasis
  9.1.1 Decreased respiratory rate (16,17)
  9.1.2 Resolution of fever (2,18)
  9.1.3 Normal pulse rate (14)
  9.1.4 Absent crackles (rales) (20) or presence of or improvement in previously absent or diminished breath sounds
  9.1.5 Normal chest x-ray (2)
  9.1.6 Improved arterial oxygen tension (PaO_2) and decreased alveolar-arterial oxygen tension gradient, or $P(A–a)O_2$ (1,3,4,9,10)
  9.1.7 Increased VC and peak expiratory flows (4,16,17)
  9.1.8 Return of functional residual capacity (FRC) or VC to preoperative values (4,15–17) in absence of lung resection
9.2 Improved inspiratory muscle performance
  9.2.1 Attainment of preoperative flow and volume levels (1)
  9.2.2 Increased forced vital capacity (FVC)

IS 11.0 MONITORING:

Direct supervision of every patient performance is not necessary once the patient has demonstrated mastery of technique (6,16,23); however, preoperative instruction, volume goals, and feedback are essential to optimal performance.

11.1 Observation of patient performance and utilization
>**11.1.1** Frequency of sessions (16)
>**11.1.2** Number of breaths/session (16)
>**11.1.3** Inspiratory volume or flow goals achieved (16) and 3- to 5-second breath-hold maintained
>**11.1.4** Effort/motivation (16)

11.2 Periodic observation of patient compliance with technique, (6,16,23) with additional instruction as necessary

11.3 Device within reach of patient (5) and patient encouraged to perform independently

11.4 New and increasing inspiratory volumes established each day

11.5 Vital signs

Reprinted with permission from *Respiratory Care* 1991; 36: 1402–1405. The complete AARC Clinical Practice Guidelines are available from the AARC Web site (http://www.aarc.org), from the AARC Executive Office, or from *Respiratory Care* journal.

AARC Clinical Practice Guideline: Intermittent Positive-Pressure Breathing

IPPB 4.0 INDICATIONS:

4.1 The need to improve lung expansion
>**4.1.1** The presence of clinically important pulmonary atelectasis when other forms of therapy have been unsuccessful (incentive spirometry, chest physiotherapy, deep breathing exercises, positive airway pressure) or the patient cannot cooperate (9–14)
>**4.1.2** Inability to clear secretions adequately because of pathology that severely limits the ability to ventilate or cough effectively and failure to respond to other modes of treatment (13)

4.2 The need for short-term ventilatory support for patients who are hypoventilated as an alternative to tracheal intubation and continuous ventilatory support (12–21)

4.3 The need to deliver aerosol medication (We are not addressing aerosol delivery for patients on long-term mechanical ventilation.) (4)
>**4.3.1** Although some authors oppose the use of IPPB in the treatment of severe bronchospasm (acute asthma, unstable or status asthmaticus, exacerbated COPD), (6,22–24) we recommend a careful, closely supervised trial of IPPB when treatment using other techniques (metered dose inhaler [MDI] or nebulizer) has been unsuccessful (1,25–33)
>**4.3.2** IPPB may be used to deliver aerosol medications to patients with fatigue as a result of ventilatory muscle weakness (e.g.,

failure to wean from mechanical ventilation, neuromuscular disease, kyphoscoliosis) or chronic conditions in which intermittent ventilatory support is indicated (e.g., ventilatory support for home care patients and the more recent use of nasal IPPV for respiratory insufficiency) (1,15–21)

IPPB 5.0 CONTRAINDICATIONS:
Although no absolute contraindications to the use of IPPB therapy (except the oft-cited tension pneumothorax) have been reported, the patient with any of the following should be carefully evaluated before a decision is made to initiate IPPB therapy.
>**5.1** Intracranial pressure (ICP) >15 mm Hg
>**5.2** Hemodynamic instability
>**5.3** Recent facial, oral, or skull surgery
>**5.4** Tracheoesophageal fistula
>**5.5** Recent esophageal surgery
>**5.6** Active hemoptysis
>**5.7** Nausea
>**5.8** Air swallowing
>**5.9** Active untreated tuberculosis
>**5.10** Radiographic evidence of bleb
>**5.11** Singulation (hiccups)

IPPB 6.0 HAZARDS/COMPLICATIONS:
>**6.1** Increased airway resistance (34)
>**6.2** Barotrauma, pneumothorax (34)
>**6.3** Nosocomial infection (34)
>**6.4** Hypocarbia (4,35)
>**6.5** Hemoptysis (4,35)
>**6.6** Hyperoxia when oxygen is the gas source (34)
>**6.7** Gastric distention (34)
>**6.8** Impaction of secretions (associated with inadequately humidified gas mixture) (34)
>**6.9** Psychological dependence (34)
>**6.10** Impedance of venous return (34)
>**6.11** Exacerbation of hypoxemia
>**6.12** Hypoventilation
>**6.13** Increased mismatch of ventilation and perfusion
>**6.14** Air trapping, auto-PEEP, overdistended alveoli

IPPB 8.0 ASSESSMENT OF NEED:
>**8.1** Presence of atelectasis
>**8.2** Reduced pulmonary function as evidenced by reduction in timed volumes and vital capacity (e.g., FEV_1 <65% predicted, FVC <70% predicted, MVV <50% predicted, 60 or VC <10 ml/kg) precluding an effective cough
>**8.3** Neuromuscular disorders or kyphoscoliosis with associated decreases in lung volumes and capacities
>**8.4** Fatigue or muscle weakness with impending respiratory failure

(Continued)

(CPG Continued)

8.5 Presence of acute severe bronchospasm or exacerbated COPD that fails to respond to other therapy

> **8.5.1** Regardless of the type of delivery device used (MDI with spacer or small-volume, large-volume, or ultrasonic nebulizer), it is important to recognize that the dose of the drug needs to be titrated to give the maximum benefit. (37,39)
>
> **8.5.2** Based on proven therapeutic efficacy, variety of medications, and cost-effectiveness, the MDI with accessory device should be the first method to consider for administration of aerosol. (42,55–59,61,62)

8.6 With demonstrated effectiveness, the patient's preference for a positive-pressure device should be honored.

IPPB 9.0 ASSESSMENT OF OUTCOME:

9.1 Tidal volume during IPPB greater than during spontaneous breathing (by at least 25%)

9.2 FEV_1 or peak flow increase

9.3 Cough more effective with treatment

9.4 Secretion clearance enhanced as a consequence of deep breathing and coughing

9.5 Chest x-ray improved

9.6 Breath sounds improved

9.7 Favorable patient subjective response

IPPB 11.0 MONITORING:

Items from the following list should be chosen as appropriate for the specific patient:

11.1 Performance of machine trigger sensitivity, peak pressure, flow setting, FIO_2 inspiratory time, expiratory time, plateau pressure, PEEP

11.2 Respiratory rate and volume

11.3 Peak flow or FEV_1/FVC

11.4 Pulse rate and rhythm from ECG if available

11.5 Patient subjective response to therapy — pain, discomfort, dyspnea

11.6 Sputum production — quantity, color, consistency, and odor

11.7 Mental function

11.8 Skin color

11.9 Breath sounds

11.10 Blood pressure

11.11 Arterial hemoglobin saturation by pulse oximetry (if hypoxemia is suspected)

11.12 Intracranial pressure (ICP) in patients for whom ICP is of critical importance

11.13 Chest radiograph

Reprinted with permission from *Respiratory Care* 1993; 38: 1189–1195. The complete AARC Clinical Practice Guidelines are available from the AARC Web site (http://www.aarc.org), from the AARC Executive Office, or from *Respiratory Care* journal.

HYPERVENTILATION MODALITIES

Incentive Spirometry

Incentive spirometry is a modality that utilizes the patient's own muscular effort to accomplish hyperinflation of the lungs. A device commonly called an *incentive spirometer* is used to provide biofeedback on the degree of patient inspiratory effort. The patient is then encouraged to perform a voluntary maximal inspiration with a 3- to 5-second inspiratory hold before exhalation is begun.

Intermittent Positive-Pressure Breathing

Intermittent positive-pressure breathing (IPPB) is a therapeutic modality utilizing a ventilator to deliver positive pressure during the inspiratory phase of breathing. The expiratory phase is passive and the patient exhales to ambient pressure. Typically, the breathing circuit includes a nebulizer to deliver a medication during the treatment. IPPB is a short-term therapeutic modality and is not a means of continuous ventilatory support.

Intrapulmonary Percussive Ventilation

Intrapulmonary percussive ventilation (IPV) is applied using a high-frequency ventilator. The delivery of small volumes of gas at a high frequency (100 to 250/min) to the airways via a mouthpiece serves to increase mean airway pressures, while the pulsed gas flow helps to break up secretions and to distribute ventilation more evenly. Coughing following IPV therapy further helps to mobilize and clear secretions. The capability to deliver a dense aerosol during therapy allows administration of bronchodilators or mucokinetic or vasoactive agents to promote bronchial hygiene further.

GOALS OF AND INDICATIONS FOR HYPERINFLATION THERAPY

Although the hyperinflation modalities are different, frequently their clinical goals and indications for therapy are similar.

Reversal of Atelectasis

Postoperative pain and the effects of anesthetics and analgesics reduce the depth of breathing and the frequency of coughing even in relatively normal patients. Often the result is atelectasis and, potentially, pneumonia.

The three hyperinflation modalities provide methods for expanding a patient's lungs. Incentive spirometry relies on a patient's own muscular effort to accomplish the task. To use this modality effectively, the patient must be alert, cooperative, and able to follow directions well. IPPB utilizes a ventilator to assist the patient. All hyperinflation methods can be equally effective in preventing postoperative pulmonary complications (Indihar, Forsberg, & Adams, 1982).

Improvement of the Cough or Cough Mechanism

An increase in tidal volume will enable the patient to generate greater flows and volumes during a cough. The greater the flow, the more effective a cough will be in expelling secretions.

All hyperinflation modalities provide methods for increasing inspiratory volumes. Incentive spirometry can generate large intrapleural pressures. These pressures help to maintain airway patency and to prevent atelectasis. It has also been suggested that hyperinflation stimulates the type II alveolar cells to produce surfactant, a fluid that reduces alveolar surface tension. IPPB may assist some patients by providing augmented volumes to facilitate more effective coughing (American Thoracic Society [ATS], 1980).

Medication Delivery

IPPB is unique among the three hyperinflation modalities in its ability to deliver medication. Aerosol deposition with volume-oriented IPPB delivery has been found to be equal to that achieved with more simple methods of aerosol therapy (Mihailoff & Gentry, 1985). Additionally, some patients who have difficulty coordinating their respiratory pattern may receive more effective bronchodilator therapy with IPPB than with other, simpler methods of aerosol therapy (ATS, 1980).

HAZARDS AND COMPLICATIONS OF HYPERVENTILATION THERAPY

Hypocapnea Induced by Hyperventilation

Hyperventilation may occur as a result of any hyperinflation modality. Each results in the patient's taking deeper breaths than normal.

Commonly reported signs and symptoms are dizziness, a feeling of light-headedness, a tingling sensation, loss of balance, and headache. These adverse reactions can be prevented to some extent by providing frequent rest periods during therapy sessions. Allow the patient to rest for about 1 minute after five to seven breaths.

Interruption of Hypoxic Drive

Patients with severe chronic obstructive lung disease are stimulated to breathe because with this disease, the body senses a need for oxygen. The normal response to increased CO_2 levels—the hypoxic drive—is absent. If such patients are given too much oxygen, that stimulation to breathe may diminish or cease. Patients with chronic lung disease receiving oxygen therapy must be closely monitored with serial blood gas determinations or oximetry.

IPPB therapy is administered with compressed gas. Departmental policy and the availability of compressed air often determine whether air or oxygen is used. Most hospitals have oxygen piped into almost every room, making its administration convenient. When IPPB is administered with oxygen, the delivered oxygen concentration will range from approximately 64% to 90% if the air-mix mode is used during inspiration (McPherson, 1995). This concentration of oxygen may be very hazardous to the patient with severe chronic obstructive lung disease. If oxygen administration is required, an oxygen blender may be used to regulate precisely the concentration being delivered.

If in doubt, use compressed air as the source gas to power the ventilator. IPPB therapy may be administered safely in this way without the interruption of the hypoxic drive.

Decreased Cardiac Output

The application of IPPB increases the mean intrathoracic pressure during inspiration. The applied pressure is contained within the thoracic cavity, increasing the intrathoracic pressure above normal levels. IPPB therapy, if improperly administered, can compress the mediastinum enough to impede the venous return from the periphery through the vena cava. Impedance of venous return, combined with the squeezing effect on the mediastinum, will result in a markedly decreased cardiac output and a fall in blood pressure. The risk of these abnormalities is especially high if the patient is hypovolemic.

This hazard may be alleviated by maintaining the inspiratory-to-expiratory ratio (I:E ratio) within normal limits or greater. A normal I:E ratio in a spontaneously breathing person is 1:2—if inspiration occurs in 1 second, expiration will take 2 seconds. If IPPB is administered with an I:E ratio of 1:2 or greater, adequate time will be available to allow the great vessels and the heart to fill with blood. The expiratory phase in IPPB therapy is passive, with no positive pressure applied. This lack of positive pressure will allow the intrathoracic pressure to return to normal levels.

The I:E ratio may be manipulated during IPPB therapy by the adjustment of the inspiratory flow control (if available) or by proper patient instruction.

Increased Intracranial Pressure

The increased intrathoracic pressure combined with decreased cardiac output may cause an increased intracranial pressure. Impedance of venous return results in backup of blood flow in the cranium. The skull is quite rigid, and expansion due to an increased volume is not possible. If venous return is impeded severely enough, intracranial pressure may go up significantly. Patients with already elevated intracranial pressures, due to head trauma or other causes, are more susceptible to development of increased intracranial pressure from IPPB therapy.

Increased intracranial pressure may be avoided by maintaining the I:E ratio during IPPB therapy at 1:2 or greater. This allows adequate filling of the great vessels and heart between the applications of positive pressure.

Pneumothorax

The incidence of pneumothorax resulting from IPPB therapy is low (Ziment, 1984). If IPPB is administered using excessive volumes, caution should be exercised and the patient should be closely monitored.

Application of pressures exceeding 25 cm H_2O should be approached with caution. Ensure that the I:E ratio is maintained within normal ranges and carefully monitor exhaled volumes. Some patients may be able to tolerate this pressure, but others will not. Carefully monitor your patient when using pressures in this range. Observe your patient for the following signs or symptoms: sudden onset of chest pain and sudden onset of dyspnea. If your patient has either of these symptoms, discontinue therapy and carefully evaluate the patient.

Patients with end-stage emphysema may be especially at risk for this complication. The emphysematous lung's alveolar septa are destroyed in the disease process, leaving large blebs. These blebs trap air on expiration and are not capable of withstanding high pressures.

Untreated Pneumothorax

Administering IPPB therapy to a patient with an untreated pneumothorax is extremely hazardous and therefore contraindicated. A pneumothorax is the presence of free air in the thoracic cavity, predominantly in the pleural space. The usual treatment of the condition involves the placement of a chest tube into the pleural space and evacuation of the free air by the application of vacuum or suction.

Administering IPPB therapy to a patient with an untreated pneumothorax could cause a tension pneumothorax to develop. A tension pneumothorax is the presence of free air in the thoracic cavity at a pressure greater than ambient pressure. The pressure difference will cause lung collapse on the affected side with compression of the heart and great vessels, impeding the ability of the heart to circulate blood. If the pressure continues, eventual circulatory collapse may result.

If you suspect a tension pneumothorax has developed during IPPB therapy, auscultate and percuss the chest. With pneumothorax, auscultation on the affected side will indicate absent or diminished breath sounds. Percussion on the affected side will yield a hyperresonant percussion tone. You may be able to observe deviation of the trachea to the unaffected side as a result of the compression caused by the pressure in the thoracic cavity from the tension pneumothorax. IPPB must be terminated and the pneumothorax must be treated immediately, as it is a life-threatening condition.

If a patient has a patent operating chest tube in place, IPPB therapy may be safely administered.

INCENTIVE SPIROMETERS

Voldyne Volumetric Exerciser

The Voldyne is a single-patient-use, disposable incentive spirometer manufactured by Sherwood Medical, St. Louis, MO. The Voldyne is a relatively simple device consisting of a vertical tube with a piston that indicates the inspired volume and a yellow float to indicate inspiratory flow. Figure 17-1 is a photograph of a Voldyne Volumetric Exerciser. As the patient inhales deeply, a negative pressure is created above the inspiratory float and the piston. The piston rises, indicating the maximum inspired

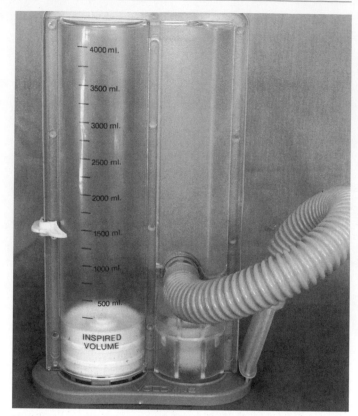

Figure 17-1 *The Voldyne Volumetric Exerciser*

volume. The yellow float will remain suspended as long as inspiratory flow exists. The patient is encouraged to inhale as deeply as possible and to achieve a maximal inspiratory volume. During the maneuver, you should also encourage the patient to keep the yellow float suspended at all times. A movable marker may be raised or lowered, indicating the desired volume for the patient to achieve.

Monaghan Spirocare

Two models of Spirocare are in clinical use. The larger earlier model uses 115 V AC power. The more recently developed battery-powered unit is smaller. Both devices work on the same principle.

Both spirometers rely on an electronic flow-sensing device. Within the handheld mouthpiece is a clear plastic tube containing a small turbine suspended on the longitudinal axis of the tube. As the patient inhales, the turbine spins. The convolutions on the turbine interrupt a light beam in the handheld mouthpiece. The greater the number of interruptions of the light beam, the faster the air flows through the mouthpiece. This flow is electronically converted to a volume inside the spirometer. As the volume increases, a series of indicators light up in sequence. When the patient inhales a greater volume, more lights on the indicator panel light up. Thus the patient can be encouraged to take deeper and deeper breaths. Figure 17-2 is a photograph of a Monaghan Spirocare.

Built into the spirometer is a counter indicating the number of times a preset volume has been achieved.

The front of the older unit has a counter on one side where you can set a desired number of volumes to be

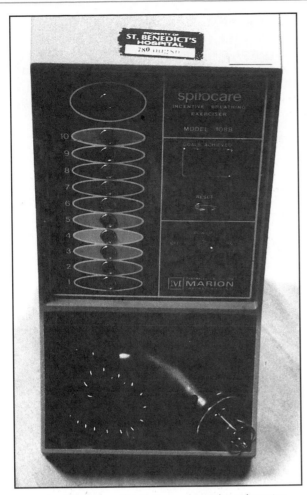

Figure 17-2 *The Monaghan Spirocare incentive spirometer*

achieved. You can then encourage the patient to match that number by working independently on his or her own. As the patient achieves the desired volume, the counter increases in increments of 1. Desired volumes may be set either inside the side panel on the spirometer, on the older unit, or under the indicator panel, on the newer unit.

The Spirocare devices also have a light indicator to encourage an inspiratory hold. When a volume is reached, a large light on the top of the spirometer illuminates and stays lit for 3 seconds. Patients should be encouraged not to exhale until the light goes out.

THE BIRD MARK 7 VENTILATOR

The Bird Mark 7 is a pressure-limited patient- or time-cycled ventilator used in IPPB therapy. It is pneumatically powered, requiring a 50 psi compressed gas source for operation. Because of its pneumatic characteristics and delivered tidal volume, flow rate and oxygen concentration tend to change as the patient's respiratory status changes.

The Bird Mark 7 is a small, portable ventilator, which may be powered with compressed gas cylinders or hospital piping systems. The Mark 7 is frequently used in the emergency and transport settings. Structurally the device may be divided into three main components: the ambient chamber on the left, made of a transparent green

plastic; the center body in the middle, machined from an aluminum alloy; and the pressure chamber on the right, slightly smaller than the ambient chamber and made from a transparent green plastic.

Control Function

The controls on the Bird Mark 7 are numbered. Each control is discussed in sequence in this section. If a Bird Mark 7 ventilator is available, refer to it as you read.

1: Pressure

The pressure control regulates the amount of pressure that must build up in the breathing circuit before inspiration is terminated. In this manner it determines the tidal volume being delivered to the patient. The pressure control, in combination with the flow rate control, determines the tidal volume, I:E ratio, and delivered oxygen concentration.

Pressure is controlled by a movable arm on the far right of the ventilator. Figure 17-3 shows the pressure control. The control determines the position of a magnet relative to a metal plate. During inspiration, pressure builds in the pressure chamber and pushes against a diaphragm attached to the center body. Eventually, the force from the pressure exceeds the magnetic pull from the pressure control adjustment and moves the diaphragm to the left. When it does, a switch attached to the diaphragm cycles the ventilator off and inspiration is terminated.

2: Air Mix

The air mix control provides a limited amount of control over the fraction of inspired oxygen (FiO_2) delivered to the patient. It is a valve that determines whether the flow delivered to the patient will be pure source gas (the gas powering the ventilator) or source gas mixed with room air. Figure 17-3 shows the air mix control, located near the bottom of the center body.

If the air mix control is pushed in to the on position, only source gas is delivered to the patient. If the source gas is oxygen, and the air mix control is pushed in, 100%

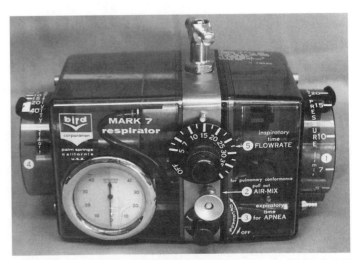

Figure 17-3 *A photograph showing the controls on the Bird Mark 7 ventilator: 1, pressure; 2, air mix; 3, expiratory timer; 4, sensitivity; 5, flow rate*

oxygen will be delivered to the patient. If the source gas is room air, the delivered gas will be air.

With the air mix control pulled to the out position, gas flow is directed through a Venturi opening in the ambient chamber. Figure 17-4 shows the Venturi. The high-velocity jet entrains ambient air, diluting the source gas concentration. When the source gas is oxygen, depending on the other control settings, the delivered oxygen concentration may range from 65% to 95%. It is important to monitor the FiO_2 frequently if specific oxygen concentrations are important.

3: Expiratory Timer

The expiratory timer is not used for IPPB therapy. It is used to cycle the ventilator on when a patient is apneic. Attempts to use it on a spontaneously breathing patient will cause asynchronous ventilation leading to increased work of breathing, as well as frustration for both the practitioner and the patient. It is located at the base of the center body. Figure 17-3 shows the expiratory timer. This control is a pneumatic timer; it controls the ventilatory rate by allowing source gas to leak out of a closed chamber. The

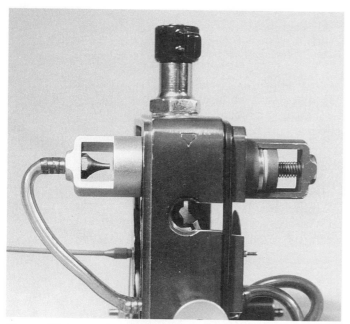

Figure 17-4 *The Venturi located on the center body inside the Bird Mark 7 ventilator*

faster the source gas leaks, the more quickly the chamber empties, increasing the ventilatory rate. Conversely, a slow leak will provide a long time interval, decreasing the rate. Attached to a diaphragm in the chamber is a rod that mechanically triggers inspiration by physically moving the metal plate in the ambient chamber, initiating inspiration.

4: Sensitivity

The sensitivity control regulates how much effort must be exerted by the patient to cycle the ventilator on for inspiration. It is controlled by a movable arm on the extreme left-hand side. Figure 17-3 shows the sensitivity control. Functionally, the sensitivity control determines the position of a magnet relative to a metal disk attached to a diaphragm on the center body. When the magnet is placed closer to the metal plate, more effort is required to initiate inspiration owing to the increased magnetic attraction. To make it easier to initiate inspiration, the sensitivity control arm is rotated toward the rear of the ventilator. This control moves the magnet farther from the metal plate, reducing magnetic attraction, and hence the effort required to initiate a breath.

5: Flow Rate

Adjustment of the flow rate determines the length of inspiration and, to some extent, the delivered tidal volume. Flow rate is adjusted by a black knob attached to a needle valve located near the top of the center body. Figure 17-3 shows the flow rate control. The flow is determined by the size of the opening created by the position of the needle valve relative to its seat.

Gas Flow through the Breathing Circuit

Inspiration

During inspiration, gas flows to the patient through both the large-bore tubing and the small-diameter tubing. This flow through both tubes begins simultaneously as inspiration is initiated. Figure 17-5 identifies the components of a disposable circuit.

The large-bore tubing is attached to the outlet of the ventilator. Figure 17-6 shows its attachment. This gas will either be pure source gas or source gas mixed with room air (determined by the air mix control).

The flow through the small-diameter tubing powers the nebulizer and closes the exhalation valve on the

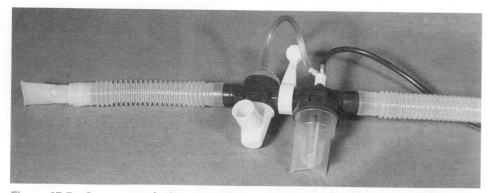

Figure 17-5 *Components of a disposable IPPB circuit configured for the Bird ventilator*

breathing circuit. This flow is pure source gas. When the flow closes the exhalation valve, gas flow through the circuit can go only in one direction — toward the patient.

Figure 17-7 is a diagram showing gas flow during inspiration.

Expiration

Whereas inspiration during IPPB occurs with the assistance of positive pressure applied to the airways, expiration is passive. The elastic recoil of the lungs and thorax allows the patient to exhale passively. During expiration, all gas flow through the breathing circuit toward the patient, as well as gas delivered to close the exhalation valve, has stopped. With no flow, the exhalation valve is open. As the patient exhales, the gas flows through the exhalation port out into the room. Figure 17-8 shows gas flow through the breathing circuit on expiration.

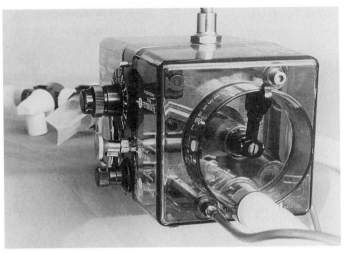

Figure 17-6 *Attachment of the circuit to the Bird ventilator*

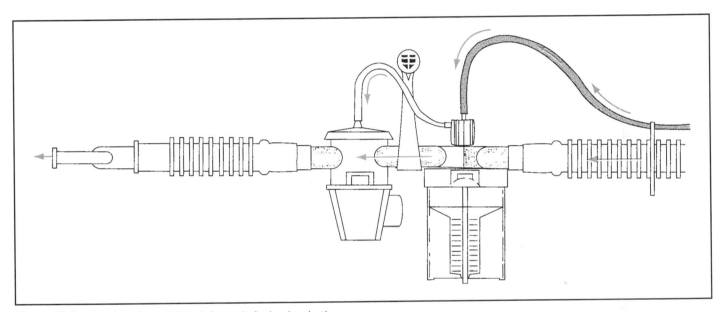

Figure 17-7 *Gas flow through the Bird circuit during inspiration*

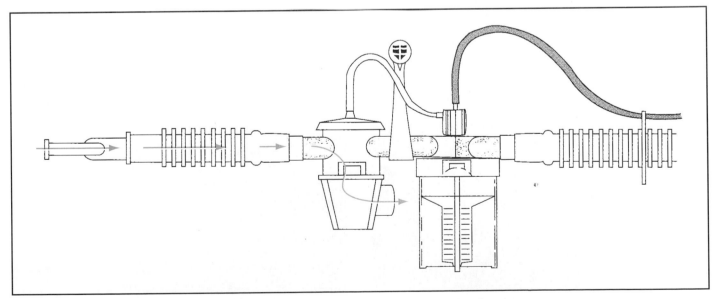

Figure 17-8 *Gas flow through the Bird circuit during expiration*

THE BENNETT PR-2 VENTILATOR

The Bennett PR-2 ventilator is a pneumatically powered, pressure-limited, time- or patient-cycled ventilator used for IPPB therapy. It requires a 50 psi compressed gas source for operation. Because of its pneumatic characteristics and delivered tidal volume, the flow rate and oxygen concentration tend to change as the patient's respiratory status changes.

The Bennett PR-2 may be powered by compressed gas cylinders or a hospital piping system. It is frequently used in the emergency and anesthesia recovery settings. Its small size and portability facilitate its use in compact spaces.

Controls
Pressure Control

The pressure control regulates the amount of pressure that must build up in the breathing circuit before inspiration is terminated. In this manner it determines the tidal volume being delivered to the patient. The pressure control is a low-pressure regulator that controls inspiratory pressure. It operates in a similar way as for the regulators discussed in Chapter 12, "Oxygen Supply Systems." It is adjustable from 0 to 45 cm H_2O pressure. The pressure control is a large black knob located at the center of the ventilator. Figure 17-9 shows the pressure control.

Air Dilution

The air dilution control on the Bennett PR-2 ventilator has a similar function to the air mix control on the Bird Mark 7 ventilator. It dilutes the source gas with ambient air by using a Venturi. If the control is pushed in, gas is diverted through the Venturi. When the control is pulled out, the ventilator operates on 100% source gas. If the source gas is oxygen, and the air dilution control is pulled out, 100% source gas will be delivered to the patient. When the ventilator is operating with oxygen as the source gas and the air dilution control pushed in, the delivered FIO_2 will range from 40% to 100%. It is important to monitor the FIO_2 delivery if the oxygen concentration is critical. This control is on the right side of the ventilator. Figure 17-10 shows its location.

Rate

The rate control is not normally used for IPPB therapy. It is a control used when the patient is apneic. Attempts to use it on a spontaneously breathing patient will cause asynchronous respiration with increased work of breathing, as well as frustration for both the practitioner and the patient.

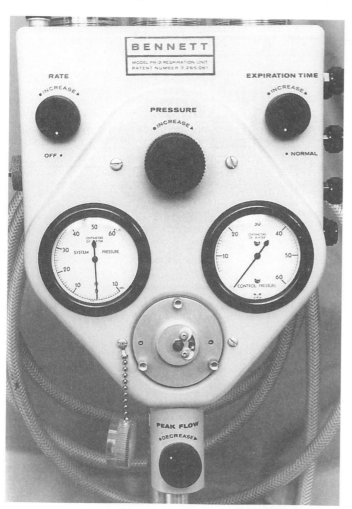

Figure 17-9 *The controls on the front of the Bennett PR-2 ventilator*

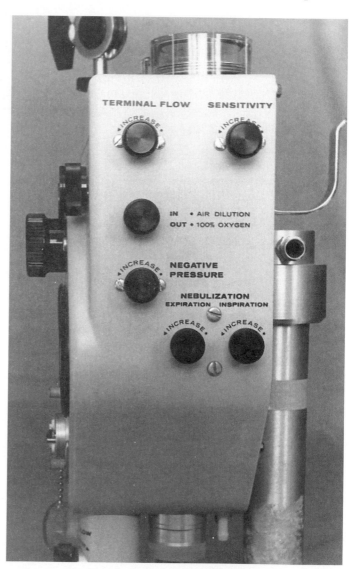

Figure 17-10 *Controls on the right side of the Bennett PR-2 ventilator*

This control is a needle valve. The flow of gas past the needle valve determines the length of expiratory time and therefore when the ventilator cycles on for inspiration. Figure 17-9 shows the rate control's location.

Expiration Time

The expiration time control is not normally used for IPPB therapy. It is a control that modifies the rate control setting by further lengthening expiratory time. By turning the control clockwise, a needle valve closes an opening, further reducing flow of gas from the rate control and lengthening expiratory time. Figure 17-9 shows the location of the expiration time control.

Nebulizer Controls: Inspiration and Expiration

The Bennett PR-2 is fairly unusual in that it provides controls for regulation of a nebulizer during both the inspiratory and the expiratory phases. The inspiration nebulizer control affects the operation of the nebulizer during the inspiratory phase. By rotating the control clockwise, a needle valve is opened, which increases the flow of gas to the nebulizer. The nebulizer is powered by 100% source gas. Its use affects the delivered FIO_2 when the ventilator is powered by compressed oxygen as a source gas, unless the ventilator is set with the dilution control on 100% oxygen.

The expiration nebulizer control provides a flow of gas during the expiratory phase to power the nebulizer. Normally, it is opened only slightly to fill the dead space between the nebulizer and the patient's mouth with aerosol in preparation for the next inspiration. Figure 17-10 shows both the inspiration and expiration nebulizer controls.

Negative Pressure Control

The negative pressure control allows for the application of up to negative 6 cm H_2O pressure to the airway during expiration. Its function is to assist the patient in evacuating inspired gas on exhalation. This control directs a 50 psi gas source to a Venturi.

The negative pressure from the Venturi is applied both to the Bennett valve (described later for the Bennett AP-5 ventilator) and to the breathing circuit. To operate properly, this control requires a special manifold cap to apply the negative pressure to the breathing circuit.

The location of this control is on the right of the ventilator, as shown in Figure 17-10. Negative pressure is seldom used with IPPB therapy.

Sensitivity

Sensitivity on the Bennett PR-2 ventilator is preset at a level of approximately 0.5 cm H_2O pressure. Use of the sensitivity control can decrease the amount of effort required of the patient to cycle the ventilator on for inspiration. It accomplishes this by directing a flow of gas against the upper drum vane in the Bennett valve. As the control is turned counterclockwise, a needle valve opens, initiating the gas flow. The farther it is opened, the higher the flow is, resulting in less effort required to cycle the ventilator on. Figure 17-10 shows its location.

Terminal Flow

This control, located on the right side of the ventilator, helps to compensate for leaks in the breathing circuit, or assists in cycling the ventilator off for expiration in delivering pressures greater than 20 to 25 cm H_2O. If a patient is unable to create a seal on the mouthpiece, the terminal flow control can help compensate for the system's leak. By turning this control, a needle valve is opened, directing flow through a Venturi that accelerates the flow of gas distal to the Bennett valve.

This control aids the closing of the Bennett valve by allowing the flow past the valve to decrease to the point where it will terminate inspiration. Figure 17-10 shows the location of this control.

It is important to note that using this control dilutes the delivered gas with room air via the Venturi used in its operation. If you are attempting to deliver 100% oxygen, this control will lower the delivered FIO_2.

Peak Flow

Peak flow delivered from the Bennett PR-2 will vary depending on the pressure in the breathing circuit. When inspiration begins, pressure in the circuit is low and the flow rate is high. As pressure in the circuit builds during inspiration, flow constantly decreases owing to the decrease in the pressure gradient across the Bennett valve. Finally, at end-inspiration, flow is minimal. In a sense, the valve is sensitive to the flow needs of the patient.

The peak flow control provides a variable orifice distal to the Bennett valve. It limits the maximum flow rate delivered from the ventilator, but not the delivered flow. By decreasing the orifice, flow is restricted. This control is not the same as the flow rate control on the Bird Mark 7 ventilator. It limits the maximum flow from the ventilator. In its fully closed position, flow is limited to 15 L/min.

The peak flow control is positioned below the Bennett valve. Figure 17-9 shows its location.

System and Control Pressure Manometers

These two manometers are located on the front of the ventilator. The one on the left indicates the system or breathing circuit pressure. The one on the right indicates the pressure set by the pressure control.

The control pressure manometer indicates the desired pressure to be delivered to the breathing circuit. It determines in part the tidal volume, I:E ratio, and FIO_2. This pressure is adjusted using the pressure control described previously.

The system pressure reflects the pressure in the breathing circuit.

BENNETT AP-5 VENTILATOR

The Puritan Bennett AP-5 ventilator is designed primarily for home use (Figure 17-11). It is electrically powered and does not require a compressed gas source for operation. The controls were designed simply so that the average patient can use the ventilator correctly and effectively.

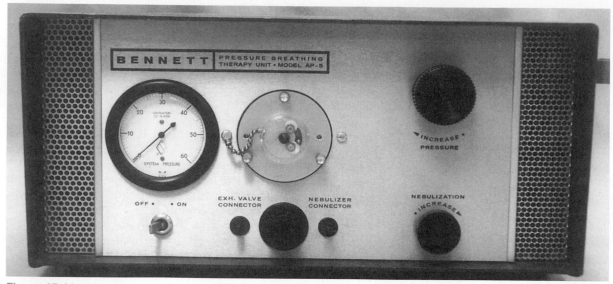

Figure 17-11 *A photograph of the Puritan Bennett AP-5 ventilator*

Controls

The controls consist of an on/off switch, a pressure control, and a nebulizer control. Airway pressure may be monitored by observing the pressure manometer.

On/Off Switch

The on/off switch controls the flow of electricity to the internal air compressor, which powers the ventilator. The AP-5 ventilator operates on 120 V alternating current (AC). Turning the switch on activates the compressor.

Pressure Control

The pressure control is the large black knob at the upper right of the control panel. Pressures may be adjusted between 0 and 30 cm H_2O. The pressure control operates using a spring-loaded disk that vents excess pressure to the atmosphere.

Flow through the pressure control is augmented by a Venturi. Ambient air is filtered by a 40-micrometer filter before entering the Venturi. The Venturi boosts the flow out of the pressure regulator, providing a flow of between 75 and 90 L/min.

Nebulizer Control

The nebulizer on the AP-5 operates continuously during both inspiration and exhalation. The nebulizer control is a needle valve. Moving the control toward the "Increase" position increases flow through the nebulizer, thus increasing the rate of nebulization.

Pressure Manometer

The pressure manometer is used to monitor the inspiratory pressure during IPPB therapy. The manometer is calibrated from 0 to 60 cm H_2O.

The Bennett Valve

The Bennett valve is analogous to an on/off switch. It controls the cycling of the ventilator. It is a flow-sensitive valve, responding to the inspiratory flow created by the patient. Little effort is required to cycle it (only 0.5 cm H_2O).

Figure 17-12 shows a simplified schematic of the Bennett valve. As the patient initiates inspiration, the negative pressure generated causes the lower vane to drop, rotating the drum. In this manner, the valve senses the flow. As the drum rotates, gas flows through the drum, rotating it farther by providing pressure above the vane. When the drum is rotated fully counterclockwise, maximum flow is occurring. Figure 17-13 depicts the inspiratory sequence.

As pressure builds in the circuit (and the patient's lungs), flow decreases. As the flow decreases, the weight on the right of the valve rotates it clockwise, closing it. When the flow reaches 1 to 3 L/min, the weight is sufficient to close the valve completely owing to gravity. Figure 17-14 shows the expiratory sequence.

Gas Flow through the Breathing Circuit

The flow through the Bennett breathing circuit is similar to that for the Bird Mark 7 breathing circuit, except that there are two small-diameter tubes.

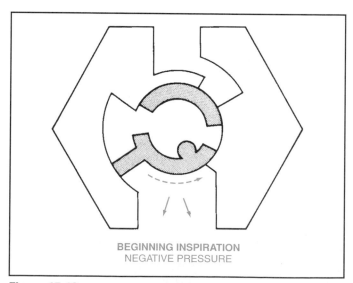

BEGINNING INSPIRATION
NEGATIVE PRESSURE

Figure 17-12 *A schematic of the Bennett valve*

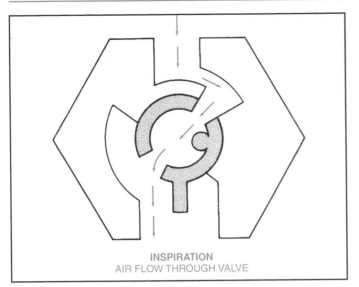

Figure 17-13 *A schematic illustrating the operation of the Bennett valve during inspiration*

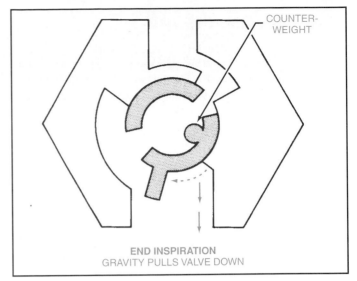

Figure 17-14 *A schematic illustrating the operation of the Bennett valve as it closes*

The large-bore tube is connected to the outlet of the ventilator. It conducts the main flow of gas to the patient.

One small-diameter line powers the exhalation valve, closing it on inspiration. In the closed position, gas can flow through the circuit only toward the patient. On expiration, no gas pressure is supplied to the exhalation valve, and the patient exhales passively to the atmospheric pressure. The second small-diameter line powers the nebulizer. The inspiration and expiration nebulizer controls determine the phase in which the nebulizer is operating. Figure 17-15 shows the breathing circuit and the flow through it.

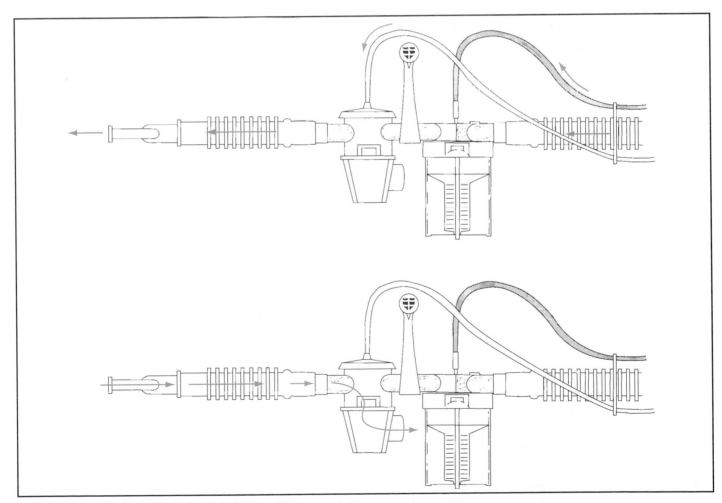

Figure 17-15 *Gas flow through the Bennett IPPB circuit*

PERCUSSIONAIRE IPV-1

The Percussionaire IPV-1 (Figure 17-16) is an acute care ventilator designed for the management of patients with cardiopulmonary disease in whom secretion mobilization is desirable. This ventilator is used to deliver IPV therapy.

Controls

Source Pressure

The source pressure control is located on the side panel behind the hinged door on the front of the ventilator. The source pressure is adjustable to between 20 and 50 psi. Source pressure determines the impact velocity of the percussive pulses. For most patients an initial setting of around 30 psi is recommended.

Impact Control

The impact control regulates the frequency of the percussive ventilatory pulses sent to the Phasitron (discussed later on). Frequencies are adjustable between 100 and 250 cycles per minute.

Manual Inspiration

By depressing the manual inspiration button, the ventilator can be set to the oscillatory mode. This feature is provided in the event that the ventilator is used for cardiopulmonary resuscitation efforts.

Phasitron

The Phasitron provides a mechanical and pneumatic interface between the IPV ventilator and the patient's airway. The Phasitron (Figure 17-17) consists of a jet, an

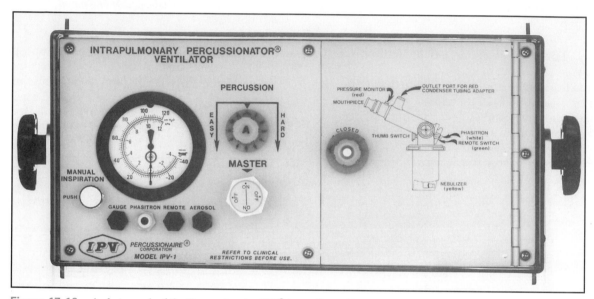

Figure 17-16 *A photograph of the Percussionaire IPV®-1 ventilator (Courtesy of* Percussionaire Corporation, Sandpoint, ID)

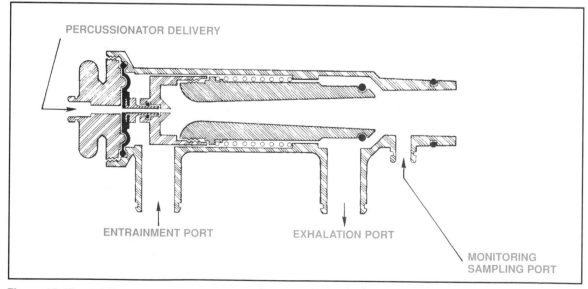

Figure 17-17 *A full section showing the Phasitron® (Courtesy of* Percussionaire Corporation, Sandpoint, ID)

orifice servo diaphragm, and a spring-loaded sliding Venturi body. Pulsed gas from the IPV ventilator enters the orifice servo diaphragm and jet of the Phasitron. As the diaphragm distorts, the sliding Venturi body advances, closing the expiratory port and delivering gas to the patient. When gas pressure is removed from the orifice diaphragm/jet, spring tension slides the Venturi body back, opening the exhalation port. A dense aerosol is drawn into the Phasitron assembly through the entrainment port adjacent to the orifice servo diaphragm.

Pulsed gas delivery from the IPV device begins when the patient depresses the thumb button. The patient actively inhales during pulsed gas delivery. The patient may release the thumb button, stopping pulsed gas delivery for exhalation, or alternatively, may exhale actively against pulsed gas delivered through the Phasitron.

Changing Tidal Volume Delivery and Ventilatory Frequency

Tidal volume delivery is determined by the setting on the source pressure control. As source pressure is increased, tidal volume delivery increases. Source pressure may be adjusted between 20 and 50 psi. It is suggested to begin therapy at around 30 psi. If chest expansion and percussive effect are inadequate at this setting, increase source pressure.

Ventilatory frequency is adjusted using the impact control. As frequency is increased, the effect of source pressure is attenuated. At lower frequencies, each pulsed gas delivery is more accentuated than with higher frequencies at the same source pressure. It is suggested that most patients start with the control at mid-position. Rotating the control to the left increases the frequency and decreases the effect of source pressure (impulse).

OBJECTIVES

At the end of this chapter, you should be able to:

* Demonstrate the use of an incentive spirometer including:
  — Patient instruction
  — Use of equipment
  — Troubleshooting of equipment
  — Emphasis of self-motivation on the part of the patient
* Demonstrate the correct operation of the Bird Mark 7, Bennett PR-2, and Bennett AP-5 ventilators; given an order for IPPB therapy using a test lung:
  — Establish the ordered pressure.
  — Establish the ordered tidal volume.
  — Establish the ordered ventilatory rate.
  — Maintain an I:E ratio of 1:2 or greater.
  — Maintain flow rates and pressures within human physiologic limits.
  — Monitor FIO_2.
* Demonstrate how to administer IPPB therapy with normal saline to a laboratory partner.
* Demonstrate the ability to evaluate the signs and symptoms of the adverse effects resulting from IPPB therapy.

* State the criteria for terminating IPPB therapy.
* Describe the appropriate action that should be taken in the event of terminating IPPB therapy, including:
  — Who should be notified
  — Correct patient assessment and monitoring
  — Correct charting of why the therapy was terminated
* Demonstrate appropriate charting following the administration of IPPB therapy.
* Demonstrate the correct operation of the Percussionaire IPV®-1 ventilator; given an order for IPV therapy using a test lung:
  — Correctly assemble the ventilator for use.
  — Establish the correct source pressure.
  — Establish the correct frequency.
* With a laboratory partner as your patient, demonstrate how to administer IPV therapy:
  — Correctly instruct your patient.
  — Correctly adjust the controls for the patient's comfort and efficacy of the therapy.

INCENTIVE SPIROMETRY

Patient Instruction

The effectiveness of any hyperinflation therapy is dependent on patient cooperation and effort. This can only be accomplished using thorough patient instruction.

Be certain to instruct the patient to inhale through the device. Most patients have a natural tendency to blow through it. A few practice trials and a demonstration on your part using exaggerated technique will help. If incentive spirometry is to be self-administered, be sure the patient can operate the device successfully without prompting.

Incentive Spirometry Equipment

To prepare the Voldyne for use, attach the large-bore tubing to the fitting on the front of the unit. Adjust the yellow pointer to the desired volume.

Instruct the patient to inhale deeply through the mouthpiece. The negative pressure generated will raise the piston from the bottom of the tube.

Troubleshooting amounts to ensuring that all fittings and connections are tight.

To prepare the Monaghan Spirocare for use, plug it into a suitable wall power outlet or ensure that the batteries are in place and in good condition. Turn the power switch on and insert a clear flow tube into the handle. Make sure the keyway matches on the flow tube and handle so that the rim of the flow tube is flush with the handle.

The operation of this device is accomplished by setting the desired goal either inside the side panel, in the old unit, or under the display panel, in the new unit. The patient is then instructed to take a breath through the mouthpiece. The volume will be indicated on the display panel by a series of lights illuminating in sequence.

Troubleshooting requirements for this spirometer are very limited. Ensure that the clear flow tube is seated properly and verify that the power requirements for the spirometer are adequate.

IPPB THERAPY

Verify the Physician's Order

Prior to administering IPPB therapy, verify the physician's order in the patient's chart. Look for the components of a complete order, including the amount and dilution of medication, frequency, goals of therapy, duration, pressure range, and desired tidal volume. If clarification is needed, contact the physician.

Scan the Chart

Check the patient's chart for the patient's history. A history of chronic obstructive pulmonary disease (COPD) (especially late-stage emphysema), pneumothorax (check for treatment), hypotension, or head injury should alert you to possible complications resulting from the administration of IPPB therapy.

A quick review of recent results of blood gas analysis will be helpful in your assessment of the patient's pulmonary status and of the need for oxygen administration. Also scan the chart for any pulmonary function test reports, laboratory data, physician's progress notes, and x-ray reports. In brief, scan the chart looking for any information that could alert you to potential complications as a result of IPPB administration.

Administration of Therapy
Patient Positioning

The ideal patient position for IPPB therapy is seated with the legs dangling at the edge of the bed or sitting upright in a chair. This position allows the chest to expand fully without restrictions. An upright position may not be possible with all patients. Full Fowler's or semi-Fowler's position is the next best. Positions may need to be modified depending on the patient's condition. Use good judgment and assess your patient for contraindications.

Appropriate Monitoring before Therapy

Current clinical practice dictates the monitoring of therapy to document its effectiveness. It is difficult to document how effective a therapeutic modality is if you do not first assess what a patient is capable of spontaneously before therapy. Before therapy you should monitor breath sounds, pulse, respiratory rate, inspiratory capacity, spontaneous tidal volume, peak expiratory flow, and blood pressure.

Ideal Breathing Pattern

The ideal breathing pattern for IPPB therapy is similar to the breathing pattern used for small-volume nebulizer therapy, discussed in Chapter 15, "Humidity and Aerosol Therapy." Instruct the patient to inhale, which will cycle the respirator on. Tell the patient to inhale with the ventilator. By actively assisting the ventilator, the patient will achieve a greater inspiratory capacity (Welch, Shapiro, Mercurio, Wagner, & Hiragamu, 1980). At the end of the inspiratory phase, instruct the patient to pause briefly before exhaling, to allow for a more even deposition of the aerosol.

This breathing pattern is unnatural, and success will require both thorough instruction by the therapist and practice by the patient. It is common for the patient to close the glottis, terminating inspiration, on first experiencing the positive pressure delivered by the ventilator. It is imperative that the patient relax on inspiration to allow the ventilator to fill the lungs.

Exhalation is passive, requiring little effort. Instruct the patient to count to three before beginning the next breath. A short pause will help to decrease the respiratory rate and preserve a more normal I:E ratio.

Monitoring the Patient during IPPB Therapy

During therapy, closely monitor the patient. Measure the pulse and respiratory rate frequently. Constantly assess the patient for any signs or symptoms of the hazards and complications discussed earlier.

Monitor the ventilator tidal volume during therapy using a portable respirometer attached to the exhalation port (Wright, Dragger, or Haloscale). Good IPPB administration will result in a ventilator tidal volume 25% greater than the maximum spontaneous inspiratory capacity (ATS, 1980). You should strive for a ventilator tidal volume approaching the spontaneous inspiratory capacity as long as undue harm is not caused to the patient. With these volumes, monitor delivered pressures closely. Frequent pressure and flow adjustments may be required to achieve a high inspiratory capacity. The physician may indicate a maximum pressure not to be exceeded during therapy.

Monitoring the Patient during Bronchodilator Administration

If you are administering a bronchodilator, it is important to monitor the patient for any side effects due to the medication. Chapter 15, "Humidity and Aerosol Therapy," discusses the most common drugs administered by aerosol and their actions and side effects. Closely monitor the patient's pulse when administering bronchodilators. If it increases by 25/min or is 50% greater than baseline (depending on the departmental policies), discontinue therapy.

Recognition of Adverse Effects of IPPB Therapy

Hyperventilation

When patients hyperventilate they may complain of light-headedness or dizziness. Some patients complain of a tingling sensation. A headache may often be precipitated. If this effect is severe, the patient may breathe rapidly and deeply without control until a loss of consciousness occurs.

Appropriate Action. If any of these signs or symptoms occurs, discontinue therapy. Allow the patient to rest, breathing spontaneously for a few minutes. If hyperventilation continues, contact the patient's attending physician or seek assistance from other personnel.

Interruption of the Hypoxic Drive

With interruption of the hypoxic drive, patients often become very lethargic and drowsy. Spontaneous respiratory rate and depth decrease markedly. If the reaction is severe, the patient may go into respiratory arrest. The administration of IPPB may precipitate an episode of hypoventilation that is not evident for some time. A patient who experiences a significant drop in tidal volume and respiratory rate following therapy, with the foregoing signs and symptoms, should be closely observed.

Appropriate Action. At the first indications of these symptoms, discontinue therapy immediately. Stay with the patient and closely monitor the respiratory rate and depth, pulse, and blood pressure. Observe the patient for signs of cyanosis. If possible, call the patient's nurse so that additional appropriate vital signs can be monitored. If respiratory arrest occurs, initiate cardiopulmonary resuscitation (CPR) and get help.

This event may be prevented by reviewing the patient's history first to identify persons at risk (due to COPD) and by administering therapy using compressed air rather than oxygen.

Decreased Cardiac Output

The effects of IPPB on the cardiovascular system may be minimized by maintaining an I:E ratio of 1:2 or greater. Decreased cardiac output is indicated by a fall in blood pressure. If the patient is in the intensive care unit, an arterial line may be present, making blood pressure monitoring easy and convenient. In the absence of these more sophisticated monitoring devices, manual blood pressure measurement is your only means of monitoring for this adverse effect. You may be able to detect cardiac rhythm changes when monitoring the pulse. Patients at risk (those who have cardiovascular disease) should be monitored closely. A drop in blood pressure may be indicated by complaints of dizziness or faintness, pallor, or diaphoresis or cyanosis.

Appropriate Action. At the first sign of cardiac compromise, discontinue therapy and monitor the patient closely. If possible, have a nurse assist you in monitoring the patient. If the blood pressure remains low and the cardiovascular system fails to recover after discontinuance of therapy, contact the physician immediately.

Increased Intracranial Pressure

Rising intracranial pressure can impair cerebral circulation and damage brain tissue. Unless the patient is at risk (owing to head trauma or neurological condition) and the intracranial pressure is already being monitored, an increase in intracranial pressure is very difficult to detect. Some affected patients exhibit bulging and experience increased pressure around the eye orbits. Other symptoms may include changes in sensorium and loss of consciousness. Most patients at risk will have an intracranial pressure monitoring line (ICP line) in place.

Appropriate Action. Patients at risk should be closely monitored. If intracranial pressure increases significantly, discontinue therapy. Try to administer therapy with the patient in semi-Fowler's or full Fowler's position, if possible, to help reduce the effects of IPPB on intracranial pressure. Frequently, the physician's order for IPPB will specify a position in these circumstances. If the patient has experienced spinal injury or multiple trauma in addition to the cranial problems, it is wise to request clarification of what position to use during IPPB therapy.

Pneumothorax

Patients with an existing pneumothorax should not receive IPPB therapy unless a chest tube is in place. One hazard of IPPB therapy is a pneumothorax occurring as the result of an air leak in the lung. The result is air in the pleural space, compressing lung tissue.

Patients experiencing a pneumothorax often complain of a sharp chest pain and shortness of breath. With a tension pneumothorax, patients are often gasping.

Appropriate Action. Terminate IPPB therapy. Quickly auscultate the chest. Absent or diminished breath sounds may indicate the presence of a pneumothorax. Percuss the chest; if hyperresonance is present and breath sounds are absent or decreased, be very suspicious. If you observe a shift in the trachea, contact a physician immediately. If possible, call the patient's nurse to assist you in monitoring the patient. Monitor the respiratory rate and depth and pulse frequently.

A STAT chest x-ray film is indicated, and if a pneumothorax is present, the physician will place a chest tube.

Do not continue therapy if the patient has a pneumothorax that has not been treated.

Post–IPPB Therapy Monitoring

Following IPPB therapy administration, monitor breath sounds, pulse, respiratory rate, spontaneous tidal volume, peak expiratory flow, and vital capacity.

Charting the Procedure

Appropriate charting includes the following: date and time of administration; medication, amount and dilution; duration of therapy; pressure; respirator tidal volume; and the patient's parameters before and after therapy.

Also indicate the ability of the patient to cooperate and follow your instructions. Indicate whether the patient's coughing was productive and what was expectorated.

In the event of adverse reactions, your charting should include why you discontinued therapy (observation of signs and symptoms). You should indicate how you monitored your patient, and what you observed. The people contacted should include the physician, nurse, and your supervisor. Indicate who was contacted, when, and what action was taken.

All charting should conform with the standards and policies of the agency in which the therapy was rendered.

INTRAPULMONARY PERCUSSIVE VENTILATION THERAPY

Verify the Physician's Order

Prior to IPV therapy administration, verify the physician's order in the patient's chart. Look for components of the order, including medication, amount and dilution, and length and frequency of therapy. If clarification is needed, contact the physician.

Scan the Chart

Check the patient's history in the medical record for any indications of untreated pneumothorax, hypotension, or head injuries (elevated intracranial pressure). These problems may be contraindications to IPV therapy because mean intrathoracic pressures will be elevated during therapy. If further clarification is required, contact the patient's physician.

Administration of Therapy

Patient Positioning

The ideal patient position for IPV therapy is seated comfortably in the upright position. If the patient is unable to comply, a high Fowler's or semi-Fowler's position is also acceptable. If you modify the patient's positioning for therapy, be certain that the position you choose does not interfere with achieving the desired clinical goals.

Appropriate Monitoring before Therapy

Prior to beginning therapy, you should monitor the patient's respiratory rate, heart rate, and breath sounds. Because IPV therapy is effective in mobilization of pulmonary secretions, an increase in sputum production is important to note. If bronchodilators are administered with IPV therapy, documentation of peak expiratory flow or FEV_1 pretherapy and posttherapy is appropriate.

Ideal Breathing Pattern

The patient should be instructed to hold the lips tightly around the mouthpiece and to depress the thumb button. Once the button has been depressed, percussive ventilation will begin. The patient should be instructed to inhale and allow the IPV ventilator to fill the lungs and to percuss them for approximately 5 seconds. After the lungs are full, the patient releases the thumb button and exhales completely through the mouthpiece. This process should be repeated until all of the medication in the nebulizer has been delivered.

Monitoring during Therapy

The patient's heart rate, respiratory rate, and breath sounds should be monitored during therapy. If portions of the patient's lungs demonstrated diminished or absent breath sounds prior to therapy, monitor these areas during therapy for improved ventilation. The pressure manometer on the control panel of the IPV ventilator may be monitored to determine peak inspiratory pressures during therapy. When the source pressure is increased, peak pressures during percussion also increase.

The patient's subjective response to therapy such as complaints of dyspnea, pain, or discomfort should be noted. Some patients require time to become accustomed to the high-frequency gas pulsations delivered by the IPV device. Often, increasing the frequency helps the patient to tolerate therapy more easily because the impact of each pulse is lessened.

Monitoring following Therapy

Following IPV therapy, the patient's heart rate, respiratory rate, and breath sounds should be assessed. Quantify sputum production and note its color and consistency and whether any odor is present. If a bronchodilator was used, assess the patient's peak expiratory flow or FEV_1 following therapy.

Charting the Procedure

Document in the patient's chart the date and time of IPV therapy. Note medications used, including amount and dilution. Document the source pressure and the patient's subjective response to therapy. Document all vital signs, breath sounds, and sputum production.

References

American Association for Respiratory Care. (1991). AARC clinical practice guideline: Incentive spirometry. *Respiratory Care, 36*(12), 1402–1405.

American Association for Respiratory Care. (1993). AARC clinical practice guideline: Intermittent positive pressure breathing. *Respiratory Care, 38*(11), 1189–1195.

American Thoracic Society. (1980). Guidelines for the use of intermittent positive pressure breathing (IPPB). *Respiratory Care, 25*(3), 365–370.

Indihar, F. J., Forsberg, D. P., & Adams, A. B. (1982). A prospective comparison of three procedures used in attempts to prevent postoperative pulmonary complications. *Respiratory Care, 27*(5), 564–568.

McPherson, S. (1995). *Respiratory therapy equipment* (5th ed.). St. Louis, MO: Mosby.

Mihailoff, M., & Gentry, M. (1985). A comparison of intrapulmonary aerosol deposition by IPPB and simple aerosol therapy. Presented in the Open Forum as an abstract during the 1985 AARC Annual Meeting.

Welch, M. A., Shapiro, B., Mercurio, P., Wagner, W., & Hiragamu, G. (1980). Methods of intermittent positive pressure breathing. *Chest, 78*(3), 463–467.

Ziment, I. (1984). Intermittent positive pressure breathing. In X. Burton, J. Hodgkin, & J. Ward (Eds.), *Respiratory Care* (pp. 546–581). Philadelphia: Lippincott.

Additional Resources

Bird Corporation. *Instructions for operating the Mark 7 Respirator, Mark 8 Respirator, Mark 10 and Mark 14 ventilators by Bird.* Palm Springs, CA: Author.

O'Donohue, W. J. (1979). Maximum volume IPPB for the management of pulmonary atelectasis. *Chest, 76*(6), 683–687.

Percussionaire Corporation. (1993). *Intrapulmonary percussive ventilation, a twelve year learning curve 1980–1993.* Sandpoint, ID: Author.

Puritan-Bennett Corporation. (1969). *Operating instructions: Bennett model PR-2 respiration unit.* Overland Park, KS: Author.

Scanlan, C., Spearman, C. B., & Sheldon, R. L. (1999). *Egan's fundamentals of respiratory therapy* (7th ed.). St. Louis, MO: Mosby.

Practice Activities: Bird Mark 7

CIRCUIT ASSEMBLY

Permanent reusable circuits as well as disposables are available for the Bird Mark 7 ventilator. In this activity set you will assemble a disposable universal IPPB circuit and correctly adapt it for the Bird Mark 7 ventilator.

Figure 17-18 shows the contents of a typical disposable universal IPPB circuit. Some of these parts are not required for the Bird Mark 7 circuit.

1. Nebulizer and exhalation valve drive line assembly
   The Bird Mark 7 employs a single small-diameter tube to drive both the nebulizer and the exhalation valve. The small adapter with the short piece of small-diameter tubing is used for this purpose. To assemble:

   a. Insert the tubing adapter onto the nebulizer nipple. Connect the other end of the small-diameter tube to the exhalation valve nipple. Figure 17-19 shows the circuit correctly configured.

   b. Next, take the longer piece of small-diameter tubing and attach it to the adapter. Figure 17-19 shows the circuit assembled. The extra piece of small-diameter tubing with the flared ends may be discarded.

2. Mouthpiece assembly

   a. Attach the short flex tube to the outlet of the manifold assembly. Attach the mouthpiece to the other end of the flex tube. Figure 17-19 shows the circuit correctly assembled.

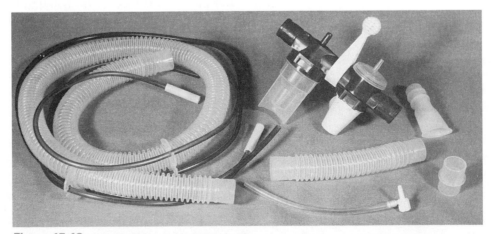

Figure 17-18 *A typical disposable IPPB circuit*

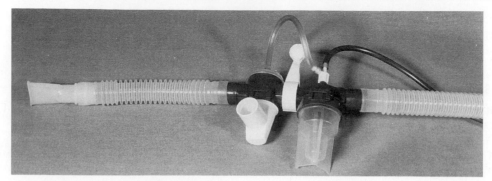

Figure 17-19 *The universal IPPB circuit correctly configured for the Bird ventilator*

3. Attachment of the circuit to the ventilator
  a. The large-bore tubing connects the ventilator to the manifold. Attach the large-bore tubing to the outlet on the right side of the ventilator. This attachment may require a 15-mm straight adapter (sometimes called a mask adapter), which may be supplied with the circuit.
  b. Attach the small-diameter tubing that powers the nebulizer and exhalation valve to the small nipple on the right side of the ventilator, next to the large-bore outlet.

OPERATION OF THE VENTILATOR
The controls on the Bird Mark 7 and 8 are numbered. These practice activities follow similar numbering. It will facilitate your learning of the controls if you think of them in sequence.

For these activities, remove the mouthpiece on the circuit; replace it with a 15-mm straight adapter (mask adapter) and a rubber test lung. Make sure that the test lung is free of leaks and the rubber strap is in good condition.

Attach the ventilator to a 50 psi compressed gas source. If the ventilator cycles on prematurely, pull out on the hand-timer rod located in the center of the sensitivity control rod. This control should cycle the ventilator off. If it does not, move the sensitivity control toward the front of the ventilator and rotate the expiratory timer control fully clockwise. Now repeat the procedure of pulling the hand-timer rod. If the ventilator continues to cycle on, ask for assistance from your laboratory instructor.

Activity 1: Pressure Control (1)
Leave the sensitivity control in its current position. Adjust the flow rate control so that the number 15 is at the twelve o'clock position. The pressure is controlled by a movable plastic arm or vernier. The manufacturer refers to this control as one of two vernier arms.

1. Adjust the pressure control so the vernier arm aligns with the number 10. Push the hand-timer rod in to initiate inspiration. Observe the pressure manometer and note at what pressure the inspiratory phase stops. Write this pressure down.
  a. Repeat this activity and time the length of the inspiratory phase. Write down your value.

2. Adjust the pressure control so the vernier arm aligns with the number 15. Initiate inspiration by pushing the

hand-timer rod in. Observe the pressure manometer and note at what pressure the inspiratory phase stops. Write this pressure down.
  a. Repeat this activity and time the length of the inspiratory phase. Write down your value.

3. Adjust the pressure control so the vernier arm aligns with the number 25. Push the hand-timer rod in to initiate inspiration. Observe the pressure manometer and note at what pressure the inspiratory phase stops. Write this value down.

Questions:
A. In activity 1, at what pressure did the ventilator terminate inspiration?
B. What effect did moving the pressure control from 10 to 25 have on the cycling pressure (pressure at which inspiration is terminated)?
C. Compare the inspiratory times for activities 1 through 3. How do you account for the increased inspiratory time when you did not manipulate the flow rate control?
D. Assume that a patient is breathing at a rate of 10 breaths per minute. Calculate the I:E ratios for activities 1 and 3.
E. If you want the pressure delivered in activity 3, but with the I:E ratio in activity 1, what control would you need to manipulate?

Activity 2: Air Mix Control (2)
This control is discussed in the section Oxygen Delivery with IPPB. Its function is highly variable with pressure, flow, and sensitivity. It will make more sense to you after you have worked with the pressure, flow, and sensitivity controls.

Activity 3: Expiratory Timer Control (3)
This control is not normally used with IPPB therapy. It is used only with the apneic patient. This control is used to set the ventilatory rate.

Activity 4: Sensitivity Control (4)
With the flow rate control set so that the number 7 is at the twelve o'clock position, adjust the pressure control on the right of the ventilator to about the eleven o'clock position.

1. Move the sensitivity control toward the back of the ventilator until it automatically cycles on, then move the control toward the front of the ventilator about ½ inch. The ventilator should be off.

a. Squeeze the test lung and release it, observing the manometer. How far did the manometer deflect into the negative pressure range?

b. Move the sensitivity control about ½ inch toward the front of the ventilator. Squeeze the test lung again, observing the manometer. How far did the manometer deflect into the negative pressure range this time?

c. Move the sensitivity control about 1 inch more toward the front of the ventilator. Squeeze the test lung and observe the manometer. How far did the manometer deflect into the negative pressure range?

Questions:

A. Which setting required the least effort (negative pressure) to initiate inspiration?

B. Which setting required the most effort (negative pressure) to initiate inspiration?

C. As a patient working hard to breathe, where do you think you would prefer to have the ventilator set?

Activity 5: Flow Rate Control (5)

Additional Equipment Required:
A watch with a sweep second hand
Set the sensitivity control to the setting you prefer. Leave the pressure control in the same position.

1. Adjust the flow rate control so that the number 5 is at the twelve o'clock position. Initiate inspiration by pushing the hand-timer rod in. Observe how long it takes to complete the inspiratory phase. Write this time down.

2. Adjust the flow rate control so that the number 15 is at the twelve o'clock position. Push the hand-timer rod in to initiate inspiration. Observe how long it takes to complete the inspiratory phase. Write this time down.

3. Adjust the flow rate control so that the number 30 is at the twelve o'clock position. Push the hand-timer rod in to initiate inspiration. Observe how long it takes to complete the inspiratory phase.

Questions:

A. In activity 1, assume the patient is breathing at a rate of 10 breaths per minute. Using the value you measured for inspiratory time, calculate the I:E ratio.

B. In activity 3, assume the patient is breathing at a rate of 10 breaths per minute. Using the value you measured for inspiratory time, calculate the I:E ratio.

C. As you progressed from activity 1 to activity 3, what effect did the flow rate control have on inspiratory time?

TIDAL VOLUME DELIVERY WITH IPPB THERAPY

A clinical goal of IPPB therapy is reversal of atelectasis. However, it is difficult to quantify how deeply a patient is breathing strictly by observation. In this activity set, you will monitor delivered tidal volumes and adjust the controls appropriately to increase or decrease the delivered tidal volume while maintaining an I:E ratio of 1:2 or greater.

Additional Equipment Required:

Watch with a sweep second hand
Portable respirometer (Wright, Dragger, or Haloscale)

Activity 1

1. Adjust the sensitivity control so the vernier arm is in the twelve o'clock position. Adjust the flow rate control so that the number 15 is in the twelve o'clock position. Adjust the pressure control so that the vernier aligns with the number 15.

2. Attach a portable respirometer to the exhalation port of the manifold assembly.

3. Push the hand-timer rod in to initiate inspiration. Measure the tidal volume. Adjust the pressure control until a tidal volume of 300 cc is reached.

4. Rotate the expiratory timer control counterclockwise until a ventilatory rate of 12 breaths per minute is established.

5. Measure the inspiratory time using your watch. Calculate the I:E ratio.

6. Adjust the flow rate control until you have an I:E ratio of 1:2 or greater.
   a. Measure the tidal volume and adjust the pressure to reach 300 cc as required.
   b. Adjust the flow rate control, as required, to maintain an I:E ratio of 1:2.
   c. Repeat the foregoing steps until the desired goal is reached.

Activity 2

1. Adjust the sensitivity control so the vernier arm is in the twelve o'clock position. Adjust the flow rate control so that the number 15 is in the twelve o'clock position. Adjust the pressure control so that the vernier aligns with the number 15.

2. Attach a portable respirometer to the exhalation port of the manifold assembly.

3. Push the hand-timer rod in to initiate inspiration. Measure the tidal volume. Adjust the pressure control until a tidal volume of 500 cc is reached.

4. Rotate the expiratory timer control counterclockwise until a ventilatory rate of 10 breaths per minute is established.

5. Measure the inspiratory time using your watch. Calculate the I:E ratio.

6. Adjust the flow rate control until you have an I:E ratio of 1:2 or greater.
   a. Measure the tidal volume and adjust the pressure to reach 500 cc as required.
   b. Adjust the flow rate control, as required, to maintain an I:E ratio of 1:2.
   c. Repeat the foregoing steps until the desired goal is reached.

7. Decrease the tidal volume to 400 cc while maintaining the same I:E ratio and ventilatory rate.

OXYGEN DELIVERY WITH IPPB THERAPY

Oxygen delivery with IPPB therapy is very common. Because the ventilator is pneumatically powered, the use of a 50 psi oxygen source will provide for oxygen delivery. However, the delivered FIO_2 is not consistent throughout the inspiratory phase. If a precise oxygen concentration is desired, it is recommended that you use a blender with a 50 psi outlet to adjust the FIO_2. When using a blender, push the air dilution control in. This will ensure delivery of 100% source gas from the blender.

If the ventilator is powered by a compressed gas cylinder, use a two-stage regulator to ensure that adequate flow rates are provided.

AIR MIX CONTROL

The air mix control is located just below the pressure control on the front of the ventilator. If the control is pulled out, air is mixed with oxygen using a Venturi inside the ventilator. With the control pushed in, 100% source gas is delivered.

Additional Equipment Required:
Oxygen analyzer
Briggs adapter

Activity 1

1. Attach the oxygen analyzer between the mouthpiece and manifold using the Brigg's adapter.

2. Replace the mouthpiece with a test lung using a 15-mm straight adapter to attach it.

3. Pull the air mix control out.

4. Measure the delivered oxygen concentration after manipulating each of the following controls. After each control has been manipulated, return it to its original position. As with any scientific experiment, manipulate only one control or variable at a time.

Activity 2

a. Set the pressure control so the vernier arm aligns with the number 15.
b. Set the flow rate control so the number 15 is in the twelve o'clock position.
c. Measure the oxygen concentration.

1. Move the flow rate control so the number 5 is in the twelve o'clock position. Measure the oxygen concentration during inspiration.

2. Move the flow rate control so the number 30 is in the twelve o'clock position. Measure the oxygen concentration during inspiration.

Activity 3

a. Set the flow rate control so the number 15 is in the twelve o'clock position.
b. Set the pressure control so the vernier arm aligns with the number 15.
c. Push the air mix control in.

1. Measure the oxygen concentration on inspiration.

2. Move the pressure control to correspond with the number 25.

3. Move the pressure control to correspond with the number 10.

Question:
A. Which control(s) affected the oxygen concentration?

Practice Activities: Puritan Bennett PR-2

CIRCUIT ASSEMBLY

Permanent and disposable IPPB circuits are available for the PR-2 ventilator. In this activity set, you will assemble a disposable universal IPPB circuit and correctly adapt it for the Bennett PR-2 ventilator.

Nebulizer Drive Line Attachment

The nebulizer on the Bennett PR-2 ventilator is driven by a single small-diameter tube with flared ends.

1. Attach the long small-diameter tube with flared ends to the nipple on top of the nebulizer in the manifold assembly. Figure 17-20 shows its correct attachment.

Exhalation Valve Drive Line Assembly

The exhalation valve on the Bennett PR-2 ventilator is driven by the single small-diameter tube without flared ends.

1. Attach the long small-diameter tube, without flared ends, to the nipple on top of the exhalation valve on the manifold assembly. Figure 17-20 shows its correct assembly.

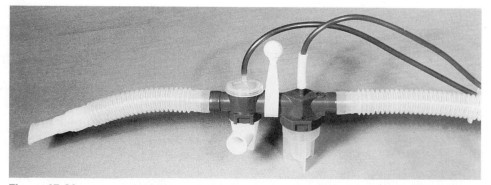

Figure 17-20 *The universal circuit correctly configured for the Bennett IPPB ventilators*

Mouthpiece Assembly

1. Attach the short flex tubing to the outlet of the manifold assembly. Attach the mouthpiece to the short section of large-bore tubing. Figure 17-20 shows the circuit correctly assembled.

Attachment of the Circuit to the Ventilator

1. Attach the large-bore tubing to the large-bore outlet found at the very bottom of the ventilator.

2. Attach the nebulizer drive line to the small-diameter nipple to the right of the large-bore outlet.

3. Attach the exhalation valve drive line to the small-diameter nipple to the left of the large-bore outlet.

OPERATION OF THE RESPIRATOR

For these activities, remove the mouthpiece on the circuit and replace it with a 15-mm straight adapter (mask adapter) and a rubber test lung. Make sure the test lung is free of leaks and the rubber strap is in good condition.

Attach the ventilator to a 50 psi compressed gas source. Initially, a compressed air source will be adequate. If the ventilator cycles on prematurely, rotate the sensitivity control fully clockwise, and rotate both the rate control and expiration time control fully counterclockwise. If the ventilator continues to autocycle, ask for assistance from your laboratory instructor.

Sensitivity Control

Adjust the pressure control until 12 cm H_2O is registered on the system pressure manometer.

1. Rotate the sensitivity control counterclockwise until the ventilator cycles automatically, then rotate it one full turn clockwise.
   a. Squeeze the test lung to initiate inspiration. Observe the system pressure manometer. How far did the needle deflect into the negative pressure range? Write this value down.
   b. Rotate the sensitivity control ½ to 1 full turn clockwise. Squeeze the test lung to initiate inspiration. Observe the system pressure manometer. How far did the needle deflect into the negative pressure range? Write this value down.
   c. Rotate the sensitivity control fully clockwise. Initiate inspiration by squeezing the test lung. Observe the system pressure manometer and note the needle's deflection into the negative pressure range. Write this value down.

Questions:
A. Which setting required the least effort (negative pressure) to initiate inspiration?
B. Which setting required the most effort (negative pressure) to initiate inspiration?
C. As a patient with difficulty breathing, where do you think you would prefer to have the ventilator sensitivity control set?

Pressure Control

Adjust the sensitivity control by rotating it fully clockwise. Rotate both the rate and expiratory time controls fully counterclockwise.

1. Adjust the pressure control until 10 cm H_2O is registered on the control pressure manometer. Squeeze the test lung to initiate inspiration and observe the system pressure manometer. At what pressure was inspiration terminated? Write this value down.

2. Adjust the pressure control until 15 cm H_2O is registered on the control pressure manometer. Squeeze the test lung to initiate inspiration and observe the system pressure manometer. At what pressure was inspiration terminated? Write this value down.

3. Adjust the pressure control until 30 cm H_2O is registered on the control pressure manometer. Squeeze the test lung to initiate inspiration and observe the system pressure manometer. At what pressure was inspiration terminated? Write this value down.

Questions:
A. In activity 1, at what pressure did the ventilator terminate inspiration?
B. Compare the inspiratory times for activities 1 and 3. How do you account for the longer inspiratory time?
C. Assume a patient is breathing at a rate of 10 breaths per minute. Calculate the I:E ratios for activities 1 and 3.
D. How can you increase the I:E ratio in activity 3 without changing the pressure setting?

Nebulizer Controls

The Bennett PR-2 ventilator has the ability to control the nebulizer function during both inspiration and expiration.

Disconnect the test lung temporarily for this activity set.

1. Fill the nebulizer with 3 ml of normal saline.
2. Turn on the inspiration nebulizer control one full turn counterclockwise.
3. Initiate inspiration by moving the Bennett valve up. Observe what happens. Turn off the ventilator using the Bennett valve and turn off the nebulizer.
4. Turn on the expiration nebulizer control one full turn counterclockwise.
5. Initiate inspiration using the Bennett valve. Observe what happens during inspiration. Turn off the ventilator using the Bennett valve. Observe what happens.
6. Turn on the inspiration nebulizer control one full turn. Initiate inspiration using the Bennett valve. Turn off the ventilator using the Bennett valve.

For most IPPB therapy protocols, the inspiration nebulizer control is adjusted to provide adequate aerosol output on inspiration. The expiration nebulizer is opened just enough to fill the dead space in the tubing with aerosol.

VOLUME DELIVERY WITH IPPB THERAPY

A clinical goal of IPPB therapy is improvement in the distribution of ventilation. This can be accomplished in part by the delivery of a deep breath by the ventilator. However, it is difficult to quantify how deeply a patient is breathing strictly by observation. In these exercises you will learn how to monitor delivered tidal volumes and to adjust the controls appropriately to increase or decrease the delivered tidal volume while maintaining an I:E ratio of 1:2 or greater.

Additional Equipment Required:
Watch with a sweep second hand
Portable respirometer (Wright, Dragger, or Haloscale)

Activity 1

1. Rotate the rate control clockwise until a rate of 12 breaths per minute is established.

2. Measure the ventilator tidal volume with the spirometer and adjust the pressure control until a tidal volume of 300 cc is reached.

3. Measure the length of inspiratory time.

4. Calculate the I:E ratio. If the I:E ratio is less than 1:2, rotate the expiratory time control until a ratio of at least 1:2 is achieved.
   a. Remeasure the tidal volume.
   b. Remeasure the rate.
   c. Adjust the controls as required to maintain a rate of 12/min and a tidal volume of 300 cc. Maintain an I:E ratio of 1:2.

Activity 2

1. Rotate the rate control clockwise until a rate of 10 breaths per minute is established.

2. Measure the ventilator tidal volume with the spirometer, and adjust the pressure control until a tidal volume of 500 cc is reached.

3. Measure the length of inspiratory time.

4. Calculate the I:E ratio. If the I:E ratio is less than 1:2, rotate the expiratory time control until a ratio of at least 1:2 is achieved.
   a. Remeasure the tidal volume.
   b. Remeasure the rate.
   c. Adjust the controls as required to maintain a rate of 10/min and a tidal volume of 500 cc. Maintain an I:E ratio of 1:2.

Questions:
A. What control was manipulated to increase the tidal volume?
B. As tidal volume increased, what happened to inspiratory time and the I:E ratio?
C. In a spontaneously breathing patient (so that no manipulation of rate or expiratory time controls is allowed), how can you increase the I:E ratio without compromising tidal volume?

OXYGEN DELIVERY WITH IPPB THERAPY

Oxygen delivery with IPPB therapy is very common. Because the ventilator is pneumatically powered, the use of a 50 psi oxygen source will provide for oxygen delivery. However, the delivered FIO_2 is not consistent throughout the inspiratory phase.

Because oxygen delivery varies, if a precise oxygen concentration is desired, it is recommended that you use a blender with a 50 psi outlet to adjust the FIO_2. When using a blender, pull the air dilution control out, which will ensure delivery of 100% source gas from the blender.

If the ventilator is powered by a compressed gas cylinder, use a two-stage regulator to ensure that adequate flow rates are provided.

AIR DILUTION CONTROL

This control is located on the right side of the ventilator. With the control pushed in, air and oxygen are mixed by means of a Venturi. If the control is pulled out, 100% source gas is delivered.

Activity 1

Additional Equipment Required:
Briggs adapter
Oxygen analyzer
Compressed oxygen source

1. Attach the oxygen analyzer in the circuit between the mouthpiece and the manifold using the Briggs adapter.

2. Replace the mouthpiece with a test lung using a 15-mm adapter to attach it.

3. Push the air mix control in.

4. Set the pressure control so that 15 cm H_2O appears on the system pressure manometer.

5. Measure the delivered oxygen concentration after manipulating each of the following controls. After each control has been manipulated, return it to its original position. As with any scientific experiment, manipulate only one control or variable at a time.
   a. Adjust the pressure control to 20 cm H_2O.
   b. Turn on the inspiration nebulizer control one full turn.
   c. Turn on the expiration nebulizer control one full turn.
   d. Turn on both nebulizer controls one full turn.
   e. Turn on the terminal flow control one full turn.

Activity 2

1. Attach the oxygen analyzer in the circuit between the mouthpiece and the manifold using the Briggs adapter.

2. Replace the mouthpiece with a test lung using a 15-mm adapter to attach it.

3. Pull the air mix control out.

4. Set the pressure control so that 15 cm H_2O appears on the system pressure manometer.

5. Measure the delivered oxygen concentration after manipulating each of the following controls. After each control has been manipulated, return it to its original position. As with any scientific experiment, manipulate only one control or variable at a time.
   a. Adjust the pressure control to 20 cm H_2O.
   b. Turn on the inspiration nebulizer control one full turn.
   c. Turn on the expiration nebulizer control one full turn.
   d. Turn on both nebulizer controls one full turn.
   e. Turn on the terminal flow control one full turn.

Questions:
A. What controls affected FIO_2 delivery?
B. Why did the terminal flow control decrease the oxygen delivery in activity 2?
C. Why did the nebulizer controls increase oxygen delivery in activity 1?

Practice Activities: Puritan Bennett AP-5

CIRCUIT ASSEMBLY

Permanent and disposable IPPB circuits are available for the AP-5 ventilator. In this activity set you will assemble a disposable universal IPPB circuit and correctly adapt it for the Bennett AP-5 ventilator.

Nebulizer Drive Line Attachment

The nebulizer on the Bennett AP-5 ventilator is driven by a single small-diameter tube with flared ends.

1. Attach the long small-diameter tube with flared ends to the nipple on top of the nebulizer in the manifold assembly. Figure 17-21 shows its correct attachment.

Exhalation Valve Drive Line Assembly

The exhalation valve on the Bennett AP-5 ventilator is driven by the single small-diameter tube without flared ends.

1. Attach the long, small-diameter tube, without flared ends, to the nipple on top of the exhalation valve on the manifold assembly. Figure 17-21 shows its correct assembly.

Mouthpiece Assembly

1. Attach the short flex tubing to the outlet of the manifold assembly. Attach the mouthpiece to the short section of the large-bore tubing. Figure 17-21 shows the circuit correctly assembled.

Attachment of the Circuit to the Ventilator

1. Attach the large-bore tubing to the large-bore outlet found at the bottom center of the ventilator's control panel.
2. Attach the nebulizer drive line to the small-diameter nipple located to the right of the large-bore outlet.
3. Attach the exhalation valve drive line to the small nipple to the left of the large-bore outlet.

Operation of the Ventilator

For this activity set, remove the mouthpiece on the circuit and replace it with a 15-mm straight adapter (mask adapter) and a rubber test lung. Make sure the test lung is free from leaks and the rubber strap is in good condition.

Connect the ventilator's power cord to a 120 V alternating current electrical outlet. Rotate the pressure control and the nebulizer control fully counterclockwise.

Pressure Control

1. Turn the ventilator on by moving the on/off switch to the on position.
2. Rotate the pressure control clockwise between ¼ and ½ of a full turn. Squeeze the test lung to initiate inspiration, and monitor the pressure manometer. Adjust the pressure control until 10 cm H_2O has been reached.
   a. At what pressure was inspiration terminated?
   b. How long did inspiration take?
3. Connect a respirometer to the exhalation port of the manifold, and measure the exhaled volume. Average the volume measured over 5 to 10 breaths.
4. Adjust the pressure control by rotating it farther clockwise. Squeeze the test lung to initiate inspiration, and monitor the pressure manometer. Adjust the pressure control until 20 cm H_2O has been reached.
   a. At what pressure was inspiration terminated?
   b. How long did inspiration take?
5. Connect a respirometer to the exhalation port of the manifold, and measure the exhaled volume. Average the volume measured over 5 to 10 breaths.

Questions:
A. What determined when the AP-5 ventilator cycled into expiration?
B. What effect does the pressure control have on inspiratory time?
C. What effect does the pressure control have on delivered volume?

Nebulizer Control

Disconnect the test lung from the ventilator for this activity set.

1. Adjust the pressure control by rotating it clockwise one full turn. Squeeze the test lung to initiate inspiration, and monitor the pressure manometer. Adjust the pressure control until 20 cm H_2O has been reached.
2. Add 2 ml of normal saline to the nebulizer.
3. Adjust the nebulizer control by rotating it fully counterclockwise. Initiate inspiration by lifting on the counterweight of the Bennett valve.
4. Observe the nebulizer's output.
5. Rotate the nebulizer control fully clockwise. Initiate inspiration by lifting on the counterweight of the Bennett valve.
6. Observe the nebulizer's output.

Question:
A. Which setting resulted in more output from the nebulizer?

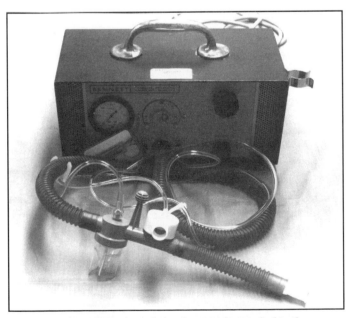

Figure 17-21 *The universal circuit correctly attached to the Bennett AP-5 ventilator*

Practice Activities: Percussionaire IPV-1 Ventilator

CIRCUIT ASSEMBLY

In this activity set, you will correctly assemble the circuit for the IPV®1 intrapulmonary percussive ventilator.

1. Open the nebulizer by rotating the nebulizer bowl counterclockwise. Add medication in the proper dilution and quantity to the nebulizer bowl, and reinstall it to the green tee cap assembly.

2. Connect the Phasitron to the nebulizer assembly by inserting the entrainment port into the nebulizer assembly.

3. Install the four-tube multicolored drive harness to the manifold assembly:
   a. Connect the white tube to the cap on the Phasitron.
   b. Connect the green tube to the socket opposite the thumb switch.
   c. Connect the red tube to the proximal monitoring port near the mouthpiece.
   d. Connect the yellow tube to the base of the nebulizer.

4. Install the four-tube multicolored drive harness to the ventilator by matching the colors of the tube to the sockets located below the pressure manometer.

5. Install the red adapter bushing onto the outlet of the Phasitron and connect the large-bore red tubing to it. This prevents the patient's clothing from becoming spattered with excess aerosolized medication.

6. Connect a 50 psi gas source to the gas inlet on the back of the IPV-1 ventilator.

OPERATION OF THE VENTILATOR

For this activity set, remove the mouthpiece on the circuit and replace it with a 15-mm straight adapter (mask adapter) and a rubber test lung. Make sure the test lung is free from leaks and the rubber strap is in good condition.

Adjust the source pressure control to 30 psi. The source pressure control is located inside the compartment behind the hinged door on the right side of the control panel.

Percussion Control

1. Rotate the percussion control fully clockwise. Activate percussive ventilation by depressing the manual inspiration button or the thumb button on the Phasitron assembly.
   a. Determine the frequency (slow, medium, or fast).
   b. Note approximately how much volume is delivered with each breath.

2. Rotate the percussion control fully counterclockwise. Activate percussive ventilation by depressing the manual inspiration button or the thumb button on the Phasitron assembly.
   a. Determine the frequency (slow, medium, or fast).
   b. Note approximately how much volume is delivered with each breath.

Questions
A. Which setting resulted in the highest ventilatory rate?
B. How did rotating the percussion control affect volume delivery?

Source Pressure Control

1. Set the percussion control to the twelve o'clock, midrange position. Decrease the source pressure to 20 psi by rotating the knob counterclockwise. Activate percussive ventilation by depressing the manual inspiration button or the thumb button on the Phasitron assembly.
   a. Determine the frequency (slow, medium, or fast).
   b. Note approximately how much volume is delivered with each breath.

2. Set the percussion control to the twelve o'clock, midrange position. Decrease the source pressure to 40 psi by rotating the knob counterclockwise. Activate percussive ventilation by depressing the manual inspiration button or the thumb button on the Phasitron assembly.
   a. Determine the frequency (slow, medium, or fast).
   b. Note approximately how much volume is delivered with each breath.

Question:
A. What effect did the source pressure have on volume delivery with each breath?

Practice Activities: Hyperinflation Therapy

1. With a laboratory partner, practice giving each other directions on how to use an incentive spirometer. Include the following information:
   a. Explain what incentive spirometry does physiologically.
   b. Explain how to use the spirometer.
   c. Explain the importance of the patient's cooperation and effort.
   Note: When a patient does not seem to do well, it usually can be attributed to poor instruction.

2. Practice incentive spirometry using a laboratory partner. Include in your practice:
   a. Correct assembly
   b. Troubleshooting
   c. Patient instructions

3. Complete the practice activities for the Bird Mark 7 and the Bennett PR-2 ventilators.

4. Practice administering IPPB with normal saline to a laboratory partner using the IPPB Therapy Check List as a guide.

Safety Precautions
A. IPPB therapy may be hazardous owing to the application of positive pressure in the lungs. Approach high

pressures and volumes (greater than 25 cm H$_2$O and 50% of the inspiratory capacity) with caution.

B. Closely monitor your laboratory partner for signs and symptoms indicating the adverse affects of IPPB therapy. If you observe any of the signs or symptoms described, terminate the therapy and notify your laboratory instructor immediately.

Check List: Incentive Spirometry

_____ 1. Verify the physician's order.
_____ 2. Scan the chart for relevant information.
_____ 3. Observe standard precautions, including handwashing.
_____ 4. Obtain and assemble your equipment.
_____ 5. Introduce yourself and explain the procedure.
6. Position the patient properly.
_____ a. Semi-Fowler's
_____ b. Full Fowler's
_____ c. Dangling
_____ 7. Assess the patient's spontaneous parameters. Some facilities require a vital capacity determination once each day.
_____ 8. Assist the patient in the performance.

_____ 9. Emphasize self-motivation. With the prevalence of television in patients' rooms, the patient can be encouraged to perform three repetitions on the spirometer during each commercial break.
_____ 10. Leave the spirometer within the patient's reach.
_____ 11. Clean up after yourself.
_____ 12. Ensure that your patient is safe and comfortable.
_____ 13. Record the procedure in the patient's chart. Include date, time, volumes achieved, vital capacity, breath sounds, and, if the cough was productive, the amount, color, and consistency of the sputum.

Check List: IPPB Therapy

_____ 1. Verify the physician's order. In the absence of a complete order, take appropriate action.
2. Scan the patient's chart.
_____ a. History
_____ b. Chest x-ray film and report
_____ c. Blood gas values, if available
_____ 3. Gather the required equipment.
_____ 4. Observe standard precautions, including handwashing.
5. During patient monitoring, measure the following:
_____ a. Pulse
_____ b. Respiratory rate
_____ c. Breath sounds
_____ d. Spontaneous inspiratory capacity
_____ e. Peak expiratory flow
_____ f. Blood pressure
_____ 6. Assemble the equipment properly.

7. Instruct the patient on:
_____ a. Proper breathing pattern
_____ b. How to initiate inspiration
_____ c. How to exhale properly
_____ d. Symptoms to be aware of
8. Administer IPPB therapy.
_____ a. Deliver a tidal volume 25% greater than the spontaneous inspiratory capacity.
9. Monitor the patient during therapy:
_____ a. Take the pulse.
_____ b. Determine respiratory rate.
_____ c. Watch for adverse signs and symptoms.
_____ d. Measure blood pressure.
_____ 10. Assist your patient with coughing.
_____ 11. Monitor the effectiveness of the therapy by measuring peak flow and vital capacity.
_____ 12. Assess the patient for adverse affects.
_____ 13. Remove all unneeded equipment.
_____ 14. Chart appropriately.

Check List: Intrapulmonary Percussive Ventilation Therapy

_____ 1. Verify the physician's order.
_____ 2. Scan the chart for relevant information.
_____ 3. Observe standard precautions, including handwashing.
_____ 4. Obtain and assemble your equipment.
_____ 5. Introduce yourself and explain the procedure.
_____ 6. Position the patient properly.
_____ 7. Assess the patient prior to therapy.

_____ 8. Instruct the patient on IPV therapy.
_____ 9. Assist and coach the patient during therapy.
_____ 10. Periodically, have the patient cough.
_____ 11. Monitor the patient during therapy.
_____ 12. Assess the patient following therapy.
_____ 13. Clean up after yourself.
_____ 14. Ensure that the patient is safe and comfortable.
_____ 15. Document the procedure in the patient's chart.

Self-Evaluation Post Test: Hyperinflation Therapy

1. A goal of incentive spirometry is:
   a. to reduce the therapist's workload.
   b. to provide means of using a patient's muscles to hyperinflate the lungs.
   c. to inflict pain and suffering.
   d. to place the patient on a fixed schedule of therapy convenient for the therapist.

2. A sign that your patient may be hyperventilating during incentive spirometry is:
   a. a complaint of feeling light-headed.
   b. a complaints of feeling dizzy.
   c. a tingling sensation.
   d. All of the above

3. Of the following, which is the most important aspect of incentive spirometry?
   a. Duration of therapy
   b. Frequency of therapy
   c. Thorough patient instruction
   d. Therapist's knowledge of the patient's diagnosis

4. Which of the following is a hazard associated with incentive spirometry?
   a. Oxygen toxicity   c. Hypoxemia
   b. Hypercapnia   d. Hypocapnia

5. The contraindications to IPPB therapy may include:
   a. untreated pneumothorax.
   b. atelectasis.
   c. pneumonia.

   d. cystic fibrosis.

6. Which of the following should be included in a complete physician's order for IPPB?
   a. Medication and dilution
   b. Frequency
   c. Desired clinical goals of therapy
   d. Duration of therapy
   e. All of the above

7. What is a contraindication to IPPB therapy?
   a. Complaints of pain
   b. Untreated pneumothorax
   c. Productive cough
   d. Urinary retention
   e. Shallow tidal volumes

8. IPPB therapy may be hazardous to the patient whose records show:
   I. possible pneumothorax.
   II. uncorrected hypotension.
   III. elevated intracranial pressure.
   a. I   d. I, II
   b. II   e. I, II, III
   c. III

9. To increase the frequency (respiratory rate) when using the Percussionaire IPV-1 ventilator, you must increase the:
   a. source pressure.   c. manual control.
   b. impact control.   d. nebulizer control.

PERFORMANCE EVALUATION: INCENTIVE SPIROMETRY

Date: Lab _____ Clinical _____ Agency _____

Lab: Pass _____ Fail _____   Clinical: Pass _____ Fail _____

Student name _____ Instructor name _____

No. of times observed in clinical _____

No. of times practiced in clinical _____

PASSING CRITERIA: Obtain 90% or better on the procedure. Tasks indicated by * must receive at least 1 point, or the evaluation is terminated. Procedure must be performed within designated time, or the performance receives a failing grade.

SCORING:
2 points — Task performed satisfactorily without prompting.
1 point — Task performed satisfactorily with self-initiated correction.
0 points — Task performed incorrectly or with prompting required.
NA — Task not applicable to the patient care situation.

TASKS:

			PEER	LAB	CLINICAL
*	1.	Verifies the physician's order	☐	☐	☐
	2.	Scans the chart	☐	☐	☐
*	3.	Obtains and assembles the required equipment	☐	☐	☐
*	4.	Observes standard precautions, including handwashing	☐	☐	☐
	5.	Introduces self and explains procedure	☐	☐	☐
*	6.	Places the patient into proper position	☐	☐	☐
*	7.	Assesses patient parameters	☐	☐	☐
*	8.	Assists in the patient's performance	☐	☐	☐
*	9.	Emphasizes the importance of self-motivation to the patient	☐	☐	☐
*	10.	Leaves the device within the patient's reach	☐	☐	☐
*	11.	Uses aseptic technique	☐	☐	☐
	12.	Removes unneeded equipment	☐	☐	☐
*	13.	Records the procedure on the patient's chart	☐	☐	☐

SCORE: Peer _____ points of possible 24; _____%

Lab _____ points of possible 24; _____%

Clinical _____ points of possible 24; _____%

TIME: _____ out of possible 20 minutes

STUDENT SIGNATURES   **INSTRUCTOR SIGNATURES**

PEER: _____   LAB: _____

STUDENT: _____   CLINICAL: _____

PERFORMANCE EVALUATION:
IPPB THERAPY

Date: Lab _____ Clinical _____ Agency _____

Lab: Pass _____ Fail _____   Clinical: Pass _____ Fail _____

Student name _____   Instructor name _____

No. of times observed in clinical _____

No. of times practiced in clinical _____

PASSING CRITERIA: Obtain 90% or better on the procedure. Tasks indicated by * must receive at least 1 point, or the evaluation is terminated. Procedure must be performed within designated time, or the performance receives a failing grade.

SCORING:
2 points — Task performed satisfactorily without prompting.
1 point — Task performed satisfactorily with self-initiated correction.
0 points — Task performed incorrectly or with prompting required.
NA — Task not applicable to the patient care situation.

TASKS:		PEER	LAB	CLINICAL
*	1. Verifies the physician's order	☐	☐	☐
	2. Scans the chart	☐	☐	☐
	3. Gathers the equipment			
*	a. Respirometer	☐	☐	☐
*	b. Ventilator	☐	☐	☐
*	c. Peak flowmeter	☐	☐	☐
*	d. Breathing circuit	☐	☐	☐
*	e. Medication	☐	☐	☐
*	4. Assembles and tests the equipment	☐	☐	☐
*	5. Observes standard precautions, including handwashing	☐	☐	☐
*	6. Positions the patient	☐	☐	☐
	7. Monitors the patient			
*	a. Pulse and respirations	☐	☐	☐
*	b. Breath sounds	☐	☐	☐
*	c. Inspiratory capacity	☐	☐	☐
*	d. Peak expiratory flow rate	☐	☐	☐
*	e. Blood pressure	☐	☐	☐
	8. Instructs the patient			
*	a. Explains correct breathing pattern	☐	☐	☐
*	b. Explains how to initiate a breath	☐	☐	☐
*	c. Explains how expiration occurs	☐	☐	☐
*	d. Explains warning signs and symptoms	☐	☐	☐

9. Administers therapy
  * a. Adjusts the ventilator as required ☐ ☐ ☐
  * b. Monitors tidal volume ☐ ☐ ☐
  * c. Monitors respiratory and heart rates ☐ ☐ ☐
  * d. Monitors blood pressure ☐ ☐ ☐
10. Assists and encourages the patient to cough ☐ ☐ ☐
11. Monitors therapy effectiveness
  * a. Inspiratory capacity ☐ ☐ ☐
  * b. Peak expiratory flow rate ☐ ☐ ☐
12. Removes unneeded equipment ☐ ☐ ☐
  * 13. Practices aseptic techniques ☐ ☐ ☐
  * 14. Records procedure on the patient's chart ☐ ☐ ☐

SCORE: Peer _____ points of possible 58; _____%

Lab _____ points of possible 58; _____%

Clinical _____ points of possible 58; _____%

TIME: _____ out of possible 15 minutes

STUDENT SIGNATURES

PEER: _____

STUDENT: _____

INSTRUCTOR SIGNATURES

LAB: _____

CLINICAL: _____

PERFORMANCE EVALUATION:
INTRAPULMONARY PERCUSSIVE VENTILATION (IPV)

Date: Lab _____ Clinical _____ Agency _____

Lab: Pass _____ Fail _____   Clinical: Pass _____ Fail _____

Student name _____ Instructor name _____

No. of times observed in clinical _____

No. of times practiced in clinical _____

PASSING CRITERIA: Obtain 90% or better on the procedure. Tasks indicated by * must receive at least 1 point, or the evaluation is terminated. Procedure must be performed within designated time, or the performance receives a failing grade.

SCORING:
2 points — Task performed satisfactorily without prompting.
1 point — Task performed satisfactorily with self-initiated correction.
0 points — Task performed incorrectly or with prompting required.
NA — Task not applicable to the patient care situation.

TASKS:

			PEER	LAB	CLINICAL
*	1.	Verifies the physician's order	☐	☐	☐
*	2.	Scans the chart for relevant information	☐	☐	☐
*	3.	Observes standard precautions, including handwashing	☐	☐	☐
	4.	Obtains and assembles the equipment	☐	☐	☐
	5.	Introduces self and explains the procedure	☐	☐	☐
	6.	Positions the patient properly	☐	☐	☐
*	7.	Assesses the patient prior to therapy	☐	☐	☐
*	8.	Instructs the patient on IPV therapy	☐	☐	☐
*	9.	Assists and coaches the patient during therapy	☐	☐	☐
	10.	Periodically, has the patient cough	☐	☐	☐
	11.	Monitors the patient during therapy	☐	☐	☐
	12.	Assesses the patient following therapy	☐	☐	☐
	13.	Cleans up	☐	☐	☐
	14.	Ensures that the patient is safe and comfortable	☐	☐	☐
	15.	Documents the procedure in the patient's chart	☐	☐	☐

SCORE:
Peer _____ points of possible 30; _____%
Lab _____ points of possible 30; _____%
Clinical _____ points of possible 30; _____%

TIME: _____ out of possible 30 minutes

STUDENT SIGNATURES   **INSTRUCTOR SIGNATURES**

PEER: _____   LAB: _____

STUDENT: _____   CLINICAL: _____

CHAPTER 18
BRONCHOSCOPY ASSISTING

INTRODUCTION

Bronchoscopy is visual examination of the tracheobronchial tree. This procedure may be performed using a rigid or a flexible fiberoptic bronchoscope. Bronchoscopy is frequently employed in the management of patients in the acute care setting and in physicians' clinics. As a respiratory care practitioner, you will be expected to understand how to assist the physician in this very important diagnostic and therapeutic procedure.

   In this chapter you will learn the indications and contraindications, hazards and complications, and technique and equipment required for the procedure, and how to correctly monitor the patient. In respiratory care practice in the acute care setting, this procedure will be most commonly performed in the short-stay outpatient area and in the intensive care unit, in both adult and pediatric patients.

KEY TERMS

- Bronchoalveolar lavage (BAL)
- Bronchoscopy
- Cytology brush
- Diagnostic bronchoscopy
- Fiberoptic bronchoscope
- Forceps
- Rigid bronchoscope
- Therapeutic bronchoscopy
- Wang needle

OBJECTIVES

At the end of this chapter, you should be able to:

- Differentiate between therapeutic and diagnostic bronchoscopy.
- Describe the indications for therapeutic and diagnostic bronchoscopy.
- Differentiate between a flexible and rigid bronchoscope and state when the use of a rigid bronchoscope is indicated.
- Describe the construction of a flexible fiberoptic bronchoscope.
- Describe the specialized instruments used during bronchoscopy.
- List the types of laboratory tests performed on samples obtained via bronchoscopy.
- List the different solutions utilized for cytological, histological, and microbiological analysis of bronchoscopy samples.

- Describe the appropriate personal protective equipment that should be worn during a bronchoscopy procedure.
- Describe the components of a designated bronchoscopy room or suite for outpatient bronchoscopy procedures.
- Describe the structure and function of both rigid and flexible bronchoscopes.
- Describe the medications utilized to provide anesthesia and analgesia for a patient prior to bronchoscopy and the potential hazards and adverse effects of these medications.
- Describe how to appropriately monitor the patient during the bronchoscopy procedure.
- Describe how bronchoscopy may be performed on a patient receiving mechanical ventilation via an endotracheal tube or tracheostomy tube.
- Describe the hazards and complications of bronchoscopy.

CLINICAL PRACTICE GUIDELINES

AARC Clinical Practice Guideline
Fiberoptic Bronchoscopy Assisting

FBA 4.0 INDICATIONS:
Indications include but are not limited to:

4.1 The presence of lesions of unknown etiology on the chest x-ray film or the need to evaluate recurrent or persistent atelectasis or pulmonary infiltrates (1–5)

4.2 The need to assess patency or mechanical properties of the upper airway (1,2,4)

4.3 The need to investigate hemoptysis, persistent unexplained cough, localized wheeze, or stridor (1–6)

4.4 Suspicious or positive sputum cytology results (1–4)

4.5 The need to obtain lower respiratory tract secretions, cell washings, and biopsies for cytologic, histologic, and microbiologic evaluation (1,2,5,7,8)

4.6 The need to determine the location and extent of injury from toxic inhalation or aspiration (1,2,4)

4.7 The need to evaluate problems associated with endotracheal or tracheostomy tubes (tracheal damage, airway obstruction, or tube placement) (1–5)

(Continued)

351

(CPG Continued)

4.8 The need for aid in performing difficult intubations (1,2,4,5)

4.9 The suspicion that secretions or mucous plugs are responsible for lobar or segmental atelectasis (1–4)

4.10 The need to remove abnormal endobronchial tissue or foreign material by forceps, basket, or laser (1)

4.11 The need to retrieve a foreign body (although under most circumstances, rigid bronchoscopy is preferred) (4,5,9)

FBA 5.0 CONTRAINDICATIONS:

Flexible bronchoscopy should be performed only when the relative benefits outweigh the risks.

5.1 Absolute contraindications include:

5.1.1 Absence of consent from the patient or his/her representative unless a medical emergency exists and patient is not competent to give permission (1)

5.1.2 Absence of an experienced bronchoscopist to perform or closely and directly supervise the procedure (1,2)

5.1.3 Lack of adequate facilities and personnel to care for such emergencies as cardiopulmonary arrest, pneumothorax, or bleeding (1,2)

5.1.4 Inability to adequately oxygenate the patient during the procedure (1)

5.2 The danger of a serious complication from bronchoscopy is especially high in patients with the disorders listed, and these conditions are usually considered absolute contraindications unless the risk-benefit assessment warrants the procedure (1,2).

5.2.1 Coagulopathy or bleeding diathesis that cannot be corrected (1,2)

5.2.2 Severe obstructive airways disease (1,2)

5.2.3 Severe refractory hypoxemia (1,2)

5.2.4 Unstable hemodynamic status including dysrhythmias (1,2)

5.3 Relative contraindications (or conditions involving increased risk), according to the American Thoracic Society Guidelines for Fiberoptic Bronchoscopy in adults (1) include:

5.3.1 Lack of patient cooperation

5.3.2 Recent myocardial infarction or unstable angina

5.3.3 Partial tracheal obstruction

5.3.4 Moderate-to-severe hypoxemia or any degree of hypercarbia

5.3.5 Uremia and pulmonary hypertension (possible serious hemorrhage after biopsy)

5.3.6 Lung abscess (danger of flooding the airway with purulent material)

5.3.7 Obstruction of the superior vena cava (possibility of bleeding and laryngeal edema)

5.3.8 Debility, advanced age, and malnutrition

5.3.9 Respiratory failure requiring mechanical ventilation

5.3.10 Disorders requiring laser therapy, biopsy of lesions obstructing large airways, or multiple transbronchial lung biopsies

5.3.11 Known or suspected pregnancy because of radiation exposure

5.4 The safety of bronchoscopic procedures in asthmatic patients is a concern, but the presence of asthma does not preclude the use of these procedures (7,10)

FBA 6.0 HAZARDS/COMPLICATIONS:

6.1 Adverse effects of medication used before and during the bronchoscopic procedure (2,5,11,12)

6.2 Hypoxemia (2,13)

6.3 Hypercarbia

6.4 Wheezing (14)

6.5 Hypotension (14)

6.6 Laryngospasm, bradycardia, or other vagally mediated phenomena (2,5,11)

6.7 Mechanical complications such as epistaxis, pneumothorax, and hemoptysis (5,11,15)

6.8 Increased airway resistance (2,16)

6.9 Death (17)

6.10 Infection hazard for health care workers or other patients (18–21) (see also Section 13)

6.11 Cross-examination of specimens or bronchoscopes (18–21)

FBA 8.0 ASSESSMENT OF NEED:

Need is determined by the presence of clinical indicators as previously described in Section 4.0, and by the presence of contraindications as described in Section 5.0.

FBA 9.0 ASSESSMENT OF OUTCOME:

Patient outcome is determined by clinical, physiologic, and pathologic assessment. Procedural outcome is determined by the accomplishment of the procedural goals as indicated in Section 4.0, and by quality assessment indicators listed in Section 11.0.

FBA 11.0 MONITORING:

The following should be monitored before, during, and/or after bronchoscopy, continuously, until the patient returns to his presedation level of consciousness.

11.1 Patient

11.1.1 Level of consciousness (30)

11.1.2 Medications administered, dosage, route, and time of delivery (30)

11.1.3 Subjective response to procedure (e.g., pain, discomfort, dyspnea) (30)

11.1.4 Blood pressure, heart rate, rhythm, and changes in cardiac status

11.1.5 SpO_2 and FiO_2 (30,31)

11.1.6 Tidal volume, peak inspiratory pressure, adequacy of inspiratory flow, and other ventilation parameters if subject is being mechanically ventilated

11.1.7 Lavage volumes (delivered and retrieved)

11.1.8 Documentation of site of biopsies and washings and tests requested on each sample

11.1.9 Periodic postprocedure follow-up monitoring of patient condition is advisable for 24–48 hours for inpatients. Outpatients should be instructed to contact the bronchoscopist regarding fever, chest pain or discomfort, dyspnea, wheezing, hemoptysis, or any new findings presenting after the procedure has been completed. Oral instructions should be reinforced by written instructions that include names and phone numbers of persons to be contacted in emergency.

11.2 Technical devices

11.2.1 Bronchoscope integrity (fiberoptic or channel damage, passage of leak test) (23)

11.2.2 Strict adherence to the recommended procedures for cleaning, disinfection, and sterilization of the devices, and the integrity of disinfection or sterilization packaging (22,23)

11.2.3 Smooth, unhampered operation of biopsy devices (forceps, needles)

11.3 Record keeping

11.3.1 Quality assessment indicators as determined appropriate by the institution's quality assessment committee

11.3.2 Documentation of monitors indicated in Sections 11.1 and 11.2

11.3.3 Identification of bronchoscope used for each patient

11.3.4 Annual assessment of the institutional or departmental bronchoscopy procedure, including an evaluation of:

11.3.4.1 Adequacy of bronchoscopic specimens (size or volume for accurate analysis, sample integrity)

11.3.4.2 Review of infection control procedures and compliance with the current guidelines for semicritical patient-care objects (22,25)

11.3.4.3 Synopsis of complications

11.3.4.4 Control washings to ensure that infection control and disinfection/sterilization procedures are adequate, and that cross-contamination of specimens does not occur

11.3.4.5 Annual review of the bronchoscopy service and all of the aforementioned records with the physician bronchoscopists

Reprinted with permission from *Respiratory Care* 1993; 38: 1173–1178. The complete AARC Clinical Practice Guidelines are available from the AARC Web site (http://www.aarc.org), from the AARC Executive Office, or from *Respiratory Care* journal.

THERAPEUTIC AND DIAGNOSTIC BRONCHOSCOPY

Bronchoscopy is commonly performed for two reasons: therapeutic and diagnostic. Therapeutic indications usually involve secretion removal, foreign body removal, or airway management problems. Diagnostic bronchoscopy is performed to identify or rule out pathologic conditions.

Therapeutic Bronchoscopy

Therapeutic bronchoscopy is performed to remove excessive pulmonary secretions or foreign material suspected of causing lobar or segmental atelectasis. By performing bronchoscopy, the material (secretions or foreign bodies) may be removed and the lobe or segment reinflated (Prakash, Offord, & Stubbs, 1991; Landa, 1978).

Therapeutic bronchoscopy may also be performed to evaluate placement of an endotracheal tube or to perform difficult intubation. Occasionally, an endotracheal tube can become dislodged or obstructed. The flexible bronchoscope provides a convenient way to assess endotracheal tube placement and to check the tube for obstruction. In some cases, difficult intubation may be performed by passing a flexible bronchoscope through the endotracheal tube and advancing it during direct visualization. The ability to direct the flexible tip of the bronchoscope facilitates the placement of the endotracheal tube (Green, 1991; Finucane & Santora, 1996).

Diagnostic Bronchoscopy

Diagnostic bronchoscopy is performed to obtain lower respiratory tract secretions or tissue samples for cytological, histological, or microbiological study (Holgate, Wilson, & Howarth, 1992). Cytological testing is frequently performed on tissue samples obtained from lesions of unknown etiology as observed on the chest x-ray (Prakash et al., 1991).

INDICATIONS FOR BRONCHOSCOPY

The indications for both therapeutic and diagnostic bronchoscopy were briefly discussed in the previous section. Table 18-1 lists the indications for both therapeutic and diagnostic bronchoscopy, as adapted from the American Association for Respiratory Care *Clinical Practice Guideline: Fiberoptic Bronchoscopy Assisting* (AARC, 1993).

TABLE 18-1: Bronchoscopy Indications

Therapeutic Indications
- Removal of secretions or mucous plugs causing lobar or segmental atelectasis
- Removal of abnormal endobronchial tissue or foreign bodies
- Evaluation of endotracheal tube placement or performance of difficult intubation

Diagnostic Indications
- Evaluation of lesions of unknown etiology as observed on chest x-ray
- Assessment of patency or mechanical properties of the upper airway
- Investigation of hemoptysis, persistent cough, localized wheezing, or stridor
- Sampling of lower respiratory tract secretions for cytological, histological, or microbiological analysis
- Investigation of suspicious or positive cytological findings
- The need to determine the location and extent of injury from toxic inhalation or aspiration

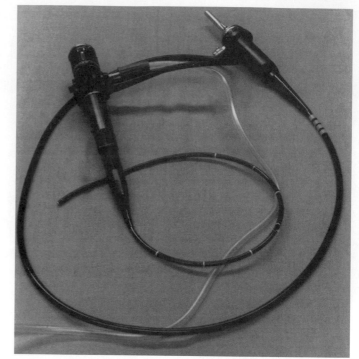

Figure 18-2   *A photograph of a flexible fiberoptic bronchoscope*

RIGID AND FLEXIBLE BRONCHOSCOPES

The *rigid bronchoscope* (Figure 18-1) has some unique advantages and disadvantages. The rigid bronchoscope is frequently used for the removal of foreign bodies. It has a much larger channel that allows the bronchoscopist to pass larger instruments, which are more effective in grasping and removing foreign objects. The larger channel also facilitates removal of large quantities of liquid or more purulent material because a greater amount of subambient pressure may be applied to the larger channel.

The disadvantages of the rigid bronchoscope are that it must be used with the patient under general anesthesia and that it provides a limited view of the tracheobronchial tree, as it cannot pass beyond the main bronchi.

The flexible *fiberoptic bronchoscope* (Figure 18-2) may be used to assess areas located more distally than the rigid bronchoscope can reach. The flexible fiberoptic bronchoscope has a control operated by the bronchoscopist's

thumb that enables maneuvering of the bronchoscope tip in a desired direction. This capability allows the bronchoscope to make the sharp bends and turns required to assess the upper lobes. Most recently, video bronchoscopy has gained popularity (Figure 18-3). The video bronchoscope incorporates a miniaturized television camera that

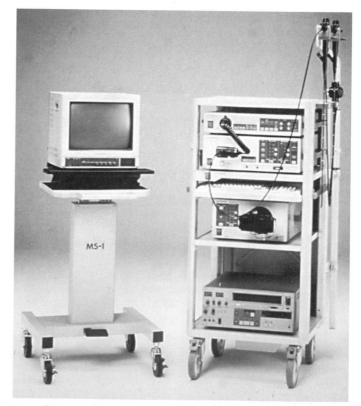

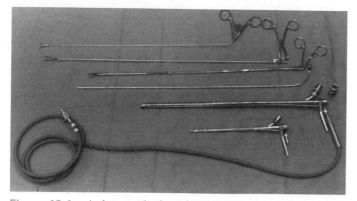

Figure 18-1   *A photograph of a rigid bronchoscope*

Figure 18-3   *A photograph of a video bronchoscope* (Courtesy of Olympus Medical Corporation, Melville, NY)

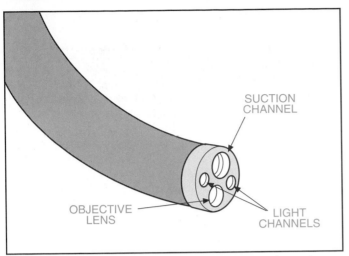

Figure 18-4 *A cross section showing the light channels, suction channel, and objective lens of a fiberoptic bronchoscope*

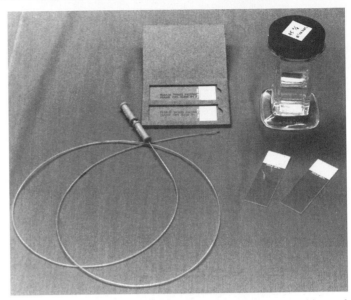

Figure 18-5 *A photograph of a cytology brush, dry slide holder, and 95% alcohol fixative*

allows the bronchoscopist to observe the procedure on a large-screen color monitor. Videotaping of the procedure can also be performed, which provides a real-time permanent record of the bronchoscopy.

Construction of a Flexible Fiberoptic Bronchoscope

The fiberoptic bronchoscope consists of several parts (Figure 18-4). The light channel conducts light from the portable light source to the bronchoscope via fiberoptic bundles. The tip of the bronchoscope is marked in centimeters to assist the bronchoscopist in determining the placement of the scope. The fiberoptic bronchoscope has one or two light channels, an objective lens, and a suction channel (see Figure 18-4). The light channels conduct light from the light source to the distal tip of the bronchoscope. The objective lens focuses the image onto a fiberoptic bundle that conducts the image to the lens set at the proximal end of the bronchoscope, where the bronchoscopist can focus the image. The suction channel is used to aspirate secretions or blood and is also used to pass specialized instruments such as the cytology brush, forceps, and basket.

TYPES OF INSTRUMENTS

The instruments used during flexible bronchoscopy include the cytology brush, Wang needle, forceps, and basket. The *cytology brush* is a small brush (Figure 18-5) that is designed to be passed through the suction channel and brushed against the location of interest in the tracheobronchial tree. Cytology brushes may be sheathed or unsheathed. A sheathed brush (Figure 18-6) is used to obtain a sample that does not become contaminated during retrieval through the suction channel. Use of the sheathed brush is described later in the chapter.

The *Wang needle* is used to sample an area of interest that lies on the opposite side of the bronchial wall from where the bronchoscope is located (Figure 18-7). The Wang needle passes through the bronchial wall and material is

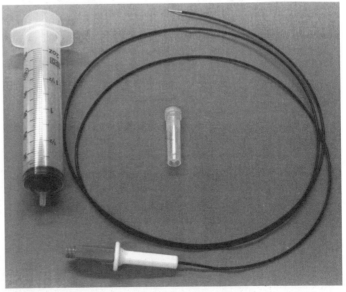

Figure 18-6 *A photograph of a sheathed or protected cytology brush and Saccomanno's solution*

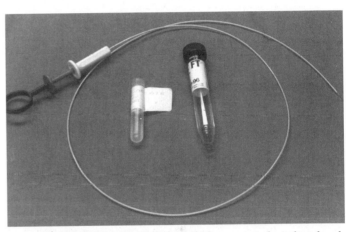

Figure 18-7 *A photograph of a Wang needle used for needle biopsy, a 20-ml syringe, and fixative solution*

then aspirated for analysis (Figure 18-8). Use of the Wang needle is discussed later in this chapter.

The *forceps* are used to sample areas of interest by "biting" off small chunks of tissue (Figure 18-9). Forceps may also be used to retrieve small foreign objects that may be easily grasped. However, once the object has been grasped, the entire bronchoscope must be withdrawn because few foreign objects will pass through the small suction channel.

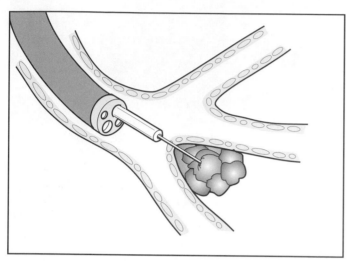

Figure 18-8 *An illustration showing the applications of the Wang needle*

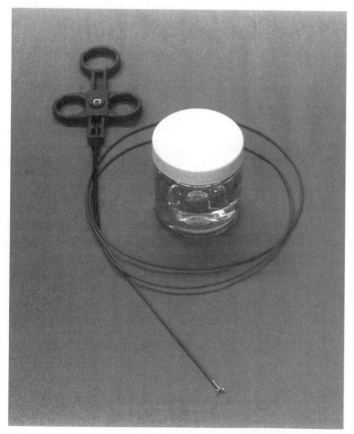

Figure 18-9 *A photograph of a pair of biopsy forceps and fixative solution*

TYPES OF SAMPLE TESTING AND ANALYSIS

Types of testing and analysis performed on samples obtained by bronchoscopy include cytological, histological, and microbiological testing. Cytological testing is performed to study a cell's structure, function, or origin. Tissue samples obtained by bronchoscopy are frequently suspected of being cancerous. Histological testing primarily focuses on the structure of cells, their composition, and how they are organized. Microbiological testing is used to identify the cause of various pulmonary infections, including those due to bacteria, viruses, fungi, and protozoans. It is important to know how the physician wishes to analyze the samples obtained during bronchoscopy because the fixative agent or treatment of the sample for the laboratory will vary depending on the tests that will be performed.

SOLUTIONS USED TO FIX OR PREPARE SAMPLES FOR TESTING

Depending on the type of tests to be performed on the samples obtained during bronchoscopy, as a respiratory care practitioner you will be expected to know how to prepare the samples properly for the pathologist. Cytological, histological, or microbiological testing determines what solutions are used to prepare the samples.

If cytological studies will be performed, the samples are usually obtained via brushing or washings. Gently streak or smear the slide with the sample brush using an S-shaped motion. Fix the slide in 95% alcohol. Alternatively, Saccomanno's solution may be used, in which case the brush may be clipped off with scissors and dropped into a test tube containing the solution (Figure 18-10).

Histological testing requires that the sample be fixed in a formalin solution. Usually, test tubes or small sample collection containers that contain formalin solution are prepared in advance. The samples are then introduced into

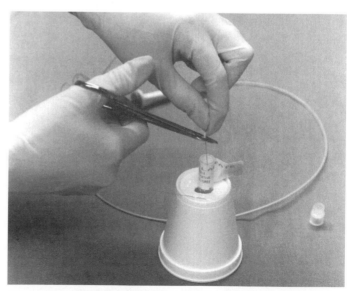

Figure 18-10 *A photograph showing the biopsy brush being clipped into a test tube of Saccomanno's solution*

the solution, capped or sealed, and sent to the laboratory for analysis.

Samples for microbiological testing may not be fixed at all. The 95% alcohol, Saccomanno's, and formalin solutions could potentially kill or seriously hamper the growth of microorganisms. Physiologic saline (0.9%) or Ringer's lactate is frequently used for preparation of microbiology samples to quantify organisms per milliliter.

PERSONAL PROTECTIVE EQUIPMENT

Bronchoscopy is an invasive procedure in which the bronchoscopist and the bronchoscopy assistant are at risk for body substance contact via splashing or direct contact; therefore, the standard precautions as recommended by the Centers for Disease Control and Prevention (CDC) should be strictly adhered to (Garner & the Hospital Infection Control Practices Committee, 1996). Personal protective equipment includes a waterproof gown, gloves, mask and goggles or full face shield or mask-shield combination, and a radiation dosimeter badge.

A waterproof gown is required because body fluids may come in contact with the bronchoscopist or the bronchoscopy assistant. Without the use of a waterproof gown, it is likely that your clothing could become soiled with the patient's secretions or body fluids during the procedure.

The use of gloves is mandatory. You will be handling instruments (brushes, forceps, or baskets) and syringes (used in sampling of bronchoalveolar lavage fluid) that have come in contact with the patient's body fluids. Therefore, a protective barrier is required to prevent these fluids from coming in contact with your skin.

A mask over your mouth and nose is worn to protect you from inhaling or aspirating aerosolized droplets that can be produced by the patient's coughing during the procedure. If the presence of acid-fast bacilli (AFB) is suspected, both the bronchoscopist and the bronchoscopy assistant should wear HEPA (high-energy particulate air) masks in accordance with CDC and Occupational Safety and Health Administration (OSHA) guidelines.

Goggles, a full face shield, or a mask-shield combination is worn to protect the eyes from splashes and aerosolized droplets. The specific type of personal protective eyewear is a matter of personal preference; however, it should be worn at all times.

A radiation dosimeter badge should also be worn because often bronchoscopy is performed under fluoroscopy so that the bronchoscopist may more accurately assess the placement of the bronchoscope. The dosimeter badge should be analyzed for radiation exposure according to both OSHA and institutional policies and procedures.

BRONCHOSCOPY ROOM OR SUITE

Frequently, outpatient bronchoscopy is performed in a specialized room or suite specifically designed for the procedure. The bronchoscopy suite has multiple banks of fluorescent lighting that provide a high degree of illumination while not producing excessive heat. Irradiation by ultraviolet (UV) lights placed high in the room is utilized to destroy AFB bacteria that may be aerosolized during coughing. The room also has special filtration and air-changing requirements, in which the air is circulated at a faster rate than in other areas. The bronchoscopy suite is also equipped with piped oxygen, air, and vacuum services that may be required to run equipment and provide supplemental oxygen for the patient during the procedure.

MEDICATIONS EMPLOYED FOR ANESTHESIA AND ANALGESIA

As a respiratory care practitioner you are expected to know how to prepare the patient properly for the bronchoscopy procedure, which includes both anesthesia and analgesia. The medications frequently used for bronchoscopy are listed in Table 18-2.

For initial preparation of the patient, 4 ml of 4% lidocaine is aerosolized using a small-volume nebulizer. A bronchodilator such as albuterol may be mixed with and aerosolized along with the lidocaine solution. Then the patient inhales the mixture and should be encouraged to exhale through the nose to help anesthetize the nasal passages more completely. The nebulizer treatment may be followed by use of Hurricane or Cetacaine spray. Upper airway reflexes and the effectiveness of topical anesthesia may be tested by using a long cotton-tipped swab to manipulate the uvula while the patient holds the mouth open widely.

The absence of the gag reflex is an encouraging sign of the effectiveness of your efforts to provide topical anesthesia.

Long cotton-tipped swabs may be used to anesthetize the nasal passages further. The swabs are dipped into lidocaine jelly (4%) and then passed into the nasal passages. Some physicians prefer to use cocaine topically because it causes the blood vessels in the nasal mucosa to constrict, opening the passage further and helping to control any bleeding.

A venous catheter (an intravenous [IV] line) may be placed to facilitate the administration of analgesics such as diazepam, midazolam, or lorazepam. Use of these medications achieves the desired analgesic effect, reducing the patient's anxiety regarding the procedure; however, these drugs may produce unwanted hazards and complications.

TABLE 18-2: Medications Used in Bronchoscopy

Medications for Anesthesia
- Lidocaine (Xylocaine) 1%, 2%, 4%; 0.5% for pediatric patients
- Benzocaine spray (Hurricane spray)
- Benzocaine-tetracaine-butamben (Cetacaine) spray

Medications for Secretion or Bleeding Management
- Atropine
- Epinephrine (1:20,000 concentration)

Medications for Sedation
- Diazepam (Valium)
- Midazolam (Versed)
- Lorazepam (Ativan)

Hazards and Complications of the Medications Used for Bronchoscopy

The lidocaine (2% distal to the vocal cords) that is aerosolized prior to the procedure, and which may also be administered during the procedure through the suction channel, has potential unwanted effects. In some patients it is possible to achieve low but measurable plasma concentrations of lidocaine from the doses given before and during bronchoscopy. Adverse effects with low plasma concentrations may include vertigo, restlessness, tinnitus, and difficulty in focusing the eyes. Further increases in plasma concentration can lead to skeletal muscle twitching and seizures (Stoelting, 1987). Therefore, with administration of this drug, the patient should be monitored for these signs and symptoms.

The use of analgesic agents such as diazepam, midazolam, and lorazepam may cause depression of the respiratory drive in some patients (Stoelting, 1987). This effect may be observed primarily as a decrease in respiratory rate and tidal volume. Patients should be closely monitored for signs and symptoms of respiratory depression when these drugs are given.

PATIENT MONITORING

Patient variables that should be monitored during bronchoscopy include blood pressure, heart rate and rhythm, SpO_2, and FiO_2. The patient's blood pressure should be measured and recorded prior to anesthetic administration. In the event of an adverse drug effect, baseline blood pressure is very helpful in patient management.

Heart rate and rhythm are easily monitored in real time by the use of electrocardiographic (ECG) monitoring equipment. Usually cardiac leads are placed and lead II is monitored. Changes in rate and rhythm may be easily assessed at any point during the procedure. Alarm limits may also be set to alert the bronchoscopist and the assistant of potential problems.

SpO_2 may be monitored using a pulse oximeter, with alarm limits set to signal impending problems. FiO_2 may

also need to be monitored if the patient is receiving high-flow oxygen or is being mechanically ventilated during the procedure.

HAZARDS AND COMPLICATIONS OF BRONCHOSCOPY

Hazards and complications of bronchoscopy include hypoxemia (Schnapf, 1991), wheezing, hypotension, bradycardia, hemoptysis, bleeding, and infection. Hypoxemia is a common complication of bronchoscopy. Many patients undergoing the procedure have underlying lung disease. The insertion of the bronchoscope and the application of subambient pressure result in the removal of oxygen from the airways, causing hypoxemia, in much the same manner as described in Chapter 20.

Wheezing may be precipitated by the irritation of the patient's airway by the bronchoscope. This stimulation can result in bronchospasm, causing wheezing. Frequently, a bronchodilator such as albuterol is mixed with the lidocaine and given prior to bronchoscopy to help to prevent this effect.

Hypotension, bradycardia, and other vagal reflex effects may be caused by the physical stimulation of the bronchoscope in the airway via the vagus nerve. The patient should be monitored for these effects; early detection is facilitated by the electrocardiographic monitor and automatic blood pressure monitoring if available.

Localized bleeding during bronchoscopy is usually controlled by the administration of 1:20,000 epinephrine through the suction channel of the bronchoscope and application of direct pressure with the tip of the bronchoscope. The patient may experience hemoptysis following the procedure as these localized areas of bleeding gradually resolve.

Because bronchoscopy is an invasive procedure, infection is always a concern. The likelihood of infection and cross-contamination may be minimized through the proper care and cleaning of the bronchoscope between patients.

OBJECTIVES

At the end of this chapter, you should be able to:

- Demonstrate how to prepare the equipment required for bronchoscopy.
- Demonstrate how to prepare the paperwork and charting forms needed for this procedure.
- Demonstrate how to prepare the medications used for the procedure.
- Demonstrate how to connect the proper monitoring equipment to the patient and set the alarms appropriately.
- Demonstrate how to start an IV line or insert a heparin lock.
- Demonstrate how to administer preoperative medications, including those for analgesia and anesthesia.

- Demonstrate how to provide supplemental oxygen during the procedure.
- Demonstrate how to assist the bronchoscopist during the procedure, including administration of medications and collection of specimens for analysis.
- Demonstrate how to properly prepare specimens for analysis by the laboratory, including those for cytological, histological, and microbiological study.
- Demonstrate how to assist the physician during a bronchioalveolar lavage (BAL).
- Correctly monitor the patient during the procedure for adverse effects.
- Demonstrate how to perform bronchoscopy on a patient who is being mechanically ventilated.

- Demonstrate how to monitor the patient after the procedure and prepare the bronchoscope for cleaning.
- Demonstrate correct documentation of the procedure, including medications administered and patient monitoring data.

- Correctly clean the bronchoscope following the procedure.
- Demonstrate how to correctly deliver the specimens obtained during the procedure to the laboratory for analysis.

EQUIPMENT PREPARATION

Bronchoscopy can progress smoothly and almost effortlessly, or it may be conducted in a tense environment in which nothing seems to go correctly. The ease of the procedure is largely dependent on how well the bronchoscopy assistant has set up and prepared for the procedure. Therefore, it is very important that you prepare everything and have all required equipment ready at hand and organized in such a way that you can easily retrieve what is required when needed.

Bronchoscope Preparation

Attach the bronchoscope to the light source and connect the light source to a suitable electrical outlet (120 V 60 Hz or 220 V 60 Hz). Turn on the light source and check to ensure that light is conducted to the distal end of the bronchoscope and that the light source is functioning properly.

If required, attach the suction valve to the bronchoscope and connect the bronchoscope to a suction source. Adjust the vacuum level to the maximum setting. It is also advisable to have a second vacuum source ready with a Yankauer suction tool attached to it. Place the bronchoscope onto the bronchoscopy cart or tray and cover it with a sterile towel.

Have a bite block at hand so that if the physician wishes to pass the bronchoscope orally the bronchoscope may be protected. The preferred route is to pass the bronchoscope nasally rather than orally. Even with the use of a bite block, an orally placed instrument can occasionally slip out of position so that the patient bites down reflexively, ruining the fiberoptics.

Medication Preparation

First, draw up 50 ml of 2% lidocaine and transfer it into a sterile container such as a urology analysis container. Label the container "2% lidocaine" and locate it on the bronchoscopy cart or tray where it can be easily reached. Have two 10-ml syringes with "slip tips" nearby for drawing up the solution as required.

Then draw up 50 ml of normal saline (0.9%) and transfer it into a sterile container such as a urology analysis container. Label the container "normal saline" and locate it on the bronchoscopy cart or tray where it can be easily reached. Have two 10-ml syringes with "slip tips" nearby for drawing up the solution as required.

Finally, draw up 20 ml of 1:20,000 epinephrine and transfer it into a sterile container such as a urology analysis container. Label the container "1:20,000 epinephrine" and locate it on the bronchoscopy cart or tray where it can be easily reached. Have two 10-ml syringes with "slip tips" nearby for drawing up the solution as required.

Also have available several unit dose containers (4 ml) of 20% acetylcysteine (Mucomyst) should the physician wish to instill it through the bronchoscope. Have available a 10-ml syringe for injecting the solution through the bronchoscope.

Sample Solution Preparation

Have slide containers with 95% alcohol, formalin, and normal saline (0.9%) available. Additionally, test tubes containing those solutions and Saccomanno's solution should be at hand. Attach blank labels to the specimen containers and have a pen readily available to label the container as to where the sample was obtained during the procedure. Clean sterile slides should be available to make smears for cytological study. Often a slide dispenser is used to prepare specimens. Dry slides are frequently used for AFB and mycological culturing. Organize your containers into groupings (cytology, histology, and microbiology) so that during the procedure you do not have to hunt to find what you need.

Emergency Equipment

Ensure that a "code cart" is in the procedure room. Check the cart for appropriate ACLS emergency medications; a manual resuscitator; a defibrillator; and intubation supplies, including a suction catheter.

Personal Protective Equipment

Check to be sure that personal protective equipment is available for all personnel participating in the procedure. This equipment includes waterproof gowns, masks (HEPA if required), gloves, and eye protection.

Equipment for the Patient

It is desirable to have certain pieces of equipment available for the patient. These items include tissues, an emesis basin, a denture cup (if required), a washcloth, and a small hand towel.

DOCUMENTATION PREPARATION

This procedure requires an informed consent form that must be signed by the patient and a witness. The form explains the procedure and the hazards and complications associated with it. It may be necessary for you to explain to the patient in nontechnical language what the form means; therefore, you should be familiar with it and what it says. If the bronchoscopy procedure is to be performed in the intensive care unit setting and the patient is unable to sign the form, a member of the patient's immediate family may give consent if such a person is available.

Have any charting forms required by your institution at hand with the patient's name and identification number imprinted or written in ink on the forms. Also have any laboratory testing request forms available and marked with the patient's name and identification number.

PATIENT PREPARATION

Prior to performing the bronchoscopy procedure, it is important to prepare the patient for the procedure. This includes establishing appropriate monitoring and administration of anesthesia and analgesia, and having the patient sign the appropriate consent forms.

Monitoring

Attach cardiac leads so that lead II may be monitored. Connect the patient to an ECG monitor and verify that heart rate and rhythm are appropriately displayed.

Measure the patient's blood pressure, and if a blood pressure cuff is available, apply it and attach it to an automatic sphygmomanometer. Set the time interval to the desired frequency of blood pressure measurement.

Initiate continuous pulse oximetry monitoring. The use of a finger or ear probe is usually best for this procedure. An ear probe is less likely to experience artifact due to patient motion during the procedure. Check the oximeter against the ECG monitor to verify that the signal is appropriate.

Anesthesia and Analgesia

Start an IV line or insert a heparin lock so that intravenous access is available for the administration of analgesic agents.

Nebulize 4 to 5 ml of 4% lidocaine and, depending on your institution's policy, add 2.5 mg albuterol to the solution to achieve bronchodilation. Have the patient inhale deeply and slowly. Request that the patient exhale through the nose to help anesthetize the upper airway more fully. Following the administration of the lidocaine, Hurricane or Cetacaine spray may be used to anesthetize the upper airway further. Evaluate the numbness of the upper airway by manipulating the uvula with a long cotton-tipped swab. If the patient does not gag, the airway has been well anesthetized.

Using long cotton-tipped swabs, apply 4% lidocaine jelly to the nasal passages and into the region of the turbinates. This will help to lubricate the airway and also to anesthetize it further.

When the physician arrives, determine whether or not analgesic medication is desired and what dose is to be administered intravenously. Draw up the medication according to the physician's instructions and administer the drug through the IV line or heparin lock.

SUPPLEMENTAL OXYGEN

Supplemental oxygen may be provided by using a nasal cannula with one prong "clipped off" or plugged, or by using a simple mask in which one side has had an opening cut into it so that the bronchoscope may be passed through it. Monitor the patient's SpO_2 and adjust the oxygen delivery to maintain saturations greater than 90% during the procedure.

BRONCHOSCOPY ASSISTING

Bronchoscopy assisting involves many skills, including medication administration, assistance with tissue sampling, and specimen preparation.

Medication Administration

The physician will advance the bronchoscope through either naris and advance it through the upper airway. If the patient begins to cough or fight the procedure, be prepared to instill 2% lidocaine upon the physician's request.

Once the bronchoscope enters the larynx, the coughing reflex is commonly encountered. Again, be prepared to administer 2% lidocaine on the physician's request. Depending on how the procedure progresses, the physician will request that you instill 2% lidocaine, normal saline, or if secretions are very thick, 20% acetylcysteine.

Tissue Sampling

Tissue sampling is frequently performed to obtain small samples for laboratory analysis. The most common instruments used are the biopsy forceps and the brush (either protected or unprotected).

Forceps

If tissue samples are required for diagnostic purposes, the physician will perform biopsy using the forceps, brush, or the Wang needle. If biopsy is to be performed, you will be requested to pass the forceps through the suction channel. Be certain that the forceps are closed when you pass them through the suction channel. Open forceps will damage the fiberoptics of the bronchoscope. The physician will then direct the tip of the scope, guiding the forceps to the desired location, and will advance the forceps near the tissue site. The physician will request "open," which means that you must open the forceps by pushing the thumb control. The physician will then push the open forceps into the tissue to be sampled and request "closed," which means you must then retract the thumb control to close the forceps. Before the procedure, manipulate the forceps so that you know which position is open and which is closed.

Brushes

Brushing is usually performed for cytological or histological analysis. The brushes used may be protected or unprotected. If protected brushing is performed, a protected brush is passed through the suction channel much like the forceps. The physician will request "out," which means that you must advance the inner brush through the wax seal, exposing it past the outer sheath, by manipulating the thumb control; then the brush is advanced. The physician will brush the desired site multiple times and request "retract" or "in," which means that you must then retract the brush once again into the protective sheath. The brush is then withdrawn, and slides are made or the brush is clipped off and dropped into the proper solution for the test.

Wang Needle

The Wang needle is used to sample areas that are on the opposite side of the bronchial wall from the bronchoscope (extrabronchial). As for the forceps, you must pass the Wang needle with the needle retracted. Failure to do so will ruin the bronchoscope's fiberoptics. The Wang needle is passed through the bronchoscope in a similar way to the forceps and brush. The physician will request "out," which means that you must advance the needle, exposing it past the sheath, by manipulating the thumb control. The physician will then "dart" the desired site multiple times and request "retract" or "in," which means that you must then retract the brush once again into the protective sheath. Often the Wang needle is used under a fluoroscope to determine its location more precisely. Suction is applied to the end of the Wang needle with a syringe to aspirate a sample for analysis. Very small samples are secured by this method, so look closely to ensure that you have obtained an adequate specimen. Prepare the sample as required for cytological or histological analysis.

Bleeding Control

Often during sampling, bleeding may occur. The physician may control bleeding by direct pressure, instillation of 1:20,000 epinephrine, or a combination of both. It is important to have good suction through the bronchoscope to protect the airway in the event of profound bleeding. If bleeding is profound, a pulmonary tamponade balloon may be inserted, inflated, and left in place to control bleeding.

SPECIMEN PREPARATION

As described earlier, it is important to have ready the different solutions that may be needed to prepare your samples for analysis. Properly prepared and labeled samples make it easier for the pathologist to achieve an accurate diagnosis. If you can make it easier for the pathologist and the pulmonologist performing the procedure through your preparation and proficiency, you are in effect marketing your services.

Label all samples with the patient's name and the anatomical location from which the samples were taken. Ask the physician to name all lobes and segments sampled, to ensure that specimens from several different areas are not inadvertently mislabeled.

If you are in doubt, ask the pulmonologist whether the sample is for cytological, histological, or microbiological analysis and prepare the sample accordingly by using the correct solution.

BRONCHOALVEOLAR LAVAGE

Bronchoalveolar lavage (BAL) is performed when the area to be sampled is distal to the segmental or subsegmental bronchi in which the bronchoscope is resting. The bronchoscopist advances the bronchoscope until it is "wedged," totally occluding the airway. The bronchoscopist will then request that you instill 30 to 50 ml of normal saline (0.9%) rapidly through the suction channel and then withdraw the syringe plunger firmly, attempting to aspirate as much of the instilled saline as possible through the bronchoscope. The concept is to lavage the area distal to the bronchoscope with saline and then to recover as much of the saline as possible. The recovered solution will contain the cells that the physician wishes to analyze. When you perform BAL, be sure to turn off the suction to the bronchoscope, or install a trap, so that if the physician occludes the suction port, the sample will not be lost to the wall suction unit! BAL may be performed several times until the physician is satisfied that the area has been adequately sampled. BAL is often performed to obtain specimens for microbiological analysis. Visually inspect the sample, observing for a foamy head, almost like that on beer, indicating that surfactant is present and that you obtained a good sample.

PATIENT MONITORING

As described earlier, the patient must be monitored for signs of hypoxemia, wheezing, hypotension, bradycardia, hemoptysis, and bleeding. Through the use of appropriate monitoring devices and paying attention to the patient, early signs may be detected. Remember that the physician is more focused on the bronchoscope and its location and may not necessarily be closely watching the patient. Therefore, it is your responsibility as the assistant to report adverse signs or symptoms. This may easily be performed using the ECG monitor, blood pressure monitor, and pulse oximeter. Your knowledge and assessment skills are what make you as a respiratory care practitioner uniquely qualified to assist in this procedure.

Following the procedure, closely monitor the patient's level of consciousness and evaluate the patient for the return of the protective reflexes of the upper airway as the local anesthetic wears off. Evidence of the return of reflexes includes coughing and appropriate swallowing. The medications used for analgesia may be reversed using agents such as naloxone or flumazenil. Before the patient is allowed to leave the area, be certain that he or she is alert enough to walk and behave appropriately. It is frequently recommended that another person drive the patient home following the procedure. It is also important to instruct the patient not to eat or drink anything for at least 2 hours following the procedure because aspiration may be likely owing to the local anesthesia.

BRONCHOSCOPY DURING MECHANICAL VENTILATION

Bronchoscopy may be performed on patients who are receiving mechanical ventilation. This is accomplished by inserting the instrument through a swivel adapter that has a soft Silastic seal, which helps to prevent volume loss in passing the bronchoscope (Figure 18-11). The bronchoscope is advanced through the endotracheal

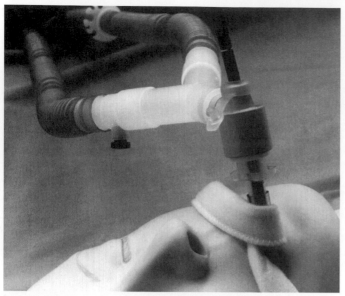

Figure 18-11 *A photograph showing how a swivel adapter is used to perform bronchoscopy on a patient on ventilatory support through an endotracheal tube*

or tracheostomy tube. If the patient is orally intubated, a bite block should be inserted to protect the bronchoscope.

Ventilator settings will need to be modified during the procedure. Usually the tidal volume is reduced, the flow rate reduced, the FIO$_2$ increased, and the respiratory rate increased. Experience is required to determine the optimal settings that still achieve adequate ventilation and oxygenation without the occurrence of ventilator pressure cycling (high-pressure alarm) with each breath.

DOCUMENTATION

Bronchoscopy assisting requires appropriate documentation of the procedure just as for other respiratory care procedures. Documentation should include the patient's baseline blood pressure, ECG strip, and SpO$_2$. The preparation of the patient, including medications used, IV access, and routes of delivery, should also be documented. Appropriate notations during the procedure of blood pressure, respiratory rate, ECG, and SpO$_2$ should also be provided.

The amount and type of medications given during the procedure should also be documented. If you know you started with 50 ml each of lidocaine and normal saline and 20 ml of 1:20,000 epinephrine, measuring what you have left and subtracting it from what you started with will tell you the amount you used. Any use of other medications such as acetylcysteine and analgesia-reversal agents should also be documented.

The location of samples obtained and the type of tests (cytological, histological, or microbiological) the samples were prepared for should also be noted. If BAL was performed, note how much aspirate was recovered and the number of attempts that were made.

The patient's recovery data, including respiratory rate, ECG, and blood pressure, should be documented. It is also important to document the return of reflexes by noting coughing, swallowing, and so forth.

CLEANING THE BRONCHOSCOPE

The bronchoscope is initially prepared for cleaning by aspirating about 100 to 200 ml of normal saline through the suction channel. A cleaning brush may be passed through the bronchoscope a few times and more saline aspirated before transporting the bronchoscope to the decontamination area.

At the decontamination area, the bronchoscope is disassembled and those parts that can be decontaminated using surgical instrument soap are washed and rinsed. The outer surface of the bronchoscope is cleaned with a disinfection solution and a soft cloth.

The bronchoscope's suction channel is cleaned by aspirating a cold disinfection agent such as Cidex or Control III through the suction channel and brushing it with the cleaning brush. Following cleaning, the bronchoscope should then be tested for leaks. The bronchoscope may then be placed into an automatic endoscope washer, in which alternately a cold disinfection solution and sterile water are passed through the bronchoscope, cleaning it. Alternatively, the bronchoscope may be immersed in a cold disinfection solution and allowed to stand for the required period of time.

Following disinfection, the bronchoscope is rinsed with sterile water and then 95% alcohol is injected through the suction channel, which promotes drying. The bronchoscope is then aseptically covered until it will be used again.

SAMPLE DELIVERY

Once the samples are labeled and properly prepared, they should be delivered to the laboratory for analysis. Any institutional slips required for testing should be filled out completely and submitted with the samples. Most laboratories require time and date stamping of when samples are received; therefore, comply with the requirements and use the stamping machine to accomplish this on the laboratory slips. Your prompt delivery and handling of the specimens will help to ensure that an accurate diagnosis may be made. Remember that you are marketing your services not only to the patient and the pulmonologist but also to the pathologist!

References

American Association for Respiratory Care. (1993). AARC clinical practice guideline: Fiberoptic bronchoscopy assisting. *Respiratory Care, 38*(11), 1173–1178.

Finucane, B. T., & Santora, A. H. (1996). *Principles of airway management* (2nd ed*.*). Philadelphia: F. A. Davis.

Garner, J. S., & the Hospital Infection Control Practices Committee. (1996). Guidelines for isolation precautions in hospitals. *American Journal of Infection Control, 24*, 24–52.

Green, C. G. (1991). Assessment of the pediatric airway by flexible bronchoscopy. *Respiratory Care, 36*(6), 555–565.

Holgate, S. T., Wilson, J. R., & Howarth, P. H. (1992). New insights into airway inflammation by endobronchial biopsy. *American Review of Respiratory Disease, 145*(2).

Landa, J. F., (1978). Indications for bronchoscopy. *Chest, 73*(5), (Suppl.).

Prakash, U. B. S., Offord, U. B., & Stubbs, S. E. (1991). Bronchoscopy in North America: The ACCP survey. *Chest, 100*(6).

Schnapf, B. M. (1991). Oxygen desaturation during fiberoptic bronchoscopy in pediatric patients. *Chest, 99*, 591–594.

Stoelting, R. (1987). *Pharmacology and physiology in anesthetic practice.* Philadelphia: Lippincott.

Additional Resources

Burton, G. G., Hodgkin, J., & Ward, J. (1997). *Respiratory care: A guide to clinical practice* (4th ed.). Philadelphia: Lippincott.

Kacmarek, R., & Pierson, D. J. (1992). *Foundations of respiratory care.* New York: McGraw-Hill.

Practice Activities: Bronchoscopy Assisting

1. Organize and set up a bronchoscopy tray or cart, including:
   a. Fixative solutions
   b. Microscope slides
   c. Instruments: biopsy forceps, brushes, and Wang needle
   d. Saline
   e. Topical anesthetics
   f. Analgesics
   g. Intravenous supplies
   h. 10-ml syringes

2. Once the cart or tray has been organized, practice bronchoscopy assisting with a lab partner, with one partner calling for a particular item and the other retrieving it.

3. Using water-soluble lubricant, practice making S-shaped smears on microscope slides with the brush. Practice evenly distributing the material throughout your smear.

4. Make a list of all of the emergency supplies that you might want when performing bronchoscopy, should an emergency situation occur.

5. Assemble the bronchoscope and test it for function:
   a. Light source
   b. Suction source

6. Practice using the biopsy forceps, protected brush, and Wang needle until you can change from the open to the closed position without having to concentrate or think about it.

7. Using an intubation mannequin for practice, practice performing the bronchoscopy procedure with a lab partner, alternating roles as the bronchoscopist and the bronchoscopy assistant.

8. Using a water-soluble lubricant as a "sample," practice preparing slides for cytology, histology, and microbiology analysis.

9. Using a lab partner as a patient, properly instrument the patient for monitoring during bronchoscopy, including blood pressure, ECG, and pulse oximetry.

10. Using your institution's charting forms, prepare the following:
    a. Informed consent
    b. Bronchoscopy charting form
    c. Laboratory testing requests

11. Using an intubation mannequin, intubate the mannequin and practice performing bronchoscopy with a lab partner using the specialized swivel adapter.

12. Disassemble the bronchoscope, and practice the cleaning procedure according to your institutional policy.

Check List: Bronchoscopy Assisting

_____ 1. Follow standard precautions, including hand-washing.
2. Gather the appropriate equipment and supplies:
_____ a. Bronchoscope and light source
_____ b. Fixative solutions
_____ c. Microscope slides
_____ d. Instruments: biopsy forceps, brushes, and Wang needle
_____ e. Saline
_____ f. Topical anesthetics
_____ g. Analgesics
_____ h. Intravenous supplies
_____ i. 10-ml syringes
_____ j. Personal protective equipment
3. Prepare the documentation for the procedure:
_____ a. Informed consent form
_____ b. Charting forms
_____ c. Laboratory request forms
_____ 4. Organize the bronchoscopy tray or cart.
_____ 5. Assemble and test the bronchoscope.

_____ 6. Correctly instrument the patient for monitoring.
_____ 7. Gown and glove for the procedure.
_____ 8. Initiate an IV line or insert a heparin lock.
9. Administer anesthesia topically:
_____ a. Small-volume nebulizer
_____ b. Cotton-tipped swabs
_____ 10. Evaluate adequacy of anesthesia.
_____ 11. Administer analgesia per physician's request.
_____ 12. Assist the physician with the procedure.
13. As required, obtain tissue samples for analysis:
_____ a. Brushing
_____ b. Biopsy specimens
_____ c. BAL
_____ 14. Assist the physician with bleeding control as required.
_____ 15. Monitor the patient during the procedure.
_____ 16. Correctly document the procedure.
_____ 17. Evaluate the patient following the procedure.
_____ 18. Properly clean and care for the bronchoscope.

Self-Evaluation Post Test: Bronchoscopy Assisting

1. Which of the following rationales is/are indicated for a therapeutic bronchoscopy?
   I. Removal of secretions or mucous plugs
   II. Assessment of the patency or mechanical properties of the upper airway
   III. Removal of abnormal endobronchial tissue or foreign bodies
   IV. Investigation of hemoptysis, persistent cough, localized wheezing, or stridor
   a. I, II   c. II, III
   b. I, III   d. II, IV

2. Which of the following rationales is/are indicated for a diagnostic bronchoscopy?
   I. Removal of secretions or mucous plugs
   II. Assessment of the patency or mechanical properties of the upper airway
   III. Removal of abnormal endobronchial tissue or foreign bodies
   IV. Investigation of hemoptysis, persistent cough, localized wheezing, or stridor
   a. I, II   c. II, III
   b. I, III   d. II, IV

3. For which of the following indications might a rigid bronchoscope be preferred over a fiberoptic bronchoscope?
   a. Removal of foreign bodies
   b. Diagnosis of peripheral lung disease
   c. Bronchoalveolar lavage
   d. Brushing for cytology

4. Which of the following may be performed on samples obtained from bronchoscopy?
   I. Cytology testing
   II. Histology testing
   III. Microbiology testing
   a. I   c. II, III
   b. I, II   d. I, II, III

5. Which of the following is/are considered appropriate personal protective equipment for bronchoscopy?
   I. Waterproof gown
   II. Gloves
   III. Eye shields or goggles
   IV. Mask or HEPA mask
   a. I   c. I, II, III
   b. I, II   d. I, II, III, IV

6. Which of the following make(s) a bronchoscopy suite or room different from the typical outpatient exam room?
   I. Air filtration rate
   II. Ultraviolet lights
   III. Increased lighting
   IV. Presence of piped gases
   a. I   c. I, II, III
   b. I, II   d. I, II, III, IV

7. Which of the following are medications employed for anesthesia?
   I. Lidocaine (Xylocaine)
   II. Lorazepam (Ativan)
   III. Benzocaine (Hurricane spray)
   IV. Midazolam (Versed)
   a. I, II   c. II, III
   b. I, III   d. II, IV

8. Which of the following are medications employed for analgesia?
   I. Lidocaine (Xylocaine)
   II. Lorazepam (Ativan)
   III. Benzocaine spray (Hurricane spray)
   IV. Midazolam (Versed)
   a. I, II
   b. I, III
   c. II, III
   d. II, IV

9. Which of the following is/are appropriate for monitoring the patient during bronchoscopy?
   I. Heart rate and rhythm
   II. Blood pressure
   III. Pulse oximetry
   IV. Respiratory rate and rhythm
   a. I
   b. I, II
   c. I, II, III
   d. I, II, III, IV

10. Which of the following may be (a) hazard(s) of bronchoscopy?
    I. Bleeding
    II. Hemoptysis
    III. Wheezing
    IV. Hypotension
    a. I
    b. I, II
    c. I, II, III
    d. I, II, III, IV

PERFORMANCE EVALUATION: BRONCHOSCOPY ASSISTING

Date: Lab _____   Clinical _____   Agency _____

Lab: Pass _____   Fail _____   Clinical: Pass _____   Fail _____

Student name _____   Instructor name _____

No. of times observed in clinical _____

No. of times practiced in clinical _____

PASSING CRITERIA: Obtain 90% or better on the procedure. Tasks indicated by * must receive at least 1 point, or the evaluation is terminated. Procedure must be performed within designated time, or the performance receives a failing grade.

SCORING:

2 points — Task performed satisfactorily without prompting.
1 point — Task performed satisfactorily with self-initiated correction.
0 points — Task performed incorrectly or with prompting required.
NA — Task not applicable to the patient care situation.

TASKS:

		PEER	LAB	CLINICAL
*	1. Observes standard precautions, including handwashing	☐	☐	☐
*	2. Prepares all documentation forms			
	a. Informed consent	☐	☐	☐
	b. Charting forms	☐	☐	☐
	c. Laboratory request slips	☐	☐	☐
*	3. Organizes and sets up a bronchoscopy tray or cart, including:			
	a. Fixative solutions	☐	☐	☐
	b. Microscope slides	☐	☐	☐
	c. Biopsy forceps, brushes, and Wang needle	☐	☐	☐
	d. Saline	☐	☐	☐
	e. Topical anesthetics	☐	☐	☐
	f. Analgesics	☐	☐	☐
	g. Intravenous supplies	☐	☐	☐
	h. 10-ml syringes	☐	☐	☐
*	4. Ensures emergency supplies are available	☐	☐	☐
*	5. Assembles the bronchoscope and tests its function	☐	☐	☐
*	6. Prepares the patient for monitoring			
	a. ECG	☐	☐	☐
	b. Blood pressure	☐	☐	☐
	c. Oximetry	☐	☐	☐
*	7. Applies personal protective equipment	☐	☐	☐
*	8. Starts an IV line or inserts a heparin lock	☐	☐	☐

 *   9. Administers local anesthesia

        a. Nebulizes 4% lidocaine   ☐   ☐   ☐

        b. Administers lidocaine jelly on swabs   ☐   ☐   ☐

 *   10. Administers analgesia per physician's request   ☐   ☐   ☐

 *   11. Assists the physician with the procedure   ☐   ☐   ☐

 *   12. Prepares samples for laboratory analysis   ☐   ☐   ☐

 *   13. Monitors the patient   ☐   ☐   ☐

 *   14. Correctly documents the procedure   ☐   ☐   ☐

 *   15. Correctly disassembles and cleans the bronchoscope   ☐   ☐   ☐

 *   16. Delivers specimens to the lab for analysis   ☐   ☐   ☐

SCORE: Peer   _____ points of possible 56; _____%

            Lab   _____ points of possible 56; _____%

            Clinical _____ points of possible 56; _____%

TIME: _____ out of possible 30 minutes

STUDENT SIGNATURES   INSTRUCTOR SIGNATURES

PEER: _____   LAB: _____

STUDENT: _____   CLINICAL: _____

CHAPTER 19
EQUIPMENT PROCESSING AND SURVEILLANCE

INTRODUCTION

A variety of methods are used for the decontamination of respiratory therapy equipment. Because of the presence of water, saline, and body secretions in warm reservoirs, respiratory therapy equipment may serve as an excellent vector for the growth and transmission of disease. A knowledge of the organisms, the general principles of microbiology, and the effects the processing methods have on microorganisms is essential to process equipment correctly. An understanding of how the different methods affect rubber and plastics is also required to prevent costly errors.

In this chapter you will have a review of basic microbiology. You will learn how the various processing methods affect microorganisms and the equipment being processed. You will also learn about bacteriological surveillance and how it is an integral part of equipment processing.

KEY TERMS

- Antisepsis
- Bacilli
- Bacteriological surveillance
- Capsule
- Cocci
- Disinfection
- Endotoxins
- Ethylene oxide
- Eukaryotic bacteria
- Gamma irradiation
- Glutaraldehyde
- Gram stain
- Pasteurization
- Prokaryotic bacteria
- Quaternary ammonium compounds
- Spirilla
- Steam autoclaving
- Sterilization

OBJECTIVES

At the end of this chapter, you should be able to:

- Differentiate between eukaryotic and prokaryotic organisms.
- Differentiate among the following bacterial shapes:
  — Cocci
  — Bacilli
  — Spirilla
- Differentiate between capsules and endospores and their significance for equipment processing.
- Differentiate between the cell wall structure of gram-positive and gram-negative bacteria.
- Describe the structural characteristics of viruses.
- Define the following terms:
  — Sterilization
  — Disinfection
  — Antisepsis
- Differentiate among the following processing methods and how they kill microorganisms:
  — Steam autoclaving

  — Pasteurization
  — Ethylene oxide processing
  — Glutaraldehyde processing
  — Exposure to quaternary ammonium compounds
  — Gamma irradiation
- Diagram and explain the rationale for the design of an equipment processing facility.
- Explain the purpose of a bacteriological surveillance program.
- Differentiate among the following sampling methods and state the most appropriate application for each:
  — Aliquot
  — Output
  — Rinse
  — Rodac plate
  — Swab
- Explain how the data from a bacteriological surveillance program are utilized.

RELATED MICROBIOLOGY

Eukaryotic and Prokaryotic Cell Types

Eukaryotic organisms have a true nucleus containing genetic material (chromosomes). The nucleus is a membrane-enclosed structure separate from other structures within the cell. The cell reproduces by *mitosis*, wherein the genetic material is duplicated and the cell

divides in two. Eukaryotic organisms are more complex than prokaryotes.

Prokaryotic bacteria have a single naked DNA molecule within the cell. Internal structures are fewer and far less complex than those of eukaryotes. Replication is accomplished by cell division, not mitosis as in eukaryotic organisms. There are significant differences in the cell wall structure, as discussed later when the Gram stain is explained.

Bacterial Shapes

Bacterial shapes further help to classify prokaryotic bacteria. The most common shapes are cocci, bacilli, and spirilla. These shapes are illustrated in Figure 19-1. The shapes are relatively constant and more or less independent of environmental influences.

Cocci are spherical in shape. A rounded shape enables this bacterial type to resist desiccation because of its smaller surface area.

Bacilli are rod-shaped. They are greater in length than in diameter. The greater surface area makes them more susceptible to desiccation but also allows these bacteria to absorb nutrients more easily from the environment.

Spirilla are spiral in configuration. A spiral shape aids in motility through fluids.

Gram Stain

The *Gram stain* is used to differentiate further among the prokaryotic bacteria. The Gram stain demonstrates differences in composition of the cell walls of bacteria. The prokaryotes are divided into *gram-positive* and *gram-negative* organisms according to their response to the Gram stain.

Gram-positive bacteria have cell walls that are composed of a single layer and are thicker than cell walls of gram-negative bacteria. The wall is composed of peptidoglycan (a material composed of two sugars and a small group of amino acids). Figure 19-2 compares the cell wall structures of gram-positive and gram-negative organisms. During the Gram stain process, the thickness of the cell wall causes the alcohol or acetone to seal it by dehydration, thereby preventing the release of the crystal violet solution. The captured stain makes the organism appear purple in color.

Gram-negative bacteria have a more complex, multilayered cell wall. These bacteria have a peptidoglycan layer

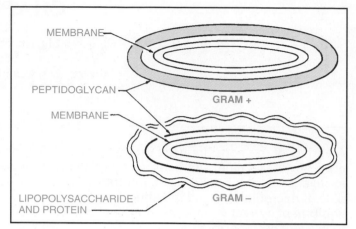

Figure 19-2   *A comparison of gram-positive and gram-negative cell wall structures*

and also a lipopolysaccharide and protein layer in their cell walls. Frequently this outer layer containing lipopolysaccharides is toxic to humans. This occurs primarily when the cell lyses and harmful substances called *endotoxins* are released from the cell wall. During the Gram stain process, the alcohol or acetone dissolves the crystal violet compound in the cell wall so that the color is washed away. As a result, gram-negative bacteria appear colorless.

Capsules and Endospores

Some bacteria secrete a slimy or gummy material on the surface of the cell wall. When this material forms a closely compacted structure, it is termed a *capsule*. These capsules are usually composed of polysaccharides, polypeptides, or polysaccharide-protein complexes (Brock, Madigan, Martinko, & Parker, 1984). Presence of a capsule brings a survival or protective advantage to the bacteria. The capsule makes it difficult for the body's phagocytes to ingest the bacteria. The presence of capsules may also cause the formation of antibodies. Generally speaking, encapsulated bacteria are more difficult to destroy.

Some prokaryotic bacteria reproduce by means of endospores. *Bacillus* and *Clostridium* are common bacteria that reproduce in this way. Genetic material within the endospore is encapsulated within the cell by a very resistant wall. Eventually, the cell lyses, releasing the endospore. The spore can lie dormant for years, surviving very unfavorable conditions. The spore is very resistant to heat, ionizing radiation, and chemicals. When conditions are right, the spore germinates, forming a new vegetative organism. Because of the resistance spores possess, special techniques for equipment processing must be employed to destroy them.

Common Causative Organisms

Table 19-1 summarizes the common organisms that are responsible for many nosocomial infections. As shown in the table, many of these organisms are present in sinks, water reservoirs, and the body's secretions. Aseptic techniques and proper decontamination and equipment processing will help to reduce the incidence of nosocomial infections.

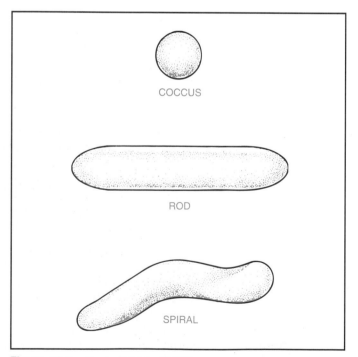

Figure 19-1   *Common bacterial shapes*

TABLE 19-1: Organisms Commonly Implicated in Nosocomial Infections

ORGANISM	DISEASE	SOURCE	FORM	PROCESSING
Haemophilus influenzae	Meningitis Pneumonia Epiglottitis	Upper respiratory tract	Gram– bacillus	Pasteurize
Klebsiella pneumoniae	*Klebsiella* pneumonia	Solutions, reservoirs	Gram– bacillus	Pasteurize
Legionella pneumophila	Legionnaires' disease	Sinks, showers, air ducts	Gram– bacillus	Pasteurize
Mycobacterium tuberculosis	Tuberculosis	Secretions, vectors	Spore	Sterilize
Neisseria	Meningitis Sexually transmitted disease (STD)	Secretions	Gram– diplococci	Pasteurize
Pseudomonas aeruginosa	*Pseudomonas* pneumonia	Secretions, reservoirs, soap, sinks	Gram– bacillus	Pasteurize
Serratia	Pneumonia	Solutions, reservoirs	Gram– bacillus	Pasteurize
Staphylococcus aureus	Staphylococcal infections	Secretions, nasal passage, vectors, wounds	Gram+ cocci	Pasteurize
Streptococcus pneumoniae	Pneumonia	Secretions	Gram+ cocci	Pasteurize

EQUIPMENT PROCESSING TERMS

Before the different methods of equipment processing are discussed, it is important to understand some of the terms used in the process. The different methods accomplish different results depending on the techniques employed and the effects the methods have on microorganisms.

Sterilization

Sterilization is the complete destruction of all forms of microorganisms, including spores. The equipment or surface is completely free of any living microorganisms. This does not imply that the equipment or surface does not have dead "carcasses" of microorganisms. They are there; however, further life is not possible, and replication does not occur when they are cultured.

Disinfection

Disinfection is the complete destruction of vegetative forms of pathogenic microorganisms. Note that spores are not included in this definition. Only vegetative, or living, forms are destroyed.

Antisepsis

Antisepsis is the application of chemical agents to a surface to inhibit microbial growth and reproduction. It does not kill organisms; it just slows them down. Typically, chemical agents may be applied to the skin or the surface of equipment to accomplish this end. For example, wiping a mouthpiece with alcohol before its use is one application of antisepsis.

EQUIPMENT PROCESSING METHODS

There are several different methods employed in equipment processing. It is important to understand whether the method sterilizes or disinfects and what effect it has on equipment that has plastic or rubber parts. Each method has its own specific equipment and procedural requirements that, if not met, will render the processing ineffective. It is important to understand each method and its requirements to ensure the destruction of harmful microorganisms. No matter what manner is used, the handling, packaging, and storage after processing have a direct effect on the cleanliness of equipment used at the patient's bedside. Also, equipment does not remain decontaminated forever. Each method of sterilization has an expiration date. This length of time will vary with the method and packaging used. Therefore, rotation of supplies is important. All processed equipment should be dated at the time processing is complete. Stock should be checked to ensure that supplies are not out of date.

Steam Autoclaving

Steam autoclaving is one of the more common methods employed in the processing of medical equipment. This method will sterilize any equipment that is properly prepared and processed.

The steam autoclave works by combining high heat, moisture, and pressure. Moist heat is more penetrating than dry heat. This may easily be understood by comparing two climates: A warm day with a temperature of 90°F is more comfortable in Salt Lake City than in Washington, DC because of the differences in moisture content of the air. A similar principle is employed in the steam autoclave. Steam (water vapor) is combined with high heat (121 to 126°C) and increased pressure (1 to 2 atm) to penetrate cellular structures effectively, thereby destroying microorganisms.

Correct preparation of equipment for this processing method is important. Equipment should be disassembled and washed in a detergent solution to remove gross particles and body secretions. The equipment is then rinsed and packaged in a porous material such as muslin, linen, kraft or brown paper, crepe paper, or Mylar (a polyester film).

The equipment must be loosely packed so that the steam can penetrate all surfaces. Any liquid containers must be loosely capped to allow penetration of the steam.

Exposure time, temperature, and pressure are critical to ensure this method's effectiveness. Before exposure, all air must first be evacuated from the autoclave and replaced by steam. A typical setting is 121°C at 15 psi for 15 minutes or 121°C at 30 psi for 3 minutes. Masking tape indicators are used to verify that exposure has been sufficient for sterilization. If the conditions and time period are correct, the indicator will change color. Similar indicators are available for use with the ethylene oxide processing method.

Autoclaving may be detrimental to some equipment. It tends to dull surgical instruments and to speed deterioration of rubber and some plastics, and cannot be used on electrical/electronic devices. If you are in doubt about the ability of equipment to withstand autoclaving, contact the equipment manufacturer before use.

Pasteurization

Pasteurization of respiratory therapy equipment is popular. Its advantages include a temperature that is not high enough to destroy many plastics (unlike the temperature in autoclaving). It uses only water so that employee exposure to chemicals does not occur and no residue is left on the equipment. Water is also less expensive than chemicals or other methods.

Pasteurization is a process that involves heating a liquid to temperatures sufficient to destroy vegetative organisms (living organisms capable of reproduction). This process is employed commercially in the processing of milk and beer. In respiratory care, equipment is immersed in a hot water bath at 77°C for 30 minutes. This is a disinfection method and does not sterilize equipment. The moist heat coagulates the cellular protein of microorganisms. Spores are not destroyed by this method, as their resistance to heat is much greater.

Correct preparation of equipment is important for this method to succeed. Equipment must be disassembled and washed in a detergent solution to remove any gross particles and body secretions, as they may protect and insulate the organism from the heat. The equipment should then be rinsed before pasteurizing. Small items are usually contained in a nylon net or mesh to prevent them from sinking to the bottom of the pasteurizer and making retrieval difficult. The pasteurizer temperature should be checked and the equipment immersed for the proper time period.

Following pasteurization, the equipment should be aseptically removed and allowed to dry in a special drying cabinet that filters bacteria and particles from the air. Following this, items should be assembled, packaged, and dated.

Ethylene Oxide Processing

Ethylene oxide is a toxic gas that is combined with moisture and heat to sterilize equipment. Its effectiveness depends on equipment preparation, gas concentration, humidity, and temperature.

Ethylene oxide works by affecting the enzymes, reproduction, and metabolism of microorganisms. It will kill spores if the method is correctly applied for the correct time period.

Equipment must be properly prepared for this processing method by disassembling and washing in detergent to remove mucus and body secretions. Because this method employs a gas, any microorganisms protected within mucus may not be affected by the gas. After washing, the equipment should be rinsed and allowed to dry. Water combines with the ethylene oxide to form ethylene glycol. This toxic chemical is potentially dangerous if inhaled or ingested through contact with medical equipment. After drying, the equipment should be packaged in porous packages such as wrapping paper, muslin or other cloth, or Mylar. A sterilization indicator is used for each package. It changes color if conditions and exposure time are correct and sterilization occurs. This indicator may be a special tape used to close the package or a device that is placed inside the package.

Gas concentration, temperature, and humidity all must be closely regulated for this method to be successful. Ethylene oxide concentration should be between 800 and 1000 mg/L. The ethylene oxide gas should be mixed with carbon dioxide or Freon to reduce the hazard of gas explosion. The temperature should range between 49 and 57°C. If the temperature becomes higher than 60°C, ethylene oxide will polymerize and become ineffective. The humidity should be maintained between 30% and 60%. Time exposure is typically 3 to 4 hours.

Following ethylene oxide exposure, the equipment should be aerated in a special cabinet to remove the gas. Aeration time may be as long as 24 hours or several days, depending on the material composition of the equipment.

This method may be harmful to some plastics because they retain and hold the gas. Polyvinyl chloride (PVC) and neoprene rubber require extended aeration times (McLaughlin, 1983). Owing to the detrimental effects on some materials and the longer time involved for processing, a larger stock of supplies is required.

Glutaraldehyde Processing

Glutaraldehyde is a chemical that is used to cold-sterilize or disinfect equipment by immersion. Cidex is an example of a glutaraldehyde preparation. Heat is not utilized in glutaraldehyde processing.

Glutaraldehyde is manufactured in both acid and alkaline forms. The pH range of these chemicals is critical in ensuring their effectiveness.

Equipment is processed by immersion in the activated chemical. The acid or alkaline environment glutaraldehyde provides destroys microorganisms. Organisms are destroyed by alkylation of enzymes.

To process equipment for the method, begin by disassembling it and washing it in detergent. Following the detergent wash, rinse the equipment and shake it dry before immersing it in the solution.

Equipment should be immersed for 10 to 20 minutes to disinfect and for 6 to 10 hours to sterilize it. After immersion, the equipment should be aseptically rinsed of any glutaraldehyde residue (it is toxic) with a sodium bisulfite solution (1 ounce to 1 gallon of water) and allowed to dry in a drying cabinet with filter elements to remove particles and microorganisms from the air. Because of glutaraldehyde's toxicity, some persons using this processing technique may show signs of dermal sensitivity or allergy to the fumes. This sensitivity may be a potential drawback.

Because this method involves the use of a liquid, it is not compatible with most electronic equipment. Rubber and plastic products seem to tolerate it without adverse effects. The life of the product ranges from 14 to 30 days, depending on the product. At the end of this time interval, it must be discarded and new solution prepared.

Processing with Quaternary Ammonium Compounds

Quaternary ammonium compounds ("quats") are special cationic detergents that destroy microorganisms by disrupting or lysing the cell membrane. Most quats are specific for one or a few types of organisms. Therefore,

quats are frequently combined to broaden their destruction of microorganisms.

These liquids are used in a way similar to that for the glutaraldehyde method. Clean equipment is immersed for 10 to 20 minutes. Equipment preparation is essentially the same as for the former method. The exposure time varies with the product being used. It is typically 10 to 20 minutes. This method accomplishes disinfection but not sterilization—spores and some viruses will survive exposure.

Most respiratory care equipment will tolerate this processing method. The exception is electronic equipment because a solution is used. Another disadvantage to this method is that the life of the solution is very short, on the order of 1 to 2 weeks. However, the cost is usually less than that for glutaraldehyde.

Gamma Irradiation

Gamma radiation is a form of ionizing radiation that destroys microorganisms by affecting the cells' enzymes and DNA. *Gamma irradiation* is a method of sterilization.

The equipment required for this method is expensive and the protective shielding is cumbersome. Its use is usually limited to manufacturers of medical equipment.

Owing to the nature of the radiation, the physical structure and composition of some materials may be altered by exposure. If your facility utilizes this method, consult the equipment manufacturer before subjecting equipment to this method.

FACILITY DESIGN FOR EQUIPMENT PROCESSING

The facility design for equipment processing is important in the maintenance of asepsis and the prevention of cross-contamination. Figure 19-3 shows a sample design of an equipment processing area. Note that the equipment

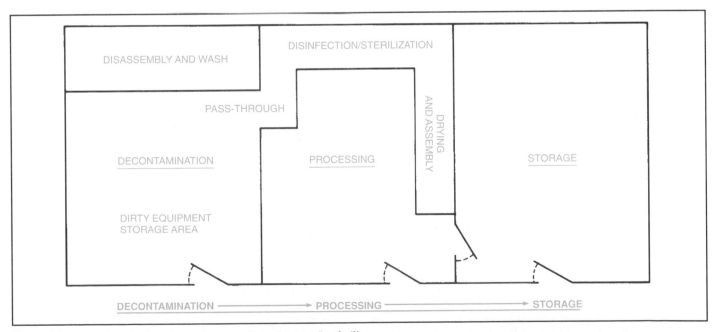

Figure 19-3 *Equipment flow pattern in an equipment processing facility*

"flows" through the facility in only one direction and that equipment in storage is physically separated from equipment being processed. The facility is divided into three main areas: decontamination, processing, and storage. The flow of equipment begins at decontamination, where it is disassembled, washed, and rinsed. Ideally, a pass-through is provided between the decontamination area and processing. The processing area is the area in which the equipment is disinfected or sterilized, reassembled, tested, and packaged for storage. As noted, the storage area should be physically separate from the other two. The design should prevent contact between clean and dirty equipment and traffic flow through the clean equipment, assembly, and storage areas.

BACTERIOLOGICAL SURVEILLANCE PROGRAMS

Bacteriological surveillance provides data on the effectiveness of disinfection and sterilization methods, equipment handling, storage procedures, and how frequently in-use equipment should be changed. Various methods are used to culture clean and in-use equipment. Each method has its advantages, disadvantages, and most suitable application.

Aliquot Culturing

Aliquot culturing is a method of culturing solutions.

A sterile sample is drawn. Then serial dilutions are made from the sample and cultured. Colony counts are made and the colonizing organisms are identified. This method is qualitative—the data obtained indicate what, but not how much, is there. Aliquot culturing is used to detect contamination in fluids.

Output Sampling

Output sampling is popular for sampling both clean and in-use equipment. Olympic Medical manufactures a special sampling device called the Aerotest device that consists of a funnel-shaped tube with a culture plate at the base of the funnel. Aerosol or gas flow is directed down the tube toward the culture plate at a specific flow rate for a specific time interval. The plate is incubated for 24 to 48 hours and colonizing organisms are then identified. If the colony count is greater than that for the ambient air, the test is considered positive. This method is quantitative, providing actual amounts as well as colony types. Output sampling is used to monitor clean and in-use equipment. Use on clean equipment can identify improper processing methods. Use on in-use equipment can assist in determining how frequently equipment changes are required.

Rinse Sampling

The rinse sampling technique involves sloshing sterile broth aseptically in respiratory therapy equipment tubing, recovering it, and allowing the broth to incubate. Colonies are then counted and colonizing organisms identified. This method is quantitative and very sensitive. Procedures must be carefully followed so as not to introduce sampling errors. This method is used primarily to culture processed equipment for assessing the effectiveness of the processing method.

Rodac Plate Sampling

Rodac plate sampling involves the use of a special raised-bed culture plate. The plate is pressed against the equipment being cultured and then incubated. This method samples a very small area and therefore may not detect contamination in other parts of the equipment. It is qualitative, providing only data on what, but not how much, is there. This method is used primarily to sample clean equipment for contamination. Because the plate is flat, its use is somewhat limited.

Swab Sampling

Swab sampling is one of the most common methods utilized in bacteriological surveillance. A special swab containing culture medium is aseptically withdrawn from its container and rubbed onto the surface being cultured. The swab is then aseptically rubbed onto a culture plate.

The plate is then incubated. Colonies are identified and counted. This method is very convenient in that small cotton-tipped applicators are used as swabs. The method is qualitative and samples only a small area.

DATA UTILIZATION

Culturing of clean equipment should be performed monthly. The data obtained will help to identify the effectiveness of processing, storage procedures, and equipment assembly practices. If positive results (indicating the presence of pathogens) are obtained, equipment handling and processing procedures must be reviewed and scrutinized to find the source of contamination. Samples at each step of the process should be cultured in an attempt to identify the point at which contamination is occurring. Once the source is identified, the procedures should be modified to eliminate the contamination problem.

In-use equipment is exposed to an environment teeming with microorganisms. Positive culture results, indicating contamination by pathogenic organisms, necessitate further investigation. If specimens from the patient using the equipment yield similar culture results, the source is the patient. If the patient's sputum culture is negative for the organism, other sources such as cross-contamination, personnel, airborne transmission, solutions, and compressed gases must be considered and investigated. The source must be identified and the contamination problem corrected.

If *Staphylococcus epidermidis* or other nonpathogenic members of the normal flora are cultured on clean or in-use equipment, the most likely contamination source is the person conducting the culturing. This is one source of sampling error. Contamination may be introduced during collection, sample handling, or culturing. Maintenance of aseptic technique during all phases is important.

OBJECTIVES

At the end of this chapter, you should be able to:

- Demonstrate how to perform output sampling on the following clean and in-use equipment:
  - Ohio Deluxe nebulizer
  - Ultrasonic nebulizer
- Demonstrate the correct technique for swab sampling.
- Demonstrate how to fill out a bacteriological surveillance record.
- Demonstrate how to decontaminate and process respiratory care equipment:

— Wash the equipment in detergent and water, removing all gross contamination.

— Rinse all equipment, removing residual detergent.

— If steam autoclaving or gas sterilizing, wrap equipment in approved wrapping material, enclosing appropriate indicators.

— Correctly sterilize or disinfect the equipment.

— Correctly assemble and package equipment following disinfection.

— Label and store the processed equipment, rotating the stock.

Not all schools or facilities will have the equipment required to perform the procedures outlined in this section. The hospital laboratory, microbiology school, or microbiology department may be willing to provide the supplies necessary to complete these activities if they are not available. Not all personnel in respiratory care will be responsible for the performance of these procedures. However, by completing these activities, you will gain a better understanding of the surveillance process.

OUTPUT SAMPLING WITH THE AEROTEST

As noted earlier in the chapter, the Aerotest device provides a convenient means of output sampling. Depending on the type of equipment being cultured, the flow rate and sampling time will vary. Follow the printed directions from the manufacturer in this regard.

Obtain the Required Supplies

Obtain the supplies required for this method of sampling. In addition to the culturing device, obtain the required paperwork for the procedure that is to be filled out on collection of the sample.

Wash Your Hands

Handwashing is important during this procedure to prevent the inadvertent introduction of microorganisms. Aseptic technique is very important to prevent sampling errors.

Prepare the Equipment for Sampling

Adjust the equipment to the correct flow, oxygen, and rate (ventilators) as specified by the manufacturer's directions.

Aseptically Use the Device

Direct the flow from the equipment down the funnel-shaped tube for the specified time period. Remove the sampling unit from the equipment being sampled. Remove the funnel-shaped tube, and using the cover you first removed, cover the agar plate and label it. Use care not to drip condensation into the device.

Transport the Plate to the Laboratory Facility

Fill out the paperwork associated with the bacteriological surveillance program and deliver the labeled plate to the laboratory facility for culturing.

SWAB SAMPLING

Obtain the Required Supplies

Obtain the supplies required for this method of sampling. In addition to the culturing device, obtain the required paperwork for the procedure that will be filled out on collection of the sample.

Wash Your Hands

Handwashing is important during this procedure to prevent inadvertent introduction of microorganisms. Aseptic technique is very important to prevent sampling errors.

Aseptically Withdraw the Swab and Sample the Area

Aseptically remove the swab from its container and rub it onto the surface being cultured. Return the swab to its container and rub it onto the culture medium. Label the swab as to what was cultured—for example, "baffle in [a particular] Ohio Deluxe nebulizer."

SURVEILLANCE RECORDS

A surveillance record should contain the information listed in Figure 19-4. It is very important that the records be correctly maintained and that all parts be completely filled out.

Transport the Plate to the Laboratory Facility

Fill out the paperwork associated with the surveillance program and deliver the labeled plate to the laboratory facility for culturing.

- Date
- Personnel who did the sample
- For in-use equipment
  — Patient's name
  — Hospital number
  — Diagnosis
  — Nursing unit or location (room number)
- Type of equipment
- Equipment number or serial number if available
- Equipment status
  — Clean
  — In-use (number of hours in service)

Figure 19-4 *Elements of the bacteriological surveillance record*

PROCESSING RESPIRATORY CARE EQUIPMENT

Washing

All equipment must be washed prior to processing. Washing removes sputum, blood or blood products, and other organic contamination. The removal of contamination is important because some processing methods (e.g., gas sterilization) may not penetrate to the surface of the equipment. Soiled parts also frequently do not function properly in an assembly, binding or not conducting gas or fluids as they should.

Equipment should be washed in water using a surgical detergent. The detergent reduces the surface tension of the water, facilitating the removal of contamination. Some detergents also have a bacteriostatic action. Use plenty of friction and water to remove stubborn contamination. Friction combined with detergent and water will remove most contamination.

Rinsing

Immediately after washing the equipment, it is important to rinse it, removing all detergent residue. The chemicals used in some processing methods (e.g., quaternary ammonium compounds and glutaraldehyde) are diluted by detergents, reducing their effectiveness.

For gas sterilization, it is important to dry the equipment before packaging and processing. Water combines with ethylene oxide to form ethylene glycol, a very toxic compound.

Packaging

Two sterilization methods—steam autoclaving and gas sterilization—require that the equipment be packaged in permeable wrapping prior to processing. The permeable wrapping allows the steam or gas to penetrate to the equipment, and helps to prevent the contamination of sterile articles following processing. A device made up of several components should be packaged loosely, to allow the steam or gas to reach all exposed surfaces.

An indicator is placed in the wrap with each piece of equipment, or special indicator tape is used to seal the wrap. The indicator will change color if sterilization conditions have been met. The color change of the indicator assures the processing technician that the processing method has met the minimum conditions for sterilization.

Processing the Equipment

Equipment processing will result in either sterilization or disinfection, depending on what method is being used. Processing in the acute care setting usually involves one of the following: (1) steam autoclaving, (2) gas sterilization, (3) use of glutaraldehydes, or (4) use of quaternary ammonium compounds. For each method, it is important to use correct temperatures, pressures, or concentrations to ensure desired results.

Package Equipment Following Disinfection

Equipment should be rinsed, dried, and packaged following processing. Aseptic procedures should be followed including a 5-minute scrub and use of a gown, shoe covers, and a hair net. Following assembly, the equipment should be checked for function and tested prior to packaging if possible. Your diligence and close attention to details may avert a crisis in the Emergency Department, operating suite, or intensive care unit.

Label and Store the Equipment

All equipment should be labeled showing the date of processing and initialed by the processing technician. The equipment should be stored with other clean equipment. All reusable equipment that has been processed should be rotated such that the most recently processed equipment is to the rear of the shelf or bin and older stock is moved forward for use.

References

Brock, T., Madigan, M., Martinko, J., & Parker, J. (1984). *Biology of microorganisms* (4th ed.). Englewood Cliffs, NJ: Prentice-Hall.

McLaughlin, A. J., Jr. (1983). *Manual of infection control in respiratory care*. Boston: Little, Brown.

Additional Resources

Burton, G. G., Hodgkin, J., & Ward, J. (1991). *Respiratory care: A guide to clinical practice* (3rd ed.). Philadelphia: Lippincott.

Eubanks, D. H., & Bone, R. (1991). *Comprehensive respiratory care* (2nd ed.). St. Louis, MO: Mosby.

Nelson, E. J. Techniques of infection control in respiratory therapy and anesthesia series: no 3: Facility design and operations of a respiratory therapy processing center. Seattle, WA: Olympic Surgical Company.

Practice Activities: Equipment Processing and Surveillance

1. Practice output sampling using an Olympic Aerotest on the following pieces of equipment:
   a. Volume ventilator
   b. Large-volume nebulizer
   c. Ultrasonic nebulizer
   d. Room humidifier
   IN YOUR PRACTICE
   (1) Obtain required supplies.
   (2) Wash your hands.
   (3) Practice aseptic technique.
   (4) Correctly prepare the equipment for sampling.
   (5) Sample for the appropriate length of time.
   (6) Label and transport the sample.
   (7) Complete all paperwork.

2. Practice swab sampling on the following equipment:
   a. Tubing dryer
   b. Oxygen humidifier
   c. Babbington nebulizer
   IN YOUR PRACTICE
   (1) Obtain required supplies.
   (2) Wash your hands.
   (3) Practice aseptic technique.
   (4) Correctly prepare equipment for sampling.
   (5) Sample for the appropriate length of time.
   (6) Label and transport sample.

(7) Complete all paperwork.

3. Obtain specimens for culture from your hands, nasal passages, and the sink in the laboratory and identify what organisms grow.

4. Practice processing respiratory care equipment, including:
   a. Washing
   b. Rinsing
      (1) Drying if required (gas sterilizing and steam autoclaving)
   c. Packaging for processing (gas sterilizing and steam autoclaving)
   d. Processing:
      (1) Steam autoclaving
      (2) Gas sterilizing
      (3) Glutaraldehyde processing
      (4) Processing with quaternary ammonium compounds
   e. Rinsing and drying if required
   f. Assembling and testing the equipment following processing.
   g. Packaging the equipment aseptically:
      (1) Labeling all equipment
   h. Stocking the equipment in the clean equipment room

Check List: Bacteriological Surveillance

_____ 1. Gather the appropriate supplies:
_____ a. Aerotest
_____ b. Sampling swabs
_____ c. Required paperwork
_____ 2. Wash your hands before obtaining a sample.
3. Prepare the equipment for sampling (if required):
_____ a. Adjust flow rate.
_____ b. Adjust FiO_2.
_____ c. Adjust rate and tidal volume.
_____ 4. Prepare a sampling device for use.
_____ 5. Aseptically obtain the sample.
_____ 6. Correctly handle the sampling device after sample collection.
_____ 7. Label and transport the sample to the lab.
_____ 8. Complete all paperwork.

Check List: Equipment Processing

_____ 1. Perform a 5-minute scrub.
2. Cover your clothing:
_____ a. Use a gown.
_____ b. Put on shoe covers.
_____ c. Put on a hair net.
_____ 3. Disassemble and wash the equipment.
_____ 4. Rinse equipment and dry it if gas sterilization is used.
5. Package equipment before processing by gas sterilization or steam autoclaving:
_____ a. Use correct wrapping material.
_____ b. Use an indicator.
6. Process the equipment correctly:
_____ a. Use the correct time exposure.
_____ b. Use the correct temperature.
_____ c. Use the correct concentration.
_____ 7. Assemble equipment following processing.
_____ 8. Test the equipment.
_____ 9. Package the equipment.
_____ 10. Label and store the equipment.

Self-Evaluation Post Test: Equipment Processing and Surveillance

1. Prokaryotic bacteria are differentiated by:
   I.   shape.   a. I, III
   II. Gram stain.   b. I, II
   III. color.   c. II, IV
   IV. size.   d. III, V
   V.   cell wall structure

2. Of eukaryotes and prokaryotes, the more complex organisms are the:
   a. prokaryotes.   b. eukaryotes.

3. The complete destruction of all microorganisms is:
   a. termed sterilization.
   b. accomplished by pasteurization.
   c. termed asepsis.
   d. termed disinfection.

4. A method of disinfection is:
   a. ethylene oxide processing.
   b. steam autoclaving.
   c. gamma irradiation.
   d. exposure to quaternary ammonium compounds.

5. Which of the following principles are incorporated into the design of an equipment processing facility?
   I.   Equipment flows in one direction.
   II. Stored and processed equipment are separated.
   III. Reassembly takes place in the decontamination area.
   IV. Disinfection/sterilization takes place in the processing area.
   a. I, III, IV   c. II, III, IV
   b. I, II, IV   d. I, II

6. An indicator is used to:
   a. establish when equipment is out of date.
   b. tell when equipment has been cleaned.
   c. identify when sterilization has occurred.
   d. tell when equipment has been contaminated.

7. Gram-negative bacteria appear:
   a. red.
   b. violet.
   c. blue.
   d. colorless.

8. Gram-positive bacteria appear:
   a. red.
   b. violet.
   c. blue.
   d. colorless.

9. The most common types of sampling methods are:
   I.   aliquot.   a. I, III
   II. output.   b. II, IV
   III. rinse.   c. I, IV
   IV. Rodac plate.   d. II, V
   V.   swab.

10. Which of the following methods are quantitative?
   a. Aliquot
   b. Rodac plate
   c. Output
   d. Swab

PERFORMANCE EVALUATION:
BACTERIOLOGICAL SURVEILLANCE

Date: Lab _____ Clinical _____ Agency _____

Lab: Pass _____ Fail _____   Clinical: Pass _____ Fail _____

Student name _____ Instructor name _____

No. of times observed in clinical _____

No. of times practiced in clinical _____

PASSING CRITERIA: Obtain 90% or better on the procedure. Tasks indicated by * must receive at least 1 point, or the evaluation is terminated. Procedure must be performed within designated time, or the performance receives a failing grade.

SCORING: 2 points — Task performed satisfactorily without prompting.
              1 point — Task performed satisfactorily with self-initiated correction.
              0 points — Task performed incorrectly or with prompting required.
              NA — Task not applicable to the patient care situation.

TASKS: PEER   LAB   CLINICAL

*   1. Gathers the appropriate equipment   ☐   ☐   ☐

*   2. Observes standard precautions, including handwashing   ☐   ☐   ☐

     3. Prepares the equipment for sampling

*   a. Sets the flow rate   ☐   ☐   ☐

*   b. Adjusts O$_2$% as required   ☐   ☐   ☐

*   c. Sets the rate and tidal volume on ventilator if required   ☐   ☐   ☐

*   4. Aseptically prepares the sampling device   ☐   ☐   ☐

*   5. Correctly samples the equipment   ☐   ☐   ☐

*   6. Correctly handles culturing device following sampling   ☐   ☐   ☐

*   7. Labels and transports sample to the laboratory for culture   ☐   ☐   ☐

*   8. Completes all required paperwork   ☐   ☐   ☐

SCORE: Peer _____ points of possible 20; _____%

           Lab _____ points of possible 20; _____%

           Clinical _____ points of possible 20; _____%

TIME: _____ out of possible 20 minutes

STUDENT SIGNATURES   INSTRUCTOR SIGNATURES

PEER: _____   LAB: _____

STUDENT: _____   CLINICAL: _____

PERFORMANCE EVALUATION: EQUIPMENT PROCESSING

Date: Lab _____ Clinical _____ Agency _____

Lab: Pass _____ Fail _____   Clinical: Pass _____ Fail _____

Student name _____   Instructor name _____

No. of times observed in clinical _____

No. of times practiced in clinical _____

PASSING CRITERIA: Obtain 90% or better on the procedure. Tasks indicated by * must receive at least 1 point, or the evaluation is terminated. Procedure must be performed within designated time, or the performance receives a failing grade.

SCORING:
2 points — Task performed satisfactorily without prompting.
1 point — Task performed satisfactorily with self-initiated correction.
0 points — Task performed incorrectly or with prompting required.
NA — Task not applicable to the patient care situation.

TASKS:

			PEER	LAB	CLINICAL
*	1.	Performs a 5-minute scrub	☐	☐	☐
*	2.	Wears appropriate attire			
		a. Gown	☐	☐	☐
		b. Shoe covers	☐	☐	☐
		c. Hair cover	☐	☐	☐
*	3.	Disassembles and washes equipment	☐	☐	☐
*	4.	Rinses equipment and dries it if gas sterilization is used	☐	☐	☐
*	5.	Packages equipment before processing if required			
		a. Uses correct packaging	☐	☐	☐
		b. Uses an indicator	☐	☐	☐
*	6.	Processes equipment correctly			
		a. Uses correct time exposure	☐	☐	☐
		b. Uses correct temperature	☐	☐	☐
		c. Uses correct concentration	☐	☐	☐
*	7.	Assembles equipment following disinfection	☐	☐	☐
*	8.	Tests equipment before packaging	☐	☐	☐
*	9.	Labels and stores equipment	☐	☐	☐

SCORE: Peer _____ points of possible 26; _____%

Lab _____ points of possible 26; _____%

Clinical _____ points of possible 26; _____%

TIME: _____ out of possible 90 minutes

STUDENT SIGNATURES   **INSTRUCTOR SIGNATURES**

PEER: _____   LAB: _____

STUDENT: _____   CLINICAL: _____

CHAPTER 20

EMERGENCY AIRWAY MANAGEMENT

INTRODUCTION

Emergency airway management is an important role of the respiratory care practitioner. Respiratory failure may result from many underlying disorders. When it occurs, a patent airway must quickly be established and ventilation resumed.

A simple method of airway management is patient positioning to relieve obstruction so that the patient's own respiratory efforts may resume. Alternatively, airway management may involve placement of an artificial airway and manual ventilation of the patient using a manual resuscitator.

It is important that you understand the rationale, techniques, and equipment for emergency airway management and the associated hazards and complications. In this chapter you will learn patient positioning to open the airway, how to use a manual resuscitator, and intubation techniques.

KEY TERMS

- Anterior mandibular displacement
- Endotracheal pilot tube and balloon
- Endotracheal tube
- Endotracheal tube cuff
- Extubation
- Head tilt
- Intubation
- Laryngeal mask airway (LMA)
- Laryngeal obstruction
- Laryngoscope
- MacIntosh blade
- Miller blade
- Nasopharyngeal airway
- Oropharyngeal airway
- Soft tissue obstruction

OBJECTIVES

THEORY

At the end of this chapter, you should be able to:

- Identify the anatomical structures of the upper airway.
- Identify the reflexes encountered in descending order from the mouth to the carina, and state the significance of these reflexes in relation to the level of consciousness.
- Explain the etiology of upper airway obstruction.
- Explain the mechanisms of the manual maneuvers utilized to open the airway:
  — Head tilt and chin lift
  — Anterior mandibular displacement
- Differentiate between a self-inflating and a flow-inflating manual resuscitator.
- Describe the types of valves commonly utilized in manual resuscitators. Explain the advantages and disadvantages of each type.
- Describe the following for the commonly utilized self-inflating manual resuscitators:
  — FiO_2 delivery with and without reservoir attachment
  — Identify those that deliver oxygen-enriched gas during spontaneous ventilation
  — Ease of cleaning aspirate
- State the importance of maintaining an I:E ratio of at least 1:2 or greater while ventilating a patient with a manual resuscitator.
- Describe the hazards and complications associated with the use of a manual resuscitator on the nonintubated patient.
- Explain the mechanism of airway maintenance with

the following devices, and state their indications, advantages, disadvantages, and associated hazards:
  — Nasopharyngeal airway
  — Oropharyngeal airway
- Describe the laryngeal mask airway (LMA) and its insertion.
- Describe the routes of intubation and their advantages and disadvantages:
  — Oral route
  — Nasal route
- Describe the two types of laryngoscopes and blades used for intubation, including:

Laryngoscopes
  — Conventional
  — Fiberoptic

Laryngoscope Blades
  — MacIntosh
  — Miller
- Describe the construction and design of a modern endotracheal tube,L and state the significance of the following components in relation to their function:
  — Murphy eye
  — Cuff
    — Bivona foam cuff
    — Standard cuff
  — Pilot tube
  — Markings
  — Pilot balloon
- Describe the early and late complications of intubation.
- List the indications for intubation and the criteria for extubation.

CLINICAL PRACTICE GUIDELINES

AARC Clinical Practice Guideline:
Resuscitation in Acute Care Hospitals

RACH 4.0 INDICATIONS:

Cardiac arrest, respiratory arrest, or the presence of conditions that may lead to cardiopulmonary arrest as indicated by rapid deterioration in vital signs, level of consciousness, and blood gas values — included in those conditions are:

4.1 Airway obstruction — partial or complete

4.2 Acute myocardial infarction with cardio-dynamic instability

4.3 Life-threatening dysrhythmias

4.4 Hypovolemic shock

4.5 Severe infections

4.6 Spinal cord or head injury

4.7 Drug overdose

4.8 Pulmonary edema

4.9 Anaphylaxis

4.10 Pulmonary embolus

4.11 Smoke inhalation

4.12 High-risk delivery

RACH 5.0 CONTRAINDICATIONS:

Resuscitation is contraindicated when:

5.1 The patient's desire not to be resuscitated has been clearly expressed and documented in the patient's medical record. (1–3)

5.2 Resuscitation has been determined to be futile because of the patient's underlying condition or disease. (4–9)

RACH 6.0 PRECAUTIONS/HAZARDS AND/OR COMPLICATIONS:

The following represent possible hazards or complications related to the major facets of resuscitation:

6.1 Airway management (10,11)

6.1.1 Failure to establish a patent airway (12)

6.1.2 Failure to intubate the trachea (12)

6.1.3 Failure to recognize intubation of the esophagus (12)

6.1.4 Upper airway trauma, laryngeal and esophageal damage (13–17)

6.1.5 Aspiration (12,13,18,19)

6.1.6 Cervical spine trauma (10,13)

6.1.7 Unrecognized bronchial intubation (18,20)

6.1.8 Eye injury (10)

6.1.9 Facial trauma (18)

6.1.10 Problems with ETT cuff (21)

6.1.11 Bronchospasm (10)

6.1.12 Laryngospasm (10)

6.1.13 Dental accidents (13,18)

6.1.14 Dysrhythmias (22)

6.1.15 Hypotension and bradycardia due to vagal stimulation (10,23)

6.1.16 Hypertension and tachycardia

6.1.17 Inappropriate tube size (18,21)

6.2 Ventilation

6.2.1 Inadequate oxygen delivery (FDO_2) (24–27)

6.2.2 Hypo- and/or hyperventilation (28–30)

6.2.3 Gastric insufflation and/or rupture (12,31)

6.2.4 Barotrauma (32–34)

6.2.5 Hypotension due to reduced venous return secondary to high mean intra-thoracic pressure (35,36)

6.2.6 Vomiting and aspiration (12)

6.2.7 Prolonged interruption of ventilation for intubation (37,38)

6.2.8 Failure to establish adequate functional residual capacity in the newborn (39–41)

6.3 Circulation

6.3.1 Ineffective chest compression (42,43)

6.3.2 Fractured ribs and/or sternum (12,13,44,45)

6.3.3 Laceration of spleen or liver (12,13, 44–49)

6.3.4 Failure to restore circulation despite functional rhythm

6.3.4.1 Severe hypovolemia (50,51)

6.3.4.2 Cardiac tamponade (51)

6.3.4.3 Hemo- or pneumothorax (50,51)

6.3.4.4 Hypoxia

6.3.4.5 Acidosis

6.3.4.6 Hyperkalemia

6.3.4.7 Massive acute myocardial infarction (50)

6.3.4.8 Hypothermia (in neonates (52,53) and children (38))

6.3.4.9 Aortic dissection (50)

6.3.4.10 Air embolus, pulmonary embolism (50)

6.4 Electrical therapy

6.4.1 Failure of defibrillator (54)

6.4.2 Shock to team members (55)

6.4.3 Inappropriate countershock

6.4.3.1 Muscle burn (56,57)

6.4.3.2 Infantile hematomyelia (58)

6.4.4 Induction of malignant dysrhythmias (59,60)

6.4.5 Interference with implanted pacemaker function (61)

6.4.6 Fire hazard (62)

6.5 Drug administration

6.5.1 Inappropriate drug or dose

6.5.2 Idiosyncratic or allergic response to drug

6.5.3 Endotracheal-tube drug-delivery failure (63–65) — The endotracheal tube dose should be 2 to 2.5 times the normal I.V. or intraosseous dose, diluted in 10 ml of normal saline (or distilled water). The drug should be instilled via endobronchial catheter to ensure distribution beyond central airways.

RACH 8.0 ASSESSMENT OF NEED:

8.1 Assessment of patient condition

8.1.1 Prearrest — Identification of patients (including the fetus) in danger of imminent arrest and in whom consequent early intervention may prevent arrest and improve outcome. These are patients with conditions that may lead to cardiopulmonary arrest as indicated by rapid deterioration in vital signs, level of consciousness, blood gas values, or fetal monitoring data (see Section 4.00).

8.1.2 Arrest — Absence of spontaneous breathing and/or circulation

8.1.3 Postarrest — Once a patient has sustained an arrest, the likelihood of additional life-threatening problems is high and continued vigilance and aggressive action using this Guideline are indicated. Control of the airway and cardiac monitoring must be continued and optimal oxygenation and ventilation ensured.

RACH 9.0 ASSESSMENT OF PROCESS AND OUTCOME:

9.1 Timely, high-quality resuscitation improves patient outcome in terms of survival and level of function. Despite optimal resuscitation performance, outcomes are affected by patient-specific factors. Patient condition postarrest should be evaluated from this perspective.

9.2 Documentation and evaluation of the resuscitation process (e.g., system activation, team member performance, functioning of equipment, and adherence to guidelines and algorithms) should occur continuously and improvements be made. (66–70)

RACH 11.0 MONITORING:

11.1 Patient

11.1.1 Clinical assessment — Continuous observation of the patient and repeated clinical assessment by a trained observer provide optimal monitoring of the resuscitation process. Special consideration should be given to the following:

11.1.1.1 Level of consciousness

11.1.1.2 Adequacy of airway

11.1.1.3 Adequacy of ventilation

11.1.1.4 Peripheral/apical pulse and character

11.1.1.5 Evidence of chest and head trauma

11.1.1.6 Pulmonary compliance and airway resistance

11.1.1.7 Presence of seizure activity

11.1.2 Assessment of physiologic parameters — Repeat assessment of physiologic data by trained professionals supplements clinical assessment in managing patients throughout the resuscitation process. Monitoring devices should be available, accessible, functional, and periodically evaluated for function. These data include but are not limited to: (66)

11.1.2.1 Arterial blood gas studies (although investigators have suggested that such values may have a limited role in decision making during CPR (124))

11.1.2.2 Hemodynamic data (119, 125–127)

11.1.2.3 Cardiac rhythm (38:2236, 120,121)

11.1.2.4 Ventilatory frequency, tidal volume, and airway pressure (66,67,87)

11.1.2.5 Exhaled CO_2 (110–114)

11.1.2.6 Neurologic status

11.2 Resuscitation process — Properly performed resuscitation should improve patient outcome. Continuous monitoring of the process will identify areas needing improvement. Among these areas are response time, equipment function, equipment availability, team member performance, team performance, complication rate, and patient survival and functional status.

Reprinted with permission from *Respiratory Care* 1993; 38: 1179–1188. The complete AARC Clinical Practice Guidelines are available from the AARC Web site (http://www.aarc.org), from the AARC Executive Office, or from *Respiratory Care* journal.

AARC Clinical Practice Guideline
Management of Airway Emergencies

MAE 4.0 INDICATIONS:

4.1 Conditions requiring management of the airway, in general, are impending or actual (1) airway compromise, (2) respiratory failure, and (3) need to protect the airway. Specific conditions include but are not limited to:

4.1.1 Airway emergency prior to endotracheal intubation

4.1.2 Obstruction of the artificial airway

4.1.3 Apnea

(Continued)

(CPG Continued)

4.1.4 Acute traumatic coma (1)

4.1.5 Penetrating neck trauma (2)

4.1.6 Cardiopulmonary arrest and unstable dysrhythmias (3)

4.1.7 Severe bronchospasm (4–8)

4.1.8 Severe allergic reactions with cardiopulmonary compromise (9,10)

4.1.9 Pulmonary edema (11,12)

4.1.10 Sedative or narcotic drug effect (13)

4.1.11 Foreign body airway obstruction (3)

4.1.12 Choanal atresia in neonates (14)

4.1.13 Aspiration

4.1.14 Risk of aspiration

4.1.15 Severe laryngospasm (15)

4.1.16 Self-extubation (16,17)

4.2 Conditions requiring emergency tracheal intubation include, but are not limited to:

4.2.1 Persistent apnea

4.2.2 Traumatic upper airway obstruction (partial or complete) (18–20)

4.2.3 Accidental extubation of the patient unable to maintain adequate spontaneous ventilation (16,17)

4.2.4 Obstructive angioedema (edema involving the deeper layers of the skin, subcutaneous tissue, and mucosa) (21–23)

4.2.5 Massive uncontrolled upper airway bleeding (2,24)

4.2.6 Coma with potential for increased intracranial pressure (25)

4.2.7 Infection-related upper airway obstruction (partial or complete):

4.2.7.1 Epiglottitis in children or adults (26,27)

4.2.7.2 Acute uvular edema (28)

4.2.7.3 Tonsillopharyngitis or retropharyngeal abscess (29)

4.2.7.4 Suppurative parotitis (30)

4.2.8 Laryngeal and upper airway edema (31)

4.2.9 Neonatal- or pediatric-specific:

4.2.9.1 Perinatal asphyxia (32,33)

4.2.9.2 Severe adenotonsillar hypertrophy (34,35)

4.2.9.3 Severe laryngomalacia (36,37)

4.2.9.4 Bacterial tracheitis (38–40)

4.2.9.5 Neonatal epignathus (41,42)

4.2.9.6 Obstruction from abnormal laryngeal closure due to arytenoid masses (43)

4.2.9.7 Mediastinal tumors (44)

4.2.9.8 Congenital diaphragmatic hernia (45)

4.2.9.9 Presence of thick and/or particulate meconium in amniotic fluid (46–48)

4.2.10 Absence of airway protective reflexes

4.2.11 Cardiopulmonary arrest

4.2.12 Massive hemoptysis (49)

4.3 The patient in whom airway control is not possible by other methods may require surgical placement of an airway (needle or surgical cricothyrotomy). (20,50,51)

4.4 Conditions in which endotracheal intubation may not be possible and in which alternative techniques may be used include but are not limited to:

4.4.1 Restriction of endotracheal intubation by policy or statute

4.4.2 Difficult or failed intubation in the presence of risk factors associated with difficult tracheal intubations (52) such as:

4.4.2.1 Short neck, (53) or bull neck (54)

4.4.2.2 Protruding maxillary incisors (53)

4.4.2.3 Receding mandible (53)

4.4.2.4 Reduced mobility of the atlanto-occipital joint (55)

4.4.2.5 Temporomandibular ankylosis (55)

4.4.2.6 Congenital oropharyngeal wall stenosis (56)

4.4.2.7 Anterior osteophytes of the cervical vertebrae, associated with diffuse idiopathic skeletal hyperostosis (57)

4.4.2.8 Large substernal and/or cancerous goiters (58)

4.4.2.9 Treacher Collins syndrome (59)

4.4.2.10 Morquio-Brailsford syndrome (60)

4.4.2.11 Endolaryngeal tumors (61)

4.4.3 When endotracheal intubation is not immediately possible

MAE 5.0 CONTRAINDICATIONS:

Aggressive airway management (intubation or establishment of a surgical airway) may be contraindicated when the patient's desire not to be resuscitated has been clearly expressed and documented in the patient's medical record or other valid legal document. (62–64)

MAE 6.0 PRECAUTIONS/HAZARDS AND/OR COMPLICATIONS:

The following represent possible hazards or complications related to the major facets of management of airway emergencies:

6.1 Translaryngeal intubation or cricothyrotomy is usually the route of choice. It may be necessary occasionally to use a surgical airway. Controversy exists as to whether intubation is hazardous in the presence of an unstable injury to the cervical spine. In one series the incidence of serious cervical spine injury in a severely injured population of blunt trauma patients was relatively low, and commonly used methods of precautionary airway management rarely led to neurologic deterioration. (65–67)

6.1.1 Failure to establish a patent airway (68–70)

6.1.2 Failure to intubate the trachea (68,69)

6.1.3 Failure to recognize intubation of esophagus (25,68,71–81)

6.1.4 Upper airway trauma, laryngeal, and esophageal damage (82)

6.1.5 Aspiration (70,74,82,83)

6.1.6 Cervical spine trauma (67,84,85)

6.1.7 Unrecognized bronchial intubation (25,68,72,82,86,87)

6.1.8 Eye injury (70)

6.1.9 Vocal cord paralysis (88)

6.1.10 Problems with ETT tubes:

    6.1.10.1 Cuff perforation (89)

    6.1.10.2 Cuff herniation (89)

    6.1.10.3 Pilot-tube-valve incompetence (90)

    6.1.10.4 Tube kinking during biting (70,89)

    6.1.10.5 Inadvertent extubation (17, 25,68,72,86,91–93)

    6.1.10.6 Tube occlusion (17,72, 82,89,93,94)

6.1.11 Bronchospasm (68,70,74)

6.1.12 Laryngospasm (72)

6.1.13 Dental accidents (70)

6.1.14 Dysrhythmias (94)

6.1.15 Hypotension and bradycardia due to vagal stimulation (94)

6.1.16 Hypertension and tachycardia (94,95)

6.1.17 Inappropriate tube size (89,96–99)

6.1.18 Bleeding

6.1.19 Mouth ulceration (82)

6.1.20 Nasal-intubation specific:

    6.1.20.1 Nasal damage including epistaxis

    6.1.20.2 Tube kinking in pharynx

    6.1.20.3 Sinusitis (100–102) and otitis media

6.1.21 Tongue ulceration

6.1.22 Tracheal damage including tracheo-esophageal fistula, tracheal innominate fistula, tracheal stenosis, and tracheomalacia (103–107)

6.1.23 Pneumonia (108)

6.1.24 Laryngeal damage with consequent laryngeal stenosis, (82,101,107,109,110) laryngeal ulcer, granuloma, polyps, synechia

6.1.25 Surgical cricothyrotomy or tracheostomy-specific (111,112)

    6.1.25.1 Stomal stenosis (82,113)

    6.1.25.2 Innominate erosion (113)

6.1.26 Needle cricothyrotomy–specific (114–118)

    6.1.26.1 Bleeding at insertion site with hematoma formation

    6.1.26.2 Subcutaneous and mediastinal emphysema (117)

    6.1.26.3 Esophageal perforation

6.2 Emergency ventilation

    6.2.1 Inadequate oxygen delivery (119–121)

    6.2.2 Hypo- or hyperventilation (122–124)

    6.2.3 Gastric insufflation and/or rupture (125,126)

    6.2.4 Barotrauma (127–129)

    6.2.5 Hypotension due to reduced venous return secondary to high mean intrathoracic pressure (130–132)

    6.2.6 Vomiting and aspiration (125)

    6.2.7 Prolonged interruption of ventilation for intubation (3,126)

    6.2.8 Failure to establish adequate functional residual capacity in the newborn (133–135)

    6.2.9 Movement of unstable cervical spine (more than by any commonly used method of endotracheal intubation) (136)

    6.2.10 Failure to exhale due to upper airway obstruction during percutaneous transtracheal ventilation (118,136)

MAE 8.0 ASSESSMENT OF NEED:

The need for management of airway emergencies is dictated by the patient's clinical condition. Careful observation, the implementation of basic airway management techniques, and laboratory and clinical data should help determine the need for more aggressive measures. Specific conditions requiring intervention include:

8.1 Inability to adequately protect airway (e.g., coma, lack of gag reflex, inability to cough) with or without other signs of respiratory distress

8.2 Partially obstructed airway. Signs of a partially obstructed upper airway include ineffective patient efforts to ventilate, paradoxical respiration, stridor, use of accessory muscles, patient's pointing to neck, choking motions, cyanosis, and distress. Signs of lower airway obstruction may include the above and wheezing.

8.3 Complete airway obstruction. Respiratory efforts with no breath sounds or suggestion of air movement are indicative of complete obstruction.

8.4 Apnea. No respiratory efforts are seen. May be associated with cardiac arrest.

8.5 Hypoxemia, hypercarbia, and/or acidemia seen on arterial blood gas analysis, oximetry, or exhaled gas analysis.

8.6 Respiratory distress. Elevated respiratory rate, high or low ventilatory volumes, and signs

(Continued)

(CPG Continued)

of sympathetic nervous system hyperactivity may be associated with respiratory distress.

MAE 9.0 ASSESSMENT OF PROCESS AND OUTCOME:

Timely intervention to maintain the patient's airway can improve outcome in terms of survival and level of function. Under rare circumstances, maintenance of an airway by nonsurgical means may not be possible. Despite optimal maintenance of the airway, patient outcomes are affected by patient-specific factors. Lack of availability of appropriate equipment and personnel may adversely affect patient outcome. Monitoring and recording are important to the improvement of the process of emergency airway management. Some aspects (e.g., frequency of complications of tracheal intubation or time for establishment of a definitive airway) are easy to quantitate and can lead to improvement in hospitalwide systems. Patient condition following the emergency should be evaluated from this perspective.

MAE 11.0 MONITORING:

11.1 Patient

11.1.1 Clinical signs — Continuous observation of the patient and repeated clinical assessment by a trained observer provide optimal monitoring of the airway. Special consideration should be given to the following: (174)

11.1.1.1 Level of consciousness

11.1.1.2 Presence and character of breath sounds

11.1.1.3 Ease of ventilation

11.1.1.4 Symmetry and amount of chest movement

11.1.1.5 Skin color and character (temperature and presence or absence of diaphoresis)

11.1.1.6 Presence of upper airway sounds (crowing, snoring, stridor)

11.1.1.7 Presence of excessive secretions, blood, vomitus, or foreign objects in the airway

11.1.1.8 Presence of epigastric sounds

11.1.1.9 Presence of retractions

11.1.1.10 Presence of nasal flaring

11.1.2 Physiologic variables — Repeated assessment of physiologic data by trained professionals supplements clinical assessment in managing patients with airway difficulties. Monitoring devices should be available, accessible, functional, and periodically evaluated for function. These data include but are not limited to: (142,175)

11.1.2.1 Ventilatory frequency, tidal volume, and airway pressure

11.1.2.2 Presence of CO_2 in exhaled gas

11.1.2.3 Heart rate and rhythm

11.1.2.4 Pulse oximetry

11.1.2.5 Arterial blood gas values

11.1.2.6 Chest radiograph

11.2 Endotracheal tube position — Regardless of the method of ventilation used, the most important consideration is detection of esophageal intubation.

11.2.1 Tracheal intubation is suggested but may not be confirmed by:

11.2.1.1 Bilateral breath sounds over the chest, symmetrical chest movement, and absence of ventilation sounds over the epigastrium (174,175,177)

11.2.1.2 Presence of condensate inside the tube, corresponding with exhalation (174,176,177)

11.2.1.3 Visualization of the tip of the tube passing through the vocal cords

11.2.1.4 Esophageal detector devices may be useful in differentiating esophageal from tracheal intubation (178,179)

11.2.2 Tracheal intubation is confirmed by detection of CO_2 in the exhaled gas, (180–182) although cases of transient CO_2 excretion from the stomach have been reported. (183)

11.2.3 Tracheal intubation is confirmed by endoscopic visualization of the carina or tracheal rings through the tube.

11.2.4 The position of the endotracheal tube (i.e., depth of insertion) should be appropriate on chest radiograph.

11.3 Airway management process — A properly managed airway may improve patient outcome. Continuous evaluation of the process will identify components needing improvement. These include response time, equipment function, equipment availability, practitioner performance, complication rate, and patient survival and functional status.

Reprinted with permission from *Respiratory Care* 1995; 40(7): 749–760. The complete AARC Clinical Practice Guidelines are available from the AARC Web site (http://www.aarc.org), from the AARC Executive Office, or from *Respiratory Care* journal.

ANATOMY OF THE UPPER AIRWAY

Tongue

The tongue is the first structure you will see as you open the patient's mouth to look down the airway. The tongue falling back against the posterior pharynx is a common cause of upper airway obstruction. In the unconscious patient, it is amazing how flaccid the tongue is.

Figure 20-1 shows what you will see when looking down the airway. Refer to this illustration as you read the description of the structures.

Vallecula

The vallecula is a notch between the base of the tongue and the epiglottis. When a MacIntosh laryngoscope blade is used, the distal tip is placed in the vallecula. The vallecula may be found by advancing the blade along the tongue until advancement terminates.

Epiglottis

The epiglottis is a lidlike cartilaginous structure that serves as a cover over the trachea. When closed, it protects the trachea from food or other foreign material. The structure is located superiorly as you look down the airway. When the Miller (straight) laryngoscope blade is used, the epiglottis is lifted. This is the farthest a laryngoscope blade is ever advanced down the airway.

Arytenoid Cartilages

The arytenoid cartilages are fairly large structures having right and left sides just beyond the epiglottis. These are oval-shaped structures in the lower portion of your field of view.

Vocal Cords

The vocal cords are your target when you are orally intubating a patient. The paired cords appear as a white

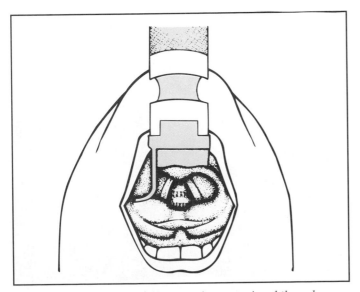

Figure 20-1 *Anatomy of the upper airway as viewed through a laryngoscope*

inverted *V* near the top of your field of view. As you advance the endotracheal tube, aim for these. You should be able to visualize the tube passing through the vocal cords.

The vocal cords will move with inspiration and expiration. It may be necessary to wait until the vocal cords open before passing the endotracheal tube through them.

REFLEXES OF THE UPPER AIRWAY

The upper airway is protected by a variety of reflexes. The presence of foreign substances or irritation stimulates various reflexes at different levels. These protective reflexes help to maintain airway patency and protect it from obstruction. They also serve to protect the lower airways from foreign objects and noxious gases or fumes.

Swallow

The first reflex encountered in the upper airway, in progressing from the mouth toward the lower airway, is the swallow reflex. Toward the posterior portion of the oropharynx are nerve receptors termed *swallowing receptors*. Stimulation of this area by food or a foreign object will cause an involuntary reflex, resulting in pharyngeal muscle contractions that propel the food or object posteriorly toward the esophagus. Lack of the swallow reflex may allow oral secretions to pool in the posterior oral pharynx. The integrity of the remaining reflexes are essential to prevent aspiration of these secretions.

A patient without the swallow reflex needs oral suctioning frequently. Positioning the patient lying on the side with the head turned toward the lower shoulder will allow the secretions to drain out of the mouth.

Gag

Toward the posterior oropharynx are vagal receptors that will cause gagging with sufficient stimulation. The gag reflex may induce vomiting, further compromising the patency of the airway. The gag reflex is a strong reflex, with some patients being more susceptible to gagging than others. The reflex may be depressed with central nervous system (CNS) depression, anesthesia, or drug overdose, or it may be intentionally depressed using lidocaine topically. Topical lidocaine is frequently used prior to bronchoscopy to depress the protective reflexes. A patient awakening from anesthesia may gag on an oropharyngeal airway as the patient returns to consciousness. While the patient is under anesthesia, the airway may be used without reflex stimulation. However, few patients can tolerate these airways when conscious.

Laryngeal

Stimulation of the larynx will cause the epiglottis to slam shut and the vocal cords to approximate (come together). The approximation of the vocal cords causes *laryngospasm*. All of us have experienced this reflex when food "goes down the wrong pipe." Other causes for laryngospasm are anaphylaxis and epiglottitis. Under these circumstances, the laryngospasm may be severe enough to totally occlude the airway.

Tracheal

Stimulation of the trachea will induce a cough. The trachea is very sensitive to stimulation by foreign material. The presence of secretions mobilized by air flow is sufficient to stimulate a cough. The placement of an artificial airway into the trachea may also stimulate a cough by irritation.

Carinal

The carina, which is where the trachea branches into the right and left mainstem bronchi, is extremely sensitive to stimulation. Stimulation of this area causes a cough reflex.

Reflexes and Loss of Consciousness

As a person loses consciousness, the reflexes protecting the airway are lost, in descending order, from the swallow reflex to the carinal reflex. The level of consciousness is reflected in the presence or absence of the reflexes. As you are intubating a patient, observe for the presence of reflexes. The presence of reflexes at one or more levels will indicate the patient's level of consciousness. Conversely, reflexes are regained in ascending order from the carinal reflex to the swallow reflex. This information is also useful in evaluating coma, and in assessing the need for intubation in neurologically depressed patients, such as those suffering from drug intoxication.

UPPER AIRWAY OBSTRUCTION

Causes

Upper airway obstruction may result from soft tissue or laryngeal obstruction. Contributing factors include CNS depression as the result of drug overdose or anesthesia; cardiac arrest; loss of consciousness; space-occupying lesions such as tumors; edema; and the presence of foreign material, aspirate, vomitus, or blood in the airway. The most common cause is soft tissue obstruction from the loss of muscle tone resulting in the tongue slipping back against the soft palate. *Laryngeal obstruction* is more commonly the result of muscle spasm (laryngospasm), edema from croup, epiglottitis, or the presence of foreign material. Laryngeal obstruction resulting from laryngeal spasm may occur as a result of anaphylactic reaction, postintubation, or foreign body aspiration, or in the near-drowning victim.

Clinical Findings

Upper airway obstruction is often accompanied by very noisy inspiratory efforts. The noise may vary from a mild snoring sound to a roar. Silence may indicate total obstruction. Generally speaking, the louder the noise is, the worse the obstruction. Frequently in severe obstruction, you may observe retraction of the intercostal muscles accompanied by sternal and clavicular retraction. Retractions are more easily observed in the infant or child. If prolonged, upper airway obstruction can lead to hypoxemia and hypercapnia. Total airway obstruction may lead to death in 5 to 10 minutes.

Positional Maneuvers to Open the Airway

The goal of airway management is the prompt restoration of airway patency. The majority of upper airway obstructions can be relieved using simple positional maneuvers. Once an airway is established, evaluate the adequacy of ventilation. Often, relief of the airway obstruction will allow spontaneous respirations to resume.

In the clinical setting, patients at risk for airway obstruction should be positioned to prevent its occurrence. Patients who have CNS depression, or who are under anesthesia or are comatose, should be placed on their side with the head tilted toward the lower shoulder to prevent aspiration. The placement of an artificial airway (as tolerated), such as a nasopharyngeal or an oropharyngeal airway, will also help to prevent airway obstruction.

Head Tilt

The *head tilt* maneuver involves tilting the head back to relieve *soft tissue obstruction* from the tongue and soft palate. It may be accomplished in one of two ways. One maneuver involves the placing of one hand under the neck and the palmar surface of the other hand against the forehead. One hand lifts the neck, while the other hand tilts the head back. The other maneuver is most easily performed while you are standing behind the patient. Using both hands, place one hand on the forehead and push back; with the other hand, lift the mandible. Performance of this maneuver is effective and rapid. Figure 20-2 shows the proper hand placement and patient position. In the event of obvious trauma, as from a motor vehicle accident, use of this maneuver may be contraindicated. If the vertebral column has been involved in the trauma, permanent nerve damage may be caused by this maneuver. In such cases, a better choice of technique is anterior mandibular displacement.

Anterior Mandibular Displacement

Anterior mandibular displacement is performed by grasping the jaw at the ramus on each side and lifting the jaw

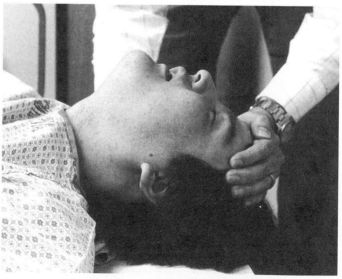

Figure 20-2 *The head tilt maneuver to relieve upper airway obstruction*

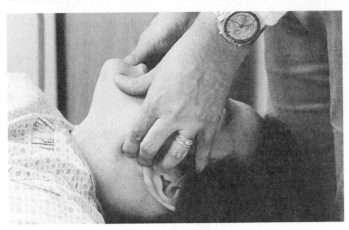

Figure 20-3 *Anterior mandibular displacement to relieve airway obstruction*

forward. This maneuver can be accomplished without tilting or moving the head, making it the treatment of choice in suspected vertebral column trauma. Figure 20-3 shows the maneuver to open the airway.

Triple Airway Maneuver

The triple airway maneuver is a combination of the head tilt, anterior mandibular displacement, and the separation of the teeth to open the mouth.

RESUSCITATORS

Once a patent airway has been restored, the adequacy of spontaneous respirations must be evaluated. Ventilatory assistance may be administered with a manual resuscitator.

There are two main types of manual resuscitators: self-inflating and flow-inflating. Each has advantages and disadvantages. Owing to the differences in operation, the technique for using each is also different. As a respiratory care practitioner, you will be expected to be thoroughly familiar with each type.

A self-inflating resuscitator, as the name implies, will automatically inflate after the bag is squeezed for inspiration. These resuscitators are constructed so that the walls have a stiffness or rigidity to them that causes the bag to return to its original shape after compression. Because of the stiffer wall design, it may be difficult to feel the compliance of a patient's lungs and thorax. Because of the structure of the bag, it is easily operated with one hand as you hold the mask to the patient's face with the other hand. These resuscitators are useful in the emergency

setting because they do not require a compressed gas source for operation. Compressed oxygen may be added to them to deliver an oxygen-enriched atmosphere.

A flow-inflating resuscitator, as the name implies, depends on the flow of source gas to inflate. This resuscitator will not operate without a compressed gas source. The construction of this resuscitator is such that the bag is very floppy and compliant. This makes it easy to assess the compliance of a patient's lungs and thorax. It is possible to deliver 100% oxygen with this resuscitator. Use of this device with a resuscitation mask is more difficult and requires considerable practice.

Gas-Powered Resuscitators

Gas-powered resuscitators are available that operate using a 50 psi oxygen source. A gas-powered resuscitator works as either a pressure-limited resuscitator, delivering a pre-set pressure (usually no more than 50 cm H_2O), or as a demand valve, so that the patient is able to initiate the inspiration. These resuscitators have a standardized patient connection (15 mm inner diameter and 22 mm outer diameter) that enables them to be used with a resuscitation mask or an artificial airway. An advantage of these devices is that 100% oxygen is delivered and some fatigue from prolonged manual ventilation is relieved. Before using this type of device, verify that it has a safety popoff valve to prevent delivery of excessive pressures. Verify that it works.

Valve Types Used in Self-Inflating Manual Resuscitators

The purpose of all valves used in manual resuscitators is to deliver gas to the patient during inspiration and to allow the patient to exhale to the ambient atmosphere on exhalation. Additional criteria used in the design of these valves include sensitivity to the patient's inspiratory efforts, ease of cleaning should they become fouled with vomitus, compact size, and ease of disassembly for cleaning and parts replacement.

Several types of valves and different valve combinations are used to accomplish the stated objectives. Figure 20-4 shows the different types of valves used for manual resuscitators. Table 20-1 compares the characteristics of these valve types with one another.

Besides having a working knowledge of the valves used in the self-inflating manual resuscitators, you should also be aware of the different capabilities of each device (FiO_2 delivery, spontaneous ventilation from the reservoir). Table 20-2 compares the different manual resuscitators.

TABLE 20-1: Types of Self-Inflating Manual Resuscitation Valves			
TYPE	**EASE OF CLEANING**	**EASE OF DISASSEMBLY**	**SENSITIVITY**
Diaphragm (leaf)	Good	Good	Good
Spring and disk or spring and ball	Good	Good	Poor
Duck bill	Good	Good	Good

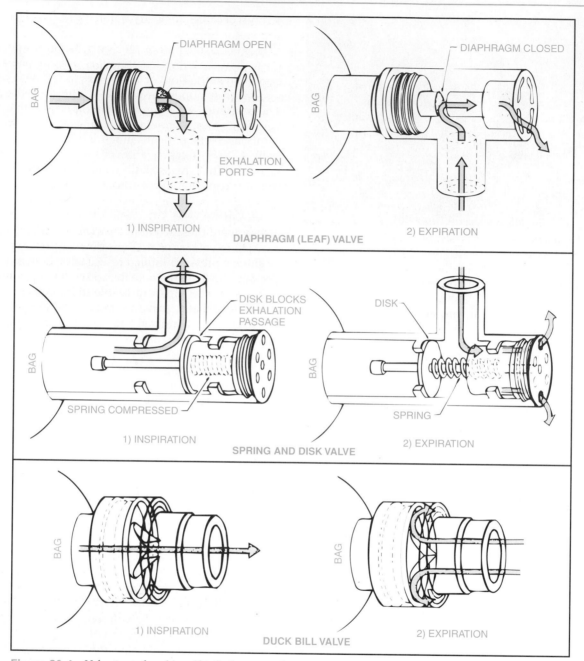

Figure 20-4 *Valve types found in self-inflating manual resuscitators*

TABLE 20-2: Comparison of Self-Inflating Manual Resuscitators

RESUSCITATOR	VALVE TYPE	SPONTANEOUS VENTILATION FROM BAG	FiO₂ WITH RESERVOIR	FiO₂ WITHOUT RESERVOIR
Ambu NR	Leaf diaphragm	Yes	59–90%	53–86%
Ambu Mark III	Diaphragm	Yes	Up to 100%	Above 40%
Hope	Spring and disk	No	55–66%	33–65%
Hope II	Spring and ball	No	70–99%	29–42%
Laerdal II	Duck bill	Yes	82–100%	32–41%
PMR 2	Diaphragm	Yes	Up to 100%	28–42%
Pulmanex	Duck bill	Yes	89–94%	34–42%

IMPORTANCE OF INSPIRATORY-EXPIRATORY RATIO DURING RESUSCITATION

The use of a manual resuscitator involves applying pressure or squeezing the bag and forcing gas into the airway to ventilate the patient's lungs. This method of ventilation is similar in principle to intermittent positive-pressure breathing (IPPB) and therefore the hazards and complications are similar. You may want to review the effects of positive intrathoracic pressure found in Chapter 17, "Hyperinflation Therapy."

Increased intrathoracic pressure can decrease venous return to the heart through the vena cava. Decreased venous return, combined with the compression of the mediastinum, can lead to a significant decrease in cardiac output. In an emergency situation, one of the primary goals is the improvement of circulation.

The adverse affects may be avoided by ventilating the patient using an inspiratory-expiratory (I:E) ratio of 1:2 or greater. An I:E ratio of 1:2 will allow sufficient time for the heart to fill during the expiratory phase when there is no positive pressure in the thoracic cavity.

Hazards of Manual Resuscitation

The major hazards associated with manual resuscitation include gastric distention, aspiration, and diminished cardiac output. Gastric distention can result when inflation pressures open the esophagus, admitting air into the stomach. The etiology of decreased cardiac output has been previously discussed.

Another hazard is inadequate ventilation due to poor technique or an ill-fitting mask. Equipment malfunctions may also reduce effective ventilation.

Pharyngeal Airways in Manual Resuscitation

Pharyngeal airways are specialized devices employed to maintain a patent airway. This is accomplished through bypassing the site of the obstruction or preventing the tongue from slipping back against the soft palate. The most common airways used in ventilating a nonintubated patient with a manual resuscitator are the nasopharyngeal and oropharyngeal airways and laryngeal mask airways (LMAs).

Pharyngeal airways are not tolerated well once the patient is awake or alert. They do not provide a direct passage to the lower airway, and they do not protect the patient from aspiration in the case of diminished protective reflexes as intubation would. These airways are intended for short-term management.

Nasopharyngeal Airway

The *nasopharyngeal airway* is often referred to as a nasal horn or trumpet, names acquired due to its shape. Figure 20-5 shows a nasal trumpet. The nasopharyngeal airway is inserted through one of the nares of the nose and past the turbinates with the tip separating the tongue from the posterior soft palate. Figure 20-6 shows the airway in proper position. This airway is far from stable, but it is usually well tolerated. Its position at the opening of the naris should be checked frequently to ensure it has not slipped anteriorly, or worse, posteriorly. Some styles have a means to secure the airway to the patient's face, using tape or a tie of some type.

Oropharyngeal Airway

The *oropharyngeal airway* is larger than the nasopharyngeal airway. It is designed to be inserted into the mouth and then rotated with the tip resting against the base of the tongue. It is designed to separate the tongue from the posterior palate. It does not provide a tube for the patient to breathe through, so its fit is essential to accomplish the job. This airway is not tolerated well by the conscious patient. It may cause a severe gag reflex and vomiting. Figure 20-7 shows the airway and its proper insertion.

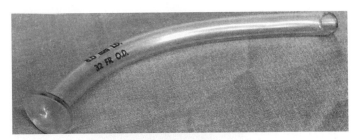

Figure 20-5   *A photograph of a nasopharyngeal airway*

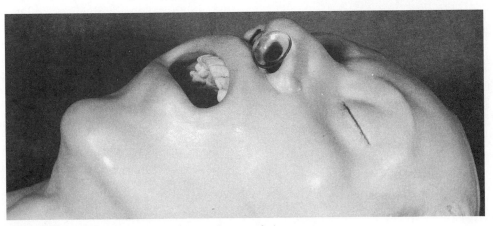

Figure 20-6   *Correct placement of a nasopharyngeal airway*

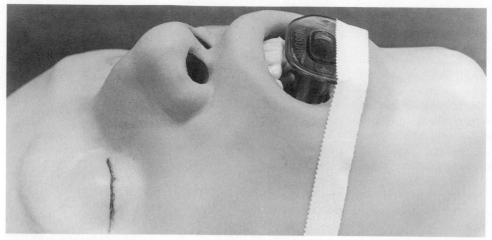

Figure 20-7 *Correct use of an oropharyngeal airway*

Like the nasopharyngeal airway, this airway is unstable. Patients with this airway in place should not be left alone. Gagging and vomiting as well as displacement of the airway are common complications. It is easy for the patient to manipulate the airway with the tongue, often spitting it out.

Several types of these airways are available. Figure 20-8 shows some of the varieties that are manufactured.

Laryngeal Mask Airway (LMA)

The *laryngeal mask airway (LMA)* is illustrated in Figure 20-9. It is a small triangular-shaped inflatable mask that is secured to a tube, similar in size to an endotracheal tube. The LMA is designed to be inserted such that once the

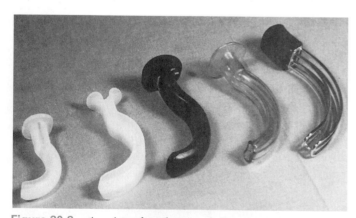

Figure 20-8 *A variety of oropharyngeal airways*

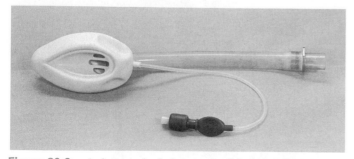

Figure 20-9 *A photograph of a laryngeal mask airway (LMA)*

mask is inflated, the tip rests against the upper esophageal sphincter and the sides face into the pyriform fossae, lying just under the base of the tongue. This device is designed to seal the esophagus, preventing gastric aspiration while providing a patent airway for positive-pressure ventilation to the trachea.

INTUBATION: WHAT IS IT?

There are several criteria utilized in making a decision to intubate a patient. One or more of these criteria is justification for the intubation of a patient. Figure 20-10 lists these criteria.

Intubation involves the placement of an endotracheal tube into the trachea. There are two routes: oral and nasal. Each route has its inherent advantages and disadvantages. Ultimately, the endotracheal tube passes down the posterior pharynx, past the epiglottis, through the vocal cords with the distal tip resting 1.5 inches above the carina. With the endotracheal tube in place, the patient is said to be intubated.

Oral Route

The oral route of intubation is the fastest and most direct. It is usually the first route learned by most respiratory care practitioners. During the procedure, the vocal cords are directly visualized by the use of a laryngoscope while the endotracheal tube is inserted. If the cords are visualized, the chances of esophageal intubation are minimized. The size of the upper airway permits the use of a larger endotracheal tube, minimizing the resistance through the

* Failure of other artificial airways to maintain a patent airway
* Need for repeated deep tracheal suctioning
* Need for long-term mechanical ventilation
* Protection of the airway

Figure 20-10 *Criteria for intubation*

artificial airway (Poiseuille's law). When the procedure is properly performed, trauma to the oral and laryngeal structures is minimal. If the first attempt does not meet with success, a repeat attempt may be made after allowing sufficient time for reventilation and oxygenation before the repeat attempt.

There are disadvantages to the oral route of intubation. Oral care is difficult owing to the presence of the large endotracheal tube. The presence of tape or other supportive materials also hampers access to the oral cavity for care. A conscious patient will often gag or cough from movement of the tube in the airway. Because of the size of the oral cavity in relationship to the endotracheal tube and the presence of copious oral secretions, it is difficult to stabilize the endotracheal tube securely.

Nasal Route

Some facilities do not allow respiratory care practitioners to perform nasal intubation of the patient. This description is provided so that the respiratory care practitioner may better assist the physician performing this procedure.

Patients may be intubated nasally if they have experienced oral or facial trauma, making the oral intubation route impossible or impractical. An anesthesiologist will often nasally intubate patients during the administration of general anesthesia. Nasal intubation is common enough that the respiratory care practitioner should be familiar with the technique and know how to secure the endotracheal tube properly after the procedure has been performed.

There are several advantages to this route of intubation. As mentioned, if a patient has suffered trauma to the mouth or face making the oral route impractical, the patient may still be intubated nasally. Generally speaking, conscious patients tolerate nasal intubation better than oral intubation because the gag reflex is not as strongly stimulated. The absence of the endotracheal tube in the mouth makes oral care much easier, allowing sufficient access. The naris of the nose provides a natural anatomical structure to stabilize the endotracheal tube. Just a small amount of tape to prevent the tube from moving in or out is all that is required.

There are several disadvantages to the nasal route. Owing to the size of the nasal passage, a smaller tube, which increases resistance, must be used. This can be significant during mechanical ventilation and in weaning the patient because of the increased work of breathing. Smaller tubes may also make suctioning the airway more difficult. During nasal intubation, the vocal cords are not directly visualized, making this procedure "blind." The length of time taken for the procedure is longer. The tube must be first inserted through the nasal passages and then advanced down through the lower airway. Sometimes, this procedure is performed using a laryngoscope and Magill forceps to visualize the distal end of the tube and guide the tube through the vocal cords. The long-term placement of an endotracheal tube through the nasal passages may result in necrosis of the nasal tissue caused by the pressure of the tube decreasing the blood flow through the capillaries.

Equipment for Endotracheal Intubation
Laryngoscopes

There are two main types of laryngoscopes in use. One is termed conventional and the other fiberoptic.

The conventional *laryngoscope* is the most common type in use today. It consists of a handle containing batteries, a switch, and a socket into which different blades can be snapped in place. It works much like a flashlight. To turn it on, position the blade at a right angle to the handle by snapping it up. A blade is inserted by holding the handle vertically and aligning the socket on the blade with the handle socket. Pull each part together as if trying to pull each past the other. Figure 20-11 shows a laryngoscope with a Miller blade and its assembly.

The fiberoptic laryngoscope utilizes fiberoptics to transmit light to its distal tip. It has a self-contained battery pack and a flexible fiberoptic bundle that takes the place of a conventional blade. Owing to its small diameter and flexibility, it may be inserted into the endotracheal tube, and together the two can be advanced into position. An advantage of this laryngoscope is the ability to visualize the carina once the tube is in place. Exercise caution in the use of this equipment. Fiberoptics are fragile. Biting down on the laryngoscope by the patient could cause permanent damage to it.

Blades

There are two types of laryngoscope blades commonly used: the Miller and the MacIntosh. The *Miller blade* is the straight blade. Figure 20-12 shows several sizes of Miller blades. When using this blade, the epiglottis is physically lifted. The *MacIntosh blade* is a curved blade. It is inserted into the vallecula. As the laryngoscope is lifted, the epiglottis will follow, exposing the vocal cords and laryngeal structures. Many practitioners find it easier to visualize the cords with this blade.

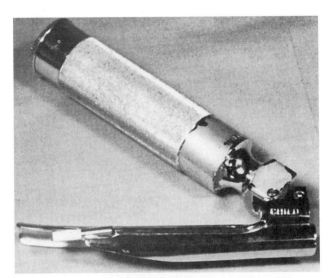

Figure 20-11 *A conventional laryngoscope with a Miller blade attached*

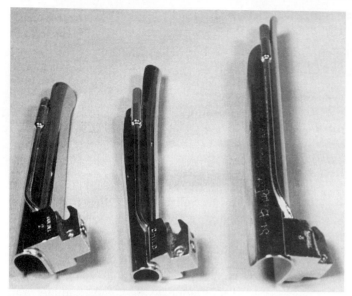

Figure 20-12 *Different sizes of Miller laryngoscope blades*

Characteristics of Endotracheal Tubes

Modern endotracheal tubes are made of polyvinyl chloride (PVC), which is inert and nontoxic to tissue. The polymer is semirigid and is molded into a gentle curve that matches the curve of the airway. If you look closely at an *endotracheal tube*, you will see a stripe that runs almost the full length of the tube. This stripe is radiopaque and will show as a white band on the radiograph, helping to locate the exact position of the tip. Figure 20-13 shows an endotracheal tube. These tubes come in different diameters and are cut to an approximate length.

Murphy Eye Endotracheal Tube

A Murphy endotracheal tube has an eye or opening opposite the bevel on the distal end of the tube. Figure 20-14 shows this eye. In the event the distal tip becomes occluded, air flow may still pass through this eye (although resistance will be significantly greater).

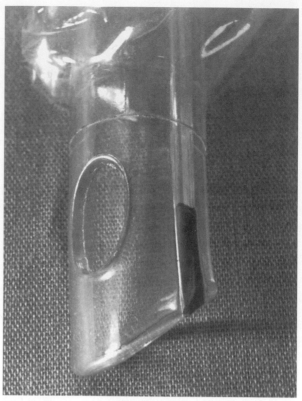

Figure 20-14 *The Murphy eye on an endotracheal tube*

Endotracheal Tube Cuff

The *endotracheal tube cuff* is an inflatable balloon near the tip of the tube. It creates a seal against the tracheal wall. An inflated cuff permits the application of positive pressure to the lungs and protects the airway from aspiration. It is best to use a high-volume, low-pressure cuff. This will distribute the pressure over a greater area, minimizing damage to the mucosa.

One type of cuff is designed not to be inflated. It is the Bivona foam cuff. To use this cuff, first evacuate all of the air and seal it with the stopper provided. Once the tube is

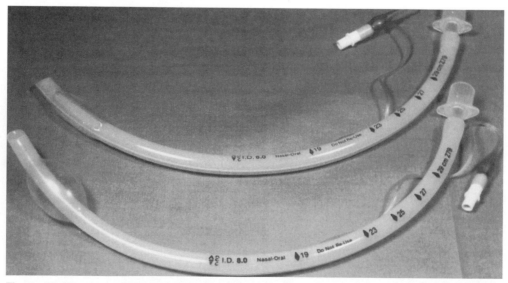

Figure 20-13 *A contemporary endotracheal tube*

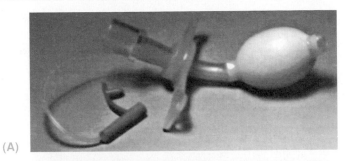

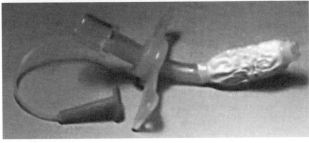

(A)

(B)

Figure 20-15 *The pilot line is open, allowing the foam in the cuff to expand (A). Air has been withdrawn from the cuff and the pilot line capped, deflating it (B).*

in place, open the pilot tube to atmospheric pressure. The foam in the cuff will reexpand, exerting minimal pressure to the tracheal wall. Figure 20-15 shows two Bivona cuffs, one evacuated and one expanded.

Pilot Tube and Balloon

The *endotracheal pilot tube* conducts air to the cuff of the tube. Be careful not to inadvertently cut the pilot tube. If you do so, the patient will need to be reintubated.

If the pilot tube on a Bivona endotracheal tube is cut, you will be unable to deflate the cuff to extubate the patient. Sometimes a needle from a syringe may be carefully inserted into the inside of the pilot tube. This then allows a syringe to be attached. However, this procedure is difficult and it often requires luck for a successful result.

The endotracheal pilot balloon is located on the proximal end of the pilot tube. It will indicate whether air is present in the endotracheal tube cuff. The larger the balloon is, the more air (volume) is in the cuff. It is advisable to measure cuff volume and cuff pressure twice each shift.

Markings

The proximal end of an endotracheal tube is conveniently marked in centimeter increments. This can provide a rough guide as to how far a tube has been advanced. However, it is best to rely on a chest x-ray film to determine tube placement in relation to the carina. After a chest x-ray has verified the position, the markings may be used to establish whether it has slipped in or out from the original location.

COMPLICATIONS OF INTUBATION

The complications of intubation may be divided into early and late complications. Early complications generally occur during the procedure itself, whereas late complications occur hours or days after intubation.

Early Complications

One of the most common early complications is esophageal intubation. This may be assessed by auscultating the chest and by a chest x-ray. On auscultation, breath sounds will be diminished or absent. End-tidal CO_2 may also be used to confirm esophageal intubation. If the esophagus is intubated, the exhaled CO_2 will quickly fall to zero. Observe the abdomen while ventilating the patient. If the esophagus is intubated, the abdomen will rise and fall. Auscultate the abdomen: if sounds are present on inspiration, esophageal intubation is likely. A chest x-ray will ultimately confirm that the tube is improperly placed. However, often you cannot afford the time required for an x-ray in an emergency situation.

Trauma to the dentition or the oral cavity may result from a difficult intubation. If the patient is conscious, administration of a fast-acting paralytic agent (such as succinylcholine) by a physician or a nurse anesthetist will facilitate intubation and minimize trauma. At the very least, a conscious patient should receive intravenous diazepam to decrease anxiety and to facilitate the procedure.

If the endotracheal tube is advanced too far, the right or left mainstem bronchus will be intubated. Advance the endotracheal tube only a short distance past the vocal cords. After placement, obtain a chest x-ray to verify that its position is 1.5 inches above the carina.

On intubation, there is a possibility of kinking the tube, making the resistance to air flow very high. If you suspect the tube has kinked, try to pull it out slightly and then try to ventilate the patient again. If required, extubate the patient and insert another endotracheal tube.

Vomiting and aspiration may occur during the procedure. Have both a Yankauer (tonsil tip) and a suction catheter readily available to clear vomitus. Clear the oropharynx with the Yankauer suction first, and then intubate.

Late Complications

Vocal cord damage may occur as a result of the cord being approximated by the endotracheal tube and the friction resulting from it. It is not uncommon for a patient to sound hoarse for several hours after extubation.

Tracheal stenosis—narrowing of the trachea by scar tissue—may be a long-term complication of intubation. The decrease of capillary circulation combined with the irritation of the tube itself may cause tracheal damage. The best way to manage this condition is to prevent it.

If cuff pressure is maintained at a level greater than 25 cm H_2O for extended periods, capillary circulation will be impeded, resulting in tissue necrosis. It is best to keep cuff pressures at 20 cm H_2O or lower. Another method to determine cuff inflation is to establish a *minimal occlusion volume* (MOV). To perform this technique, inflate the lungs with positive pressure while simultaneously inflating the cuff. Stop cuff inflation just when the airway is occluded and escaping air is no longer heard. If cuff pressure is measured, it will generally be 25 cm H_2O or lower. If pressures are much greater, it is likely that too small an endotracheal tube was inserted. With the *minimal leak technique*, a slight leak is allowed during inspiration. To perform this technique, inflate the cuff under positive pressure. Stop cuff inflation when a small leak is heard at the mouth during inspiration.

Infection is a common complication from intubation. The introduction of bacteria into the lower airway is probably due to the bypassing of the upper airway defense mechanisms.

Extubation

Once the patient is able to manage secretions or the underlying cause for intubation has been resolved, *extubation* may be performed. Nelson, Hunter, and Morton (1983) have listed the criteria for extubation in *Critical Care Respiratory Therapy: A Laboratory and Clinical Manual* (Figure 20-16).

The complications of extubation are associated primarily with edema, laryngospasm, and aspiration.

The artificial airway is irritating to the tracheal and laryngeal structures. Following its removal, the tissue frequently swells in response to the irritation, narrowing the lumen of the airway. Laryngospasm may occur in some patients as the endotracheal tube is withdrawn through the larynx. Aspiration may occur when the cuff is deflated and secretions that have pooled above the cuff drain inferiorly down the trachea. The epiglottis may not function normally for a few hours, also increasing the risk of aspiration.

Knowledge of these potential complications can help you to avoid them. Edema may be relieved by the application of cool aerosol following extubation. Aspiration complications may be avoided by complete suctioning prior to extubation and keeping the head elevated by placing the patient in a semi-Fowler's position. Epiglottitis and edema may be treated by the administration of racemic epinephrine via small-volume nebulizer following extubation to reduce mucosal edema by stimulating the alpha receptors in the mucosal circulatory system.

- Vital capacity greater than 15 to 18 ml per kg of ideal body weight, or 3 × normal predicted tidal volume
- Spontaneous minute ventilation less than 10 L/min
- Maximum inspiratory force greater than –25 cm H_2O
- Inspired oxygen concentration less than 0.4
- Arterial blood gas values within clinically acceptable range
- Mechanical ventilatory support no longer required
- Airway protection mechanisms present
- Underlying reason for intubation resolved

Figure 20-16 *Criteria for extubation* (Reprinted with permission from Nelson, E. J., Hunter, P., & Mouton, E. *Critical care respiratory therapy: A laboratory and clinical manual*, Table 6–1. ©1983 by Little, Brown and Company)

PROFICIENCY OBJECTIVES

At the end of this chapter, you should be able to:

- Demonstrate the manual maneuvers to open the airway.
- Using an intubation mannequin, demonstrate the correct use of an oropharyngeal and a nasopharyngeal airway.
- Demonstrate how to assemble and prepare for use, including testing for function prior to use, a self-inflating manual resuscitator.
- Using a self-inflating manual resuscitator and a mask, maintain a patent airway and ventilate a resuscitation mannequin for 3 minutes, according to the following criteria:
  — Maintain an I:E ratio of 1:2 or greater
  — Maintain a rate of 12 breaths per minute
  — Observe the patient for the following:
    — Vomiting
    — Skin color
    — Chest expansion
    — Gastric distention

- Using an intubated resuscitation mannequin, demonstrate the use of a flow-inflating resuscitator, ventilating the mannequin according to the following criteria:
  — Maintain an I:E ratio of 1:2 or greater.
  — Maintain a rate of 12 breaths per minute.
  — Observe the "patient" for the following:
    — Skin color
    — Chest expansion

- Demonstrate oral intubation of a resuscitation mannequin using first a Miller and then a MacIntosh laryngoscope blade.

- Discuss the rationale for hyperinflation and oxygenation prior to intubation.

- Describe the procedure used for nasal intubation, and demonstrate how to secure a nasal endotracheal tube.

- Using an orally intubated mannequin, demonstrate how to extubate the mannequin.

PATIENT POSITIONING TO RELIEVE UPPER AIRWAY OBSTRUCTION

The positional maneuvers employed to relieve upper airway obstruction are discussed earlier in this chapter. The procedures and techniques are not covered here. It is suggested that you review this portion of the chapter before proceeding.

AIRWAY INSERTION

Insertion of the Nasopharyngeal Airway

Nasopharyngeal airways come in different diameters and lengths. They are made from a soft rubber or plastic. Some manufacturers shape and mark them for use in the right or left naris.

Use of a nasopharyngeal airway is contraindicated in patients receiving anticoagulant therapy or those who have bleeding disorders. The insertion of this airway may cause trauma to the nasopharynx with associated bleeding.

For proper sizing of a nasopharyngeal airway, place the distal end of the airway at the tragus of the ear. The length of the airway should span from the tragus of the ear to the tip of the nose. As a general rule, use the largest-diameter tube that can easily be inserted without undue force or trauma.

The technique of nasopharyngeal airway insertion begins with lubrication of the entire length of the airway with a water-soluble lubricant. Insert the airway gently through the nostril, parallel to the floor of the nasal cavity, matching the curve of the airway with the patient's airway. If the airway has a beveled distal tip, the bevel should face medially. The nasal passage progresses posteriorly along the floor of the nasal cavity, then inferiorly. Do not attempt to insert the airway up the nose toward the eyes. Gently advance the airway. If resistance is encountered, redirect or rotate the airway slightly. Do not force the insertion of the airway. If you cannot successfully insert an airway in one naris, try the other rather than attempting insertion by force. The tip of the airway should be just past the level of the posterior tongue, separating it from the posterior oropharynx. Once the airway is in place, the flared end will help to prevent further advancement of the airway down the nasal passage. However, check its placement frequently. Figure 20-6 shows the airway's placement.

You may not be able to insert this airway into a patient with a deviated septum. The use of this airway under this circumstance is not indicated.

Potential complications of using this type of airway include hearing problems caused by irritation of the eustachian tubes and mucosal irritation and trauma. The airway should be changed every 8 hours, and the new airway should be inserted into the alternate naris.

Insertion of the Oropharyngeal Airway

The airway is inserted by rotating the tip so that it is directed toward the hard palate. The airway is advanced toward the rear of the oropharynx and then rotated 180° so the tip now points down toward the throat. The rotation of the airway displaces the tongue forward and opens the passage between the tongue and the posterior pharynx. Figure 20-7 shows the airway's placement.

This airway should not be used if its placement stimulates gagging and vomiting. The patient should be positioned to minimize aspiration and should be closely watched.

PREPARATION OF MANUAL RESUSCITATORS

This section describes the preparation of manual resuscitators for use with a resuscitation mask. Any of the manual resuscitators may be used directly on an endotracheal tube or tracheostomy tube by removing the resuscitation mask. The patient connection on all of these devices is standardized, having an inside diameter of 15 mm and an outside diameter of 22 mm. It provides a direct connection with endotracheal tubes, tracheostomy tubes, masks, and manual resuscitators.

Check the valves for correct assembly and operation. Visually inspect the valve to ensure that it is assembled correctly and squeeze the bag several times to verify valve operation.

Attach the reservoir assembly to the manual resuscitator. Attach the oxygen connecting tubing to an oxygen flowmeter and set the flow to 10 to 15 L/min. Reassess the operation of the valves by squeezing the bag several times. Occlude the patient outlet, and squeeze the bag. Pressure should be maintained within the bag, indicating that the valve(s) are functioning properly.

To assemble a flow-inflating manual resuscitator, you will need the following components: an anesthesia elbow with an oxygen inlet, a 3- or 5-liter anesthesia bag (cut off the very tip of the distal end), a length of oxygen connecting tubing, and an oxygen flowmeter. Attach the anesthesia bag to the anesthesia elbow. This may require the use of a mask adapter (22-mm outside diameter, 15-mm inside diameter). Attach the oxygen connecting tubing between the anesthesia elbow and the flowmeter. Figure 20-17 shows the completed assembly.

VENTILATION WITH A MANUAL RESUSCITATOR

Patient Positioning

Place the patient in a supine position and open the airway using one of the manual maneuvers. It is easiest to ventilate a patient in this position. It also allows for the observation of chest expansion and gastric distention. This position also permits cardiac compression, if it is required.

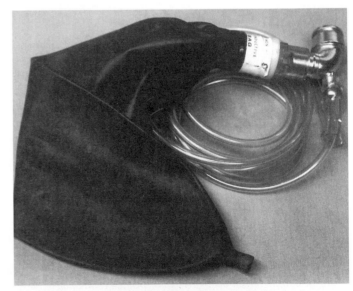

Figure 20-17 *Assembly of a flow-inflating manual resuscitator*

Mask Placement

Place the mask on the patient's face, applying the mask to the bridge of the nose first and then securing a tight seal below the lower lip. With a little practice, the mask's position can be maintained with the thumb and index finger of one hand, freeing the third, fourth, and fifth fingers on that hand to hook under the mandible, displacing it anteriorly to maintain a patent airway. Figure 20-18 shows the mask placement and finger positions. The other hand is free to compress the bag, inflating the lungs. The maintenance of an absolutely tight seal between the mask and face is required at all times for a flow-inflating manual resuscitator.

Ventilation

If the patient is apneic, ventilation may begin immediately. Ventilate the patient at a rate of 8 to 16 breaths per minute. Watch for chest expansion to ensure you are delivering adequate volumes. Ventilate the patient with an I:E ratio of at least 1:2 or better to minimize the effects of positive intrathoracic pressure on the cardiovascular system.

It is important not to hyperventilate your patient. Often the rush of the emergency setting may cause health care personnel to become overly zealous. Hyperventilation will cause a rapid change in $PaCO_2$ in patients who have been hypoventilating for long time periods. Hyperventilation of these patients may potentially result in seizures.

If the patient has spontaneous respiratory efforts, match your ventilation efforts with the patient's efforts. When the patient begins inspiration, deliver a breath with the manual resuscitator. Knowledge of which resuscitators allow spontaneous ventilation is helpful under these circumstances.

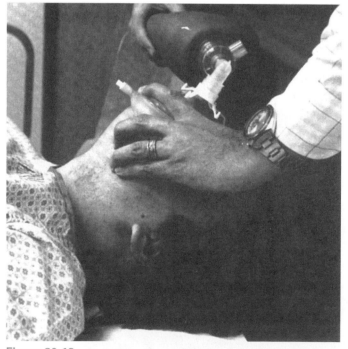

Figure 20-18 *Correct use of a mask for manual ventilation of the patient*

Ventilation with a flow-inflating manual resuscitator requires that you pinch the distal end of the bag during compression. With exhalation, you must release the distal end to allow the exhaled gas to exit the bag. Oxygen flow will flush the exhaled CO_2 from the bag. A person unfamiliar with the operation of a flow-inflating bag will frequently have the flow set too high. A high oxygen flow will cause the bag to balloon, making it very difficult to manage with one hand. Either turn down the flow rate or compress the bag from the middle portion, decreasing the volume of the bag (as long as minute ventilation and tidal volume are adequate).

Patient Assessment during the Procedure

As mentioned previously, observe the patient for chest expansion, which indicates adequate volume delivery. Note the amount of resistance you encounter as you are ventilating the patient. This resistance is a direct reflection of the compliance of the lungs and thorax. If resistance is increased, it may indicate decreased compliance or a partial obstruction of the airway. Reassess the airway patency and continue ventilation. This is easier to assess with use of a flow-inflating manual resuscitator. Another person, if available, should auscultate the chest to assess ventilation.

Observe the patient frequently for signs of cyanosis. Watch for any signs of gastric distention. Gastric insufflation is a dangerous potential complication of bag and mask ventilation, as it may result in vomiting and aspiration. Decompression may be accomplished by the insertion of a nasogastric tube. If long-term resuscitation is expected, the early insertion of a nasogastric tube is recommended. Do not attempt to decompress the stomach by pushing on it until the patient is intubated. This maneuver may result in the patient's vomiting, with the aspirate being driven into the tracheobronchial tree by the positive-pressure ventilation.

Assess the patient's pulse frequently. Another advantage of using the third, fourth, and fifth fingers to displace the mandible is that the last two fingers may assess the pulse, using the facial artery just anterior to the angle of the mandible. Other health care personnel available should assess carotid and femoral pulses to ensure adequate circulation. Cardiopulmonary complications may be minimized by using an I:E ratio of 1:2 or greater.

EQUIPMENT PREPARATION AND ASSEMBLY FOR INTUBATION

The equipment required for endotracheal intubation may be conveniently stored on a small tray or in a small fishing tackle box. The supplies needed are listed in Figure 20-19.

Preparation of the Laryngoscope

The laryngoscope should be assembled and a blade attached. Check the light for operation. If the light fails to illuminate, change the batteries and the bulb. If this fails to render it operational, change handles and repair the first unit later when time permits.

- Gloves, goggles, or face shield
- Laryngoscope
- Laryngoscope blades
- Spare batteries
- Spare bulbs
- Oropharyngeal airways (several sizes)
- Yankauer suction (tonsil tip)
- Endotracheal tubes sized from 6.5-mm to 10-mm inner diameter
- 10-ml (or larger) syringe
- Cloth first-aid tape
- Water-soluble lubricant
- Magill forceps
- Stylet

Figure 20-19 *Equipment needed for intubation*

Oropharyngeal Airways

Lay out the airways in a convenient way that allows you to grab one quickly as the need arises. For female adult patients, small to medium sizes should be used. A male patient usually requires a medium to large airway size. The airway is sized properly when the flange rests on the patient's lips and the distal tip keeps the posterior tongue separated from the soft palate.

Yankauer Suction

Connect the Yankauer suction (tonsil tip) to a vacuum gauge and suction trap. Adjust your vacuum level to –120 mm Hg. Have the suction ready at hand where you may instantly pick it up. Have a 14 French sterile suction catheter or suction kit handy for use after the patient is intubated.

10-ml (or Larger) Syringe

Fill the syringe with 6 to 9 cc of air. Have it ready for attachment to the pilot balloon after the patient is intubated.

Cloth First-Aid Tape

Tear several strips about 15 inches long from a roll of 1-inch cloth first-aid tape. You will need this later to secure the tube. Stick the tape on a nearby wall or other surface where it will be handy and will not tangle.

Water-Soluble Lubricant

Squeeze out some lubricant onto a sterile 4 × 4-inch gauze pad for lubricating the endotracheal tube prior to insertion.

Magill Forceps

Keep these handy in case the patient needs to be nasally intubated.

Endotracheal Tubes

Check the cuff on the endotracheal tube prior to insertion by inflating it with about 10 cc of air (depending on cuff size, use more or less). Make sure the cuff is not torn and is capable of withstanding the pressure. Endotracheal tube

sizes for female adult patients range from 7.5- to 8.5-mm inner diameter, whereas male patients' sizes range from 8.5- to 9.5-mm inner diameter. Nasal intubation requires a longer-length tube than that needed for oral intubation.

Stylet

The stylet is a flexible metal wire used to stiffen the endotracheal tube. This will help during insertion of the tube to keep the tip anterior and guide it into the trachea.

General Notes

If the patient has been hypoxic for an extended period, or if it is an emergency situation, the person with the most intubation experience should make the attempt. Because you are at this point a new respiratory care practitioner, it is best for you to gain experience under more controlled circumstances. Ideally, this occurs in the operating room under the supervision of an anesthesiologist or a nurse anesthetist.

No more than 30 seconds should elapse from the time the laryngoscope enters the mouth until the endotracheal tube has been inserted. If the tube has not been inserted in this time frame, withdraw the laryngoscope and ventilate the patient with a manual resuscitator for 1 or 2 minutes and reattempt the intubation. For intubation of a patient in the clinical setting, no more than three attempts should be made. If you cannot insert the tube, ventilate the patient and get someone who can.

Patient Positioning

The patient should be positioned supine with a small roll under the shoulders and the head slightly hyperextended. Imagine walking up to a rosebush to sniff the roses, and visualize your head position as you extend your neck to get your nose closer to the blossom. That is the position you want your patient to assume. Figure 20-20 shows a patient in the "sniffing" position. Figure 20-21 shows what happens to the anatomy of the upper airway in this position versus having the head at a right angle to the body.

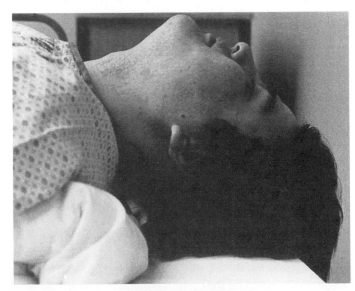

Figure 20-20 *A patient in the "sniffing" position*

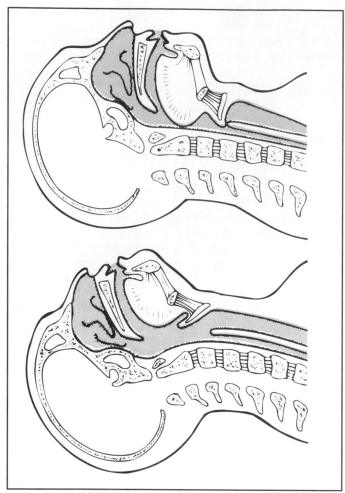

Figure 20-21 *A comparison of the airway of a patient in two supine positions*

Hyperinflation and Oxygenation

Intubation is an emergency procedure often performed on apneic, hypoxic patients. The procedure may stimulate the vagus nerve, causing bradycardia and the cough reflex if present. Two or three minutes of vigorous resuscitation with 100% oxygen will enable patients to tolerate the procedure better with fewer complications.

INTUBATION TECHNIQUES

Oral Intubation

First, prepare all of your equipment as described previously in the section on preparation.

Position your patient in the "sniffing" position, slightly hyperextending the head. Insert an airway and manually ventilate the patient on 100% oxygen for 2 to 3 minutes. After ventilation, remove the airway.

Miller Blade (Straight Blade)

The Miller blade is inserted into the mouth at a slight angle. As you face the patient, standing at the top of the head, insert the tip of the blade in the right corner of the mouth. Advance the tip of the blade at an angle toward

the lower left of the tongue; then slide the handle and blade to the left. This will lift and displace the tongue to the left side of the mouth, allowing you to visualize the airway. Continue to advance the blade until the epiglottis is visualized. Pick up the epiglottis with the tip of the blade by lifting straight up. The vocal cords should now be visualized.

MacIntosh Blade (Curved Blade)

The MacIntosh blade is inserted into the mouth in the same way as the Miller blade. The difference lies in the advancement of the blade. The blade is advanced until the epiglottis is visualized. At this point, the tip of the blade should be in the vallecula. Lift straight up. As you lift, the epiglottis will also be lifted, allowing you to visualize the vocal cords.

Evaluation

Once the tube is in place, remove the blade and attach the resuscitator to the patient connection. Inflate the cuff and ventilate the patient with several breaths. Watch for chest expansion and auscultate the chest for bilateral breath sounds. It is important to realize that at this point the endotracheal tube is highly unstable. You should hold on to it at all times until it is permanently secured.

Once bilateral breath sounds are confirmed, tape the tube in place. The use of tincture of benzoin will help the adhesive tape adhere to the skin better. Figure 20-22 shows one technique of taping a tube. Obtain a chest x-ray to verify tube placement. Adjust the tube placement as required, and secure it more thoroughly using tape or a commercial harness as shown in Figure 20-23.

Nasal Intubation

Nasal intubation is a more difficult procedure than oral intubation. Usually it is performed by a physician, with the respiratory care practitioner assisting.

Begin by assembling and testing all of the equipment as described in the section on equipment preparation.

Position the patient in a "sniffing" position. Manually ventilate the patient for 2 or 3 minutes using 100% oxygen.

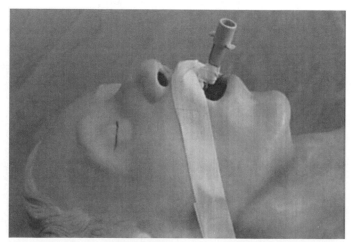

Figure 20-22 *One method of securing an oral endotracheal tube with adhesive tape*

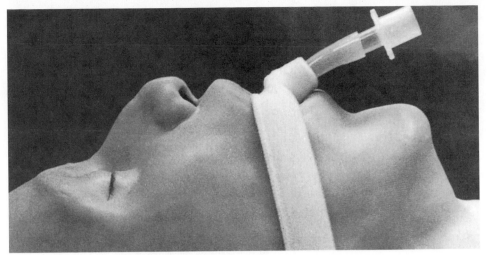

Figure 20-23   *Use of a commercially made harness to secure an oral endotracheal tube*

Anesthetize the nasal passage with lidocaine, cocaine, or both.

Lubricate the endotracheal tube well with water-soluble lubricant. Advance the tube down the nasal passage. If the patient is breathing spontaneously, wait for the inspiratory phase, and try to advance the tube past the epiglottis into the trachea. This is termed *blind intubation.*

It may be necessary to use a laryngoscope to visualize the airway. Either a Miller or a MacIntosh blade may be used. Forceps may be required to direct the tube into the trachea.

Note the position of the tube by the markings on it. Inflate the cuff and ventilate the patient with a manual resuscitator. Auscultate the chest for bilateral breath sounds. Obtain a chest x-ray to verify correct tube placement.

Secure the tube using 1-inch-wide cloth first-aid tape. Tear off two lengths approximately 9 inches long. Tear the tape in half lengthwise for about 4 inches. Secure the wide end next to the nose above the upper lip. Wrap one small tail around the tube and secure the other tail to the upper lip. Repeat the process on the other side. Figure 20-24 shows the tube secured this way.

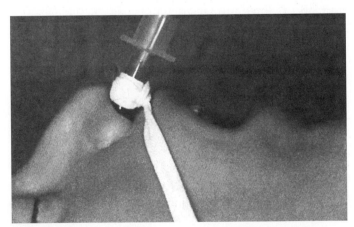

Figure 20-24   *One method of securing the tube of a nasally intubated patient*

EXTUBATION

Extubation Technique

Extubation is one of the highlights of being a respiratory care practitioner. Your patient has finally become well enough that the artificial airway is no longer needed. Removal of the endotracheal tube is easier than insertion, but care must be taken not to contaminate the lower airway. Whenever a patient is extubated, always have the supplies needed to intubate the patient again if required.

Position the patient in full Fowler's position.

Hyperinflate and oxygenate the patient with a manual resuscitator. Suction the airway prior to removing the endotracheal tube.

Attach the syringe to the pilot balloon. Wrap the catheter around the fourth and fifth fingers of your dominant hand (the one wearing the sterile glove for suctioning), allowing the distal 4 inches of the catheter to rest in the oropharnyx. Hold the syringe between the third finger and the first segment of the fourth finger. Position the endotracheal tube between the second and third fingers. Figure 20-25 shows this seemingly complex hand position.

Inflate the lungs using the manual resuscitator. Apply an end-inspiratory hold, while simultaneously withdrawing air from the endotracheal tube cuff by extending your thumb to pull out the plunger on the syringe and remove air from the cuff. This positive pressure jets out around the tube, propelling secretions into the mouth where the catheter evacuates them, preventing them from sliding back down the airway. Now extubate the patient by removing the endotracheal tube. After the tube is removed, instruct the patient to cough vigorously. Administer supplemental oxygen as ordered by the physician.

Monitoring after Extubation

Following extubation, careful monitoring is important to ensure that the patient is able to maintain adequate ventilation and to control secretions effectively. Auscultate the

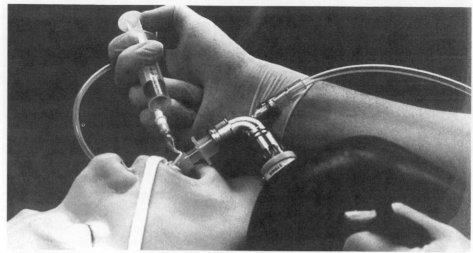

Figure 20-25 *Use of a flow-inflating manual resuscitator, suction catheter, and a syringe during extubation*

chest to ensure that the lungs are clear. Assess the patient's breathing for stridor, which may indicate laryngospasm or edema. Ensure that the patient's swallow reflex is intact. Inform the patient that although speaking is now permissible, the patient will be hoarse for a while and should minimize speech for about 8 hours. Also, do not administer liquids by mouth for 8 hours or until the swallow reflex is fully regained.

References

American Association for Respiratory Care. (1993). AARC clinical practice guideline: Resuscitation in acute care hospitals. *Respiratory Care, 38*(11), 1179–1188.

American Association for Respiratory Care. (1995). AARC clinical practice guideline: Management of airway emergencies. *Respiratory Care, 40*(7), 749–760.

Nelson, E. J., Hunter, P., & Morton, E. (1983). *Critical care respiratory therapy: A laboratory and clinical manual.* Boston: Little, Brown.

Additional Resources

Barnes, T. A., & Watson, M. E. (1982). Oxygen delivery performance of four adult resuscitation bags. *Respiratory Care, 27*(2), 139–146.

Barnes, T. A., & Watson, M. (1983). Oxygen delivery performance of old and new designs of the Laerdal, Vitalograph, and Ambu adult manual resuscitators. *Respiratory Care, 28*(9), 1121–1128.

Burton, G. G., Hodgkin, J., & Ward, J. (1991). *Respiratory care* (3rd ed.). Philadelphia: Lippincott.

Fitzmaurice, M. W., & Barnes, T. A. (1980). Oxygen delivery performance of three adult resuscitation bags. *Respiratory Care, 25*(9), 928–933.

LeBouef, L. L. (1980). 1980 assessment of eight adult manual resuscitators. *Respiratory Care, 25*(11), 1136–1142.

Shapiro, B. A., Harrison, R., Kacmarek, R., & Cane, R. (1991). *Clinical application of respiratory care* (4th ed.). Chicago: Year Book Medical.

Practice Activities: Manual Resuscitation

1. Using a laboratory partner as your patient, place the patient in a supine position and open the airway using the following positional maneuvers:
   a. Head tilt, chin lift
   b. Anterior mandibular displacement

2. Using an intubation mannequin, practice the insertion of the following airways:
   a. Nasopharyngeal
   b. Oropharyngeal

3. Practice assembling, testing for function, and troubleshooting the following self-inflating manual resuscitators:
   a. Ambu Mark III
   b. Hope or Hope II
   c. Laerdal II
   d. Hudson Life Saver II
   e. PMR 2

4. Attach a portable respirometer (Wright, Dragger, Halo-scale) to a manual resuscitator and measure the tidal volume you can deliver using one hand and then using both hands.

5. Practice ventilating a resuscitation mannequin using the following self-inflating manual resuscitators:
   a. Ambu Mark III
   b. Hope or Hope II
   c. Laerdal II
   d. Hudson Life Saver II
   e. PMR 2
   Include the following:
   (1) Ventilate the mannequin with a I:E ratio of 1:2 or greater.
   (2) Maintain a rate of 12 breaths per minute.
   (3) Observe for chest expansion, gastric distention, and skin color.

6. Using the following manual resuscitators and a respirometer, measure the tidal volume delivered using one hand and then using both hands to compress the bag:
   a. Ambu Mark III
   b. Hope or Hope II
   c. Laerdal II
   d. Hudson Life Saver II
   e. PMR 2
   Calculate the following:
   (1) Using the stroke volume measured, calculate the minute volume you would deliver if you were ventilating a patient at a rate of 12 breaths per minute.
   (2) Using the stroke volume measured, calculate the minute volume you would deliver if you were ventilating a patient at a rate of 20 breaths per minute.

7. Assemble, test for function, and troubleshoot a flow-inflating manual resuscitator.

8. Using an intubated resuscitation mannequin, practice ventilating the mannequin with a flow-inflating manual resuscitator, including the following:
   a. Maintain an I:E ratio of 1:2 or greater.
   b. Maintain a rate of 12 breaths per minute.
   c. Observe the following:
      (1) Chest expansion
      (2) Gastric distention
      (3) Skin color

9. Using a laboratory partner as a patient, practice assisting the patient's ventilation with a self-inflating manual resuscitator.

INTUBATION PRACTICE ACTIVITIES

1. Assemble all of the equipment required for intubation.

2. Assemble the laryngoscope and test it for proper operation.

3. Check the self-inflating manual resuscitator for proper operation.

4. Place an intubation mannequin or a laboratory partner in proper position for intubation.
   a. Supine
   b. "Sniffing" position

5. Using an intubation mannequin, practice using both the Miller (straight) blade and the MacIntosh (curved) blade.
   a. Miller blade:
      (1) Hold the laryngoscope in your left hand.
      (2) Insert it at an angle and slide it left into position.
      (3) Slowly advance the blade.
      (4) Pick up the epiglottis with the tip of the blade.
   b. MacIntosh blade:
      (1) Hold the laryngoscope in your left hand.
      (2) Insert the blade at an angle and slide it left into position.
      (3) Slowly advance the blade.
      (4) When the epiglottis is visualized, lift straight up, exposing the vocal cords.

6. Using an intubation mannequin, practice oral intubation, including the following steps:
   a. Equipment assembly and testing
   b. Patient positioning
   c. Hyperinflation and oxygenation with 100% oxygen
   d. Correct laryngoscope use
   e. Insertion of the endotracheal tube within 15 seconds
   f. Stabilization of the endotracheal tube until secured with tape
   g. Ventilation of the patient with adequate volumes and I:E ratio
   h. Auscultation of the chest for tube placement
   i. Securing the endotracheal tube with first-aid tape

7. Using an intubation mannequin, insert an endotracheal tube nasally and secure it properly with first-aid tape.

8. Orally intubate an intubation mannequin and practice the extubation procedure, including the following:
   a. Positioning the patient
   b. Hyperinflation and oxygenation
   c. Aspirating the airway prior to removal
   d. Deflation of the cuff under positive pressure
   e. Aspirating expelled secretions
   f. Removal of the endotracheal tube
   g. Monitoring the patient

Check List: Manual Resuscitation

_____ 1. Wash your hands.

2. Gather the appropriate equipment:
_____ a. Manual resuscitator
_____ b. Oxygen flowmeter
_____ c. Resuscitation mask
_____ d. Oxygen connecting tubing
_____ e. Artificial airway
_____ f. Personal protective equipment (gloves, goggles, or face shield)

3. Assemble and check equipment function.
_____ a. Check valve assembly.
_____ b. Assemble the resuscitator.
_____ c. Attach:
_____ (1) Mask
_____ (2) Connecting tubing
_____ (3) Flowmeter set at 10 to 15 L/min
4. Apply the mask to the patient:
_____ a. Apply to bridge of nose first.
_____ b. Obtain a good seal.

_____ c. Anteriorly displace mandible with free fingers.
5. Ventilate the patient.
_____ a. Deliver adequate volume.
_____ b. Ventilate with an I:E ratio of 1:2 or greater.
6. Assess the patient during the procedure for:
_____ a. Cyanosis
_____ b. Vomiting/gagging
_____ c. Gastric distention
_____ d. Airway placement
_____ 7. Following procedure, clean up the area.

Check List: Intubation

1. Assemble all needed equipment:
_____ a. Laryngoscope
_____ b. Laryngoscope blades
_____ c. Spare batteries
_____ d. Oropharyngeal airways
_____ e. Yankauer suction and supplies
_____ f. 10-ml (or larger) syringe
_____ g. Stylet
_____ h. Cloth first-aid tape
_____ i. Water soluble lubricant
_____ j. Magill forceps
_____ k. Self-inflating manual resuscitator
_____ l. Oxygen flowmeter
_____ m. Endotracheal tubes sized 6.5 mm to 10 mm
_____ n. Personal protective equipment (gloves, goggles, or face shield)
_____ 2. Test all equipment to ensure proper function.

_____ 3. Hyperinflate and oxygenate the patient using a manual resuscitator prior to attempting intubation.
4. Position the patient properly.
_____ a. Supine
_____ b. "Sniffing" position
_____ 5. Use the laryngoscope properly.
_____ 6. Insert the endotracheal tube within 30 seconds.
7. Ventilate the patient with a manual resuscitator, using:
_____ a. Adequate volume delivery
_____ b. I:E ratio of at least 1:2
_____ 8. Stabilize the tube at all times until it is taped securely.
_____ 9. Auscultate the chest for tube placement.
_____ 10. Obtain a chest x-ray film.
_____ 11. Tape the tube securely.

Check List: Extubation

_____ 1. Verify the physician's order.
_____ 2. Scan the chart to ensure the patient is ready for extubation.
_____ 3. Measure spontaneous parameters and blood gases.
4. Gather the required equipment:
_____ a. Intubation tray
_____ b. 20-ml syringe
_____ c. Suction supplies
_____ d. Oxygen/aerosol equipment
_____ e. Personal protective equipment (gloves, goggles, or face shield)
_____ 5. Wash your hands.
_____ 6. Introduce yourself and explain the procedure.

_____ 7. Position the patient in full Fowler's position.
_____ 8. Suction the patient thoroughly.
_____ 9. Oxygenate the patient with 100% oxygen using a flow-inflating manual resuscitator.
_____ 10. Deflate the cuff while the patient is exhaling forcefully and withdraw the tube.
_____ 11. Have the patient cough several times and speak to allow you to assess for hoarseness and to clear the airway.
_____ 12. Administer cool aerosol as ordered.
_____ 13. Evaluate the patient following extubation.
_____ 14. Clean up the area.
_____ 15. Chart the procedure.

Self-Evaluation Post Test: Emergency Airway Management

1. When using a flow-inflating bag, you should:
   a. connect it to a 50 psi oxygen source.
   b. pinch the tail of the bag when delivering a breath.
   c. release the tail during the expiratory phase.
   d. Both b and c

2. The most commonly used airway for ventilating a patient with a manual resuscitator is the:
   a. nasopharyngeal airway.
   b. oropharyngeal airway.
   c. nasal trumpet.
   d. tracheostomy tube.

3. Patient observation during manual resuscitation should include:
   I. skin color.
   II. chest expansion.
   III. gastric distention.
   IV. the presence of vomiting.
   a. I, II
   b. I, II, III
   c. II, III, IV
   d. I, II, III, IV

4. Two advantages of a flow-inflating manual resuscitator are:
   I. size.
   II. its self-inflation characteristics.
   III. oxygen delivery.
   IV. ease of assessing patient compliance.
   V. ease of using it with a resuscitation mask.
   a. I, II
   b. II, IV
   c. III, IV
   d. IV, V

5. A common complication of manual resuscitation is:
   a. vagal stimulation.
   b. bradycardia.
   c. gastric distention.
   d. pneumothorax.

6. When using a Miller (straight) laryngoscope blade, you should:
   a. insert the tip of the blade into the vallecula.
   b. insert the tip of the blade through the vocal cords.
   c. lift the epiglottis with the tip of the blade.
   d. insert the tip of the blade into the larynx.

7. Attempts to insert the endotracheal tube should be limited to:
   a. 10 seconds.
   b. 15 seconds.
   c. 20 seconds.
   d. 30 seconds.

8. The first thing you should do to assess the placement of an endotracheal tube is to:
   a. auscultate the chest.
   b. order a chest x-ray film.
   c. check for cyanosis.
   d. observe the stomach expanding on inspiration.

9. The best way to prevent equipment malfunction is to:
   a. use new equipment.
   b. carefully check equipment before use.
   c. have all supplies ready.
   d. Both b and c

10. The last reflex a patient loses when progressing into unconsciousness is the:
    a. gag reflex.
    b. laryngeal reflex.
    c. tracheal reflex.
    d. carinal reflex.

PERFORMANCE EVALUATION:
MANUAL RESUSCITATION

Date: Lab _____ Clinical _____ Agency _____

Lab: Pass _____ Fail _____   Clinical: Pass _____ Fail _____

Student name _____ Instructor name _____

No. of times observed in clinical _____

No. of times practiced in clinical _____

PASSING CRITERIA: Obtain 90% or better on the procedure. Tasks indicated by * must receive at least 1 point, or the evaluation is terminated. Procedure must be performed within designated time, or the performance receives a failing grade.

SCORING: 2 points — Task performed satisfactorily without prompting.
                1 point — Task performed satisfactorily with self-initiated correction.
                0 points — Task performed incorrectly or with prompting required.
                NA — Task not applicable to the patient care situation.

TASKS:		PEER	LAB	CLINICAL
*	1. Observes standard precautions, including handwashing	☐	☐	☐
	2. Obtains the required equipment			
*	a. Oxygen flowmeter	☐	☐	☐
*	b. Manual resuscitator	☐	☐	☐
*	c. Resuscitation mask	☐	☐	☐
*	d. Oxygen connecting tubing	☐	☐	☐
*	e. Artificial airway	☐	☐	☐
*	f. Gloves, goggles, or face shield	☐	☐	☐
*	3. Assembles and checks the equipment	☐	☐	☐
	4. Applies the mask			
*	a. Seats mask on bridge of nose first	☐	☐	☐
*	b. Obtains a good seal	☐	☐	☐
*	c. Lifts the mandible with fingers	☐	☐	☐
	5. Ventilates the patient appropriately			
*	a. Maintains I:E ratio of 1:2 or greater	☐	☐	☐
*	b. Delivers adequate volumes	☐	☐	☐
	6. Reassesses the patient for			
*	a. Cyanosis	☐	☐	☐
*	b. Vomiting	☐	☐	☐
*	c. Gastric distention	☐	☐	☐
*	7. Ventilates for an appropriate time period	☐	☐	☐
*	8. Removes the equipment after the procedure	☐	☐	☐

SCORE: Peer   _____ points of possible 36; _____%

           Lab   _____ points of possible 36; _____%

           Clinical   _____ points of possible 36; _____%

TIME: _____ out of possible 5 minutes

STUDENT SIGNATURES   INSTRUCTOR SIGNATURES

PEER: _____   LAB: _____

STUDENT: _____   CLINICAL: _____

PERFORMANCE EVALUATION: INTUBATION

Date: Lab _____ Clinical _____ Agency _____

Lab: Pass _____ Fail _____   Clinical: Pass _____ Fail _____

Student name _____   Instructor name _____

No. of times observed in clinical _____

No. of times practiced in clinical _____

PASSING CRITERIA: Obtain 90% or better on the procedure. Tasks indicated by * must receive at least 1 point, or the evaluation is terminated. Procedure must be performed within designated time, or the performance receives a failing grade.

SCORING:
2 points — Task performed satisfactorily without prompting.
1 point — Task performed satisfactorily with self-initiated correction.
0 points — Task performed incorrectly or with prompting required.
NA — Task not applicable to the patient care situation.

TASKS:

			PEER	LAB	CLINICAL
*	1.	Observes standard precautions, including handwashing	☐	☐	☐
	2.	Obtains the required equipment			
*		a. Oxygen flowmeter	☐	☐	☐
*		b. Manual resuscitator	☐	☐	☐
*		c. Resuscitation mask	☐	☐	☐
*		d. Laryngoscope and blades	☐	☐	☐
*		e. Artificial airways	☐	☐	☐
*		f. 10-ml (or larger) syringe	☐	☐	☐
*		g. Endotracheal tubes	☐	☐	☐
*		h. Stylet	☐	☐	☐
*		i. Lubricant	☐	☐	☐
*		j. Tape	☐	☐	☐
*		k. Suctioning supplies	☐	☐	☐
*		l. Gloves, goggles, or face shield	☐	☐	☐
*	3.	Assembles and checks the equipment	☐	☐	☐
*	4.	Positions the patient	☐	☐	☐
*	5.	Hyperinflates and oxygenates the patient	☐	☐	☐
*	6.	Correctly uses the laryngoscope	☐	☐	☐
*	7.	Inserts the tube within 15 seconds	☐	☐	☐
*	8.	Ventilates following intubation			
*		a. Gives adequate volumes	☐	☐	☐
*		b. Maintains I:E ratio greater than 1:2	☐	☐	☐
*	9.	Stabilizes tube until taped	☐	☐	☐
*	10.	Auscultates for tube position	☐	☐	☐

*   11. Tapes tube ☐ ☐ ☐
*   12. Orders chest x-ray film ☐ ☐ ☐
*   13. Cleans up patient area afterward ☐ ☐ ☐
*   14. Uses aseptic technique ☐ ☐ ☐

SCORE: Peer   _____ points of possible 52; _____%

            Lab   _____ points of possible 52; _____%

            Clinical   _____ points of possible 52; _____%

TIME: _____ out of possible 10 minutes

STUDENT SIGNATURES   INSTRUCTOR SIGNATURES

PEER: _____   LAB: _____

STUDENT: _____   CLINICAL: _____

PERFORMANCE EVALUATION: EXTUBATION

Date: Lab _____ Clinical _____ Agency _____

Lab: Pass _____ Fail _____   Clinical: Pass _____ Fail _____

Student name _____   Instructor name _____

No. of times observed in clinical _____

No. of times practiced in clinical _____

PASSING CRITERIA: Obtain 90% or better on the procedure. Tasks indicated by * must receive at least 1 point, or the evaluation is terminated. Procedure must be performed within designated time, or the performance receives a failing grade.

SCORING:
2 points — Task performed satisfactorily without prompting.
1 point — Task performed satisfactorily with self-initiated correction.
0 points — Task performed incorrectly or with prompting required.
NA — Task not applicable to the patient care situation.

TASKS:

			PEER	LAB	CLINICAL
*	1.	Verifies the physician's order	☐	☐	☐
*	2.	Scans the chart to ensure the patient is ready for extubation	☐	☐	☐
*	3.	Measures spontaneous parameters and blood gases	☐	☐	☐
*	4.	Gathers the required equipment			
		a. Intubation tray	☐	☐	☐
		b. 20-ml syringe	☐	☐	☐
		c. Suction supplies	☐	☐	☐
		d. Oxygen/aerosol equipment	☐	☐	☐
		e. Gloves, goggles, or face shield	☐	☐	☐
*	5.	Observes standard precautions, including handwashing	☐	☐	☐
	6.	Introduces self and explains the procedure	☐	☐	☐
*	7.	Positions the patient in full Fowler's position	☐	☐	☐
*	8.	Suctions the patient thoroughly	☐	☐	☐
*	9.	Oxygenates the patient with 100% oxygen using a flow-inflating manual resuscitator	☐	☐	☐
*	10.	Deflates the cuff under positive pressure and withdraws the tube	☐	☐	☐
*	11.	Has the patient cough several times and speak to assess hoarseness and clear the airway	☐	☐	☐
*	12.	Administers cool aerosol	☐	☐	☐
*	13.	Evaluates the patient	☐	☐	☐
*	14.	Cleans up the area	☐	☐	☐
*	15.	Charts the procedure	☐	☐	☐

SCORE: Peer   _____ points of possible 38; _____%

           Lab   _____ points of possible 38; _____%

           Clinical   _____ points of possible 38; _____%

TIME: _____ out of possible 20 minutes

STUDENT SIGNATURES   INSTRUCTOR SIGNATURES

PEER: _____   LAB: _____

STUDENT: _____   CLINICAL: _____

CHAPTER 21

ARTIFICIAL AIRWAY CARE

INTRODUCTION

As a respiratory care practitioner, you will be responsible for the routine care of the artificial airway. Artificial airway care includes humidification (Chapter 15), suctioning, cuff care, and for tracheostomy tubes, stoma care. This routine care is necessary to ensure a patent airway and protection of the lower airway from aspirated secretions and infection. Stoma care is needed to prevent the accumulation of secretions or exudate at the stoma site. You will be expected to perform these procedures correctly and safely.

KEY TERMS

- Closed suction system
- Decannulation
- Fenestrated tracheostomy tube
- Minimal leak technique
- Minimal occlusion volume (MOV) technique
- Passy-Muir valve
- Suction catheters
- Suctioning
- Tracheostomy
- Tracheostomy button
- Wash-out volume

OBJECTIVES

At the end of this chapter, you should be able to:

- State the rationale for nasotracheal and artificial airway aspiration (suctioning).
- Compare and contrast the functional characteristics of the following suction catheters and the advantages of each:
  — Whistle tip
  — Coudé tip
  — Argyle Aeroflow
  — Closed suction systems
- State the rationale for application of intermittent versus continuous suction.
- State the complications of airway aspiration and describe how to minimize them.
- State the rationale for the use of hyperinflation and oxygenation before and after suctioning.
- Describe the use of a mechanical ventilator (volume ventilator) to oxygenate and hyperinflate the patient for suctioning.
- Explain the importance of maintaining cuff pressures below 25 cm H_2O.

- List the indications for a tracheostomy.
- Explain the purpose of tracheostomy and stoma care, and state the associated hazards and complications.
- Identify the following types of tracheostomy cannulas, and describe their clinical application:
  — Single cuff tracheostomy tube
  — Single cuff tracheostomy tube with a disposable inner cannula
  — Single cuff fenestrated tracheostomy tube
  — Silver Hollinger or Jackson tracheostomy tube
  — Bivona foam cuff
- Identify the following specialized tracheostomy tubes and tracheostomy appliances, and describe their clinical application:
  — Pitt Speaking Tube/Communi-Trach
  — Trach button
  — Kistner button
  — Passy-Muir valve
  — Olympic Trach-Talk

CLINICAL PRACTICE GUIDELINES

**AARC Clinical Practice Guideline:
Nasotracheal Suctioning**

NTS 4.0 INDICATIONS:
The need to maintain a patent airway and remove secretions or foreign material from the trachea in the presence of:

4.1 Inability to clear secretions (6)

4.2 Audible evidence of secretions in the large/central airways that persist in spite of patient's best cough effort (4,7,8–10)

NTS 5.0 CONTRAINDICATIONS:
Listed contraindications are relative unless marked as absolute.

5.1 Occluded nasal passages

5.2 Nasal bleeding

5.3 Epiglottitis or croup (absolute)

5.4 Acute head, facial, or neck injury

5.5 Coagulopathy or bleeding disorder (2)

5.6 Laryngospasm (2)

(Continued)

(CPG Continued)

    5.7 Irritable airway
    5.8 Upper respiratory tract infection

NTS 6.0 HAZARDS/COMPLICATIONS:
    6.1 Mechanical trauma (10–15)
        6.1.1 Laceration of nasal turbinates (5,7,16)
        6.1.2 Perforation of the pharynx (17)
        6.1.3 Nasal irritation/bleeding (16,18)
        6.1.4 Tracheitis
        6.1.5 Mucosal hemorrhage (13)
    6.2 Hypoxia/hypoxemia (1,14,19–21)
    6.3 Cardiac dysrhythmias/arrest (3,7,14,15)
    6.4 Bradycardia (1,19,22–24)
    6.5 Increase in blood pressure (1,19,21)
    6.6 Hypotension (1,19)
    6.7 Respiratory arrest (7)
    6.8 Uncontrolled coughing (1,15,18)
    6.9 Gagging/vomiting (18,25)
    6.10 Laryngospasm (1,2,7)
    6.11 Bronchoconstriction/bronchospasm (1,14,15)
    6.12 Pain (18)
    6.13 Nosocomial infection (15,16,23)
    6.14 Atelectasis (5,14)
    6.15 Misdirection of catheter (15,18)
    6.16 Increased intracranial pressure (ICP) (21, 26,27)
        6.16.1 Intraventricular hemorrhage (21)
        6.16.2 Exacerbation of cerebral edema

NTS 8.0 ASSESSMENT OF NEED:
    8.1 Personnel should auscultate chest for indications for NT suctioning. (1,29)
    8.2 Personnel should assess effectiveness of cough.

NTS 9.0 ASSESSMENT OF OUTCOME:
    9.1 Effectiveness of NTS should be reflected by improved breath sounds.
    9.2 Effectiveness of NTS should be reflected by removal of secretions.

NTS 11.0 MONITORING:
The following should be monitored during and following the procedure:
    11.1 Breath sounds
    11.2 Skin color (36)
    11.3 Breathing pattern and rate
    11.4 Pulse rate, dysrhythmia, ECG if available
    11.5 Color, consistency, and volume of secretions
    11.6 Presence of bleeding or evidence of physical trauma
    11.7 Subjective response including pain (25)
    11.8 Cough
    11.9 Oxygenation (pulse oximeter if available)
    11.10 Intracranial pressure (ICP), if equipment is available

Reprinted with permission from *Respiratory Care* 1992; 37: 898–901. The complete AARC Clinical Practice Guidelines are available from the AARC Web site (http://www.aarc.org), from the AARC Executive Office, or from *Respiratory Care* journal.

AARC Clinical Practice Guideline Endotracheal Suctioning of Mechanically Ventilated Adults and Children with Artificial Airways

ETS 4.0 INDICATIONS:
    4.1 The need to remove accumulated pulmonary secretions as evidenced by one of the following:
        4.1.1 Coarse breath sounds by auscultation or "noisy" breathing
        4.1.2 Increased peak inspiratory pressures during volume-controlled mechanical ventilation or decreased tidal volume during pressure-controlled ventilation
        4.1.3 Patient's inability to generate an effective spontaneous cough
        4.1.4 Visible secretions in the airway
        4.1.5 Changes in monitored flow and pressure graphics
        4.1.6 Suspected aspiration of gastric or upper airway secretions
        4.1.7 Clinically apparent increased work of breathing
        4.1.8 Deterioration of arterial blood gas values
        4.1.9 Radiologic changes consistent with retention of pulmonary secretions
    4.2 The need to obtain a sputum specimen to rule out or identify pneumonia or other pulmonary infection or for sputum cytology
    4.3 The need to maintain the patency and integrity of the artificial airway
    4.4 The need to stimulate a patient cough in patients unable to cough effectively secondary to changes in mental status or the influence of medication
    4.5 Presence of pulmonary atelectasis or consolidation, presumed to be associated with secretion retention

ETS 5.0 CONTRAINDICATIONS:
Endotracheal suctioning is a necessary procedure for patients with artificial airways. Most contraindications are relative to the patient's risk of developing adverse reactions or worsening clinical condition as a result of the procedure. When indicated, there is no absolute contraindication to endotracheal suctioning because the decision to abstain from suctioning in order to avoid a possible adverse reaction may, in fact, be lethal.

ETS 6.0 HAZARDS/COMPLICATIONS: (1,2)
    6.1 Hypoxia/hypoxemia (16–23)
    6.2 Tissue trauma to the tracheal and/or bronchial mucosa (19,24)
    6.3 Cardiac arrest (22,25)
    6.4 Respiratory arrest (21)
    6.5 Cardiac dysrhythmias (2,19,24)
    6.6 Pulmonary atelectasis (17,19,21)
    6.7 Bronchoconstriction/bronchospasm (19)

6.8 Infection (patient and/or caregiver) (19,26,27)
6.9 Pulmonary hemorrhage/bleeding (19,24)
6.10 Elevated intracranial pressure (28–30)
6.11 Interruption of mechanical ventilation (18)
6.12 Hypertension (31)
6.13 Hypotension (31)

ETS 8.0 ASSESSMENT OF NEED:

Qualified personnel should assess the need for endotracheal suctioning as a routine part of a patient/ventilator system check.

ETS 9.0 ASSESSMENT OF OUTCOME:

9.1 Improvement in breath sounds
9.2 Decreased peak inspiratory pressure (PIP) with narrowing of PIP — Plateau; decreased airway resistance or increased dynamic compliance; increased tidal volume delivery during pressure-limited ventilation
9.3 Improvement in arterial blood gas values (ABGs) or saturation as reflected by pulse oximetry (SpO$_2$)
9.4 Removal of pulmonary secretions

ETS 11.0 MONITORING:

The following should be monitored prior to, during, and after the procedure:
11.1 Breath sounds
11.2 Oxygen saturation
    11.2.1 Skin color
    11.2.2 Pulse oximeter, if available
11.3 Respiratory rate and pattern
11.4 Hemodynamic parameters
    11.4.1 Pulse rate
    11.4.2 Blood pressure, if indicated and available
    11.4.3 ECG, if indicated and available
11.5 Sputum characteristics
    11.5.1 Color
    11.5.2 Volume
    11.5.3 Consistency
    11.5.4 Odor
11.6 Cough effort
11.7 Intracranial pressure, if indicated and available
11.8 Ventilator parameters
    11.8.1 Peak inspiratory pressure and plateau pressure
    11.8.2 Tidal volume
    11.8.3 Pressure, flow, and volume graphics, if available
    11.8.4 FiO$_2$
11.9 Arterial blood gases, if indicated and available

Reprinted with permission from *Respiratory Care* 1993; 38: 500–504. The complete AARC Clinical Practice Guidelines are available from the AARC Web site (http://www.aarc.org), from the AARC Executive Office, or from *Respiratory Care* journal.

SUCTIONING

Rationale for Suctioning

The cough is one of the normal defense mechanisms that protects the airway. It rids the airway of foreign matter and expels excess secretions. This reflex is essential in the maintenance of life (Guyton, 1984). An effective cough is dependent on the ability to close the glottis, to generate high intrathoracic pressure. The sudden opening of the glottis results in forceful expulsion of gas, which is the cough. Patients with respiratory disabilities or disease may have excessive secretions that they are unable to manage. Because excessive secretions provide an excellent medium for bacterial growth, pneumonia may result, with subsequent atelectasis, hypoxemia, and increased work of breathing.

The cough reflex may be depressed, bypassed, or even absent for a variety of reasons. These may include central nervous system (CNS) depression (such as with drug overdose), brainstem injury, cerebrovascular accident (CVA), pain, and muscle weakness. The presence of an artificial airway precludes effective utilization of the cough mechanism. In these instances and others, it may be necessary to intervene by suctioning the secretions from the airway. This intervention is known as airway aspiration or suctioning.

What Is Suctioning?

Suctioning is an invasive procedure that involves the insertion of a small catheter into the airway and the application of a vacuum (subambient pressure) to aspirate secretions or foreign material. Once in place, a vacuum is applied, and the catheter is withdrawn, evacuating secretions.

Because this is an invasive procedure, scrupulous aseptic technique should be observed at all times to prevent the inadvertent introduction of bacteria into the tracheobronchial tree.

Suction Catheter Designs

With advances in pulmonary medicine and in the practice of respiratory care, an evolution has occurred in the design of *suction catheters*. Generally, advancements have improved efficiency, reduced mucosal trauma, and improved cost containment.

Whistle Tip

The whistle tip catheter design incorporates an eye on the side of the catheter proximal to the distal opening. Figure 21-1 shows a whistle tip design. The advantage of this design is that if the tip comes in contact with the mucosa, the eye provides a relief for the applied vacuum. In this manner, inadvertent "biopsy" of mucosal tissue is prevented.

Coudé Tip

The Coudé tip is an angled tip design. This design permits the selective entry into the right or left mainstem bronchus. Figure 21-2 shows an example of the Coudé tip design. To maximize the usefulness of this catheter design, you must pay close attention to the tip position on entering the patient's airway or an artificial airway. By advancing the catheter and selectively rotating the tip right or left, the chance of entering the desired bronchus is increased. Guaranteed 100% entry is not possible; however, the likelihood of accurate entry is greater with this design than with a straight-tipped catheter.

Argyle Aeroflow

The Argyle Aeroflow device constitutes a fairly recent evolution in catheter design. The tip of the catheter is designed with an open end and a raised ring or bead surrounding the opening. Additionally, several small holes are drilled proximal to the ring. Figure 21-3 shows the Argyle Aeroflow catheter.

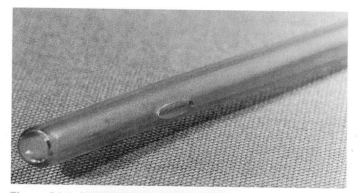

Figure 21-1   The whistle tip suction catheter

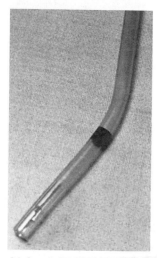

Figure 21-2   A Coudé tip suction catheter

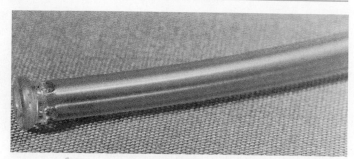

Figure 21-3   The Argyle Aeroflow suction catheter

The special tip design keeps the proximal holes away from the mucosa. Should the distal opening become occluded, the proximal openings will allow the applied vacuum pressure to be vented, preventing mucosal damage at the tip. When it was introduced, this design resulted in less mucosal trauma than that noted for other conventional designs available at that time (Sackner, Landa, Greeneltch, & Robinson, 1973).

Closed Suction Systems

The Trach Care Suction System is an example of a multiple-use *closed suction system* catheter design, manufactured by Ballard Medical, Inc., Salt Lake City, UT. Figure 21-4 shows the Trach Care catheter. The catheter is encased in a sealed plastic protective sheath. The distal end is attached to a modified aerosol T and the proximal end is attached to a control valve. The suction system is a replaceable item, and the manufacturer recommends changing it with the ventilator circuit.

The system is unique in that disconnection from mechanical ventilation or the patient's oxygen source is not required for suctioning (owing to the design of the modified aerosol T).

Most facilities incorporate this system into the ventilator circuit and change the Trach Care system with the ventilator circuit. Whenever the patient requires suctioning, the same catheter is used. A question was raised regarding infection control and the possible introduction of bacteria resulting from the use of this system. Investigators found no significant difference in colony counts between the multiple-use catheter system and a conventional design (Ritz, Coyle, & Scott, 1984). This design improves convenience, prevents physiological problems associated with ventilator disconnection, and reduces costs to the patient.

Continuous versus Intermittent Suction

The application of continuous versus intermittent suction on withdrawal of the suction catheter is a debate that continues today in respiratory care. There has not been any recent research to support either method decisively (Fluck, 1985). The application of continuous suction is thought to provide more efficient removal of secretions, to prevent the retention of mucous plugs, and to allow less vacuum application due to mucus in the catheter. Advocates of intermittent suction during catheter withdrawal claim less mucosal trauma and lessening of hypoxia from the evacuation of oxygen from the lung as advantages of this method.

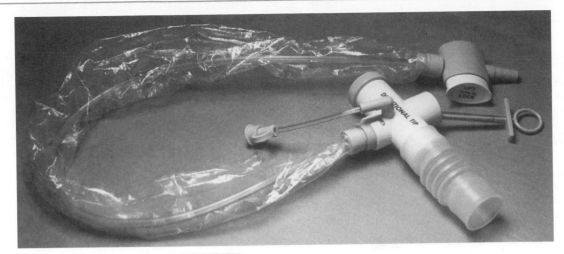

Figure 21-4 ❧ *The Trach Care Suction System*

Complications and Hazards of Suctioning

Various investigators have studied the complications of suctioning. The complications identified include tissue trauma, hypoxemia, microatelectasis, cardiac arrhythmias, and nosocomial infection (mainly associated with nasotracheal aspiration) (Demers, 1982).

Tissue Trauma

Tissue trauma caused by suctioning usually involves the invagination (infolding) of airway mucosal tissue into the catheter tip or Murphy eye (Jung & Gottlieb, 1976; Sackner et al., 1973). The applied vacuum may be strong enough to draw the mucosal tissue into the openings. Minimal trauma may result in a slight reddening of the tissue, representing an area of irritation. More severe trauma results in petechiae, or in actual inadvertent "biopsy" of tissue.

Trauma may be minimized in three ways. First, set the vacuum level between –80 and –120 mm Hg maximum pressure (Nelson, Hunter, & Morton, 1983); second, apply vacuum only intermittently (Jung & Gottlieb, 1976). Last, limit the suction attempt to no more than 15 seconds (Jung & Gottlieb, 1976; Nelson et al., 1983).

Hypoxemia

It has been shown that tracheobronchial suction will induce hypoxemia (Fell & Cheney, 1971; Naigow & Powaser, 1977; Skelley, Deeren, & Powaser, 1980). Hypoxemia is the result of the evacuation of oxygen from the tracheobronchial tree. A controlled clinical study demonstrated an average reduction in arterial oxygen tension (PaO_2) of 33 mm Hg following 15 seconds of endotracheal suction (Skelley et al., 1980). In current clinical practice, similar effects may be easily observed with oximetry.

Hypoxemia may be prevented by preoxygenation and postoxygenation and hyperinflation of the lungs with 100% oxygen (Fell & Cheney, 1971; Naigow & Powaser, 1977; Skelley et al., 1980). It is very important to perform these procedures before and after suctioning to prevent hypoxemia and to reverse atelectasis.

The selection of the proper catheter size is important in suctioning the artificial airway so that the inadvertent application of excessive vacuum is prevented. A good general rule to follow is that the outside diameter of the catheter should not exceed one-half of the inside diameter of the artificial airway. Using a catheter that is too large could cause the application of excessive vacuum, resulting in atelectasis or, worse, the collapse of a total segment of the lung.

Cardiac Arrhythmias

Cardiac arrhythmias are common during suctioning of the unstable patient in the intensive care unit (ICU). They may be induced by vagal stimulation or hypoxemia. The vagus nerve innervates the trachea and the carinal areas. Stimulation may result in bradycardia and premature ventricular contractions (PVCs). These and other arrhythmias are also associated with hypoxemia. Those patients who have a predisposing condition of hypoxemia or cardiac irritability should be carefully monitored while being suctioned. Careful attention should be paid to preoxygenation and postoxygenation. If nasotracheal suction is performed, excessive manipulation of the catheter should be avoided.

Pneumonia

Pneumonia as a complication of bronchoscopy has been documented (Pereia et al., 1975). The introduction of bacteria into the lower airway is a hazard of suctioning. The catheter passing through the nasal or oral pharynx will transport bacteria to the lower airway. This hazard may be minimized by applying aseptic technique during the procedure. It is also important to prevent cross-contamination in patients at risk for pulmonary infections.

Oxygenation and Hyperinflation Using Mechanical Ventilation

It is a common practice in the critical care setting to use the ventilator for hyperinflation and oxygenation in patients who are receiving ventilatory support. This involves increasing the ventilation oxygen level to 100% and administering either sigh (refer to Chapter 26) or normal tidal volume breaths in succession. This regimen is then followed by suctioning the patient. It is easy to overlook the effects of *wash-out volume* of the ventilator circuit prior to suctioning. Failure to keep this concept in mind may result in inadequate preoxygenation.

Wash-Out Volume

If the volume ventilator is used for preoxygenation and hyperinflation prior to suctioning the patient, you must wait up to 2 minutes, depending on the ventilator and the patient's tidal volume and respiratory rate after the FiO_2 is set to 1.00, before the patient actually receives 100% oxygen (Benson & Pierson, 1979). Furthermore, following the guidelines of oxygenation for 1 minute prior to suctioning (Fell & Cheney, 1971), you should wait at least 3 minutes before beginning the procedure when using a volume ventilator for oxygenation.

Positive End-Expiratory Pressure

Patients receiving positive end-expiratory pressure (PEEP) are more susceptible to hypoxemia when they are disconnected from mechanical ventilation for suctioning. The sudden removal of PEEP will often result in a dramatic fall in PaO_2. Also, once PEEP is removed and then resumed again, it may take some time to regain the level of oxygen saturation the patient had before disconnection of PEEP (Demajo, 1985). One group of investigators found that oxygenation using the mechanical ventilator and suctioning through an open swivel adapter produced a smaller decrease in PaO_2 (Baker, Baker, & Koen, 1983). Other investigators studied the Trach Care system, suctioning without oxygenation or disconnection from PEEP or mechanical ventilation, and found that there was no significant drop in oxygen saturation (Demajo, 1985).

These studies indicate that the best way to suction patients on PEEP is not to disconnect them from mechanical ventilation, if at all possible. The Trach Care system is a convenient and cost-effective means to provide artificial airway care for these patients without disconnecting them from PEEP.

Indications for a Tracheostomy

There are several indications for a tracheostomy. These indications are summarized in Figure 21-5.

CUFF PRESSURE MONITORING

Cuff pressures in excess of 25 cm H_2O have been shown to cause mucosal damage to the tracheal tissues (Scanlan, Spearman, & Sheldon, 1995; Stauffer & Silvestri, 1982). Higher pressures exerted against the tracheal wall result in decreased circulation, edema, and if prolonged, tracheal necrosis. Therefore, it is important to monitor cuff pressures, maintaining them below 25 cm H_2O.

- To provide a patent airway following intubation or when intubation is contraindicated
- To protect the lower airway from aspiration
- To permit frequent aspiration of secretions
- To allow long-term mechanical ventilation
- To reduce anatomical dead space

Figure 21-5 *Indications for a tracheostomy*

In some patients this may not be possible if cuff pressures below 25 cm H_2O cannot effectively seal the trachea during positive-pressure ventilation. For these patients, keep the cuff inflated enough that a slight leak is heard during inspiration. This is termed the *minimal leak technique*.

TRACHEOSTOMY AND STOMA CARE

Purpose of Tracheostomy and Stoma Care

Tracheostomy and stoma care is essential to prevent infection and to preserve the patency of the airway. A *tracheostomy* is created by a surgical procedure requiring, like other surgical procedures, that the incision be kept clean and dry to promote healing and to reduce the likelihood of infection. A tracheostomy is a particularly dirty area owing to the expectoration of secretions through the tracheostomy tube and seepage around it. Secretions, if not removed from the tube and airway by suctioning and periodic cleaning, may become encrusted, reducing or compromising the lumen of the airway. Administration of adequate humidification aids liquefaction of secretions. Accumulated secretions may also become colonized by bacteria, infecting the lower airway.

Hazards and Complications of Tracheostomy Care

Displacement and Decannulation of the Tracheostomy Tube

In performing tracheostomy care, it is essential that the tracheostomy tube be stabilized at all times. This is especially true if the surgical procedure to create the tracheostomy was performed in the previous 24 hours (a "fresh trach"). Displacement of the tracheostomy tube from the trachea may result in its lodging in the subcutaneous tissue, thus compromising the airway. Loss of ventilation and subcutaneous emphysema may result from this complication.

If the tracheostomy is fresh, a surgeon should be immediately consulted to replace the tracheostomy tube. It is very difficult to locate the incision in the trachea early after a tracheostomy is performed. Later on, the stoma becomes more established and it is easier to reinsert the tracheostomy tube.

Decannulation is the removal of the tracheostomy tube. This may occur accidentally during tracheostomy care or as a result of a strong cough or other movements by the patient if the tube is not well secured.

Like tracheostomy tube displacement, decannulation of a fresh trach requires the immediate services of a surgeon. If the stoma is well established, a practitioner may easily reinsert the tracheostomy tube.

Infection

A tracheostomy is created by a surgical procedure. Because of the nature of the surgical site, infection is a potential complication. Infection may be minimized by adequate maintenance of the airway (suctioning) and proper tracheostomy care. Initially, tracheostomy care may be required every 4 hours. As the tracheostomy begins to heal, tracheostomy care may be reduced to once every shift and may eventually be performed on a daily basis, depending on the patient's condition.

Types of Tubes
Single Cuff Tracheostomy Tube

The single cuff disposable single patient use tracheostomy tube is the most common type of tube used. Figure 21-6 shows this type of tube. It is generally made of polyvinyl chloride (PVC), which is a nontoxic type of plastic. These tubes do not have a removable inner cannula; therefore, it is recommended that they be changed every 7 days to preserve the patency of the airway.

Single Cuff Tracheostomy Tube with a Disposable or Removable Inner Cannula

This type of tube is similar to the single cuff tracheostomy tube with the exception of the removable inner cannula. Figure 21-7 shows a double lumen tube with a removable inner cannula. By removing the inner cannula, cleaning is facilitated and it becomes easier to maintain the patency of the airway. Some of these tubes have disposable inner cannulas, whereas others are cleaned and then reinserted. This cleaning eliminates the need to change the tracheostomy tube periodically.

Single Cuff Fenestrated Tracheostomy Tube

The *fenestrated tracheostomy tube* has a fenestration or window in the outer cannula. Figure 21-8 shows a single cuff fenestrated tracheostomy tube. By removing the inner cannula and deflating the cuff, the patient can breathe through the upper airway. This will facilitate weaning the patient from the tracheostomy appliance. Cleaning is facilitated by the removal of the inner cannula. If the patient's upper airway becomes obstructed or if mechanical ventilation is needed, the inner cannula may be inserted and the cuff reinflated. The fenestrated tube then is functionally similar to a single cuff tube with a removable inner cannula.

Silver Holinger Tracheostomy Tube

The silver Holinger or Jackson tube is a nondisposable, reusable tracheostomy tube with a removable inner cannula. Figure 21-9 shows this tracheostomy tube. This tube is cuffless and has a removable inner cannula. These tubes are made of sterling silver. This type of tube is commonly used in long-term tracheostomy patients because of its superior durability and ease of cleaning.

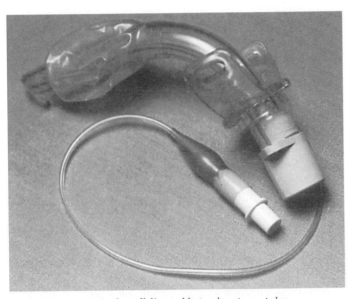

Figure 21-6   *A single cuff disposable tracheostomy tube*

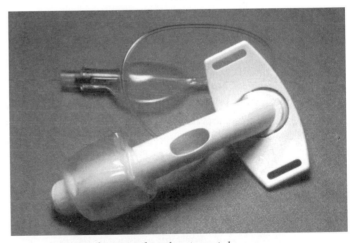

Figure 21-8   *A fenestrated tracheostomy tube*

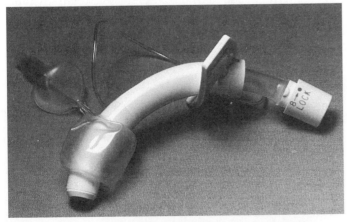

Figure 21-7   *A single cuff disposable tracheostomy tube with a removable inner cannula*

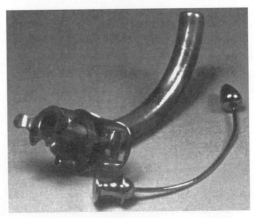

Figure 21-9   *A Jackson tracheostomy tube*

A tube of like construction, but shorter, is called a *laryngectomy tube* and may be encountered in patients who have had a laryngectomy performed.

Bivona Foam Cuff

The Bivona foam cuff tube has a foam cuff that self-inflates. Once the tube is in position, the pilot tube is opened to the atmosphere. The foam then expands, sealing the airway. The cuff is designed to exert no more than 25 mm Hg of pressure against the tracheal wall.

It is important never to inflate this type of cuff, as this makes it a high-pressure cuff.

Specialized Tracheostomy Tubes and Appliances

Communi-Trach

This tracheostomy tube is similar to the Pitt Speaking Tube. A fitting is provided that directs a flow of oxygen above the cuff of the tube. When the patient occludes a thumb port, gas flows up and through the vocal cords, allowing the patient to speak. Figure 21-10 shows this device. Speech is accomplished without deflating the cuff. The phonation is rather hoarse, but the patient may be understood. It takes some coordination to attempt speech independent of diaphragmatic motion.

Tracheostomy Button

A *tracheostomy button* is a useful device that facilitates weaning the patient from a tracheostomy. Figure 21-11 shows an Olympic Trach button. Spacer rings are provided to adjust the length of the button to accommodate various neck sizes. An intermittent positive-pressure breathing (IPPB) adapter may be inserted into the button to facilitate attachment of devices for ventilation, or a plug may be inserted to allow the patient to breathe through the upper airway.

The tracheostomy button is inserted into the stoma with the distal tip resting just inside the trachea. Figure 21-12 shows a cross section of the airway and the tracheostomy button's placement. With the plug or IPPB adapter removed, the airway may be suctioned, facilitating airway management.

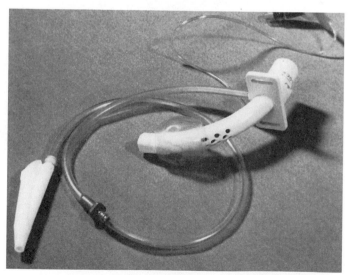

Figure 21-10 *The Communi-Trach tracheostomy tube*

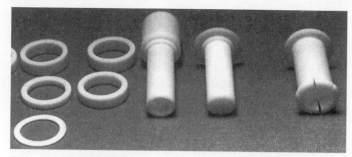

Figure 21-11 *An Olympic Trach button with spacer rings, plug, and IPPB adapter*

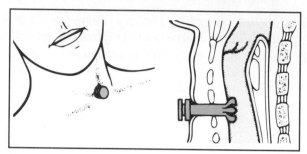

Figure 21-12 *Anatomical placement of a tracheostomy button*

Kistner Button

The Kistner tracheostomy tube is a plastic tube that is somewhat similar to the Olympic Trach button in its use and placement. Figure 21-13 shows this appliance. This device is inserted into the stoma with the distal end resting just inside the trachea. A plastic cap containing a one-way valve is then inserted over the tube. With the cap in place, the patient may inhale through the tube; on exhalation the one-way valve closes, forcing air up through the upper airway. With this device, the patient may speak and develop sufficient intrathoracic pressures to cough effectively.

Olympic Trach-Talk

Olympic Trach-Talk is a modified aerosol T with a one-way valve. Figure 21-14 is a photograph of this device. When the device is used, the cuff of the tracheostomy tube is deflated and the Trach-Talk is then placed on the tube. When the patient inhales, the one-way valve opens, allowing gas to flow into the lower airway. On exhalation, the valve closes, forcing air up through the upper airway. Like the Kistner trach tube, this device facilitates speech and effective coughing. The Olympic Trach-Talk should be

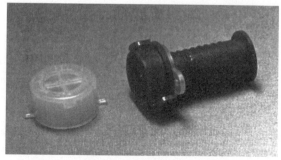

Figure 21-13 *A Kistner button*

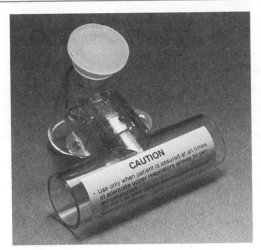

Figure 21-14 *The Olympic Trach-Talk*

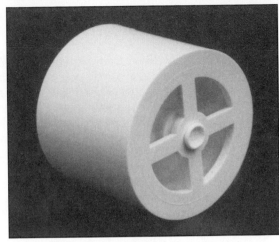

Figure 21-15 *A photograph of the Passy-Muir valve (Courtesy of* Passy-Muir, Inc., Irvine, CA)

used only in alert patients who are capable of managing their own secretions.

Passy-Muir Valve

The *Passy-Muir valve* is a tracheostomy valve manufactured by Passy-Muir, Inc., Irvine, CA (Figure 21-15). This device consists of a leaf or diaphragm valve, which during inspiration allows the patient to inhale through the tracheostomy tube and which during exhalation closes and forces air through the upper airway. When this device is used, it is important to deflate the cuff of the tracheostomy tube prior to installing the Passy-Muir valve onto the airway.

PROFICIENCY OBJECTIVES

At the end of this chapter, you should be able to:

- Assemble the equipment required for airway aspiration and test it for proper operation before use.
- Using an intubation mannequin, demonstrate nasotracheal suctioning.
- Using an intubated mannequin, demonstrate artificial airway aspiration.
- Using an intubated intubation mannequin or a tracheostomy mannequin, demonstrate cuff deflation and inflation and how to check cuff pressure.
- Demonstrate the proper procedure for cleaning a double cannula tracheostomy tube.
- Using a tracheostomy mannequin, demonstrate how to perform stoma care.
- Verbally describe the action to be taken in the event of accidental decannulation or tube displacement.

SUCTIONING PROCEDURE

Equipment Needed for Suctioning

The equipment needed for suctioning may be assembled individually, or a suction kit may be used. The kit is very convenient and contains the majority of the supplies required. Figure 21-16 lists the equipment required for suctioning. The first three items—suction catheter, gloves, and goggles—are normally contained in most suction kits. The packaging wrapper serves as a convenient sterile field for preparing the equipment.

Equipment Preparation

Assemble and test the manual resuscitator for proper operation and set the oxygen flowmeter between 10 and 15 L/min.

After assembling your equipment, connect the vacuum regulator or suction pump and set the vacuum level between −80 and −120 mm Hg. Do this by occluding

- Sterile suction catheter
- Sterile gloves
- Goggles or face shield
- Sterile basin or container
- Sterile normal saline for irrigation
- Sterile distilled water to clean the catheter
- Vacuum regulator or pump with suction trap
- Flow-inflating or self-inflating manual resuscitator
- Water-soluble lubricant

Figure 21-16 *Equipment needed for suctioning*

the suction line and observing the gauge. Do not exceed –120 mm Hg vacuum. Place the vacuum line within easy reach.

Open the package of gloves and catheter or open the suctioning kit. To prepare the suctioning kit, open the package so it lies flat. Pop open the irrigation container and fill it with sterile distilled water. Have the gloves and catheter arranged on the inside of the package, which has become your sterile field, so you may easily reach them. Squeeze a little water-soluble lubricant onto the sterile field where you can later lubricate the catheter.

Unit dose packages of normal saline usually used in aerosol therapy are also convenient for irrigation. The packages are sterile and each contains between 2.5 and 5 ml of fluid. If these are not available, draw up 10 ml of sterile normal saline into a syringe for irrigation of the artificial airway.

Open the sterile distilled water container and pour some into the sterile basin to irrigate the suction line following suctioning. Arrange all of your irrigation fluids so they are convenient and easily accessible.

Positioning for Artificial Airway Aspiration

The two preferred patient positions for artificial airway aspiration are semi-Fowler's and supine. The artificial airway ensures that the catheter will enter the airway, so positioning is less critical. The semi-Fowler's position affords better chest expansion for hyperinflation, and if the patient gags and vomits, the airway is somewhat more protected.

Preaspiration Patient Assessment

Auscultate the chest, paying close attention near the large airways. The presence of crackles is a good indication for suctioning. In some patients the use of a stethoscope will not be required. When these patients breathe, they will have very noisy, gurgling respirations.

Suctioning should be performed only if secretions are present. In clinical practice, you will find suctioning ordered every hour or at some given time interval. Assess the patient at this interval and chart your findings. If suctioning is needed, perform the procedure, but do not suction the patient's airway just because it's ordered at that time interval.

Oxygenation and Hyperinflation of the Patient's Lungs

Using a flow-inflating or self-inflating manual resuscitator, oxygenate and hyperinflate the patient's lungs for 1 or 2 minutes prior to suctioning. An advantage of using a flow-inflating manual resuscitator is that the patient may breathe spontaneously from the bag, receiving 100% oxygen. Some self-inflating manual resuscitators also allow for spontaneous breathing of supplemental oxygen from the bag. Refer to Table 20-2 in Chapter 20, "Emergency Airway Management."

If you are using a mechanical ventilator for this task, and the patient has an artificial airway in place, turn the oxygen percentage control to 100%. Allow at least an additional 2 minutes to compensate for the ventilator wash-out volume.

Nasotracheal Suctioning Procedure

Two common patient positions are used in nasotracheal suctioning: semi-Fowler's and supine with a roll under the shoulders. The latter position is often referred to as the "sniffing" position. Both of these positions facilitate entry into the airway.

Glove your dominant hand using sterile technique. Pick up the catheter with your gloved hand, wrapping it around your fingers to maintain its cleanliness and keep it under control at all times. Figure 21-17 shows the catheter coiled in this way. Expose approximately 8 to 10 inches of the distal end of the catheter and lubricate it with water-soluble lubricant.

Gently insert the catheter into one of the nares with your gloved hand, matching the droop of the catheter with the natural curve of the airway. Slowly advance the catheter. If resistance is encountered, withdraw and gently redirect the catheter. Do not use force.

After inserting approximately 8 to 10 inches of the catheter, listen at the control port for the inspiratory phase. The objective is to slip the catheter past the epiglottis into the trachea. During inspiration, the epiglottis is open. If this does not work, instruct your patient to cough and slip the catheter into the larynx. Sometimes having the patient say "E" during expiration will help.

You will be able to tell when the catheter is inserted into the trachea because the patient will be coughing violently. The patient's color will often turn red and then almost ashen. As soon as the catheter has entered the trachea, connect the vacuum and apply intermittent suction while withdrawing the catheter. As you withdraw the catheter, if you feel resistance or pulling, release vacuum by lifting your thumb off the control port. Withdraw the catheter 1 or 2 cm and reapply vacuum. Limit the application of vacuum to no more than 15 seconds.

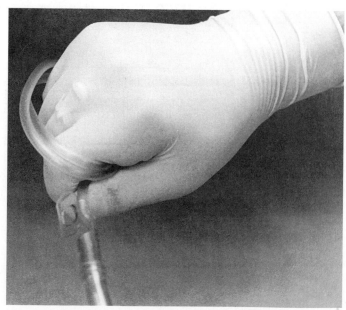

Figure 21-17 *The suction catheter wrapped around the gloved hand*

Withdraw the catheter to approximately the uvular level. Disconnect the vacuum line and oxygenate the patient. Before attempting to suction again, oxygenate the patient for 1 or 2 minutes. By withdrawing the catheter only to the uvula, you are minimizing trauma caused by inserting the catheter through the nose and turbinates repeatedly. By disconnecting the vacuum line, suction is not applied at the distal end of the catheter, withdrawing oxygen from the airway.

After oxygenating the patient, advance the catheter into the trachea as required to clear the airway. In some instances, it may be necessary to instill normal saline into the catheter to thin the thick secretions. The unit dose saline vials and the tip of the syringe conveniently fit the proximal end of the catheter where the vacuum line is connected. Never instill saline through a needle. Cover the control port with your thumb and instill 3 ml of saline down the catheter. Following instillation, suction the airway, applying intermittent suction as outlined previously.

Following the procedure, oxygenate and hyperinflate the patient for 1 or 2 minutes. If the patient is alert, you may use a nonrebreathing mask and instruct the patient to take slow, deep breaths. Otherwise, a manual resuscitator may be used. After each suctioning attempt and after the procedure is completed, it is important to oxygenate the patient to prevent a fall in PaO_2.

Return the patient to any previous oxygen therapy. Using your stethoscope, assess the patient to ensure that the airway has been cleared.

Following the procedure, dispose of your equipment and clean up the area. Clear the vacuum line by aspirating sterile distilled water. Reassure the patient and ensure that the patient is safe and comfortable.

Use of a Nasopharyngeal Airway

Patients needing frequent nasotracheal suctioning may benefit from placement of a nasopharyngeal airway. The airway will facilitate repeated suctioning while minimizing trauma to the nose and nasopharynx.

Artificial Airway Aspiration

The artificial airway provides a direct passage to the airway below the larynx. Normal physiological protective mechanisms are bypassed. Introduction of pathogenic bacteria into the airway could possibly result in pneumonia, an extended hospital stay, or death.

Glove your dominant hand. Pick up the catheter with your gloved hand, wrapping it around your fingers to control it and to preserve its cleanliness. Connect the proximal end to the vacuum line.

If the secretions are thick, instill 3 ml of normal saline down the artificial airway and hyperinflate the patient's lungs for several breaths. A flow-inflating manual resuscitator may be used with one hand while suctioning the patient. Figure 21-18 shows the correct use of the aseptic gloved hand, with the other hand hyperinflating the patient, while preserving aseptic technique.

Gently insert the catheter down the airway until resistance is felt. Withdraw the catheter 1 to 2 cm and apply intermittent suction. If you feel resistance or pulling on the catheter, release vacuum by lifting your thumb off the control port. Withdraw the catheter 1 to 2 cm, and reapply vacuum. Limit your suctioning to a total of 15 seconds. As you withdraw the catheter, wrap it around your gloved hand, or roll it up and hold it between your fingers.

Oxygenate the patient for 1 or 2 minutes, using a manual resuscitator or a mechanical ventilator.

Repeat the suctioning procedure as required to clear the airway. Clear the catheter and the suction line by aspirating sterile distilled water before repeating your suction attempt.

Following the procedure, oxygenate and hyperinflate the patient's lungs for 1 or 2 minutes. These measures are

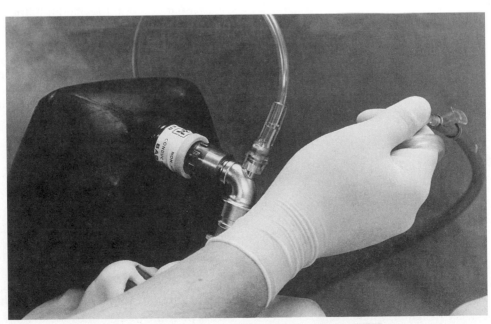

Figure 21-18 *Use of the flow-inflating manual resuscitator while suctioning*

important to prevent drastic changes in PaO_2 following suctioning.

Assess the patient by auscultating the chest to ensure the airways are clear.

Clean up the area and dispose of your equipment appropriately. Ensure that the patient is safe and comfortable and return the patient to oxygen therapy.

Use of a Closed Suction System

The Trach Care catheter is much easier to use than a conventional catheter in that aseptic technique is facilitated by the design of the system.

Connect the control valve to a vacuum source set between –80 and –120 mm Hg.

Perform oxygenation and hyperinflation of the lungs for 1 or 2 minutes prior to suctioning the patient's airway. If the patient is receiving ventilatory support, the ventilator may be used for oxygenation. Investigators have found that oxygenation is not required if the patient is not disconnected from mechanical ventilation for suctioning (Demajo, 1985). In these two studies, desaturation was less using the Trach Care system. However, some desaturation still occurred in most cases.

Advance the catheter into the airway, compressing the protective sheath as the catheter is advanced. Intermittently apply the vacuum when withdrawing the catheter. If resistance or pulling is felt, withdraw the catheter 1 to 2 cm and apply vacuum. Limit total suctioning time to 15 seconds or less.

Oxygenate the patient with 100% oxygen between suction attempts.

Should irrigation with normal saline be required, there is a special connection on the modified aerosol T for this purpose. Attach a syringe (without a needle) or unit dose normal saline vial and instill the saline. Following suctioning, the same port may be used to clear the catheter and vacuum line.

Repeat the suctioning procedure as required to clear the airway.

Following the procedure, oxygenate the patient for 1 or 2 minutes.

Assess the patient by auscultating the chest to ensure that you have cleared the airway of secretions.

Turn off the control valve on the Trach Care system to prevent the inadvertent application of vacuum.

Return the patient to previous oxygen therapy regimen.

CUFF PRESSURE MEASUREMENT

Measurement of cuff pressures and the inflation of the cuff may be performed using either of two methods: the *minimal occlusion volume (MOV) technique* and the *minimal leak technique*.

Pressure Manometer and Three-Way Stopcock

Cuff pressures are measured using a pressure manometer calibrated in cm H_2O. A small-diameter tube, a three-way stopcock, and a syringe are attached as shown in

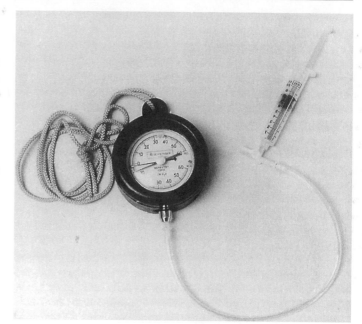

Figure 21-19 *A photograph of a cuff pressure manometer*

Figure 21-19. By rotating the valve of the stopcock, you choose which ports are open to one another. By pointing the valve toward the patient's pilot tube, the syringe and pressure manometer are open to one another and the pilot tube is off. When the valve is rotated opposite to the syringe, all three ports (patient, pressure manometer, and syringe) are open to one another.

To inflate the cuff to obtain MOV pressure, first turn the valve so that the open port (patient) is off. Pressurize the manometer and tubing to 18 cm H_2O by adding air from the syringe. Attach the cuff manometer to the pilot tube by pushing the connectors together. Rotate the valve so that it is opposite the syringe. Add or subtract air using the syringe just until no leak is heard at the patient's mouth. Measure the cuff pressure.

To inflate the cuff to obtain minimal leak pressure, first turn the valve so that the open port (patient) is off. Pressurize the manometer and tubing to 18 cm H_2O by adding air from the syringe. Attach the cuff manometer to the pilot tube by pushing the connectors together. Rotate the valve so it is opposite the syringe. Add or subtract air using the syringe just until a small leak is heard at the patient's mouth during a positive-pressure breath. Measure the cuff pressure.

Posey Cufflator

The Posey Cufflator combines the functions of a syringe, stopcock, and pressure manometer into one single unit (Figure 21-20). The silver port is connected to the pilot tube of the artificial airway. Once they are connected, cuff pressure is recorded on the manometer. If there is insufficient air in the cuff, you may squeeze the bulb, adding air into the cuff. If too much pressure is present, the red toggle valve on the side of the device may be depressed, venting excess pressure to the atmosphere. Both addition and subtraction of pressure may be accomplished using one hand.

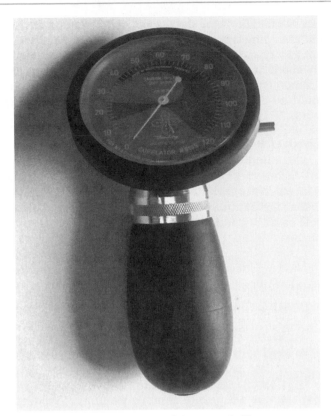

Figure 21-20 *A photograph of the Posey Cufflator*

Either the MOV or minimal leak technique may be employed with this device.

TRACHEOSTOMY CARE PROCEDURE

Equipment Required for Tracheostomy Care

The equipment requirements for tracheostomy and stoma care are minimal. Often, most of the required equipment is contained in a disposable single-use tracheostomy care kit. Figure 21-21 is a listing of the required supplies.

- *• Sterile cotton applicators
- *• Sterile 4 × 4-inch gauze pads
- *• Fabric tracheostomy ties
- *• Sterile brush or cotton pipe cleaners
- *• Sterile gloves
- • Sterile water
- • Hydrogen peroxide (3%)
- • Scissors
- • Supplemental oxygen source
- • Spare sterile tracheostomy tube
- • Self-inflating or flow-inflating resuscitator
- • Syringe
- • Cuff pressure manometer

*The first five items are usually contained in a disposable tracheostomy care kit.

Figure 21-21 *Equipment needed for tracheostomy care*

Cuff Deflation and Inflation

The deflation and inflation of a tracheostomy cuff constitute a routine part of caring for a tracheostomy.

Before deflating the cuff, suction the airway to ensure it is clear and free from secretions. Following airway aspiration, suction the oropharynx. Leave the suction catheter positioned at the posterior portion of the oropharynx and deflate the cuff while simultaneously applying positive pressure to the airway with a manual resuscitator. This will expel any secretions pooled above the cuff into the mouth where they may be suctioned.

Inflate the cuff to MOV. Using a pressure manometer, measure the cuff pressure. Ensure that the cuff pressure is less than 25 cm H_2O.

Components of Tracheostomy Care Procedure

Physician's Order for Care

Often, a physician's order will not include tracheostomy care. Tracheostomy care is a routine procedure performed on any patient following a tracheostomy. It is always prudent, however, to check the respiratory care department's policy and procedure manual to ensure that this clinical procedure is covered by departmental policies.

Auscultate the Chest

It is necessary to auscultate the chest prior to performing tracheostomy care for two reasons: (1) to determine if the patient's lungs are clear of secretions, and (2) if secretions are present, to determine whether suctioning is required prior to performing tracheostomy care. You will feel very frustrated if you neglect this part of the procedure if, after performing tracheostomy care, the patient coughs a large amount of secretions over your work, necessitating that you repeat it. Listen for equal bilateral breath sounds. This will provide a rough indicator as to the placement of the tracheostomy tube. If the tube is accidentally displaced during the procedure, breath sounds after completion of tracheostomy care will be diminished, absent, or unequal.

Prepare a Sterile Field and Apply Sterile Gloves

Tracheostomy care is treated as a sterile procedure. It is essential that you perform this procedure as aseptically as possible. Begin the procedure by unfolding the sterile towel supplied in the tracheostomy care kit to prepare a sterile field. All of the sterile supplies should be placed on this sterile field, arranged so they are convenient and accessible. Pour the sterile water and hydrogen peroxide into the two basins. You are now ready to put on the sterile gloves.

Gloves are worn for this procedure to protect both you and the patient. Treat the stoma site as an incision or a surgical site. It should be considered the *clean* area. All cleansing motions should originate at the stoma site and then progress outward, in a radiating pattern.

Remove and Clean the Inner Cannula

Using one hand, stabilize the tracheostomy tube by holding the flange. With the other hand, remove the inner cannula by twisting the lock or rotating it to the unlocked position and removing it. If the patient requires mechanical ventilation, insert a tracheostomy adapter and reconnect the patient to the ventilator. If supplemental oxygen is required, a tracheostomy mask may be used to provide oxygen while the inner cannula is being cleaned.

Soak the inner cannula in the hydrogen peroxide and scrub it with a brush or cotton applicator. Remove any dried or inspissated secretions both inside and outside of the cannula. Ensure that the lumen is unobstructed. Thoroughly clean the area that mates with the flange and ensure that the locking mechanism is free of secretions.

Rinse the inner cannula in sterile water and shake it dry. If you attempt to reinsert the inner cannula without removing the excess water, any water dripping down the trachea may stimulate a cough reflex.

Reinsert the Inner Cannula

Using a similar two-handed technique, replace the inner cannula. Following the replacement of the cannula, return the patient to the previous mode of therapy (mechanical ventilation or supplemental oxygen as required).

STOMA CARE PROCEDURE

Tracheostomy care and stoma care are usually performed together as one procedure. In this text, each is identified as a separate procedure for the sake of clarity. Both procedures are sterile procedures and should be performed as aseptically as possible. Stoma care involves the cleaning of the stoma site and the application of clean tracheostomy ties and a dressing.

Assess the Tracheostomy Tube Position

If this procedure is performed separately, auscultate the chest to assess the breath sounds before performing the procedure. Determine whether the patient requires suctioning, and listen for bilateral breath sounds.

Remove the Old Dressing and Ties

After determining that all supplies are at hand and prepared, stabilize the tracheostomy tube with one hand and remove the old dressing. Then cut and remove the old ties.

It is essential, once the ties are cut, that the tube be stabilized at all times. It is very easy for accidental decannulation to occur once the ties are removed. A sudden movement or cough may be all that is required for displacement of the tube or decannulation. A spare tube should be available for immediate use if decannulation occurs.

Clean the Stoma Site

Initially, it may be necessary to clean the stoma area with 4 × 4-inch gauze pads dipped in hydrogen peroxide if a large amount of secretions are present. Begin cleaning at the stoma and move out from the site. Use each pad for a single pass only, and discard used pads by placing them in your dirty area. Carefully observe the stoma for unusual redness, swelling, or pulsation of the tracheostomy tube.

Following the removal of the majority of the secretions, use cotton-tipped applicators dipped in hydrogen peroxide for the detail cleaning. Clean very carefully around the stoma and the flanges of the tracheostomy tube.

After completing the cleaning using hydrogen peroxide, rinse the site using gauze pads dipped in sterile water. Pat the area dry with sterile gauze pads.

In some facilities, a small amount of povidone-iodine ointment is applied to help retard the growth of any microorganisms. This is not a universal practice and may require a physician's order. Check your hospital procedure manual to verify whether the ointment is used. Care should be exercised not to apply any non–water-soluble ointments around the stoma site.

Apply a Clean Dressing and New Ties

Never cut a gauze pad to make a dressing. Small cotton filaments separate from the gauze and may be absorbed into the healing stoma and later cause an abscess. A clean dressing may be constructed using a sterile 4 × 4-inch gauze pad if a dressing is not supplied in the tracheostomy care kit. Figure 21-22 shows how to fold the dressing for use. A variety of feltlike materials are used for commercial stoma dressings.

Apply new ties. The ties should be cut prior to performing the procedure so that the tube may be stabilized at all times. Tie a square knot to secure the tracheostomy tube. Never use a bow knot, as it is too easy to untie.

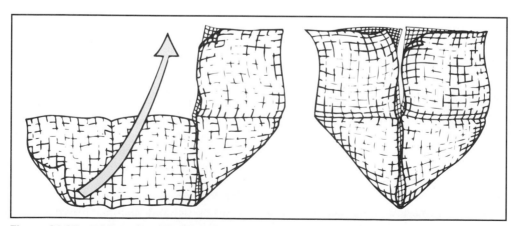

Figure 21-22 *Folding a 4 × 4-inch gauze pad to make a tracheostomy dressing*

A square knot is secure and easy to untie if necessary. A square knot may be tied by passing the right tie over the left, forming a half-hitch and then passing the left tie over the right, forming another half-hitch. Figure 21-23 shows how to tie this knot.

Alternatively, the new ties may be threaded through the flange and tied prior to removing the old ties. Using this technique, the chance of decannulation is minimized because the old ties help to secure the tracheostomy tube while the new ties are being placed. The disadvantage of this technique is that the old ties and secretions may soil the new ties with the patient's secretions.

Reassess the Tracheostomy Tube Position

Auscultate the chest following the procedure to assess the tube position. If the placement of the tube is in doubt, assess the adequacy of the patient's ventilation. If the patient is not in distress, summon help and attempt to reinsert the tube (unless the trach is less than 24 hours old).

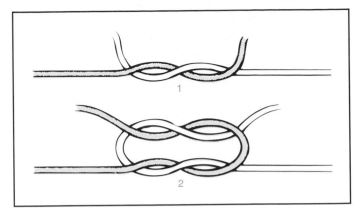

Figure 21-23 *How to tie a square knot*

If the patient is in distress, cover the stoma site with a sterile 4 × 4-inch gauze pad and ventilate the patient by mouth until a physician arrives to assist in reinserting the tube.

References

American Association for Respiratory Care. (1992). AARC clinical practice guideline: Nasotracheal suctioning. *Respiratory Care, 37*(8), 898–901.

American Association for Respiratory Care. (1993). AARC clinical practice guideline: Endotracheal suctioning of mechanically ventilated adults and children with artificial airways. *Respiratory Care, 38*(5), 500–504.

Baker, P. O., Baker, J., & Koen, P. (1983). Endotracheal suctioning techniques in hypoxemic patients. *Respiratory Care, 28*(12), 1563–1568.

Benson, M. S., & Pierson, D. J. (1979). Ventilator wash-out volume: A consideration in endotracheal suction preoxygenation. *Respiratory Care, 24*(9), 832–835.

Demajo, W. (1985). Effects of suctioning patients without interruption of ventilation. Toronto General Hospital, Surgical Intensive Care Unit. Photocopy.

Demers, R. R. (1982). Complications of endotracheal suctioning procedures. *Respiratory Care, 27*(4), 453–457.

Fell, T., & Cheney, F. W. (1971). Prevention of hypoxia during endotracheal suction. *Annals of Surgery, 174*(1), 24–28.

Fluck, R. R., Jr. (1985). Suctioning — intermittent or continuous? *Respiratory Care, 30*(10), 837–838.

Guyton, A. C. (1984). *Physiology of the human body.* Philadelphia: Saunders.

Jung, R., & Gottlieb, L. S. (1976). Comparison of tracheobronchial suction catheters in humans. *Chest, 69*(2), 179–181.

Naigow, D., & Powaser, M. M. (1977). The effect of different endotracheal suction procedures on arterial blood gases in a controlled experimental model. *Heart and Lung, 6*(5), 808–815.

Nelson, E. J., Hunter, P., & Morton, E. (1983). *Critical care respiratory therapy: A laboratory and clinical manual.* Boston: Little, Brown.

Pereia, W., Kovnat, D. M., Khan, M. A., Iacovino, J. R., Spivack, M. L., & Snider, G. L. (1975). Fever and pneumonia after flexible fiberoptic bronchoscopy. *American Review of Respiratory Disease, 112,* 59–64.

Ritz, R., Coyle, M., & Scott, L. (1984). A comparison of bacteriological contamination of a multiple use suction system versus a disposable suction system: A pilot study. *Respiratory Care, 29*(10), 1048.

Sackner, M. A., Landa, J. F., Greeneltch, N., & Robinson, M. J. (1973). Pathogenesis and prevention of tracheobronchial damage with suction procedures. *Chest, 64*(3), 284–290.

Scanlan, C., Spearman, C., & Sheldon, R. (1995). *Egan's fundamentals of respiratory therapy* (6th ed.). St. Louis, MO: Mosby.

Skelley, B., Deeren, S. M., & Powaser, M. M. (1980). The effectiveness of two preoxygenation methods to prevent endotracheal suction-induced hypoxemia. *Heart and Lung, 9*(2), 316–323.

Stauffer, J. L., & Silvestri, R. (1982). Complications of endotracheal intubation, tracheostomy and artificial airways. *Respiratory Care, 27*(4), 417.

Additional Resources

Bonner, J. T., & Hall, J. R. (1985). *Respiratory intensive care of the adult patient.* St. Louis, MO: Mosby.

Burton, G. C., Hodgkin, J., & Ward, J. (1997). *Respiratory care: A guide to clinical practice* (4th ed.). Philadelphia: Lippincott.

Eubanks, D. H., & Bone, R. (1991). *Comprehensive respiratory care* (2nd ed.). St. Louis, MO: Mosby.

Lyons, R. J. (1979). *Tracheostomy care.* Pleasanton, CA: Shiley.

Practice Activities: Suctioning

1. Assemble the equipment required for airway aspiration, including the following:
   a. Sterile catheter
   b. Sterile gloves
   c. Goggles or face shield
   d. Sterile basin or container
   e. Sterile distilled water
   f. Sterile normal saline
   g. Flow-inflating or self-inflating manual resuscitator
   h. Vacuum gauge or pump and suction trap
   i. Water-soluble lubricant

2. Verify the operation of the vacuum gauge or pump and set the vacuum level between −80 and −120 mm Hg.

3. Assemble and test the manual resuscitator for proper operation.

4. With a laboratory partner as your patient, position the patient for:
   a. Nasotracheal suctioning
      (1) Semi-Fowler's
      (2) Supine in "sniffing" position
   b. Artificial airway aspiration
      (1) Semi-Fowler's
      (2) Supine in "sniffing" position

5. Using an intubation mannequin or a laboratory partner, practice oxygenation and hyperinflation:
   a. Without an artificial airway
   b. With an artificial airway

6. Using an intubation mannequin, practice nasotracheal and artificial airway aspiration using the following criteria:
   a. Equipment assembly and testing
   b. Patient assessment
   c. Preoxygenation and hyperinflation using a self-inflating or flow-inflating manual resuscitator
   d. Suctioning
      (1) Vacuum range between −80 and −120 mm Hg
      (2) Application of vacuum limited to 15 seconds
      (3) Vacuum is applied intermittently
      (4) Sterile technique is maintained
   e. Oxygenation following airway aspiration
   f. Normal saline instillation as required
   g. Airway aspiration repeated as required
   h. Oxygenation and hyperinflation following the procedure
   i. Patient assessment following the procedure

7. Using an intubated intubation mannequin, practice using the Trach Care suctioning system, including the following:
   a. Patient assessment
   b. Preoxygenation and hyperinflation
   c. Suctioning
      (1) Vacuum range between −80 and −120 mm Hg
      (2) Application of vacuum limited to 15 seconds
      (3) Vacuum applied intermittently
   d. Oxygenation and hyperinflation following aspiration
   e. Normal saline instillation as required
   f. Aspiration repeated as required
   g. Oxygenation and hyperinflation following the procedure
   h. Patient assessment following procedure
   i. Control valve is turned off

8. Using an intubated intubation mannequin, practice measuring cuff pressures with the following techniques:
   a. MOV technique
   b. Minimal leak technique

Practice Activities: Tracheostomy and Stoma Care

1. Practice preparing a sterile field:
   a. Glove using sterile technique
   b. Arrange supplies without contamination

2. Using a tracheostomy mannequin, practice tracheostomy care:
   a. Auscultate the chest.
   b. Prepare a sterile field and supplies.
   c. Remove and clean inner cannula.
      (1) Use hydrogen peroxide.
      (2) Clean the inner cannula thoroughly.
      (3) Rinse the inner cannula in sterile water.
      (4) Provide supplemental oxygen or ventilation as required.

3. Check for tube placement by auscultating the chest.

4. Using a tracheostomy mannequin, practice stoma care:
   a. Auscultate the chest.
   b. Perform procedure aseptically.

c. While stabilizing the tube at all times:
   (1) Remove old dressing and ties.
   (2) Clean the stoma site.
      (a) Use 4 × 4-inch gauze pad and hydrogen peroxide to clean large amounts of secretions.
      (b) Use cotton-tipped applicators for detail cleaning.
      (c) Rinse the area with sterile water using 4 × 4-inch gauze pads.
      (d) Apply povidone-iodine ointment as required.
      (e) Replace tracheostomy ties.
      (f) Replace the dressing.
d. Evaluate breath sounds to determine tracheostomy tube placement.

Check List: Nasotracheal Suctioning

_____ 1. Assemble equipment.
        2. Prepare and test equipment.
_____   a. Arrange a sterile field.
_____   b. Check the vacuum level.
_____   c. Pour the solutions.
_____ 3. Properly position the patient.
        4. Assess the patient.
_____   a. Auscultate the trachea.
_____   b. Auscultate around the large airways.
        5. Oxygenate and hyperinflate the patient for 1 or 2 minutes on 100% oxygen.
        6. Suction the patient.
_____   a. Vacuum range between −80 and −120 mm Hg

_____   b. Application of vacuum limited to 15 seconds
_____   c. Vacuum applied intermittently
_____   d. Sterile technique maintained
_____ 7. Oxygenate following aspiration.
_____ 8. Instill saline as required.
_____ 9. Repeat suctioning until the airway is clear.
_____ 10. Oxygenate and hyperinflate the patient for 1 or 2 minutes on 100% oxygen following the procedure.
_____ 11. Reassess the patient.
_____ 12. Return the patient to previous oxygen therapy.
_____ 13. Clean up the area.
_____ 14. Record the procedure in the chart.

Check List: Artificial Airway Aspiration

_____ 1. Assemble the required equipment.
        2. Prepare and test the equipment.
_____   a. Check the vacuum level.
_____   b. Arrange a sterile field.
_____   c. Pour the solutions.
_____ 3. Position the patient.
_____ 4. Assess the patient by auscultation.
        5. Oxygenate and hyperinflate the patient:
_____   a. Using a manual resuscitator
_____   b. Using the mechanical ventilator, allowing for wash-out volume
        6. Suction the patient.
_____   a. Vacuum range between −80 and −120 mm Hg

_____   b. Application of vacuum limited to 15 seconds
_____   c. Vacuum applied intermittently
_____   d. Sterile technique maintained
_____ 7. Oxygenate following aspiration.
_____ 8. Instill normal saline as required.
_____ 9. Repeat aspiration until airway is clear.
_____ 10. Oxygenate following the procedure with 100% oxygen for 1 or 2 minutes.
_____ 11. Assess the patient following the procedure.
_____ 12. Return the patient to previous oxygen therapy.
_____ 13. Clean up the area.
_____ 14. Record the procedure in the chart.

Check List: Cuff Pressure Monitoring

_____ 1. Assemble and test the equipment needed prior to measurement of cuff pressures.
_____ 2. Follow standard precautions including handwashing.
_____ 3. Pressurize the manometer and tubing to 18 cm H_2O.
_____ 4. Attach the manometer to the pilot tube by pushing the connectors together.
        5. Measure the cuff pressure:

_____   a. MOV technique
_____   b. Minimal leak technique
_____ 6. Turn off the stopcock to the pilot tube.
_____ 7. Disconnect the cuff manometer from the pilot tube.
_____ 8. Remove any unneeded equipment.
_____ 9. Assess the patient's breath sounds.
_____ 10. Record your findings in the chart.

Check List: *Tracheostomy and Stoma Care*

_____ 1. Verify the order or policy and review the chart for pertinent information.

_____ 2. Explain the procedure.

_____ 3. Assemble the required equipment.

4. Auscultate the chest.

_____   a. Determine tube placement.

_____   b. Determine the need for suctioning and suction as required.

_____ 5. Prepare a sterile field and arrange all supplies aseptically.

_____ 6. Using sterile technique, glove for the procedure.

7. Remove and clean the inner cannula.

_____   a. Use hydrogen peroxide.

_____   b. Rinse in sterile water.

_____   c. Provide supplemental oxygen or ventilation as required.

_____   d. Stabilize the tube at all times.

_____ 8. Replace the inner cannula.

9. While stabilizing the tube at all times:

_____   a. Remove old ties and dressing.

  b. Clean the stoma area.

_____   (1) Use 4 × 4-inch gauze pad.

_____   (2) Use cotton applicators for fine detail.

_____   (3) Rinse stoma site with sterile water.

_____   c. Replace ties.

_____   d. Replace dressing.

_____ 10. Evaluate breath sounds following the procedure.

_____ 11. Remove the supplies and clean up the area.

_____ 12. Reposition the patient as required.

_____ 13. Record the procedure in the patient's chart.

Self-Evaluation Post Test: *Artificial Airway Care*

1. When suctioning a patient, you should limit the suctioning time to:
   a. no more than 10 seconds.
   b. no more than 15 seconds.
   c. no more than 20 seconds.
   d. no more than 25 seconds.
   e. no more than 30 seconds.

2. The level of vacuum on the vacuum gauge should be set at:
   a. −80 to −120 mm Hg.
   b. 120 to 150 mm Hg.
   c. less than 80 mm Hg.
   d. 70 to 80 cm H_2O.
   e. 100 cm H_2O.

3. During nasotracheal suctioning, mucosal irritation can be reduced by:
   a. using a larger catheter.
   b. leaving the catheter in place.
   c. leaving the catheter in place and disconnecting it from the vacuum source.
   d. not applying suction at all.
   e. ensuring the vacuum is greater than 150 mm Hg.

4. The advantages of the Trach Care system include:
   I. cost effectiveness.
   II. the ability to suction without disconnection.
   III. decreased mucosal trauma.
   IV. selective entry into right or left bronchi.
   a. I, II
   b. I, III
   c. I, IV
   d. I, II, IV
   e. II, IV

5. Which of the following are complications of suctioning?
   I. Tissue trauma
   II. Decreased cardiac output
   III. Hypoxemia
   IV. Cardiac arrhythmias
   V. Infection
   a. I, II, V
   b. II, III, V
   c. I, III, IV
   d. I, III, IV, V
   e. I, V

6. A potential complication of stoma care is:
   a. obturator occlusion.
   b. inner cannula obstruction.
   c. decannulation.
   d. hypoventilation.
   e. hypercapnia.

7. Tracheostomy tube displacement is most rapidly assessed by:
   a. chest x-ray.
   b. fluoroscopy.
   c. auscultation.
   d. percussion.
   e. arterial blood gas analysis.

8. The purpose of tracheostomy and stoma care is:
   a. to keep the stoma site clean and dry.
   b. to keep the airway patent.
   c. to remove secretions from the stoma site.
   d. to reduce the chance of nosocomial infection.
   e. All of the above

9. When using a gauze pad to make a dressing, you should:
   a. cut the dressing to fit.
   b. never use gauze for a dressing.
   c. fold the dressing to fit.
   d. use a lot of tape to hold the dressing.
   e. not use a dressing at all.

10. Before performing tracheostomy and stoma care you should:
    I. auscultate the chest.
    II. take the respiratory rate.
    III. draw specimens for ABG analysis.
    IV. suction the patient if needed.
    a. I, II
    b. I, III
    c. I, IV
    d. II, IV
    e. III, IV

PERFORMANCE EVALUATION:
NASOTRACHEAL SUCTIONING

Date: Lab _____ Clinical _____ Agency _____

Lab: Pass _____ Fail _____   Clinical: Pass _____ Fail _____

Student name _____ Instructor name _____

No. of times observed in clinical _____

No. of times practiced in clinical _____

PASSING CRITERIA: Obtain 90% or better on the procedure. Tasks indicated by * must receive at least 1 point, or the evaluation is terminated. Procedure must be performed within designated time, or the performance receives a failing grade.

SCORING:
2 points — Task performed satisfactorily without prompting.
1 point — Task performed satisfactorily with self-initiated correction.
0 points — Task performed incorrectly or with prompting required.
NA — Task not applicable to the patient care situation.

TASKS:		PEER	LAB	CLINICAL
*	1. Follows standard precautions, including handwashing	☐	☐	☐
	2. Obtains required equipment			
*	a. Suction kit or	☐	☐	☐
	(1) Sterile catheter	☐	☐	☐
	(2) Sterile gloves	☐	☐	☐
	(3) Sterile basin	☐	☐	☐
	(4) Eye protection (goggles or face shield)	☐	☐	☐
*	b. Manual resuscitator	☐	☐	☐
*	c. Sterile water	☐	☐	☐
*	d. Water-soluble lubricant	☐	☐	☐
*	e. Vacuum gauge or pump and trap	☐	☐	☐
*	3. Assembles and checks equipment	☐	☐	☐
*	4. Positions the patient	☐	☐	☐
*	5. Assesses the need for suctioning	☐	☐	☐
*	6. Hyperinflates and oxygenates the patient	☐	☐	☐
*	7. Inserts the catheter	☐	☐	☐
	8. Suctions the airway			
*	a. Vacuum level of –80 to –120 mm Hg	☐	☐	☐
*	b. Application of vacuum limited to no more than 15 seconds	☐	☐	☐
*	c. Sterile technique maintained	☐	☐	☐
*	9. Oxygenates following suctioning	☐	☐	☐
*	10. Instills saline as required	☐	☐	☐
*	11. Repeats aspiration as required	☐	☐	☐
*	12. Repositions the patient	☐	☐	☐

*   13. Returns the patient to previous oxygen therapy   ☐   ☐   ☐

*   14. Cleans up the area after the procedure   ☐   ☐   ☐

*   15. Records the procedure in the patient's chart   ☐   ☐   ☐

SCORE: Peer   _____ points of possible 44; _____%

            Lab   _____ points of possible 44; _____%

            Clinical   _____ points of possible 44; _____%

TIME: _____ out of possible 20 minutes

STUDENT SIGNATURES   **INSTRUCTOR SIGNATURES**

PEER: _____   LAB: _____

STUDENT: _____   CLINICAL: _____

PERFORMANCE EVALUATION:
ENDOTRACHEAL SUCTIONING

Date: Lab _____ Clinical _____ Agency _____

Lab: Pass _____ Fail _____   Clinical: Pass _____ Fail _____

Student name _____ Instructor name _____

No. of times observed in clinical _____

No. of times practiced in clinical _____

PASSING CRITERIA: Obtain 90% or better on the procedure. Tasks indicated by * must receive at least 1 point, or the evaluation is terminated. Procedure must be performed within designated time, or the performance receives a failing grade.

SCORING:
2 points — Task performed satisfactorily without prompting.
1 point — Task performed satisfactorily with self-initiated correction.
0 points — Task performed incorrectly or with prompting required.
NA — Task not applicable to the patient care situation.

TASKS:	PEER	LAB	CLINICAL
* 1. Follows standard precautions, including handwashing	☐	☐	☐
2. Obtains required equipment			
* a. Suction kit or	☐	☐	☐
(1) Sterile catheter	☐	☐	☐
(2) Sterile gloves	☐	☐	☐
(3) Sterile basin	☐	☐	☐
(4) Eye protection (goggles or face shield)	☐	☐	☐
* b. Manual resuscitator	☐	☐	☐
* c. Sterile water	☐	☐	☐
* d. Water-soluble lubricant	☐	☐	☐
* e. Vacuum gauge or pump and trap	☐	☐	☐
* 3. Assembles and checks equipment	☐	☐	☐
* 4. Positions the patient	☐	☐	☐
* 5. Assesses the need for suctioning	☐	☐	☐
6. Hyperinflates and oxygenates the patient			
* a. Uses a manual resuscitator, or	☐	☐	☐
* b. Uses a ventilator allowing for wash-out volume	☐	☐	☐
* 7. Inserts the catheter	☐	☐	☐
8. Suctions the airway			
* a. Vacuum level of −80 to −120 mm Hg	☐	☐	☐
* b. Application of vacuum limited to no more than 15 seconds	☐	☐	☐
* c. Sterile technique maintained	☐	☐	☐

9. Oxygenates following suctioning

*   a. Uses a manual resuscitator, or   ☐   ☐   ☐

*   b. Uses a ventilator allowing for wash-out volume   ☐   ☐   ☐

*   10. Instills saline as required   ☐   ☐   ☐

*   11. Repeats aspiration as required   ☐   ☐   ☐

*   12. Oxygenates and hyperinflates for 1 or 2 minutes following the procedure   ☐   ☐   ☐

*   13. Repositions the patient   ☐   ☐   ☐

*   14. Returns the patient to previous oxygen therapy   ☐   ☐   ☐

*   15. Cleans up the area after the procedure   ☐   ☐   ☐

*   16. Records the procedure in the patient's chart   ☐   ☐   ☐

SCORE: Peer   _____ points of possible 50; _____%

            Lab   _____ points of possible 50; _____%

            Clinical   _____ points of possible 50; _____%

TIME: _____ out of possible 20 minutes

STUDENT SIGNATURES   INSTRUCTOR SIGNATURES

PEER: _____   LAB: _____

STUDENT: _____   CLINICAL: _____

PERFORMANCE EVALUATION: MONITORING CUFF PRESSURES

Date: Lab _____ Clinical _____ Agency _____

Lab: Pass _____ Fail _____   Clinical: Pass _____ Fail _____

Student name _____ Instructor name _____

No. of times observed in clinical _____

No. of times practiced in clinical _____

PASSING CRITERIA: Obtain 90% or better on the procedure. Tasks indicated by * must receive at least 1 point, or the evaluation is terminated. Procedure must be performed within designated time, or the performance receives a failing grade.

SCORING:
2 points — Task performed satisfactorily without prompting.
1 point — Task performed satisfactorily with self-initiated correction.
0 points — Task performed incorrectly or with prompting required.
NA — Task not applicable to the patient care situation.

TASKS:

			PEER	LAB	CLINICAL
*	1.	Assembles and tests equipment	☐	☐	☐
*	2.	Follows standard precautions, including handwashing	☐	☐	☐
*	3.	Pressurizes the manometer and tubing to 18 cm H_2O	☐	☐	☐
*	4.	Attaches the manometer to the pilot tube	☐	☐	☐
*	5.	Measures the cuff pressure			
		a. MOV technique	☐	☐	☐
		b. Minimal leak technique	☐	☐	☐
*	6.	Turns off the stopcock to the pilot tube	☐	☐	☐
*	7.	Disconnects the cuff manometer	☐	☐	☐
	8.	Removes any unneeded equipment	☐	☐	☐
*	9.	Auscultates the chest	☐	☐	☐
*	10.	Charts the procedure	☐	☐	☐

SCORE:

Peer _____ points of possible 22; _____%

Lab _____ points of possible 22; _____%

Clinical _____ points of possible 22; _____%

TIME: _____ out of possible 15 minutes

STUDENT SIGNATURES   **INSTRUCTOR SIGNATURES**

PEER: _____   LAB: _____

STUDENT: _____   CLINICAL: _____

PERFORMANCE EVALUATION:
TRACHEOSTOMY AND STOMA CARE

Date: Lab _____ Clinical _____ Agency _____

Lab: Pass _____ Fail _____   Clinical: Pass _____ Fail _____

Student name _____   Instructor name _____

No. of times observed in clinical _____

No. of times practiced in clinical _____

PASSING CRITERIA: Obtain 90% or better on the procedure. Tasks indicated by * must receive at least 1 point, or the evaluation is terminated. Procedure must be performed within designated time, or the performance receives a failing grade.

SCORING: 2 points — Task performed satisfactorily without prompting.
            1 point — Task performed satisfactorily with self-initiated correction.
            0 points — Task performed incorrectly or with prompting required.
            NA — Task not applicable to the patient care situation.

TASKS:

			PEER	LAB	CLINICAL
*	1.	Verifies order or policy	☐	☐	☐
*	2.	Scans the chart for pertinent information	☐	☐	☐
*	3.	Introduces self	☐	☐	☐
	4.	Explains the procedure	☐	☐	☐
*	5.	Gathers the appropriate equipment	☐	☐	☐
*	6.	Follows standard precautions, including handwashing	☐	☐	☐
*	7.	Auscultates the chest	☐	☐	☐
*	8.	Suctions the patient as required	☐	☐	☐
*	9.	Prepares a sterile field	☐	☐	☐
*	10.	Gloves aseptically	☐	☐	☐
	11.	Removes the inner cannula			
*		a. Stabilizes the tube	☐	☐	☐
*		b. Provides supplemental oxygen or ventilation as required	☐	☐	☐
	12.	Cleans the inner cannula			
*		a. Uses hydrogen peroxide	☐	☐	☐
*		b. Cleans inside and outside	☐	☐	☐
*		c. Rinses with sterile water and shakes dry	☐	☐	☐
*	13.	Reinserts the inner cannula	☐	☐	☐
*	14.	Removes the old dressing and ties	☐	☐	☐
	15.	Performs stoma care			
*		a. Stabilizes tube at all times	☐	☐	☐
*		b. Cleans from stoma out	☐	☐	☐
*		c. Uses hydrogen peroxide	☐	☐	☐
*		d. Rinses with sterile water	☐	☐	☐

*	16. Applies new ties and dressing	☐	☐	☐
*	17. Auscultates the chest	☐	☐	☐
*	18. Cleans up the area and removes the supplies	☐	☐	☐
*	19. Returns the patient to previous therapy	☐	☐	☐
*	20. Records the procedure in the patient's chart	☐	☐	☐

Score: Peer   _____ points of possible 52; _____%

              Lab   _____ points of possible 52; _____%

              Clinical   _____ points of possible 52; _____%

TIME: _____ out of possible 20 minutes

STUDENT SIGNATURES

PEER: _____

STUDENT: _____

INSTRUCTOR SIGNATURES

LAB: _____

CLINICAL: _____

CHAPTER 22
CHEST TUBES

INTRODUCTION

Caring for the acutely ill patient will require that you understand how to manage and troubleshoot chest tubes. As a respiratory care practitioner, you may be required to assist the physician in the placement of chest drains or chest tubes and then to maintain them once they are placed. In this chapter, you will learn about what chest tubes are and what they do, how to assist the physician in placing these tubes, and how to maintain and troubleshoot them once they are placed.

KEY TERMS

- Chest drain
- Chest tube
- Collection chamber
- Suction control chamber
- Trocar
- Water seal chamber

OBJECTIVES

At the end of this chapter, you should be able to:

- State the indications for placement and the purpose of chest tubes.
- Differentiate between a chest drain and a chest tube.
- Describe why a chest tube might be placed anteriorly or posteriorly in the thoracic cavity.
- Describe the function of the three components of a disposable chest drainage system:
  — Collection chamber
  — Water seal chamber

  — Suction control chamber
- Describe the consequences of the presence of too much or too little water in the water seal chamber.
- Describe the consequences of the presence of too much or too little water in the suction control chamber.
- Describe how to assess whether the vacuum source is correctly regulated.
- Describe how to assess the chest drainage system for leaks and how to correct them.

CHEST TUBES: BASIC PRINCIPLES

Indications for Chest Tube Placement

Chest tubes are indicated to remove blood, pus, pleural fluid, or air from the thoracic cavity (McMahon-Parkes, 1997). Chest drains may be placed in the mediastinal space or the pleural space.

Mediastinal drain placement may be indicated postoperatively (as after coronary artery bypass grafting or open heart surgery) to remove blood or to remove air (pneumopericardium). Mediastinal drains are important in the prevention of postoperative cardiac tamponade, which may cause the cardiac output to fall to dangerous levels. Once the postoperative bleeding has resolved, the drains are then removed.

Pleural drains may be placed to remove blood, pleural fluid, pus, or air from the pleural space. Air or fluid in the pleural space will cause a loss of lung volume on the affected side. Often the patient will present with dyspnea, a fall in oxygen saturation, and dullness or hyperresonance to percussion (depending upon whether the problem is air or fluid). Often when a drain is placed to remove air from the pleural space (pneumothorax), it is called a chest tube. Chest tubes may be indicated following trauma or postoperatively (thoracic surgery), or to manage barotrauma from mechanical ventilation.

Chest Drains versus Chest Tubes

Frequently the terms *chest tube* and *chest drain* are used interchangeably. A drain is a device that has the purpose of removing fluid. In this textbook, the term *chest tube* will be used to describe drains (placed for fluid removal) as well as tubes placed to remove air. In the case of thoracic applications, fluids may include blood, pleural fluid, or pus. A chest tube is placed in the pleural space to remove air (pneumothorax). Figure 22-1 is a photograph of a chest tube. Note the trocar in the photograph (lower solid piece).

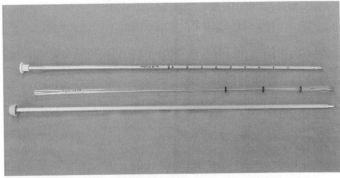

Figure 22-1 *A photograph of a chest tube with the trocar (lower solid piece). Note that the trocar can be inserted into the chest tube, providing rigidity for insertion.*

The *trocar* is a rigid metal rod that is inserted into the chest tube for insertion. The trocar provides stiffness to the otherwise flexible polyvinyl chloride (PVC) tube (made of the same material as for endotracheal tubes), allowing it to be advanced into place by separating tissue. Once the tube is properly positioned, the trocar is removed, leaving the hollow chest tube to perform its function.

Rationale for Placement

Chest tubes or pleural drains are placed either anteriorly high in the thoracic cavity or posteriorly in the thoracic cavity. The rationale for placement depends on whether the tube is to function as a chest drain or as a chest tube. Note that gravity will cause the fluid to collect in the lowest part of the thorax, owing to its greater density. Therefore, to act as a drain, a drain is placed posteriorly along the base of the lung to remove fluid as it is collected (Figure 22-2).

Air will migrate preferentially to the least gravity-dependent (highest) area owing to its decreased density. Therefore, chest tubes are placed anteriorly near the apex of the lung to remove the free pleural air (see Figure 22-2).

CHEST DRAINAGE SYSTEM

Components of a Chest Drainage System

There are currently seven different brands of disposable chest drainage systems on the market (Carroll, 2000; Schiff, 2000). Even though brands vary, all of the disposable systems have common components. The collection system is divided into three parts: the collection chamber, the water seal chamber, and the suction control chamber (Figure 22-3).

The *collection chamber* is the part of the drainage system that collects fluids from the patient. It is calibrated in milliliters (ml) and is commonly subdivided into columns of 600 to 1000 ml per column. By observing the collection chamber, you can assess the amount of drainage, and its color and consistency, over time. You can mark the collection chamber using a piece of tape or marking pen, noting the amount and date and time of measurement, to detect trends in fluid drainage (McMahon-Parkes, 1997).

The *water seal chamber* is the center portion of the collection system (see Figure 22-3). The water seal chamber acts as a one-way valve, allowing air to escape from the

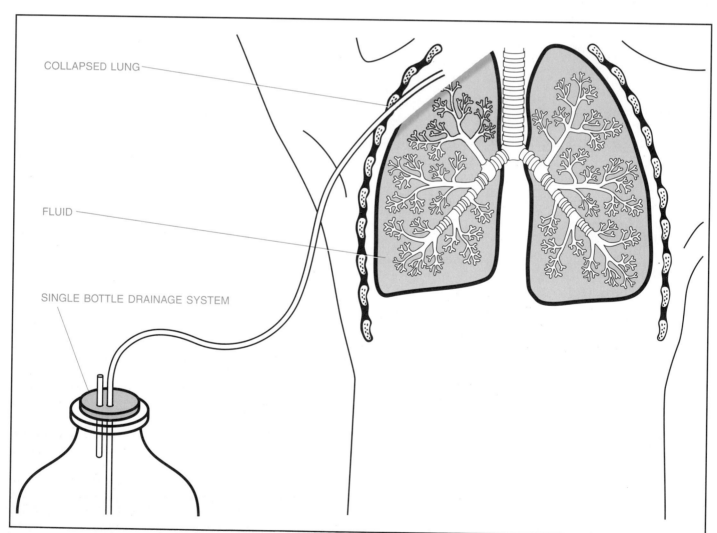

COLLAPSED LUNG

FLUID

SINGLE BOTTLE DRAINAGE SYSTEM

Figure 22-2 *An illustration showing placement of a chest tube. The chest tube is placed anteriorly near the apex of the lung to capture air as it migrates away from the gravity-dependent areas.*

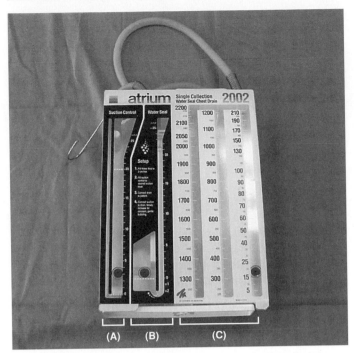

Figure 22-3 *An illustration of the three parts of a chest drainage system: the suction control chamber (A), the water seal chamber (B), the collection chamber (C)*

pleural or mediastinal space but not allowing it to enter those spaces from the atmosphere. To appreciate the principle of operation, immerse one end of a drinking straw in a glass of water. You can blow air through the straw into the glass, but you cannot draw air in through the straw if it is below the level of the liquid. Typically, the water seal chamber is filled only to a depth of 2 cm. This allows air to freely escape the pleural or mediastinal space while protecting the patient from drawing ambient air into those areas (Smith, Fallentine, & Kessel, 1995).

The *suction control chamber* is the chamber most distal from the patient's chest tube (see Figure 22-3). The purpose of this chamber is to regulate the amount of vacuum applied to the chest tube and thus to the patient's thoracic cavity. For most adult patients, the suction control chamber is filled to a depth of 20 cm. This depth provides application of continuous vacuum at a pressure of 20 cm H_2O below ambient pressure. If the depth is increased (to, say, 25 cm), a pressure of 25 cm H_2O below ambient pressure would be applied. The level of vacuum that is applied is directly proportional to the depth in the suction control chamber. If it is low, less vacuum is applied and conversely, if it is high, more vacuum is applied.

Important Principles of Operation
Effects of Water Level in the Water Seal Chamber

Maintenance of the correct water level in the water seal chamber is important. If too little water is in the chamber (less than 2 cm), there is increased risk that with a deep breath (increased subambient pressure in the thorax), air could be drawn into the thoracic cavity. Conversely, too much water in the water seal chamber (greater than 2 cm)

will inhibit air from leaving the thoracic cavity because it must overcome a greater pressure (depth in the chamber) to escape (Smith et al., 1995).

Effects of Water Level in the Suction Control Chamber

As for the water seal chamber, proper regulation of the amount of water in the suction control chamber is also important. Too much or too little water in the suction control chamber may also adversely affect the patient. As described previously, the depth of water in the suction control chamber determines how much subambient pressure is applied to the thoracic cavity. The vacuum regulator on the wall outlet does not control the amount of subambient pressure applied; only the suction control chamber does. For most adults, 20 cm H_2O is the most commonly applied vacuum level. However, most modern drainage systems are capable of being adjusted between 5 and 25 cm H_2O, depending on how deep the chamber is filled. It is important to monitor the water level in the control chamber to ensure that the correct level of subambient pressure is being applied to the chest tube and the patient's thoracic cavity.

Vacuum Regulation

Besides the depth of water in the suction control chamber, proper adjustment of the vacuum regulator connected to the wall vacuum outlet is also important. The level in the suction control chamber regulates the amount of subambient pressure applied to the thoracic cavity, as described before. However, it is important to adjust the vacuum regulator correctly as well, to achieve continuous gentle bubbling in the suction control chamber (Smith et al., 1995). To achieve this level, decrease the vacuum level by turning down the suction regulator control until bubbling ceases. Then increase the vacuum level applied from the regulator until bubbling is continuous but gentle. If the bubbling is too vigorous, evaporation can occur in the suction control chamber, decreasing the level of subambient pressure applied to the thoracic cavity.

Assessment for Leaks

Leaks are identified by observing continuous bubbling in the water seal chamber. Normally, the water seal chamber will occasionally bubble as air is evacuated from the pleural or mediastinal space. If continuous bubbling occurs, there is an air leak either within the thorax or externally in the tubing and connections.

First, assess the patient. Determine if the patient is in distress. Auscultate and percuss the chest to determine if the pneumothorax has increased in size or if a tension pneumothorax may be present. If a tension pneumothorax has occurred, contact the patient's physician immediately.

If the patient is not in distress and appears out of any danger, assess the system for leaks. First, check all tubing connections. Connections should be tight and taped with pink surgical tape (airtight and watertight) to prevent leaks. If the leak persists, using a toothless clamp (one that won't puncture the surgical tubing), briefly clamp the tubing where it attaches to the patient's chest tube. If the bubbling stops, the leak is in the patient's chest (Carroll, 1995). Air leaks are common following many thoracic surgical procedures (e.g., pneumonectomy, lobectomy). The surgeon may wish to be notified when leaks persist following surgery; note it in the patient's chart and notify the physician as appropriate. If the leak persists when the tubing is clamped at the patient's chest tube, the leak is in the system itself. Move the clamp in short intervals, briefly

clamping each time, while moving closer to the collection chamber. If the bubbling stops, the leak is in the connecting tubing (between the chest tube and the collection chamber). The tubing has a hole and must be replaced. If you reach the collection chamber itself and clamp the tubing where it enters the chamber and the leak stops, the leak is in the drainage system and the whole unit must be replaced (Carroll, 1995).

PROFICIENCY OBJECTIVES

At the end of this chapter, you should be able to:

- Collect and assemble the equipment required to assist the physician with the placement of a chest tube.
- Demonstrate how to assist the physician with the placement of a chest tube.
- Demonstrate how to assess the placement of a chest tube radiographically.

- Demonstrate how to set up a three-chamber disposable water seal chest drainage system.
- Demonstrate how to monitor and troubleshoot a chest drainage system.
- Demonstrate how to identify and correct leaks in the system.

ASSISTING WITH CHEST TUBE PLACEMENT

Equipment Required for Chest Tube Placement

As a respiratory care practitioner, you may be required to assist the physician with the placement of a chest tube. The most common settings in which this occurs are the Emergency Department, the intensive care unit (ICU), and the surgical floor in the acute care hospital. Common equipment required includes a chest tube insertion tray, sterile gloves, chest tubes, local anesthetic, antiseptic, the chest drainage system, and a vacuum regulator for the wall suction.

The chest tube tray typically includes sterile drapes, a scalpel, suture material, cotton-tipped or sponge swabs, antiseptic (usually povidone-iodine), and a sterile dressing. The chest tube insertion tray contains most of the supplies required to insert a chest tube. You will additionally need to obtain the chest tubes, local anesthetic, syringes, and the chest drainage system.

Draw up 4% lidocaine into a syringe in preparation for the procedure. The physician will use local anesthetic at the point of insertion. The physician may also order an analgesic, such as midazolam, prior to the procedure to help relax the patient. It is helpful to draw up and prepare medications in advance in case you are required to maintain sterile technique during the procedure.

Open the chest drainage system. Fill the suction control chamber to 20 cm H_2O and fill the water seal chamber to 2 cm H_2O. Connect the vacuum regulator to the wall outlet. Connect the drainage system to the wall outlet with surgical tubing. Don't apply vacuum to the system at this time. Set everything up in preparation for the procedure.

Assisting the Physician with the Procedure

Using a bedside tray or counter space, open the sterile chest tube insertion tray. Use the packaging wrap to form

a sterile field. Assist the physician with applying sterile gloves if requested to do so.

Place the patient in a high Fowler's or semi-Fowler's position for anterior tube placement if the patient's condition permits it. You may be requested to pour or squeeze povidone-iodine solution into a sterile cup molded into the tray. The physician will apply the antiseptic to the site of the chest tube insertion. Following application of antiseptic, he or she may use disposable sterile drapes to form a sterile field. Many disposable drapes have adhesive strips to help them to stay in place and are usually applied directly to the skin. Once the site is prepped and draped, the physician will inject the site with local anesthetic.

Most chest tubes that are to drain air are inserted on the anterior chest in the second or third intercostal space along the midclavicular line. An incision is made right over the rib and will dissect up and over the rib in an angular fashion. This will aid in closing the opening when the tube is withdrawn.

Chest tubes placed to drain fluid will be placed lower in the chest, in the fourth or lower intercostal space along the midaxillary line. The patient is placed lying on the side, with the affected side superior. Once the incision is made, the chest tube will be advanced posteriorly, toward the base of the lung where gravity will draw the fluid.

Assist the physician by opening the chest tube package such that he or she can obtain it, maintaining his or her sterile technique. The physician will insert the chest tube with the trocar in place, directing it superiorly toward the apex of the lung (air moves away from the gravity-dependent areas). The patient may experience discomfort during the procedure. Considerable pressure is required to insert the tube through the muscle layers and into the pleural space.

Once the chest tube is placed, the physician will suture it into place to minimize the chance of its becoming displaced. Suturing the skin will also pull it up tight around the chest tube, helping to prevent leaks. Once it is sutured, assist the physician by opening the sterile petrolatum gauze dressing, which may be applied around the chest tube. A sterile airtight dressing is then applied over the gauze dressing to prevent dissection of air into the pleural space around the tube through the incision site.

Assessment of Chest Tube Placement

Chest tube placement is assessed by obtaining a chest x-ray. Most patients in the ICU setting will have portable anteroposterior films taken. Like endotracheal tubes, chest tubes have a radiopaque line that promotes their visibility on an x-ray. Verify that the chest tube is located properly and directed properly (superiorly for air, inferiorly for fluid).

SETUP AND MAINTENANCE OF THE CHEST DRAINAGE SYSTEM

Setting up the Drainage System

If you followed the steps outlined previously for equipment assembly, you have the drainage system's suction control and water seal chambers filled with water and the unit connected to the vacuum regulator. Using latex surgical tubing, connect the patient's chest tube to the latex tubing using a barbed connector as shown in Figure 22-4. If you anticipate a large amount of drainage, you may wish to trim the opening of the barbed connector, enlarging it so that fluids may flow more freely (Figure 22-5) (Smith et al.,

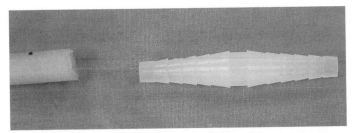

Figure 22-4 *Connecting the chest tube to the latex surgical tubing using a barbed connector*

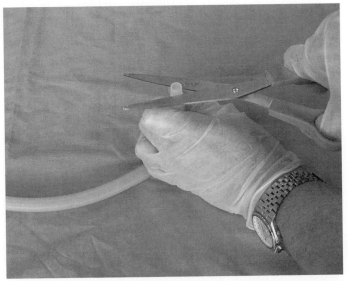

Figure 22-5 *Trimming the barbed connector, enlarging the opening*

1995). Once the connections are made at the chest tube, tape the connection using pink watertight/airtight surgical tape. Taping the connection will help to minimize the possibility of a leak at the connection.

Connect the surgical tubing to the drainage system and tape that joint as well. Make certain that there are no dependent loops in the tubing between the patient and the drainage system. Any dependent loops can collect fluid, stopping flow. You want an uninterrupted downward pathway from the chest tube to the drainage system.

Adjust the vacuum regulator until gentle continuous bubbling is observed in the suction control chamber. Gentle continuous bubbling ensures that enough vacuum is being applied (greater than the water depth in the suction control chamber). However, the depth of water in the suction control chamber is what regulates the amount of subambient pressure applied to the patient's chest tube. Gentle, not vigorous, bubbling is important. Vigorous bubbling increases water evaporation in the suction control chamber, ultimately decreasing the level of subambient pressure applied to the patient's chest tube.

Monitoring and Troubleshooting the Drainage System

Monitoring a chest drainage system involves measuring and documenting fluid collection and monitoring and maintaining water levels in the water seal chamber and suction control chamber. Fluid drainage should be monitored initially every 30 to 60 minutes (Smith et al., 1995). If the patient's drainage exceeds 100 ml per hour and appears to be increasing, notify the physician. Once the drainage slows, monitoring may be performed every 2 hours. Marking on the collection chamber with a permanent marker or using tape is helpful in detecting trends in the patient's drainage. Mark the amount, date, and time of the measurement using the marking pen or affix a piece of tape with the same information. The amount, color, and consistency of drainage should be documented.

At least every 4 hours, monitor the water levels in the suction control chamber and the water seal chamber. With time, water will evaporate from the suction control chamber, and addition of water will be required to maintain the subambient pressure level. If the chamber becomes overfilled, most drainage systems have a diaphragm or port where fluid may be removed from the suction control chamber (Pettinicchi, 1998).

Proper water level (2 cm H_2O) is very important in the water seal chamber. Too much water in the chamber makes it more difficult for air or fluid to drain, whereas too little water increases the risk of entry of atmospheric air into the patient's thoracic cavity. If the water level in the water seal chamber increases (without addition of water by yourself), too much vacuum is being applied to the system. Press and hold the negative-pressure relief valve (usually located on the top of most drainage systems) to relieve the excess pressure (Pettinicchi, 1998). Once the pressure is relieved, the water level will return to normal.

Identifying and Correcting Leaks

Leaks in the chest drainage system are potentially dangerous because ambient air may enter through leaks in the system into the patient's thoracic cavity. Therefore, it is important for you to be able to identify and correct leaks.

During normal operation, the water seal chamber will periodically bubble. As air is drawn from the pleural space, it passes through the collection chamber and then bubbles through the water seal chamber. You can even notice the water level in the water seal chamber rise and fall with ventilation. The level rises during spontaneous exhalation and falls during inspiration. This slight change in fluid level is due to changes in pressure within the thoracic cavity with ventilation. If the patient is on mechanical ventilation, during inspiration the level rises (positive intrapleural pressure) and during exhalation it will fall. This normal rise and fall of the fluid level is termed "tidaling" (Carroll, 1995).

Continuous bubbling in the water seal chamber is a sign of a leak. It is important to distinguish whether the leak is the patient's chest (intrathoracic) or in the system, external to the patient. External leaks can be corrected. To differentiate the location of the leak, momentarily clamp the chest tube where it exits the patient's chest. Only clamp the chest tube briefly, using a toothless clamp or one protected with tape or rubber guards. If the bubbling stops, the leak is within the patient's chest. Sometimes air leaks are common with some thoracic surgical procedures (e.g., bullectomies, lobectomies). If bubbling persists, now you must check the drainage system.

Move the clamp to just below the joint between the patient's chest tube and the surgical tubing. Briefly clamp this location and observe the water seal chamber. If the bubbling stops, your leak is at that joint. Remove the tape, make sure the connector is tightly inserted into both the chest tube and the surgical tubing and retape the joint. Repeat the clamp test to ensure that the leak has stopped. If bubbling persists when this location is clamped, the leak is distal to the point it was clamped.

Move distal from the patient, clamping the surgical tubing briefly in about 10-cm increments. If the bubbling stops, you have identified a leak in the tubing. Have the patient exhale and hold the breath. Clamp the chest tube about 4 to 6 cm from the point where the tube exits the patient's chest, using a protected clamp. Place a second clamp 2.5 cm distal to the first. Now you may aseptically change the tubing. Once the tubing is changed, remove the clamps and have the patient resume normal ventilation. If you progressively move along the entire length of the tubing and bubbling persists, the leak is in the drainage system.

To change the drainage system, set up a new system by initially filling the suction control and water seal chambers with water to their proper levels. Instruct the patient to exhale and then hold the breath. Clamp the chest tube with a protected or toothless clamp. Place a second padded clamp 2.5 cm distal to the first and clamp the chest tube again. Aseptically change the drainage system. Remove the clamps and instruct the patient to resume normal ventilation. Record the initial drainage and assure yourself that the new unit is functioning properly.

References

Carroll, P. (1995). Chest tubes made easy. *RN, 58*(12), 46–55.

Carroll, P. (2000). Exploring chest drain options. *RN, 63*(10), 50–52.

McMahon-Parkes, K. (1997). Management of pleural drains. *Nursing Times, 24*(52).

Pettinicchi, T. A. (1998, March). Troubleshooting chest tubes. *Nursing 1998,* 58–59.

Schiff, L. (2000). Market choices. Chest drainage systems. *RN, 63*(10), 57–58.

Smith, R. N., Fallentine, J., & Kessel, S. (1995). Underwater chest drainage bringing the facts to the surface. *Nursing '95, 25*(2), 60–63.

Practice Activities: Chest Tubes

1. Have your laboratory partner critique your aseptic technique while you prepare a chest tube insertion tray for use.

2. Properly prepare a chest drainage system for use:
   a. Fill the suction control chamber with water.
   b. Fill the water seal chamber with water.
   c. Connect the unit to a vacuum regulator.

3. Use a resuscitation mannequin as a "patient." With your laboratory partner, role play the parts of a physician inserting a chest tube and a respiratory care practitioner assisting in the procedure.
   a. Prepare the chest tube insertion tray for use.
   b. Draw up local anesthetic (4% lidocaine).
   c. Assist the physician with surgical prep and draping.
   d. Assist the physician by passing instruments.
   e. Assist the physician with placement of the sterile airtight dressings.
   f. Assist the physician by connecting the newly placed chest tube with the drainage system.

4. With your laboratory instructor, view several chest x-rays of patients who have chest tubes placed. Determine if the tube is for a pneumothorax, pleural drainage, or mediastinal drainage.

5. Monitor a chest drainage system:
   a. Drainage
   b. Suction control chamber water level
   c. Water seal chamber water level

6. Using a resuscitation mannequin as a patient, practice troubleshooting a chest drainage system:

   a. Determine if the leak is within the patient's thorax or the drainage system.
   b. Troubleshoot the system for leaks.

7. Using a blank sheet of paper, practice what you would chart when monitoring a chest drainage system. When you have finished, have your laboratory instructor critique your charting.

Check List: Chest Tubes

_____ 1. Wash your hands.
2. Assemble the required equipment:
_____ a. Chest tube insertion tray
_____ b. Local anesthetic and syringes
_____ c. Chest tubes
_____ d. Chest drainage system
_____ e. Vacuum regulator
3. Prepare the chest drainage system for use:
_____ a. Fill the suction control chamber.
_____ b. Fill the water seal chamber.
_____ c. Connect the vacuum regulator to a wall source.
_____ d. Connect the chest drainage system to the vacuum regulator and check the system for operation.
4. Prepare the chest tube insertion tray for use:
_____ a. Aseptically open the tray, creating a sterile field.
_____ b. Draw up topical anesthetics.
_____ c. Organize supplies for easy retrieval and access.

5. Assist the physician with the procedure:
_____ a. Assist with surgical prep and draping.
_____ b. Assist by passing instruments.
_____ c. Assist with placement of the sterile airtight dressings.
_____ d. Assist by connecting the newly placed chest tube with the drainage system.
6. Monitor the drainage system:
_____ a. Drainage output
_____ b. Water level in the suction control chamber
_____ c. Water level in the water seal chamber
7. Assess the chest drainage system for leaks:
_____ a. Determine if the leak is intrathoracic (patient) or in the chest drainage system.
_____ b. If the leak is in the drainage system, systematically identify it.
_____ 8. Following the procedure, clean up the area by disposing of unused and opened supplies.
_____ 9. Wash your hands.
_____ 10. Document the procedure in the patient's chart.

Self-Evaluation Post Test: Chest Tubes

1. Indications for placement of a chest drainage system for fluid drainage include:
   I.   coronary artery bypass graft surgery.
   II. pleural effusion.
   III. pneumothorax.
   IV. blunt chest trauma.
   a. I
   b. I, II
   c. III
   d. III, IV

2. Indications for placement of a chest tube for removal of air include:
   I.   coronary artery bypass graft surgery.
   II. pleural effusion.
   III. pneumothorax.
   IV. blunt chest trauma.
   a. I
   b. I, II
   c. III
   d. III, IV

3. A chest tube placed for evacuation of air would be:
   I.   placed at the second or third intercostal space.
   II. placed at the fourth or lower sixth intercostal space.
   III. directed superiorly toward the apex.
   IV. directed inferiorly toward the base.

   a. I, III
   b. I, IV
   c. II, III
   d. II, IV

4. A chest tube placed for fluid evacuation would be:
   I.   placed at the second or third intercostal space.
   II. placed at the fourth or lower sixth intercostal space.
   III. directed superiorly toward the apex.
   IV. directed inferiorly toward the base.
   a. I, III
   b. I, IV
   c. II, III
   d. II, IV

5. Which of the following chambers regulates the amount of subambient pressure applied to the patient's chest?
   a. Collection chamber
   b. Water seal chamber
   c. Suction control chamber
   d. Vacuum regulator

6. Which of the following chambers prevents ambient air from entering the patient's thoracic cavity?
   a. Collection chamber
   b. Water seal chamber
   c. Suction control chamber
   d. Vacuum regulator

7. When monitoring the chest drainage system for a postoperative thoracotomy patient, you find the water seal chamber is filled to 8 cm H_2O. As a respiratory care practitioner, you should:
   a. ignore it because the levels should range between 5 and 20 cm H_2O.
   b. press and hold the negative-pressure relief valve.
   c. ensure that the chamber is filled to 2 cm H_2O.
   d. Both b and c.

8. Too much water in the water seal chamber:
   I. inhibits air/fluid from being evacuated from the chest.
   II. facilitates evacuation of air/fluid from the chest.
   III. causes more pressure having to be generated for air/fluid to be removed.
   IV. causes less pressure having to be generated for air/fluid to be removed.

   a. I, III
   b. I, IV
   c. II, III
   d. II, IV

9. Vigorous bubbling in the suction control chamber:
   a. is required to maintain adequate subambient pressure.
   b. may result in excess subambient pressure being applied to the chest.
   c. may cause increased evaporation of water.
   d. None of the above.

10. Constant bubbling in the water seal chamber:
    a. is normal and should be ignored.
    b. is a sign of a leak.
    c. indicates that too much pressure is being applied at the vacuum regulator.
    d. indicates that the suction control chamber is filled too much.

PERFORMANCE EVALUATION:
CHEST TUBES

Date: Lab _____ Clinical _____ Agency _____

Lab: Pass _____ Fail _____   Clinical: Pass _____ Fail _____

Student name _____ Instructor name _____

No. of times observed in clinical _____

No. of times practiced in clinical _____

PASSING CRITERIA: Obtain 90% or better on the procedure. Tasks indicated by * must receive at least 1 point, or the evaluation is terminated. Procedure must be performed within designated time, or the performance receives a failing grade.

SCORING:

2 points — Task performed satisfactorily without prompting.
1 point — Task performed satisfactorily with self-initiated correction.
0 points — Task performed incorrectly or with prompting required.
NA — Task not applicable to the patient care situation.

TASKS:	PEER	LAB	CLINICAL
1. Washes hands	☐	☐	☐
2. Assembles the required equipment			
a. Chest tube insertion tray	☐	☐	☐
b. Local anesthetic and syringes	☐	☐	☐
c. Chest tubes	☐	☐	☐
d. Chest drainage system	☐	☐	☐
e. Vacuum regulator	☐	☐	☐
* 3. Prepares the chest drainage system for use			
a. Fills the suction control chamber	☐	☐	☐
b. Fills the water seal chamber	☐	☐	☐
c. Connects the regulator to a wall source	☐	☐	☐
d. Connects the chest drainage system to the vacuum regulator and checks the system for operation	☐	☐	☐
4. Prepares the chest tube insertion tray for use			
a. Opens the tray, creating a sterile field	☐	☐	☐
b. Draws up topical anesthetics	☐	☐	☐
c. Organizes supplies for easy retrieval	☐	☐	☐
5. Assists the physician with the procedure			
a. Assists with surgical prep and draping	☐	☐	☐
b. Assists by passing instruments/supplies	☐	☐	☐
c. Assists with placing the dressings	☐	☐	☐
d. Connects the chest tube to the drainage system	☐	☐	☐

6. Monitors the drainage system
   a. Drainage output ☐ ☐ ☐
   b. Water level in the suction control chamber ☐ ☐ ☐
   c. Water level in the water seal chamber ☐ ☐ ☐
7. Assesses the chest drainage system for leaks
   a. Determines if the leak is intrathoracic or in the chest drainage system ☐ ☐ ☐
   b. Identifies the leak's location in the system ☐ ☐ ☐
8. Cleans up the area ☐ ☐ ☐
9. Washes hands ☐ ☐ ☐
10. Documents the procedure in the patient's chart ☐ ☐ ☐

SCORE: Peer _____ points of possible 50; _____%

Lab _____ points of possible 50; _____%

Clinical _____ points of possible 50; _____%

TIME: _____ out of possible 45 minutes

STUDENT SIGNATURES.

PEER: _____

STUDENT: _____

INSTRUCTOR SIGNATURES

LAB: _____

CLINICAL: _____

CHAPTER 23

INSERTION AND MAINTENANCE OF INTRAVENOUS LINES

Stephen S. Pitts
David A. Field

INTRODUCTION

The insertion and maintenance of peripheral intravenous (IV) catheters constitute an advanced skill practiced by many respiratory care practitioners today. For safe and effective technique in clinical practice, both an understanding of the theory of IV administration and a comprehensive training program are necessary.

In this chapter you will learn the theory behind IV therapy as well as the specifics of IV insertion and maintenance and associated complications.

KEY TERMS

- Air embolism
- Butterfly catheter
- Catheter shear or catheter fragment embolism
- Cellulitis
- Chevron
- gtt
- Hypertonic solution
- Hypotonic solution
- Infiltration
- Infusion pumps
- Isotonic solution
- KVO
- Over-the-needle catheter
- Patency
- Phlebitis
- prn
- Thrombus
- TKO
- Wheal

OBJECTIVES

At the end of this chapter, you should be able to:

- Explain the rationale(s) for the insertion of intravenous (IV) needles, to include:
  - The administration of medications on a continuous or prn (as needed) basis
  - The administration of fluids to maintain normal hydration of the patient
  - The administration of fluids in the presence of shock
  - The administration of blood and blood products
- Differentiate among isotonic, hypertonic, and hypotonic solutions, and explain their effects on the vascular system and the cells of the body.
- Describe the procedure for locating an acceptable anatomical site for the insertion of an IV needle.
- Describe the complications associated with the insertion and maintenance of an IV line.
- Explain the steps associated with the maintenance of an existing IV line and how to correct problems with the line.
- Perform calculations necessary to run a solution at the prescribed rate.

This section deals with the reasoning and indications for intravenous catheter placement and the maintenance of the solutions that can be infused through them.

THE PRINCIPLES OF INTRAVENOUS THERAPY

Intravenous access is established in a patient for a variety of reasons. These include the administration of medications over a long-term period as an infusion, or as a single dose given as needed (*prn*). Both methods of medication administration are made easier and more comfortable for the patient if an indwelling intravenous catheter is in place. The existence of this catheter eliminates the necessity of repeated injections that can be both painful and frightening to the patient.

Another reason for the establishment of an IV line is to help maintain the normal fluid status of the patient. It is not uncommon for a patient who is unable to eat or drink normally to become dehydrated and need the assistance of intravenous "feedings." Patients who are under long-term care and continue to be unable to maintain normal caloric intake can be given intravenous infusions that include all of the necessary electrolytes, fatty acids, and carbohydrates, as well as fluid to maintain a homeostatic state.

In the presence of shock, whether it be from hypovolemia, sepsis, anaphylaxis, or any other cause, normal tissue perfusion can be drastically altered and in severe cases cease completely. With the aid of the IV line, fluids, blood, and blood products can be infused to assist in returning the body to its normal state.

Blood and blood products, such as plasma, packed red blood cells, and platelets, can also be administered through an established IV line. In the case of a patient who may require many such transfusions, the presence of a patent catheter makes such procedures very easy and expedient.

INTRAVENOUS FLUID PROPERTIES

There are numerous types of IV fluids that are available for both direct undiluted infusion, and as the diluent in medication administration. Examples of these include D₅W (5% dextrose in water), lactated Ringer's solution (which contains electrolytes and lactate as a buffer), normal (physiologic) saline (0.9% sodium chloride [NaCl] in water), and many combinations of these, such as D₅–0.45% NaCl and D₅–LR.

Many medications will become inactivated or their action decreased if they are mixed in the incorrect solution. Proper use of these medications requires that they be mixed only in a specific solution. For example, the anticoagulant heparin is mixed with D₅W for administration to the patient.

Most of the IV solutions that are used for mixing medications and for fluid replacement are isotonic with extracellular fluid (that is, they have the same tonicity as measured by solute concentration). With the administration of an *isotonic solution*, there is very little if any net movement of fluid into or out of the cells. This is most desirable for maintaining a normal environment for cellular function. A *hypertonic solution* will cause water to be drawn from inside the cell and into the vascular space. This effect may be desirable in cases of cerebral edema or fluid retention due to renal failure or overhydration. An example of a hypertonic solution is mannitol, which is used in some head injury cases. A *hypotonic solution*, which has a solute concentration lower than that of the fluid inside the cells, will result in a net movement of water from the vascular space to inside the cell. This effect may be helpful in cases of severe dehydration where the function of cells is hampered owing to the absence of necessary intracellular fluid. A 0.225% NaCl solution is considered a hypotonic solution.

LOCATING ACCEPTABLE SITES FOR INTRAVENOUS NEEDLE PLACEMENT

In assessing a possible site for IV needle insertion, several factors must be taken into consideration. Many times, the IV line will remain for an extended period of time. This may be dictated by the length of stay of the patient, hospital policy regulating the length of time that an IV may remain in place, the failure of an IV to remain patent, or any combination of the above. When the IV site is chosen, it should be assumed that the site will remain for an extended period of time, and the location chosen accordingly.

A basic knowledge of the location of the major superficial veins that are generally used for IV cannulation is very helpful. Figure 23-1 shows the location of many of these vessels and where they are located on the lower

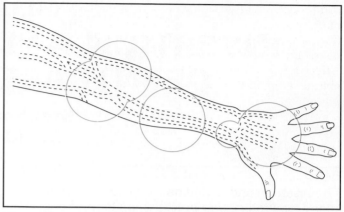

Figure 23-1 *The major veins of the forearm are good sites for insertion of IV catheters. The areas within the circles are common sites that are used.*

portion of the arm. Although IV catheters can be placed in the leg or foot in adults, and in a scalp vein in newborns and infants, these sites carry their own special considerations and are not addressed here.

In choosing a site, it is preferable to select the nondominant hand or arm of the patient (i.e., the left arm of a right-handed patient). This will allow the patient to be less restricted in performing normal daily functions. It is also suggested that the catheter be placed in a location that does not "stick out" or extend away from the extremity in such a manner that it will be constantly bumped or jarred and consequently disrupt the *patency* of the IV.

Areas directly over joints and bony prominences are less desirable sites, as it is possible to make contact with the bone during insertion of the IV needle. This can lead to infection and is also quite painful. Catheter positions on the inside of a joint, or in the area that forms the "crease" in a joint, are also not the first sites of consideration owing to problems created when the joint is moved. This could lead to "kinking" of the catheter, which could restrict or stop the flow of fluids. These sites also limit the range of motion for the patient.

Another consideration is the amount of pain experienced by the patient during the procedure of inserting the catheter into the vein. Generally, the underside of the lower arm and the inside of the wrist are more sensitive than the back of the hand, the anterior and inferior portions of the lower arm, and the inside of the elbow. Although some institutions require the use of a local anesthetic, this is not always the case, so consideration for the comfort of the patient is of importance.

With some medical conditions, a tourniquet cannot be applied to the patient's arm. These include the placement of a shunt for renal dialysis and a previous mastectomy. The extremity opposite the side affected by these conditions should be selected.

A tourniquet is applied above or proximal to the site that is selected for the insertion of the catheter. This restrictive band is usually made of rubber and can be either a flat band or a tubular piece of latex, such as a Penrose drain. Generally, a wider band of 1 inch to 1½ inches is more comfortable than a narrower ¼-inch or ½-inch band. A blood pressure cuff can also be used to occlude venous flow. The cuff is inflated so that it reads 20 to 30 mm Hg below the systolic number of the patient's blood pressure. After the placement of the tourniquet, you should be able to palpate the radial pulse distal to the tourniquet placement site.

To hold the tourniquet in place temporarily, make a loop around the patient's arm with one free end of the band. This end is then folded over itself and tucked under the other end of the tourniquet. It is important to leave the free end of the folded-over section exposed so that it may be grasped and pulled free to loosen the tourniquet when you desire to do so (Figure 23-2).

Once the tourniquet has been properly applied, the restriction of venous flow will cause the veins of the arm to distend and become engorged with blood. Visualization and palpation of the vessels will make the selection of a proper site possible. Select a site that is relatively straight and free of palpable "knots" or "Ys." These "knots" are valves in the vein that help to maintain the flow of blood in the correct direction; they will not allow the passage of the IV catheter. The bifurcations or "Ys" are junctions of two vessels and should be avoided.

The vessel should be large enough to accept the catheter that has been chosen. In situations where the IV line is being established strictly for the administration of medications, a smaller catheter may be acceptable. When large amounts of fluids or blood products will be given, a larger catheter may be desired, and a larger vessel is chosen. Again, the comfort of the patient should be taken into consideration, and a catheter no larger than necessary should be chosen for performing the procedure.

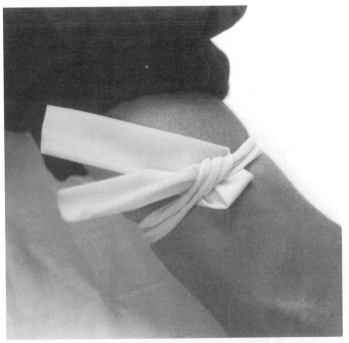

Figure 23-2 *This method of tying the tourniquet allows easy removal by grasping the end of the folded-over section and pulling quickly.*

COMPLICATIONS OF INTRAVENOUS THERAPY

With the practice of good aseptic technique and attention to detail in proper IV needle insertion, most "starts" will be accomplished without a great deal of difficulty. However, there are certain problems inherent to this procedure that may be unavoidable, and recognition of their existence is important to both the comfort and the safety of the patient.

Infiltration

Infiltration occurs when the fluid or medication that is being infused leaks out of the blood vessel that was cannulated. This results in a swelling at the site, which can be quite painful. This problem may be caused by a small laceration or puncture to the vessel incurred during the process of inserting the needle, or may be due simply to the vessel's inability to maintain its integrity owing to previous medications (i.e., steroids) or the structure of the vessel itself. In some circumstances, the IV line will continue to function, but this is not usually the case. The infusion should be discontinued, the IV catheter removed, direct pressure applied to the site for at least 5 minutes, and a new site selected for reinsertion of the IV.

Infiltration may also occur prior to attaching the IV fluids if the needle has been passed entirely through the vessel during the insertion, so that blood flows out of the puncture site. Many times, this will appear as a hematoma or bruise that is visible beneath the skin. Again, in this case, the catheter should be removed, direct pressure and a bandage applied, and another site chosen.

Thrombosis

After the successful introduction of an IV catheter, it is possible for a blood clot to form at the site of insertion, at the end of the catheter or in the cannulated vessel. This *thrombus* could break free and potentially become an embolus that may lodge in a smaller vessel of the lung or brain, creating the symptoms of pulmonary embolism or cerebrovascular accident (CVA or stroke).

Any complaint of pain, tenderness, or swelling at the IV site should be investigated thoroughly and evaluated for the possibility of thrombus formation. Gentle palpation at the site may reveal a mass or lump around or near the end of the catheter. Under many circumstances, the IV infusion will have slowed dramatically or stopped altogether. Under no circumstances should the clot be "flushed" or cleared by application of pressure to the IV bag or by use of a fluid-filled syringe to force the clot out of the catheter. A syringe can be attached to the IV tubing and negative pressure applied by drawing back on the plunger of the syringe to attempt to draw the clot out of the catheter and into the syringe. This technique should be attempted gently; if it is unsuccessful, discontinue the infusion, remove the catheter, dress the site appropriately, and obtain IV access elsewhere.

Phlebitis and Cellulitis

Phlebitis, or inflammation of the vein, may occur simply owing to the presence of a foreign body such as the IV catheter. *Cellulitis*, or an inflammation of the surrounding tissues, may also occur. These problems are not necessarily an indication of poor technique or infection. Both can be present with symptoms of tenderness, swelling, and possibly heat at the site. In these cases, the intravenous infusion may continue to run at its normal rate. However, if either is suspected, it is much better to discontinue the infusion, decannulate the vessel, dress the site, and attempt to locate another site for the infusion to be started.

Air Embolism

The infusion of approximately 50 cc of air into an IV line may be fatal to the normal adult. Care must be taken when assembling the tubing to the bag, and the subsequent flushing of the line, to ensure that all air is removed before the tubing is connected to the catheter. Maintaining the IV bag in an upright (vertical orientation) position at all times will also reduce the possibility of air entering the tubing, causing an *air embolism*. Most modern infusion pumps are equipped to detect the presence of air in the tubing and will alarm if the condition exists.

It is also possible for air to enter the tubing at any of the connections in the circuit, such as at the connection between the catheter and the tubing, or at the connection between an extension set and the primary IV tubing. If these connections are loose, air can be drawn into the circuit by the Venturi effect. Proper technique in assembling the IV tubing and any of its components, as well as ensuring that the tubing is attached tightly to the IV catheter, will help to prevent the aspiration of air into the circuit.

Catheter Shear or Catheter Fragment Embolism

During the placement of an IV needle, it is possible for the flexible catheter to become slightly bent or distorted after the metal stylet is removed. For this reason, the metal needle should never be reinserted or advanced back into the catheter. This may cut off or "shear" the end of the catheter, which may subsequently enter the vascular system, leading to problems discussed earlier. This complication is termed *catheter shear* or *catheter fragment embolism*.

MAINTENANCE OF INTRAVENOUS INFUSIONS

Once an IV infusion has been established, it is important that the site, the fluid level in the bag, and the rate of infusion be monitored. This will ensure that the site remains patent and that the IV infusion is running at the prescribed rate. With the widespread use of *infusion pumps*, the rate and the desired amounts to be given to the patient are easily programmed and then monitored by the pump. The indwelling catheter, however, must be visually inspected by the technician.

Each institution specifies predetermined lengths of time for which IV catheters may remain in place. This period of time varies, but is typically between 24 and 72 hours. You should become familiar with the policies in your facility that dictate this period of time. At the site of insertion, the date and time of the start, and your name or initials should be recorded on a piece of tape. This allows for easy identification of how long the IV line has been in place.

Inspection of the site should include looking to ensure that the infusion has not infiltrated, and that there are no signs of phlebitis or cellulitis. This visualization should include looking for any swelling, redness, or tenderness around the catheter. The infusion should be running at the correct rate, and the IV bag should contain the correct fluid and any additives that have been prescribed. If any problems are discovered, you should report them immediately to the person in charge of the patient's care.

DRIP RATE CALCULATIONS

In some instances, it may be necessary or desirable to run an IV infusion without the assistance of an infusion pump. It is therefore necessary that you be able to perform the appropriate calculations and run the infusion at the prescribed rate.

The terms *TKO* (to keep open) and *KVO* (keep vein open) can be used interchangeably and refer to a rate that is just fast enough to keep the infusion running and to prevent a clot from forming in the catheter. The type of infusion set that is being used will determine the correct rate. You should become familiar with the type and brand of sets in use at your institution, and with the number of drops (*gtt*) in the drip chamber that equal 1 ml for each type. Common drip sets and their drops per milliliter (gtt/ml) rates are minidrips, which produce 60 drops per milliliter, and macrodrips, which produce 10, 12, or 15 drops per milliliter. The sterile packages that contain the sets should have information printed on them to indicate the gtt/ml rate. Some sets have the number printed on the tabs next to the drip chamber. Rates of 10 to 15 drops per minute (gtt/min) with a 60 gtt/ml set will ensure that the vein will remain open and that the infusion will continue to run. Five to eight drops per minute is appropriate with the other administration sets.

There are two ways in which IV infusions are commonly ordered. The first is to infuse a set amount over a given period of time (e.g., 1 liter over 4 hours). The second is to run the infusion at a set rate per hour (e.g., 100 ml per hour). The formulas for calculating the infusion rate are very similar in both cases.

In the first instance, the *drops per minute* will equal the volume to be infused multiplied by the gtt/ml of the infusion set. The product is then divided by the total time the infusion is to run in minutes.

Example:

1 liter of 0.9% NaCl over 3 hours.

The administration set delivers 15 gtt/ml.

gtt/minute = 1000 ml × 15 gtt/ml/180 minutes
= approximately 84 gtt/ml

To figure a rate in *milliliters per hour*, the drops per minute equals the volume to be infused multiplied by the gtt/ml of the infusion set; the product is then divided by 60 minutes.

Example:

Lactated Ringer's to run at 100 ml per hour.

The administration set delivers 15 gtt/ml.

gtt/minute = 100 ml × 15 gtt/ml/60 minutes
= 25 gtt/ml

These simple formulas will work for all rates of infusion and administration sets, and the respiratory care practitioner should be familiar with them and be able to perform the calculations quickly.

OBJECTIVES

At the end of this chapter, you should be able to:

- Collect and assemble all of the equipment necessary for starting an intravenous infusion.

- Using a lab partner or a mannequin arm for simulation, demonstrate proper technique for the application of a tourniquet and selection of an appropriate IV insertion site.

- Demonstrate, using aseptic technique and standard precautions, the insertion of an intravenous needle and establishment of a patent IV.

- Demonstrate proper technique for securing the intravenous needle and the administration set to the patient.
- Demonstrate the proper disposal of all used and unused supplies.
- Demonstrate the calculations necessary to run the IV infusion at the prescribed rate, and adjust the flow of the IV accordingly.
- Demonstrate the steps for maintenance of an ongoing intravenous infusion.
- Demonstrate the steps for discontinuing an intravenous infusion.

A physician's order is required for this procedure to be performed. This order may be in the form of a protocol or given as the result of a consultation or examination. You should be familiar with the type of system in place in your facility.

SUPPLIES NEEDED FOR INTRAVENOUS CANNULATION

Prior to beginning the venipuncture technique, it is necessary to select and gather all of the necessary equipment to perform the procedure.

Needle Selection

An understanding of the numbering system for the size of IV catheters is necessary to help you select a range of catheters of appropriate size when planning to establish an IV line. The gauge of the portion of the catheter that remains in the vein is used. Catheters can range from as small as a tiny 27-gauge butterfly to a much larger 14-gauge polytetrafluoroethylene (Teflon) or plastic over-the-needle catheter. An easy rule to remember is the larger the number, the smaller the catheter.

There are several different types of intravenous needles available. Each type has its advantages and disadvantages and many have very specific uses in the clinical setting. This chapter deals only with the hollow butterfly needle and the over-the-needle types of catheters.

The *butterfly needle*, so named because of the plastic tabs that extend away from the needle much like a butterfly's wings, has a fairly limited use. Because the needle that remains in the vein is metal, it is possible for the vein to become lacerated or punctured with any movement or contact. These needles are also typically very small, for example, 25-gauge or 27-gauge. Their primary use is in infants and the elderly, who have very small veins and in whom the desired infusion rate of the IV is typically very slow. The needle must be secured in a very stable manner; an arm board can also be used to ensure that minimal movement of the extremity around the needle is allowed. These needles can also be used in the tiny scalp veins of infants.

The *over-the-needle catheter* is a plastic or Teflon sleeve that has a hollow metal needle running through its length. This allows for the use of the metal needle to initiate the insertion and obtain access to the lumen of the vein, but after the removal of this metal stylet, the only remaining portion is the flexible, relatively blunt catheter. These needles typically range in size from the very small 24-gauge up to a large-bore 14-gauge. The needle is usually two gauges smaller than the plastic catheter (e.g., an 18-gauge IV catheter uses a 20-gauge needle/stylet). Figure 23-3 shows a typical butterfly and an over-the-needle catheter.

When selecting the catheter to be used for the insertion, remember that the needle must be small enough to fit into the vein but large enough to allow the infusion to run at the prescribed rate. Experience, institution policy, and the advice of experienced coworkers will help in these decisions.

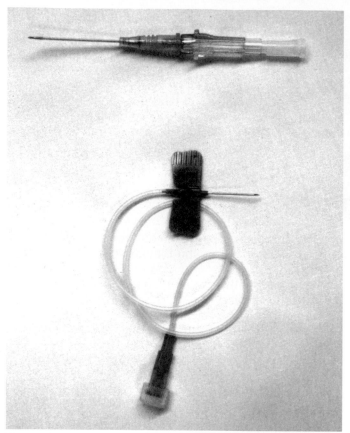

Figure 23-3 *Two common types of catheters are the butterfly (in the lower half of the figure), shown with the small tubing attached, and the over-the-needle type of catheter.*

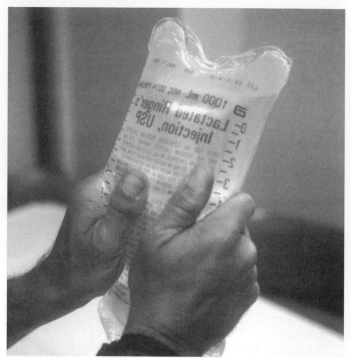

Figure 23-4 *Firmly squeezing the IV solution bag allows for the detection of any small holes in the container.*

Other Supplies

Preparation of all necessary equipment prior to the actual performance of the venipuncture will aid in making the process go smoothly. Knowledge of your institution's policies and procedures will help you to assemble correctly the administration set, including any extension tubing or T-connectors, and to perform the preferred method for anchoring the IV catheter to the patient.

If at all possible, the IV fluid and administration set should be prepared outside of the patient's room. This will help to avoid creating anxiety in the patient.

The prescribed fluid bag should be obtained. Prior to opening, confirm that the correct fluid is being selected, such as 0.9% NaCl (physiologic saline). The expiration date of the fluid should be visible through the opaque or transparent covering. Open the protective covering by tearing at the precut tab.

Inspect the integrity of the bag by squeezing it firmly to look for any small leaks (Figure 23-4). The fluid inside should be clear and free from particulate matter. At this time if there are any medications that need to be added, they can be injected into the port with the yellow rubber stopper, located either on the bottom of the bag or in the lower front portion.

Select the proper administration set. If an infusion pump will be used, make sure that the set is compatible with the pump to be used. Occlude the tubing by either closing the roller clamp or using one of the small slide clamps.

Remove the protective cap from the end with the drip chamber attached. Remove the protective cap from the IV bag. Insert the "spike" from the administration set into the port on the IV bag (Figure 23-5). Care must be used, as the plastic spike is very sharp and it is possible to push the spike through the side of the port where it may injure your hand or fingers.

Fill the drip chamber halfway by squeezing the chamber once or twice. Allow the flow to stop before unclasping the tubing, to help reduce the number of small air bubbles that enter the tubing. In the event that the chamber becomes overfilled, simply invert the chamber and the bag and then squeeze some of the fluid back into the bag.

Flush the administration tubing by releasing the roller or slide clamp. It may be necessary to remove the protective cap from the end of the set to allow the fluid to flow more freely. Care must be taken to not touch the end of the tubing, however, as it is sterile. Hold the end of the tubing lower than the bag to allow the fluid to flow. If a cassette for an infusion pump is in line, this portion of the tubing may have to be held inverted to clear all air and allow for proper function.

Once the entire tubing has been flushed, replace the protective cap on the male end, if it has been removed.

Another type of administration set that may be used is a heparin or saline lock. This allows for the administration of prn medications, without having a solution bag and administration tubing attached. The set consists of a male adapter plug that can be directly attached to the IV catheter or a short T-connector. The plug and any tubing

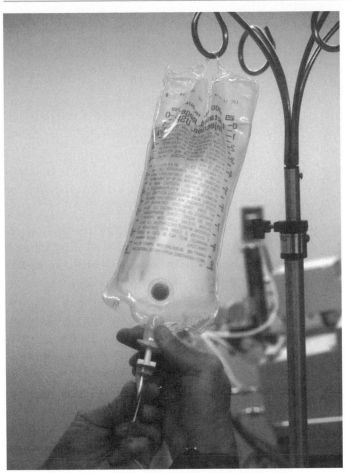

Figure 23-5 *Insertion of the spike of the administration set into the fluid bag allows fluid to flow into the tubing. Care must be taken, as the spike is sharp and can cause injury.*

attached to it must be flushed using a syringe filled with either normal saline solution or a very dilute heparin solution used specifically for heparin locks. Again, check with institution policy to see which is preferred.

There are commercial IV start kits that may be available. These kits include all of the necessary supplies except for gloves and the catheter itself.

If you need to assemble the necessary supplies yourself, here is a list of what you will need:

1. Protective gloves
2. Mask
3. Protective eyewear (in case of inadvertent splashing of blood)
4. A selection of IV catheters
5. Tape
6. Tourniquet
7. 2 × 2-inch gauze
8. Alcohol swabs
9. Povidone-iodine swabs
10. Sterile, transparent dressing for covering the insertion site
11. Local anesthetic, if required
12. Approved sharps container

Take all supplies to the patient's bedside. Organize the supplies in such a manner that all can be reached easily.

VENIPUNCTURE PROCEDURE

With practice, venipuncture can be accomplished quickly and professionally. Developing a plan or system that suits your preferences will help ensure success.

Standard Precautions

Blood and blood products are body fluids that require adherence to standard precautions. It is important to wear protective gloves, a mask, and eyewear to minimize the risk of acquiring an illness owing to inadvertent exposure to these fluids.

General Considerations

A physician's order is required before the performance of intravenous cannulation. The patient's chart should be reviewed for such an order. If your institution has established protocols covering IV insertion, you should be familiar with them.

The patient should be educated about the procedure and any questions answered prior to beginning. Many people have a fear of needles, and a professional, knowledgeable manner will help to alleviate some of this anxiety.

The patient should be asked about any allergies relating to iodine products and tape. There are many different types of tape that can be used to lessen reactions due to sensitivity or allergy. Alcohol only can be used if the patient has had previous reactions to iodine products.

It may be necessary to shave the arm of the patient with a safety razor, to remove hair that would interfere with securing the IV. An area approximately 2 inches square should be shaved around the planned insertion site.

Local Anesthetic Use

Many institutions require that a local anesthetic be used prior to the insertion of an IV needle. The puncture site should be prepared in the same manner as for IV insertion described later in the chapter. Draw up 0.1 to 0.2 ml of 2% lidocaine, without epinephrine, into a tuberculin syringe with a 25-gauge needle. Puncture the skin at the site chosen for IV placement. The needle should be in the dermal layer. Draw back on the plunger. If blood appears, the needle has entered a vessel and should be removed and moved to another location.

Slowly inject the anesthetic into the skin to produce a *wheal* at the site. The wheal should be approximately 1 cm in diameter. Withdraw the needle and dab any blood that may appear with a 2 × 2-inch gauze sponge. Allow 1 or 2 minutes before performing the venipuncture.

Do not recap the syringe. Place the used syringe in an approved sharps container.

Site Preparation

Once the equipment has been assembled and the procedure explained to the patient, a site for insertion of the catheter can be chosen. Wash your hands and don protective gloves.

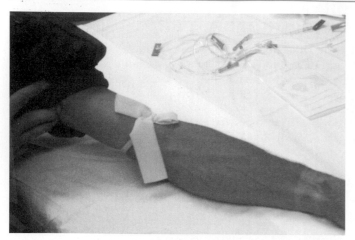

Figure 23-6 *The tourniquet is used to occlude venous flow, which distends the veins with blood. This allows for visualization and palpation of the vein to determine its usefulness for venipuncture.*

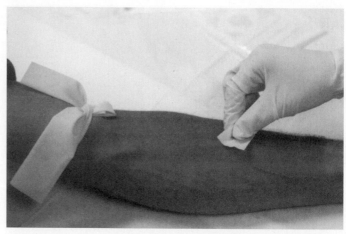

Figure 23-8 *The povidone-iodine is removed using an alcohol swab. When the site cleansing is complete, an area approximately 2 inches square will have been prepped.*

Apply the tourniquet above the location on the arm where you will be looking for an acceptable vein. In most cases the tourniquet can be placed above the elbow (Figure 23-6). This allows evaluation of the entire lower arm for suitable vessels. However, the tourniquet can be placed above the wrist or in the middle of the forearm.

After the application of the tourniquet, palpate for a radial pulse to ensure that arterial blood flow has not been occluded. Have the patient place the arm in a dependent position. The patient can also be asked to clench the fist several times, to aid in distending the veins.

Visually locate a vein that appears suitable. Gently palpate the vein with your finger for any valves or bifurcations. The distended vein should rebound quickly when palpated. If local anesthetic will be used, release the tourniquet, cleanse the area appropriately, and inject the anesthetic. After 1 or 2 minutes, reapply the tourniquet.

Cleanse the area chosen for insertion with the povidone-iodine solution. This should be done in a circular motion (Figure 23-7), beginning at the center and moving outward.

The povidone-iodine is removed using an alcohol swab (Figure 23-8). Begin at the top center of the area and wipe

toward the hand. Move to the side of the area just cleansed, and again wipe the swab from top to bottom. Continue this process until the entire area has been cleansed. The site chosen for insertion should be roughly in the center of this clean area.

Technique

Select an IV catheter of the appropriate size and remove the protective sleeve (Figure 23-9). Grasp the catheter in your dominant hand (Figure 23-10) with your fingers located on the plastic of the stylet. Do not grasp the hub of the catheter, as it will simply slide off of the needle when insertion is attempted. The bevel of the metal needle should be facing directly upward. In a well-lit room, the light will reflect off the bevel (Figure 23-11).

Using your other hand, apply gentle traction to the skin by pulling it toward the patient's hand. This will help to stabilize the vein and will prevent the skin from bunching up as the needle is inserted.

With the needle held at an angle of approximately 10° to 30° up from the skin (Figure 23-12), enter the skin with

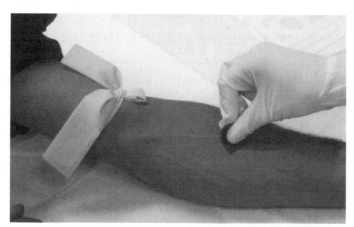

Figure 23-7 *The site chosen for venipuncture is cleansed with a povidone-iodine solution. This should be performed beginning at the center and proceeding outward in ever-widening circles.*

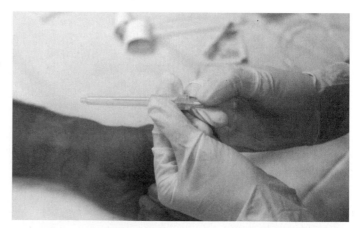

Figure 23-9 *Grasping the plastic portion of the catheter in one hand and the protective cover in the other, remove the cover by pulling in opposite directions.*

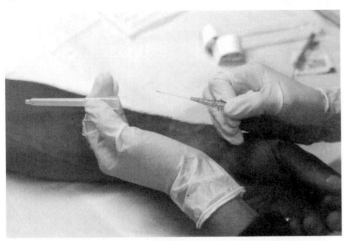

Figure 23-10 *After removal of the protective cover, maintain your fingers on the plastic portion of the stylet. Begin looking for the bevel of the needle.*

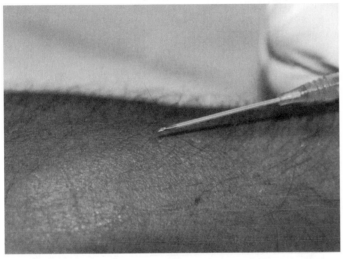

Figure 23-11 *With proper lighting, the bevel of the needle can be easily located and should be kept facing directly up from the patient's skin.*

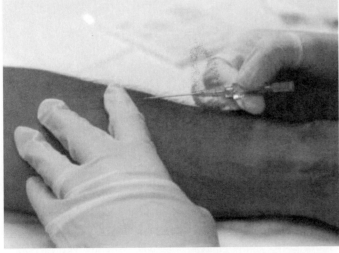

Figure 23-12 *The correct angle of insertion between the patient's skin and the needle is between 10° and 30°.*

a quick, firm motion (Figure 23-13). Remember that you are attempting not to enter the vein at this point but simply to get through the dermal layers.

While maintaining the same or slightly shallower angle from the skin, advance the needle toward the vein. A "flash" of blood in the clear chamber of the catheter (Figure 23-14) indicates that the vessel has been entered. It is also common to feel a slight "pop" as the needle enters the vein. Advance the entire needle approximately 5 to 10 mm to ensure that the catheter has also entered the vein. Care must be taken at this point so that the needle is not allowed to go through the opposite wall of the vein, resulting in infiltration. The angle of the needle can be lowered to help prevent this.

The nondominant hand can now release traction on the skin and grasp the hub of the catheter. Gently slide the catheter off of the needle/stylet and advance it until the front part of the hub is in contact with the skin. Do not withdraw

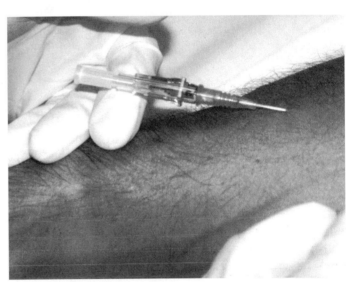

Figure 23-13 *The initial step of insertion is to get the needle through the dermal layers of the skin, not directly into the vein.*

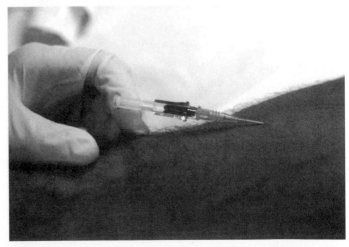

Figure 23-14 *As the needle enters the vein, blood will appear in the flash chamber of the needle. The entire unit should then be advanced about 1 cm.*

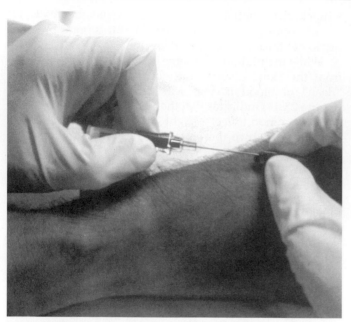

Figure 23-15 *After the hub of the catheter has been advanced so that it is touching the skin, remove the stylet with one hand while applying pressure on the skin over the end of the catheter with the other hand.*

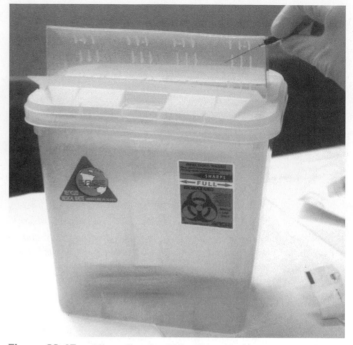

Figure 23-17 *All needles should be disposed of in an approved sharps container.*

the needle as you are doing this (Figure 23-15), as it provides direction and stabilization for the flexible catheter.

With the nondominant hand, reach up and grasp the folded-over end of the tourniquet, and with a quick pull, remove the tourniquet.

After the catheter is in place, with the hub against the skin, one or two fingers of the nondominant hand should be firmly placed on the skin (Figure 23-16), over the area where the end of the plastic catheter is lying. This will help to prevent a rush of blood out of the catheter when the needle is removed.

Remove the needle/stylet with the dominant hand and place it in the sharps container (Figure 23-17). Place a 2 × 2-inch gauze sponge under the hub of the catheter to catch any blood that may leak out. Grasp the end of the administration set or male adapter plug and remove the protective cover. (This may sound like you need three hands, but with practice, it can be done with two quite easily.)

Insert the end of the tubing or plug into the hub of the catheter and, with a slight twisting motion, push the two together (Figure 23-18).

While holding the catheter in place, open the roller clamp slowly. Watch the drip chamber for evidence of flow. If it appears that the IV infusion is not running, the catheter tip may be against the vessel wall, impeding the flow. Slowly withdraw the catheter, up to 1 cm, while watching

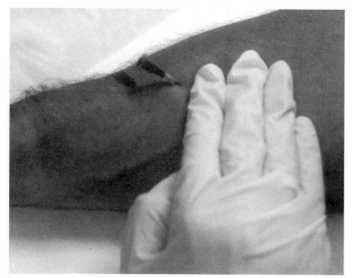

Figure 23-16 *Firm pressure applied over the end of the catheter with your fingertips will prevent the free flow of blood from the end of the catheter.*

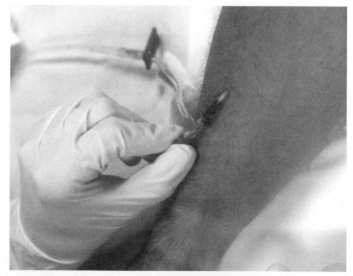

Figure 23-18 *Attach the end of the administration set tubing into the hub of the catheter. This can be done with a slight twisting motion to ensure a patent, leak-free connection.*

the drip chamber. When good flow is obtained, discontinue withdrawing the catheter and hold it in position.

Cover the site with the sterile, transparent dressing. The dressing should cover only the hub of the catheter and the actual puncture site (Figure 23-19). Do not cover the end of the administration tubing. This allows for easy change of the tubing if necessary without the risk of disengaging the catheter from the vessel.

During the next steps, care must be taken that the patient does not move the extremity. Explain to the patient that you are going to tape the IV catheter in place. Gross movement may dislodge the IV, as it is being kept in place only by the transparent dressing.

Slide a ½-inch-wide piece of tape, approximately 3 inches long, under the end of the tubing where it connects to the catheter, sticky side facing up, centering the tubing and hub in the piece of tape. Cross one end of the tape over the tubing and stick the tape to the patient's skin. Cross the remaining end over and stick it to the skin. This taping pattern, called a *chevron*, helps to secure the end of the tubing and the hub of the catheter in place (Figure 23-20). Place a 2-inch piece of tape over the chevron, securing it to the patient. Approximately 1 to 2 inches from the first piece of tape, place another 2-inch piece of tape across the tubing.

Make either a half loop or a full loop out of the administration tubing (Figure 23-21), and secure it with tape. This excess tubing serves as a safety device in case the tubing is inadvertently pulled. The loop changes the direction of pull so that the catheter is not pulled in the opposite direction in which it was inserted.

At this time, either place the cassette in the pump and begin administering the fluids, or adjust the roller clamp so that the fluid flows at the prescribed rate. The calculations necessary should have been performed prior to the beginning of the insertion procedure.

If it is necessary to place an arm board to prevent the catheter from being occluded secondary to patient movement, do so at this time. The board should be padded for patient comfort and should be long enough to extend both above and below the insertion site far enough to prevent movement. When taping the board in place, do so in a manner that does not restrict the flow of blood or the fluid infusing from the IV.

An important element to remember in securing the tubing and catheter in place is that tape should not cover any of the Y injection ports located in the tubing. These sites are for administration of medications into the tubing and should be left uncovered.

Explain to the patient that the procedure is complete. Educate the patient about signs and symptoms that may indicate that an infiltration, phlebitis, or cellulitis is beginning. Have the patient alert the care provider of any pain, swelling, or redness that may occur. Also give the patient time to address any questions or concerns that he or she may have.

Make sure that all used needles have been placed in an approved container. Collect all used supplies and their wrappers, protective covers, and so on, and place them in the appropriate waste containers. Clean up any spilled

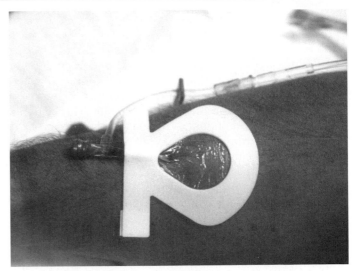

Figure 23-19 *A sterile transparent dressing should cover the site of insertion. This allows for continuing inspection of the site for any redness or swelling.*

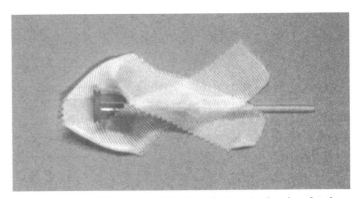

Figure 23-20 *A chevron results when the tape is placed under the catheter hub sticky side up and the ends of the tape are then criss-crossed over the catheter hub.*

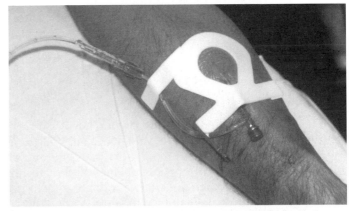

Figure 23-21 *Reserving a loop of tubing secured adequately with tape will help to prevent the inadvertent dislodging of the catheter.*

blood with the approved antiseptic cleaner. Remember that any items contaminated with blood or body fluids should be placed in a biohazard waste container. Remove your gloves, wash your hands, and record the procedure in the patient's chart. Local policy will dictate the manner in which this is done.

MAINTENANCE OF INTRAVENOUS INFUSIONS

The IV infusion line should be checked on a regular basis to ensure that the infusion is running properly, that the fluid level in the bag is appropriate, and that there are no signs of impending problems with the site. These checks also allow for the changing of tubing as it is required.

When performing the maintenance of IV infusions, attempt to develop a routine that will allow you to perform these checks in a timely and efficient manner. In this routine, the fluid level of the IV solution should be checked. If it is necessary to change the fluid, obtain a new bag of solution and confirm that it is clear, not outdated, and the correct type of fluid. Open the protective bag and remove the solution. Clamp the administration set tubing with either the roller clamp or a slide clamp. Remove the protective plug or cap from the new bag. Holding the drip chamber in an upright position, tip the solution bag upside down and pull the drip chamber "spike" from the bag. Inverting the solution bag will prevent any remaining fluid from running out when the drip chamber is removed. Reinsert the drip chamber spike into the new solution bag. Hang the bag and reset the correct drip rate using the roller clamp.

Ensure that the administration set tubing does not need to be changed. Many institutions use color-coded labels or dated labels to track how long a tubing has been in use. If the tubing need to be changed, obtain a new administration set that matches the one currently being used. Prepare a small syringe, 1 ml or 3 ml, by filling it with the same fluid that is being infused into the patient. This can be done by withdrawing the fluid from one of the ports on the side or bottom of the IV solution bag. Remove the needle, dispose of it in the sharps container, and set the syringe aside where it can be easily reached. Take care not to contaminate the syringe hub. A male adapter plug can be used in place of the syringe, if this adheres to hospital policy. Remember that the plug must be flushed with solution to remove any air before it is used. Wash your hands and put on protective gloves, a mask, and eye protection.

After clamping the tubing closed, begin to remove the tape from the tubing beginning at the end nearer the solution bag. As you get closer to the hub of the catheter and the end of the tubing, take care that you do not inadvertently pull the catheter from the vein. Once all of the tape has been removed from the tubing, gently pull the end of the tubing from the hub of the catheter. While you are doing this, use one or two fingers to apply pressure to the skin over the end of the catheter to prevent the flow of blood from the catheter hub. Place the syringe or male adapter plug into the hub of the catheter.

Invert the solution bag, remove the old administration set, and dispose of it in a biohazard waste container. Remove the protective cover from the "spike" of the new set and insert it into the solution bag. Squeeze the drip chamber until it is half full and flush the air from the tubing by opening the clamp and allowing the solution to flow. Reattach the tubing to the catheter hub, after removing the syringe or plug, and retape the tubing to secure it to the patient. Clean up any spilled fluid or blood; remove your gloves, mask, and eyewear; and wash your hands again.

DISCONTINUING INTRAVENOUS THERAPY

IV therapy can be discontinued for any number of reasons. You should be familiar with how to remove the catheter and dress the site to minimize patient discomfort, prevent unnecessary hematoma formation, and help prevent infection.

Once the decision has been made to remove the catheter, the procedure is quite simple. Aseptic technique and standard precautions should be observed.

After washing your hands and putting on protective gloves, a mask, and eyewear, clamp the IV tubing to discontinue the flow of the solution. Open one or two packages of sterile 2 × 2-inch gauze sponges and have them easily accessible. Begin untaping the tubing from the patient's arm. When the tape is removed, carefully peel the edges of the transparent dressing away from the patient's skin. It is not necessary to remove the dressing from the hub of the catheter, as attempting to do so may inadvertently pull the catheter out.

Once the tubing and catheter are no longer secured to the patient, place a folded 2 × 2-inch sponge over the insertion site and press gently. Grasp the hub of the catheter and quickly pull it from the skin. Continue to press firmly over the insertion site to help minimize bleeding both at the skin and at the vessel. You should continue to hold pressure over the site for at least 5 minutes.

Inspect the catheter that has been removed to ensure that it is intact. If you suspect that a portion of the catheter was not removed, immediately notify the person in charge of the patient's care.

After ensuring that the site is not actively bleeding, place a different folded 2 × 2-inch sponge over the site and secure it with a piece of tape. In some institutions it is acceptable to use an adhesive strip-type bandage in place of the 2 × 2-inch sponge.

Clean up the area that has been used and dispose of all supplies, including the IV bag, tubing, and catheter, in a biohazard waste container. Remove your gloves and wash your hands.

References

American Heart Association. (1994). *Advanced cardiac life support*. Dallas, TX: Author.

Caroline, N. L. (1993). *Emergency care in the streets* (3rd ed.). Boston: Little, Brown.

Grant, H. D., O'Keefe, M., Limmer, D., Murry, R., & Bergeron, J. (1990). *Brady emergency care*. Englewood Cliffs, NJ: Prentice-Hall.

Additional Resources

Bruner, P. M., Sineltzer, S., & Bare, B. (1984). *Textbook of medical-surgical nursing*. Philadelphia: Lippincott.

Potter, P. (1987). *Basic nursing theory and practice*. St. Louis, MO: Mosby.

Saxton, D. F., Pelikan, P. K., Nugent, P. M., & Hyland, P. A. (1983). *Addison-Wesley manual of nursing practice*. Menlo Park, CA: Addison-Wesley.

Practice Activities: Intravenous Line Insertion and Maintenance

1. Prepare IV solution to be used:
   a. Identify proper solution per physician order.
   b. Open package (save package/bag).
   c. Recheck proper solution and expiration date.
   d. Gently squeeze bag to ensure there are no leaks.
   e. Remove the protective covering from the outlet port of the fluid bag.
   f. Hang the fluid bag on an IV pole or hook (use anything applicable).
   g. Remove protective covering from the spike/sharp end of the infusion tubing.
   h. Insert the sharp end of the infusion tubing into the uncovered port of the fluid bag (make sure that it is snug).
   i. Fill the infusion tubing drip chamber by squeezing it several times until the drip chamber is half filled.
   j. Remove the protective covering from the patient end of the infusion tubing, being careful not to touch this end and keeping it sterile.
   k. Making use of gravity and using the package/bag that the solution came in to catch the drips, allow the IV solution to flow freely out the patient end until all bubbles are cleared from the infusion tubing (*note*: watch for bubbles that collect in injection ports upstream).

2. Prepare and gather IV supplies:
   a. Lay all supplies needed close to where you will be performing the procedure:
      (1) IV pole with solution and tubing
      (2) Tourniquet
      (3) Razor
      (4) Povidone-iodine swab
      (5) Alcohol-based swab
      (6) IV catheter
      (7) Securing tape/holder

3. Prepare your patient:
   a. Set patient at ease.
   b. Explain what you are going to do.
   c. Explain why you are doing it.
   d. Position yourself and the patient comfortably.

4. Using a laboratory partner as your patient, perform the following for the listed venous puncture sites:
   a. Properly position the patient.
   b. Locate the probable insertion site.
   c. Palpate the site.
   Puncture sites:
      (1) Medial vein of the forearm
      (2) Radial vein in the wrist
      (3) Cephalic vein on the back of the hand

5. Apply a tourniquet to the arm to cause venous distention.
   a. Place a tourniquet 10 cm or 5 inches above the insertion site.
   b. Have partner clench and unclench fist several times.
   c. Palpate insertion site.
   d. Practice tying and releasing tourniquet several times.

6. Prepare insertion site:
   a. Wash your hands.
   b. Don latex gloves.
   c. Scrub area directly over the vein using a povidone-iodine swab. Move swab in ever-widening circles away from center of puncture site, out approximately 4 cm.
   d. Scrub area directly over the vein using an alcohol-based swab. Move the swab in ever-widening circles away from center of puncture site, out approximately 4 cm.

7. Prepare the IV catheter.
   a. Open the catheter in a manner that preserves its sterility. (Follow manufacturer's directions.)
   b. Remove catheter from the package using the two to three fingers that you will use to insert the catheter (take care not to touch the needle end of the catheter with your fingers).

8. Using a venous arm simulator:
   a. Practice preparing the IV solution to include when flushing the infusion tubing.
   b. Practice accumulating the supplies you will need.
   c. Observe standard precautions and aseptic technique.
   d. Practice placement of the tourniquet.
   e. Practice holding the catheter with your fingers.
   f. Practice the angle of catheter insertion.
   g. Practice your insertion skill.
   h. Practice removing the tourniquet.
   i. Practice hooking up the infusion tubing.
   j. Practice the proper disposal of sharps and waste.
   k. Practice the proper securing of the catheter.

Check List: Peripheral IV Insertion

1. Verify physician's order.
2. Check patient's chart for contraindications and pertinent information.
3. Gather supplies:
   a. Latex gloves
   b. Razor
   c. Povidone-iodine swab
   d. Alcohol-based swab
   e. Tourniquet
   f. IV fluid
   g. IV solution
   h. IV catheter of appropriate size
   i. Tape or securing system
   j. Sharps container
   k. Waste container
4. Wash your hands.
5. Don latex gloves.
6. Explain procedure to patient.
7. Position patient.
8. Position yourself.
9. Palpate arm for appropriate site:
   a. Medial vein of the forearm
   b. Radial vein of the wrist
   c. Cephalic vein on the back of the hand
10. Apply tourniquet.
11. Repalpate arm and choose a specific site.
12. Prep the site:
    a. Use a razor if hair will interfere.
    b. Use povidone-iodine swab.
    c. Use alcohol-based swab.
13. Open catheter package using sterile technique and position catheter for insertion.
14. Perform the IV puncture:
    a. Use correct angle (10° to 30° and aligned with vein).
    b. Ensure bevel is up.
    c. Penetrate skin.
    d. Advance needle to flashback.
    e. Advance catheter only into vein.
    f. Remove needle and place in sharps container.
    g. With free hand, apply firm pressure with fingers directly to the cannulated vein at least 2 cm above the hub.
15. Insert the infusion tubing into the hub of the catheter snugly.
16. Release tourniquet.
17. Release finger pressure of the free hand.
18. Secure catheter hub using sterile transparent dressing.
19. Secure infusion tubing to arm.
20. Run solution per physician's order.
21. Observe for complications:
    a. Infiltration
    b. Impaired flow of solution
22. Document procedure:
    a. Time
    b. Date
    c. Catheter size
    d. Site
    e. Number of attempts
    f. Solution used
    g. Rate of infusion

Self-Evaluation Post Test: Intravenous Line Insertion and Maintenance

1. Complications of peripheral IV insertion include:
   a. hematoma.
   b. air embolus.
   c. cellulitis.
   d. infection.
   e. All of the above

2. It is acceptable to have a few air bubbles left in your infusion tubing before hooking it up to the patient/catheter.
   a. True
   b. False

3. All of the following supplies will be required to insert an IV catheter except:
   a. scalpel.   d. tape.
   b. povidone-iodine swab.   e. sedative.
   c. IV catheter.

4. A tourniquet should be placed:
   a. between the puncture site and the shoulder.
   b. 6 to 12 cm above the puncture site.
   c. below the site.
   d. 5 to 10 cm above the puncture site.
   e. 3 to 4 cm above the puncture site.

5. Upon insertion, the bevel of the needle should be:
   a. up.
   b. down.
   c. to the side.

6. The proper angle of the IV insertion is:
   a. 30° to 60° and aligned with the vein.
   b. 10° to 30° degrees and aligned with the vein.
   c. 60° and aligned with the vein.
   d. 45° and aligned with the vein.
   e. <10° and aligned with the vein.

7. Which of the following is an indicator confirming that you are in the vein and that it is patent?
   a. Good flashback
   b. Little resistance to advancing catheter
   c. Free-running IV solution
   d. No infiltration into surrounding tissues
   e. All of the above

8. It is considered acceptable to take off one of your gloves to get a better feel for the vein.
   a. True
   b. False

9. After catheter insertion, but before tourniquet removal, finger pressure on the cannulated vein allows:
   a. for pain control.
   b. time for the infusion tubing to be attached before blood flow begins to back up.
   c. time to flush infusion tubing to get it ready.
   d. time for disposal of sharps.
   e. All of the above

10. When documenting an IV insertion, you should include:
    a. date/time.
    b. catheter/size.
    c. number of attempts.
    d. site.
    e. All of the above

Date: Lab _____ Clinical _____ Agency _____

Lab: Pass _____ Fail _____   Clinical: Pass _____ Fail _____

Student name _____ Instructor name _____

No. of times observed in clinical _____

No. of times practiced in clinical _____

PASSING CRITERIA: Obtain 90% or better on the procedure. Tasks indicated by * must receive at least 1 point, or the evaluation is terminated. Procedure must be performed within designated time, or the performance receives a failing grade.

SCORING:
2 points — Task performed satisfactorily without prompting.
1 point — Task performed satisfactorily with self-initiated correction.
0 points — Task performed incorrectly or with prompting required.
NA — Task not applicable to the patient care situation.

TASKS:

			PEER	LAB	CLINICAL
*	1.	Verifies physician's order	☐	☐	☐
	2.	Scans the chart	☐	☐	☐
*	3.	Gathers necessary supplies			
		a. Latex gloves	☐	☐	☐
		b. Razor	☐	☐	☐
		c. Iodine-based swab	☐	☐	☐
		d. Alcohol-based swab	☐	☐	☐
		e. Tourniquet	☐	☐	☐
		f. IV catheter	☐	☐	☐
		g. Securing tape/transparent sterile dressing	☐	☐	☐
		h. IV solution	☐	☐	☐
		i. Infusion tubing	☐	☐	☐
*	4.	Follows standard precautions, including handwashing	☐	☐	☐
*	5.	Dons gloves, mask, and protective eyewear	☐	☐	☐
*	6.	Prepares IV solution	☐	☐	☐
*	7.	Prepares infusion tubing without bubbles	☐	☐	☐
	8.	Positions self and patient	☐	☐	☐
	9.	Explains procedure to patient	☐	☐	☐
*	10.	Palpates probable sites	☐	☐	☐
*	11.	Applies tourniquet	☐	☐	☐
*	12.	Repalpates and chooses specific site	☐	☐	☐
*	13.	Prepares insertion site			
		a. Preps area with iodine-based swab	☐	☐	☐
		b. Cleans area with alcohol-based swab	☐	☐	☐

14. Prepares IV catheter
   - a. Opens package maintaining sterile catheter ☐ ☐ ☐
   - b. Holds catheter in fingers ☐ ☐ ☐

* 15. Inserts IV catheter
   - a. Bevel is up ☐ ☐ ☐
   - b. Correct angle is at 10° to 30° ☐ ☐ ☐
   - c. Advances to flashback ☐ ☐ ☐
   - d. Advances catheter into vein ☐ ☐ ☐
   - e. Removes needle to sharps container ☐ ☐ ☐
   - f. Applies finger pressure to vein proximal to site ☐ ☐ ☐

* 16. Inserts infusion tubing ☐ ☐ ☐

* 17. Removes tourniquet ☐ ☐ ☐

* 18. Secures catheter hub with tape ☐ ☐ ☐

* 19. Secures infusion tubing with tape ☐ ☐ ☐

* 20. Runs solution per physician's order ☐ ☐ ☐

* 21. Watches for complications ☐ ☐ ☐

22. Cleans up area and removes unused supplies ☐ ☐ ☐

* 23. Documents procedure ☐ ☐ ☐

SCORE: Peer _____ points of possible 70; _____%

Lab _____ points of possible 70; _____%

Clinical _____ points of possible 70; _____%

TIME: _____ out of possible 20 minutes

STUDENT SIGNATURES

PEER: _____

STUDENT: _____

INSTRUCTOR SIGNATURES

LAB: _____

CLINICAL: _____

CHAPTER 24
INTRA-AORTIC BALLOON PUMPING

Darren Powell

INTRODUCTION

Since its inception more than 30 years ago, intra-aortic balloon pumping (IABP) has become a powerful tool in the treatment of patients with cardiovascular disease. The role of IABP therapy is to provide left ventricular support to the critically ill patient. The environment in which IABP is utilized is often stressful. A solid understanding of the principles and steps involved in IABP will help you to perform the tasks required in this stressful critical care environment.

KEY TERMS

- Afterload
- Cardiac output
- Coronary artery disease
- Counterpulsation
- Intra-aortic balloon
- Intra-aortic balloon pump
- Left heart
- Left ventricular dysfunction
- Myocardial contractility
- Preload
- Right heart
- Valvular pathology

OBJECTIVES

At the end of this chapter, you should be able to:

- Describe the cardiac anatomy and physiology.
- Define how changes in preload, afterload, and myocardial contractility affect the cardiac output.
- Differentiate between myocardial oxygen supply and demand.
- Identify pathological states requiring intra-aortic balloon pumping therapy.

CARDIAC ANATOMY

The Pump

The heart is a four-chambered organ designed to receive, pressurize, and pump blood through the body (Figure 24-1). It is really two pumps tied together by the vascular system. One side is dedicated to pumping blood to the lungs—this is the "right heart." The other side—the "left heart"—pumps blood to the rest of the body.

Veins

Veins are vessels that return blood to the heart. They are commonly associated with "blue blood," but this is not always the case. The pulmonary veins return blood to the left atrium from the lungs. The blood returning from the proximal pulmonary veins is the most oxygen-rich in the body.

Arteries

Arteries are vessels that transport blood from the heart. The pulmonary artery arises from the right ventricle. The aorta arises from the left ventricle.

Atria

Atrium literally means "receiving chamber." In the heart the atria receive blood from the veins. The right atrium receives deoxygenated blood from the body through the vena cava and coronary sinus. The left atrium receives oxygenated blood from the lungs through the four pulmonary veins. Blood flow is fairly constant into the atria.

Ventricles

The right ventricle receives blood from the right atrium during diastole and pumps into the pulmonary artery during systole. The left ventricle receives blood from the left atrium during diastole and pumps into the aorta during systole.

Cardiac Valves

The intracardiac valves are all one-way valves allowing blood to move forward only. Their purpose is to separate the ventricles from the atria and arteries at the appropriate time during the cardiac cycle. The valves can be divided into two sets.

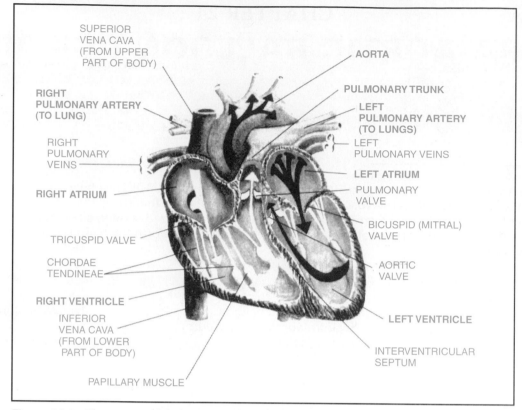

Figure 24-1 *The anatomy of the heart*

Atrioventricular valves separate ventricles from atria. They are open during diastole and closed during systole. Atrioventricular valves include the tricuspid valve for the right heart and the mitral (bicuspid) valve for the left heart.

Semilunar valves separate the ventricles from the arteries. These valves are open during systole and closed during diastole. They include the pulmonic for the right heart and the aortic for the left heart.

Right Heart

The *"right heart"* pumps blood through the pulmonary vasculature. There is very low resistance to blood flow in the lungs; thus, the pressure required to move blood through the pulmonary arteries is low. The right ventricle and atrium are designed to operate at low pressures; therefore, they are thin-walled, with a low muscle mass. Thus, the right heart is essentially a volume pump, not a pressure pump.

Left Heart

The *"left heart"* serves the systemic vasculature. There is 10 to 20 times more resistance to blood flow in the systemic circulation than in the pulmonary circulation. The majority of this resistance is generated as the blood moves through the arterioles. The arterioles have the ability to regulate blood flow to a region by vasoconstriction or vasodilation. Because there is higher resistance in the systemic system, the left heart operates at much higher pressures; therefore, the left ventricle is a pressure pump. Problems with left ventricular performance lead to serious compromise of cardiac function.

CARDIAC PHYSIOLOGY

A familiarity of the variables involved with cardiac physiology is paramount to understanding how IABP can be beneficial to the patient with compromised cardiac function. The following brief review touches on the important concepts.

Cardiac Output

Cardiac output is the amount of blood the heart pumps each minute and is expressed as liters per minute (L/min). Normal resting cardiac output for an adult is about 5.0 L/min. To express a cardiac output accurately for each patient, it is important to index the cardiac output, relating it to the body surface area (BSA). This is done by dividing the cardiac output by the BSA (Dubois, 1936); the result is termed the *cardiac index*, as shown in the following equation:

$$\text{Cardiac index} = \frac{\text{cardiac output}}{\text{body surface area}}$$

The units for cardiac index are $L/min/m^2$. Using the cardiac index allows accurate comparison of cardiac function among people of different body sizes. Trained athletes can increase their cardiac output by a factor of 6. The difference between resting and maximal cardiac output is termed the *cardiac reserve*. Patients with impaired cardiac function demonstrate a diminished cardiac reserve; however, their resting cardiac output may be maintained by compensatory mechanisms. There are many variables affecting cardiac output. Biofeedback response mechanisms adjust the cardiac output to meet metabolic needs. The primary cardiovascular response to these signals is to adjust the stroke volume or the heart rate, or both. The stroke volume is the amount of blood pumped per beat and is expressed as milliliters per beat (ml/beat). The cardiac output can be expressed as the sum of the stroke volume multiplied by the heart rate:

$$\text{Cardiac output} = \text{stroke volume} \times \text{heart rate}$$

A typical stroke volume of 70 ml and a heart rate of 70 bpm yield a normal cardiac output of 4900 ml/min, expressed as 4.9 L/min.

Preload

Preload is defined as the amount of diastolic stretch applied to the ventricular myocardium before systole. The importance of preload is related to a special property of myocardium. This property is described by the Starling principle, or Starling's law (Figure 24-2). Simply stated, the more you stretch the myocardium, the harder it will contract. The myocardium can be likened to a rubber band. The more it is stretched, the more it will snap back. Preload is how far the ventricle is stretched prior to diastole. As can be seen by examining the Starling curve, we can get better performance by optimizing the preload. Too much preload is not good and can impede cardiac performance, as indicated on the right side of the graph (see Figure 24-2). If the myocardium is overstretched, the myocardium loses performance, just as a rubber band will break if it is stretched too far. Starling's law describes how the heart adjusts for variations in venous return, and with differing lengths of diastole as seen with arrhythmias such as atrial fibrillation or premature ventricular contractions (PVCs).

Preload is evaluated separately for the left and right sides of the heart. Clinically, left ventricular preload is measured as the left ventricular end-diastolic pressure (LVEDP). This may also be obtained by measuring the pulmonary capillary wedge pressure (PCWP). LVEDP and PCWP are interchangeable. Either represents the filling pressure of the left ventricle. The central venous pressure (CVP) is the filling pressure of the right heart. The concept of preload is important because by optimizing the stretch of the ventricles, it is possible to obtain a more powerful contraction from them. Thus, the heart will have an improved stroke volume, increasing the cardiac output. Clinically, the way preload is altered is to adjust the patient's vascular volume. By infusing volume, preload may be increased. If the patient has too much volume, the heart loses the Starling benefit, with resulting edema and risk of heart failure. Therefore, the hypervolemic patient may be given diuretics, which are used to decrease vascular volume and ventricular preload.

Afterload

Afterload is defined as the resistance the ventricle must overcome to eject blood. To continue the rubber band analogy, the afterload is equivalent to the load the rubber band must lift. The preload is how far the rubber band is stretched, while the afterload is how heavy the object is that it must lift. An increased afterload on the ventricle leads to a reduced ejection of blood. Afterload in physiological terms has three components: (1) the diastolic pressure in the artery the ventricle must overcome to begin ejection, (2) the vascular resistance the ventricle must overcome to complete the ejection, and (3) the viscosity of the blood to be moved. Clinically, left ventricular afterload is measured as the systemic vascular resistance (SVR) or the diastolic pressure in the aorta. To improve ventricular performance, afterload is reduced by the administration of vasoactive medications that relax the arterioles, such as nitrates.

Myocardial Contractility

Myocardial contractility is defined as how forcefully the heart contracts during systole. To use the rubber band analogy one more time, contractility is equivalent to the thickness of the rubber band. A thicker rubber band will lift a heavier load and therefore will do more work. A hypercontractile state of the myocardium leads to an increased stroke volume even against an increased afterload. Contractile state is measured in the cardiac catheterization laboratory by recording intracardiac left ventricular pressure. From the left ventricle we measure the slope of the left ventricular pressure during isovolumetric contraction; this is represented as dP/dT. A more forceful contraction leads to a steep upslope. There is no good direct way to measure this parameter at the bedside. Clinically, the contractile state of the ventricles is managed by giving positive inotropic drugs, such as digitoxin.

Myocardial Oxygen Supply

Myocardial oxygen supply is composed of four variables: coronary blood flow, dissolved oxygen in the blood, pH of the blood, and perfusion pressure. The heart needs fuel to work. The coronary arteries are the

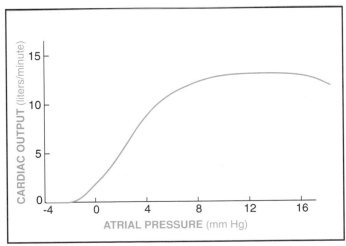

Figure 24-2 *A Starling curve showing the effect of preload on cardiac output. Note that the more the myocardium is stretched, the harder it will contract.* (*Courtesy of* Guyton. [1984], *A textbook of medical physiology*, Philadelphia: Saunders)

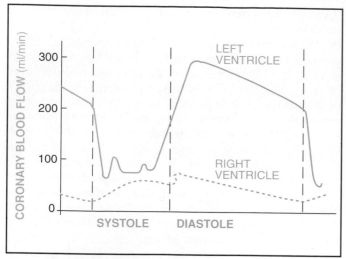

Figure 24-3 *The phasic flow of blood through the coronary arteries of the right and left ventricles (Courtesy of* Guyton [1984], *A textbook of medical physiology*, Philadelphia: Saunders)

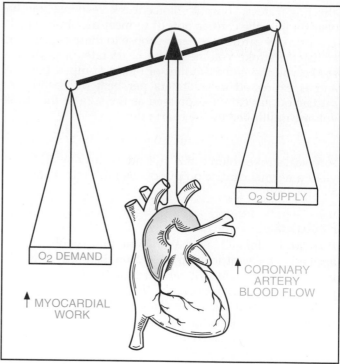

Figure 24-4 *An increase in myocardial work increases oxygen demand. As a result, coronary artery vasodilation may occur as a compensatory mechanism to increase perfusion and oxygen supply to the myocardium. (Courtesy of* Berne, R., & Levy, M. [1992], *Cardiovascular Physiology*, St. Louis, MO: Mosby–Year Book)

fuel lines to the cardiac muscle. The majority of blood flow to the cardiac muscle occurs during diastole (Figure 24-3). This is because the tension in the wall surrounding the coronary arteries increases during systole, increasing resistance to blood flow. The fact that most of the coronary perfusion occurs during diastole is an important point to remember—as you will learn later, IABP helps to increase the diastolic pressure in the aorta.

Patients may become ischemic if there is an intrinsically low PaO$_2$ even in the absence of coronary artery disease. If the blood pH is not within normal range, the availability of oxygen to the cell may become impeded due to the shift of the oxyhemoglobin dissociation curve.

Perfusion pressure is measured as the difference between the pressure going into and that coming out of an arterial system. For the coronary arteries these points are the aorta and the right atrium. Lowering the aortic or raising the right atrial pressure will inhibit coronary artery perfusion.

Myocardial Oxygen Demand

Myocardial oxygen demand is determined by the metabolic rate of the cardiac tissue. Most of the energy requirements occur during isovolumetric contraction. This is the phase of the cardiac cycle when the ventricles are building pressure to open the semilunar valves, to begin ejection. Oxygen supply and demand is a balance between opposing forces (Figure 24-4).

Phases of the Cardiac Cycle

A review of the phases of the cardiac cycle will be helpful. The cardiac cycle is generally broken into two periods: systole and diastole. Systole is the period of ventricular ejection and diastole is the period of ventricular filling.

Electrocardiographic Events

The P wave marks atrial contraction. The QRS complex initiates ventricular systole. The T wave represents ventricular repolarization and approximates the beginning of diastole.

Isovolumetric Contraction

The ventricular wave form is rectangular in shape. The ECG QRS complex initiates rapid depolarization of the ventricular myocardium. This leads to the rapid rise of the left ventricular pressure. As the left ventricular pressure exceeds the left atrial pressure, the mitral valve closes. From the time the mitral valve is closed and until the aortic valve opens, there is no volume change within the left ventricle and the pressure is rising. This is the period of isovolumetric contraction, where the majority of cardiac energy expenditure occurs.

Systolic Ejection

As the left ventricular pressure exceeds the aortic pressure, the aortic valve opens and ejection occurs until the left ventricular pressure falls below the aortic pressure. At this point the aortic valve closes, which marks the end of systole.

Isovolumetric Relaxation

From the time the aortic valve closes and until the left ventricular pressure falls below the left atrial pressure and the mitral valve opens, there is no volume change within the left ventricle. This period is called the isovolumetric relaxation phase.

Diastolic Filling Period

From the time the mitral valve opens until it is closed by the left ventricular pressure exceeding the left atrial pressure, the left ventricle is filling. This is termed the diastolic filling period.

CARDIAC PATHOLOGY

It is important to understand the pathologic processes affecting the heart, and to know which conditions may benefit from IABP therapy. A limited review of cardiac pathology leading to the need for IABP therapy follows.

Coronary Artery Disease

Obstructive *coronary artery disease* is the most important and common pathologic condition responsible for reducing the oxygen available to the myocardium. Blood flow will generally be inhibited, causing symptoms if the vessels are reduced by 50% or greater in cross-sectional diameter. Coronary arterioles distal to a stenosis or obstruction will dilate to reduce resistance and thus increase flow. Another compensatory mechanism to help maintain myocardial perfusion is the development of collateral circulation. The myocardium needs a steady supply of oxygen. Myocardial muscle is aerobic; therefore, there can be no oxygen debt. If the myocardium is deprived of oxygen, the tissue becomes ischemic. Ischemic myocardium does not contract or conduct impulses efficiently. Ischemia is reversible by the restoration of the oxygen supply and demand balance. If the oxygen deprivation is prolonged, the tissue can undergo infarction. A myocardial infarction will result in the death of myocardial tissue and permanent loss of contractile and conductive properties. The size and consequences of an infarct are directly related to which coronary artery is involved.

The left coronary artery is the most important. The left coronary artery perfuses the anterior and lateral walls of the left ventricle. These walls make up about two-thirds of the total left ventricle. An obstruction of any part of the left coronary artery will result in a loss in left ventricular performance. The right coronary artery perfuses the inferior wall of the left ventricle.

IABP can play an important role in the management of these patients when the left ventricular performance is compromised by myocardial infarction.

Left Ventricular Dysfunction

Left ventricular dysfunction can occur through several disorders, including hypovolemia, hypervolemia, and loss of contractility.

In hypovolemia, the vascular volume is low, and there will not be enough preload to elicit a forceful contraction. With hypovolemia the heart is working on the far left of the Starling curve. Hemorrhage or diuresis can lead to

hypovolemia. IABP would not be helpful for this cause of reduced ventricular function.

In hypervolemia, the vascular and ventricular volumes are high and the ventricle will be forced to work from the far right of the Starling curve, where the myocardial fibers are stretched too far to contract efficiently. IABP can be helpful in patients suffering from volume overload. IABP reduces cardiac afterload, allowing for a larger stroke volume. With a larger stroke volume, more of the blood in the ventricle will be ejected. If more is ejected, less will remain at the end of the contraction. So reducing the afterload also reduces the preload.

It is common for the heart to lose contractility following an ischemic event or infarction. After an ischemic event or infarction, the left ventricular wall motion abnormalities are defined as regional. The segment of muscle supplied by the coronary artery that was pathologically involved will be affected. If this area is large the remaining functional muscle may not be able to maintain cardiac output without some assistance. IABP is helpful here because it reduces the afterload and increases the coronary perfusion pressure, thus reducing oxygen demand while increasing supply.

Ventricular Septal Defect

Ventricular septal defects (VSDs) can be congenital or acquired. An acquired VSD can be associated with an infarct of the interventricular septum with subsequent muscular rupture. Infarcted tissue becomes weaker following necrosis. The etiology for post–septal rupture is the great pressure difference between the left and the right ventricles. The VSD allows a left to right shunt to occur from the left ventricle to the right ventricle. This has the effect of increasing pulmonary circulation and decreasing systemic circulation. IABP will be employed to reduce the left heart preload and afterload. This reduces the pressure gradient between the left and right ventricles. If the pressure gradient is reduced, there will be less shunting.

Valve Pathology

Valve pathology may involve blockage or leakage. A valve that restricts forward flow by increasing resistance is termed *stenotic*. With valvular stenosis, blood pressure will build in the proximal chamber or vascular system. A valve that leaks is termed *incompetent* or *regurgitant*. With valvular regurgitation, volume overload proximal to the valve will result. In a closed system a volume increase leads to a pressure increase, so these mechanisms of pathology are tied together.

Stenotic Valves

IABP therapy is not commonly used for patients with stenotic valves unless heart failure develops secondary to the stenosis.

Mitral Regurgitation

IABP therapy may alleviate the symptoms from mitral regurgitation. This is accomplished by reducing the preload and afterload of the left ventricle, thus reducing the systolic force required by the left ventricle to complete ejection. Mitral regurgitation is a systolic event. A reduction in left ventricular systolic force will reduce the mitral regurgitation and associated symptoms of pulmonary congestion.

Aortic Insufficiency

IABP therapy will augment the diastolic pressure in the aorta. Aortic insufficiency is a diastolic event. Therefore, IABP therapy would exacerbate the symptoms of aortic insufficiency and is contraindicated.

OBJECTIVES

At the end of this chapter, you should be able to:

- List the indications, contraindications, and complications with IABP therapy.
- State the hemodynamic benefits of IABP therapy.
- List the steps and equipment required to insert an intra-aortic balloon catheter.
- Identify the electrocardiographic and arterial pressure wave forms utilized to trigger the inflation and deflation of the intra-aortic balloon.

- List the steps required to initiate balloon counterpulsation.
- Describe how to identify and correct early or late inflation and deflation of an intra-aortic balloon.
- Describe the care and assessment of a patient undergoing IABP therapy.
- Explain how to wean a patient from IABP.
- Describe how to remove a balloon/sheath assembly from a patient's femoral artery and how to establish hemostasis.

FUNDAMENTAL PRINCIPLES OF IABP THERAPY

There are several technical and procedural considerations involved in IABP therapy. Special attention to balloon insertion, placement, and timing is critical. There are minor variations between different balloon pumps and catheters. Refer to each balloon and equipment operator manual specific to your institution. It is also important for you to be familiar with and utilize the policy and procedure manual for your institution regarding IABP therapy.

The Intra-aortic Balloon

The *intra-aortic balloon* (IAB) is a large-caliber dual lumen balloon catheter. One lumen runs through the catheter to the end hole. This lumen is used to advance the catheter over a wire into the descending aorta and to measure pressures once the catheter is placed. The other lumen is in communication with the balloon. This lumen is used to rapidly conduct helium into and out of the balloon. Helium is chosen because of its low molecular weight and inertia. The volume of the balloon is usually 40 cc for an adult (Figure 24-5).

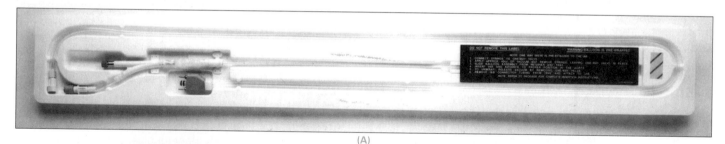

(A)

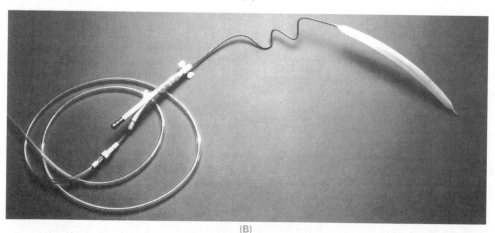

(B)

Figure 24-5 *An intra-aortic balloon catheter packaged in its sterile tray (A); the intra-aortic balloon catheter (B). Note the flexibility demonstrated in the shaft, which allows placement through very tortuous vascular systems.* (Courtesy of Arrow International, Reading, PA)

The Intra-aortic Balloon Pump

The *intra-aortic balloon pump* (IAB pump) is a mobile console used to conduct helium into and out of the IAB. This gas movement is triggered by an ECG R wave sensor. The balloon is inflated during diastole and deflated for systole. These events occur rapidly, so the pump must conduct the helium rapidly. The common features of IAB pumps are listed below. (Refer to the operator's manual of your specific device.)

1. The console has a monitor that displays three signals: ECG, arterial pressure tracing, and balloon inflation status.
2. There will be two balloon timing adjustments: inflation timing and deflation timing. Each of these can be adjusted earlier or later in the cardiac cycle.
3. Balloon volume adjustment is used to increase or decrease the amount of helium conducted to the balloon.
4. The assist ratio may be adjusted at 1:1, 1:2, 1:4, or 1:8. The assist ratio is the ratio of balloon inflation to the heart rate (Figure 24-6).

Hemodynamic Benefits

The IAB pump is a left ventricular assist device. The IAB is placed into the descending aorta. The distal tip is positioned just distal to the origin of the left subclavian artery.

The proximal balloon needs to be positioned proximal to the origin of the renal arteries. The balloon is inflated during diastole and deflated during systole (Figure 24-7). Counterpulsation of the balloon will effectively separate the systemic circulation into two compartments. Proximal arteries, organs, and tissues will benefit from an increased diastolic perfusion pressure. Most important, the brain and heart will benefit from this increased perfusion pressure. All tissues will benefit from the increased cardiac output afforded by IABP therapy.

Balloon Inflation

Balloon inflation is adjusted to coincide with the beginning of diastole. This occurs at the dicrotic notch of the arterial pressure trace (Figure 24-8). Figure 24-9 illustrates the augmentation in arterial pressure afforded by IABP therapy. As the balloon is inflated, it will hold the blood in the proximal vascular compartment, creating an increased diastolic pressure known as *diastolic augmentation*. Note the difference in mean pressures following the dicrotic notch illustrated in Figures 24-8 and 24-9. This increased diastolic pressure enhances the perfusion of myocardium. Remember that the majority of myocardial perfusion occurs during diastole. This supercharged diastolic flow dramatically increases the oxygen supply to the myocardium to alleviate the effects of ischemia.

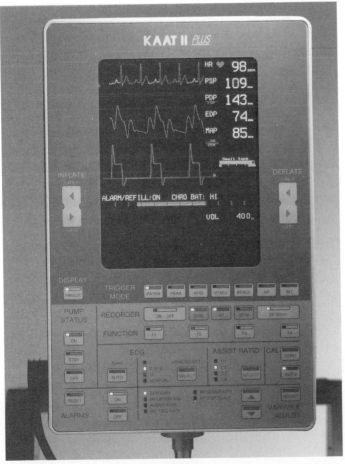
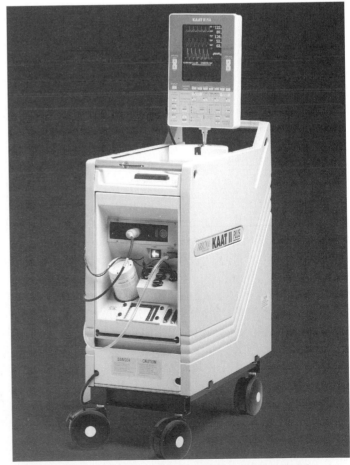

Figure 24-6 *Intra-aortic balloon pump console display screen (left) and console control panel (right) (Courtesy of Arrow International, Reading, PA)*

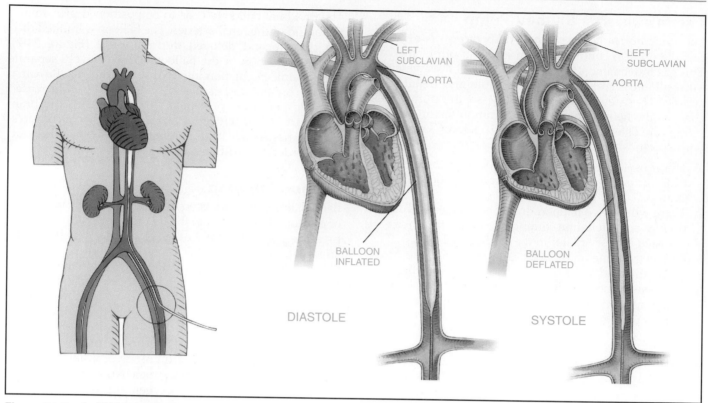

Figure 24-7 *An illustration showing the correct placement of the intra-aortic balloon catheter (Courtesy of* Arrow International, Reading, PA)

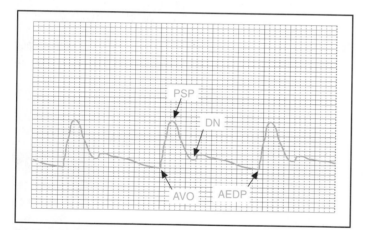

Figure 24-8 *The arterial pressure wave-form landmarks: AVO, aortic valve opens, indicating the beginning of systole; AEDP, aortic end-diastolic pressure; PSP, peak systolic pressure (65–75% of the stroke volume has been delivered); DN, dicrotic notch (closure of the aortic valve and start of diastole, with the last 25–35% of stroke volume having been delivered) (Courtesy of* Arrow International, Reading, PA)

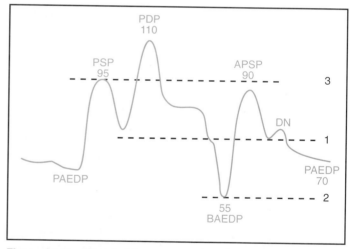

Figure 24-9 *The arterial pressure tracing showing diastolic augmentation. The "Timing Three": (1) Inflation just prior to the dicrotic notch (DN). If inflation occurs greater than 40 ms before DN, then it is early inflation. If the DN is exposed, inflation is late. (2) Deflation: The balloon aortic end-diastolic pressure (BAEDP) must be less than the patient aortic end-diastolic pressure (PAEDP). If PAEDP > BAEDP, then the deflation is late. (3) Deflation: The assisted peak systolic pressure (APSP) should be greater than the peak systolic pressure (PSP). If PSP > APSP, then deflation is too early.*

Balloon Deflation

Balloon deflation is R wave triggered by the pump and adjusted to occur during isovolumetric contraction of the left ventricle. Balloon deflation occurs an instant before systole. As the balloon displacement decreases by the pump's removal of helium, there is a sudden volume and pressure decrease in the aorta. This creates a pronounced drop in the aortic end-diastolic pressure, which allows the ventricle to open the aortic valve and begin ejection with less effort. This effectively causes a reduction of afterload. As the balloon deflation reduces afterload, the myocardial oxygen demand is reduced. When the afterload is reduced, there will be a more complete emptying of the ventricle in the form of an increased stroke volume. If the stroke volume is increased, the cardiac output will increase. Increased stroke volume means there is a reduced preload by virtue of the enhanced emptying of the ventricle. Preload is measured as the left ventricular end-diastolic or pulmonary capillary wedge pressure (LVEDP or PCWP). By reducing the preload, we can minimize the amount of pulmonary edema commonly associated with heart failure. By increasing the stroke volume, we can allow the heart rate to drop and still maintain cardiac output. As the heart rate decreases, there is a longer time period for diastole. As time for diastole increases, myocardial perfusion also increases.

There are many hemodynamic benefits gained with the use of IABP therapy. Table 24-1 summarizes these benefits.

Indications, Contraindications, and Complications with IABP Therapy
Indications

Indications for IABP therapy include:

- Refractory unstable angina
- Cardiogenic shock
- Hemodynamic instability at the time of cardiac surgery
- Acute myocardial infarction complicated by mitral regurgitation or ventricular septal defect
- Intractable ventricular tachycardia secondary to myocardial ischemia
- High-risk percutaneous coronary angioplasty or valvuloplasty

TABLE 24-1: Benefits of Intra-aortic Balloon Pumping: Inflation and Deflation Modes

	INFLA-TION	DEFLA-TION
Decreased signs of myocardial ischemia: angina, ST segment changes, ventricular arrhythmias	XX	XX
Increased coronary artery blood flow	XX	
Decreased afterload		XX
Decreased MVO$_2$ and demand		XX
Increased cardiac output	X	XX
Increased urine output	X	XX
Decreased preload (PCWP, CVP)	X	XX
Decreased pulmonary congestion, improved arterial oxygenation, improved breath sounds, clearing chest x-ray	X	XX
Improved mentation	XX	X
Decreased heart rate	XX	XX
Decreased lactic acidosis	X	XX
Increased pulse rate and increased pulse pressure	XX	X

Courtesy of Arrow International, Reading, PA

Contraindications

The following list summarizes the contraindications to IABP therapy:

- Aortic regurgitation
- Anatomical abnormality of the iliac-femoral arteries
- Aortic aneurysm or dissection
- Presence of a large patent ductus arteriosus
- Bleeding diathesis
- Sepsis

Complications

The following list summarizes the potential complications of IABP therapy:

- Primarily vascular complications, including:
  — Pulse loss
  — Limb ischemia
  — Thromboembolism
  — Compartment syndrome
  — Aortic dissection
- Local injury "entry wound"
- Infection

Insertion Technique

This section is not intended to be a comprehensive review of the skills and variables required to acquire vascular access and navigate in the arterial circulation. For a thorough discussion refer to *Cardiac Catheterization, Angeography, and Intervention* by Grossman and Baim.

The most common hospital locations for IABP insertion are the cardiac catheterization laboratory, the cardiovascular surgical theater, and the coronary or intensive care unit.

Procedure Setup

To prepare properly for IABP insertion, you should complete the following tasks.

Arrange for the radiology department to staff and supply a high-quality portable C-arm fluoroscopic unit with lead aprons for three or four staff members.

Arrange for the patient to be transferred to a fluoroscopy bed in the nursing unit's designated procedure room.

Set up a sterile procedure table according to your hospital's policy and procedure manual. This should include a heparinized flush basin, syringes, gowns and gloves, needles, hand towels, cotton 4 × 4-inch gauze pads, patient prep and drape supplies, and the equipment required for a femoral access.

Verify the patient's informed consent status, and if required, complete the paperwork and have the patient and witnesses sign the informed consent.

Procedural Steps

Turn on power to the IAB pump console. Attach a good electrocardiographic lead system and prepare a transducer for the arterial line input. These two physiological monitoring parameters provide a redundant trigger backup. Both the ECG and arterial blood pressure wave forms will be utilized during the initiation process.

Prep and drape the patient's femoral artery sites bilaterally in a sterile fashion. Because this procedure is invasive, it is important to maintain and practice the procedure as aseptically as possible. Assist the physician with vascular access into the femoral artery usually using the Seldinger technique.

Prepare the IAB per the manufacturer's instructions and assist the physician with IAB placement. Fluoroscopic guidance may be utilized to ensure correct placement of the catheter and balloon. The balloon will be advanced over a wire through a sheath (sheathless balloons are also available).

Confirm proper placement, with the distal tip of the balloon in the descending thoracic aorta. The IAB should not encroach into the aortic arch, and the proximal balloon body should be positioned to lie proximal to the renal arteries. The balloon should not overlie the renal arteries; otherwise, it will occlude renal blood flow during inflation.

The balloon may need to be unfurled before initiation of counterpulsation. This is generally accomplished by turning the shaft of the intra-aortic balloon catheter in a counterclockwise rotation. (Refer to specific manufacturer's instructions.)

Connect the arterial pressure line to the central lumen of the catheter and connect the helium shuttle tube from the console to the balloon port.

Initiation of IABP Therapy

You should now be ready to initiate IABP therapy. This is an exciting and fast-paced procedure. For the patient to receive maximum hemodynamic benefit, speed is of the essence.

Initiation of Counterpulsation

It is important to understand the different components of a normal arterial pressure tracing (see Figure 24-8). It is important to identify two points of interest: (1) the dicrotic notch and (2) the end-diastolic pressure.

The IAB will be inflated in diastole at point 1 (the dicrotic notch) and deflated in systole at point 2 (the end-diastolic pressure). Figure 24-9 exhibits a balloon pumping at a 1:2 ratio, which is used to adjust timing. Figure 24-10 illustrates the safe and unsafe inflation time periods.

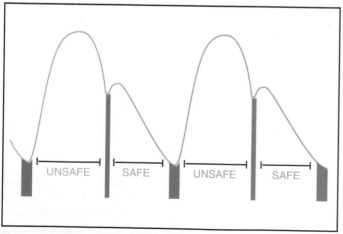

Figure 24-10 *A pressure graph illustrating safe and unsafe balloon timing* (*Courtesy of* Quaal, S. J. [1993], *Comprehensive intra-aortic balloon counterpulsation* (2nd ed.), St. Louis, MO: Mosby–Year Book)

Encroachment of balloon inflation into systole will have serious deleterious effects. If the balloon is inflated during any part of systole, there will be severe increases in myocardial workload because the left ventricle will be forced to pump against increased resistance.

To set the proper IAB timing, a two-phase approach is described. First, set the parameters close to the ECG signal. The ECG signal will be highlighted on the console where the balloon will inflate. Initially adjust the inflation to occur on the down slope of the ECG T wave. Deflation will be set to occur just before the ECG R wave. Once this is set, it is time to turn on the pump at a ratio of one assist (inflation) for every two heartbeats; this is the 1:2 assist ratio.

Next, fine-tune the timing to perfection using the arterial pressure tracing at an assist ratio of 1:2. This 1:2 ratio will allow you to see the effects of timing adjustments (see Figures 24-8, 24-9, and 24-10).

Inflation Parameters

Remember that the balloon inflation must not encroach upon systole. Systole ends at the point of the dicrotic notch on the arterial pressure tracing. It is best to move the inflation timing later until you can see the dicrotic notch and then slowly move the inflation timing earlier until you can see a distinct "V" at the point of the dicrotic notch (Figure 24-11).

Deflation Parameters

You want the balloon to be deflated before systole begins (Figure 24-12). Systole begins just at the point in diastole before the pressure begins to rise rapidly. Move the deflation timing early until you can see a flat bottom on the tracing just before the next systole. Then adjust the deflation later until you have a sharp, deep "V"; this will coincide with the balloon-assisted end-diastolic pressure. It is important to maintain this pressure as low as possible because this pressure is equivalent to the afterload of the left ventricle. The left ventricle will benefit from a reduced afterload.

Early or Late Inflation and Deflation

Of the four variables of improper timing, two are dangerous and two merely fail to optimize the hemodynamic benefits of IABP. The two dangerous mistakes are those that allow the balloon inflation to encroach upon systole: early inflation and late deflation.

Early Inflation.   Early inflation causes the ventricle to eject through increased resistance. This will exacerbate ischemia. Notice how the inflation rides up on the systolic ejection pressure during early inflation (Figure 24-13).

Late Inflation.   Late inflation does not harm the patient; rather, it fails to help as much as possible. Notice the exposed dicrotic notch. This is a sign that the inflation is late (Figure 24-14).

Early Deflation.   Early deflation results in a lesser hemodynamic benefit of IABP. Notice the flat plateau in diastole just before the systolic upstroke. The deflation should encroach upon the upstroke of systole to form a pronounced "V" (Figure 24-15).

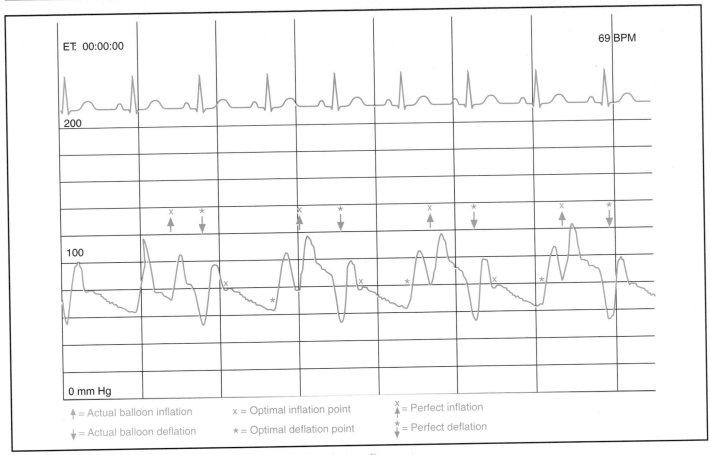

Figure 24-11 *ECG and arterial pressure tracings illustrating inflation adjustment*

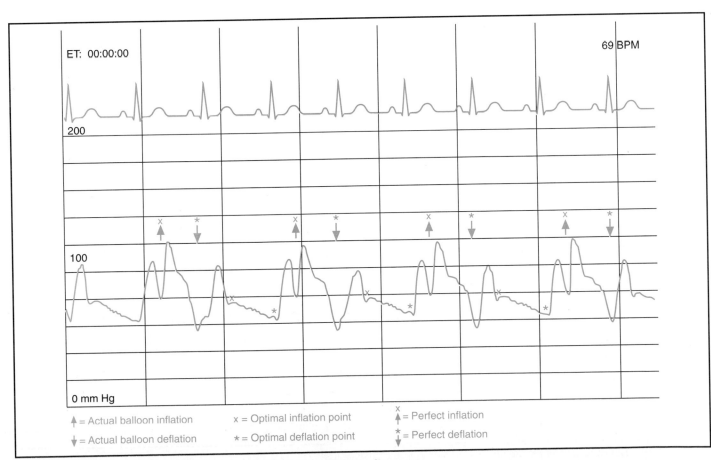

Figure 24-12 *ECG and arterial pressure tracings illustrating deflation adjustment*

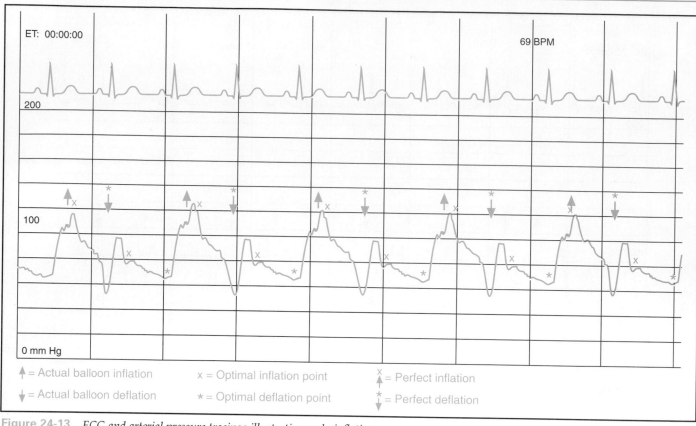

Figure 24-13   *ECG and arterial pressure tracings illustrating early inflation*

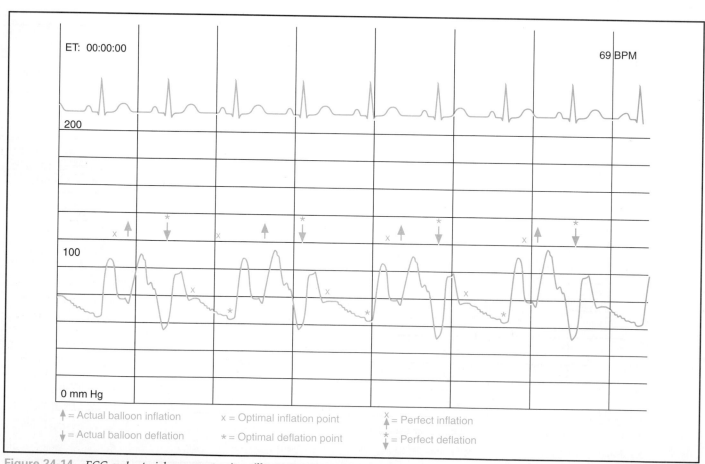

Figure 24-14   *ECG and arterial pressure tracings illustrating late inflation*

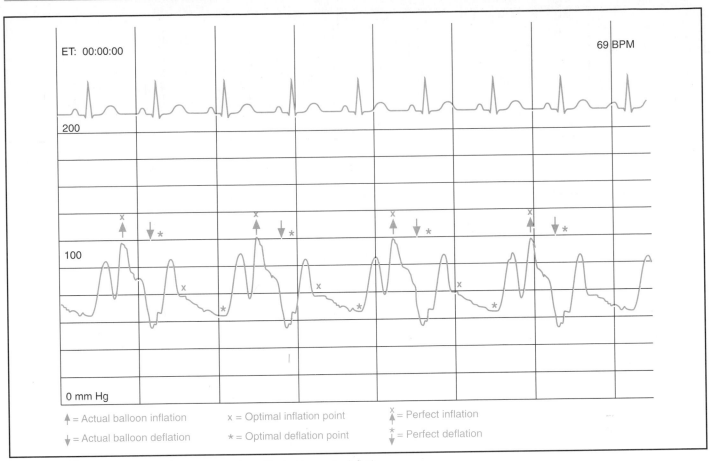

Figure 24-15 *ECG and arterial pressure tracings illustrating early deflation*

Late Deflation.
Late deflation encroaches into systole. This is a costly error in terms of myocardial oxygen demand. This causes the ventricle to eject against an increased resistance during late deflation (Figure 24-16).

Care of the IABP Patient

Anticoagulation Therapy

The patient must be kept adequately anticoagulated for the duration of IABP therapy. This is accomplished with a heparin bolus and drip to maintain the clotting times at twice-normal values (George, 1988). A heparin bolus of 5000 units followed by a heparin drip at 600 to 1000 units/hour to maintain a partial thromboplastin time of between 50 and 60 seconds has been recommended (Miller, 1986).

Limb Ischemia

The circulation distal to the IAB insertion needs to be closely monitored for signs of ischemia. Monitoring should include pulse, capillary refill, color, and ankle-brachial index. Monitoring data must be compared with preinsertion peripheral circulatory evaluation data.

Hemodynamic Assessment

The patient's cardiac output, cardiac index, arterial systolic blood pressure, and left ventricular filling pressures must be carefully monitored.

Infection

Proper aseptic care of the IAB entry site must be maintained. Only through careful asepsis can inadvertent infections be prevented.

Patient Positioning

The patient must be prevented from bending the affected leg at the hip. This usually means tying the affected ankle to the bed and having the patient lie flat in bed with no more than 15° of head elevation.

Weaning from the Pump

Once the underlying cause for IABP initiation has been corrected, the patient will need to be weaned from IABP support. IABP therapy cannot be abruptly terminated. The left ventricle becomes accustomed to the IABP pump, so its support must be slowly removed. This is accomplished by reducing the pumping frequency. All pumps have the feature of variable pumping ratios. First, begin at a ratio of 1:2 and assess the patient's response. If the hemodynamic response is satisfactory, the pumping ratio can be reduced further to 1:4 and then 1:8. Figures 24-17 and 24-18 illustrate tracings for weaning ratios of 1:4 and 1:8, respectively. The rate of weaning is dependent on the patient's satisfactory response to the reduced support. Each phase of the weaning process usually lasts 4 hours. Another method of weaning the patient is gradually reducing the amount

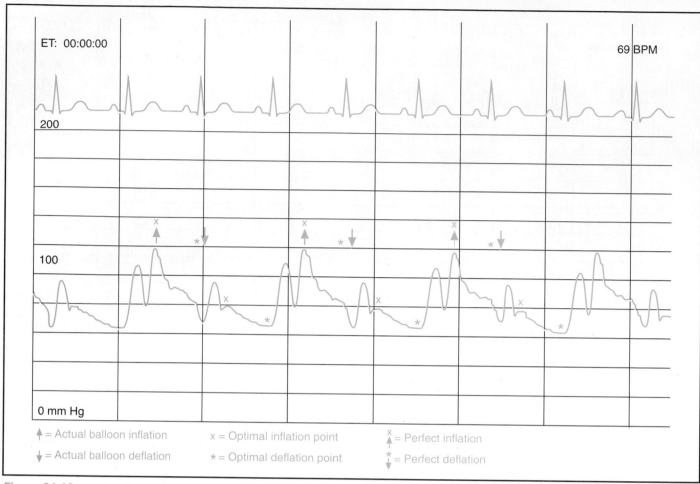

ET: 00:00:00

69 BPM

200

100

0 mm Hg

↑ = Actual balloon inflation   x = Optimal inflation point   ˣ↑ = Perfect inflation

↓ = Actual balloon deflation   * = Optimal deflation point   *↓ = Perfect deflation

Figure 24-16 *ECG and arterial pressure tracings illustrating late deflation*

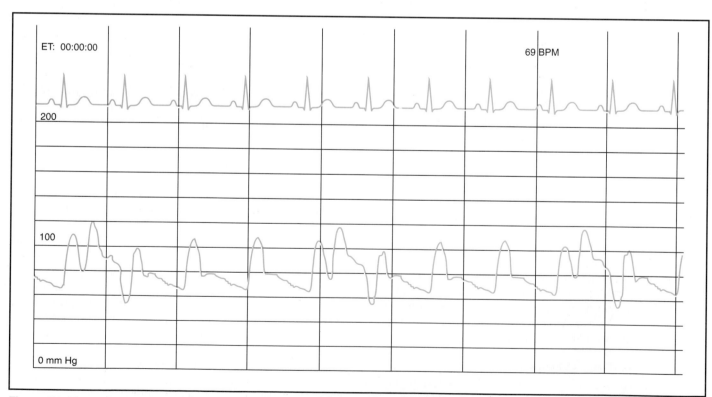

ET: 00:00:00

69 BPM

200

100

0 mm Hg

Figure 24-17 *ECG and arterial pressure tracings illustrating weaning with a pumping ratio of 1:4*

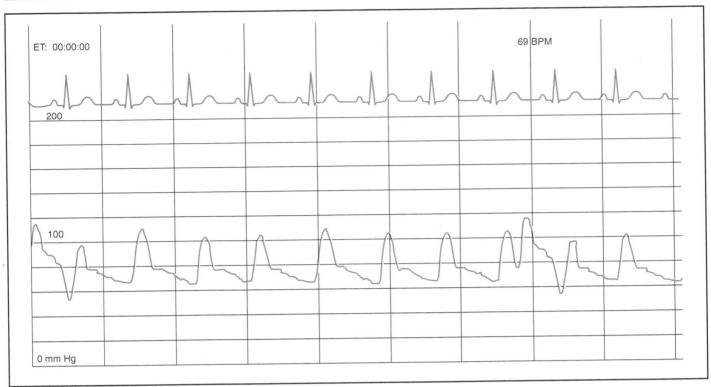

Figure 24-18 *ECG and arterial pressure tracings illustrating weaning with a pumping ratio of 1:8*

of helium shuttled. Once the balloon is turned off, it must be removed, as a risk of thrombus formation exists with a static balloon.

Removal of Balloon/Sheath—Hemostasis

The heparin drip should be stopped 2 to 4 hours before the balloon is turned off and the sheath is removed. The balloon should not be allowed to remain in place without pumping because it carries a risk of thrombus formation. At this point it would be prudent to verify the physician's orders to remove the balloon/sheath and that the patient's hemodynamic status has stabilized.

Removing the IAB/Sheath

First, prepare to pull this sheath from the femoral artery in the usual manner. There are two special areas requiring your undivided attention during this process. The IAB is a large-caliber device that has been inserted into a heavily anticoagulated patient, so be prepared for a lengthy time frame before the insertion site has sufficiently closed. Have a relief person or hemostatic device nearby in the event you become fatigued. It is not uncommon for pressure to be applied for at least 45 minutes to achieve hemostasis.

There may be a thrombus on or near the sheath, depending on how long the patient has been on IABP support. A modified arterial device removal technique is advised. When the sheath is removed, it is suggested to occlude the distal flow and allow a healthy 1- or 2-second spurt of blood to exit the entry site. This should remove

any thrombus. After this spurt, resume normal arterial puncture hemostatic measures.

Patient Instructions

The patient needs to be informed of some basic arterial puncture precautions. Providing the rationale for the instructions promotes the patient's compliance with these precautions.

The patient should remain in bed for at least 6 hours after hemostasis. This allows the clot at the arterial puncture site to harden enough to bear the increased strain of ambulation.

An important precaution is to keep the affected leg straight so that the clot is not dislodged. With movement, the artery will flex while the clot does not. Sitting up in bed is prohibited, for the same reason, and only 15° of head elevation is permitted. Instruct the patient to protect the puncture site if coughing or sneezing by the application of firm hand pressure over the dressing. Tell the patient to call an attendant or caregiver immediately if he or she suspects bleeding. The symptoms to look for include lightheadedness, nausea, bulging tension, and warmth in the groin. The bleeding will not stop on its own; the patient will need help if bleeding persists.

Finally, the patient must not lift the head from the pillow. This act would pull on the muscles surrounding the puncture site and could dislodge the clot.

If the patient bleeds, you must start the 6-hour clock again (6 hours of bed rest). This usually solicits the patient's compliance if the previous instructions have not already.

References

Berne, R. M., & Levy, M. (1992). *Cardiovascular physiology* (5th ed.). St. Louis, MO: Mosby–Year Book.

Dubois, E. F. (1936). *Basal metabolism in health and disease*. Philadelphia: Lea & Febiger.

George, B. S. (1988). Thrombolysis and intra-aortic balloon pumping following acute myocardial infarction—experience in four TAMI studies. *Cardiac Assists, 4,* 1.

Grossman, W., & Baim, D. (1995). *Cardiac catheterization, angiography, and intervention* (5th ed.). Philadelphia: Lea & Febiger.

Miller, L. W. (1986). Emerging trends in the treatment of acute myocardial infarction and the role of intra-aortic balloon pumping. *Cardiac Assists, 3,* 1.

Quaal, S. J. (1993). *Comprehensive intra-aortic balloon counterpulsation* (2nd ed.). St. Louis, MO: Mosby–Year Book.

Additional Resources

Aroesty, J. M. (1979). Cardiogenic shock. In E. Donoso & S. Cohen (Eds.), *Critical cardiac care*. New York: Stratton Intercontinental Medical Book Corp.

Dunkman, W. B., Leinbach, R. C., Buckley, M. J., Mundth, E. D., Austen, W. G., & Kantrowitz, A. R. (1972). Clinical and hemodynamic results of intra-aortic balloon pumping and surgery for cardiogenic shock. *Circulation, 46,* 465.

Gold, H. K., Leinbach, R. C., Sanders, C. A., Buckley, M. J., Mundth, E. D., & Austen, W. G. (1973). Intra-aortic balloon pumping for interventricular septal defect or mitral regurgitation complicating acute myocardial infarction. *Circulation, 47,* 1191.

Guyton, A. (1984). *Textbook of medical physiology*. Philadelphia: Saunders.

Hanson, E. C. (1978). Control of post infarction ventricular irritability with intra-aortic balloon pump. *Circulation, 62*(Suppl. I), 130.

Introduction to intra-aortic balloon pumping. (1995). Reading, PA: Arrow International.

Kern, M. (1994). *The cardiac catheterization handbook* (2nd ed.). St. Louis, MO: Mosby–Year Book.

Leinbach, R. C., Gold, H. K., Harper, R. W., Buckley, M. J., & Austen, W. G. (1978). Early intra-aortic balloon pumping for anterior myocardial infarction without shock. *Circulation, 58,* 204.

Sturm, J. T., McGee, M. G., Fuhrman, T. M., Davis, G. L., Turner, S. A., Edelman, S. K., & Norman, J. C. (1980). Treatment of postoperative low output syndrome with intra-aortic balloon pumping: Experience with 419 patients. *American Journal of Cardiology, 45,* 1033.

Weintraub, R. M., Aroesty, J. M., Paulin, S., Levine, F. H., Markis, J. E., & LaRaia, P. J. (1979). Medically refractory unstable angina pectoris: Long term follow-up of patients undergoing intra-aortic balloon counterpulsation and operation. *American Journal of Cardiology, 43,* 877.

Practice Activities: Intra-aortic Balloon Pumping

1. Review the operator's manual for the make and mode of balloon pump used in your institution.

2. Review the package insert for the IAB catheter.

3. Practice the setup of the IAB pump:
   a. Connect an ECG signal generator to the console to simulate proper ECG timing.

4. Contact the supplier of your IAB pump and arrange to borrow an interactive pressure generator to simulate the arterial effects of your timing adjustments.

5. Practice changing the helium cylinder on the IAB pump console.

6. Practice setting up and calibrating an arterial pressure transducer.

7. Hemodynamically assess several patients in the cardiac care unit, including:
   a. Cardiac output (thermal dilution)
   b. Pulmonary vascular resistance
   c. Systemic vascular resistance
   d. Cardiac filling pressures

8. Practice arterial hemostasis techniques by removing arterial lines for patients with femoral cannulations.

9. Practice correct aseptic technique, site preparation, and draping for catheter insertion.

Check List: Insertion of the Intra-aortic Balloon

_____ 1. Set up an IAB procedure table according to hospital policy.

_____ 2. Prepare IAB according to manufacturer's specifications.

_____ 3. Prep and drape femoral artery insertion site.

4. Assist the physician:

_____ a. With securing vascular access

_____ b. Insertion of IAB

_____ c. Connection of IAB to console

Check List: Initiation and Timing of IABP

_____ 1. Prepare IABP console.
_____ 2. Obtain accurate ECG and arterial blood pressure signals on the console monitor for timing.
_____ 3. Initiate IABP at 2:1 ratio and adjust inflation and deflation timing.

_____ 4. Recognize errors in timing.
_____ 5. Troubleshoot the pump/balloon:
_____   a. Low helium
_____   b. Kinked tubing
_____   c. Trigger/sensing problems

Check List: IABP Patient Assessment and Weaning

1. Evaluate the effectiveness of counterpulsation:
_____   a. Cardiac output
_____   b. Pulmonary capillary wedge pressure
_____   c. Mean arterial pressure
_____   d. Peripheral pulses
2. Evaluate the patient for adequate cardiovascular response to the weaning process:
_____   a. Cardiac output
_____   b. Pulmonary capillary wedge pressure
_____   c. Mean arterial pressure
_____   d. Peripheral pulses

_____ 3. Wear personal protective equipment and follow standard precautions.
_____ 4. Assess lower limb pulses before decannulation.
_____ 5. Pull sheath, allowing proximal clots to eject.
_____ 6. Maintain pressure until hemostasis is achieved.
_____ 7. Apply appropriate dressing.
_____ 8. Instruct patient as to 6-hour recovery period.
_____ 9. Document procedure in patient record.

Self-Evaluation Post Test: Intra-aortic Balloon Pumping

1. Trained athletes can increase their cardiac output by a factor of 6. The difference between resting and maximal cardiac output is called:
a. cardiac index.
b. stroke work.
c. cardiac reserve.
d. afterpotential.

2. Preload on a ventricle is analogous to the stretch of a rubber band. Clinically, we measure this preload as:
a. mean arterial pressure.
b. left ventricular end-diastolic pressure.
c. cardiac output divided by body surface area.
d. cardiac output.

3. The majority of coronary blood flow occurs during which phase of the cardiac cycle?
a. Diastole
b. Isovolumetric contraction
c. Systole
d. Rapid filling

4. Myocardial metabolism can operate in an anaerobic fashion for short durations just as skeletal muscle does.
a. True
b. False

5. A definite contraindication to IABP therapy is the presence of:
a. aortic insufficiency.
b. mitral regurgitation.
c. coronary artery disease.
d. tortuous iliac arteries.

6. Balloon inflation is triggered to occur:
a. at the beginning of diastole.
b. at the beginning of systole.

7. Balloon deflation is adjusted to occur:
a. at the beginning of diastole.
b. at the beginning of systole.

8. Of the following four IABP timing errors, name the two that can cause serious deleterious effects:
I. Early inflation
II. Early deflation
III. Late inflation
IV. Late deflation
a. I, II
b. II, III
c. I, IV
d. II, III

9. When initiating balloon counterpulsation, you can best evaluate the effect of your timing adjustments by initially setting the assist ratio at:
a. 1:1.
b. 1:2.
c. 1:4.
d. 1:8.

10. How long should a patient's arterial puncture site normally be held to establish hemostasis following removal of the IAB system?
a. 9 minutes
b. 15 minutes
c. 25 minutes
d. 45 minutes

11. When pressure is applied to an artery following arterial catheterization, the pressure you apply with your hand should be firm enough to:
a. leave the artery downstream widely patent so a good pulse is felt.
b. not quite occlude the artery so a faint pulse is felt.
c. completely occlude the artery downstream, so no pulse is felt.
d. completely occlude it—in fact, as hard as you can push.

PERFORMANCE EVALUATION:
INSERTION OF THE INTRA-AORTIC BALLOON

Date: Lab _____ Clinical _____ Agency _____

Lab: Pass _____ Fail _____   Clinical: Pass _____ Fail _____

Student name _____ Instructor name _____

No. of times observed in clinical _____

No. of times practiced in clinical _____

PASSING CRITERIA: Obtain 90% or better on the procedure. Tasks indicated by * must receive at least 1 point, or the evaluation is terminated. Procedure must be performed within designated time, or the performance receives a failing grade.

SCORING: 2 points — Task performed satisfactorily without prompting.
1 point — Task performed satisfactorily with self-initiated correction.
0 points — Task performed incorrectly or with prompting required.
NA — Task not applicable to the patient care situation.

TASKS: PEER   LAB   CLINICAL

*   1. Sets up an IAB procedure table according to hospital policy   ☐   ☐   ☐

*   2. Prepares IAB according to manufacturer's specifications   ☐   ☐   ☐

*   3. Preps and drapes femoral artery insertion site   ☐   ☐   ☐

*   4. Assists the physician

           a. Securing vascular access   ☐   ☐   ☐

           b. Inserting IAB   ☐   ☐   ☐

           c. Connecting IAB to console   ☐   ☐   ☐

*   5. Documents the procedure in the patient record   ☐   ☐   ☐

SCORE: Peer   _____ points of possible 14; _____%

                Lab   _____ points of possible 14; _____%

                Clinical   _____ points of possible 14; _____%

TIME: _____ out of possible 30 minutes

STUDENT SIGNATURES   **INSTRUCTOR SIGNATURES**

PEER: _____   LAB: _____

STUDENT: _____   CLINICAL: _____

PERFORMANCE EVALUATION:
INITIATION AND TIMING OF IABP

Date: Lab _____ Clinical _____ Agency _____

Lab: Pass _____ Fail _____   Clinical: Pass _____ Fail _____

Student name _____ Instructor name _____

No. of times observed in clinical _____

No. of times practiced in clinical _____

PASSING CRITERIA: Obtain 90% or better on the procedure. Tasks indicated by * must receive at least 1 point, or the evaluation is terminated. Procedure must be performed within designated time, or the performance receives a failing grade.

SCORING:
2 points — Task performed satisfactorily without prompting.
1 point — Task performed satisfactorily with self-initiated correction.
0 points — Task performed incorrectly or with prompting required.
NA — Task not applicable to the patient care situation.

TASKS:		PEER	LAB	CLINICAL
*	1. Prepares IAB console	☐	☐	☐
*	2. Obtains an accurate ECG and arterial blood pressure signals on the console monitor for timing	☐	☐	☐
*	3. Initiates IABP at 2:1 ratio and adjusts inflation and deflation timing	☐	☐	☐
*	4. Recognizes errors in timing	☐	☐	☐
*	5. Troubleshoots the pump/balloon			
	a. Low helium content	☐	☐	☐
	b. Kinked tubing	☐	☐	☐
	c. Trigger/sensing problems	☐	☐	☐
*	6. Documents the procedure in the patient record	☐	☐	☐

SCORE: Peer _____ points of possible 16; _____%

Lab _____ points of possible 16; _____%

Clinical _____ points of possible 16; _____%

TIME: _____ out of possible 10 minutes

STUDENT SIGNATURES   INSTRUCTOR SIGNATURES

PEER: _____   LAB: _____

STUDENT: _____   CLINICAL: _____

PERFORMANCE EVALUATION:
IABP PATIENT ASSESSMENT AND WEANING

Date: Lab _____ Clinical _____ Agency _____

Lab: Pass _____ Fail _____   Clinical: Pass _____ Fail _____

Student name _____ Instructor name _____

No. of times observed in clinical _____

No. of times practiced in clinical _____

PASSING CRITERIA: Obtain 90% or better on the procedure. Tasks indicated by * must receive at least 1 point, or the evaluation is terminated. Procedure must be performed within designated time, or the performance receives a failing grade.

SCORING: 2 points — Task performed satisfactorily without prompting.
1 point — Task performed satisfactorily with self-initiated correction.
0 points — Task performed incorrectly or with prompting required.
NA — Task not applicable to the patient care situation.

TASKS:	PEER	LAB	CLINICAL
* 1. Evaluates the effectiveness of counterpulsation			
a. Cardiac output	☐	☐	☐
b. Pulmonary capillary wedge pressure	☐	☐	☐
c. Mean arterial pressure	☐	☐	☐
d. Peripheral pulses	☐	☐	☐
* 2. Evaluates the patient for adequate cardiovascular response to the weaning process:			
a. Cardiac output	☐	☐	☐
b. Pulmonary capillary wedge pressure	☐	☐	☐
c. Mean arterial pressure	☐	☐	☐
d. Peripheral pulses	☐	☐	☐
* 3. Wears personal protective equipment and follows standard precautions	☐	☐	☐
* 4. Assesses lower limb pulses before decannulation	☐	☐	☐
* 5. Pulls sheath allowing proximal clots to eject	☐	☐	☐
* 6. Maintains pressure until hemostasis is achieved	☐	☐	☐
* 7. Applies appropriate dressing	☐	☐	☐
* 8. Instructs patient as to 6-hour recovery period	☐	☐	☐
* 9. Documents procedure in patient record	☐	☐	☐

CHAPTER 25

NONINVASIVE POSITIVE-PRESSURE VENTILATION

INTRODUCTION

Noninvasive positive-pressure ventilation (NPPV) is the application of positive pressure via the upper respiratory tract for the purpose of augmenting alveolar ventilation (American Respiratory Care Foundation [ARCF], 1997). For the purposes of this chapter, NPPV is further defined as the application of positive-pressure ventilation to the upper respiratory tract using either a nasal or full-face mask as the ventilator-patient interface. NPPV is not new, but has been utilized for many years (Pierson, 1997). Application of NPPV is becoming more common.

Ventilators used for NPPV include any of the acute care ventilators employed in the intensive care setting. However, the ventilators most commonly applied for this purpose are the portable pressure-targeted ventilators (PTVs) such as *continuous positive airway pressure* (CPAP) and *bi-level positive airway pressure* (BiPAP) ventilators (Kacmarek, 1997). Recent advances in technology have improved the monitoring capabilities of these ventilators. These advances, combined with concurrent advances in ECG, oximetry and blood pressure monitoring, have reduced some of the risks associated with managing patients using NPPV.

KEY TERMS

- Bi-level positive airway pressure (BiPAP)
- Continuous positive airway pressure (CPAP)
- Expiratory positive airway pressure
- Full-face mask
- Inspiratory positive airway pressure
- Nasal mask
- Nasogastric tube
- Pressure-targeted ventilation (PTV)
- Rapid-shallow-breathing index
- Spacers
- Spontaneous breath
- Timed breath

OBJECTIVES

At the end of this chapter, you should be able to:

- Define noninvasive positive-pressure ventilation (NPPV).
- List the indications for NPPV.
- Describe the assessment of a patient for NPPV.
- Compare and contrast the advantages and disadvantages of nasal and full-face masks as the patient-ventilator interface.
- State the hazards and complications associated with NPPV.
- Describe the effects of changes in resistance and compliance on volume delivery with pressure-targeted ventilation (PTV).
- Describe the modes of NPPV.
- Explain how to provide supplemental oxygen.
- State what monitoring devices should be used when a patient is receiving NPPV.

DEFINITION OF NONINVASIVE POSITIVE-PRESSURE VENTILATION

Noninvasive positive-pressure ventilation (NPPV) is the application of positive pressure via the upper respiratory tract for the purpose of augmenting alveolar ventilation (ARCF, 1997). NPPV is increasingly used to provide improved alveolar ventilation to those patients in acute respiratory failure, especially when intubation is not desirable (Brochard et al., 1995; Wunderink & Hill, 1997). By using a nasal or full-face mask as the interface between the patient and the ventilator, the associated complications of intubation may be avoided. Advantages of avoiding intubation include better ability of the patient to communicate and the ability to take fluids and medications orally.

INDICATIONS FOR NONINVASIVE POSITIVE-PRESSURE VENTILATION

The indications for NPPV are summarized in Table 25-1.

Many authors have investigated the efficacy of NPPV in acute respiratory failure (Brochard et al., 1995; Kramer, Meyer, Meharg, Cece, & Hill, 1995; Martin et al., 2000). The greatest number of patients in which this modality has been utilized is acute exacerbation of chronic obstructive

TABLE 25-1: Indications for NPPV in Acute Respiratory Failure

Acute exacerbation of chronic obstructive pulmonary disease

Acute hypoxemic respiratory failure

Acute cardiogenic pulmonary edema

Weaning from ventilatory support

Community-acquired pneumonia

Postoperative respiratory failure

Severe acute asthma

Do not resuscitate/do not intubate orders

pulmonary disease (COPD). NPPV can be effective in augmenting alveolar ventilation with the goals of reducing $PaCO_2$, increasing PaO_2, increasing SpO_2, and normalizing arterial pH. Intubation and mechanical ventilation may accomplish many of these same goals; however, NPPV avoids the hazards and complications of intubation as described in Chapter 20.

Patients with COPD benefit from NPPV by avoiding intubation (Brochard et al., 1995; Wunderink & Hill, 1997). Often, once intubated, these patients tend to have an extended ventilator course and may be difficult to wean and extubate. NPPV may help the patient through the period of acute respiratory failure, allowing time for antibiotics, diuretics, and other medications to work, so that intubation is avoided.

Hypoxic respiratory failure may also be an indication for NPPV. This is especially true in cases in which the patient or the patient's family has requested not to intubate or resuscitate. In these cases, NPPV may assist the patient through the acute respiratory failure phase, giving other medications time to work. NPPV can temporarily reverse the hypoxemia and hypercarbia associated with acute respiratory failure.

NPPV may also play a role in acute cardiogenic pulmonary edema (Mehta et al., 1997). NPPV can again provide augmented alveolar ventilation until other medications have time to work (diuretics and cardiac medications). NPPV helps the patient through the period of acute respiratory failure, and once the pulmonary edema resolves, the patient may resume spontaneous respiration.

In some cases, the patient fails initial weaning and extubation from mechanical ventilation. NPPV can provide a means of augmenting alveolar ventilation without reintubation and initiation of conventional ventilation. NPPV can again provide time, permitting the patient to gain ventilatory strength and to complete the weaning process successfully.

Community-acquired pneumonia can lead to ventilatory failure and corresponding hypercapnia and hypoxemia. In these cases, NPPV may provide the muscle unloading and ventilatory assistance required, overcoming the patient's short-term ventilatory failure. The potential benefits of short-term NPPV include avoidance of intuba-

tion and providing time (ventilatory support) for the antibiotics and other medications to work.

NPPV may also be helpful in postoperative respiratory failure. Postoperative respiratory failure is characterized by hypoxemia and hypercarbia. NPPV can provide ventilatory assistance without intubation, supporting these patients until the underlying cause of respiratory failure has resolved.

NPPV has been successfully used in asthma and status asmaticus (Meduri et al., 1991; Pollack, Torres, & Alexander, 1996). Asthma is one of the diseases classified as a chronic obstructive pulmonary disease. In asthma, the patient may present with hypercarbia and hypoxemia. NPPV can support the patient's ventilation without intubation and therefore has been shown to have benefit.

Many patients with chronic disease have made the determination, with or without family consensus, to not be intubated and mechanically ventilated when they become terminally ill. NPPV has been used to provide ventilatory support in these patients, potentially allowing time to overcome the cause of ventilatory failure.

ASSESSMENT OF THE PATIENT FOR NONINVASIVE POSITIVE-PRESSURE VENTILATION

Patient assessment for NPPV is similar to assessment of patients for intubation and continuous mechanical ventilation. Assessment should include determination of ventilatory parameters, arterial blood gases, oxygen saturation, and work of breathing and detection of changes in the patient's vital signs.

Ventilatory parameters include tidal volume, minute volume, frequency, and the rapid-shallow-breathing index. Tidal volumes of less than 3 to 5 ml/kg are indicative of impending ventilatory failure. A patient cannot move sufficient volume (greater than dead space volume) to sustain ventilatory needs when the tidal volume falls to this level. A minute volume in excess of 10 L/min is also indicative of impending failure. Excessive muscle work is required to sustain this level of ventilation, and therefore it can't be maintained for long periods of time. A respiratory rate of greater than 35 per minute is also indicative of impending failure. Like increased minute ventilation, increased ventilatory rates require more muscle effort to sustain, and therefore can't be maintained for long periods of time. The *rapid-shallow-breathing index* is often used as a weaning criterion (Krieger, Isber, Breitenbucher, Throop, & Ershowsky, 1997). The rapid-shallow breathing index (RSBI) is the frequency divided by the tidal volume (in liters).

$$RSBI = \frac{frequency}{tidal\ volume\ (L)}$$

An index of 130 or greater is an indication of impending failure. The rapid-shallow-breathing index quantifies the relationship between the ventilatory rate (frequency) and the tidal volume.

Arterial blood gas analysis is also used to identify impending ventilatory failure. The pH, $PaCO_2$, and PaO_2

are measured and compared with the patient's baseline values to determine impending ventilatory failure. A pH of less than 7.25, a $PaCO_2$ greater than 55 mm Hg (except in chronic hypercapnia), and a PaO_2 of less than 50 mm Hg on an FIO_2 (fraction of inspired oxygen) greater than 0.5 are indicative of impending failure. It is important to trend results of arterial blood gas analysis against the patient's normal values. Taking these values and using them as absolute guidelines in the chronically ill patient may often lead to the wrong conclusion about the patient's condition.

A declining oxygen saturation or a saturation of less than 90% is also not a good sign. Oxygen saturation as measured by pulse oximetry (SpO_2) is widely used to determine oxygenation. In using pulse oximetry, it is important to ensure that the signal strength is adequate and to compare the pulse rate with the heart monitor. If both are adequate, the reading will probably be valid as well.

Work of breathing is best assessed by inspection (refer to Chapter 3). Use of accessory muscles, retractions, and pursed-lip breathing all are signs of increased ventilatory work. Careful inspection combined with the patient's subjective comments regarding the perceived work of breathing combined with the ventilatory parameters will complete the picture of the patient's actual work of breathing.

Impending ventilatory failure will also result in changes in the patient's vital signs. Hypoxemia, hypercapnia, and increased ventilatory work all have an impact on the vital signs. Typically tachycardia, arrhythmias, and hypertension will present concomitantly with the changes in ventilatory status.

PATIENT-VENTILATOR INTERFACE IN NONINVASIVE POSITIVE-PRESSURE VENTILATION

The interface of the ventilator with the patient—the mask and headgear—is critical to the success of NPPV (Turner, 1997). Patient comfort is important in tolerance of NPPV. Therefore, the type of mask (nasal versus full-face), type of harness, and the fit of the mask are imperative to the success of NPPV. A patient who is uncomfortable wearing the mask will tear it off the face if he or she is able to do so. As a clinician you must decide what type, size, and fit are best for the patient.

Patients who are claustrophobic often tolerate a *nasal mask* better. The nasal mask fits over the nose and upper lip, leaving the mouth relatively free (Figure 25-1). Advantages of the nasal mask include decreased risk of aspiration, ability to eat and drink, and improved verbal communication. The cushion that seals the mask should be of very soft, nonallergenic material. When the mask is fitted properly, little force should be required by the harness to maintain a good seal.

The *full-face mask* fits over the entire mouth and nose (Figure 25-2). The face mask has the advantage of lower resistance to flow than with the nasal mask (Turner, 1997). However, the full-face mask carries the risk of increased aspiration. Therefore, a *nasogastric tube* is often placed to decompress the stomach and reduce the risk of aspiration. Other disadvantages of the full-face mask include the inability of the patient to take any food or liquids by mouth and decreased ability to communicate verbally.

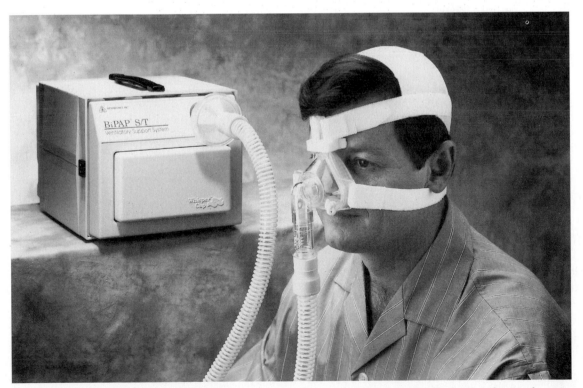

Figure 25-1 *The nasal mask used for NPPV. Note how it fits over the nose and upper lip, leaving the mouth relatively free.* (*Courtesy of* Respironics, Inc., Pittsburgh, PA)

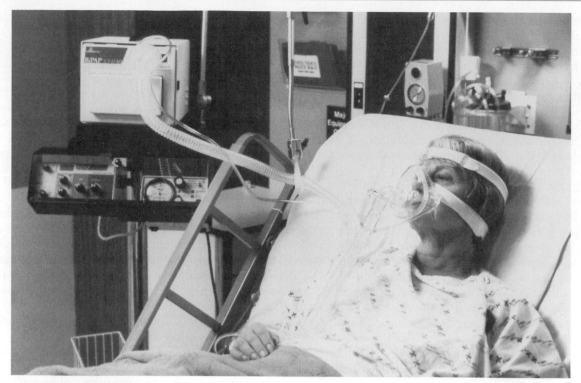

Figure 25-2 *The full-face mask. Note how it fits, covering both the mouth and nose. (Courtesy of* Respironics, Inc., Pittsburgh, PA)

HAZARDS AND COMPLICATIONS OF NONINVASIVE POSITIVE-PRESSURE VENTILATION

Hazards and complications of NPPV include leaks, nasal or sinus pain or discomfort, gastric insufflation, eye irritation, barotrauma, aspiration pneumonia, mucous plugging, and hypoxemia (Hill, 1997).

Leaks in the circuitry used in NPPV are common. Most ventilators used for NPPV are able to tolerate and compensate for some amount of leak. However, too much of a leak will result in decreased ventilation (lower pressure), leading to hypoxemia and hypercarbia. The fit of the mask and harness is important to minimize leaks. Your skill as a clinician in fitting the mask and adjusting the harness is important to the success of NPPV. Therefore, it is important for you to become proficient and to have a variety of masks available for use.

Nasal or sinus pain is a frequent complaint of patients being ventilated by mask. The increased flow and pressure through the sinuses from the ventilator cause this discomfort. If possible, initiate NPPV at lower pressures and gradually work toward the desired target pressure to achieve the desired tidal volume and minute ventilation. Pressure sores and ulcerations may also occur owing to excessive pressure of the mask against the face. The bridge of the nose is the most common site for these pressure sores. Again, proper mask fit is imperative to the success of NPPV.

Gastric insufflation is often reported as a consequence of NPPV. Gastric insufflation occurs because the pressure and flow from the ventilator may be transmitted to the esophagus as well as the trachea. Like IPPB, NPPV can result in gastric insufflation. Sometimes a nasogastric tube is used in conjunction with NPPV to decompress the stomach, preventing gastric insufflation.

Eye irritation occurs because of flow around the mask up into the eyes. This flow is caused by leaks. If the mask fits properly, eye irritation can be minimized. Use of *spacers*, proper mask fit, and correct adjustment of the headgear or harness can minimize leaks, correcting this problem.

Barotrauma may result from the application of too much pressure in ventilating a patient with NPPV. Like IPPV, NPPV has the potential to cause a pneumothorax by rupturing a bleb in a patient with bullous lung disease.

Aspiration pneumonia is a potential complication of NPPV. Because the airway is not as secure as with an endotracheal or a tracheostomy tube, aspiration into the lower airway is possible. If the patient's protective reflexes are compromised or absent, intubation and conventional ventilation should be considered.

NPPV ventilators often are used without humidification. The increased flow of relatively dry air may result in drying of the respiratory mucosa and mucous plugging. Adequate patient hydration and maintenance of adequate cough and pulmonary clearance are important to minimize this potential complication.

Hypoxemia can occur with NPPV. Not all NPPV ventilators are capable of providing supplemental oxygen concentrations. Many NPPV ventilators require the clinician to bleed in oxygen to achieve the desired SpO_2 levels. If NPPV fails to achieve the desired oxygenation outcomes, intubation and conventional ventilation should be considered.

HOW RESISTANCE AND COMPLIANCE AFFECT NONINVASIVE POSITIVE-PRESSURE VENTILATION

NPPV is really *pressure-targeted ventilation* (Kacmarek, 1997). In pressure-targeted ventilation, a set pressure is applied to achieve a desired tidal volume. NPPV ventilators do not have tidal volume controls or adjustment capability as in most acute care ventilators. Rather, the clinician selects an inspiratory pressure that is then delivered by the ventilator to achieve the desired tidal volume. Volume and flow both vary during inspiration, and are not adjustable or set by the clinician. Volume delivery therefore varies, just as volume delivery varies with IPPB.

Changes in resistance affect inspiratory time. Increases in airway resistance (R_{AW}) result in increased inspiratory times, in that pressure rises more slowly to the target level (Strumpf, Carlisle, Millman, Smith, & Hill, 1990). With increased R_{AW}, volumes may also concomitantly decrease during the typical 1- to 2-second inspiratory times during ventilation.

Changes in compliance have a profound effect on volume delivery at a set pressure. Decreased compliance (from a stiffer lung or thorax) causes decreased volume delivery for a given pressure. Increased compliance results in greater volume delivery for a given set pressure.

Because both R_{AW} and compliance affect volume delivery, it is important to monitor delivered tidal volumes, SpO_2, and blood gases to ensure that the patient is being adequately ventilated. Volume delivery will vary breath by breath depending on how the patient's condition changes.

MODES OF NONINVASIVE POSITIVE-PRESSURE VENTILATION

The modes of NPPV ventilation include pressure adjustment, spontaneous, spontaneous/timed, and timed ventilation. Pressure adjustment entails adjusting both inspiratory and expiratory pressures. Inspiratory pressure is often named *inspiratory positive airway pressure* (IPAP) in bilevel pressure ventilation. IPAP is the peak inspiratory pressure that is achieved when the ventilator delivers a breath. IPAP is typically adjustable between 4 and 40 cm H_2O depending on the unit. *Expiratory positive airway pressure* (EPAP) is the pressure level maintained in the circuit during the expiratory phase. EPAP may be adjusted between 4 and 20 cm H_2O depending on the ventilator.

Spontaneous mode is what the name implies. The ventilator senses the patient's inspiratory effort (flow) and initiates a ventilator-supported breath (pressure delivery). Inspiratory flow rapidly increases and the desired pressure is maintained for the set inspiratory time (% IPAP). During exhalation, pressure delivery decreases and the EPAP pressure is maintained during the expiratory phase until the ventilator senses the next *spontaneous breath.* If the patient becomes apneic, no breath delivery will occur in this mode. All breath delivery is dependent on the patient's intact respiratory drive.

Spontaneous/timed mode is like the spontaneous mode just described but has a backup breath (timed) delivery. As long as the patient is breathing spontaneously, the ventilator delivers breaths in response to the patient's effort. If the patient becomes apneic, the ventilator reverts to the timed mode and delivers breaths at the set rate. Breath rates may be set between 4 and 40 breaths per minute, depending on the ventilator.

Timed mode is a mode in which breath delivery is determined by the breath rate control. The breath rate control is simply a timer that determines the start of inspiration. At a rate of 10 breaths per minute, every 6 seconds a time-triggered breath will be initiated. The inspiratory time is determined by the % IPAP or inspiratory time control. Spontaneous respiratory efforts by the patient will not trigger inspiration in this mode.

SUPPLEMENTAL OXYGEN DELIVERY

The PTV ventilators used in NPPV were originally employed in the home setting for treatment of sleep apnea. As such, they were designed initially to run on household electrical power and be independent of any gas source. As the application of these ventilators was expanded into the acute care setting, the need for supplemental oxygen delivery became required. Some ventilators now provide for the adjustment of oxygen concentrations (% oxygen) just as with other acute care ventilators. However, if this adjustment is not available, oxygen must be bled into the circuit.

Often, supplemental oxygen is provided by bleeding in oxygen through an adapter at the outlet of the ventilator (Figure 25-3). Alternatively, oxygen may be provided by bleeding it into a port on the nasal mask. SpO_2 and arterial blood gases should be monitored to ensure that the patient's oxygenation needs are being met. Additionally, tidal volumes should be monitored to ensure that they are also adequate to meet the patient's needs and have not changed owing to the addition of supplemental oxygen.

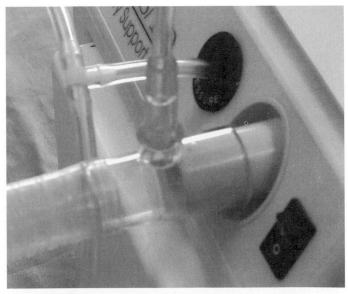

Figure 25-3 *Supplemental oxygen being bled into the circuit at the ventilator outlet*

PATIENT MONITORING

Patients on NPPV require careful monitoring and considerable one-on-one care during initiation of NPPV. Monitors used should include oxygen saturation, cardiac, blood pressure, and oxygen analysis monitors.

Oximetry is important in determining whether NPPV is meeting the patient's oxygenation requirements. Oximeters with alarms (set off by low SpO_2) are helpful in signaling a decrease in the patient's oxygen saturation. When you use an oximeter, the measured heart rate should be compared with the patient's heart rate (as monitored or palpated), and the signal strength should also be verified when you are taking readings.

Heart monitors are important in detecting arrythmias and changes in heart rate. Critically ill patients should be monitored closely for cardiac complications. Continuous ECG monitoring is the standard of care for these patients.

Blood pressure may be monitored by the use of noninvasive blood pressure monitors. At set intervals, the automated blood pressure cuff inflates and the readings are obtained. Hypotension from NPPV is a rare complication (Hill, 1997). Appropriate blood pressure monitoring will alert you to changes in the patient's status.

Oxygen analyzers are used to monitor the FiO_2 delivered when supplemental oxygen is used. Monitoring may be performed continuously by placing the sensor in-line with the patient circuit or by periodically checking the FiO_2. As always, in using an oxygen analyzer, it is important to calibrate the device periodically (once each shift).

PROFICIENCY OBJECTIVES

At the end of this chapter, you should be able to:

- Demonstrate the assessment of a patient for the need for NPPV:
  — Respiratory frequency
  — Tidal volume
  — Minute ventilation
  — Rapid-shallow-breathing index
  — Vital capacity
  — SpO_2
  — Arterial blood gases
- Demonstrate how to assemble and test an NPPV ventilator prior to use.
- Demonstrate how to select a mask for NPPV:
  — Demonstrate the use of both nasal and full-face masks.
  — Demonstrate how to use the harness/headgear correctly.

- — Demonstrate how to size the mask correctly for the patient's face.
- Demonstrate how to establish appropriate ventilator settings:
  — IPAP
  — EPAP
  — % IPAP
  — Mode
  — FiO_2
  — Alarms
- Demonstrate how to establish appropriate monitoring for the patient on NPPV.
  — ECG monitoring
  — Oximetry
  — Noninvasive blood pressure monitoring
  — Oxygen analysis
- Demonstrate how to chart NPPV in the patient's flow sheet or chart.

PATIENT ASSESSMENT FOR NPPV

Prior to initiation of NPPV, the patient must be closely assessed to determine the need for ventilation. This assessment may include physical assessment, oximetry, arterial blood gas analysis, and determination of ventilatory parameters.

Physical assessment and spontaneous parameters are described in previous chapters (Chapters 4 and 5). The acutely ill patient may be hypoxemic and hypercapneic; therefore, caution and common sense are required when the mechanics of ventilation are assessed. The patient may require supplemental oxygen to maintain adequate oxygen saturation even without any undue stress. Arterial blood gas analysis is important in establishing the patient's baseline pH, $PaCO_2$, and PaO_2 prior to NPPV. Periodically, repeat arterial blood gases may be obtained following commitment to NPPV to determine whether the patient is being adequately ventilated.

ASSEMBLY AND TESTING OF THE VENTILATOR

The ventilator circuit required for NPPV is relatively simple (Figure 25-4). Connection and assembly of the circuit are described for the NPPV ventilators in the practice activity section of this chapter.

Testing of the circuit's integrity can be accomplished by blocking the mask interface and placing the ventilator into the timed mode with a set rate. Observe for the pressure to rise to the set IPAP level for the appropriate percentage of the inspiratory time. If the pressure fails to rise to the IPAP level, you have a leak. Check all connections for leaks and make sure all connections are tight.

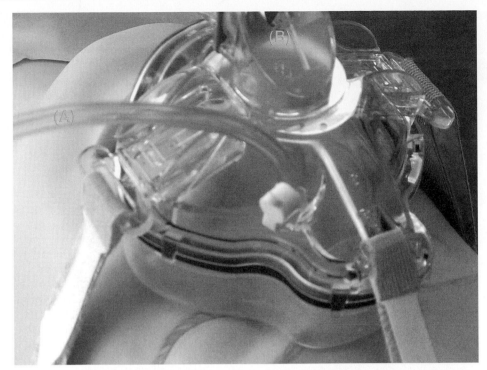

Figure 25-4   *A schematic of the NPPV ventilator circuit. Note the proximal pressure line (A), main circuit tubing (B), and mask interface.*

MASK SELECTION

Mask selection and fitting constitute one of the most important determinants of success with NPPV. Selection and fitting of the mask require both knowledge and skill. As a new respiratory care practitioner, you will need time and practice under the supervision of a seasoned practitioner to master this skill.

Fitting of nasal masks can be facilitated using the size guide rings (Figure 25-5). Once the patient's nose is matched to the size, a mask can then be selected. Besides size, the type of cushion is also important to the correct mask fit. If a mask is correctly selected, minimal pressure will be required to make it seal. Figure 25-6 shows a nasal mask correctly fitted to the patient's face.

Full-face masks must cover both the nose and the mouth. Sizes vary from small to large. The cushion is important as well as the size to obtain the proper seal. Once the correct mask size is selected, the four-point harness is used to hold the mask in position. As with the nasal mask, if it is fitted correctly, minimal pressure will be required to secure the full-face mask. Figure 25-7 shows the full-face mask correctly fitted to the patient.

The head gear or straps are important in securing the mask and keeping it in place. A common mistake made by inexperienced respiratory care practitioners is to tighten the straps too much. Too much tension can cause pressure sores to develop quickly, making the mask very uncomfortable for the patient. Remember that if the mask is correctly fitted, little pressure will be required to seal it.

Spacers may be used in conjunction with the nasal mask to relieve pressure on the bridge of the nose. Spacers

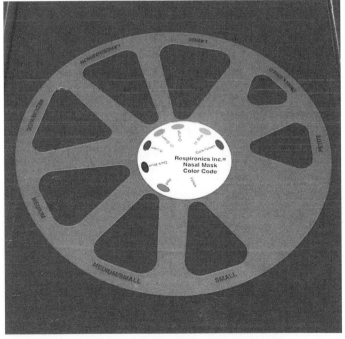

Figure 25-5   *A sizing ring being utilized to determine the correct manufacturer's mask size for a patient (Courtesy of* Respironics, Inc., Pittsburgh, PA)

generally rest against the forehead, reducing pressure along the apex of the mask. Spacers come in varying thickness and materials. Choose the spacer that fits the patient the best and helps to improve the mask fit and patient comfort.

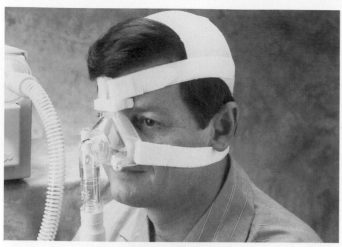

Figure 25-6 *A photograph of a nasal mask correctly fitted and secured to a patient's face* (*Courtesy of* Respironics, Inc., Pittsburgh, PA)

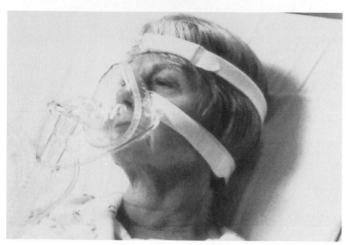

Figure 25-7 *The full-face mask correctly fitted to the patient's face* (*Courtesy of* Respironics, Inc., Pittsburgh, PA)

VENTILATOR SETTINGS

The physician may order specific pressures (IPAP and EPAP), rate, and FiO_2 for NPPV. Alternatively, the physician may order a desired tidal volume range; in this case, as a clinician you must adjust the IPAP and EPAP to achieve it. In either case, you must be able to adjust both IPAP and EPAP controls as well as the inspiratory time (% IPAP) to achieve the desired ventilation.

Most often, spontaneous/timed mode is utilized for NPPV. This allows the ventilator to detect the patient's spontaneous efforts, triggering ventilator-supported breaths. In this mode, if the patient fails to initiate a breath, the ventilator's backup rate will ensure ventilation.

FiO_2 levels may be adjusted by "bleeding in" oxygen or by setting the % oxygen control. In either case, monitoring the FiO_2 using an oxygen analyzer must be done to confirm the correct settings.

Alarms will vary depending on the NPPV ventilator that is used. The simplest type of alarm is a pressure disconnect alarm. In the event of a severe leak or tubing disconnect, pressure will fall and the alarm will sound. Other NPPV ventilators have more sophisticated alarm and monitoring systems. Alarm systems specific to NPPV ventilators will be discussed later in the practice activities portion of this chapter.

PATIENT MONITORING

The ECG leads should be placed and connected to the patient monitor. Verify that the ECG wave form is correct and that the leads have been correctly placed.

Connect the patient to a continuous oximeter monitor. Verify that the heart rate display matches the ECG heart rate. Also ensure that the signal strength is adequate for a good reading. Patient motion, bright ambient light, fingernail polish, and other factors can influence the accuracy of pulse oximeters.

If noninvasive blood pressure monitoring is desired, connect the blood pressure cuff to the patient's arm and program the unit for the desired blood pressure measurement interval. Press the manual pressure measurement button to verify that it is connected correctly and working properly.

If continuous oxygen (FiO_2) monitoring is desired, connect the oxygen analyzer in-line at the ventilator outlet. If oxygen is bled into the circuit, where you bleed in the oxygen and where you place the monitor is important. Don't place the monitor upstream from the point of oxygen addition and expect to have an accurate reading. If oxygen is bled into the system, you may wish to consider spot checks of FiO_2 rather than continuous monitoring.

PATIENT CHARTING

At a minimum, patient charting should include breath sounds, heart rate, SpO_2, work of breathing, IPAP, EPAP, mode, ventilatory rate, tidal volume, estimated leak, ventilator rate (backup), and FiO_2. Often a flow sheet is used to record the data in a checklist format. Monitoring may be performed as frequently as every hour or more often, depending on the patient's status. At initiation of NPPV, it takes considerable time to fit the mask, make the ventilator adjustments, and work with the patient to relieve anxiety and to faciliatate getting used to the NPPV system.

References

American Respiratory Care Foundation. (1997). Consensus conference: Noninvasive positive pressure ventilation. *Respiratory Care, 42*(4), 364–369.

Brochard, L., Mancebo, J., Wysocki, M., Lofaso, F., Conti, G., Rauss, A., Simonneau, G., Benito, S., Gasparetto, A., & Lemaire, F. (1995). Noninvasive ventilation for acute exacerbations of chronic obstructive pulmonary disease. *New England Journal of Medicine, 333,* 817–822.

Hill, N. (1997). Complications of noninvasive positive pressure ventilation. *Respiratory Care, 42*(4), 432–442.

Kacmarek, R. M. (1997). Characteristics of pressure-targeted ventilators used for noninvasive positive pressure ventilation. *Respiratory Care, 42*(4), 380–388.

Kramer, N., Meyer, T. J., Meharg, J., Cece, R. D., & Hill, N. S. (1995). Randomized, prospective trial of noninvasive positive pressure ventilation in acute respiratory failure. *American Journal of Respiratory and Critical Care Medicine, 151,* 1799–1806.

Krieger, B. P., Isber, J., Breitenbucher, A., Throop, G., & Ershowsky, P. (1997). Serial measurements of the rapid-shallow-breathing index as a predictor of weaning outcome in elderly medical patients. *Chest, 112*(4), 1029–1034.

Martin, T. J., Hovis, J. D., Costantino, J. P., Bieman, M. I., Donahoe, M. P., Rogers, R. M., Kreit, J. W., Sciurba, F. C., Stiller, R. A., & Sanders, M. H. (2000). A randomized, prospective evaluation of noninvasive ventilation for acute respiratory failure. *American Journal of Respiratory and Critical Care Medicine, 161,* 807–813.

Meduri, G. U., Abou-Shala, N., Fox, R. C., Jones, C. B., Leeper, K. V., & Wunderink, R. G. (1991). Noninvasive positive pressure ventilation via face mask: First-line intervention in patients with acute hypercapnia and hypoxemic respiratory failure. *Chest, 100*(2), 445–454.

Mehta, S., Jay, G. D., Woolard, R. H., Hipona, R. A., Connolly, E. M., Cimini, D. M., Drinkwine, J. H., & Hill, N. S. (1997). Randomized, prospective trial of bilevel versus continuous positive airway pressure in acute pulmonary edema. *Critical Care Medicine, 25,* 620–628.

Pierson, D. J. (1997). Noninvasive positive pressure ventilation: History and terminology. *Respiratory Care, 42*(4), 370–379.

Pollack, C., Jr., Torres, M. T., & Alexander, L. (1996). Feasibility study of the use of bi-level positive airway pressure for respiratory support in the emergency department. *Annals of Emergency Medicine, 27*(2), 189–192.

Strumpf, D. A., Carlisle, C. C., Millman, R. P., Smith, K. W., & Hill, N. S. (1990). An evaluation of the respironics BiPAP bi-level CPAP device for delivery of assisted ventilation. *Respiratory Care, 35*(5), 415–422.

Turner, R. (1997). NPPV: Face versus interface. *Respiratory Care, 42*(4), 389–393.

Wunderink, R. G., & Hill, N. S. (1997). Continuous and periodic applications of noninvasive positive pressure ventilation in respiratory failure. *Respiratory Care, 42*(4), 394–402.

Practice Activities: Respironics S/T-D BiPAP Ventilator

CIRCUIT ASSEMBLY

Figure 25-8 illustrates the Respironics S/T-D circuit that is assembled and ready to attach to the ventilator. Note the circuit consists of two pieces of tubing, the patient tubing (22-mm diameter) and the proximal pressure line. The tubing must terminate at the patient end with a Whisper Swivel. The Whisper Swivel is equivalent to an exhalation valve, allowing the patient to exhale to the ambient air, and acts as a one-way valve during inspiration. The mask (nasal or full-face) attaches to the Whisper Swivel.

Connect the patient tubing (22 mm) to the ventilator outlet. If you are not using the remote control unit, connect the proximal line to the proximal connector on the front of the unit. If the remote control unit is being used, connect a T adapter to the proximal line, connecting one end to the ventilator and the other to the pressure monitor, as shown in Figure 25-9.

VENTILATOR PREPARATION

On the rear of the ventilator, verify that the correct voltage is selected for the line power in your facility. Verify that the on/off switch is in the off position, and connect the power cord to an appropriate power outlet.

VENTILATOR OPERATION VERIFICATION

Turn the ventilator on, and set the controls to the following settings:

IPAP:	4 cm H2O
EPAP:	4 cm H2O
Mode:	Timed
BPM:	10
% IPAP:	30%

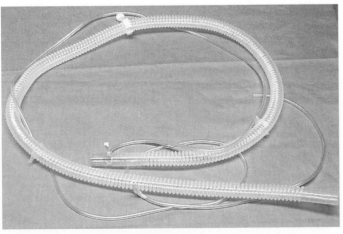

Figure 25-8 *The S/T-D patient circuit*

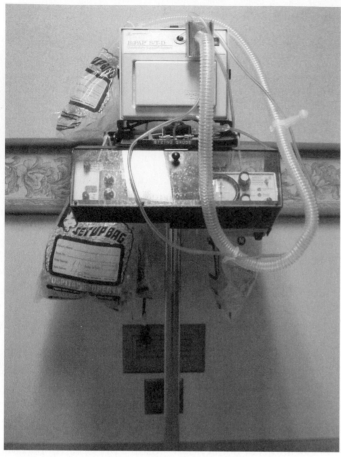

Figure 25-9 *The circuit connected to the ventilator. Note how a T adapter is used on the proximal pressure line to connect both the ventilator and the monitoring alarm.*

1. Occlude the mask outlet on the circuit and verify that the pressure reading on the manometer is 4 cm H_2O. If you are using the remote control panel with its monitor, verify the digital display of the IPAP control.

2. Increase the IPAP setting to 10, 15 and 20 cm H_2O, verifying each pressure level.

3. Turn the IPAP control to its maximum setting.

4. Adjust the EPAP control to 10, 15, and 20 cm H_2O, verifying each pressure level.

5. Adjust the EPAP control to 4 cm H_2O and the IPAP control to 10 cm H_2O.

6. Set the Mode control to Spontaneous mode:
   a. Open the mask port to simulate a breath.
   b. Verify that the ventilator cycles into inspiration and observe that the IPAP control light illuminates.
   c. Verify that the inspiratory time lasts between 2 and 3 seconds before cycling into EPAP (exhalation).

7. Set the Mode control to Spontaneous/Timed mode:
   a. Verify that the Spontaneous/Timed LED is illuminated.
   b. Adjust the BPM to 10 and occlude the mask port.
   c. Verify that the rate is 10/minute.
   d. Adjust the BPM control to 15 and verify the rate.
   e. Open the mask port and verify that the ventilator cycles into inspiration.

8. Set the Mode control to Timed mode:
   a. Verify that the Timed LED is illuminated.
   b. Adjust the BPM to 10 and occlude the mask port.
   c. Verify that the rate is 10/minute.
   d. Adjust the BPM control to 15 and verify the rate.
   e. Set the BPM control to 10 and adjust the % IPAP time to 50%. Verify that the IPAP time increases appropriately.

ACTIVITIES

To complete these practice exercises, it is recommended that you use a lung analog/simulator such as a Medishield or Manley test lung. With these units, you may easily adjust resistance (R_{AW}) and compliance for the following exercises to simulate changes in the patient's condition.

Exercise 1: Resistance and Compliance

Initial Settings
    Mode: Spontaneous/Timed
    BPM: 10
    IPAP: 15 cm H_2O
    EPAP: 4 cm H_2O
    % IPAP: 30%

1. Connect the ventilator to the test lung. Have the resistance control set at zero and the compliance set with only one spring.

2. Note the following:
   a. Tidal volume (digital display) (or use the measurement on the test lung bellows)
   b. Inspiratory time
   c. Ventilatory rate

3. Change the resistance to 50, increasing the R_{AW}.

4. Note the following:
   a. Tidal volume (digital display) (or use the measurement on the test lung bellows)
   b. Inspiratory time
   c. Ventilatory rate

Questions:
A. What happened to the tidal volume delivery?
B. What happened to the inspiratory time?

5. Return the R_{AW} control to zero.

6. Decrease the compliance by adding an additional spring onto the bellows of the test lung.

7. Note the following:
   a. Tidal volume (digital display) (or use the measurement on the test lung bellows)
   b. Inspiratory time
   c. Ventilatory rate

Questions:
A. What happened to the tidal volume delivery?
B. What happened to the inspiratory time?

8. Change the controls to the following:
    BPM: 10
    IPAP: 20 cm H_2O
    EPAP: 8 cm H_2O
    % IPAP: 20%

9. Repeat steps 3 through 7.

10. Note the following:
    a. Tidal volume (digital display) (or use the measurement on the test lung bellows)
    b. Inspiratory time
    c. Ventilatory rate

Questions:
A. What happened to the tidal volume delivery?
B. What happened to the inspiratory time?

Exercise 2: Oxygen Addition

1. Assemble the Respironics S/T-D ventilator and a circuit.

2. Attach an O_2 enrichment adapter (an aerosol T with a small-diameter nipple on it) to the ventilator outlet. Using oxygen tubing, connect a flowmeter to the O_2 enrichment adapter.

3. Connect the circuit to the O_2 enrichment adapter.

4. Place an oxygen analyzer in-line at the Whisper Swivel and connect the ventilator to a test lung.

5. Set the ventilator to the following settings:
   Mode: Spontaneous/Timed
   BPM: 10
   IPAP: 15 cm H_2O
   EPAP: 4 cm H_2O
   % IPAP: 30%

6. Without adding oxygen, verify that the FiO_2 reads 0.21.

7. Turn the oxygen flowmeter to 3 L/min. Measure the FiO_2 after three breaths.

8. Turn off the flowmeter, and allow the test lung to purge any oxygen for about 2 minutes.

9. Turn the oxygen flowmeter to 10 L/min. Measure the FiO_2 after three breaths.

Question:
A. What changes in FiO_2 did you observe?

Exercise 3: NPPV Application

Identify a laboratory partner who will act as your patient. With your laboratory instructor observing you, complete the following exercise.

1. Assemble the Respironics S/T-D ventilator and attach a clean circuit.

2. Using standard precautions, select the correct nasal mask for your patient and the appropriate headgear and spacers.

3. Connect the mask to the circuit, and set the ventilator to the following settings:
   Mode: Spontaneous/Timed
   IPAP: 15 cm H_2O
   IPAP: 4 cm H_2O
   BPM: 10/min
   % IPAP: 20%

4. Fit the mask to your patient, using the spacer(s) and the headgear.

5. Observe the pressure manometer and the LEDs for correct operation.

6. Note the following:
   a. Tidal volume
   b. Inspiratory time
   c. Ventilatory rate

7. Change the IPAP to 10 cm H_2O.

8. Note the following:
   a. Tidal volume
   b. Inspiratory time
   c. Ventilatory rate

Questions:
A. What happened to the tidal volume when the IPAP was changed?
B. What happened to the inspiratory time when the IPAP was changed?

Practice Activities: Respironics BiPAP Vision

CIRCUIT ASSEMBLY

The circuit for the BiPAP Vision is similar to that employed with the S/T-D ventilator. Figure 25-10 illustrates the Respironics Vision circuit that is assembled and ready to attach to the ventilator. Note the circuit consists of two pieces of tubing; the patient tubing (22-mm diameter) and the proximal pressure line. The tubing must terminate at the patient end with a Whisper Swivel. The Whisper Swivel is equivalent to an exhalation valve, allowing the patient to exhale to the ambient air, and acts as a one-way valve during inspiration. The mask (nasal or full-face) attaches to the Whisper Swivel.

VENTILATOR PREPARATION

1. Connect a main flow bacteria filter to the ventilator outlet. A standard bacteria filter commonly employed with acute care ventilators will work for this application.

2. Connect the large-diameter (22 mm) tubing to the ventilator's outlet and connect the proximal pressure line to the proximal pressure port above it.

3. Connect the ventilator to a 50 psi oxygen source using a high-pressure hose and the DISS adapter located on the rear of the ventilator.

4. Verify that the voltage is set correctly for your facility by checking the voltage setting window above the AC power connection on the rear of the ventilator.

5. Verify that the Start/Stop switch is in the Stop position. Connect the power cord to your facility's AC electrical outlet.

6. Move the Start/Stop switch to the Start position. The BiPAP Vision will conduct a 15-second self-test on initial start-up.

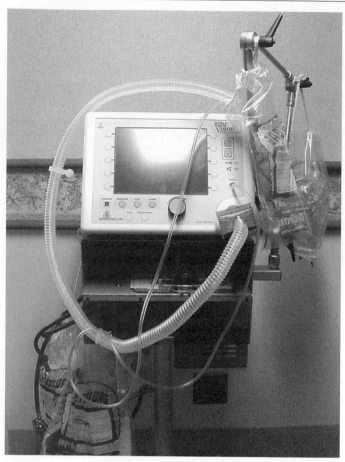

Figure 25-10 *A photo of the circuit assembly for the Respironics BiPAP Vision*

7. Press the "Test Exh Port" soft key on the upper left part of the display screen. This will begin the exhalation port test. It is important to perform this test before each use and following each circuit change. This test will calculate the leak in the circuit, allowing monitoring for patient leaks and of tidal volume delivery.
   a. Occlude the mask port on the patient circuit.
   b. Press the "Start Test" soft key at the upper right of the screen.
   c. The test will take about 15 seconds to complete.
   d. In the event that the ventilator detects a problem, follow the prompts on the screen, checking the circuit or proximal line, and repeat the test by pressing the "Start Test" soft key.

8. Press the "Monitoring" key on the lower left corner of the control panel. The ventilator is now ready for use.

VENTILATOR OPERATION VERIFICATION

Prior to using the ventilator, as a clinician you should verify that it is functioning properly. The self- and exhalation port tests are designed to check the majority of the ventilator's systems. By checking the modes and pressure settings, you can be assured of the ventilator's operation.

1. Complete steps 1 through 8 in the ventilator preparation section.

2. Occlude the patient circuit and press the "Options" soft key at the lower right corner of the monitoring screen. If an alarm is active, press the "Reset" hard key (one with the two diagonal slashes at the upper right part of the control panel).

3. Press the "Test Alarms" soft key located in the middle of the left-hand side of the display screen. This test will verify the function of the audible and visual alarms. The "Vent Inop" and "Check Vent" icons will illuminate below the "Reset" hard key.

4. Press the "Mode" key (center hard key to the right of the "Monitoring" key), and select S/T (Spontaneous/ Timed) mode key. Set the ventilator to the following settings:
IPAP:	15 cm H_2O
EPAP:	5 cm H_2O
Rate:	16/min
Timed Inspiration:	1.0 second
Rise Time:	0.1 second

5. Press the "Alarms" hard key and make the following alarm settings:
Hi Pressure:	20 cm H_2O
Low Pressure:	10 cm H_2O
Low Pressure Delay:	20 seconds
Apnea:	Disabled
Low Minute Ventilation:	0 L/min
High Rate:	40/minute
Low Rate:	10/minute

6. Press the "Monitoring" key and return to the monitoring screen. Occlude the circuit outlet port and verify IPAP, EPAP, rate, and inspiratory time.

7. Create a small leak at the circuit outlet. Verify that the ventilator cycles into inspiration. Once the breath is triggered, occlude the port again.

8. Press the "Alarms" hard key to obtain the current alarm settings. Change the high pressure alarm to 10 cm H_2O. Verify that the high pressure alarm activates on the next breath cycle (with the outlet port occluded). Reset the alarm to 20 cm H_2O.

9. Open the circuit outlet simulating a patient disconnect. Wait about 30 seconds to verify that the low pressure alarm activates. Occlude the circuit outlet and press the "Alarm Reset" key.

10. Press the "Apnea" soft key on the lower left portion of the display screen. Adjust the apnea parameter to 20 seconds. Keep the circuit outlet occluded and verify that the alarm activates. Readjust the "Apnea" parameter to Disabled and press the "Alarm Reset" key.

ACTIVITIES

To complete these practice exercises, it is recommended that you use a lung analog/simulator such as a Medishield or Manley test lung. With these units, you may easily adjust resistance (R_{AW}) and compliance for the following exercises to simulate changes in the patient's condition.

Exercise 1: Continuous Positive Airway Pressure (CPAP) Mode

CPAP mode is a spontaneous mode; there is no backup ventilatory support. If the patient fails to take a breath, the ventilator will not respond by providing one. When performing this exercise, you must provide the test lung with a spontaneous effort by expanding the bellows, simulating inspiration.

The active controls are CPAP (pressure) and % O_2.

1. Assemble the ventilator's circuit and prepare the ventilator for operation as described above.

2. Press the "Mode" key (lower left part of the control panel), and select CPAP mode by pressing its soft key.

3. Adjust the CPAP level to 10 cm H_2O by pressing the CPAP soft key and rotating the adjustment knob adjacent to the ventilator outlet.

4. Select the "Activate New Mode" soft key at the lower right corner of the display screen. CPAP mode and a pressure of 10 cm H_2O have now been selected and activated.

5. Simulate spontaneous breathing by moving the test lung's bellows. Observe the display screen and the data it presents (pressure, volume and flow graphics, rate, and pressure level).

6. Supplemental oxygen can be provided by selecting the % O_2 soft key, rotating the adjustment knob to the desired FiO₂ and pressing the "Activate New Mode" soft key.

7. Alarms may be adjusted by depressing the "Alarm" hard key next to the adjustment knob. The alarm setup page is then displayed on the display screen. From this page you may adjust the following alarms:
   a. High pressure limit (cm H_2O)
   b. Low pressure limit (cm H_2O)
   c. Low pressure alarm delay (seconds)
   d. Apnea
   e. Low minute ventilation (L/min)
   f. High rate
   g. Low rate

Exercise 2: CPAP Application

Identify a laboratory partner who will act as your patient. With your laboratory instructor observing you, complete the following exercise.

1. Assemble the Respironics BiPAP Vision ventilator and attach a clean circuit.

2. Using appropriate universal precautions, select the correct nasal mask for your patient and the appropriate headgear and spacers.

3. Connect the mask to the circuit, and set the ventilator to the following settings:
   Mode: CPAP
   CPAP: 10 cm H_2O
   % O_2: 21%

4. Fit the mask to your patient, using the spacer(s) and the headgear.

5. Observe the pressure manometer and the LEDs for correct operation.

6. Note the following:
   a. Graphics (pressure, volume, flow)
   b. Breath rate
   c. % O_2
   d. CPAP setting

7. Set the following alarms:
   a. High pressure limit: 15 cm H_2O
   b. Low pressure limit: 5 cm H_2O
   c. Low pressure alarm delay: 20 seconds
   d. Low minute ventilation: 3 L/min
   e. High rate: +8 BPM above patient rate
   f. Low rate: −8 BPM below patient rate

8. Have your patient hyperventilate and hypoventilate to observe the alarm functions.

9. Increase the CPAP setting to 15 cm H_2O and readjust the alarms appropriately.

Questions:
A. What happened to the tidal volume when the CPAP setting was changed?
B. What happened to the inspiratory time when the CPAP setting was changed?

Exercise 3: Spontaneous/Timed (S/T) Mode

1. Assemble the ventilator's circuit and prepare the ventilator for operation as described above.

2. Press the "Mode" key (lower left part of the control panel), and Spontaneous/Timed mode by pressing its soft key (S/T).

3. The following are the active controls:
   * IPAP
   * EPAP
   * Rate
   * Timed Inspiration
   * % O_2
   * IPAP Rise Time

4. Set the controls to the following settings by selecting the appropriate soft key and then rotating the adjustment knob to the desired setting.
   IPAP: 15 cm H_2O
   EPAP: 5 cm H_2O
   Rate: 10 BPM
   Timed Inspiration: 0.1 second
   % O_2:   21%
   IPAP Rise Time: 0.1 second

   Once the adjustments have been made, push the "Activate New Mode" soft key to initiate the new settings.

5. Connect the patient outlet port to the test lung, and observe the following:
   a. Graphics (pressure, volume, flow)
   b. Breath rate
   c. % O_2
   d. IPAP and EPAP pressures

6. Change the resistance to 50, increasing the R_{AW}.

7. Note the following:
   a. Tidal volume (digital display)
   b. Graphics (pressure, volume, and flow)
   c. Inspiratory time

Questions:
A. What happened to the tidal volume delivery?
B. What happened to the inspiratory time?

8. Return the R_{AW} control to zero.

9. Decrease the compliance by adding an additional spring onto the bellows of the test lung.

10. Note the following:
    a. Tidal volume (digital display)
    b. Graphics (pressure, volume, and flow)
    c. Inspiratory time

Questions:
A. What happened to the tidal volume delivery?
B. What happened to the inspiratory time?

11. Change the controls to the following:
    BPM: 10
    IPAP: 20 cm H_2O
    EPAP: 8 cm H_2O
    % IPAP: 20%

12. Repeat steps 6 through 8.

13. Note the following:
    a. Tidal volume (digital display)
    b. Graphics (pressure, volume, and flow)
    c. Inspiratory time

Questions:
A. What happened to the tidal volume delivery?
B. What happened to the inspiratory time?

Exercise 3: Spontaneous/Timed (S/T) Mode Application

Identify a laboratory partner who will act as your patient. With your laboratory instructor observing you, complete the following exercise.

1. Assemble the Respironics BiPAP Vision ventilator and attach a clean circuit.

2. Using standard precautions, select the correct nasal mask for your patient and the appropriate headgear and spacers.

3. Connect the mask to the circuit, and set the ventilator to the following settings:
   Mode: Spontaneous/Timed
   IPAP: 15 cm H_2O
   IPAP: 4 cm H_2O
   BPM: 10/min
   Timed Inspiration: 0.1 second
   % O_2:   21%
   IPAP Rise Time: 0.1 second

   Once the settings are established, activate the new mode.

4. Fit the mask to your patient, using the spacer(s) and the headgear.

5. Note the following:
   a. Tidal volume (digital display)
   b. Graphics (pressure, volume, and flow)
   c. Inspiratory time

6. Adjust the alarms appropriately for your patient's volumes, pressures, and rate.

7. Change the IPAP to 10 cm H_2O.

8. Note the following:
   a. Tidal volume (digital display)
   b. Graphics (pressure, volume, and flow)
   c. Inspiratory time

Questions:
A. What happened to the tidal volume when the IPAP pressure was changed?
B. What happened to the inspiratory time when the IPAP pressure was changed?

Check List: Initiation of NPPV

_____ 1. Verify the physician's order.
_____ 2. Scan the patient's chart as time permits.
_____ 3. Wash hands before seeing the patient.
          4. Assess the patient:
_____   a. Respiratory rate
_____   b. Tidal volume
_____   c. Minute ventilation
_____   d. Rapid-shallow-breathing index
_____   e. Vital capacity
_____   f. SpO_2
_____   g. Arterial blood gases
          5. Gather the required equipment:
_____   a. NPPV ventilator
_____   b. Circuit
_____   c. Masks and fitting guide
_____   d. Spacers and headgear
_____   e. Oxygen analyzer

_____   f. Oximeter monitor
_____   g. ECG monitor
_____   h. Noninvasive blood pressure monitor
_____ 6. Assemble the circuit and test the NPPV ventilator.
_____ 7. Adjust the ventilator to the ordered settings.
_____ 8. Fit the mask/headgear to the patient.
_____ 9. Connect the NPPV ventilator to the patient.
_____ 10. Work with the patient to promote comfort and adjustment to mask ventilation.
_____ 11. Readjust the mask/headgear as required for optimal comfort and minimal leaks.
          12. Monitor the following:
_____   a. IPAP
_____   b. EPAP
_____   c. Rate

_____   d. Tidal volume
_____   e. Minute volume
_____   f. Inspiratory time
_____   g. Graphics (if available)
_____   h. SpO$_2$
_____   i. Breath sounds and work of breathing

_____   j. FIO$_2$
_____   13. Set the alarms appropriately.
_____   14. Record all parameters in the patient's chart.
_____   15. Clean up the area, discarding any disposable packaging.
_____   16. Wash hands upon leaving the area.

Self-Evaluation Post Test: Noninvasive Positive-Pressure Ventilation (NPPV)

1. Indications for NPPV include which of the following?
   I. Acute exacerbation of COPD
   II. Acute pulmonary edema
   III. Acute hypercapneic respiratory failure
   IV. Acute asthma
   a. I
   b. I, II
   c. I, II, III
   d. I, II, III, IV

2. Advantages of ventilation without intubation include which of the following?
   a. Use of lower pressures
   b. Ability to communicate better
   c. Ability to take fluids/medications orally
   d. Both b and c

3. Which of the following should be assessed prior to commitment to NPPV?
   I. SpO$_2$
   II. Respiratory rate and tidal volume
   III. Blood gases
   IV. Rapid-shallow-breathing index
   a. I
   b. I, II
   c. I, II, III
   d. I, II, III, IV

4. When assessing your patient, you note the following:
   Respiratory rate: 35/min
   Tidal volume: 0.27 L
   SpO$_2$: 85%
   FIO$_2$: 0.50
   The patient's rapid-shallow-breathing index is:
   a. 130.
   b. 7.7.
   c. 350.
   d. 43.

5. Advantages of the nasal mask include which of the following?
   I. Ability to communicate verbally
   II. Ability to eat or drink
   III. Less confining (to prevent claustrophobia)
   IV. Covers only the mouth
   a. I
   b. I, II
   c. I, II, III
   d. I, II, III, IV

6. The increased risks associated with use of a full-face mask include:
   I. increased chance of gastric insufflation.
   II. increased risk of aspiration.
   III. perception of claustrophobia.
   IV. increased pressure required to seal the mask.
   a. I
   b. I, II
   c. I, II, III
   d. I, II, III, IV

7. Hazards and complications of NPPV include which of the following?
   I. Nasal/sinus pain or discomfort
   II. Eye irritation
   III. Barotrauma
   IV. Mucous plugging
   a. I
   b. I, II
   c. I, II, III
   d. I, II, III, IV

8. With use of NPPV, decreased compliance may result in which of the following changes?
   I. Increased tidal volume
   II. Decreased tidal volume
   III. Increased inspiratory time
   IV. Decreased inspiratory time
   a. I, III
   b. I, IV
   c. II, III
   d. II, IV

9. With use of NPPV, increased airway resistance (R$_{AW}$) may result in which of the following changes?
   I. Increased tidal volume
   II. Decreased tidal volume
   III. Increased inspiratory time
   IV. Decreased inspiratory time
   a. I, III
   b. I, IV
   c. II, III
   d. II, IV

10. Which of the following modes allows sensing of patient effort and delivery of assisted ventilation with a backup rate in case of apnea?
    a. Spontaneous
    b. Timed
    c. Spontaneous/timed
    d. Mandatory

PERFORMANCE EVALUATION: INITIATION OF NONINVASIVE POSITIVE-PRESSURE VENTILATION (NPPV)

Date: Lab _____ Clinical _____ Agency _____

Lab: Pass _____ Fail _____   Clinical: Pass _____ Fail _____

Student name _____ Instructor name _____

No. of times observed in clinical _____

No. of times practiced in clinical _____

PASSING CRITERIA: Obtain 90% or better on the procedure. Tasks indicated by * must receive at least 1 point, or the evaluation is terminated. Procedure must be performed within designated time, or the performance receives a failing grade.

SCORING:
2 points — Task performed satisfactorily without prompting.
1 point — Task performed satisfactorily with self-initiated correction.
0 points — Task performed incorrectly or with prompting required.
NA — Task not applicable to the patient care situation.

TASKS:		PEER	LAB	CLINICAL
*	1. Verifies the physician's order	☐	☐	☐
*	2. Reviews the patient's chart	☐	☐	☐
*	3. Washes hands	☐	☐	☐
*	4. Gathers the equipment	☐	☐	☐
	5. Assesses the patient			
*	a. Respiratory rate	☐	☐	☐
*	b. Tidal volume	☐	☐	☐
*	c. Minute volume	☐	☐	☐
*	d. Rapid-shallow-breathing index	☐	☐	☐
*	e. Vital capacity	☐	☐	☐
*	f. SpO$_2$	☐	☐	☐
*	g. Arterial blood gases	☐	☐	☐
	6. Gathers the required equipment:			
*	a. NPPV ventilator	☐	☐	☐
*	b. Masks and fitting guide	☐	☐	☐
*	c. Spacers and headgear	☐	☐	☐
*	d. Oxygen analyzer	☐	☐	☐
*	e. Oximeter monitor	☐	☐	☐
*	f. ECG monitor	☐	☐	☐
*	g. Blood pressure monitor	☐	☐	☐
*	7. Assembles circuit and tests NPPV ventilator	☐	☐	☐
*	8. Adjusts the ventilator to ordered settings	☐	☐	☐
*	9. Correctly fits mask/headgear	☐	☐	☐

*   10. Connects the patient to the NPPV ventilator   ☐ ☐ ☐

*   11. Assists the patient with fit/comfort   ☐ ☐ ☐

*   12. Readjusts mask/headgear as needed   ☐ ☐ ☐

     13. Monitors the patient

*   a. IPAP   ☐ ☐ ☐

*   b. EPAP   ☐ ☐ ☐

*   c. Rate   ☐ ☐ ☐

*   d. Tidal volume   ☐ ☐ ☐

*   e. Minute volume   ☐ ☐ ☐

*   f. Inspiratory time   ☐ ☐ ☐

*   g. Graphics (flow, volume)   ☐ ☐ ☐

*   h. SpO_2 ☐ ☐ ☐

*   i. Breath sounds   ☐ ☐ ☐

*   j. FiO_2 ☐ ☐ ☐

*   k. Sets the alarms appropriately   ☐ ☐ ☐

*   l. Records all parameters in chart   ☐ ☐ ☐

*   14. Cleans up the area, discarding disposable supplies   ☐ ☐ ☐

*   15. Washes hands before leaving   ☐ ☐ ☐

SCORE: Peer   _____ points of possible 76; _____%

             Lab   _____ points of possible 76; _____%

             Clinical   _____ points of possible 76; _____%

TIME: _____ out of possible 40 minutes

STUDENT SIGNATURES   INSTRUCTOR SIGNATURES

PEER: _____   LAB: _____

STUDENT: _____   CLINICAL: _____

CHAPTER 26
CONTINUOUS MECHANICAL VENTILATION

INTRODUCTION

As a respiratory care practitioner, you will work with several different types of mechanical ventilators. You will be expected to assemble, test, and operate these ventilators safely and effectively.

Mechanical ventilation involves more than simply knowing how to operate the equipment safely. Mechanical ventilation may result in serious adverse effects on the pulmonary and cardiovascular systems. Knowledge of these effects and how to monitor the patient to assess them is essential.

In this chapter you will learn the concept of mechanical ventilation, the indications for mechanical ventilation, how to identify patients at risk for respiratory failure, and the complications of mechanical ventilation.

KEY TERMS

- Assist/control mode
- Barotrauma
- Continuous mechanical ventilation
- Control mode
- Dynamic compliance

- Expiratory retard
- Inspiratory hold
- Pontoppidan's criteria
- Pressure control ventilation
- Pressure limit

- Sigh mode
- SIMV/IMV mode
- Static compliance
- Tubing compliance
- Volume ventilation

OBJECTIVES

At the end of this chapter, you should be able to:

- Define the term *continuous mechanical ventilation*.
- Differentiate between volume-cycled and pressure-cycled ventilation, and the implications of each modality for patient management.
- State the indications for mechanical ventilation.
- List the criteria for implementation of mechanical ventilation, including the following:
  — Mechanics of ventilation
  — Oxygenation
    — PaO_2
    — $P(A-a)O_2$
  — Ventilation
    — $PaCO_2$
    — pH
- Differentiate among the following modes of mechanical ventilation:
  — Control
  — Assist/control
  — IMV
  — Sigh
- Describe the complications of mechanical ventilation:
  — Barotrauma
  — Cardiovascular complications
  — Effects on other organ systems

CLINICAL PRACTICE GUIDELINES

AARC Clinical Practice Guideline
Patient-Ventilator System Checks

MV-SC 4.0 INDICATIONS:
A patient-ventilator system check must be performed on a scheduled basis (which is institution-specific) for any patient requiring mechanical ventilation for life support. In addition, a check should be performed:
  4.1 Prior to obtaining blood samples for analysis of blood gases and pH
  4.2 Prior to obtaining hemodynamic or bedside pulmonary function data
  4.3 Following any change in ventilator settings

  4.4 As soon as possible following an acute deterioration of the patient's condition (this may or may not be heralded by a violation of ventilator-alarm thresholds)
  4.5 Any time that ventilator performance is questionable (9)

MV-SC 5.0 CONTRAINDICATIONS:
There are no absolute contraindications to performance of a patient-ventilator system check. If disruption of PEEP or FDO_2 results in hypoxemia, bradycardia, or hypotension, portions of the check requiring disconnection of the patient from the ventilator may be contraindicated. (10,11)

(Continued)

(CPG *Continued*)

MV-SC 6.0 HAZARDS/COMPLICATIONS:

6.1 Disconnecting the patient from the ventilator during a patient-ventilator system check may result in hypoventilation, hypoxemia, bradycardia, and/or hypotension. (10,11)

6.2 Prior to disconnection, preoxygenation and hyperventilation may minimize these complications. (12–19)

6.3 When disconnected from the patient, some ventilators generate a high flow through the patient circuit that may aerosolize contaminated condensate, putting both the patient and clinician at risk for nosocomial infection. (20)

MV-SC 8.0 ASSESSMENT OF NEED:

Because of the complexity of mechanical ventilators and the large number of factors that can adversely affect patient-ventilator interaction, routine checks of patient-ventilator system performance are mandatory.

MV-SC 9.0 ASSESSMENT OF OUTCOME:

Routine patient-ventilator system checks should prevent untoward incidents, warn of impending events, and ensure that proper ventilator settings, according to physician's order, are maintained.

MV-SC 11.0 MONITORING:

In order to ensure that patient-ventilator system checks are being performed according to these guidelines, an indicator should be created to monitor this activity as part of the appropriate department's quality improvement program. Specific criteria for the indicator should include at least items 2.4 and 12.0 of this guideline.

Reprinted with permission from *Respiratory Care* 1992; 37: 882–886. The complete AARC Clinical Practice Guidelines are available from the AARC Web site (http://www.aarc.org), from the AARC Executive Office, or from *Respiratory Care* journal.

AARC Clinical Practice Guideline
Ventilator Circuit Changes

VCC 4.0 INDICATIONS:

The decision to change a ventilator circuit should be governed by:

4.1 Length of time the existing circuit has been in use (1–11)

4.2 Type of circuit and humidification device in use (1,3,6–20)

4.3 Circuit function (presence of a malfunctioning circuit or a circuit that leaks)

4.4 Appearance of ventilator circuit (Circuits that are not clean in appearance should be replaced.)

VCC 5.0 CONTRAINDICATIONS:

5.1 Presence of conditions in the patient's cardiopulmonary or neurologic status that might make tolerance of disconnection from mechanical ventilation hazardous to the patient

5.2 Inability to safely and effectively ventilate or maintain patient during the ventilator circuit change

5.3 Absence of a clean and functional circuit to use as a replacement

VCC 6.0 HAZARDS/COMPLICATIONS:

6.1 Patient's condition may predispose him or her to harm or injury during the changing process:

6.1.1 Hemodynamic instability

6.1.2 Hypo- or hyperoxia with sequelae

6.1.3 Hyper or hypocapnia

6.1.4 Airway obstruction

6.1.5 Artificial airway displacement

6.1.6 Contamination of patient or staff from exposure to material in circuit (8,21)

6.2 Patient may not be safely maintained during disconnection from the ventilator:

6.2.1 Inappropriate or inadequate ventilation (f and/or V_t)

6.2.2 Inappropriate or inadequate oxygenation (FIO_2 and/or PEEP)

6.2.3 Inappropriate increase in work of breathing

6.2.4 Airway obstruction

6.3 Inability to ensure that the replacement circuit has been safely and effectively disinfected and that it is operationally sound (29,30)

6.3.1 Transmission of pathogens to patient and to health care personnel

6.3.2 Hazards of exposure to residual toxic disinfectants or associated disinfectant by-products (30)

6.3.3 Malfunctioning or suboptimally functioning ventilator or circuit

6.3.4 Failure to ensure proper ventilator function with patient reconnection (i.e., correct settings, absence of leaks, functioning alarms, proper valve placement (31))

6.3.5 Potential for patient-ventilator disconnection (31)

6.4 Manipulation and disconnection of the ventilator tubing can cause contaminated ventilator condensate to spill into the patient's airway, exposing the patient to further risk of infection (8,21–24,26–28)

6.5 Changing ventilator circuits more frequently than is necessary may increase the risk of nosocomial pneumonia. (8,23)

6.6 Failure to ensure proper ventilator function prior to reinstituting mechanical ventilation may endanger patient. (31)

VCC 8.0 ASSESSMENT OF NEED:

8.1 Objective—limiting the transmission of infection

8.1.1 Reliance on published Centers for Disease Control and Prevention (CDC) recommendations (25–29)

8.1.2 Reliance on institutional standards established by monitoring and surveillance and/or published research

8.2 Objective—to prevent malfunction and to maintain optimal performance

8.2.1 Competency of the circuit should be monitored for tubing leaks.

8.2.2 In-line filters should be assessed for increased resistance. (33–37)

8.2.3 Equipment affected over time by water (e.g., spirometers) should be monitored.

8.3 Objective — to maintain a circuit clean in appearance: Inspect appearance of circuit.

Reprinted with permission from *Respiratory Care* 1994; 39(8): 797–802. The complete AARC Clinical Practice Guidelines are available from the AARC Website (http://www.aarc.org), the AARC Executive Office, or from *Respiratory Care* journal.

AARC Clinical Practice Guideline
Long-Term Invasive Mechanical Ventilation in the Home

HIMV 4.0 INDICATIONS:

4.1 Patients requiring invasive long-term ventilatory support have demonstrated:

    4.1.1 An inability to be completely weaned from invasive ventilatory support or

    4.1.2 A progression of disease etiology that requires increasing ventilatory support

4.2 Conditions that met these criteria may include but are not limited to ventilatory muscle disorders, (4,5,10,11,14,16–19,21,26,27,33,35,38, 42,43,46,52,54–62) alveolar hypoventilation syndrome, (4,5,10,17,18,19,23,33,34,42,43,46,47,59, 60) primary respiratory disorders, (4,10,17,18, 19,23,42,46,59,60) obstructive diseases, (5,10,57, 58) restrictive diseases, (5,10,16,43,46,56) and cardiac disorders including congenital anomalies. (17,19,23,42,46,59)

HIMV 5.0 CONTRAINDICATIONS:

Contraindications to HIMV include:

5.1 The presence of a physiologically unstable medical condition requiring higher level of care or resources than available in the home. (4–7,10, 14,16,17,19,20,21,23,26,29,33,52,59) Examples of indicators of a medical condition too unstable for the home and long term care setting are:

    5.1.1 FiO_2 requirement > 0.40 (4,5,10,16,35)

    5.1.2 PEEP > 10 cm H_2O (4,5,10,12,16,35)

    5.1.3 Need for continuous invasive monitoring in adult patients (4,6,16)

    5.1.4 Lack of mature tracheostomy

5.2 Patient's choice not to receive home mechanical ventilation (5,10,16,19,23,26,39,42,52,56,58, 63,64)

5.3 Lack of an appropriate discharge plan (4,5, 8,11,13,18,33,34,38,39,46,48,51,65)

5.4 Unsafe physical environment as determined by the patient's discharge planning team (10,13,66)

    5.4.1 Presence of fire, health, or safety hazards including unsanitary conditions. (39,51)

5.4.2 Inadequate basic utilities (such as heat, air conditioning, electricity) (4,5,10,19, 22,33,38,39,52,67)

5.5 Inadequate resources for care in the home:

    5.5.1 Financial (9,10,13,14,16,18,19,23,25, 26,33,35,38–40,44,52,55,56,59,68,69)

    5.5.2 Personnel

        5.5.2.1 Inadequate medical follow-up (13,14,16,18,29,33,36,38,39,50,61)

        5.5.2.2 Inability of VAI to care for self, if no caregiver is available (5,16)

        5.5.2.3 Inadequate respite care for caregivers (17,19,26)

        5.5.2.4 Inadequate numbers of competent caregivers (5,13,21,23,25, 26,30,38,39,52,68)

HIMV 6.0 HAZARDS AND COMPLICATIONS:

6.1 Deterioration or acute change in clinical status of VAI. Although ventilator-associated complications in the home are poorly documented, experience in other sites can be extrapolated. The following may cause death or require rehospitalization for acute treatment:

    6.1.1 Medical: Hypocapnia, respiratory alkalosis, (70) hypercapnia, respiratory acidosis, (70) hypoxemia, barotrauma, (5,64,70) seizures, hemodynamic instability, (21) airway complications (stomal or tracheal infection, mucous plugging, tracheal erosion or stenosis), (5) respiratory infection (tracheobronchitis, pneumonia), (57,70,71) bronchospasm, (5) exacerbation of underlying disease, or natural course of the disease

    6.1.2 Equipment-related: Failure of the ventilator, malfunction of equipment, (10) inadequate warming and humidification of the inspired gases, inadvertent changes in ventilator settings, accidental disconnection from ventilator, (27) accidental decannulation

    6.1.3 Psychosocial: Depression, (5,10,43) anxiety, (4,10,43) loss of resources — caregiver or financial, (10,19,25,40,43) detrimental change in family structure or coping capacity (5,10,19,25,34,38,54,55,56,71,72)

HIMV 8.0 ASSESSMENT OF NEED:

8.1 Determination that indications are present and contraindications are absent

8.2 Determination that the goals listed in 2.1 can be met in the home

8.3 Determination that no continued need exists for higher level of services

8.4 Determination that frequent changes in the plan of care will not be needed

(Continued)

(CPG Continued)

HIMV 9.0 ASSESSMENT OF OUTCOME:

At least the following aspects of patient management and condition should be evaluated periodically as long as the patient receives HIMV:

9.1 Implementation and adherence to the plan of care

9.2 Quality of life

9.3 Patient satisfaction

9.4 Resource utilization

9.5 Growth and development in the pediatric patient

9.6 Unanticipated morbidity, including need for higher level site of care

9.7 Unanticipated mortality

HIMV 11.0 MONITORING:

The frequency of monitoring should be determined by the ongoing individualized care plan and be based upon the patient's current medical condition. The ventilator settings, proper function of equipment, and the patient's physical condition should be monitored and verified: (1) with each initiation of invasive ventilation to the patient, including altering the source of ventilation, as from one ventilator or resuscitation bag to another ventilator; (2) with each ventilator setting change; (3) on a regular basis as specified by individualized plan of care. (35)

All appropriately trained caregivers should follow the care plan and implement the monitoring that has been prescribed. These caregivers may operate, maintain, and monitor all equipment and perform all aspects of care required by the VAI after having been trained and evaluated on their level of knowledge for that equipment and the VAI's clinical response to each of the interventions.

11.1 Lay caregivers should monitor the following regularly:

11.1.1 Patient's physical condition: respiratory rate, heart rate, color changes, chest excursion, diaphoresis, lethargy, blood pressure, and body temperature

11.1.2 Ventilator settings: The frequency at which alarms and settings are to be checked should be specified in the plan of care.

11.1.2.1 Peak pressures

11.1.2.2 Preset tidal volume

11.1.2.3 Frequency of ventilator breaths

11.1.2.4 Verification of oxygen concentration setting

11.1.2.5 PEEP level (if applicable)

11.1.2.6 Appropriate humidification of inspired gases

11.1.2.7 Temperature of inspired gases (if applicable)

11.1.2.8 Heat and moisture exchanger function

11.1.3 Equipment function: (10,13)

11.1.3.1 Appropriate configuration of ventilator circuit (82)

11.1.3.2 Alarm function

11.1.3.3 Cleanliness of filter(s) — according to manufacturer's recommendation

11.1.3.4 Battery power level(s) — both internal and external

11.1.3.5 Overall condition of all equipment

11.1.3.6 Self-inflating manual resuscitator — cleanliness and function

11.2 A Level-II practitioner should perform a thorough, comprehensive assessment of the patient and the patient-ventilator system on a regular basis as prescribed by the plan of care. In addition to the variables listed in 11.1.1–11.1.3, the Level-II practitioner should implement, monitor, and assess results of other interventions as indicated by the clinical situation and anticipated in the care plan.

11.2.1 Pulse oximetry — should be used in patients requiring a change in prescribed oxygen levels or in patients with a suspected change in condition. (10,35)

11.2.2 End-tidal CO_2 — may be useful for establishing trends in CO_2 levels during weaning. (10,23,33,35,59,83,84)

11.2.3 Specimen collection (and analysis as applicable) as prescribed by physician — including but not limited to sputum and blood work (e.g., arterial blood gas analysis and complete blood counts) (5,10,32,37)

11.2.4 Cardiorespiratory monitoring (electrocardiogram, heart rate trending) (10)

11.2.5 Pulmonary function testing

11.2.6 Ventilator settings

11.2.7 Exhaled tidal volume

11.2.8 Analysis of fraction of inspired oxygen

11.3 Level-II personnel are also responsible for maintaining interdisciplinary communication concerning the plan of care.

11.4 Level-II personnel should integrate respiratory plan of care into the patient's total care plan. (10) Plan of care should include:

11.4.1 All aspects of patient's respiratory care (66) and

11.4.2 Ongoing assessment and education of the caregivers involved

Reprinted with permission from *Respiratory Care* 1995; 40(12): 1313–1320. The complete AARC Clinical Practice Guidelines are available from the AARC Web site (http://www.aarc.org), from the AARC Executive Office, or from *Respiratory Care* journal.

WHAT IS CONTINUOUS MECHANICAL VENTILATION?

Continuous mechanical ventilation (CMV) is the support of a patient's ventilatory needs by artificial means. A patient in respiratory failure or approaching respiratory failure may be ventilated mechanically until the disease state or underlying cause for respiratory failure has been resolved and the patient's ventilatory efforts have adequately resumed.

The mechanical ventilator applies positive pressure to the airway during inspiration until either a preset pressure, volume, or time is reached. The patient is allowed to exhale passively to ambient pressure, and then the cycle is repeated. Figure 26-1 graphically depicts this pattern.

Two common types of ventilators that may be utilized to ventilate adult patients are pressure-limited and volume-limited ventilators. The volume-limited ventilator is more commonly used in the critical care setting because it reliably delivers a preset volume regardless of changes in the patient's condition. The pressure-limited ventilator is more commonly used for short-term support as it is more difficult to manage with an unstable patient.

A pressure-limited ventilator, as the name implies, delivers a breath using positive pressure and then terminates inspiration when a preset pressure is reached. This is the same principle as for intermittent positive-pressure breathing (IPPB), discussed in Chapter 17, "Hyperinflation Therapy." Delivered volume will vary with the patient's condition and lung compliance. As either changes, volume will also vary; constant monitoring of the patient is required to ensure adequate ventilation. Examples of this type of ventilator are a Bird Mark 7 and a Puritan–Bennett PR-2.

A volume-limited ventilator, as the name implies, delivers a breath using positive pressure and terminates inspiration after a preset volume has been delivered. Pressure will vary with these ventilators, while the delivered volume will remain constant. Changes in the patient's condition or lung compliance will not appreciably affect volume delivery. Comparatively speaking, it is easier to manage a patient ventilated with this device than with a pressure-limited ventilator. Tidal volume and minute volume may be maintained within a consistent range very easily.

INDICATIONS FOR MECHANICAL VENTILATION

Respiratory failure and the ensuing need for ventilatory support may occur for a variety of reasons. Mechanical ventilation will not cure the condition that precipitated respiratory failure. It is strictly a supportive measure, providing the physician and the health care team time to resolve the underlying cause.

An extended time period may be required to correct the underlying cause of respiratory failure. Furthermore, a large staffing and financial commitment is involved in sustaining a patient on mechanical ventilation. The decision to initiate mechanical ventilation should not be taken lightly. This supportive therapy should be initiated only upon a physician's order. The patient should be carefully evaluated and assessed prior to ventilator commitment. In some instances, mechanical ventilation may prolong life, without any hope of resolving the underlying cause of respiratory failure. Under these circumstances the decision to initiate mechanical ventilation involves serious moral, legal, and ethical considerations.

Figure 26-2 summarizes some of the pathological conditions that may precipitate respiratory failure. The mechanism leading to respiratory failure for each of these entities is briefly reviewed in the following discussion.

Neuromuscular Conditions

Muscular Dystrophy

Muscular dystrophy is a disease that affects the motor neurons and peripheral nerves. It is usually a hereditary disorder. The onset of respiratory failure is usually gradual over a period of years. As the dysfunction of the muscles progresses to the point where ventilation is compromised, serial vital capacity measurements are helpful in assessing when to commit the patient to mechanical ventilation. The patient and family must be closely involved in the

---

1. Neuromuscular conditions
   a. Muscular dystrophy
   b. Poliomyelitis
   c. Idiopathic polyneuritis (Guillain-Barré syndrome)
   d. Drug overdose, sedation, anesthesia
   e. Head injury
   f. Spinal injury
2. Skeletal or multiple trauma
   a. Flail chest
   b. Multiple trauma
3. Conditions affecting gas exchange
   a. Pulmonary embolism
   b. ARDS
   c. Gram-negative sepsis
   d. Left ventricular failure and pulmonary edema

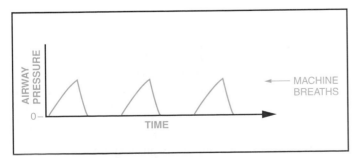

Figure 26-1 *A graphic representation of positive-pressure ventilation*

Figure 26-2 *Pathological conditions that may cause respiratory failure*

decision. Mechanical ventilation in this situation is strictly supportive. An absolute cure for the underlying condition has not been discovered.

Poliomyelitis

Poliomyelitis is a communicable disease, preventable through immunization. In the late 1940s and early 1950s a large epidemic swept the United States. The advent of the Salk vaccine alleviated the outbreak. Since that time, poliomyelitis has received little attention in the media. In many people's minds, the condition is extinct. This is not true. Immunization is still important to control further outbreaks of the disease.

The symptoms of acute poliomyelitis include headache, pain in muscles (especially around the head and neck), vomiting, and fever. Paralysis progresses quite rapidly over a period ranging from a few hours to two or three days. The paralysis usually affects the limbs, but may also impair the ability to swallow (management of secretions) and respiratory muscle function. Serial vital capacities are useful in determining the point at which ventilatory assistance is indicated.

Idiopathic Polyneuritis (Guillain-Barré Syndrome)

Guillain-Barré syndrome is a paralysis of unknown origin. Recent studies suspect the cause to be viral in nature. This condition is usually preceded by an upper respiratory infection several weeks earlier. The paralysis occurs in ascending fashion. The patient may first become clumsy, experiencing difficulty walking. As the paralysis progresses, the legs can no longer support the body weight. It is usually at this point that the patient appears in the emergency room. Paralysis continues to ascend, eventually involving the respiratory muscles. Serial vital capacities are useful in determining the point of ventilator commitment. The majority of cases will resolve completely. Ventilator support, physical therapy, and range of motion exercises are essential to the patient's complete recovery.

Drug Overdose, Sedation, Anesthesia

Drug overdose, sedation, and anesthesia all affect the central nervous system, which may result in depression of respiration. In mild cases this may result in hypoventilation, hypoxemia, and hypercapnia. In more severe cases, apnea may result. These patients should be monitored closely. Protective reflexes of the upper airway may be absent, with impairment of the ability to manage secretions and possible aspiration. In the event of apnea or severe hypoventilation, ventilator commitment may be necessary. The time required for the underlying cause to resolve is usually quite short. The use of the drug naloxone (Narcan) may aid in the reversal of the effects of narcotics.

Head Injury

Severe head injury results in deep coma, hypoventilation, or apnea. Blood gases and measurements of ventilatory mechanics may be used to assess the need for mechanical ventilation. The physician may order hyperventilation of patients with head injuries. Maintaining an arterial carbon dioxide tension ($PaCO_2$) of around 30 mm Hg will help decrease cerebral blood flow and reduce intracranial pressure (Cooper & Morrow, 1984). Often it is desirable to avoid stimulation of the cough and gag reflexes for the same reason. These patients may be unstable for the first 48 hours. Their condition may suddenly worsen owing to increased intracranial pressure, edema, or hemorrhage.

Spinal Injuries

Spinal injuries may cause damage to the spinal cord, inflicting paralysis. The level of the injury determines the affected areas. Injury at the level of the second or third cervical vertebra (C2 or C3) will result in the total loss of use of the muscles of ventilation. In this case, complete ventilatory support is required to maintain life. A lower-level injury (C5 to C6) will compromise ventilation. At this level, the diaphragm is functional, but the abdominal muscles and intercostals are paralyzed. The injury may extend up and down the spinal cord owing to edema and hemorrhage. Measurement of vital capacity, peak inspiratory force, and blood gases is useful in determining the need for ventilator commitment.

Patients with compromised function should receive vigorous pulmonary toilet to prevent the occurrence of pneumonia or other secondary respiratory infections. The patient's cough may be severely compromised, impairing the ability to manage secretions. Often, successful management of secretions is the key to keeping these patients out of respiratory failure.

Skeletal or Multiple Trauma
Flail Chest

A flail chest occurs as the result of an injury to a large area of the chest wall. In this injury, two or more ribs are broken in more than one place, causing the affected section of the chest to function independently from the thoracic cage. This results in paradoxical chest wall motion. The condition ultimately results in hypoventilation, hypoxemia, and hypercapnia. Ventilator assistance may be required until the flail chest and lung contusions resolve. Minimizing patient effort reduces the flail effect. Careful adjustment of the ventilator sensitivity and the use of paralytic drugs will help to minimize patient effort.

Multiple Trauma

Severe multiple traumatic injuries, including fractures of long bones of the pelvis, may result in release of fat emboli from the bone marrow. These may lodge in the lung as pulmonary emboli, or in the brain, producing a cerebrovascular accident (CVA). Multiple trauma may involve head injuries, severe blood loss and corresponding fall in blood pressure, aspiration of gastric contents, sepsis, or the circulation of endotoxins. Any of these factors alone or in combination may result in respiratory failure and adult respiratory distress syndrome (ARDS). Mechanical ventilation may be required as a supportive measure until the underlying cause is resolved.

Conditions Affecting Gas Exchange
Pulmonary Embolism

A pulmonary embolus may be fat, air, thrombus, or bacteria. The most common cause is venous thrombosis. In massive pulmonary embolism, circulation to a large segment of the lung is affected. Mechanical ventilation may be required to maintain arterial oxygen tension (PaO_2) and $PaCO_2$ within normal limits. The administration of heparin or other anticoagulants will help to prevent further venous thrombosis from occurring.

Adult Respiratory Distress Syndrome

ARDS is a serious condition with a high mortality rate. The causes of ARDS may include massive trauma, multiple transfusions, multiple organ failure, blunt chest trauma, and any severe pulmonary abnormality. The syndrome is characterized by a thickening of the alveolar capillary membrane, interstitial edema, pulmonary capillary congestion, and localized atelectasis. The cumulative result is a decrease in gas exchange and functional residual capacity. Affected patients have persistent hypoxemia in spite of oxygen therapy. Mechanical ventilation using high tidal volumes or positive end-expiratory pressure (PEEP), or both, may be required to sustain these patients. Careful attention must be paid to fluid/electrolyte balance, cardiovascular support, and nutritional status.

Gram-Negative Sepsis

Gram-negative septicemia is defined as the colonization of the blood by gram-negative bacteria. This is a serious condition with a high mortality rate. The bacteria and the endotoxins they produce result in increased pulmonary capillary permeability, eventual filling of the alveoli with fluid, and shock. Gas exchange in the lungs is impaired, with a resulting increase in the alveolar-arterial oxygen gradient ($P[A-a]O_2$). After culture specimens are obtained, vigorous antibiotic therapy should be initiated. These patients frequently develop high-output cardiac failure. They may breathe well, but metabolic demand is too high for the respiratory system to support. Ventilator support may be required to maintain PaO_2 and $PaCO_2$ levels within normal limits. Serial blood gases and measurement of the mechanics of ventilation are useful in determining ventilator commitment. Patients with gram-negative sepsis, which may occur in conditions such as ARDS, are very difficult to manage clinically.

Left Heart Failure and Pulmonary Edema

Failure of the left heart results in the backup of blood in the pulmonary vasculature. The increased pressure drives fluid across the alveolar-capillary membrane, leading to pulmonary edema. This condition may result from support by an intra-aortic balloon pump, coronary artery bypass grafting, mitral valve disease, or myocardial infarction. If the alveoli become filled, gas exchange is impaired. The application of mechanical ventilation and/or PEEP aids in maintaining gas exchange and in driving the fluid back into circulation.

CRITERIA FOR MECHANICAL VENTILATION

Various criteria are used to determine the need for mechanical ventilation. These criteria are frequently referred to as *Pontoppidan's criteria*, after the investigator who performed much of the original research. Assessment of the mechanics of ventilation, oxygenation, and ventilation is used to determine the need for mechanical ventilation. Table 26-1 is a summary of these criteria, including normal values and values that indicate the need for

TABLE 26-1: Criteria for Mechanical Ventilation

MEASUREMENT	NORMAL	NEED FOR MECHANICAL VENTILATION
I. Mechanics of Ventilation		
Minute volume	5–6 liters/minute	>10 liters/minute
Respiratory rate	12–20/minute	>35/minute
Tidal volume	5–7 ml/kg	<5 ml/kg normal body weight
Vital capacity	65–75 ml/kg	<15 ml/kg normal body weight
Maximum inspiratory force (MIF)	80–100 cm H_2O	< –25 cm H_2O
II. Oxygenation		
PaO_2	75–100 mm Hg	<50 mm Hg (with FiO_2 of 0.50)
$P(A-a)O_2$	25–65 mm Hg	>350 mm Hg
III. Ventilation		
$PaCO_2$	35–45 mm Hg	>55 mm Hg except in chronic conditions
pH	7.35–7.45	<7.25

Reprinted by permission from David J. Pierson, Indications for mechanical ventilation in acute respiratory failure, Respiratory Care, 28(5) (1983), 571.

mechanical ventilation. These criteria are not absolute; and their application must involve careful clinical evaluation of the patient and the prognosis.

Note: The mechanics of ventilation are discussed in Chapter 5, "Pulmonary Function Testing: Bedside Monitoring and Basic Spirometry."

Oxygenation
PaO₂

The goal of ventilation is to provide adequate oxygenation. Measurement of O_2 content of blood by evaluation of PaO_2 and hemoglobin saturation and arterial oxygen concentration (CaO_2) provides the bottom line assessment of the adequacy of oxygenation. PaO_2 is a measurement of the amount of oxygen dissolved in the plasma of arterial blood. The relative proportion of blood that is transported dissolved in the plasma is relatively small under normal circumstances. For example, in 100 ml of whole blood, 0.0031 ml of oxygen is carried dissolved in the plasma for each PaO_2 torr (mm Hg) unit. Assuming that the PaO_2 is 90 mm Hg, the actual amount of oxygen dissolved in the plasma is 0.279 ml (0.0031 ml/mm Hg × 90 mm Hg). It becomes obvious that PaO_2 indicates only a small portion of oxygen that is carried in the blood.

Besides the dissolved oxygen contained in the plasma, oxygen is also carried chemically attached to the hemoglobin. It has been determined that 1.34 ml of oxygen is carried for every gram of hemoglobin in each 100 ml of blood. The oxygen saturation (SaO_2) of the hemoglobin must also be accounted for in this determination. The following formula is used to calculate the oxygen content (CaO_2).

$$\text{ml of } O_2 \text{ carried} = 1.34 \times (\text{g of Hb}/100 \text{ ml}) \times SaO_2$$

Many critically ill patients are anemic and therefore have impaired oxygen transport capabilities. Also, oxygen consumption may be increased owing to the underlying cause of respiratory failure. Therefore, a marginal oxygen content may not be sufficient to meet the patient's metabolic needs.

The dissolved oxygen (PaO_2) and the oxygen carried chemically combined with the hemoglobin together is termed *total oxygen content*.

Most contemporary blood gas labs provide co-oximetry in conjunction with arterial blood gas analysis. Co-oximetry provides a measurement of oxygen content expressed in ml/100 ml. This is a very useful indicator of the oxygen carried in arterial blood.

P(A–a)O₂

The alveolar-arterial oxygen gradient, or $P(A–a)O_2$, is really a measurement of pulmonary efficiency. It is the difference between the oxygen tension in the alveoli and the oxygen tension in the pulmonary capillary. In theory, if the lungs are working perfectly, there would be little difference between the alveolar oxygen tension and the tension in the arterial blood. However, some gradient must exist for diffusion to occur.

Normally, humans breathing room air have a $P(A–a)O_2$ of between 25 and 75 mm Hg. A study may be performed to correlate $P(A–a)O_2$ with shunt volume by having the patient breathe 100% oxygen for at least 15 minutes and then drawing an arterial blood sample and calculating the $P(A–a)O_2$. For each 15 to 20 mm Hg $P(A–a)O_2$, approximately 1% shunt exists (Kacmarek, Craig, & Dimas, 1979). This percentage represents a crude approximation of how much blood bypasses the lungs without gas exchange.

A $P(A–a)O_2$ of greater than 350 mm Hg may indicate the need for mechanical ventilation. The lungs are operating very inefficiently, and respiratory failure may be impending.

Table 26-2, reproduced from *Respiratory Care: A Guide to Clinical Practice*, estimates both PaO_2 and $P(A–a)O_2$, according to age, at sea level with the patient breathing room air. Table 26-3, reproduced from *Comprehensive Respiratory Care*, estimates PaO_2 in persons breathing room air at different ages at different altitudes.

Measurement of Ventilation
PaCO₂

The arterial partial pressure of CO_2 ($PaCO_2$) is a direct indication of the adequacy of alveolar ventilation. One of the functions of the lungs is to eliminate CO_2 produced by the body's metabolism. An increase in $PaCO_2$ indicates that the lungs are not secreting CO_2 effectively or that the

TABLE 26-2: Normal, Upright PaO₂ and P(A–a)O₂ Values (Sea Level)

AGE (in years)	PaO₂ (mm Hg)	P(A–a)O₂ (mm Hg)
20	96–104	<5
30	92–100	<9
40	88–96	<13
50	84–92	<17
60	79–87	<22
70	75–83	<26
80	71–79	<30
90	66–74	<35

Reprinted by permission from George Burton and John E. Hodgkin, Respiratory care: A guide to clinical practice *(2nd ed.), Table 12-1. © 1991 by J. B. Lippincott Company.*

TABLE 26-3: Range of Normal PaO₂ in mm Hg

ALTITUDE	AGES 10–60	UNDER AGE 10, OVER AGE 60
Sea level	84–110	>70
2000 feet	78–104	>67
4000 feet	73–98	>64
6000 feet	66–92	>61
8000 feet	60–86	>58

Reprinted by permission from Eubanks and Bone, Comprehensive respiratory care, *Table 8-11. © 1985 by C. V. Mosby Company.*

production of CO_2 is excessive. Because diffusion block does not affect the ability of CO_2 to leave the blood, it may be assumed that hypoventilation is the cause. Patients with chronic obstructive pulmonary disease (COPD) have a high level of $PaCO_2$, which is "normal" for their condition. However, if hypoventilation is acute, a fall in pH may result, leading to respiratory acidosis. A $PaCO_2$ greater than 55 in combination with a disturbance in the mechanics of ventilation and oxygenation may indicate the need for mechanical ventilation.

pH

As noted, acute hypoventilation, if not compensated for by the kidneys, will result in respiratory acidosis. Acidosis may also occur as a result of renal failure or diabetes. A fall in pH to lower than 7.25 is life-threatening and mechanical ventilation should be initiated.

MODES OF MECHANICAL VENTILATION

The goals of mechanical ventilation include supporting the pulmonary system, providing the ventilatory support required to sustain life, manipulating the ventilatory pattern and gas distribution, decreasing the work of breathing and myocardial work, and improving oxygenation.

Various modes of ventilation are available to accomplish these goals. The modes include control, assist/control, intermittent mandatory ventilation (IMV), and sigh. Depending on the specific goal and on the patient's condition, either volume ventilation or pressure ventilation may be ordered by the physician.

Volume Ventilation

With *volume ventilation*, tidal volume, rate, and inspiratory flow are determined by the practitioner when making initial ventilator settings. In this mode of gas delivery, volume delivery is constant at a preset flow for a preset inspiratory time. Pressure during this mode of ventilation is variable, and depends upon the compliance and resistance of the patient's lungs and how readily they accept gas delivery.

Control

Control mode, as the name implies, totally controls the patient's ventilation. In the control mode, only the ventilator can initiate inspiration. This mode should be used only on patients with no spontaneous respiratory efforts, or who have been paralyzed with a neuromuscular blocking agent (pancuronium bromide [Pavulon], succinylcholine chloride [Anectine], vecuronium). Ventilating a patient with spontaneous efforts using control mode will cause asynchronous respiration and increased work of breathing. Figure 26-3 graphically depicts the control mode.

Assist/Control

Assist/control mode is a mode of mechanical ventilation that allows the patient's spontaneous efforts to initiate a breath. Each spontaneous effort the patient generates will

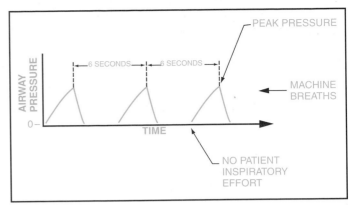

Figure 26-3   *A graphic representation of the control mode*

cycle the ventilator into the inspiratory phase, delivering a mechanical breath. A backup respiratory rate may be set to ensure a minimum rate for ventilation should the patient fail to initiate a breath spontaneously. The spontaneous effort is sensed by the ventilator as a slight negative pressure (usually –1 to –2 cm H_2O). Figure 26-4 shows this mode of ventilation graphically.

(Synchronized) Intermittent Mandatory Ventilation

Intermittent mandatory ventilation (IMV)—also called synchronous mechanical ventilation (SIMV), when mandatory (ventilation) breaths are synchronized with the patient's spontaneous efforts—is a mode of ventilation that allows the patient to breathe spontaneously from a heated nebulizer/humidifier between mechanical breaths. A machine rate is set that will guarantee adequate ventilation. Between machine breaths the patient is allowed to breathe spontaneously without the assistance of positive pressure. The *SIMV/IMV mode* is ideal for maintenance of respiratory muscle strength and for weaning from mechanical ventilation. The ventilator rate may be gradually tapered, with an increasing share of the patient's ventilation being assumed by the patient's own muscles. Figure 26-5 shows this mode graphically.

Sigh

The *sigh mode* is an artificial way to provide periodic deep breaths, emulating the normal physiological sigh. When

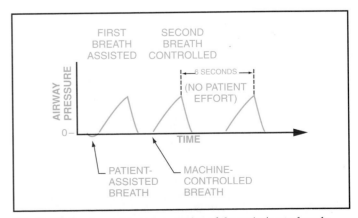

Figure 26-4   *A graphic representation of the assist/control mode*

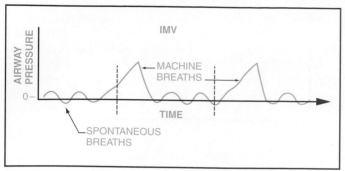

Figure 26-5 *A graphic representation of the SIMV mode*

the ventilator cycles into sigh mode, a series of breaths are given at a volume greater than the normal machine tidal volume. Most ventilators with sigh modes can be adjusted for sigh frequency (times/hour), how many sighs are given (sigh multiple), sigh volume, and sigh pressure limit (safety feature). The effectiveness of sigh is controversial. In the proficiency section of this chapter, general guidelines are given on how to set the sigh mode.

Pressure Ventilation

With *pressure ventilation*, the practitioner sets an inspiratory pressure limit, rate, and inspiratory time. During this form of ventilation, pressure rises to a preset value and is maintained for the duration of the inspiratory time. Flow rate varies, with flow initially high and then tapering as the lungs fill (Figure 26-6). Volume delivery during this mode of ventilation is also variable and depends upon the compliance and resistance of the patient's lungs (Brochard, 1996).

Typical goals of pressure ventilation include the control and maintenance of inspiratory pressure, often at a level lower than that of volume ventilation modes. By controlling inspiratory pressures, often barotrauma may be reduced.

Pressure Control Ventilation

Pressure control ventilation is a form of pressure ventilation in which the patient does not initiate any spontaneous

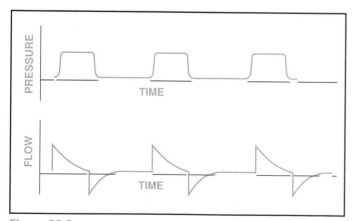

Figure 26-6 *A graphic representation of pressure control ventilation. Note how pressure remains constant for the duration of the inspiratory time while the flow rate begins at a high value and decelerates throughout the inspiratory phase.*

breaths, similar to control mode. The patient's ventilatory rate is a function of the respiratory rate established by the practitioner when making the initial ventilator settings. The patient's ventilatory drive may be intentionally suppressed (through sedation) or may be absent owing to the pathophysiology of the patient's respiratory failure. If the patient does have spontaneous respiratory efforts, pressure control ventilation may cause asynchrony and adversely increase the patient's work of breathing.

Assisted Pressure Control Ventilation

Assisted pressure control ventilation allows the patient to initiate ventilator-assisted breaths in response to a spontaneous effort (Figure 26-7). Some ventilators will trigger an assisted breath in response to a pressure change (pressure-triggered), whereas other ventilators will deliver an assisted breath in response to a flow change (flow-triggered). In either case, when the ventilator senses the patient's spontaneous effort, a mandatory or ventilator-assisted breath is delivered at the set inspiratory pressure and inspiratory time.

Pressure Control Ventilation with SIMV

Pressure control ventilation with SIMV is a form of pressure ventilation in which the mandatory breaths are pressure controlled (preset inspiratory pressure and inspiratory time) and the patient is allowed to breathe spontaneously between mandatory breaths (Figure 26-8). The ventilator may be pressure or flow triggered for breath delivery during both spontaneous and synchronized mandatory breaths.

Pressure Support Ventilation

Pressure support ventilation (PSV) is a mode in which the patient's spontaneous breaths are augmented by a pressure plateau. Once the spontaneous breath is triggered

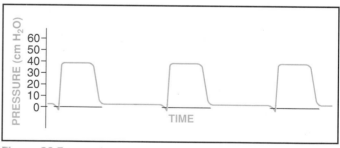

Figure 26-7 *A graphic representation of pressure control ventilation, with each breath being pressure triggered*

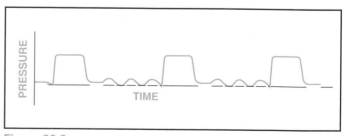

Figure 26-8 *A graphic representation of pressure control ventilation with SIMV*

(pressure or flow), that breath is augmented at a fixed pressure level. The breath is terminated when the inspiratory flow drops to 25% of the peak value (or other predetermined percentage of peak flow) (White, 1999).

Pressure support ventilation is classified as a pressure-controlled (pressure is measured and used as a control variable), pressure-triggered or flow-triggered (spontaneous breath type), and pressure-limited breathing mode.

Volume-Assisted Pressure Support

Volume-assisted pressure support is similar to pressure support, except that a minimum volume is assured with each pressure support breath. Inspiration is maintained until the assured volume level has been reached.

Airway Pressure Release Ventilation

Airway pressure release ventilation is a mode of ventilation in which the patient is allowed to breathe spontaneously at two different pressure levels. During inspiration, pressure is at one level; during expiration, the pressure falls to a lower level. The exhalation time period ranges between 1 and 2 seconds.

Mandatory breaths may also be delivered during airway pressure release ventilation. The breath may be pressure or flow triggered. Once the breath is initiated, the pressure rises to the higher level and is maintained throughout inspiration. Once inspiration ends, the pressure falls to the lower level for exhalation.

HAZARDS AND COMPLICATIONS OF MECHANICAL VENTILATION

Like IPPB, mechanical ventilation involves the application of positive intrathoracic pressure. The hazards and complications may be divided into three categories: barotrauma, cardiovascular complications, and effects on other organ systems. Patients requiring ventilatory support are frequently more unstable and ill; hence, any complications that develop may be more severe, and hazardous to the patients' recovery.

Barotrauma

Barotrauma is a category of complications that result directly from the application of pressure. These complications may include pneumothorax, pneumomediastinum, subcutaneous emphysema, tracheal rupture, and interstitial emphysema. Usually these complications result from the application of high pressures or PEEP. Patients on mechanical ventilation should be frequently assessed for evidence of barotrauma.

Cardiovascular Complications

The application of positive intrathoracic pressure may result in a decrease in venous return, which, combined with the squeezing effect on the mediastinum, will result in a decrease in cardiac output and a fall in blood pressure. The maintenance of an inspiratory-expiratory ratio (I:E) of 1:2 or greater will help to prevent these changes.

Effects on Other Organ Systems

Renal Dysfunction

Renal dysfunction and a decrease in urine output are common complications of mechanical ventilation. Two possible causes have been suggested, including an increase in production of antidiuretic hormone and a decrease in renal blood flow. The effect of these changes is an increase in fluid volume and increased intrathoracic water, yielding interstitial edema, decreased PaO_2, and increased $P(A-a)O_2$.

Gastrointestinal Bleeding

Gastrointestinal (GI) bleeding is a common complication of mechanical ventilation. It is thought that the positive pressure interferes with circulation to the spleen and GI tract. This may result in mucosal ischemia and increased effects of acid in the GI tract. GI bleeding can be a serious complication with patients on continuous mechanical ventilation. Administration of antacids will reduce the effects of this complication.

OBJECTIVES

At the end of this chapter, you should be able to:

- Demonstrate the assessment of a patient to determine the need for mechanical ventilation:
  - Assess the mechanics of ventilation:
    - Respiratory frequency
    - Minute volume
    - Vital capacity
    - Maximal inspiratory force
    - Peak expiratory flow
  - Given the following information, assess the need for mechanical ventilation:
    - PaO_2
    - $P(A-a)O_2$
    - $PaCO_2$
    - pH
- Given a simulated physician's order, demonstrate how to initiate mechanical ventilation. Establish the ordered ventilator parameters using a test lung or lung analog:
  - Assemble and test the required equipment for function.
  - Establish ordered ventilator settings.
  - Monitor the patient-ventilator system.
- Demonstrate how to change a ventilator circuit while the patient is on continuous mechanical ventilation.

ASSESSING THE PATIENT FOR MECHANICAL VENTILATION

As a respiratory care practitioner, you will frequently be involved in the assessment of the patient prior to the initiation of mechanical ventilation. This may include physical assessment of the chest, blood gas determination, and the measurement of the mechanics of ventilation. Physical assessment, arterial blood gas analysis, and bedside monitoring are discussed in previous chapters.

A critically ill patient often is hypoxemic, hypercapnic, and hypoventilating, with unstable cardiovascular status. Caution and common sense are required to assess the mechanics of ventilation. The patient may be receiving supplemental oxygen to maintain adequate arterial oxygen concentrations. It is very important to oxygenate the patient with a manual resuscitator before and after each measurement. Do not hyperventilate the patient; rather, simply provide an "edge" that will allow the patient to tolerate being removed from supplemental oxygen long enough to make your measurements.

Assessment of Oxygenation and Ventilation

Drawing arterial blood gas specimens and the calculation of the $P(A–a)O_2$ can indicate the adequacy of oxygenation and ventilation. The significance of PaO_2, $PaCO_2$, arterial pH, and $P(A–a)O_2$ is discussed earlier in this chapter. Comparison of the patient's values with those listed in Table 26-1 will indicate whether continuous mechanical ventilation is indicated.

Assessment of Cardiovascular Function

A rapid way to assess cardiovascular function is to observe the bedside cardiac monitor in the critical care setting. Heart rate and rhythm may be rapidly assessed. The presence of cardiac arrhythmias will also appear on the oscilloscope display.

In the absence of a cardiac monitor, the pulse may be taken. When measuring the pulse, note the rhythm and contour of the pulse. For review, read Chapter 2, "Basic Patient Assessment: Vital Signs and Breath Sounds."

Determination of blood pressure is also a way to assess general cardiovascular function. The blood pressure is an indicator of the body's ability to deal with changes in vascular volume, cardiac output, and general vascular tone.

Specialized Monitoring Techniques

Central venous pressure (CVP) monitoring is an invasive procedure that provides very useful information. Many patients in the critical care setting are monitored with either a CVP line or a Swan-Ganz catheter. A CVP catheter is usually inserted into a subclavian vein and threaded into a resting position in the vena cava or right atrium. The CVP measures right atrial pressure. This gives an indicator of the right ventricular end-diastolic pressure and overall performance of the right ventricle. The pressures may be monitored by means of a transducer connected to an oscilloscope monitor, continuously measuring pressure displayed as a wave form. Alternatively, pressure may be monitored intermittently using a water manometer placed at the level of the heart. These catheters provide an indicator of vascular volume and are useful in fluid management in the critically ill patient.

The Swan-Ganz catheter is usually inserted into a subclavian vein and threaded into position in the pulmonary artery. As with CVP monitoring, this is an invasive procedure. The catheter design incorporates several features, including an inflatable balloon at the tip, a thermal sensor at the tip, a central pressure measuring lumen, a lumen for intravenous infusion, and a lumen for instillation of cold sterile normal saline. Figure 26-9 shows an enlargement of the catheter with these parts identified.

By inflating the balloon during catheter insertion, the catheter is carried by the blood flow up the pulmonary artery until it becomes lodged in the vessel. Once it is lodged in a pulmonary artery, the catheter is said to be "wedged." In this wedged position, pressure is measured through the central lumen, which reflects the pressure in the left atrium and left ventricular end-diastolic pressure. This is very useful in fluid management. The higher the wedge pressure is, the more fluid or volume is in circulation.

Most Swan-Ganz catheters have a thermal sensor at the catheter tip. By injecting cold sterile normal saline (0°C), and measuring the time for the temperature to drop at the sensor, cardiac output can be calculated. Most new cardiac monitors in the critical care setting have the thermal dilution computer built into its many functions. This type of computer uses thermodilution to measure cardiac output. This measurement is technique-dependent, and three trials are normally performed to obtain a reading.

Ventilator Commitment

After the objective data have been gathered (mechanics of ventilation, oxygenation, and cardiovascular assessment), the patient's clinical condition is once again assessed. If respiratory failure appears imminent, the patient's condition can be expected to deteriorate, or the patient will become unable to sustain spontaneous ventilation. The decision to maintain the patient on continuous mechanical ventilation must be made. Mechanical ventilation should sustain the patient's pulmonary needs without compromising the function of the cardiovascular system or other organ systems. It is best to decide early on to commit the patient to mechanical ventilation. Generally, the earlier mechanical ventilation is initiated, the sooner the patient is able to be weaned.

Once the decision has been made, the patient should be intubated and an appropriate ventilator should be selected. The ventilator should allow variable oxygen concentrations, tidal volumes, respiratory rates, and flow rates. Alarms should be available for patient disconnect, excessive pressure, and oxygen concentration limits.

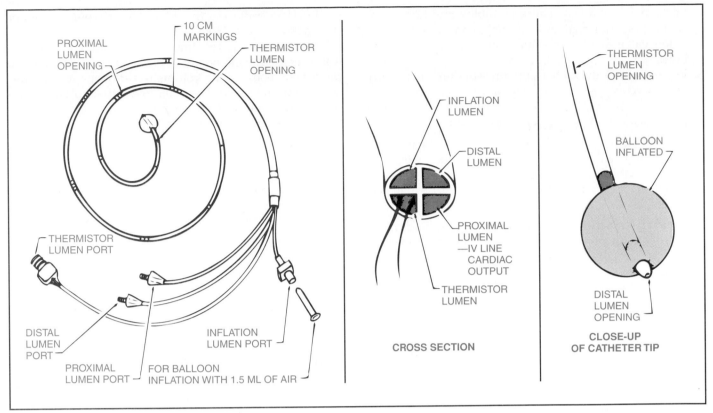

Figure 26-9 *A diagram identifying the components of a Swan-Ganz catheter*

EQUIPMENT REQUIREMENTS

There are several pieces of equipment required for initiating mechanical ventilation. Figure 26-10 is a list of the required equipment.

Equipment Preparation

A variety of ventilators are utilized in the clinical setting. The assembly of the circuitry for the more common ventilators is discussed in the practice activities. The following text describes how to test the ventilator and circuit prior to initiating mechanical ventilation.

- Ventilator
- Ventilator circuit
- Humidifier
- Spirometer (if the ventilator does not have one)
- Oxygen analyzer
- Thermometer
- Manual resuscitator and oxygen flowmeter
- Sterile water
- Suctioning supplies
- Ventilator flow sheets
- External disconnect alarm if one is not provided

Figure 26-10 *Equipment required for mechanical ventilation*

Testing for Circuit Leaks

Prior to initiation of continuous mechanical ventilation, the circuit should be checked for leaks. Set the controls on the ventilator to values listed in Table 26-4.

Perform the following steps:

1. Using a sterile gauze or sterile plastic wrap (inside the wrapping in which the circuit was packaged), occlude the patient wye (Y-connector) completely.
2. When the ventilator cycles on, pinch the exhalation valve drive line or occlude the outlet from the exhalation valve with your other hand. This will hold pressure in the circuit.
3. Observe the pressure manometer. Pressure should drop slightly and then plateau without dropping further. If the manometer does not remain at a steady value, but continues to show a pressure drop, you have a leak.

TABLE 26-4: Settings for Circuit Leak Testing and Circuit Compliance

Tidal volume	200 ml
Respiratory rate	12/min
Flow rate	40 L/min
Pressure limit	Maximum setting

4. In the event of a leak, check all tubing and humidifier connections (internal and external), and examine exhalation valve diaphragms and tubing for small tears or holes.
5. Repeat steps 1 through 4 until pressure remains steady in the circuit.

Measuring Tubing Compliance

Tubing compliance should be calculated for each circuit used to ventilate the patient. It takes very little time and is useful in establishing an accurate corrected tidal volume delivered to the patient. To calculate tubing compliance, complete the following steps:

1. Attach a respirometer to the outlet of the tubing circuit or exhalation valve to measure the exhaled volume.
2. Set the controls on the ventilator to the values listed in Table 26-4.
3. Using a sterile gauze or sterile plastic wrap (inside the wrapping in which the circuit was packaged), occlude the patient wye completely.
4. As the ventilator cycles, note the pressure reading on the pressure manometer. It may take several breaths to record the pressure accurately.
5. Read the respirometer and record the tidal volume delivered with each breath. This volume represents the volume compressed in the circuit because no volume was actually delivered.
6. Compliance is defined as a volume change per unit of force (in this case, pressure). To calculate compliance perform the following calculation:

$$\text{Tubing compliance} = \frac{\text{tidal volume}}{\text{peak inspiratory pressure}}$$

ESTABLISHING ORDERED VENTILATOR SETTINGS

The initiation of continuous mechanical ventilation requires a physician's order. It is the responsibility of the respiratory care practitioner to establish the settings as ordered on the ventilator. Occasionally, a physician will be unfamiliar with ventilator protocol or appropriate settings. In these instances, general guidelines are given that may be offered as suggestions.

Mode

The mode of mechanical ventilation in the majority of cases will be assist/control or SIMV. Some special clinical conditions may require the use of control mode. The most common mode utilized is assist/control. This mode will allow patients to regulate their own $PaCO_2$ levels, if the ventilator rate is set too low.

Tidal Volume

The machine tidal volume control adjusts the volume delivered to the patient with each machine breath. A general rule to use is to set the tidal volume to deliver 8 to 10 ml per kilogram (kg) of normal body weight. For example, if a male patient weighing 75 kg is initiated on

mechanical ventilation, the tidal volume would be set for 675 ml (9 ml/kg × 75 kg = 675 ml).

It is important to remember that even though the control is set for 900 ml, not all of that volume is delivered to the patient. Some of the volume is lost owing to compression in the circuit. To determine the actual volume delivered to the patient (corrected tidal volume), you must perform the following calculation:

$$V_t \text{ corrected} = V_t - (\text{PIP} \times Ct)$$

where

V_t corrected = corrected tidal volume
V_t = measured tidal volume
PIP = peak inspiratory pressure
Ct = tubing compliance

Assume in our example that the volume control is set at 1100 ml, and 1000 ml is measured at the exhalation port. The peak inspiratory pressure is 25 cm H_2O, and the tubing compliance is 4 ml/cm H_2O. Using the formula, you arrive at a corrected tidal volume of 900 ml.

$$\text{Corrected tidal volume} = 1000\,\text{ml} - (25\,\text{cm}\,H_2O \times 4\,\text{ml/cm}\,H_2O)$$
$$= 900\,\text{ml}$$

The tidal volume control should be adjusted so that the corrected tidal volume is within 50 ml of the ordered tidal volume.

Respiratory Rate

Ideally, the patient should be allowed to establish his or her own respiratory rate using assist/control mode, which allows the patient to initiate inspiration spontaneously. Adjust the sensitivity control so that an effort of −1 to −2 cm H_2O will initiate inspiration. The sensitivity control should be set so that work of breathing is slight and so that the machine does not cycle on without patient effort. Normally, the rate is set slightly lower than the patient's spontaneous respiratory rate. If the patient is tachypneic, set the rate between 8 and 12 breaths per minute.

Flow Rate

For the adult patient, the flow rate control is set between 40 and 60 L/min. Set the flow rate control and time the inspiratory phase. Determine the respiratory rate and the total time allowed for each breath (inspiration and expiration). Calculate the I:E ratio.

The I:E ratio should be maintained at 1:2 or greater. This will allow sufficient time for venous return, to minimize cardiovascular complications.

FiO₂

Set the FiO_2 (fraction of inspired oxygen) at 1.0 unless otherwise ordered (Martz, Joiner, & Shepherd, 1984). Once a baseline is established, the FiO_2 will be adjusted according to results of blood gas analysis.

Pressure Limit

The *pressure limit* control is like a safety valve on a pressure cooker. This control does not determine the pressure used to deliver a volume. It sets a maximum pressure that will be delivered. If excessive pressures are delivered, the inspiration will be immediately terminated and an alarm will sound. Changes in the patient's condition affecting compliance or increased airway resistance can affect the delivered pressure. This control will prevent the administration of dangerous pressures and will alert you to changes in the patient's condition. Set the control 10 to 15 cm H_2O greater than the peak inspiratory pressure.

Humidifier Temperature

Contemporary humidifiers incorporate heating elements to increase humidity output. Some are controlled by a thermostat, whereas others use a servocontroller. Adjust the humidifier temperature to maintain 35 to 37°C at the patient wye, where the temperature should be monitored.

SPECIAL VENTILATORY FUNCTIONS

Sigh

If sigh mode is ordered, adjust the sigh volume to 1.5 to 2 times greater than the ordered tidal volume (Martz et al., 1984). This will ensure the delivery of a greater than normal breath, but not compromise respiratory function with excessive volumes. Set the sighs per hour control to four per hour (one sigh every 15 minutes), or as ordered. Adjust the sigh pressure limit 10 to 15 cm H_2O greater than the peak inspiratory pressure during sigh mode. Set the sigh multiple to 2 (this will deliver two consecutive sighs every 15 minutes).

Inspiratory Hold

Inspiratory hold may be ordered to help reduce micro atelectasis. This control may be set from zero to 2 seconds (depending on the ventilator). The use of this control may increase intrathoracic pressures and compromise cardiac output. This control should be used only with a physician's order.

Expiratory Retard

Expiratory retard slows the flow on exhalation, decreasing the effect of air trapping. It is similar to exhaling through pursed lips. As with pursed-lip breathing, a back pressure in the thorax is generated. This back pressure (increased intrathoracic pressure) may cause a decrease in cardiac output. Like the inspiratory hold, expiratory retard should be used only with a physician's order.

ALARMS

The alarms available will vary depending on the ventilator being used. However, the alarms may be classified into several different types depending on their function.

Pressure Alarm

The pressure limit is a safety feature that will limit the amount of pressure delivered to the patient. If the pressure limit setting is exceeded, inspiration will be terminated and an alarm will sound. Causes for this alarm may include kinks in the tubing, the patient's lying on the tubing, airway secretions causing an increase in resistance, a pneumothorax, and coughing.

I:E Ratio Alarm

The I:E ratio alarm is a safety feature to prevent the inadvertent delivery of inverse I:E ratios (inspiration longer than expiration). If the I:E ratio is less than 1:1, inspiration will terminate and an alarm will sound. Some ventilators allow this feature to be disabled in order to ventilate patients with unusual conditions.

Tidal Volume Alarm

This is an alarm designed to alert you if the tidal volume changes from what is desired. If the tidal volume falls below a preset level, an alarm will sound. This alarm may be connected to internal or external monitoring devices. This alarm may be triggered by a patient disconnect or leaks in the patient-ventilator system (humidifier, tubing connections, artificial airway cuff).

Patient Disconnect Alarm

If the patient inadvertently becomes disconnected from the ventilator circuit, this alarm will alert you to the condition. Without an operating disconnect alarm, you or other health care personnel may not notice that the patient has become disconnected and is no longer being ventilated. This alarm may monitor either inspiratory pressure or exhaled volume.

PEEP Alarm

The PEEP alarm is provided to alert the clinician of loss of PEEP pressure during exhalation. Tubing disconnects, circuit leaks, humidification leaks, and endotracheal tube cuff leaks may all potentially cause loss of PEEP pressure. The PEEP alarm is typically set 2 to 5 cm H_2O lower than the selected PEEP level.

Source Gas Pressure Alarms

Most ventilators provide alarms for source gas pressure. If the line or inlet pressure falls below a 40 to 45 psi working pressure level, an alarm will sound. These are pressure sensors, not oxygen analyzers.

Ventilator Failure Alarm

Most ventilators have a ventilator inoperative alarm that will sound in the event of a mechanical failure. Some of these alarms are battery powered so that if an electrical failure occurs, the alarm will still function.

MONITORING THE PATIENT-VENTILATOR SYSTEM

The purpose of monitoring the patient-ventilator system is to identify changes in the patient's condition and to verify that the ventilator is operating properly and maintaining the ordered settings.

Position the patient supine. All ventilator monitoring should be performed in a consistent way. Variations in technique and patient positioning will affect the measured values.

The Patient

Your first and primary concern is the care of your patient. Any time the ventilator system is checked, the patient's well-being should be the first item on your agenda. A thorough assessment of your patient should be performed, and then the ventilator should be monitored.

Pulmonary

Auscultate the patient's chest. Are the airways clear or does the patient need suctioning? If suctioning is required, perform the procedure and then proceed. Listen for the distribution of breath sounds. Pay close attention when comparing sounds bilaterally. A sudden increase in inspiratory pressure combined with a localized decrease in breath sounds may signify a pneumothorax.

Check for recent results of arterial blood gas analysis. Are the PaO_2, $PaCO_2$, and pH being maintained within acceptable limits? Observe the patient's skin color and level of consciousness.

Observe for the use of accessory muscles if the patient is able to assist ventilation with spontaneous respiratory efforts. Use of accessory muscles indicates that the sensitivity may be set too high, or that there is an obstruction in the airway or circuit, increasing the effort required to initiate a breath.

Cardiac

Observe the heart monitor. Check heart rate and rhythm. Observe for any arrhythmias.

If the patient has a CVP or Swan-Ganz catheter in place, observe monitor display for the CVP, pulmonary artery pressure, and pulmonary artery wedge pressure. If an oscilloscope is not being used, look at the nurse's flow sheet for these values.

Neurological

Is the patient alert and oriented? The patient will be unable to speak owing to the presence of the artificial airway. However, you may communicate with the patient and reassure the patient that what you are doing is normal procedure. Observe the respiratory pattern for any irregularities.

The Ventilator

Monitoring the ventilator consists of verifying that the ventilator is operating within the ordered settings and also calculating some patient values.

Drain the ventilator tubing of any condensate and fill the humidifier to the proper level. Attention to these small details will ensure consistency in measuring the ventilatory parameters.

Figure 26-11 shows a typical ventilator flow sheet. The following discussion reviews how each item on the flow sheet is obtained.

DOCUMENTATION OF VENTILATOR SETTINGS

Mode

This is simply the mode the ventilator is operating in. The modes of ventilation include control, assist/control, and IMV. Note on the flow sheet what mode is ordered and in what mode the ventilator is operating.

Tidal Volume

Note in this space where the tidal volume control is set.

Frequency

Note in this space where respiratory frequency control is set. If the patient is in control mode, the frequency may be timed using your watch. However, if the patient is in assist/control mode, the frequency may vary from what is set.

Pressure Limit

Note in this space where the pressure limit control is set. This control should be adjusted 10 to 15 cm H_2O above the peak inspiratory pressure.

FIO_2

Analyze the FIO_2 delivered from the ventilator. This is best accomplished by analyzing the gas before it enters the humidifier. Monitoring humidified gases may have detrimental effects on some oxygen analyzers. Adjust the control to the prescribed oxygen level if it is out of adjustment. The oxygen percentage should be adjusted to within 2% of the ordered FIO_2.

Flow Rate

Note in this space where the inspiratory flow rate control is set.

I:E Ratio

Calculate the I:E ratio or measure it using the internal monitor provided on some ventilators.

Inspiratory Hold/Expiratory Retard

Note the positions of these controls if they are being utilized.

Sigh Volume

In this space note where the sigh volume is set.

Sigh Interval/Sigh Multiple

Note in this space where the sighs per hour and the sigh multiple controls are set.

Temperature

Measure the temperature at the patient wye or note the temperature indicated on the servocontroller.

Alarms

Note the settings for the pressure limit, low pressure, and low volume alarms.

Date:												
Time:												

VENTILATOR SETTINGS

Mode												
FiO_2												
Tidal Volume V_t (L)												
Sigh Volume (L)												
Rate (BPM)												
Inspiratory Flow (LPM)												
PEEP/CPAP (cm H_2O)												
Alarms (check)												

PATIENT PARAMETERS — ON VENTILATOR

Minute Volume (L)												
Rate (Total BPM)												
Tidal Volume (controlled)												
Corrected Tidal Volume (L)												
Sigh Volume (L)												
Peak Pressure (cm H_2O)												
Plateau Pressure												
Compliance (cc/cm H_2O)												
E.T. Tube Length (cm)												
Cuff Pressure (cm H_2O)												
Circuit Temp.												

PATIENT PARAMETERS — OFF VENTILATOR

Minute Volume (L)												
Rate (BPM)												
Tidal Volume (L)												
Vital Capacity (L)												
M.I.F. (Neg. cm H_2O)												
M.V.V. (LPM)												
Therapist												

Figure 26-11 *A typical ventilator flow sheet (Courtesy of St. Benedict's Hospital, Ogden, UT)*

DOCUMENTATION OF PATIENT VALUES

Peak Pressure

Note in this space the peak inspiratory pressure delivered during each machine breath.

End-Expiratory Pressure

If the patient is not on PEEP, this should be zero.

Sigh Pressure

If the patient is on sigh mode, note the peak inspiratory pressure when a sigh is delivered. This may be measured by manually sighing the patient for one or two breaths.

Plateau Pressure

The plateau pressure or static pressure is measured when there is no air flow in the patient-ventilator circuit. Explain to the patient what you are doing and that a momentary period of holding the breath will be required. This pressure is measured by pinching the exhalation valve tubing during an inspiratory cycle, occluding the exhalation port momentarily after a breath is delivered, or temporarily adjusting the inspiratory pause control between 1 and 2 seconds. Do not delay in measuring your plateau pressure value. A delay may result in stacking breaths and increasing intrathoracic pressure above safe limits.

Observe the pressure manometer. The manometer will indicate the peak inspiratory pressure and then fall slightly (5 to 15 cm H_2O) and stabilize. It is this latter pressure you want to measure. Note this pressure on the flow sheet.

Measured Tidal Volume

Using a portable respirometer or the ventilator spirometer (not a Bennett bellows spirometer), measure a minute volume. Divide the minute volume (exhaled) by the frequency to obtain an average machine tidal volume ($V_E/f = V_t$).

Tubing Compression Volume

This is calculated by multiplying the peak inspiratory pressure by the tubing compliance.

Corrected Tidal Volume

The corrected tidal volume is calculated by subtracting the tubing compression volume from the measured tidal volume. The corrected tidal volume should be adjusted to within 50 ml of the ordered tidal volume.

Dynamic Compliance

Dynamic compliance is the compliance of the lungs, thorax, and the patient-ventilator circuit. It is measured during gas flow conditions. To measure this value, divide the corrected tidal volume by the peak inspiratory pressure minus PEEP: dynamic compliance = V_t corr/(PIP − PEEP).

Static Compliance

Static compliance is an indicator of the compliance of the lungs and thorax. It is calculated by dividing the corrected tidal volume by the plateau pressure minus PEEP: static compliance = V_t corr/(plateau pressure − PEEP).

Airway Resistance

Airway resistance may be easily calculated once the peak and plateau pressures are known. The formula to calculate the airway resistance is as follows:

$$R_{AW} = \frac{\text{peak pres} - \text{plateau pres}}{\text{flow}}$$

where

R_{AW} = airway resistance
peak pres = peak airway pressure
plateau pres = plateau pressure
flow = flow rate setting in liters per second

As the pressure difference becomes greater, airway resistance increases. Airway resistance may be lowered by administering bronchodilators or anti-inflammatory agents and by keeping the airway suctioned.

Frequency

Note in this space the respiratory rate that you counted when you measured the minute volume.

IMV

In this section of the flow sheet, the patient's spontaneous efforts between machine breaths are recorded. This mode of ventilation is discussed in Chapter 27, "Special Ventilatory Procedures."

Arterial Blood Gases

When arterial blood gases are drawn, the results should be noted on the ventilator flow sheet. Note the date, time, FIO_2, and ventilator settings. If the ventilator settings are changed, 20 minutes should be allowed for the patient to equilibrate to the new settings before arterial blood gases are drawn.

CHANGING A VENTILATOR CIRCUIT

Changing the ventilator circuit is important to prevent bacterial colonization in the tubing, so that the patient does not acquire a nosocomial infection. The interval at which the ventilator circuit is changed varies between clinical facilities. The recommended interval varies from 24 to 72 hours. As a respiratory care practitioner, you must know how to change a circuit while the patient is being mechanically ventilated.

Equipment Requirements

The equipment required is summarized in Figure 26-12.

Patient Assessment

Auscultate the chest. If suctioning is indicated, perform the procedure. Note the patient's respiratory rate and rhythm. Note if the patient is assisting or is able to breathe spontaneously for a brief period. Note the peak pressure and tidal volume before beginning the procedure.

Preparing the Manual Resuscitator for Use

Connect the manual resuscitator to the oxygen flowmeter and turn on the flow to 10 to 15 L/min. Verify that the resuscitator is functioning properly. Obtain assistance. One person will ventilate the patient and the other will change the circuit.

Disconnecting All Ventilator Alarms

The disconnecting of the alarms is an important step. Failure to do so will allow the alarms to sound, startling you, the health care team, and the patient. Also take the time now to drain the circuit of any condensate.

Removing the Patient from the Ventilator

Remove the patient from the ventilator and manually ventilate the patient using a manual resuscitator. Try to

---

- Gloves, goggles, or face shield
- Ventilator circuit
- Humidifier
- Bacteria filter(s)
- Test lung
- Sterile distilled water
- Manual resuscitator and oxygen flowmeter
- Plastic bag
- Respirometer

Figure 26-12 *Equipment needed to change a ventilator circuit*

approximate the machine rate and tidal volume. If the patient is assisting, match the ventilation with the patient's own breathing rate. Closely observe the patient for signs of restlessness, tachycardia, arrhythmias, and use of accessory muscles.

Changing the Circuit

Quickly strip the ventilator of the old circuit and humidifier. As the parts are removed, place them into a plastic bag to prevent the spread of contamination. Never place dirty parts on the floor, counters, or the patient's bed.

Resetting All Alarms

Reset all alarms to the appropriate values. Ensure their proper operation and function. Measure the tidal volume and peak pressure. Compare them with the values obtained before the circuit was changed.

Disposing of Equipment Appropriately

Contain all dirty equipment in a plastic bag and transport it to the equipment processing area in your department. Ensure that the patient area is safe and free from debris left from the procedure.

References

American Association for Respiratory Care. (1991). AARC clinical practice guidelines: Patient-ventilator system checks. *Respiratory Care, 37*(8), 882–886.

American Association for Respiratory Care. (1994). AARC clinical practice guidelines: Ventilator circuit changes. *Respiratory Care, 39*(8), 797–802.

American Association for Respiratory Care. (1995). AARC clinical practice guidelines: Long-term invasive mechanical ventilation in the home. *Respiratory Care, 40*(12), 1313–1320.

Brochard, L. (1996). Pressure-limited ventilation. *Respiratory Care, 41*(5), 447–455.

Burton, G. G., Hodgkin, J. E., & Ward, J. (1991). *Respiratory care: A guide to clinical practice* (3rd ed.). Philadelphia: Lippincott.

Cooper, K. R., & Morrow, C. F. (1984). Pulmonary complications associated with head injury. *Respiratory Care, 29*(3), 263.

Eubanks, D. H., & Bone, R. C. (1991). *Comprehensive respiratory care* (2nd ed.). St. Louis, MO: Mosby.

Kacmarek, R. M., Craig, M. W., & Dimas, S. (1979). *The essentials of respiratory therapy*. Chicago: Year Book Medical Publishers.

Martz, K. V., Joiner, J. W., & Shepherd, R. M. (1984). *Management of the patient-ventilator system: A team approach* (2nd ed.). St. Louis, MO: Year Book–Mosby.

McPherson, S. P., & Spearman, C. B. (1995). *Respiratory therapy equipment* (5th ed.). St. Louis, MO: Year Book–Mosby.

White, G. C. (1999). *Equipment theory for respiratory care* (3rd ed.). Clifton Park, NY: Delmar Learning.

Additional Resources

7200 Series ventilator, options and accessories, operator's manual. (1990). Carlsbad, CA: Puritan-Bennett.

8400ST volume ventilator instruction manual. (1990). Palm Springs, CA: Bird Products.

BEAR 3 instruction manual. (1992). Riverside, CA: Bear Medical Systems.

BEAR 1000 ventilator instruction manual. (1994). Riverside, CA: Bear Medical Systems.

Demers, R. R., Pratter, M. R., & Irwin, R. S. (1981). Use of the concept of ventilator compliance in the determination of static total compliance. *Respiratory Care, 26*(7), 644.

Gillette, M. A., & Hess, D. R. (2001). Ventilator-induced lung injury and the evolution of lung-protective strategies in acute respiratory distress syndrome. *Respiratory Care, 46*(2), 130–148.

Headley-Whyte, J. (1976). *Applied physiology of respiratory care*. Boston: Little, Brown.

Nelson, E. J., Hunter, P. M., & Morton, E. (1983). *Critical care respiratory therapy: A laboratory and clinical manual*. Boston: Little, Brown.

Servo Ventilator 300 — operating manual. (1993). Solona, Sweden: Siemens-Elema AB.

Shapiro, B. A., Harrison, R. A., Kacmarek, R. M., & Cane, R. D. (1985). *Clinical application of blood gases*. Chicago: Year Book Medical Publishers.

Practice Activities: BEAR 1, BEAR 2, and BEAR 3

Not all respiratory care programs or hospitals will have all mechanical ventilators in their inventory. A representative sampling of ventilators is included in these practice activities to provide a broad spectrum of what is currently used in clinical practice or available to schools and programs. These ventilators include the BEAR 1, 2, 3, 5, and 1000; the Bird Products Corporation 8400 ST; the Lifecare PLV-102; the Nellcor-Puritan-Bennett 7200ae and Puritan-Bennett MA-1 and MA-2; and the Siemens Elema Servo 900C and Servo 300.

By completing the practice activities for the ventilators available locally, you will gain a working knowledge of their controls, settings, and operation.

CIRCUIT ASSEMBLY

Figure 26-13 shows the BEAR 1, BEAR 2, and BEAR 3 assembled and ready for the initiation of mechanical ventilation.

1. Facing the front of the ventilator, attach a main flow bacteria filter to the outlet of the ventilator.

2. Fill the humidifier with water and attach it to the heating element on the side of the machine. Attach the angled connector to the filter outlet and to the humidifier.

3. Assemble the circuit as shown in Figure 26-14 and attach it to the support arm using the fitting on the manifold assembly.

4. Attach the inspiratory side of the circuit to the outlet of the humidifier.

5. Attach the expiratory flow tube to the exhalation port on the manifold assembly using a rubber adapter.

6. Attach the exhalation valve tubing to the exhalation valve fitting on the front of the ventilator. Attach the proximal pressure line to the small water trap on the front of the ventilator.

7. Connect the ventilator to a 50 psi source of oxygen and air. Connect the ventilator power cord to a suitable 110 V outlet.

8. Attach a test lung and proceed with leak testing and calculation of circuit compliance.

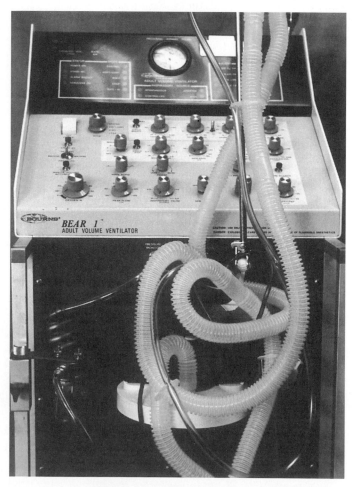

(A)

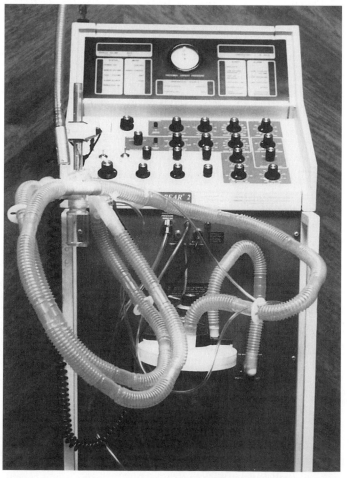

(B)   *(Continued)*

Figure 26-13 *Photos of the BEAR® 1 (A), BEAR® 2 (B), and BEAR® 3 (C) volume ventilators*

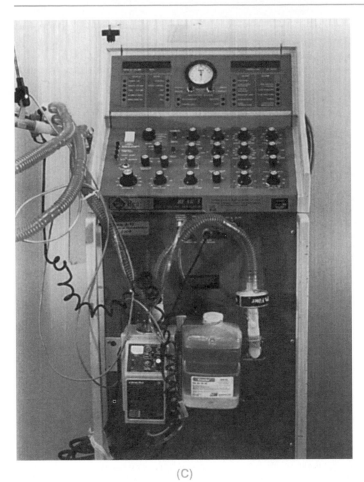

(C)

Figure 26-13 *Continued*

SYSTEM LEAK TEST

1. Set the controls to the following settings:
   a. Normal Tidal Volume   200 ml
   b. Respiratory Rate   12/min
   c. Flow Rate   40 L/min
   d. Normal Pressure Limit   maximum setting

2. Using a sterile gauze or sterile plastic wrap (inside of wrapping that the circuit was packaged in), occlude the patient wye completely.

3. When the ventilator cycles on, pinch the exhalation valve drive line or occlude the outlet for the exhalation valve with your other hand and a sterile wrap. This will hold pressure in the circuit.

4. Observe the pressure manometer. Pressure should drop slightly and then plateau without dropping further. If the manometer does not remain at a steady value but continues to drop, you have a leak.

5. In the event of a leak, check all tubing connections, humidifier connection (internal and external), exhalation valve diaphragm, and tubing for small holes.

6. Repeat steps 1 through 5 until pressure remains steady in the circuit.

TUBING COMPLIANCE

1. Set the controls to the values listed under system leak test.

2. Using a sterile gauze or sterile plastic wrap (inside of wrapping that the circuit was packaged in), occlude the patient wye completely.

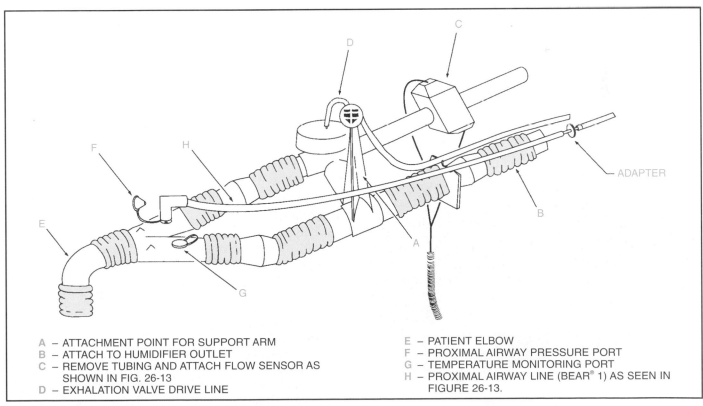

A – ATTACHMENT POINT FOR SUPPORT ARM
B – ATTACH TO HUMIDIFIER OUTLET
C – REMOVE TUBING AND ATTACH FLOW SENSOR AS SHOWN IN FIG. 26-13
D – EXHALATION VALVE DRIVE LINE

E – PATIENT ELBOW
F – PROXIMAL AIRWAY PRESSURE PORT
G – TEMPERATURE MONITORING PORT
H – PROXIMAL AIRWAY LINE (BEAR® 1) AS SEEN IN FIGURE 26-13.

Figure 26-14 *The BEAR® ventilator circuit correctly assembled for use*

3. As the ventilator cycles, note the pressure reading on the pressure manometer. It may take several breaths to record the pressure accurately.

4. Read the respirometer and record the tidal volume delivered with each breath. This volume represents the volume compressed in the circuit, since no volume was actually delivered.

5. Calculate the tubing compliance using the following formula:

$$\text{Tubing compliance} = \frac{\text{tidal volume}}{\text{peak inspiratory pressure}}$$

ACTIVITIES

To complete these practice exercises, it is recommended that you use a lung analog/simulator such as a Medishield Lung Ventilator Performance Analyzer or Retec Respirator Teaching Console. Both of these devices or other similar devices can alter resistance and compliance, simulating changes in patient condition.

If these devices are not available, a patient wye and two test lungs may be used as shown in Figure 26-15. Exercise caution. Volumes and pressures may exceed the limits of the test lungs. Resistance may be altered by adapting different sizes of endotracheal tubes and compliance may be altered by the addition of rubber bands to the test lungs.

INITIAL SETTINGS

a.	Mode	Assist/control
b.	Peak Flow	40 L/min
c.	Sensitivity	12 o'clock position
d.	Normal Pressure Limit	maximum setting
e.	Normal Tidal Volume	500 ml
f.	Normal Rate	12/min
g.	All Sigh Controls	off
h.	Oxygen Concentration	21%
i.	Wave Form	square
j.	Nebulizer	off
k.	Inspiratory Pause	0
l.	PEEP	fully counterclockwise
m.	Alarms	off
n.	Inverse Ratio Limit	off

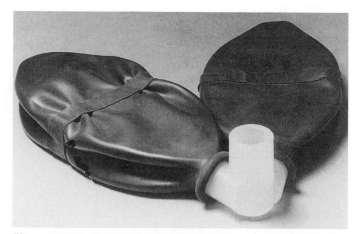

Figure 26-15 *Two test lungs assembled for use during the practice procedures*

Manipulate only one control at a time and note the result in the space provided on the flow sheet. Answer the questions that follow each of the activities.

Adjust the tidal volume control so that the corrected tidal volume is 500 ml, using the following formulas.

Tubing loss = peak inspiratory pressure × tubing compliance

Corrected tidal volume = measured tidal volume − tubing loss

PEAK FLOW CONTROL

1. Adjust the peak flow control to 20 L/min.
   a. Measure inspiratory time.
   b. Measure peak pressure.
   c. Calculate corrected tidal volume.
   d. Record the I:E ratio.

2. Adjust the peak flow control to 100 L/min.
   a. Measure inspiratory time.
   b. Measure peak pressure.
   c. Calculate corrected tidal volume.
   d. Record the I:E ratio.

Questions:

A. How do you account for the differences in inspiratory time?
B. Why were there differences in peak inspiratory pressure (PIP)?
C. Why did corrected tidal volume vary?
D. Why did the I:E ratio vary between the two exercises?

3. Return the peak flow control to 40 L/min.

NORMAL TIDAL VOLUME CONTROL

1. Set the controls to the following settings:
Peak Flow	40 L/min
Normal Tidal Volume	500 ml
Rate	12/min
   a. Measure inspiratory time.
   b. Measure peak inspiratory pressure.
   c. Calculate corrected tidal volume.
   d. Record the I:E ratio.

2. Turn the normal tidal volume control to 1500 ml.
   a. Measure inspiratory time.
   b. Measure peak inspiratory pressure.
   c. Calculate corrected tidal volume.
   d. Record the I:E ratio.

Questions:

A. Why did the pressure increase?
B. Why did the inspiratory time increase?
C. How do you account for the decrease in I:E ratio?

3. Return the normal volume control to 500 ml.

NORMAL RATE CONTROL (CYCLES OR BREATHS PER MINUTE)

Set the controls to the following settings:
Peak Flow	40 L/min
Normal Pressure Limit	maximum
Normal Tidal Volume	1000 ml
Rate	12/min

1. With the controls set as above, perform the following:
   a. Measure peak inspiratory pressure.
   b. Measure inspiratory time.
   c. Calculate corrected tidal volume.
   d. Record the I:E ratio.

2. Turn the rate control to 40 breaths/min.
   a. Measure peak inspiratory pressure.
   b. Measure inspiratory time.
   c. Calculate corrected tidal volume.
   d. Record the I:E ratio.

Questions:
A. What alarm was triggered and why?
B. What was the I:E ratio?
C. Why was the I:E ratio so low?

3. Return the rate control to 12/min.

CHANGES IN RESISTANCE AND COMPLIANCE

1. Set the controls to the following settings:

Peak Flow Control	40 L/min
Normal Pressure Limit	10 to 15 cm H_2O greater than peak pressure
Normal Tidal Volume	500 ml
Rate	12/min

   a. Measure peak inspiratory pressure.
   b. Measure inspiratory time.
   c. Calculate corrected tidal volume.
   d. Record the I:E ratio.

2. Decrease the compliance by ⅓ by adjusting the spring tension or manipulating the compliance control on the lung analog.
   a. Measure peak inspiratory pressure.
   b. Measure inspiratory time.
   c. Calculate corrected tidal volume.
   d. Record the I:E ratio.

Questions:
A. Why did the corrected tidal volume decrease?
B. Did the I:E ratio vary? If it did, why?
C. Why did the peak inspiratory pressure increase?

3. Return the compliance to the original value on the lung analog.

4. Increase the resistance by ⅓ by adjusting the resistance control on the lung analog.
   a. Measure peak inspiratory pressure.
   b. Measure inspiratory time.
   c. Calculate corrected tidal volume.
   d. Record the I:E ratio.

Questions:
Compare your values with the original values in this activity.
A. Why did the inspiratory pressure increase?
B. Why did the I:E ratio vary?
C. How do you account for differences in the corrected tidal volume?
D. Can you think of human physiological conditions that could produce similar results?

5. Return the resistance control to the original value on the lung analog.

6. Set the pressure limit control to 10 cm H_2O greater than the cycling pressure.

7. Decrease the compliance by ⅔ by adjusting spring tension or adjusting the compliance control on the lung analog.

Questions:
A. What event(s) occurred?
B. Can you think of a patient situation that could cause this?
C. What is the purpose of the normal pressure limit control?

SENSITIVITY CONTROL

Adjust the ventilator to the following settings:

Mode	Assist/control
Peak Flow	40 L/min
Sensitivity	fully counterclockwise
Normal Pressure Limit	10 cm H_2O greater than PIP
Normal Tidal Volume	500 ml
Rate	8 breaths/min
Sigh Controls	off
Oxygen Concentration	21%
Inspiratory Pause	off
PEEP	fully counterclockwise

1. Attach a mouthpiece to the patient wye and attempt to initiate a breath. Observe the pressure manometer.

2. Adjust the sensitivity control to the 12 o'clock position and initiate a breath. Observe the pressure manometer.

3. Turn the sensitivity control fully clockwise and initiate a breath. Observe the pressure manometer.
   a. Record the negative pressure when the ventilator cycled on.
   b. Observe the control panel for any changes.

4. Rotate the mode control to the control position and repeat activities 1 through 3 in this section.

Questions:
A. When you were able to initiate an assisted breath, what event(s) occurred?
B. Where would you want to set the sensitivity control for assist/control mode?
C. What happened when the mode control was in the control position?

SIGH CONTROLS

1. Set the controls to the following settings and attach the ventilator to a test lung or lung analog:

Peak Flow	40 L/min
Normal Pressure Limit	10 cm H_2O greater than PIP
Normal Tidal Volume Control	500 ml
Rate	12/min
Sigh Pressure Limit	60 cm H_2O
Sigh Volume	1000 ml
Sigh Rate	30 per hour
Multiple Sigh	3

2. Wait a few minutes and observe the control panel.

3. When the ventilator initiates the sigh mode, measure sigh volume and peak inspiratory pressure.
   a. Calculate the corrected sigh volume.

Questions:
A. What occurred when the ventilator initiated sigh mode?
B. What could occur if the patient had copious airway secretions and required suctioning?

ALARM FUNCTIONS

The BEAR® ventilators have several built-in alarms that are very helpful in the management of critically ill patients. It is important to set the alarms properly so that changes in the patient's condition will be readily apparent.

If you are using the BEAR 2 or BEAR 3, following the activities on alarm functions, press the visual reset button on the left of the control panel. Once the alarm condition has been corrected, the visual display will still indicate which alarm sounded. Pressing the reset button will clear the display.

Set the controls to the following settings and attach the ventilator to a test lung or lung analog:

Mode	Assist/control
Normal Tidal Volume	1000 ml
Normal Rate	12 breaths/min
Normal Pressure Limit	80 cm H_2O
Peak Flow	70 L/min
Sigh Controls	off
Wave Form	square
Nebulizer	off
Sensitivity	2 o'clock position
Inverse Ratio Limit	off
Oxygen Concentration	21%
Inspiratory Pause	off
PEEP	fully counterclockwise
Alarms	off

Low Pressure Alarm

Adjust the low pressure to 10 cm H_2O below the PIP (peak inspiratory pressure).

1. Loosen the jar of the Cascade humidifier, creating a leak in the circuit. Observe the pressure manometer and the control panel.

2. Tighten the Cascade humidifier.

3. Disconnect the patient wye from the test lung or lung analog. Observe the pressure manometer and the control panel.

Question:
A. What event(s) occurred?

Low Exhaled Volume

Set the controls to the same settings as in the low inspiratory pressure activity.

1. Adjust the low exhaled volume control 200 ml higher than the indicated exhaled volume on the control panel. Observe the pressure manometer and control panel.

2. Adjust the low exhaled volume control 200 ml lower than the indicated exhaled volume on the control panel.

Create a leak by loosening the Cascade humidifier jar or adjusting the leak control on the lung analog. Observe the pressure manometer and control panel.

Questions:
A. What event(s) occurred?
B. Can you think of patient care situations that may trigger this alarm?

Detection Delay (BEAR 2 and BEAR 3)

This alarm may be set from 1 to 5 breaths. In other words, 1 to 5 breaths will be delivered prior to the alarm's sounding. This provides an alarm response from rapid to several seconds or a minute (depending on rate). The lower detection delays are appropriate for patients on CPAP or IMV modes.

Apneic Period (BEAR 2 and BEAR 3)

This is an adjustable time delay for apnea. When the control is set at 2 seconds, a period of apnea for 2 seconds or more in the patient will activate the alarm. This delay may be set up to 20 seconds. It is best in clinical practice to set this alarm to a period slightly longer than the guaranteed rate set on the ventilator.

High Rate Alarm (BEAR 2 and BEAR 3)

This alarm will alert you when the patient is breathing at a respiratory rate higher than that set on the alarm. This alarm is useful for IMV and CPAP modes.

Oxygen Alarm

Set the controls for the following settings:

Peak Flow	40 L/min
Sensitivity	fully counterclockwise
Normal Pressure Limit	maximum
Normal Tidal Volume	500 ml
Rate	12 breaths/min
Oxygen Concentration	40%

1. Disconnect the ventilator from the 50 psi oxygen source.

2. Connect the oxygen line to a 50 psi air source.

Questions:
A. What event(s) occurred?
B. Do you suspect that this alarm is an oxygen analyzer?

INSPIRATORY PAUSE

This control is used to provide a slight inspiratory pause prior to exhalation. It holds pressure in the lungs for the number of seconds set on the control after the completion of the inspiratory phase.

1. Set the controls to the same settings used in the alarm section and attach the ventilator to a test lung or lung analog.

2. Turn the inspiratory pause control to 1 second. Observe the pressure manometer.

3. Turn the inspiratory pause control to 2 seconds. Observe the pressure manometer.

Question:
A. What happened by activating this control?

ADDITIONAL ACTIVITIES

Establish the following tidal volumes, rates, and FiO₂ levels. All volumes are assumed to be corrected volumes and all FiO₂ levels must be adjusted to ±2%. Verify all respiratory rates by using your watch and timing a 1-minute interval.

1. Tidal Volume   1000 ml
    Rate   10/min
    FiO₂   0.40
    Flow Rate   40 L/min

2. Tidal Volume   1200 ml
    Rate   8/min
    FiO₂   0.35
    Flow Rate   60 L/min

3. Tidal Volume   800 ml
    Rate   14/min
    FiO₂   0.50
    Flow Rate   70 L/min

Practice Activities: BEAR 5 Ventilator

CIRCUIT ASSEMBLY

Figure 26-16 shows the BEAR 5 assembled and ready for the initiation of mechanical ventilation.

1. Attach two high-pressure hoses. One is for oxygen and the other is for air. Connect them to a 50 psi source.

2. Check the tightness of the exhalation valve assembly and attach and tighten the water collection jar.

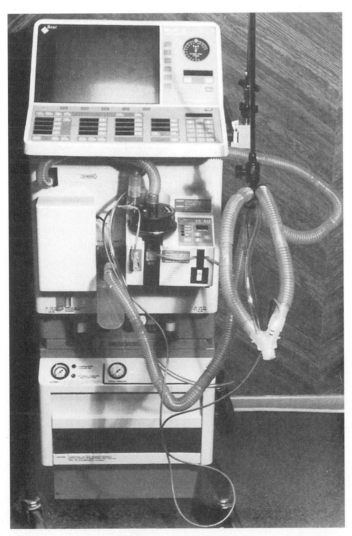

Figure 26-16 *The BEAR® 5 assembled and ready for use*

3. Install the flow tube and the external flow sensor in the temperature control chamber on the left below the control panel.

4. Connect the crossover tube between the exhalation valve and the flow tube.

5. Close the door of the temperature control chamber.

6. Connect the collector vial to the fitting on the exhalation filter and swing the door closed.

7. Attach the humidifier according to the manufacturer's specifications.

8. Assemble the adult circuit. Attach the bacteria filter between the ventilator outlet and the humidifier.

9. Connect the power cord to a suitable 115 V AC source.

TESTING THE VENTILATOR BEFORE USE
Power-up Diagnostics

Each time the power switch is turned on, a power-on self test will automatically be initiated. This test lasts for 12 seconds, during which time all display windows will be blank unless previous settings are in memory. This test is built into the microprocessor of the ventilator and requires no input from the operator. If the ventilator successfully passes its self test, it will begin operation automatically.

Operator Diagnostics

This is an extended diagnostic test built into the microprocessor of this ventilator. This test takes 3 to 5 minutes. During this test an adult patient circuit and appropriate air and oxygen lines must be connected to the ventilator. It is recommended that this test be performed on a monthly basis.

To initiate OPERATOR DIAGNOSTICS push the test key and follow the prompts given on the CRT. After each condition requested has been met, press the Enter key. Refer to the operator's manual for further information on this diagnostic test.

Using the Keyboard Entry System

The BEAR® 5 uses a pressure-sensitive keyboard to make mode, parameter, and alarm changes. Using the keyboard requires a two-step process. First, the desired parameter must be selected by pressing that key. The current value in memory (current ventilator setting) will appear in the message display window adjacent to the parameter selected. If this is not the desired value, enter the correct value by using the numeric keypad (the entered value will now appear in the keypad window). Check the window to be certain that this is the desired value. If the value is correct, press Enter. The entered value will now be stored in memory and will become the current ventilator setting during the next cycle.

If you make an error, pressing the Clear key will clear the keypad window and the ventilator will continue to cycle using the value stored in memory. After you have corrected your error, pressing the Enter key will input your new value.

SYSTEM LEAK TEST

1. Set the controls to the following settings:
   a. Mode   CPAP (zero pressure)
   b. Peak Flow   20 L/min
   c. Inspiratory Pause   2.0 seconds
   d. Sigh Volume   200 ml
   e. Sigh On   on
   f. Peak Sigh Pressure Limit 140 cm H_2O

2. Using a sterile gauze or sterile plastic wrap (inside of wrapping that the circuit was packaged in), occlude the patient wye completely.

3. Deliver a manual sigh. Observe the proximal airway pressure gauge. The pressure should read 60 to 80 cm H_2O. The pressure should fall no more than 10 cm H_2O during the 2-second pause.

4. In the event of a leak, check all tubing connections and humidifier connections (internal and external), and examine the exhalation valve diaphragm and tubing for small holes.

5. Repeat steps 1 through 4 until pressure remains steady in the circuit.

TUBING COMPLIANCE

1. Set the controls to the values listed in system leak test.

2. Using a sterile gauze or sterile plastic wrap (inside of wrapping that the circuit was packaged in), occlude the patient wye completely.

3. Deliver a manual sigh and observe the proximal airway pressure gauge. The peak pressure should be between 60 and 80 cm H_2O.

4. As the ventilator cycles, note the pressure reading on the pressure manometer. It may take several breaths to record the pressure accurately.

5. Divide the preset sigh volume by the plateau pressure.

6. Repeat steps 1 through 5 for sigh volumes of 300 ml and 400 ml. Plot these values graphically with compliance factor on the y axis and peak inspiratory pressure on the x axis.

7. To input the tubing compliance, press the C Comp button adjacent to the Tidal Vol button. Enter the cal-culated value. Tubing loss will be added to each tidal volume automatically after this entry has been made.

CRT INTERFACE

The CRT display provides information on alarms, ventilator settings, and graphics. Individual pages or displays are selected by using the horizontal and vertical soft keys surrounding the CRT display.

When the power is turned on, the mechanics page is displayed automatically. To select other pages, follow the prompts on the bottom of the screen and press the corresponding soft keys below the prompt.

The alarm page will display the current values for tidal volume, minute volume, respiratory rate, inspiratory time, I:E ratio, and peak inspiratory pressure. Appropriate alarms may be selected by using the vertical soft keys along the right of the CRT display.

The graphics page will display real-time graphs depicting proximal airway pressure, inspiratory and expiratory flow, and inspiratory and expiratory volume. To change the display, press one of the top three vertical soft keys. The horizontal soft keys will be relabeled. Press the parameter horizontal soft key, and you will then be able to change the top graph between volume, pressure, and flow. Sweeps may be altered between a 15-second and a 6-second sweep rate.

ACTIVITIES

To complete these practice activities, it is recommended that you use a lung analog/simulator such as a Medishield Lung Ventilator Performance Analyzer or Retec Respirator Teaching Console. Both of these devices or other similar devices can alter resistance and compliance simulating changes in patient condition.

If these devices are not available, a patient wye and two test lungs may be used as shown in Figure 26-15. Exercise caution. Volumes and pressures may exceed the limits of the test lungs. Resistance may be altered by adapting different sizes of endotracheal tubes, and compliance may be altered by the addition of rubber bands to the test lungs.

INITIAL SETTINGS

   a. Mode   CMV
   b. Peak Flow   40 L/min
   c. Assist Sensitivity   −2 cm H_2O
   d. High Pressure Limit   120 cm H_2O
   e. Tidal Volume   500 ml
   f. Normal Rate   12/min
   g. All Sigh Controls   off
   h. Oxygen Concentration 21%
   i. Wave Form   square
   j. Nebulizer   off
   k. Inspiratory Pause   0
   l. PEEP   0
   m. Alarms   off

Manipulate only one control at a time and note the result in the space provided on the ventilator flow sheet. Answer the questions that follow each of the activities.

PEAK FLOW CONTROL

1. Set the peak flow to 20 L/min.
   a. Measure inspiratory time.
   b. Measure peak pressure.
   c. Record corrected tidal volume.
   d. Record the I:E ratio.

2. Adjust the peak flow to 100 L/min.
   a. Measure inspiratory time.
   b. Measure peak pressure.
   c. Record corrected tidal volume.
   d. Record the I:E ratio.

Questions:
A. How do you account for the differences in inspiratory time?
B. Why were there differences in peak inspiratory pressure?
C. Why did the corrected tidal volume vary?
D. Why did the I:E ratio vary between the two activities?

3. Return the peak flow to 40 L/min.

TIDAL VOLUME CONTROL

1. Set the controls to the following settings:

Peak Flow	40 L/min
Tidal Volume	500 ml
Rate	12/min
All other settings	set to the values in the peak flow activity

   a. Measure inspiratory time.
   b. Measure peak inspiratory pressure.
   c. Record corrected tidal volume.
   d. Record the I:E ratio.

2. Adjust the tidal volume to 1500 ml.
   a. Measure inspiratory time.
   b. Measure peak inspiratory pressure.
   c. Record corrected tidal volume.
   d. Record the I:E ratio.

Questions:
A. Why did the pressure increase?
B. Why did the inspiratory time increase?
C. How do you account for the decrease in I:E ratio?

3. Return the tidal volume to 500 ml.

NORMAL RATE CONTROL (CYCLES OR BREATHS PER MINUTE)

Set the controls to the following settings:

Peak Flow	40 L/min
High Pressure Limit	120 cm H_2O
Tidal Volume	500 ml
Rate	12/min
Alarm settings	set to autoset values (see alarm section)

1. With the controls set as above, perform the following:
   a. Measure peak inspiratory pressure.
   b. Measure inspiratory time.
   c. Record corrected tidal volume.
   d. Record the I:E ratio.

2. Adjust the rate to 40 breaths/min.
   a. Measure peak inspiratory pressure.
   b. Measure inspiratory time.
   c. Record corrected tidal volume.
   d. Record the I:E ratio.

Questions:
A. What alarm was triggered and why?
B. What was the I:E ratio?
C. Why was the I:E ratio so low?

3. Return the rate control to 12/min.

CHANGES IN RESISTANCE AND COMPLIANCE

1. Set the controls to the following settings:

Peak Flow Control	40 L/min
High Pressure Limit	120 cm H_2O
Tidal Volume	500 ml
Rate	12/min
Alarm settings	set to autoset values (see alarm section)

   a. Measure peak inspiratory pressure.
   b. Measure inspiratory time.
   c. Record corrected tidal volume.
   d. Record the I:E ratio.

2. Decrease the compliance by $\frac{1}{3}$ by adjusting the spring tension or manipulating the compliance control on the lung analog:
   a. Measure peak inspiratory pressure.
   b. Measure inspiratory time.
   c. Record corrected tidal volume.
   d. Record the I:E ratio.

Questions:
A. Why did the corrected tidal volume decrease?
B. Did the I:E ratio vary? If so, why?
C. Why did the peak inspiratory pressure increase?

3. Return the compliance to the original value on the lung analog.

4. Increase the resistance by $\frac{1}{3}$ by adjusting the resistance control on the lung analog.
   a. Measure peak inspiratory pressure.
   b. Measure inspiratory time.
   c. Record corrected tidal volume.
   d. Record the I:E ratio.

Questions:
Compared with the original values in this activity:
A. Why did the inspiratory pressure increase?
B. Did the I:E ratio vary?
C. How do you account for differences in the corrected tidal volume?
D. Can you think of human physiological conditions that could produce similar results?

5. Return the resistance control to the original value on the lung analog.

6. Set the pressure limit to 10 cm H_2O greater than the cycling pressure.

7. Decrease the compliance by $\frac{2}{3}$ by adjusting spring tension or adjusting the compliance control on the lung analog.

Questions:

A. What event(s) occurred?

B. Can you think of a patient situation that could cause this?

C. What is the purpose of the normal pressure limit control?

SENSITIVITY CONTROL

Adjust the ventilator to the following settings:

Mode	CMV
Peak Flow	40 L/min
Sensitivity	fully counterclockwise
High Pressure Limit	10 cm H_2O greater than PIP
Tidal Volume	500 ml
Rate	8 breaths/min
Sigh Controls	off
Oxygen Concentration	21%
Inspiratory Pause	off
PEEP	fully counterclockwise

1. Attach a mouthpiece to the patient wye and attempt to initiate a breath. Observe the pressure manometer.

2. Set the sensitivity to –2 cm H_2O and initiate a breath. Observe the pressure manometer.

3. Adjust the sensitivity to –5 cm H_2O and initiate a breath. Observe the pressure manometer.
   a. Record the negative pressure when the ventilator cycled on.
   b. Observe the control panel for any changes.

Questions:

A. When you were able to initiate an assisted breath, what event(s) occurred?

B. Where would you want to set the sensitivity control for assist/control mode?

SIGH CONTROLS

1. Set the controls to the following settings and attach the ventilator to a test lung or lung analog:

Mode	CMV and automatic sigh
Wave Form	square
Peak Flow	40 L/min
High Pressure Limit	10 cm H_2O greater than PIP
Tidal Volume Control	500 ml
Rate	12/min
Sigh Pressure Limit	60 cm H_2O
Sigh Volume	1000 ml
Sigh Rate	15 per hour
Multiple Sigh	3
Alarm settings	set to autoset values (see alarm section)

2. Wait a few minutes and observe the control panel.

3. When the ventilator initiates the sigh mode, measure sigh volume and peak inspiratory pressure (PIP).
   a. Measure the corrected sigh volume.

Questions:

A. What occurred when the ventilator initiated sigh mode?

B. What could occur if the patient had copious airway secretions and required suctioning?

ALARM FUNCTIONS

The BEAR® 5 has several built-in alarms that are very helpful in the management of critically ill patients. It is important to set the alarms properly so that changes in the patient's condition will be readily apparent.

The vertical and horizontal soft keys below and to the right of the CRT display are used to set the alarms on the ventilator. Prompts or messages on the CRT display indicate which keys are used to set the various alarms.

AUTOSET ALARMS

The BEAR® 5 has the capability of setting all alarms automatically. The autoset parameters are listed in Table 26-5. The autoset alarm feature is selected by pressing the horizontal soft key below the CRT display "Autoset."

OTHER ALARM FUNCTIONS

Set the controls to the following settings and attach the ventilator to a test lung or lung analog:

Mode	CMV
Wave Form	square
Tidal Volume	800 ml
Rate	12 breaths/min
High Pressure Limit	80 cm H_2O
Peak Flow	70 L/min
Nebulizer	off
Sensitivity	–2 cm H_2O
Oxygen Concentration	21%
Inspiratory Pause	0
PEEP	0
Alarms	off

LOW MANDATORY AND LOW SPONTANEOUS VOLUME ALARMS

Low Mandatory Volume Alarm

Press the uppermost vertical soft key to the right of the CRT display. After this key is pressed, two prompts will appear at the lower right corner of the CRT display. These prompts are Set Low Mand and Set Low Spont.

TABLE 26-5: Autoset Alarm Settings

ALARM	SETTING
Low Exhaled Tidal Volume	* –20% or 150 ml
High/Low Exhaled Minute Volume	* ±20% or 2000 ml
High/Low Breath Rate	±3 BPM
High/Low Inspiratory Time	±20% or 0.1 second
High Peak or Sigh Pressure	10 cm H_2O greater than PIP
Low Peak Normal Pressure	* –5 cm H_2O or PEEP
High Mean Airway Pressure	5 cm H_2O
Low Mean Airway Pressure	* –5 cm H_2O or 20%
Low PEEP/CPAP Pressure	* –5 cm H_2O or 20%
High PEEP/CPAP Pressure	±5 cm H_2O
1:1 Ratio Limit	Set to previous setting

Items with an asterisk denote whichever value is greater or less.

By pressing the soft key below Set Low Mand, you may adjust the setting for the low mandatory exhaled tidal volume alarm. Once this key is pressed, the display below Low Mandatory Volume on the CRT will flash, indicating that the request for the change has been accepted. The designations for the right two horizontal soft keys will also go blank.

Enter the new alarm setting using the keypad on the right of the control panel. Select the desired value and then press Enter. The new value will be displayed on the CRT under Low Mand Vol.

1. Adjust the value of the Low Mandatory Volume to 700 ml.

Low Spontaneous Volume Alarm

The low spontaneous volume alarm is set in a similar way to that for the low mandatory volume alarm. Press the uppermost vertical soft key to select this alarm.

Press the right horizontal soft key under the prompt Set Low Spont. Enter the new desired alarm value using the keypad and pressing Enter.

1. Set the low spontaneous volume alarm to 200 ml.

ACTIVITY

1. Loosen a joint or section of the humidifier, creating a leak in the circuit. Observe the pressure manometer and the control panel for at least 1 minute.

2. Tighten the joint loosened previously on the humidifier.

3. Disconnect the patient wye from the test lung or lung analog. Observe the pressure manometer and the control panel.

Question:

A. What event(s) occurred?

LOW EXHALED AND HIGH EXHALED MINUTE VOLUME ALARMS

The BEAR® 5 has the ability to monitor the exhaled minute volume. Alarms are provided to alert you in the event of hypoventilation or hyperventilation. This feature is very helpful in weaning patients from mechanical ventilation.

1. Set the controls to the same settings found under other alarm functions.

Low Exhaled Minute Volume Alarm

This alarm is set in a similar way as the mandatory and spontaneous tidal volume alarms.

Press the vertical soft key adjacent to the display High Vol on the right of the CRT page. As with the previous alarm, the right two horizontal soft key prompts will change. The new prompts will read Set Low Vol and Set High Vol.

Press the soft key below Set Low Vol. Adjust this alarm by using the keypad and pressing Enter after you have selected the desired value.

2. Set the low minute volume alarm to 8.5 L/min.

High Minute Volume Alarm

Press the vertical soft key adjacent to the display High Vol. Press the horizontal soft key below the prompt Set High

Vol. Adjust the alarm setting using the keypad and pressing Enter after the desired value has been selected.

3. Set the high minute volume alarm to 10.2 L/min.

ACTIVITY

1. Create a leak in the circuit by loosening a connection or causing a leak in the humidifier. Observe the control panel for at least 1 minute.

2. Manually trigger several breaths by creating a slight negative pressure in the test lung or lung analog. Maintain a rate of at least 20 breaths/min. Observe the control panel for at least 1 minute.

Questions:

A. What event(s) occurred?
B. Can you think of patient care situations that may trigger this alarm?

LOW RATE AND HIGH RATE ALARMS

Adjust this alarm by pressing the vertical soft key adjacent to the display High Rate. As with the other previous alarms, the prompts above the two right horizontal soft keys will change. The new prompts read Set Low Rate and Set High Rate.

Low Rate Alarm

Set the low rate alarm by pressing the appropriate vertical soft key. Press the horizontal soft key below the Set Low Rate prompt. Adjust the alarm setting using the keypad and pressing Enter after the desired value has been selected.

1. Set the low rate alarm to 10 breaths/min.

High Rate Alarm

Press the vertical soft key adjacent to the CRT display High Rate. Press the horizontal soft key below the prompt Set High Rate. Adjust the alarm using the keypad and pressing Enter after the desired value has been selected.

2. Set the high rate alarm to 14 breaths/min.

ACTIVITY

1. Adjust the rate control on the control panel to 6 breaths/min. Observe the control panel and CRT display for at least 1 minute.

2. Set the rate control to 12 breaths/min.

3. Initiate spontaneous breaths by manually creating a negative pressure in the test lung or lung analog. Maintain a rate of 16 breaths/min. Observe the control panel and CRT display for at least 1 minute.

Questions:

A. What event(s) occurred?
B. Can you think of patient care situations that may trigger this alarm?

INSPIRATORY TIME ALARMS

Low and high inspiratory time alarms are available when the ventilator is operating in the time cycled mode. Time-cycled ventilation is not commonly used in adults. The alarms are set in a similar fashion to the other alarms.

This alarm will be covered in Chapter 27 on special ventilatory procedures.

I:E RATIO LIMIT ALARM

This alarm will alert the practitioner when the I:E ratio drops below a 1:1 ratio. If this alarm is enabled and a ratio of less than 1:1 is encountered, inspiration will be terminated, and an audible and visual alarm will result.

If this alarm is overridden, a ratio of up to 3:1 is allowed. This will allow you to set inverse I:E ratios.

To enable the ratio limit, press the vertical soft key just above the bottommost soft key. If the ratio limit was previously overridden, the two prompts on the lower right of the CRT display will change. The new prompt will read Enable.

Press the horizontal soft key below the Enable display to activate the alarm. The CRT display will now read Limit Enabled and the horizontal soft key will be relabeled Override.

To change the setting back to the override state, press the horizontal soft key below the prompt Override. The CRT display will now read Limit Overridden and the horizontal soft key prompt will read Enable.

PRESSURE ALARMS

Pressure alarms for low peak pressure, high normal pressure, and high sigh pressure are available on the BEAR 5 ventilator. These alarms are set using the vertical and horizontal soft keys.

1. Set the controls to the same settings listed under other alarm functions.

Low Peak Pressure Alarm

To set this alarm, press the lowest vertical soft key. This will relabel the three right horizontal soft key displays. The new prompts will read Start Scan, Set Display, and Set Alarms.

Press the horizontal soft key below Set Display. The horizontal soft keys will again be relabeled Set Low Peak, Set High Norm, and Set High Sigh. Press the soft key below Set Low Peak.

The alarm may be adjusted using the keypad and pressing Enter after the desired value has been selected.

2. Set this alarm to 15 cm H_2O lower than the peak inspiratory pressure.

High Normal Pressure Alarm

To set this alarm, press the lowest vertical soft key. Press the horizontal soft key below the prompt Set Display.

Press the horizontal soft key below the prompt Set High Norm. Adjust the alarm setting using the keypad and pressing Enter after the desired value has been selected.

3. Set this alarm to 15 cm H_2O greater than the peak inspiratory pressure.

High Sigh Pressure

This alarm has a similar function to that of the high normal pressure alarm except that it works only during sigh breaths. This serves as a sigh pressure limit.

1. Create a leak in the circuit. Observe the control panel and CRT display for at least 1 minute.

2. Correct the leak you created in number 1.

3. Obstruct the patient wye with a wad of tape or 2 × 2-inch gauze pad. Observe the control panel and CRT display for at least 1 minute.

Questions:
A. What event(s) occurred?
B. Can you think of patient care situations that could cause this alarm to be activated?

LOW MEAN AND HIGH MEAN AIRWAY PRESSURE ALARMS

Low and high mean airway pressure alarms are available on the BEAR 5 ventilator. They are set in a similar way as the other alarms using the vertical and horizontal soft keys.

To set the mean airway pressure alarms, press the lowest vertical soft key.

Press the horizontal soft key below the prompt Set Alarms. The two left horizontal soft key prompts will change to Set Low Mean and Set High Mean. These settings may now be adjusted using the keypad.

LOW AND HIGH PEEP/CPAP PRESSURE ALARMS

Low and high PEEP pressure alarms are available to alert you to changes in the PEEP/CPAP pressures. They are set in a similar way as the other alarms. Should a leak or obstruction in the circuit occur, the alarm would alert you to the condition.

To set these alarms, press the lowest vertical soft key. Press the horizontal key under Set alarms twice. The last two horizontal prompts should now read Set Low PEEP and Set High PEEP.

The alarm limits may now be adjusted using the keypad. Set the alarm limits plus and minus 10 to 15 cm H_2O greater and less than the PEEP/CPAP level.

OTHER NONSELECTABLE ALARMS
Low Pressure Oxygen Inlet Alarm

Set the controls for the following settings:

Peak Flow	40 L/min
Sensitivity	−2 cm H_2O
Normal Pressure Limit	maximum
Normal Tidal Volume	500 ml
Rate	12 breaths/min
Oxygen Concentration	40%

1. Disconnect the ventilator from the 50 psi oxygen source.

Questions:
A. What event(s) occurred?
B. Do you suspect that this alarm is an oxygen analyzer?

Low Pressure Air Inlet Alarm

1. Set the controls to the settings for the low oxygen pressure inlet alarm practice activities.

2. Disconnect the ventilator from the high pressure air source.

Questions:
A. What event(s) occurred?
B. Do you suspect that this alarm is an oxygen analyzer?

INTERNAL AND EXTERNAL FLOW SENSOR ALARMS

These alarms indicate a loss of a signal from these sensors or if the flow sensor is installed improperly. A ventilator inoperative alarm will also accompany these alarms because the ventilator is dependent upon information from these sensors.

OTHER CONTROLS: INSPIRATORY PAUSE

This control is used to provide a slight inspiratory pause prior to exhalation. It will hold pressure in the lungs for the number of seconds set on the control after the completion of inspiration.

1. Set the controls to the same settings used in the alarm section and attach the ventilator to a test lung or lung analog.

2. Set the inspiratory pause control to 1 second. Observe the pressure manometer.

3. Set the inspiratory pause control to 2 seconds. Observe the pressure manometer.

Question:
A. What happened by activating this control?

ADDITIONAL ACTIVITIES
Establish the following tidal volumes, rates, and FIO_2 levels. All volumes are assumed to be corrected volumes and all FIO_2 levels must be adjusted to ±2%. Verify all respiratory rates by using your watch and timing a minute interval.

1. Tidal Volume   1000 ml
   Rate   10/min
   FIO_2 0.40
   Flow Rate   40 L/min

2. Tidal Volume   1200 ml
   Rate   8/min
   FIO_2 0.35
   Flow Rate   60 L/min

3. Tidal Volume   800 ml
   Rate   14/min
   FIO_2 0.50
   Flow Rate   70 L/min

Practice Activities: BEAR 1000

CIRCUIT ASSEMBLY

Figure 20-17 shows the BEAR 1000 with the optional graphics display module assembled and ready for initiation of mechanical ventilation.

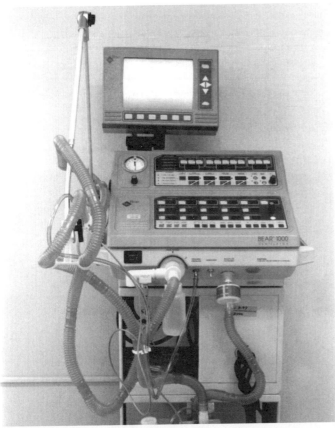

Figure 26-17 *A photograph of the BEAR® 1000 ventilator with the optional graphics display module*

1. Attach the two high-pressure hoses, one to 50 psi air and the other to 50 psi oxygen.

2. Connect the power cord to a suitable alternating current (AC) grounded outlet.

3. Attach the exhalation valve diaphragm to the exhalation valve assembly and check it for leaks. Install the exhalation valve diaphragm assembly into its seat by rotating the mounting to lock it into place. Attach the condensate collection jar assembly and the expiratory flow sensor.

4. Connect a bacteria filter to the ventilator outlet and connect it to the humidifier using a short length of 22-mm-diameter aerosol tubing.

5. Connect the inspiratory limb of the patient circuit to the humidifier and the expiratory limb to the condensate collection jar assembly.

6. Connect the proximal airway line to the proximal pressure fitting on the front of the ventilator.

TESTING THE VENTILATOR BEFORE USE (QUICK CHECKOUT)

Prior to using the ventilator for patient care, the quick checkout procedure should be performed to verify that all major subsystems are operational. This test takes approximately 2.5 minutes.

1. Turn the optional graphics display module off. Failure to do so will result in an error code d2, which may be a false indication.

2. With an adult circuit attached, press and hold the Test key on the control panel located on the front panel in the lower right-hand corner while simultaneously turning on the power switch located on the right rear of the ventilator.

3. Verify that the operator diagnostics mode has been activated by observing that the RUN DIAGNOSTICS LED is illuminated.

4. Adjust the PEEP pressure to zero by rotating the PEEP control located adjacent to the pressure manometer fully counterclockwise.

5. Observe that ALL appears in the Pres Sup/Insp Press display window; this indicates that all seven diagnostics tests will be performed.
   a. If ALL does not appear, depress the Pres Sup/Insp Pres key and rotate the green SET knob until ALL appears.

6. Plug the patient wye using a cap or other secure occlusion device.

7. Depress the Manual Breath key located at the lower center part of the control panel. The automated self test will begin and will take approximately 2.5 minutes.

8. When all diagnostics tests have been passed, a "P" will be displayed in the Assist Sensitivity display window.

SYSTEM LEAK TEST

1. Set the controls to the following settings:

Mode	Assist CMV
Peak Flow	20 L/min
Inspiratory Pause	2.0 seconds
Tidal Volume	200 ml
Peak Insp Pressure	140 cm H_2O
Rate	10/min

2. Using a sterile gauze or a sterile plastic wrap, occlude the patient wye completely.

3. Observe the pressure manometer. The pressure should read between 60 and 80 cm H_2O. The pressure should fall no more than 10 cm H_2O.

4. In the event of a leak, check all tubing connections, the humidifier, and exhalation valve diaphragm.

5. Repeat steps 1 through 4 until pressure remains steady.

TUBING COMPLIANCE

1. Set the controls to the values listed in the system leak test, and occlude the patient wye as described previously.

2. Observe and record the pressure and exhaled tidal volume readings during inspiration.

3. Divide the exhaled volume by the peak pressure.

4. Depress the Compliance Comp key located at the lower center of the control panel and enter the calculated value by rotating the SET knob and depressing the key once again.

ACTIVITIES

To complete these practice activities, it is recommended that you use a lung analog/simulator such as a Medishield Lung Ventilator Performance Analyzer or other similar device in which resistance and compliance may be easily controlled and altered.

INITIAL SETTINGS

Mode	Assist CMV
Peak Flow	40 L/min
Assist Sensitivity	2.0 cm H_2O
High Pressure Limit	120 cm H_2O
Tidal Volume	500 ml
Rate	12/min
O_2 %	21%
Wave Form	square
Nebulizer	off
Inspiratory Pause	0.0 seconds
PEEP	0.0 cm H_2O
Alarms	off

Manipulate only one control at a time and record your results on a sheet of paper. Answer the questions that follow each activity, recording each answer on your paper. If you have difficulty, ask your laboratory instructor for assistance.

PEAK FLOW CONTROL

1. Set the peak flow to 20 L/min.
   a. Measure the inspiratory time using a watch with a second hand or a stopwatch.
   b. Measure the peak pressure by depressing the Peak Pressure key on the monitoring panel.
   c. Record the corrected tidal volume (exhaled tidal volume).
   d. Record the I:E ratio by depressing the I:E ratio key and observing the display.

2. Adjust the peak flow to 100 L/min.
   a. Measure the inspiratory time using a watch with a second hand or a stopwatch.
   b. Measure the peak pressure by depressing the Peak Pressure key on the monitoring panel.
   c. Record the corrected tidal volume (exhaled tidal volume).
   d. Record the I:E ratio by depressing the I:E ratio key and observing the display.

Questions:

A. How do you account for the differences in inspiratory time?

B. Why were there differences in peak inspiratory pressure?

C. Why did the corrected tidal volume vary?

D. Why did the I:E ratio vary between the two activities?

3. Return the peak flow control to 40 L/min.

TIDAL VOLUME CONTROL

1. Set the controls to the following settings:

Peak Flow	40 L/min
Tidal Volume	500 ml
Rate	12/min

Leave all other controls set at the same values you established for the peak flow activity.
   a. Measure the inspiratory time using a watch with a second hand or a stopwatch.
   b. Measure the peak inspiratory pressure.
   c. Record the exhaled tidal volume.
   d. Record the I:E ratio.

2. Adjust the tidal volume to 1200 ml.
   a. Measure the inspiratory time using a watch with a second hand or a stopwatch.
   b. Measure the peak inspiratory pressure.
   c. Record the exhaled tidal volume.
   d. Record the I:E ratio.

Questions:
A. Why did the pressure increase?
B. Why did the inspiratory time increase?
C. How do you account for the decrease in I:E ratio?

3. Return the tidal volume control to 500 ml.

RATE CONTROL

1. Set the controls to the following settings:

   Peak Flow   40 L/min
   High Pressure Limit   120 cm H_2O
   Tidal Volume   500 ml
   Rate   12/min
   I:E Override   depressed and activated

2. With the controls as set above, perform the following:
   a. Measure the inspiratory time using a watch with a second hand or a stop watch.
   b. Measure the peak inspiratory pressure.
   c. Record the exhaled tidal volume.
   d. Record the I:E ratio.

3. Adjust the rate control to 40 breaths/min.
   a. Measure the inspiratory time using a watch with a second hand or a stopwatch.
   b. Measure the peak inspiratory pressure.
   c. Record the exhaled tidal volume.
   d. Record the I:E ratio.

Questions:
A. What was the I:E ratio?
B. Why was the I:E ratio so low?

TRIGGERING

In this section you will explore both pressure and flow triggering. It is helpful to use the graphics display panel and to select the Pressure Volume loop to view how changes affect inspiratory work.

Pressure Triggering

Adjust the ventilator to the following settings:

   Mode   Assist CMV
   Peak Flow   40 L/min
   Assist Sensitivity 5.0 cm H_2O
   Peak Insp Pressure 10 cm H_2O greater than PIP
   Tidal Volume   500 ml
   Rate   8 breaths/min
   O_2 %   21%
   Inspiratory Pause   0.0 seconds
   PEEP   0.0 cm H_2O

1. Attach a mouthpiece to the patient wye and attempt to initiate a breath. Observe both the pressure manometer and the Pressure Volume loop on the graphics display panel.

2. Set the assist sensitivity to 0.2 cm H_2O. Again using a mouthpiece, initiate a breath while observing the pressure manometer and the Pressure Volume loop.

Questions:
A. When were you able to most easily initiate a breath?
B. Where would you prefer, as a patient, to have the assist sensitivity control set?
C. What changes did you observe on the Pressure Volume loop between the two settings?

Flow Triggering

Adjust the ventilator to the following settings:

   Mode   Assist CMV
   Peak Flow   40 L/min
   Base Flow   10 L/min
   Flow Trigger   3 L/min
   Peak Insp Pressure 10 cm H_2O greater than PIP
   Tidal Volume   500 ml
   Rate   8 breaths/min
   O_2 %   21%
   Inspiratory Pause   0.0 seconds
   PEEP   0.0 cm H_2O

1. Attach a mouthpiece to the patient wye and attempt to initiate a breath. Observe both the pressure manometer and the Pressure Volume loop on the graphics display panel.

2. Adjust the base flow to 18 L/min, and again initiate a breath using a mouthpiece and observe the pressure manometer and the Pressure Volume loop.

3. Return the base flow to 10 L/min and adjust the flow trigger level to 8 L/min. Initiate a breath using a mouthpiece and observe the pressure manometer and the Pressure Volume loop on the graphics display panel.

Questions:
A. Which setting would you prefer as a patient?
B. Which setting was easiest for you?
C. What changes did you observe on the graphics display panel?
D. How can you use the Pressure Volume loop and the graphics display panel to minimize inspiratory work?

PRESSURE CONTROL VENTILATION

Set the controls to the following settings and attach the ventilator to the test lung:

   Mode   Pressure Control
   Inspiratory Pressure 30 cm H_2O
   Inspiratory Time   1.0 second
   Assist Sensitivity 5.0 cm H_2O
   Rate   12 breaths/min
   O_2 %   21%
   PEEP   0.0 cm H_2O

INSPIRATORY PRESSURE CONTROL

1. Measure and record the following using the display panel:
   a. Exhaled tidal volume
   b. I:E ratio
   c. Peak pressure
   d. Mean pressure

2. Adjust the inspiratory pressure level to 50 cm H_2O. Measure the following using the display panel:
   a. Exhaled tidal volume
   b. I:E ratio
   c. Peak pressure
   d. Mean pressure

Questions:
A. How did the change in pressure affect the I:E ratio?
B. How did the change in pressure affect the exhaled tidal volume?

INSPIRATORY TIME CONTROL

1. Set the ventilator to the following settings:

Mode	Pressure Control
Inspiratory Pressure	30 cm H_2O
Inspiratory Time	1.0 second
Assist Sensitivity	5.0 cm H_2O
Rate	6 breaths/min
O_2 %	21%
PEEP	0.0 cm H_2O

2. Measure the following using the display panel:
   a. Exhaled tidal volume
   b. I:E ratio
   c. Peak pressure
   d. Mean pressure

3. Change the inspiratory time to 3.0 seconds, and measure and record the following:
   a. Exhaled tidal volume
   b. I:E ratio
   c. Peak pressure
   d. Mean pressure

Questions:
A. How did the inspiratory time change affect the I:E ratio?
B. How did the inspiratory time change affect tidal volume delivery?
C. How did the inspiratory time change affect the inspiratory pressure?

ALARM SYSTEMS
Total Minute Volume
Set the ventilator to the following settings:

Mode	Assist CMV
Peak Flow	40 L/min
Assist Sensitivity	2.0 cm H_2O
Tidal Volume	500 ml
Rate	8 breaths/min
O_2 %	21%
Inspiratory Pause	0.0 seconds
PEEP	0.0 cm H_2O

1. Depress the Up arrow below the total minute volume alarm indicator and adjust the control to 6 L/min.

2. Using the test lung, simulate a respiratory rate of 20/min.

Questions:
A. What occurred?
B. How could you set the alarm appropriately for a patient rate of 20/min?

3. Set the alarm's upper limit to 6 L/min and lower limit to 4 L/min.

Total Breath Rate
1. Depress the Up arrow below the total breath rate alarm display and set the rate to 10 breaths/min.

2. Using the test lung, simulate a rate of 20 breaths/min.

Questions:
A. What occurred?
B. How could you set the alarm appropriately for a patient rate of 20/min?

3. Set the alarm's upper limit to 12 breaths/min and lower limit to 6 breaths/min.

Peak Inspiratory Pressure
1. Depress the Up arrow below the peak inspiratory pressure display and set it for 15 cm H_2O above the peak inspiratory pressure. Depress the Down arrow, and set its limit 15 cm H_2O below the peak inspiratory pressure.

2. Simulate a cough by rapidly squeezing the test lung.

Questions:
A. What occurred?
B. Was the alarm set appropriately?
C. What other conditions might cause this alarm to be activated?

Baseline Pressure
Set the controls to the following values:

Mode	Assist CMV
Peak Flow	40 L/min
Assist Sensitivity	4.0 cm H_2O
Tidal Volume	500 ml
Rate	8 breaths/min
O_2 %	21%
Inspiratory Pause	0.0 seconds
PEEP	5.0 cm H_2O

1. Depress the Down arrow key below the baseline pressure display and set it for 3 cm H_2O.

2. Simulate a patient effort by expanding the test lung's bellows to trigger a breath.

Questions:
A. What occurred?
B. How could you change the control settings to prevent this?
C. Is the alarm set appropriately for this level of PEEP?

3. Readjust your baseline pressure alarm to bracket the PEEP level by 3 cm H_2O.

Practice Activities: Bird 8400ST

CIRCUIT ASSEMBLY

Figure 26-18A and B shows the Bird 8400ST ventilator and a drawing of its control panel.

1. Attach the two high-pressure hoses, one to 50 psi air and the other to 50 psi oxygen to the external blender located below the ventilator. Ensure that the blender outlet is connected to the gas inlet on the back of the ventilator.

2. Connect the power cord to a suitable AC grounded outlet.

3. Install the exhalation valve diaphragm onto the ventilator exhalation valve port. Next install the exhalation valve body onto the port, ensuring that the spring-loaded safety tab is engaged.

4. Connect a bacteria filter to the ventilator outlet and connect it to the humidifier using a short length of 22-mm-diameter aerosol tubing.

5. Connect the inspiratory limb of the patient circuit to the humidifier and the expiratory limb to the exhalation valve body assembly.

6. Attach the exhalation flow transducer assembly to the ventilator's right front panel by inserting the gray fitting into the female receptacle and rotating it clockwise, locking it into place. Connect the opposite end to the exhalation valve body.

PREOPERATIONAL PERFORMANCE CHECK

Prior to using the ventilator for patient care, you should complete a performance check. This will ensure

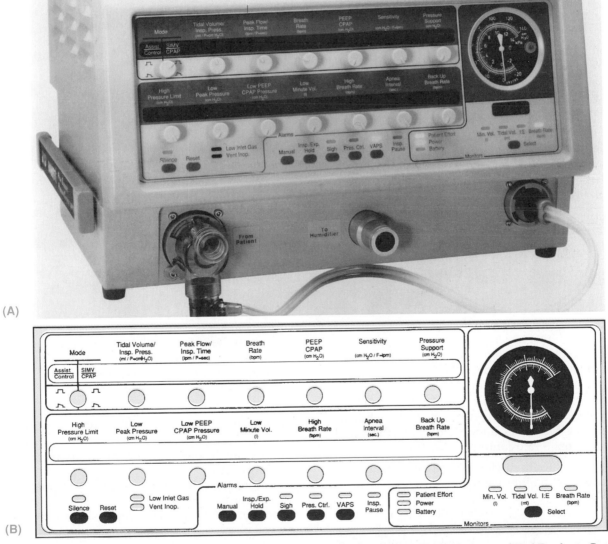

(A)

(B)

Figure 26-18 *A photograph of the Bird 8400ST ventilator (A); a drawing of the control panel (B) (Courtesy of* Bird Products Corporation, Palm Springs, CA)

that all systems and subsystems are operational before patient use.

Power-up Self Test

1. Turn the power switch on the rear of the ventilator into the ON position.
2. The ventilator will perform a 5-second test when powered up.
   a. The Power LED on the front panel illuminates and a brief audible alarm can be heard.
   b. The front panel LEDs will display segmentally in unison.
   c. The microprocessors will confirm communication links.
   d. The exhalation and flow control valves perform checks.
   e. A second audible alarm will briefly sound.
   f. Front panel LEDs will illuminate and the ventilator is ready for use.

Performance Check

Set the ventilator to the following settings.

Ventilator Settings

Mode	Assist/control (Square Wave)
Tidal Volume	500 ml
Peak Flow	60 L/min
Breath Rate	12/min
PEEP/CPAP	5 cm H_2O
Assist Sensitivity	off
Pressure Support	off

Alarm Settings

High Pressure Limit	5 cm H_2O above peak inspiratory pressure
Low Peak Pressure	10 cm H_2O below peak inspiratory pressure
Low PEEP/CPAP	2 cm H_2O below baseline pressure
High Breath Rate	14/min
Low Minute Volume	4 L/min
Apnea Interval	20 seconds
Backup Breath Rate	12/min

1. Complete a circuit pressure test:
   a. Set the breath rate to zero.
   b. Attach a test lung to the patient wye.
   c. Press and hold the Inspiratory Hold button.
   d. Press the Manual Breath button.
   e. Circuit pressure should rise and hold. If the circuit leaks, check all fittings, connections, and the humidifier for possible causes, and repeat steps a through d.
   f. Reset the breath rate control to 12/min.
2. Allow the ventilator to run for about 2 minutes and verify the following monitor values:

Minute Volume	6 L ± 0.6 L
Tidal Volume	500 ml ± 7.5 ml
I:E Ratio	1:5.7 ± 5%
Breath Rate	12/min ± 2/min

3. Verify the following alarms and their function:
   a. Power failure (Disconnect the power cord.)
   b. High pressure limit (Manually restrict the test lung.)
   c. Low peak pressure, low PEEP/CPAP (Disconnect the test lung from the patient wye.)
   d. Low minute volume (Set the breath rate control at 6/min.)
   e. High breath rate (Set the breath rate control at 15/min.)
   f. Apnea interval/apnea backup ventilation (Set the breath rate control at zero.)
   g. Flow transducer alarm (Disconnect the flow transducer from the front of the ventilator.)
   h. "CIRC" alarm and display (Disconnect the expiratory limb from the exhalation valve assembly and occlude it with your hand.)

PRACTICE ACTIVITIES

To complete these practice activities, it is recommended that you use a lung analog/simulator such as a Medishield Lung Ventilator Performance Analyzer or other similar device in which resistance and compliance may be easily controlled and altered.

INITIAL SETTINGS

Mode	Assist/control
Peak Flow	40 L/min
Sensitivity	2.0 cm H_2O
High Peak Pressure	120 cm H_2O
Tidal Volume	500 ml
Breath Rate	12/min
O_2 %	21%
Wave Form	square
PEEP	0.0 cm H_2O
Alarms	off

Manipulate only one control at a time and record your results on a sheet of paper. Answer the questions that follow each activity, recording each answer on your paper. If you have difficulty, ask your laboratory instructor for assistance.

PEAK FLOW CONTROL

1. Set the peak flow to 20 L/min.
   a. Measure the inspiratory time using a watch with a second hand or a stopwatch.
   b. Measure the peak pressure by observing the pressure manometer.
   c. Record the exhaled tidal volume. (Depress the Tidal Volume button below the pressure manometer.)
   d. Record the I:E ratio by depressing the I:E ratio key and observing the display.
2. Adjust the peak flow to 100 L/min.
   a. Measure the inspiratory time using a watch with a second hand or a stopwatch.
   b. Measure the peak pressure by observing the pressure manometer.
   c. Record the exhaled tidal volume. (Depress the Tidal Volume button below the pressure manometer.)
   d. Record the I:E ratio by depressing the I:E ratio key and observing the display.

Questions:

A. How do you account for the differences in inspiratory time?

B. Why were there differences in peak inspiratory pressure?

C. Why did the corrected tidal volume vary?

D. Why did the I:E ratio vary between the two activities?

3. Return the peak flow control to 40 L/min.

TIDAL VOLUME CONTROL

1. Set the controls to the following settings:

Peak Flow	40 L/min
Tidal Volume	500 ml
Breath Rate	12/min

Leave all other controls set at the same values you established for the peak flow activity.

a. Measure the inspiratory time using a watch with a second hand or a stop watch.

b. Measure the peak inspiratory pressure.

c. Record the exhaled tidal volume.

d. Record the I:E ratio.

2. Adjust the tidal volume to 1200 ml.

a. Measure the inspiratory time using a watch with a second hand or a stop watch.

b. Measure the peak inspiratory pressure.

c. Record the exhaled tidal volume.

d. Record the I:E ratio.

Questions:

A. Why did the pressure increase?

B. Why did the inspiratory time increase?

C. How do you account for the decrease in I:E ratio?

3. Return the tidal volume control to 500 ml.

RATE CONTROL

1. Set the controls to the following settings:

Peak Flow	40 L/min
High Peak Pressure	120 cm H_2O
Tidal Volume	500 ml
Breath Rate	12/min

2. With the controls as set above, perform the following:

a. Measure the inspiratory time using a watch with a second hand or a stopwatch.

b. Measure the peak inspiratory pressure.

c. Record the exhaled tidal volume.

d. Record the I:E ratio.

3. Adjust the rate control to 25 breaths/min.

a. Measure the inspiratory time using a watch with a second hand or a stop watch.

b. Measure the peak inspiratory pressure.

c. Record the exhaled tidal volume.

d. Record the I:E ratio.

Questions:

A. What was the I:E ratio?

B. Why was the I:E ratio so low?

TRIGGERING

In this section you will explore how the Bird 8400ST triggers breaths when the patient has a spontaneous effort.

Pressure Triggering

Adjust the ventilator to the following settings:

Mode	Assist/control
Peak Flow	40 L/min
Sensitivity	10.0 cm H_2O
High Peak Pressure	10 cm H_2O greater than PIP
Tidal Volume	500 ml
Breath Rate	8 breaths/min
O_2 %	21%
PEEP	0.0 cm H_2O

1. Attach a mouthpiece to the patient wye and attempt to initiate a breath. Observe the pressure manometer.

2. Set the assist sensitivity to 1.0 cm H_2O. Again using a mouthpiece, initiate a breath while observing the pressure manometer and the Pressure Volume loop.

Questions:

A. When were you able to most easily initiate a breath?

B. Where would you prefer as a patient to have the assist sensitivity control set?

C. What changes did you observe on the Pressure Volume loop between the two settings?

Flow Triggering

To complete the practice activities on flow triggering, you must install the special flow triggering flow sensor. When the sensor is installed, a bias flow of 10 L/min will pass through the circuit and flow sensitivities of 1 to 10 L/min may be set.

Adjust the ventilator to the following settings:

Mode	Assist/control
Peak Flow	40 L/min
Flow Sensitivity	3 L/min
High Peak Pressure	10 cm H_2O greater than PIP
Tidal Volume	500 ml
Rate	8 breaths/min
O_2 %	21%
PEEP	0.0 cm H_2O

1. Attach a mouthpiece to the patient wye and attempt to initiate a breath. Observe the pressure manometer.

2. Adjust the flow sensitivity level to 8 L/min. Initiate a breath using a mouthpiece and observe the pressure manometer.

Questions:

A. Which setting would you prefer as a patient?

B. Which setting was easiest for you?

C. What changes did you observe on the graphics display panel?

D. How can you use the Pressure Volume loop and the graphics display panel to minimize inspiratory work?

PRESSURE CONTROL VENTILATION

Set the controls to the following settings and attach the ventilator to the test lung:

Mode	Assist/control (Depress Pres. Ctrl. button)
Inspiratory Pressure	30 cm H_2O (Tidal Volume/Insp. Press.)
Inspiratory Time	1.0 second (Peak Flow/Insp. Time)
Sensitivity	5.0 cm H_2O
Breath Rate	12 breaths/min
O_2 %	21%
PEEP	0.0 cm H_2O

INSPIRATORY PRESSURE CONTROL

1. Using a test lung, measure and record the following using the display panel and manometer:
   a. Exhaled tidal volume
   b. I:E ratio
   c. Peak pressure

2. Adjust the inspiratory pressure level to 50 cm H_2O. Measure the following using the display panel and manometer:
   a. Exhaled tidal volume
   b. I:E ratio
   c. Peak pressure

Questions:

A. How did the change in pressure affect the I:E ratio?
B. How did the change in pressure affect the exhaled tidal volume?

INSPIRATORY TIME CONTROL

1. Set the ventilator to the following settings:

Mode	Assist/control (Depress the Pres. Ctrl. button)
Inspiratory Pressure	30 cm H_2O (Tidal Volume/Insp. Press. control)
Inspiratory Time	1.0 second (Peak Flow/Insp. Time control)
Sensitivity	5.0 cm H_2O
Rate	6 breaths/min
O_2 %	21%
PEEP	0.0 cm H_2O

2. Using a test lung, measure the following using the display panel and manometer:
   a. Exhaled tidal volume
   b. I:E ratio
   c. Peak pressure

3. Change the inspiratory time to 3.0 seconds, and measure and record the following:
   a. Exhaled tidal volume
   b. I:E ratio
   c. Peak pressure

Questions:

A. How did the inspiratory time change affect the I:E ratio?
B. How did the inspiratory time change affect tidal volume delivery?
C. How did the inspiratory time change affect the inspiratory pressure?

ALARM SYSTEMS

Set the ventilator to the following settings:

Mode	Assist/control
Peak Flow	40 L/min
Sensitivity	2.0 cm H_2O
Tidal Volume	500 ml
Breath Rate	8 breaths/min
O_2 %	21%
PEEP	0.0 cm H_2O

High Pressure Limit and Low Peak Pressure

1. Set the pressure limit for 15 cm H_2O above the peak inspiratory pressure.

2. Set the low peak pressure control to 15 cm H_2O below the peak inspiratory pressure.

3. Simulate a cough by rapidly squeezing the test lung.

Questions:

A. What occurred?
B. Was the alarm set appropriately?
C. What other conditions might cause this alarm to be activated?

4. Decrease the tidal volume to 250 ml.

Questions:

A. What occurred?
B. Was the alarm set appropriately?
C. What other conditions might cause this alarm to be activated?

Baseline Pressure

Set the controls to the following values:

Mode	Assist/control
Peak Flow	40 L/min
Sensitivity	4.0 cm H_2O
Tidal Volume	500 ml
Rate	8 breaths/min
O_2 %	21%
PEEP	5.0 cm H_2O

1. Set the Low PEEP/CPAP pressure alarm for 3 cm H_2O.

2. Simulate a patient effort by expanding the test lung's bellows to trigger a breath.

Questions:

A. What occurred?
B. How could you change the control settings to prevent this?
C. Is the alarm set appropriately for this level of PEEP?

3. Readjust your baseline pressure alarm to 3 cm H_2O.

Low Minute Volume

1. Set the low minute volume alarm indicator and adjust the control to 3 L/min.

Questions:

A. What occurred?
B. How could you set the alarm appropriately for the current ventilator settings?

2. Set the alarm's upper limit to 6 L/min and lower limit to 4 L/min.

High Breath Rate

1. Set the high breath rate alarm to 10 breaths/min.

2. Using the test lung, simulate a rate of 20 breaths/min.

Questions:

A. What occurred?
B. How could you set the alarm appropriately for a patient rate of 20/min?
C. Set the alarm's upper limit to 12 breaths/min and lower limit to 6 breaths/min.

Practice Activities: Lifecare PLV-102 Volume Ventilator

CIRCUIT ASSEMBLY

Figure 26-19 shows the Lifecare PLV-102 ventilator. The Lifecare PLV-102 is a small, compact ventilator that is frequently used in the home or extended care facilities. It is capable of being powered by 110 V AC, an internal battery, or an external 12 V direct current (DC) battery. To complete the circuit assembly, refer to Figure 26-20.

1. Fill the humidifier with water and ensure that the humidifier has a power source.

2. Connect the shorter length of large-bore tubing between the humidifier and the ventilator inlet.

3. Connect the longer length of large-bore tubing to the humidifier outlet and the patient manifold.

4. Attach the exhalation valve drive line to the exhalation valve fitting on the front panel of the ventilator.

5. Attach PAP (proximal airway pressure) adapter to the patient manifold. Connect the proximal airway line to the PAP adapter and the PAP fitting on the front panel of the ventilator.

6. Attach a 6-inch length of large-bore tubing between the PAP adapter and the patient's airway.

7. Connect the ventilator to a 110 V 60 Hz outlet or external 12 V DC battery, or power the ventilator with the internal 12 V battery. The POWER indication panel will inform you as to which you have selected.

8. Attach a test lung and proceed with leak testing and calculation of circuit compliance.

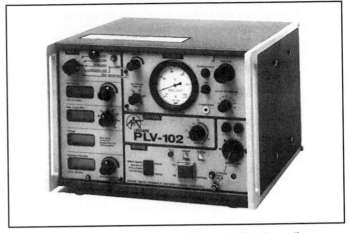

Figure 26-19 *A photograph of the Lifecare PLV-102 ventilator (Courtesy of* Lifecare, Inc., Lafayette, CO)

SYSTEM LEAK TEST

1. Set the controls to the following settings:

Tidal Volume	200 ml
Rate	12/min
Inspiratory Flow Rate	40 L/min
Airway Pressure Limit	maximum

2. Using a sterile gauze or sterile plastic wrap, occlude the patient wye completely.

3. When the ventilator cycles, pinch the exhalation valve drive line.

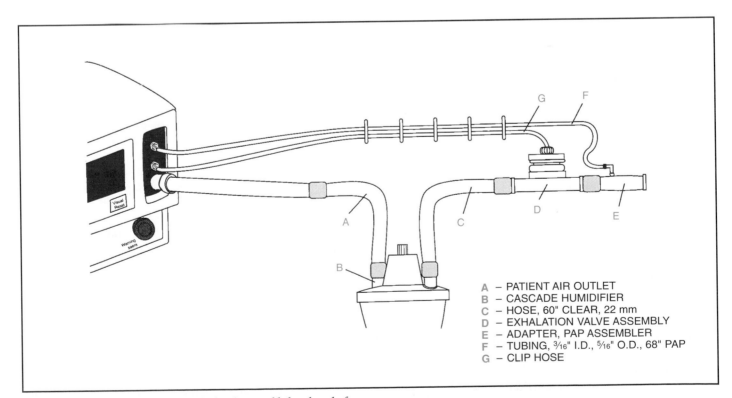

A – PATIENT AIR OUTLET
B – CASCADE HUMIDIFIER
C – HOSE, 60" CLEAR, 22 mm
D – EXHALATION VALVE ASSEMBLY
E – ADAPTER, PAP ASSEMBLER
F – TUBING, 3/16" I.D., 5/16" O.D., 68" PAP
G – CLIP HOSE

Figure 26-20 *The Lifecare PLV-102 circuit assembled and ready for use*

4. Observe the pressure manometer. The pressure should drop slightly and then plateau without dropping further. If the pressure drops, check the circuit connections and humidifier for tightness or any potential leaks.

5. Attach a portable respirometer to the exhalation valve and measure the exhaled volume when the patient wye is occluded. Measure the peak inspiratory pressure.

6. Calculate the tubing compliance using the following formula:

$$\text{Tubing compliance} = \frac{\text{tidal volume}}{\text{peak pressure}}$$

ACTIVITIES

To complete these practice activities, it is recommended that you use a lung analog/simulator such as a Medishield Lung Ventilator Performance Analyzer, Retec Respiratory Teaching Console, or a Biotech VT-2 Ventilator Performance Tester. These devices will allow you to alter resistance and compliance easily to observe how the ventilator performance changes.

If these devices are not available, a patient wye and two test lungs may be used, as shown in Figure 26-15. Exercise caution. Volumes and pressures may exceed the limits of the test lungs. Resistance may be altered by adapting different sizes of endotracheal tubes, and compliance may be altered by the addition of rubber bands to the test lungs.

CONTROL MODE
Initial Settings

Mode	Control
Airway Pressure Limit	maximum
Tidal Volume	500 ml
Rate	12/min
Inspiratory Flow Rate	40 L/min

Manipulate only one control at a time and note the result on the space provided on the flow sheet. Answer the questions that follow each of the exercises.

Adjust the tidal volume so that the corrected tidal volume is 500 ml, using the following formulas:

Tubing loss = peak pressure × tubing compliance
Corrected tidal volume = measured tidal volume − tubing loss

TIDAL VOLUME CONTROL

1. Set the controls to the initial settings.
   a. Measure inspiratory time.
   b. Record the I:E ratio.
   c. Calculate corrected tidal volume.

2. Adjust the tidal volume to 1500 ml.
   a. Measure inspiratory time.
   b. Record the I:E ratio.
   c. Calculate corrected tidal volume.

3. Return the tidal volume control to 500 ml.

Questions:
A. Why did the pressure increase?
B. Why did the inspiratory time increase?
C. What happened to the I:E ratio? Why did the I:E ratio change?
D. How could you increase the tidal volume and maintain the same I:E ratio?

RATE CONTROL
Set the controls to the following settings:

Tidal Volume	200 ml
Rate	12/min
Inspiratory Flow Rate	40 L/min
Airway Pressure Limit	maximum

1. At the above settings, perform the following:
   a. Measure inspiratory time.
   b. Record the I:E ratio.
   c. Calculate the corrected tidal volume.

2. Adjust the rate to 20 L/min.
   a. Measure inspiratory time.
   b. Record the I:E ratio.
   c. Calculate corrected tidal volume.

Questions:
A. What happened to the I:E ratio?
B. If you increase the rate, how could you maintain a similar I:E ratio?
C. Did the tidal volume vary?

FLOW RATE
Set the controls to the following settings:

Tidal Volume	200 ml
Rate	12/min
Inspiratory Flow Rate	40 L/min
Airway Pressure Limit	maximum

1. At the above settings, perform the following:
   a. Measure inspiratory time.
   b. Record the I:E ratio.
   c. Calculate corrected tidal volume.

2. Adjust the flow rate to 20 L/min.
   a. Measure inspiratory time.
   b. Record the I:E ratio.
   c. Calculate corrected tidal volume.

Questions:
A. What happened to the I:E ratio?
B. What happened to the inspiratory time?
C. Did the tidal volume vary?
D. How can the flow rate control be used in conjunction with the tidal volume control to maintain a desired I:E ratio?

ASSIST/CONTROL MODE
Set the controls to the following settings:

Tidal Volume	200 ml
Rate	12/min
Inspiratory Flow Rate	40 L/min
Airway Pressure Limit	maximum

SENSITIVITY

1. Rotate the sensitivity control counterclockwise until you can initiate inspiration by simulating a breath with the test lung exerting only −2 cm H_2O of inspiratory effort.

2. Rotate the control clockwise ¼ turn from the position in step number 1.
   a. Observe the pressure manometer during a simulated inspiration.

Questions:

A. What happened after you adjusted the control ¼ turn beyond its initial position?

B. Where do you think this control should be set?

CHANGES IN RESISTANCE AND COMPLIANCE

1. Set the controls to the following settings:

Mode	Assist/control
Tidal Volume	800 ml
Rate	15/min
Flow Rate	50 L/min
Peak Pressure	maximum

   a. Measure peak inspiratory pressures.
   b. Measure inspiratory time.
   c. Calculate corrected tidal volume.
   d. Record the I:E ratio.

2. Decrease the compliance by ⅓ by adjusting the spring tension or manipulating the compliance control on the lung analog.

   a. Measure peak inspiratory pressures.
   b. Measure inspiratory time.
   c. Calculate corrected tidal volume.
   d. Record the I:E ratio.

Questions:

A. Why did the corrected tidal volume decrease?

B. Did the I:E ratio vary? If so, why?

C. Why did the peak pressure increase?

3. Return the compliance value to norm on the lung analog.

4. Increase the resistance by ⅓ by adjusting the resistance control on the lung analog.

   a. Measure peak inspiratory pressures.
   b. Measure inspiratory time.
   c. Calculate corrected tidal volume.
   d. Record the I:E ratio.

Questions:

A. When compared with the original values listed in number 1, why did the inspiratory pressure increase?

B. Why did the I:E ratio vary?

C. How do you account for differences in the corrected tidal volume?

D. Can you think of a pathological pulmonary condition that could cause this?

5. Return the resistance control to its initial setting.

6. Decrease the compliance by ⅔ by adjusting spring tension or adjusting the lung analog.

   a. What event(s) occurred?
   b. Can you think of a disease that may cause this?
   c. What is the purpose of the pressure limit control?

VENTILATOR ALARMS

Pressure Limit

Set the controls to the following settings:

Tidal Volume	200 ml
Rate	12/min
Inspiratory Flow Rate	40 L/min

1. Turn the control fully counterclockwise. Turn the control clockwise until the ventilator no longer alarms during inspiration.

2. Increase the tidal volume to 700 ml.

Questions:

A. What happened when you increased the tidal volume?

B. Why did the ventilator alarm?

Low Pressure

Set the controls to the following settings:

Tidal Volume	500 ml
Rate	12/min
Inspiratory Flow Rate	40 L/min
Airway Pressure Limit	maximum

1. Adjust the low pressure limit control to 5 cm H_2O greater than the peak pressure.

   a. Observe what occurs.

2. Adjust the low pressure limit control to 5 cm H_2O less than the peak pressure.

   a. Observe what occurs.

Questions:

A. What happened?

B. What purpose would the low pressure alarm be good for?

C. What event(s) may cause this alarm?

I:E Ratio and Increased Inspiratory Flow

Adjust the ventilator to the following settings:

Tidal Volume	500 ml
Rate	12/min
Inspiratory Flow Rate	40 L/min
Airway Pressure Limit	maximum

1. Increase the tidal volume to 800 ml and decrease the flow rate to 10 L/min.

   a. Observe the I:E ratio display.

2. Increase the flow rate to 50 L/min.

   a. Observe the I:E ratio display.

Questions:

A. What did you observe on the I:E ratio display?

B. Is it possible to deliver inverse I:E ratio ventilation with this ventilator?

Other Alarm Conditions

Other alarm conditions are summarized as follows:

   Low internal battery
   Low external battery
   Reverse external battery connection (polarity for DC current)
   Switch to battery
   Power failure
   Ventilator malfunction

ADDITIONAL ACTIVITIES

Establish the following tidal volumes and rates. All volumes are assumed to be corrected volumes. Verify all rates and volumes using a watch and a respirometer.

1.

Tidal Volume	1000 ml
Rate	10/min
I:E ratio (desired)	1:2

2.

Tidal Volume	800 ml
Rate	14/min
I:E ratio	1:3

Practice Activities: Puritan-Bennett MA-1 and MA-2

CIRCUIT ASSEMBLY

Figure 26-21 shows the MA-1 and MA-2+2 ventilators assembled and ready for the initiation of mechanical ventilation.

MA-1

1. Facing the front of the ventilator, open the door on the lower half of the machine. Insert a larger bacteria filter through the hole in the upper left of the compartment and attach it using the clamp provided. Attach a piece of flex tubing between the bacteria filter and the outlet in the upper center of the compartment.

2. Fill the humidifier with water and attach it to the heating element on the side of the machine. Attach the angled connector to the filter outlet and to the humidifier. An MA-2+2 will also have a temperature sensor that connects to the humidifier to act as a servocontroller.

3. Assemble the circuit as shown in Figure 26-22 and attach it to the support arm using the fitting on the manifold assembly.

4. Attach the inspiratory side to the outlet of the humidifier.

5. Attach the expiratory side to the water trap and fit the water trap onto the spirometer pole.

6. Attach the exhalation valve tubing to the exhalation valve fitting on the side of the ventilator. An MA-2+2 will also have a proximal pressure line to connect to its appropriate fitting on the side of the ventilator.

7. Assemble the spirometer and attach it to the spirometer pole. Attach the small-diameter tubing from the spirometer to the black fitting labeled Spirometer.

8. Attach any external alarms utilized by your facility in accordance with recommended policies and procedures.

9. Connect the ventilator to a 50 psi source of oxygen and air (MA-2). Connect the ventilator power cord to a suitable 110 V outlet.

10. Attach a test lung and proceed with leak testing and calculation of circuit compliance.

SYSTEM LEAK TEST

1. Set the controls to the following settings:
   a. Tidal Volume   200 ml
   b. Respiratory Rate   12/min
   c. Flow Rate   40 L/min
   d. Pressure Limit   maximum setting

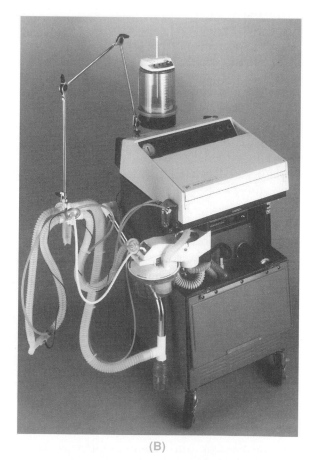

(A) (B)

Figure 26-21 *Photos of the Puritan–Bennett MA-1 (A) and Puritan–Bennett MA-2+2 (B) ventilators assembled and ready for use* (*Courtesy of* Puritan-Bennett Corporation, Carlsbad, CA)

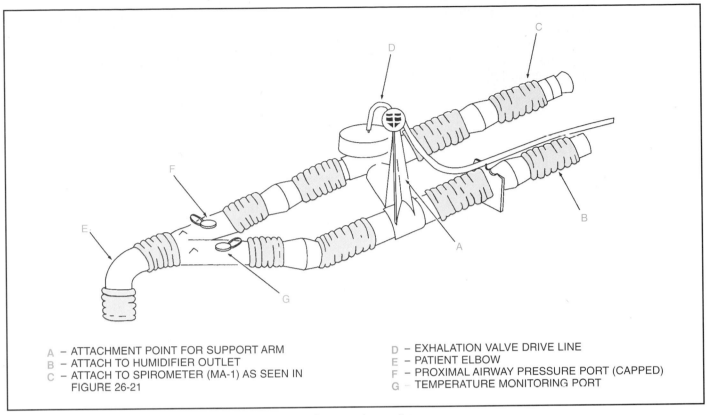

A – ATTACHMENT POINT FOR SUPPORT ARM
B – ATTACH TO HUMIDIFIER OUTLET
C – ATTACH TO SPIROMETER (MA-1) AS SEEN IN
    FIGURE 26-21

D – EXHALATION VALVE DRIVE LINE
E – PATIENT ELBOW
F – PROXIMAL AIRWAY PRESSURE PORT (CAPPED)
G – TEMPERATURE MONITORING PORT

Figure 26-22 *The MA-1 circuit assembled and ready for attachment to the ventilator*

2. Using a sterile gauze or sterile plastic wrap (inside of wrapping that the circuit was packaged in), occlude the patient wye completely.

3. When the ventilator cycles on, pinch the exhalation valve drive line or occlude the outlet for the exhalation valve with your other hand and a sterile wrap. This will hold pressure in the circuit.

4. Observe the pressure manometer. Pressure should drop slightly and then plateau without dropping further. If the manometer does not remain at a steady value but continues to drop, you have a leak.

5. In the event of a leak, check all tubing connections, humidifier connections (internal and external), exhalation valve diaphragm, and tubing for small holes.

6. Repeat steps 1 through 5 until pressure remains steady in the circuit.

TUBING COMPLIANCE

1. Set the controls to the values listed in system leak test.

2. Attach a respirometer to the outlet of the tubing circuit or exhalation valve to measure the exhaled volume.

3. Using a sterile gauze or sterile plastic wrap (inside of wrapping that the circuit was packaged in), occlude the patient wye completely.

4. As the ventilator cycles, note the pressure reading on the pressure manometer. It may take several breaths to record the pressure accurately.

5. Read the respirometer and record the tidal volume delivered with each breath. This volume represents the volume compressed in the circuit, since no volume was actually delivered.

6. Calculate the tubing compliance using the following formula:

$$\text{Tubing compliance} = \frac{\text{tidal volume}}{\text{peak inspiratory pressure}}$$

ACTIVITIES

To complete these practice activities, it is recommended that you use a lung analog/simulator such as a Medishield Lung Ventilator Performance Analyzer or Retec Respirator Teaching Console. Both of these devices or other similar devices can alter resistance and compliance simulating changes in patient condition.

If these devices are not available, a patient wye and two test lungs may be used as shown in Figure 26-15. Exercise caution. Volumes and pressures may exceed the limits of the test lungs. Resistance may be altered by adapting different sizes of endotracheal tubes, and compliance may be altered by the addition of rubber bands to the test lungs.

INITIAL SETTINGS

a. Peak Flow	40 L/min
b. Sensitivity	turn fully counterclockwise
c. Pressure Limit	maximum setting
d. Normal Volume	500 ml
e. Rate	12/min
f. All Sigh Controls	off
g. Oxygen Concentration	21%
h. Expiratory Resistance	turn fully counterclockwise

Manipulate only one control at a time and note the result in the space provided on the flow sheet. Answer the questions that follow each of the activities.

Adjust the tidal volume control so that the corrected tidal volume is 500 ml, using the following formulas:

$$\text{Tubing} = \text{peak pressure} \times \text{tubing compliance}$$
$$\text{Corrected tidal volume} = \text{measured tidal volume} - \text{tubing loss}$$

PEAK FLOW CONTROL

1. Adjust the peak flow control to 20 L/min.
   a. Measure inspiratory time.
   b. Measure peak inspiratory pressure.
   c. Calculate corrected tidal volume.
   d. Calculate the I:E ratio.

2. Adjust the peak flow control to 100 L/min.
   a. Measure inspiratory time.
   b. Measure peak inspiratory pressure.
   c. Calculate corrected tidal volume.
   d. Calculate the I:E ratio.

Questions:
A. How do you account for the differences in inspiratory time?
B. Why were there differences in peak inspiratory pressure?
C. Why did corrected tidal volume vary?
D. Why did the I:E ratio vary between the two exercises?

3. Return the peak flow control to 40 L/min.

NORMAL VOLUME CONTROL (TIDAL VOLUME)

1. Set the controls to the following settings:
   Peak Flow   40 L/min
   Normal Volume   500 ml
   Rate   12/min
   a. Measure inspiratory time.
   b. Measure peak inspiratory pressure.
   c. Calculate corrected tidal volume.
   d. Calculate the I:E ratio.

2. Turn the normal volume control to 1500 ml.
   a. Measure inspiratory time.
   b. Measure peak inspiratory pressure.
   c. Calculate corrected tidal volume.
   d. Calculate the I:E ratio.

Questions:
A. Why did the pressure increase?
B. Why did the inspiratory time increase?
C. How do you account for the decrease in I:E ratio?

3. Return the normal volume control to 500 ml.

RATE CONTROL (CYCLES OR BREATHS PER MINUTE)
Set the controls to the following settings:
   Peak Flow   40 L/min
   Pressure Limit   fully clockwise
   Normal Volume   500 ml
   Rate   12/min

1. With the controls set as above, perform the following:
   a. Measure peak inspiratory pressure.
   b. Measure inspiratory time.
   c. Calculate corrected tidal volume.
   d. Calculate the I:E ratio.

2. Turn the rate control to 40 breaths/min.
   a. Measure peak inspiratory pressure.
   b. Measure inspiratory time.
   c. Calculate corrected tidal volume.
   d. Calculate the I:E ratio.

Questions:
A. What alarm was triggered and why?
B. What was the I:E ratio?
C. Why was the I:E ratio so low?

3. Return the rate control to 12/min.

CHANGES IN RESISTANCE AND COMPLIANCE

1. Set the controls to the following settings:
   Peak Flow Control   40 L/min
   Normal Pressure   fully counterclockwise
   Normal Volume   500 ml
   Rate   12/min
   a. Measure peak inspiratory pressure.
   b. Measure inspiratory time.
   c. Calculate corrected tidal volume.
   d. Calculate the I:E ratio.

2. Decrease the compliance by ⅓ by adjusting the spring tension or manipulating the compliance control on the lung analog.
   a. Measure peak inspiratory pressure.
   b. Measure inspiratory time.
   c. Calculate corrected tidal volume.
   d. Calculate the I:E ratio.

Questions:
A. Why did the corrected tidal volume decrease?
B. Why did the I:E ratio vary?
C. Why did the peak inspiratory pressure increase?

3. Return the compliance to the original value on the lung analog.

4. Increase the resistance by ⅓ by adjusting the resistance control on the lung analog.
   a. Measure peak inspiratory pressure.
   b. Measure inspiratory time.
   c. Calculate corrected tidal volume.
   d. Calculate the I:E ratio.

Questions:
Compared with the original values in this activity:
A. Why did the inspiratory pressure increase?
B. Why did the I:E ratio vary?
C. How do you account for differences in the corrected tidal volume?
D. Can you think of human physiological conditions that could produce similar results?

5. Return the resistance control to the original value on the lung analog.

6. Set the pressure limit control to 10 cm H_2O greater than the cycling pressure.

7. Decrease the compliance by ⅔ by adjusting spring tension or adjusting the compliance control on the lung analog.

Questions:
A. What event(s) occurred?
B. Can you think of a patient situation that could cause this?
C. What is the purpose of the normal pressure limit control?

SENSITIVITY CONTROL

Adjust the ventilator to the following settings:

Peak Flow	40 L/min
Sensitivity	fully counterclockwise
Normal Pressure Limit	10 cm H_2O greater than PIP
Normal Volume	500 ml
Rate	8 breaths/min
Sigh Controls	off
Oxygen Concentration	21%
Expiratory Resistance	off

1. Attach a mouthpiece to the patient wye and attempt to initiate a breath. Observe the pressure manometer.

2. Adjust the sensitivity by turning it clockwise until the ventilator auto-cycles. Turn the sensitivity counterclockwise from this point one full turn.

3. Attempt to initiate another breath while observing the pressure manometer.
   a. Record the negative pressure when the ventilator cycled on.
   b. Observe the control panel for any changes.

Questions:
A. If you wanted the patient in control mode, how would you set the sensitivity control?
B. When you were able to initiate an assisted breath, what event(s) occurred?
C. Where would you want to set the sensitivity control for assist/control mode?

SIGH CONTROLS

1. Set the controls to the following settings:

Peak Flow	40 L/min
Normal Pressure Limit	10 cm H_2O greater than PIP
Normal Volume Control	500 ml
Rate	12/min
Sigh Pressure Limit	60 cm H_2O
Sigh Volume	1000 ml
Sigh Rate	15 per hour
Sigh Multiple	3

2. Wait a few minutes and observe the control panel.

3. When the ventilator initiates the sigh mode, measure sigh volume and PIP.
   a. Calculate the corrected sigh volume.

Questions:
A. What occurred when the ventilator initiated sigh mode?
B. What could occur if the patient had copious airway secretions and required suctioning?

ALARM FUNCTIONS
Oxygen Alarm
Set the controls for the following settings:

Peak Flow	40 L/min
Sensitivity	fully counterclockwise
Normal Pressure Limit	maximum
Normal Volume	500 ml
Rate	12 breaths/min
Oxygen Concentration	40%

1. Disconnect the ventilator from the 50 psi oxygen source.

2. Connect the oxygen supply line to a 50 psi air source.

Questions:
A. What event(s) occurred?
B. Do you suspect that this alarm is an oxygen analyzer?

Spirometer Alarm
Set the controls to the same settings as in the oxygen alarm activity. Connect the ventilator to a test lung or lung analog.

1. Disconnect the exhalation tubing from the water collection trap.

2. Turn the spirometer on by moving the slide switch.

3. Adjust the spirometer alarm by raising the white metering stick until 425 ml is registered where the stick is inserted into the tube at the top of the spirometer.

4. Press and release the test button. Slowly raise the bellows by raising the spirometer post until 600 ml is indicated by the level of the diaphragm. The alarm should cease.

5. Reconnect the exhalation tube to the water collection trap.

6. Disconnect the patient wye from the test lung or lung analog and observe what event(s) occur.

Expiratory Resistance
Set the controls to the same settings used in the oxygen alarm activity. Attach the ventilator to a test lung or lung analog.

1. Rotate the expiratory resistance control fully clockwise. Observe the pressure manometer.

2. Rotate the control counterclockwise in ½-turn increments until the control is off. Observe the pressure manometer.
   a. Measure inspiratory time.
   b. Measure expiratory time.
   c. Calculate corrected tidal volume.

3. Turn the control clockwise one full turn. Increase the rate to 40 breaths/min. Observe what occurs.

Questions:
A. What did this control do?
B. What happened when you decreased resistance?
C. Can you think of any patient care situations that would require caution in the use of this control?

ADDITIONAL ACTIVITIES

Establish the following tidal volumes, rates, and FIO_2 levels. All volumes are assumed to be corrected volumes and all FIO_2 levels must be adjusted to ±2%. Verify all respiratory rates by using your watch and timing a 1-minute interval.

1. Tidal Volume   1000 ml
   Rate   10/min
   FIO_2 0.40
   Flow Rate   40 L/min

2. Tidal Volume   1200 ml
   Rate   8/min
   FIO_2 0.35
   Flow Rate   60 L/min

3. Tidal Volume   800 ml
   Rate   14/min
   FIO_2 0.50
   Flow Rate   70 L/min

Practice Activities: Puritan-Bennett 7200ae

CIRCUIT ASSEMBLY

Figure 26-23 shows the 7200ae assembled and ready for the initiation of mechanical ventilation.

1. Install a heated exhalation bacteria filter by rotating the filter clamp located underneath the pressure-sensitive keyboard on the left of the ventilator toward you. Push the clean filter into place and lock it securely in place by rotating the clamp over the clamp catch (Figure 26-24).

2. Attach the condensation collection jar to the inlet of the heated bacteria filter using the silicone "T" assembly.

3. Attach the humidifier jar to the heating element and fill the humidifier to the correct level with sterile distilled water.

4. Open the hinged door to the right of the numeric keyboard and connect the main flow bacteria filter. Connect the filter to the inlet of the humidifier with a short piece of tubing (Figure 26-25).

5. Attach the patient circuit to the support arm and proceed to connect the tubing to the ventilator.

6. Connect the inspiration side of the circuit to the outlet of the humidifier.

7. Connect the exhalation valve tubing to the exhalation valve nipple on the ventilator.

8. If the circuit is equipped with a nebulizer, connect the nebulizer drive line to the nebulizer nipple on the ventilator.

9. Connect the proximal airway pressure line to the patient airway pressure nipple on the ventilator (the use of a small bacteria filter is recommended).

Figure 26-23 *The Puritan-Bennett 7200ae ventilator (Courtesy of Puritan-Bennett Corporation, Carlsbad, CA)*

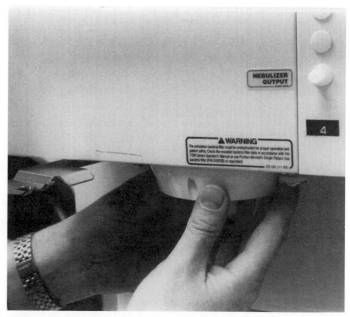

Figure 26-24 *Attachment of the expiratory filter by rotating the filter clamp closed*

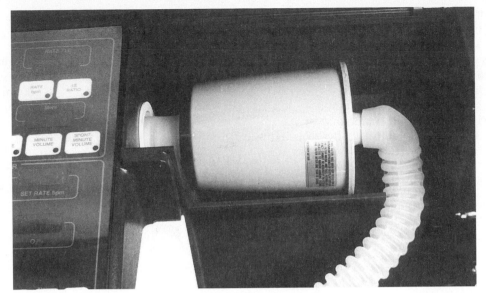

Figure 26-25 *Installation of the main flow bacteria filter*

10. Connect the servo temperature sensor for the humidifier (if so equipped) to the patient wye.

11. Connect the exhalation side of the patient circuit to the collection trap located below the keyboard.

12. Connect the high-pressure hoses to suitable outlets for air and oxygen.

13. Connect the power cord to a suitable 115 V AC source.

TESTING THE VENTILATOR BEFORE USE
Power-on Self Test
Each time the power switch is turned on or a momentary interruption of power occurs, a power-on self test (POST) will automatically be initiated. This test lasts for 10 seconds during which time the safety valve will open (allowing spontaneous breathing if a patient is connected). This test is built into the microprocessor of the ventilator and requires no input from you the operator. If the ventilator successfully passes its POST, it will begin operation automatically.

If the ventilator fails the POST, Backup Ventilator will illuminate on the alarm display and an audible alarm will sound. If this event occurs, do not use the ventilator! Contact your service representative and have it repaired before further use.

Extended Self Test (EST)
This is an extended diagnostic test built into the microprocessor of this ventilator. This test takes between 3 and 5 minutes. During this test the ventilator must be disconnected from the patient and the patient wye must be plugged.

To initiate the EST, press the EST button on the side of the ventilator, and follow the prompts given in the display window. After each condition requested has been met, press the Enter key. Refer to the operator's manual for further information on this diagnostic test.

As a part of the EST, tubing compliance and area ratio across the exhalation port are calculated and entered in the microprocessor memory in the ventilator. This feature eliminates the manual calculations to determine tubing compliance, volume loss to tubing expansion, and corrected tidal volume while monitoring mechanical ventilation.

An updated EST software program was released in February 1986. This updated EST is more user-friendly and allows the operator to bypass noncritical failures in the EST. The new program also allows completion of the EST in a much shorter time frame, permitting more rapid initiation of mechanical ventilation.

Lamp Test
By depressing this key, all lamps in the ventilator status section of the keyboard are tested. If a lamp fails to illuminate, contact your service representative to have it replaced.

USING THE KEYBOARD ENTRY SYSTEM
The Puritan-Bennett 7200ae uses a pressure-sensitive keyboard to make mode, parameter, and alarm changes. Using the keyboard requires a two-step process. First, the desired parameter must be selected by pressing that key. The current value in memory (current ventilator setting) will appear in the message display window. If this is not the desired value, enter the correct value by using the numeric keypad (the entered value will now appear in the message display window). Check the window to be certain that this is the desired value. If the value is correct, press Enter. The entered value will now be stored in memory and will become the current ventilator setting during the next cycle.

If you make an error, pressing the Clear key will clear the display window and the ventilator will continue to cycle using the value stored in memory. After you have corrected your error, pressing the Enter key will input your new value.

A safety feature is built into the keyboard. Once you select a mode or wave form that you want to change, if you do not complete the change within 10 seconds by pressing Enter, the ventilator will revert to its previous setting.

VENTILATOR DISPLAYS

Operating the ventilator displays is similar to operating the keyboard entry features of the ventilator. Ventilator settings are constantly displayed in the LED windows above the numeric keyboard.

Patient data or parameters may be selected by depressing the appropriate key, and the desired value will be displayed in the LED window or analog display. All volumes displayed are corrected (volume actually delivered to the patient).

ACTIVITIES

To complete these practice activities, it is recommended that you use a lung analog/simulator such as a Medishield Lung Ventilator Performance Analyzer or Retec Respirator Teaching Console. Both of these devices or other similar devices can alter resistance and compliance simulating changes in patient condition.

If these devices are not available, a patient wye and two test lungs may be used as shown in Figure 26-15. Exercise caution. Volumes and pressures may exceed the limits of the test lungs. Resistance may be altered by adapting different sizes of endotracheal tubes, and compliance may be altered by the addition of rubber bands to the test lungs.

INITIAL SETTINGS

a.	Mode	CMV
b.	Peak Flow	40 L/min
c.	Sensitivity	−2 cm H$_2$O
d.	High Pressure Limit	120 cm H$_2$O
e.	Tidal Volume	500 ml
f.	Respiratory Rate	12/min
g.	All Sigh Controls	off
h.	Oxygen Concentration	21%
i.	Wave Form	square
j.	Nebulizer	off
k.	Inspiratory Pause	0
l.	PEEP	fully counterclockwise
m.	Alarms	adjust to match settings

Manipulate only one control at a time and note the result in the space provided on the flow sheet. Answer the questions that follow each of the activities.

PEAK FLOW CONTROL

1. Set the peak flow to 20 L/min.
   a. Measure inspiratory time.
   b. Measure peak pressure.
   c. Record corrected tidal volume.
   d. Record the I:E ratio.

2. Adjust the peak flow to 60 L/min.
   a. Measure inspiratory time.
   b. Measure peak pressure.
   c. Record corrected tidal volume.
   d. Record the I:E ratio.

Questions:

A. How do you account for the differences in inspiratory time?
B. Why were there differences in peak inspiratory pressure?
C. Why did corrected tidal volume vary?
D. Why did the I:E ratio vary between the two activities?

3. Return the peak flow control to 40 L/min.

TIDAL VOLUME CONTROL

1. Set the controls to the following settings:
   Peak Flow   40 L/min
   Tidal Volume   500 ml
   Rate   12/min
   a. Measure inspiratory time.
   b. Measure peak inspiratory pressure.
   c. Record corrected tidal volume.
   d. Record the I:E ratio.

2. Set normal tidal volume control to 1500 ml.
   a. Measure inspiratory time.
   b. Measure peak inspiratory pressure.
   c. Record corrected tidal volume.
   d. Record the I:E ratio.

Questions:

A. Why did the pressure increase?
B. Why did the inspiratory time increase?
C. How do you account for the increase in I:E ratio?

3. Return the normal volume control to 500 ml.

NORMAL RATE CONTROL (CYCLES OR BREATHS PER MINUTE)

Set the controls to the following settings:
   Peak Flow   40 L/min
   High Pressure Limit 120 cm H$_2$O
   Tidal Volume   500 ml
   Rate   12/min

1. With the controls set as above, perform the following:
   a. Measure peak inspiratory pressure.
   b. Measure inspiratory time.
   c. Record corrected tidal volume.
   d. Record the I:E ratio.

2. Adjust the rate control to 40 breaths/min.
   a. Measure peak inspiratory pressure.
   b. Measure inspiratory time.
   c. Record corrected tidal volume.
   d. Record the I:E ratio.

Questions:

A. What alarm was triggered and why?
B. What was the I:E ratio?
C. Why was the I:E ratio so high?

3. Return the rate control to 12/min.

CHANGES IN RESISTANCE AND COMPLIANCE

1. Set controls to the following settings:
   Peak Flow Control   40 L/min
   High Pressure Limit 120 cm H$_2$O
   Tidal Volume   500 ml
   Rate   12/min
   a. Measure peak inspiratory pressure.
   b. Measure inspiratory time.
   c. Record corrected tidal volume.
   d. Record the I:E ratio.

2. Decrease the compliance by ⅓ by adjusting the spring tension or manipulating the compliance control on the lung analog.

a. Measure peak inspiratory pressure.
b. Measure inspiratory time.
c. Record corrected tidal volume.
d. Record the I:E ratio.

Questions:
A. Why did the corrected tidal volume decrease?
B. Why did the I:E ratio vary?
C. Why did the peak inspiratory pressure increase?

3. Return the compliance to the original value on the lung analog.

4. Increase the resistance by ⅓ by adjusting the resistance control on the lung analog.
   a. Measure peak inspiratory pressure.
   b. Measure inspiratory time.
   c. Record corrected tidal volume.
   d. Record the I:E ratio.

Questions:
Compared with the original values in this activity:
A. Why did the inspiratory pressure increase?
B. Why did the I:E ratio vary?
C. How do you account for differences in the corrected tidal volume?
D. Can you think of human physiological conditions that could produce similar results?

5. Return the resistance control to the original value on the lung analog.

6. Set the pressure limit control to 10 cm H_2O greater than the cycling pressure.

7. Decrease the compliance by ⅔ by adjusting spring tension or adjusting the compliance control on the lung analog.

Questions:
A. What event(s) occurred?
B. Can you think of a patient situation that could cause this?
C. What is the purpose of the normal pressure limit control?

SENSITIVITY CONTROL
Adjust the ventilator to the following settings:

Mode	CMV
Peak Flow	40 L/min
Sensitivity	–2 cm H_2O
High Pressure Limit	10 cm H_2O greater than PIP
Tidal Volume	500 ml
Rate	8 breaths/min
Sigh Controls	off
Oxygen Concentration	21%
Inspiratory Pause	0
PEEP	fully counterclockwise

1. Attach a mouthpiece to the patient wye and attempt to initiate a breath. Observe the pressure manometer.

2. Set the sensitivity control to –2 cm H_2O and initiate a breath. Observe the pressure manometer.

3. Adjust the sensitivity control to –20 cm H_2O and initiate a breath. Observe the pressure manometer.

a. Record the negative pressure when the ventilator cycled on.
b. Observe the control panel for any changes.

Questions:
A. When you were able to initiate an assisted breath, what event(s) occurred?
B. Where would you want to set the sensitivity control for assist/control mode?

SIGH CONTROLS
1. Set the controls to the following settings and attach the ventilator to a test lung or lung analog:

Mode	CMV and automatic sigh
Wave Form	square
Peak Flow	40 L/min
High Pressure Limit	10 cm H_2O greater than PIP
Tidal Volume Control	500 ml
Rate	12/min
Sigh Pressure Limit	60 cm H_2O
Sigh Volume	1000 ml
Sigh Rate	15 per hour
Multiple Sigh	3

2. Wait a few minutes and observe the control panel.

3. When the ventilator initiates the sigh mode, measure sigh volume and peak inspiratory pressure (PIP).
   a. Calculate corrected sigh volume.

Questions:
A. What occurred when the ventilator initiated sigh mode?
B. What could occur if the patient had copious airway secretions and required suctioning?

PRESSURE CONTROL VENTILATION
Set the controls to the following settings and attach the ventilator to the test lung:

Mode	Pressure Control
Inspiratory Pressure	30 cm H_2O
I:E Ratio	Press Clear (this holds Insp. Time constant)
Inspiratory Time	1.0 second
Sensitivity	5.0 cm H_2O
Rate	12 breaths/min
O_2%	21%
PEEP	0.0 cm H_2O

INSPIRATORY PRESSURE CONTROL
1. Using a test lung, measure and record the following using the display panel and manometer:
   a. Exhaled tidal volume
   b. I:E ratio
   c. Peak pressure

2. Adjust the inspiratory pressure level to 50 cm H_2O. Measure the following using the display panel and manometer:
   a. Exhaled tidal volume
   b. I:E ratio
   c. Peak pressure

Questions:

A. How did the change in pressure affect the I:E ratio?

B. How did the change in pressure affect the exhaled tidal volume?

INSPIRATORY TIME CONTROL

1. Set the ventilator to the following settings:

Mode	Pressure Control
Inspiratory Pressure	30 cm H_2O
Inspiratory Time	1.0 second
Sensitivity	5.0 cm H_2O
Breath Rate	6 breaths/min
O_2%	21%
PEEP	0.0 cm H_2O

2. Using a test lung, measure the following using the display panel and manometer:
   a. Exhaled tidal volume
   b. I:E ratio
   c. Peak pressure

3. Change the inspiratory time to 3.0 seconds, and measure and record the following:
   a. Exhaled tidal volume
   b. I:E ratio
   c. Peak pressure

Questions:

A. How did the inspiratory time change affect the I:E ratio?

B. How did the inspiratory time change affect tidal volume delivery?

C. How did the inspiratory time change affect the inspiratory pressure?

I:E RATIO CONTROL

1. Set the ventilator to the following settings:

Mode	Pressure Control
Inspiratory Pressure	30 cm H_2O
I:E Ratio	1:4
Inspiratory Time	Press Clear (this holds I:E ratio constant)
Sensitivity	5.0 cm H_2O
Breath Rate	6 breaths/min
O_2%	21%
PEEP	0.0 cm H_2O

2. Using a test lung, measure the following using the display panel and manometer:
   a. Exhaled tidal volume
   b. I:E ratio
   c. Peak pressure

3. Change the I:E ratio to 2:1, and measure and record the following:
   a. Exhaled tidal volume
   b. I:E ratio
   c. Peak pressure

Questions:

A. What happened to the inspiratory time when you changed the I:E ratio?

B. Under what circumstances would it be beneficial to hold the I:E ratio constant?

ALARM FUNCTIONS

The Puritan–Bennett 7200ae has several built-in alarms that are very helpful in the management of critically ill patients. It is important to set the alarms properly so that changes in the patient's condition will be readily apparent. Ventilator status, standard, and nonstandard alarms are summarized in Figure 26-26.

Alarm conditions may be corrected in several ways. Your first concern is your patient. Assess the patient, and if required, manually ventilate the patient until the alarm condition can be corrected.

If the patient's condition permits, determine what alarm has been activated and take corrective action.

The alarms may be reset by depressing the Reset key. If the condition that caused the original alarm has been corrected, the ventilator will revert to normal operation.

Depressing the Alarm Silence key will silence the audible alarm for 2 minutes. If the alarm condition does not correct itself or if you do not correct it, the alarm will resume after 2 minutes.

VENTILATOR STATUS ALARMS

Alarm

This display will illuminate whenever an alarm or emergency condition exists.

Caution

This display will illuminate following an alarm condition. During a standard alarm, the Alarm section of the Alarm Summary Display and the specific alarm key are illuminated. If the condition that initiated the alarm corrects itself or is corrected by the practitioner, the alarm display on the Alarm Summary switches off and the Caution section illuminates. This display alerts you to any previous alarm conditions. For example, if a patient coughs and exceeds the high pressure limit, causing an alarm, but in the next cycle is breathing within the set alarm parameters, the alarm will reset. The Caution indicator and the alarm key will remain illuminated to alert you to the previous condition.

VENTILATOR STATUS ALARMS

Alarm	Safety valve open
Normal	Backup ventilator
Caution	

STANDARD ALARMS

Low exhaled tidal volume	High respiratory rate
Low inspiratory pressure	Exhalation valve leak
Low exhaled minute volume	Apnea
Low PEEP/CPAP pressure	

NONSTANDARD ALARMS

High pressure limit	I:E
Low pressure O_2 inlet	Low battery
Low pressure air inlet	

Figure 26-26 *Puritan-Bennett 7200ae alarms*

Backup Ventilator

This indicator is illuminated when the ventilator switches to emergency mode. This occurs when a system failure or error exists. If this illuminates, replace the ventilator and contact your service representative.

Safety Valve Open

This condition may occur when AC power or both gas supplies are interrupted, when a fault is detected, or when POST is running. This is a safety feature that allows the patient to breathe spontaneously without ventilator assistance. If this is an emergency condition, replace the ventilator, and contact your service representative.

Normal

When this display is illuminated, no alarm, caution, or emergency exists. The ventilator is operating normally.

STANDARD ALARMS

Set the controls to the following settings and attach the ventilator to a test lung or lung analog:

Mode	CMV
Wave Form	square
Tidal Volume	800 ml
Rate	12 breaths/min
High Pressure Limit	80 cm H_2O
Peak Flow	70 L/min
Nebulizer	off
Sensitivity	−2 cm H_2O
Oxygen Concentration	21%
Inspiratory Pause	0
PEEP	0
Alarms	adjust for settings

Low Inspiratory Pressure Alarm

Adjust the low pressure to 10 cm H_2O below the PIP.

1. Loosen the jar of the Cascade humidifier, creating a leak in the circuit. Observe the pressure manometer and the control panel.
2. Tighten the Cascade humidifier.
3. Disconnect the patient wye from the test lung or lung analog. Observe the pressure manometer and the control panel.

Question:

A. What event(s) occurred?

Low Exhaled Tidal Volume Alarm

Set the controls to the same settings as in the low inspiratory pressure activity.

1. Adjust the low exhaled tidal volume control 200 ml higher than the indicated exhaled volume on the control panel. Observe the pressure manometer and control panel.
2. Adjust the low exhaled volume control 200 ml lower than the indicated exhaled volume on the control panel. Create a leak by loosening the Cascade humidifier jar or adjusting the leak control on the lung analog. Observe the pressure manometer and control panel.

Questions:

A. What event(s) occurred?
B. Can you think of patient care situations that may trigger this alarm?

Low Exhaled Minute Volume Alarm

1. Depress the minute volume key on the patient data portion of the control panel and record that value.
2. Adjust the minute volume alarm to 300 ml greater than the value recorded for the preceding step.

Questions:

A. What event(s) occurred?
B. Can you think of patient care situations that may trigger this alarm?

Low PEEP/CPAP Pressure Alarm

This alarm will be covered in Chapter 27, "Special Ventilatory Procedures."

High Respiratory Rate Alarm

This alarm will alert the practitioner when the patient is breathing at a respiratory rate higher than that set on the alarm. This alarm is useful for IMV and CPAP modes.

Exhalation Valve Leak

This alarm alerts you when the flow of gas to the exhalation valve is 10% of the tidal volume or 50 ml. This condition may be simulated by loosening the exhalation valve drive line to create a leak of sufficient magnitude to trigger the alarm.

NONSTANDARD ALARMS
High Pressure Limit

1. Set the controls to the settings for the standard alarms practice activities.
2. Adjust the high pressure limit alarm to 10 cm H_2O less than the peak inspiratory pressure (PIP).

Questions:

A. What event(s) occurred?
B. Can you think of patient care situations that could cause this alarm to be activated?

Low Pressure Oxygen Inlet Alarm

Set the controls for the following settings:

Peak Flow	40 L/min
Sensitivity	−2 cm H_2O
Normal Pressure Limit	70 cm H_2O
Normal Tidal Volume	500 ml
Rate	12 breaths/min
Oxygen Concentration	40%

1. Disconnect the ventilator from the 50 psi oxygen source.

Questions:

A. What event(s) occurred?
B. Do you suspect that this alarm is an oxygen analyzer?

Low Pressure Air Inlet Alarm

1. Set the controls to the settings for the low oxygen pressure inlet alarm practice activities.
2. Disconnect the ventilator from the high-pressure air source.

Questions:

A. What event(s) occurred?
B. Do you suspect that this alarm is an oxygen analyzer?

I:E Alarm

1. Set the controls to the settings for the standard alarm practice activities.
2. Adjust the peak inspiratory flow to 10 L/min.

Questions:

A. What event(s) occurred?
B. How can you correct this condition?
C. What do you suspect caused the condition?

Low Battery

This alarm condition exists when the internal battery pack does not have enough charge to sustain the audible alarm for 1 hour. If this occurs, charge or replace the battery pack (refer to the operator's manual).

Plateau

This control is used to provide a slight inspiratory pause prior to exhalation. It holds pressure in the lungs for the number of seconds set on the control after the completion of inspiration.

1. Set the controls to the same settings used in the alarm section and attach the ventilator to a test lung or lung analog.
2. Set the inspiratory pause control to 1 second. Observe the pressure manometer.

3. Set the inspiratory pause control to 2 seconds. Observe the pressure manometer.

Question:

A. What happened by activating this control?

ADDITIONAL ACTIVITIES

Establish the following tidal volumes, rates, and FIO_2 levels. All volumes are assumed to be corrected volumes and all FIO_2 levels must be adjusted to ±2%. Verify all respiratory rates by using your watch and timing a minute interval.

1. Tidal Volume — 1000 ml
   Rate — 10/min
   FIO_2 — 0.40
   Flow Rate — 40 L/min

2. Tidal Volume — 1200 ml
   Rate — 8/min
   FIO_2 — 0.35
   Flow Rate — 60 L/min

3. Tidal Volume — 800 ml
   Rate — 14/min
   FIO_2 — 0.50
   Flow Rate — 70 L/min

Practice Activities: Siemens Servo 900C

CIRCUIT ASSEMBLY

Figure 26-27 shows the Servo 900C assembled and ready for the initiation of mechanical ventilation.

1. Fill the humidifier with water and attach it to the heating element on the side of the machine. Attach the angled connector to the filter outlet and to the humidifier.

2. Assemble the circuit as shown in Figure 26-28 and attach it to the support arm. The Servo circuit does not have an exhalation valve incorporated into it. Two scissor valves (servo-controlled) inside of the ventilator control inspiration and expiration.

3. Attach the inspiratory side of the circuit to the outlet of the humidifier.

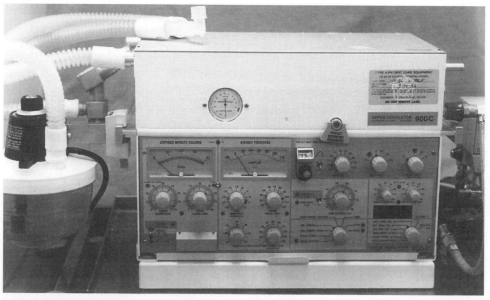

Figure 26-27 *A photograph of the Siemens Elema Servo 900C ventilator*

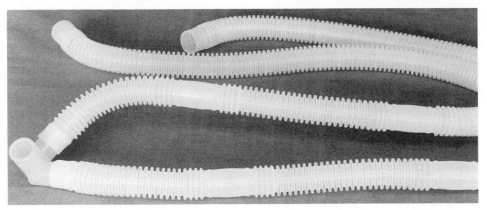

Figure 26-28 *The Siemens Elema Servo 900C circuit ready to attach to the ventilator*

4. Attach the expiratory side to the expiration channel on the side of the ventilator (the fitting that is angled down).

5. Connect the ventilator blender to a 50 psi source of oxygen and air. Connect the ventilator power cord to a suitable 110 V outlet.

6. Adjust the working pressure control until a preset working pressure of 60 cm H_2O is recorded on the working pressure gauge.

7. Attach a test lung and proceed with leak testing and calculation of circuit compliance.

SYSTEM LEAK TEST

1. Set the controls to the following settings:
   a. Mode   Volume control
   b. Minute Volume   1.0 L
   c. Normal Breath Rate   20/min
   d. Upper Pressure Limit   80 cm H_2O

2. Using a sterile gauze or sterile plastic wrap (inside of wrapping that the circuit was packaged in), occlude the patient wye completely.

3. Press the Inspiratory Pause Hold button on the lower left part of the control panel. This will hold pressure in the circuit.

4. Observe the pressure manometer. Pressure should drop slightly and then plateau without dropping further. If the manometer does not remain at a steady value but continues to drop, you have a leak.

5. In the event of a leak, check all tubing connections and humidifier connections (internal and external), and examine the tubing for small holes.

6. Repeat steps 1 through 5 until pressure remains steady in the circuit.

TUBING COMPLIANCE

1. Set the controls to the values listed in system leak test.

2. Using a sterile gauze or sterile plastic wrap (inside of wrapping that the circuit was packaged in), occlude the patient wye completely.

3. As the ventilator cycles, note the pressure reading on the pressure manometer. It may take several breaths to record the pressure accurately.

4. Rotate the multiposition switch on the lower right of the control panel to Exp Tidal Volume. This will display the expired tidal volume. Read the respirometer and record the tidal volume delivered with each breath. This volume represents the volume compressed in the circuit, because no volume was actually delivered.

5. Calculate the tubing compliance using the following formula:

$$\text{Tubing compliance} = \frac{\text{tidal volume}}{\text{peak inspiratory pressure}}$$

ACTIVITIES

To complete these practice activities, it is recommended that you use a lung analog/simulator such as a Medishield Lung Ventilator Performance Analyzer or Retec Respirator Teaching Console. Both of these devices or other similar devices can alter resistance and compliance simulating changes in patient condition.

If these devices are not available, a patient wye and two test lungs may be used as shown in Figure 26-15. Exercise caution. Volumes and pressures may exceed the limits of the test lungs. Resistance may be altered by adapting different inlet tubing sizes, and compliance may be altered by the addition of rubber bands to the test lungs.

INITIAL SETTINGS

   a. Mode   Volume control
   b. Working Pressure   60 cm H_2O
   c. Preset Minute Volume   6.0 L
   d. Upper Pressure Limit   80 cm H_2O
   e. Breaths Per Minute   12
   f. Inspiratory Time   25%
   g. Pause Time   0
   h. Trigger Sensitivity   −2
   i. Oxygen Concentration   21%
   j. Wave Form   square
   k. Alarms   off
   l. PEEP   off
   m. Inspiratory Pressure
      Above PEEP   off
   n. Alarms   off
   o. Inverse Ratio Limit   off

Manipulate only one control at a time and note the result in the space provided on the ventilator flow sheet. Answer the questions that follow each of the activities.

CALCULATION OF TIDAL VOLUME

Tidal volume is calculated by dividing the minute volume by the rate (Ve/rate = tidal volume).

Adjust the minute volume control so that the corrected tidal volume is 500 ml, using the following formula:

$$\text{Corrected tidal volume} = \text{measured tidal volume} - (\text{peak inspiratory pressure} \times \text{tubing compliance})$$

MINUTE VOLUME CONTROL

1. Adjust the minute volume control to 24 L/min.
   a. Calculate tidal volume.
   b. Calculate the corrected tidal volume.
   c. Adjust the corrected tidal volume to the calculated value by manipulating the minute volume control.

2. Adjust the minute volume control to 6 L/min.
   a. Calculate tidal volume.
   b. Calculate the corrected tidal volume.
   c. Adjust the corrected tidal volume to the calculated value by manipulating the minute volume control.

Questions:

A. How do you account for the differences in tidal volume between the two activities?
B. Why were there differences in peak inspiratory pressure?
C. Why did corrected tidal volume vary?

NORMAL RATE CONTROL

1. Set the controls to the settings for the previous activity.
   a. Measure tidal volume.
   b. Measure peak inspiratory pressure.
   c. Calculate corrected tidal volume.

2. Turn the rate control to 6 breaths/min.
   a. Measure tidal volume.
   b. Measure peak inspiratory pressure.
   c. Calculate corrected tidal volume.

3. Turn the rate control to 24 breaths/min.
   a. Measure tidal volume.
   b. Measure peak inspiratory pressure.
   c. Calculate corrected tidal volume.

Questions:

A. What happened to the peak pressure and why?
B. Why did the inspiratory time increase?
C. How do you account for the increase in tidal volume?

4. Return the normal rate control to 12 breaths/min.

INSPIRATORY TIME % CONTROL

This control and the pause time % (indirectly) determine the length of the inspiratory phase of ventilation.

The rate control determines the number of breaths that will occur each minute. For example, setting the normal rate to 12 breaths/min will result in one breath being given every 5 seconds.

Setting the inspiratory time % control to 25% will result in inspiration occupying 25% of the time allotted to the ventilatory cycle. This may be calculated by multiplying the inspiratory time % by the total time allowed for each cycle (0.25 × 5 seconds = 1.25 seconds).

Questions:

For the following rates and inspiratory time % settings, calculate the inspiratory time in seconds.
   a. 12 breaths/min   Inspiratory Time % = 25%
   b. 6 breaths/min   Inspiratory Time % = 50%
   c. 24 breaths/min   Inspiratory Time % = 20%
   d. 15 breaths/min   Inspiratory Time % = 33%

PAUSE TIME % CONTROL

This control provides a momentary inspiratory pause by closing the inspiratory and expiratory valves momentarily after delivery of a breath. The pause time, like the inspiratory time %, is a percentage of the total ventilatory cycle. The total inspiratory time is the combination of inspiratory time % and pause time % (inspiratory time % + pause time %).

The pause time in seconds may be calculated by multiplying the ventilatory cycle time by the pause time %.

For example, if the normal rate is set for 12 breaths/min (one breath every 5 seconds) and the pause time % is set for 10%, the pause time in seconds is 0.5 second (0.10 × 5 seconds = 0.5 seconds).

If the inspiratory time % control is also set at 25%, the total inspiratory time is 35% (25% inspiratory time % + 10% pause time %). The total inspiratory time in seconds is 1.75 seconds [(0.25 + 0.10) × 5 seconds = 1.75 seconds].

Questions:

For the following examples, calculate the pause time in seconds and the total inspiratory time in seconds.
   a. Rate = 12/min, Inspiratory Time % = 25%, Pause Time % = 5%
   b. Rate = 20/min, Inspiratory Time % = 33%, Pause Time % = 0
   c. Rate = 10/min, Inspiratory Time % = 20%, Pause Time % = 20%

CALCULATION OF I:E RATIO

The I:E ratio is not displayed directly on the Servo 900C. It must be calculated. To calculate the I:E ratio, you must first calculate the total inspiratory time in seconds (Inspiratory Time % + Pause Time %). Once inspiratory time is known, the remaining portion of the ventilatory cycle is for expiration. For example, if the rate is 12 breaths/min, inspiratory time % is 25%, and pause time % is 5%, total inspiratory time is 30% or 1.5 seconds (0.25 + 0.05) × 5 seconds = 1.5 seconds). Expiratory time is 3.5 seconds (5 seconds − 1.5 seconds = 3.5 seconds). The I:E ratio is 1.5:3.5 or 1:2.3.

Questions:

For the following settings, calculate the I:E ratio:
   a. Normal Rate = 12, Inspiratory Time % = 25%, Pause Time % = 10%
   b. Normal Rate = 20, Inspiratory Time % = 33%, Pause Time % = 0
   c. Normal Rate = 15, Inspiratory Time % = 20%, Pause Time % = 20%

CALCULATION OF PEAK FLOW RATE
Square Wave Pattern

The Servo 900C does not have a peak flow rate control. Flow rate is determined by the settings on the minute volume, rate, and inspiratory time % controls. When the ventilator is operating in the square wave flow pattern, it is functioning as a constant flow generator. For each of the inspiratory time % settings, there is a corresponding factor used to determine peak flow (McPherson & Spearman, 1995). Table 26-6 is a reproduction of these factors for the 900C.

To calculate peak flow rate, multiply the setting on the minute volume control by the factor for the inspiratory time % setting. For example, if the minute volume is 14 L/min and the inspiratory time % is 25%, the peak flow rate is 56 L/min (14 L/min $\times$ 4 = 56 L/min).

Tapered or Sine Wave Pattern

When the ventilator is operating in this pattern, calculating the peak flow using the method discussed above will result in an average rather than peak flow (McPherson & Spearman, 1995). To calculate the peak flow in the sine wave pattern, multiply the average flow by 1.5. For example, if the minute volume is 14 L/min and the inspiratory time % is 25%, the peak flow is 84 L/min [(14 L/min $\times$ 4) $\times$ 1.5 = 84 L/min].

TRIGGER SENSITIVITY CONTROL

The trigger sensitivity control determines how much patient effort is required to initiate an assisted, SIMV, pressure support, or CPAP breath. The control is automatically indexed to any settings on the PEEP control so that readjustment is not required when initiating PEEP.

1. Set the controls to the following settings:

Working Pressure	60 cm H_2O
Mode	Volume control
Minute Volume	12 L/min
Breaths/min	12 breaths/min
Inspiratory Time %	25%
Pause Time %	0
Upper Pressure Limit	70 cm H_2O
PEEP	0
Inspiratory Pressure Above PEEP	0

2. Set the trigger sensitivity control to –2 cm H_2O. While observing the pressure manometer, initiate a breath. Record the pressure on the manometer when a breath is delivered.

3. Set the trigger sensitivity control to –10 cm H_2O. While observing the pressure manometer, initiate a breath. Record the pressure on the manometer when a breath is delivered.

Questions:

A. How can you account for the difference in the pressure (negative) required to initiate a breath?

B. Where would you normally set the sensitivity control in clinical practice?

C. As a patient, how would you want the control to be set?

TABLE 26-6: Flow Rate Calculation Factors

INSPIRATORY TIME %	FACTOR
20%	5
25%	4
33%	3
50%	2
67%	1.5
80%	1.25

Reproduced by permission from Steven P. McPherson, Respiratory therapy equipment (3rd ed.), St. Louis, 1995, C.V. Mosby Company.

UPPER PRESSURE LIMIT CONTROL

The upper pressure limit control is similar to pressure limit controls on other ventilators. When the peak pressure reaches the value set on the control, inspiration will terminate and visual and audible alarms will activate.

1. Set the controls to the settings used in the trigger sensitivity activity.

2. Set the upper pressure limit control to 10 cm H_2O greater than the cycling pressure.

3. Decrease the compliance of the lung analog by 2/3. Observe what event(s) occur.

Questions:

A. What event(s) occurred?

B. What is the purpose of the upper pressure limit control?

C. List a patient care situation that would cause a similar event in the clinical setting that you just simulated.

VOLUME CONTROL PLUS SIGH

The Servo 900C does not have separate sigh controls. Sigh volume is administered by selecting the sigh mode. The ventilator electronically delivers the sign breaths. Every 100 control breaths the inspiratory time % is doubled, doubling the volume delivered. In this mode, the upper exhaled volume alarm limit may need to be adjusted to a higher setting.

PRESSURE CONTROL MODE

When this mode is selected, the ventilator stops functioning as a volume ventilator. Breaths are delivered at a constant pressure determined by the setting on the inspiratory pressure level above PEEP control. Rate, inspiratory time %, pause time %, and trigger sensitivity may all be set in this mode. Volume delivery will vary with changes in the patient's compliance and resistance.

ALARM FUNCTIONS
Lower and Upper Expired Minute Volume Alarm
These two alarms are typically set to 20% greater and less than the preset minute volume control in adult patients (30% is recommended when ventilating in the volume control plus sigh mode). If these limits are exceeded, visual and audible alarms will activate.

Set O₂ Alarm
The Servo 900C has a built-in oxygen analyzer. Alarms are provided with both high and low settings. It is recommended that this alarm be set to 6% above and below the desired FIO_2.

Digital Display
The multiposition switch located at the lower right of the control panel allows you to select and monitor a specific parameter. The selections include mean airway pressure, pause pressure, peak pressure, expired minute volume, expired tidal volume, inspired tidal volume, oxygen concentration, and respiratory rate. Whatever is selected on this switch, the parameter is displayed in the LED window.

SPECIAL FEATURES
Inspiratory Pause Hold
Pressing this button will close both the inspiratory and expiratory scissor valves holding a breath at end inspiration.

Expiratory Pause Hold
Pressing this button will close both the inspiratory and expiratory scissor valves holding a breath at end expiration.

Gas Change
Pressing this button quickly purges the bellows, internal tubing, and patient circuit with fresh gas from the blender. This control allows for rapid FIO_2 changes (decreases ventilator wash-out time).

SIMV AND PRESSURE SUPPORT
These two modes will be discussed in Chapter 27, "Special Ventilatory Procedures."

CHANGES IN RESISTANCE AND COMPLIANCE
1. Set the controls to the following settings:

Working Pressure	60 cm H₂O
Minute Volume	8 L/min
Breaths per Minute	10 breaths/min
Inspiratory Time %	25%
Pause Time %	0
Upper Press. Limit	60 cm H₂O
Trigger Sensitivity	−2 cm H₂O
Alarms	off

   a. Measure peak inspiratory pressure.
   b. Calculate inspiratory time.
   c. Calculate corrected tidal volume.
   d. Calculate the I:E ratio.

2. Decrease the compliance by ⅓ by adjusting the spring tension or manipulating the compliance control on the lung analog.
   a. Measure peak inspiratory pressure.
   b. Calculate inspiratory time.
   c. Calculate corrected tidal volume.
   d. Calculate the I:E ratio.

Questions:
A. Why did the corrected tidal volume decrease?
B. Why did the I:E ratio vary?
C. Why did the peak inspiratory pressure increase?

3. Return the compliance to the original value on the lung analog.

4. Increase the resistance by ⅓ by adjusting the resistance control on the lung analog.
   a. Measure peak inspiratory pressure.
   b. Calculate inspiratory time.
   c. Calculate corrected tidal volume.
   d. Calculate the I:E ratio.

Questions:
Compared to the original values in this activity:
A. Why did the inspiratory pressure increase?
B. Why did the I:E ratio vary?
C. How do you account for differences in the corrected tidal volume?
D. Can you think of human physiological conditions that could produce similar results?

5. Return the resistance control to the original value on the lung analog.

6. Set the pressure limit control to 10 cm H₂O greater than the cycling pressure.

7. Decrease the compliance by ⅔ by adjusting spring tension or adjusting the compliance control on the lung analog.

Questions:
A. What event(s) occurred?
B. Can you think of a patient situation that could cause this?
C. What is the purpose of the upper pressure limit control?

ADDITIONAL ACTIVITIES
Establish the following tidal volumes, rates, and FIO_2 levels. All volumes are assumed to be corrected volumes and all FIO_2 levels must be adjusted to ±2%. Verify all respiratory rates by using your watch and timing a 1-minute interval.

1. Tidal Volume — 1000 ml
   Rate — 10/min
   FIO_2 — 0.40

2. Tidal Volume — 1200 ml
   Rate — 8/min
   FIO_2 — 0.35

3. Tidal Volume — 800 ml
   Rate — 14/min
   FIO_2 — 0.50

Practice Activities: Siemens Servo 300

CIRCUIT ASSEMBLY

Figure 26-28 shows the patient circuit for the Servo 300 ventilator, and Figure 26-29 shows the ventilator itself.

1. Connect one high-pressure hose to a 50 psi source of air and the other to a 50 psi source of oxygen.

2. Connect the power cord to a suitable grounded AC outlet.

3. Assemble the patient circuit, which consists of an inspiratory limb, patient wye, and expiratory limb.

4. Connect a bacteria filter to the ventilator outlet and connect it to the humidifier with a short length of 22-mm-diameter flexible tubing.

5. Connect the inspiratory limb to the humidifier and the expiratory limb to the expiratory inlet.

PREUSE CHECK

1. Connect the patient wye to a test lung or lung analog.

2. Set the controls to the following settings:

Range	Adult
Airway Pressure (Upper Limit)	60 cm H_2O
Pressure Control Level	0.0 cm H_2O
PEEP	40 cm H_2O
Trigger Sensitivity	–17 cm H_2O
CMV Frequency	20/min
Inspiratory Time	25%
Pause Time %	10%
Insp. Rise Time	5%
SIMV Frequency	0.5
Lower Alarm Limit	0.0 L/min
Upper Alarm Limit	60 L/min
Volume	8 o'clock position
O_2 Concentration	40%
Mode	Ventilator off/ Battery charging

3. Make sure that the yellow light at the "Ventilator off/Battery charging" and the green light "Mains" are lit.

4. Open the lid on the patient unit (lower module).

5. Perform a start-up check.
   a. Set the mode selector to "Standby" and verify the following:
   — All yellow lights are lit for a few seconds.
   — All yellow and red lights in the alarm section stay lit during an additional moment.
   — The audible alarm signal is heard.
   — The caution sound is heard.
   — The expiratory valve closes.
   — The safety valve closes with a distinctive audible sound.
   — The "Alarms and Messages" display shows "STAND BY."

6. Perform a tightness check:
   a. Set the ventilator in pressure control mode.
   b. Set the pause hold control at the expiration position.
   c. Verify that the pressure does not drop more than 10 cm H_2O.
   d. Release the pause hold control (middle position).
   e. Set the PEEP to 0 cm H_2O.

7. Check the upper pressure alarm:
   a. Set the pressure control level to 30 cm H_2O.
   b. Turn the upper pressure limit control slowly counterclockwise until the alarm is heard.
   c. Verify that the following has occurred:
   — The upper pressure limit alarm activates at ±2 cm H_2O from the set value.
   — Inspiration stops and expiration begins.
   — The red light at "Airway Pressure" illuminates.
   — The yellow light at "Airway Pressure" illuminates during expiration.
   — The "Alarms and Messages" display shows AIRWAY PRESSURE TOO HIGH.

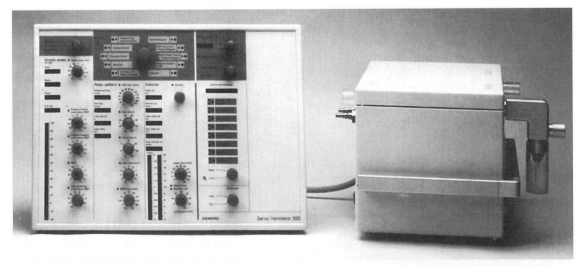

Figure 26-29 *A photograph of the Siemens Elema Servo 300 ventilator (Courtesy of Siemens Medical Systems,* Electromedical Group, Danvers, MA)

— The upper pressure limit indication on the airway bargraph flashes.

d. Set the upper pressure limit to 60 cm H_2O.

e. Set the pressure control level to zero.

f. Reset the alarm.

8. Check the minute volume alarms:

a. Set the ventilator in the volume control mode.

b. Adjust the volume control until the minute volume display reads 7.5 L/min.

— Verify that the display reads 7.5 L/min ± 0.2 L/min.

Lower Alarm Limit:

a. Turn the lower alarm limit control clockwise until it is activated, and verify the following:

— The alarm is activated once the 7.5 L/min value has been passed.

— The lower alarm limit indication on the minute volume bargraph flashes.

— The indication for the lower alarm limit on the minute volume bargraph is the same as the lower alarm limit setting ± 0.5 L/min.

— The "Alarms and Messages" display shows EXP MINUTE VOLUME TOO LOW.

— The red light at "Exp. minute volume" flashes.

b. Turn the lower alarm limit control to 0.0 L/min.

c. Reset the alarm.

Upper Alarm Limit:

a. Turn the upper alarm limit control slowly counterclockwise and verify the following:

— The alarm is activated once the 7.5 L/min value has been passed.

— The upper alarm limit indication on the minute volume bargraph flashes.

— The indication for the upper alarm limit on the minute volume bargraph is the same as the upper alarm limit setting ± 0.5 L/min.

— The "Alarms and Messages" display shows EXP MINUTE VOLUME TOO HIGH.

— The red light at "Exp. minute volume" flashes.

9. Check the apnea alarm.

a. Set the ventilator into volume support mode.

b. Wait for 20 seconds and confirm the following:

— That the apnea alarm is activated.

— The "Alarms and Messages" display shows APNEA ALARM.

— The ventilator changes from volume support to pressure regulated volume control mode.

c. Reset the alarm and make sure the ventilator switches back to volume support mode.

d. Set the ventilator into volume control mode.

10. Check the oxygen alarm system.

Lower Alarm Limit:

a. Turn and hold the "Pause Hold" at "Exp" and read the oxygen concentration value on the display "Alarms and Messages."

b. Turn the "O_2 Conc. %" clockwise and make sure of the following:

— The O_2 Concentration alarm activates when the reading is 6 ± 1% higher than the "Alarms and Messages" reading.

— The "Alarms and Messages" display reads O_2 CONC TOO LOW.

c. Set the "O_2 Conc. %" to 40%.

d. Release the "Pause Hold" button.

Upper Alarm Limit:

a. Turn and hold the "Pause Hold" at "Exp" and read the oxygen concentration value on the display "Alarms and Messages."

b. Turn the "O_2 Conc. %" counterclockwise and make sure of the following:

— The O_2 concentration alarm activates when the reading is 6 ± 1% lower than the "Alarms and Messages" reading.

— The "Alarms and Messages" display reads O_2 CONC TOO HIGH.

c. Set the "O_2 Conc. %" to 40%.

d. Release the "Pause Hold" button.

11. Check the input power alarms.

Gas Supply Pressure Alarms:

a. Disconnect the oxygen supply line from its 50 psi source and verify the following:

— The red light at "Gas supply" flashes and the "Alarms and Messages" display shows O2 SUPPLY PRESSURE TOO LOW. AIR:X.X BAR.O2: X.X BAR.

b. Connect the oxygen supply line.

c. Reset the alarm.

d. Disconnect the air supply line from its 50 psi source and verify the following:

— The red light at "Gas supply" flashes and the "Alarms and Messages" display shows AIR SUPPLY PRESSURE TOO LOW.AIR:X.X BAR.O2: X.X BAR.

e. Mute the alarm with a 2-minute reset and make sure that:

— The red display "Exp. Minute vol. L/min" still shows the same value as the green display "Minute vol. L/min" ± 0.5 L/min.

f. Disconnect the oxygen supply line from its 50 psi source so that no high pressure gas enters the ventilator and verify that the safety valve opens with a distinctive sound.

g. Reconnect both air and oxygen supply lines.

h. Reset the alarms.

12. Check the battery operation.

a. Disconnect the ventilator from its alternating current power source and verify the following:

— The yellow light at the "Ventilator off Battery Charging" and the green light "Mains" go out.

— The audible alarm is activated.

— The red light at "Battery" flashes.

— The display "Alarms and Messages" flashes BATTERY.

b. Reset the alarm and make sure that the following occurs:

— The caution sound begins.

— The yellow light at "Battery" is lit.

c. To check the internal battery, touch the touch pad at "Battery" and read the displayed text, which should normally read about 24 V.

d. Reconnect the ventilator to its AC source and ensure that the following occurs:
 — The yellow light at "Ventilator off Battery charging" and the green light "Mains" are lit.
 — The yellow light at "Battery" is no longer lit.
 — The display "Alarms and Messages" no longer shows BATTERY.
 — The caution sound stops.
e. Set the mode selector to stand by.

ACTIVITIES

To complete these practice activities, it is recommended that you use a lung analog/simulator such as a Medishield Lung Ventilator Performance Analyzer or other test lung in which resistance and compliance may be easily altered.

INITIAL VENTILATOR SETTINGS

a. Range — Adult
b. Mode — Volume control
c. Minute Volume — 6.0 L/min
d. Upper Pressure Limit — 80 cm H_2O
e. CMV Freq. — 12/min
f. Inspiratory Time % — 25%
g. Pause Time % — 0.0%
h. Trigger Sensitivity — −2 cm H_2O
i. Inspiratory Rise Time % — 1%
j. PEEP — 0 cm H_2O
k. Pressure Control — 0 cm H_2O
l. O_2 Concentration — 21%

Manipulate only one control at a time and note the results on a sheet of paper. Answer the questions following each activity on the same sheet of paper. If you encounter difficulties, ask your laboratory instructor for assistance.

VOLUME CONTROL

1. Adjust the volume control to 24 L/min.
 a. Measure and record the tidal volume.
 b. Measure the peak pressure.
 c. Using a stopwatch or second hand, measure the inspiratory time.
2. Set the volume control to 6 L/min.
 a. Measure and record the tidal volume.
 b. Measure the peak pressure.
 c. Using a stopwatch or second hand, measure the inspiratory time.

Questions:
A. Why did the tidal volume vary between the two activities?
B. How did the inspiratory pressure change?
C. Why did the inspiratory time differ between the two activities?

CMV FREQUENCY CONTROL

1. Reset the controls to the initial ventilator settings for these activities.
 a. Measure the tidal volume.
 b. Measure the peak inspiratory pressure.
 c. Measure the inspiratory time.

2. Set the CMV frequency control to 6 breaths/min.
 a. Measure the tidal volume.
 b. Measure the peak inspiratory pressure.
 c. Measure the inspiratory time.
3. Set the CMV frequency control to 20 breaths/min.
 a. Measure the tidal volume.
 b. Measure the peak inspiratory pressure.
 c. Measure the inspiratory time.

Questions:
A. What happened to the peak inspiratory pressure?
B. What happened to the tidal volume?
C. What happened to the inspiratory time?

4. Return the CMV frequency control to 12/min.

INSPIRATORY TIME % CONTROL

This control and the pause time % control determine the length of the inspiratory phase of ventilation.

The CMV frequency control determines the number of breaths that will occur each minute. For example, setting the CMV frequency control to 12 breaths/min will result in one breath being given every 5 seconds.

Setting the inspiratory time % control to 25% will result in inspiration occupying 25% of the time allotted to the ventilatory cycle. This may be calculated by multiplying the inspiratory time % control by the total time allowed for each cycle.

1. Set the ventilator to the settings at the beginning of this activity.
2. Adjust the inspiratory time % control to 50%.
 a. Measure the peak pressure.
 b. Measure the inspiratory time.
3. Adjust the inspiratory time % control to 10%.
 a. Measure the peak pressure.
 b. Measure the inspiratory time.

Questions:
A. What happened to the peak pressure?
B. What happened to the inspiratory time?

PAUSE TIME % CONTROL

This control provides a momentary inspiratory pause at the end of inspiration. The pause time % control, like the inspiratory time % control, affects the total inspiratory time. The inspiratory time is equal to the sum of the inspiratory time % and pause time %.

1. Set the ventilator to the settings at the beginning of this activity.
2. Adjust the pause time % control to 30%.
 a. Measure the peak pressure.
 b. Measure the inspiratory time.
3. Set the pause time % control to 15%.
 a. Measure the peak pressure.
 b. Measure the inspiratory time.

Questions:
A. What happened to the peak pressure?
B. What happened to the inspiratory time?

TRIGGER SENSITIVITY

The Servo 300 ventilator may be pressure or flow triggered in all modes of ventilation, allowing a high degree of flexibility.

Pressure Triggering

1. Adjust the ventilator to the settings at the beginning of these activities.

2. Attach a mouthpiece to the patient wye and attempt to initiate a breath, observing the pressure manometer.

3. Set the trigger sensitivity to 8 cm H_2O and initiate a breath, observing the pressure manometer.

4. Set the assist sensitivity to 0.5 cm H_2O. Again using a mouthpiece, initiate a breath while observing the pressure manometer.

Questions:

A. When were you able to most easily initiate a breath?
B. Where would you prefer as a patient to have the assist sensitivity control set?
C. What changes did you observe on the Pressure Volume loop between the two settings?

Flow Triggering

1. Reset the ventilator to the settings established at the start of this activity.

2. Rotate the trigger sensitivity control clockwise into the upper part of the green marked area. Attempt to initiate a breath and observe the pressure manometer.

3. Rotate the trigger sensitivity control clockwise into the upper part of the red marked area. Attempt to initiate a breath and observe the pressure manometer.

Questions:

A. Which setting would you prefer as a patient?
B. Which setting was easiest for you?
C. How can you best use the pressure manometer to set the sensitivity control?

Pressure Control Ventilation

Set the ventilator to the following settings:

Range	Adult
Mode	Pressure control
Minute Volume	6.0 L/min
Upper Pressure Limit	80 cm H_2O
CMV Freq.	12/min
Inspiratory Time %	25%
Pause Time %	0.0%
Trigger Sensitivity	−2 cm H_2O
Inspiratory Rise Time %	1%
PEEP	0 cm H_2O
Pressure Control	25 cm H_2O
O_2 Concentration	21%

PRESSURE CONTROL

1. With the ventilator in pressure control, measure the following:
   a. Peak inspiratory pressure
   b. Inspiratory time
   c. Tidal volume

2. Set the pressure control to 40 cm H_2O and measure the following:
   a. Peak inspiratory pressure
   b. Inspiratory time
   c. Tidal volume

Questions:

A. How did the pressure control affect peak inspiratory pressure?
B. How did the pressure control affect the inspiratory time?
C. How did the pressure control affect the tidal volume?

3. Set the controls back to the settings at the beginning of the pressure control ventilation activity.

INSPIRATORY TIME % AND PAUSE TIME %

Inspiratory Time % Control

1. Adjust the inspiratory time % control to 50%.
   a. Measure the peak pressure.
   b. Measure the inspiratory time.

2. Adjust the inspiratory time % control to 10%.
   a. Measure the peak pressure.
   b. Measure the inspiratory time.

Questions:

A. What happened to the peak pressure?
B. What happened to the inspiratory time?

Pause Time % Control

1. Set the ventilator to the settings at the beginning of this activity.

2. Adjust the pause time % control to 30%.
   a. Measure the peak pressure.
   b. Measure the inspiratory time.

3. Set the pause time % control to 15%.
   a. Measure the peak pressure.
   b. Measure the inspiratory time.

Questions:

A. What happened to the peak pressure?
B. What happened to the inspiratory time?

ALARM SYSTEMS

The Servo 300 ventilator has multiple alarm systems to improve patient safety and to facilitate detection of changes in the patient's condition.

Upper Pressure Alarm

1. Set the controls to the following settings:

Range	Adult
Mode	Volume control
Minute Volume	10.0 L/min
Upper Pressure Limit	80 cm H_2O
CMV Freq.	12/min
Inspiratory Time %	25%
Pause Time %	0.0%
Trigger Sensitivity	−2 cm H_2O
Inspiratory Rise Time %	1%
PEEP	0 cm H_2O

Pressure Control   0 cm H_2O
O_2 Concentration   21%

1. Adjust the upper pressure limit control to 15 cm H_2O.
   a. Observe what happens.
2. Set the upper pressure limit control 15 cm H_2O greater than the peak inspiratory pressure and quickly compress the test lung, simulating a cough.
   a. Observe what happens.

Questions:
   A. What occurred (alarms, indicators, ventilator action)?
   B. What do you feel is an appropriate setting for this alarm?

3. Reset the upper pressure limit to 80 cm H_2O.

Minute Volume Alarms
1. Set the lower alarm limit to 9.0 L/min.
2. Change the CMV frequency to 5/min and observe what occurs.
3. Set the lower alarm limit back to 9.0 L/min.
4. Set the upper alarm limit to 11 L/min.
5. Increase the CMV frequency to 15/min and observe what happens.

Questions:
   A. What happened in each situation?
   B. What is an appropriate setting for this alarm?

Apnea Alarm
1. Disconnect the test lung and wait for 30 seconds, observing what occurs.

Questions:
   A. What occurred after 20 seconds?
   B. How would this alarm be clinically useful?

Oxygen Alarm System
1. Set the O_2 concentration to 40%.
2. Set the lower alarm limit to 30% and the upper limit to 50%.
3. Turn the O_2 concentration to 60% and observe what occurs.
4. Turn the O_2 concentration to 21% and observe what occurs.

Questions:
   A. What happened?
   B. How would this alarm be clinically useful?

Check List: Initiation of Ventilation

_____ 1. Verify the order.
_____ 2. Scan the patient's chart as time permits.
_____ 3. Measure the mechanics of ventilation.
_____ 4. Assess oxygenation and cardiac status.
_____ 5. Gather the required equipment.
_____ 6. Assemble and test the equipment.
_____ 7. Adjust the ventilator to the ordered settings.
_____ 8. Connect the patient.
_____ 9. Monitor all ventilator parameters.
_____   a. Corrected tidal volume
_____   b. Rate

_____   c. FiO_2
_____   d. Adjust sensitivity.
_____   e. Adjust flow rate.
_____   f. Adjust I:E ratio to 1:2 or greater.
_____   g. Set pressure limit.
_____   h. Set all alarms.
_____   i. Record all ventilator parameters.
_____ 10. Draw arterial blood gases if ordered after 20 minutes or monitor oximetry.
_____ 11. Clean up the area.
_____ 12. Record the procedure on the patient's chart.

Check List: Monitoring Ventilation

_____ 1. Verify the physician's order.
_____ 2. Explain the procedure.
_____ 3. Assess the patient:
_____   a. Skin color
_____   b. Pulse
_____   c. Blood pressure
_____   d. Cardiac rate/rhythm
_____   e. Level of consciousness
_____   f. Breath sounds
_____ 4. Suction the patient as required.
_____ 5. Empty the condensate from the tubing.

_____ 6. Calculate corrected tidal volume.
_____ 7. Calculate static and dynamic compliance.
_____ 8. Adjust ventilator settings as required.
_____ 9. Measure FiO_2.
_____ 10. Measure circuit temperature.
_____ 11. Adjust ventilator settings and monitor as required.
_____ 12. Record all ventilator settings.
_____ 13. Use aseptic technique standard precautions.
_____ 14. Record the procedure on the patient's chart.

Check List: Changing a Ventilator Circuit

_____ 1. Verify the physician's order.
_____ 2. Explain the procedure.
_____ 3. Assemble the required equipment:
_____   a. Personal protective equipment
_____   b. New circuit and humidifier
_____   c. Manual resuscitator
_____   d. Plastic bag for disposal of old circuit
_____   e. Respirometer, if required
_____ 4. Suction the patient as required.
_____ 5. Drain the condensate from the tubing.
_____ 6. Prepare the resuscitator for use.
_____ 7. Disconnect all alarms.

_____ 8. Disconnect and manually ventilate the patient.
_____ 9. Change the circuit within 2 minutes.
_____   a. Test the new circuit.
_____   b. Measure tubing compliance.
_____   c. Check for leaks.
_____ 10. Monitor pressures and tidal volume.
_____ 11. Monitor the patient-ventilator circuit and document the findings on the ventilator flow sheet.
_____ 12. Reset all alarms.
_____ 13. Use aseptic technique standard precautions.
_____ 14. Dispose of equipment properly.
_____ 15. Record the procedure in the patient's chart.

Self-Evaluation Post Test: Continuous Mechanical Ventilation

1. The I:E ratio during mechanical ventilation should be maintained at a value of at least 1:2 because:
   a. it lowers pulmonary capillary pressure.
   b. the negative pressure can cause pulmonary capillary leaking.
   c. it allows more time for the great vessels to fill.
   d. the inspiratory time needs to be longer.

2. Which one of the following maximal inspiratory forces indicates a reduced ventilatory reserve or possible muscle weakness?
   a. -35 cm H_2O
   b. -30 cm H_2O
   c. -45 cm H_2O
   d. -25 cm H_2O

3. Which one of the following respiratory rates indicates impending respiratory failure?
   a. 12 to 15 breaths per minute
   b. 15 to 25 breaths per minute
   c. 20 to 25 breaths per minute
   d. Greater than 35 breaths per minute

4. Which one of the following vital capacities suggests that a patient may have difficulty maintaining normal ventilatory function if he or she becomes fatigued?
   a. Less than 20 ml/kg normal body weight
   b. Less than 15 ml/kg normal body weight
   c. Less than 17 ml/kg normal body weight
   d. Less than 25 ml/kg normal body weight

5. When a volume ventilator encounters increased airway resistance or changes in lung compliance, it will:
   a. continue to deliver a preset volume.
   b. fail to deliver a breath.
   c. continue to deliver a preset volume with increased airway pressures.
   d. deliver a lower volume while the peak pressure remains constant.

6. Tubing compliance factor is determined by:
   a. dividing the tidal volume by the peak pressure.
   b. dividing the peak pressure by the tidal volume.
   c. dividing the corrected tidal volume by the peak pressure.
   d. dividing the peak pressure by the corrected tidal volume.

7. Maximal inspiratory force (MIF) may be measured on an unconscious patient:
   a. by using drugs to stimulate the diaphragm.
   b. if the patient is intubated.
   c. by occluding the safety port on the MIF meter.

8. To calculate corrected tidal volume, you need:
   I.   measured tidal volume.
   II. peak inspiratory pressure.
   III. flow rate.
   IV. tubing compliance factor.
   V.   sigh volume.
   a. I, III, IV
   b. I, II, IV
   c. I, II, III, IV
   d. I, IV, V

9. With use of a volume ventilator, a decrease in total lung compliance will cause a/an:
   a. pressure decrease.
   b. decrease in respiratory rate.
   c. increase in airway pressure.
   d. decrease in delivered volume.

10. The sensitivity control should be adjusted so that the ventilator will cycle at a pressure of:
    a. -10 cm H_2O.
    b. -5 cm H_2O.
    c. -2 cm H_2O.
    d. $+3$ cm H_2O.

PERFORMANCE EVALUATION:
INITIATION OF CONTINUOUS MECHANICAL VENTILATION

Date: Lab _____ Clinical _____ Agency _____

Lab: Pass _____ Fail _____   Clinical: Pass _____ Fail _____

Student name _____   Instructor name _____

No. of times observed in clinical _____

No. of times practiced in clinical _____

PASSING CRITERIA: Obtain 90% or better on the procedure. Tasks indicated by * must receive at least 1 point, or the evaluation is terminated. Procedure must be performed within designated time, or the performance receives a failing grade.

SCORING: 2 points — Task performed satisfactorily without prompting.
1 point — Task performed satisfactorily with self-initiated correction.
0 points — Task performed incorrectly or with prompting required.
NA — Task not applicable to the patient care situation.

TASKS:		PEER	LAB	CLINICAL
*	1. Verifies the physician's order	☐	☐	☐
	2. Reviews the patient's chart	☐	☐	☐
*	3. Gathers the equipment	☐	☐	☐
*	4. Measures the mechanics of ventilation	☐	☐	☐
*	5. Assesses oxygenation and cardiac status	☐	☐	☐
*	6. Tests the equipment for function			
	a. Corrects circuit leaks	☐	☐	☐
	b. Measures circuit compliance	☐	☐	☐
*	7. Adjusts the ventilator to the ordered settings	☐	☐	☐
*	8. Connects the patient	☐	☐	☐
	9. Monitors ventilator parameters			
*	a. Rate	☐	☐	☐
*	b. Tidal volume	☐	☐	☐
*	c. FiO_2	☐	☐	☐
*	d. Sensitivity	☐	☐	☐
*	e. I:E ratio	☐	☐	☐
*	f. Pressure limit	☐	☐	☐
*	g. Circuit temperature	☐	☐	☐
*	h. Measures FiO_2	☐	☐	☐
*	i. Adjusts all alarms	☐	☐	☐
*	10. Draws blood gases or monitors oximetry	☐	☐	☐
	11. Cleans up the area	☐	☐	☐
*	12. Uses aseptic technique	☐	☐	☐
*	13. Records the procedure on the chart	☐	☐	☐

SCORE: Peer _____ points of possible 44; _____%

Lab _____ points of possible 44; _____%

Clinical _____ points of possible 44; _____%

TIME: _____ out of possible 30 minutes

PERFORMANCE EVALUATION:
MONITORING CONTINUOUS MECHANICAL VENTILATION

Date: Lab _____ Clinical _____ Agency _____

Lab: Pass _____ Fail _____   Clinical: Pass _____ Fail _____

Student name _____   Instructor name _____

No. of times observed in clinical _____

No. of times practiced in clinical _____

PASSING CRITERIA: Obtain 90% or better on the procedure. Tasks indicated by * must receive at least 1 point, or the evaluation is terminated. Procedure must be performed within designated time, or the performance receives a failing grade.

SCORING: 2 points — Task performed satisfactorily without prompting.
1 point — Task performed satisfactorily with self-initiated correction.
0 points — Task performed incorrectly or with prompting required.
NA — Task not applicable to the patient care situation.

TASKS:		PEER	LAB	CLINICAL
*	1. Verifies the physician's order	☐	☐	☐
	2. Reviews the patient's chart	☐	☐	☐
*	3. Gathers the equipment	☐	☐	☐
*	4. Explains the procedure to the patient	☐	☐	☐
	5. Assesses the patient			
*	a. Color	☐	☐	☐
*	b. Pulse	☐	☐	☐
*	c. Blood pressure	☐	☐	☐
*	d. Cardiac rate/rhythm	☐	☐	☐
*	e. Level of consciousness	☐	☐	☐
*	f. Breath sounds	☐	☐	☐
*	6. Suctions the patient as required	☐	☐	☐
*	7. Empties the condensate from the tubing	☐	☐	☐
	8. Monitors the ventilator parameters			
*	a. Rate	☐	☐	☐
*	b. Tidal volume	☐	☐	☐
*	c. FiO_2	☐	☐	☐
*	d. Sensitivity	☐	☐	☐
*	e. I:E ratio	☐	☐	☐
*	f. Pressure limit	☐	☐	☐
*	g. Circuit temperature	☐	☐	☐
*	h. Measures FiO_2	☐	☐	☐
*	i. Adjusts all alarms	☐	☐	☐
*	j. Adjusts ventilator settings	☐	☐	☐

9. Cleans up the area

☐ ☐ ☐

* 10. Uses aseptic technique

☐ ☐ ☐

* 11. Records the procedure on the chart

☐ ☐ ☐

SCORE: Peer   _____ points of possible 50; _____%

Lab   _____ points of possible 50; _____%

Clinical   _____ points of possible 50; _____%

TIME: _____ out of possible 30 minutes

STUDENT SIGNATURES

PEER: _____

STUDENT: _____

INSTRUCTOR SIGNATURES

LAB: _____

CLINICAL: _____

PERFORMANCE EVALUATION:
CHANGING A VENTILATOR CIRCUIT

Date: Lab _____ Clinical _____ Agency _____

Lab: Pass _____ Fail _____   Clinical: Pass _____ Fail _____

Student name _____   Instructor name _____

No. of times observed in clinical _____

No. of times practiced in clinical _____

PASSING CRITERIA: Obtain 90% or better on the procedure. Tasks indicated by * must receive at least 1 point, or the evaluation is terminated. Procedure must be performed within designated time, or the performance receives a failing grade.

SCORING:

2 points — Task performed satisfactorily without prompting.
1 point — Task performed satisfactorily with self-initiated correction.
0 points — Task performed incorrectly or with prompting required.
NA — Task not applicable to the patient care situation.

TASKS:

		PEER	LAB	CLINICAL
*	1. Verifies the physician's order	☐	☐	☐
	2. Reviews the patient's chart	☐	☐	☐
	3. Gathers the equipment			
	a. Gloves, goggles, or face shield	☐	☐	☐
*	b. New circuit and humidifier	☐	☐	☐
*	c. Plastic disposal bag for used circuit	☐	☐	☐
*	4. Explains the procedure to the patient	☐	☐	☐
*	5. Suctions the patient as required	☐	☐	☐
*	6. Drains the condensate from the tubing	☐	☐	☐
*	7. Disconnects all alarms	☐	☐	☐
*	8. Manually ventilates the patient	☐	☐	☐
*	9. Changes the circuit	☐	☐	☐
	10. Tests the equipment for function			
*	a. Corrects circuit leaks	☐	☐	☐
*	b. Measures circuit compliance	☐	☐	☐
*	11. Completes the procedure within 2 minutes	☐	☐	☐
*	12. Adjusts the ventilator to the ordered settings	☐	☐	☐
*	13. Connects the patient	☐	☐	☐

14. Monitors the ventilator parameters

*   a. Rate   ☐ ☐ ☐

*   b. Tidal volume   ☐ ☐ ☐

*   c. FIO_2 ☐ ☐ ☐

*   d. Sensitivity   ☐ ☐ ☐

*   e. I:E ratio   ☐ ☐ ☐

*   f. Pressure limit   ☐ ☐ ☐

*   g. Circuit temperature   ☐ ☐ ☐

*   h. Measures FIO_2 ☐ ☐ ☐

*   i. Adjusts all alarms   ☐ ☐ ☐

15. Cleans up the area   ☐ ☐ ☐

* 16. Uses aseptic technique   ☐ ☐ ☐

* 17. Records the procedure in the chart   ☐ ☐ ☐

SCORE: Peer   _____ points of possible 54; _____%

              Lab   _____ points of possible 54; _____%

              Clinical   _____ points of possible 54; _____%

TIME: _____ out of possible 30 minutes

STUDENT SIGNATURES   INSTRUCTOR SIGNATURES

PEER: _____   LAB: _____

STUDENT: _____   CLINICAL: _____

CHAPTER 27

SPECIAL VENTILATORY PROCEDURES

INTRODUCTION

Ventilation modalities have expanded from control and assist/control modes to more than a half-dozen different alternatives. As a respiratory care practitioner, you will be expected to be familiar with these modalities and their clinical applications. You may even be asked to assemble external circuitry to achieve the desired clinical goal.

Familiarity with the techniques, equipment, hazards, and complications is required to employ these special procedures successfully. In this chapter you will learn about PEEP, IMV, IMV with CPAP, CPAP, pressure support, extended mandatory minute ventilation, augmented minute ventilation, and flow triggering. You will learn the theory of these procedures and their associated hazards and complications, and how to initiate these modalities properly.

KEY TERMS

- Augmented minute ventilation (AMV)
- Continuous positive airway pressure (CPAP)
- Positive end-expiratory pressure (PEEP)
- Pressure support
- SIMV with CPAP

OBJECTIVES

At the end of this chapter, you should be able to:

- Differentiate between PEEP and CPAP.
- Describe the physiological effects of PEEP/CPAP on the following:
  — Functional residual capacity (FRC)
  — Cardiac output
  — Hepatic function
  — Renal function
  — Gastrointestinal function
- Differentiate among the following weaning methods and modes of ventilation and their clinical application:
  — T-piece weaning
  — IMV
  — SIMV
  — Pressure support
  — Extended mandatory minute volume
  — Augmented minute ventilation
  — Flow triggering
- Identify the criteria utilized to determine a patient's ability to be weaned from continuous mechanical ventilation:
  — Mechanics of ventilation
    — Vital capacity

  — Respiratory rate
  — Minute volume
  — Maximal inspiratory force
  — Oxygenation
    — PaO_2
    — $P(A-a)O_2$
  — Ventilation
    — $PaCO_2$
- Understand the rationale for performing the following specialized monitoring procedures:
  — Shunt studies
  — V_D/V_T ratio
  — Static and dynamic pressure-volume curves
- Discuss the physiological effects of weaning a patient from mechanical ventilation on the following:
  — $PaCO_2$
  — Right to left shunt
  — Cardiac output
  — Oxygen consumption
- Discuss the complications and hazards of weaning:
  — Decreased cardiac output
  — Hypoventilation and hypercapnia

PEEP AND CPAP

Positive End-Expiratory Pressure

Positive end-expiratory pressure (PEEP) is used in mechanical ventilation to apply positive pressure during exhalation. The application of PEEP prevents the airway pressure from reaching ambient pressure (defined as zero or atmospheric pressure) at end exhalation. Figure 27-1 illustrates

the application of PEEP. Graph *A* shows mechanical ventilation without PEEP. At the end of each exhalation, airway pressure reaches ambient pressure (zero). In graph *B*, the end-expiratory pressure is +5 cm H_2O. The airway pressure never reaches ambient pressure. The specific application is termed "+5 cm H_2O of PEEP." PEEP is useful to increase the PaO_2 when increasing the FIO_2 (fraction of inspired oxygen) is not desirable or when other methods have failed.

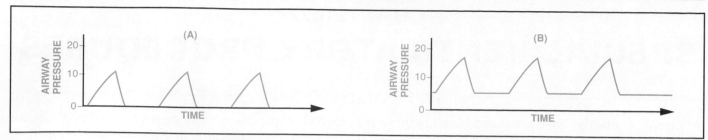

Figure 27-1 *Mechanical ventilation with PEEP illustrated graphically. Graph (A) illustrates expiration to ambient pressure; graph (B) illustrates the application of +5 cm H_2O of PEEP.*

Continuous Positive Airway Pressure

Continuous positive airway pressure (CPAP) is the application of positive pressure during inspiration and expiration to the airway during spontaneous breathing. It is similar to PEEP except that the patient is breathing spontaneously. Figure 27-2 illustrates normal spontaneous ventilation and the application of CPAP. During spontaneous ventilation as shown in graph *A*, at end exhalation the airway pressure reaches ambient pressure. With the application of CPAP, as depicted in graph *B*, pressure is applied on both inspiration and expiration. At end exhalation, pressure does not drop below +5 cm H_2O. This specific application is termed "+5 cm H_2O of CPAP."

PHYSIOLOGICAL EFFECTS OF PEEP AND CPAP

PEEP and CPAP have many beneficial effects that are helpful in the management of critically ill patients. As with other modalities, the beneficial effects are often tempered by hazards and complications. The beneficial effects primarily involve the improvement of PaO_2 by increasing the functional residual capacity (FRC). The hazards and complications are the result of pressure and its effects on the cardiovascular, renal, and gastrointestinal systems. Barotrauma, or injury due to increased intrathoracic pressure, may complicate PEEP/CPAP by leading to pneumothorax and/or subcutaneous emphysema.

Increase in Functional Residual Capacity

PEEP and CPAP cause an increase in the FRC by preventing exhalation to the normal resting expiratory level. With application of positive pressure to the airways, the alveoli are always kept slightly inflated, causing an increased volume of gas to remain in the lungs. By keeping the alveoli slightly inflated, gas exchange is improved and PaO_2 is increased without any increase in FiO_2 (Headley-Whyte, Burgess, Feeley, & Miller, 1976).

Effects on Venous Return and Cardiac Output

Positive intrathoracic pressure exerts a squeezing effect on the mediastinum and great vessels. The result of this effect is a decrease in venous return and a subsequent decrease in cardiac output. These changes are especially marked if the cardiovascular system is not able to compensate. The problem becomes especially acute in patients with cardiovascular instability or underlying cardiac complications. In these patients, the application of PEEP/CPAP must be carefully monitored.

Effects on the Renal System

Frequently, patients on PEEP/CPAP experience a decrease in urine output. This is associated with the release of antidiuretic hormone and a redistribution of intrarenal blood flow (Headley-Whyte et al., 1976). The release of antidiuretic hormone is thought to be influenced by vagal reflexes from

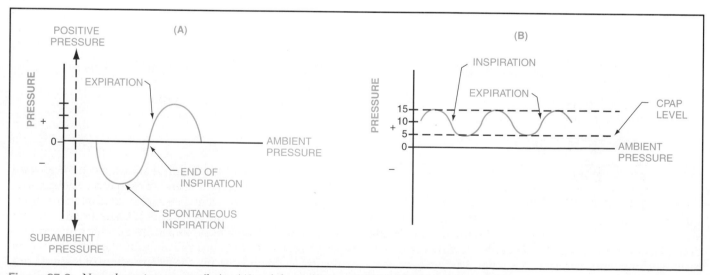

Figure 27-2 *Normal spontaneous ventilation (A) and the application of CPAP (B) illustrated graphically*

the atria (Scanlan, Spearman, & Sheldon, 1995). As pressure increases, more antidiuretic hormone is secreted by the pituitary. The effect of this is the retention of fluids and sodium. Fluid retention may increase pulmonary congestion and interfere with gas exchange. It must be closely monitored.

Effects on the Gastrointestinal System

The decrease in cardiac output results in a decrease in blood flow to the gastrointestinal (GI) tract. It is also thought that positive-pressure ventilation may result in an increase in resistance to blood flow through the GI mucosa, resulting in mucosal ischemia. Gastric ulcers are common in patients requiring long-term ventilation. Administration of antacids is helpful in reducing the incidence of ulcers (Headley-Whyte et al., 1976).

Barotrauma

Barotrauma is a common complication of PEEP/CPAP. The additional increase in airway pressure may result in a pneumothorax or subcutaneous emphysema. Careful monitoring of pressures and frequent patient monitoring of ventilator pressures will ensure that barotrauma is diagnosed early and appropriate treatment is initiated.

WEANING METHODS AND MODES OF MECHANICAL VENTILATION

T-Piece Weaning

T-piece weaning consists of removing the patient from ventilatory support and allowing the patient to breathe spontaneously from a heated aerosol T or Briggs adapter. Extubation is postponed until successful weaning has been demonstrated.

Some patients have difficulty being weaned by this method, particularly if they have required ventilatory support for an extended period of time, or if muscle weakness or excessive work of breathing is still a problem. Under these circumstances, the time without mechanical ventilation is gradually increased. Initially the patient is removed from ventilation for 10 to 15 minutes each hour. Gradually, this time is increased until the patient can sustain spontaneous ventilation and maintain adequate arterial blood gas values.

Psychological preparation is essential for patients to be weaned by this method. The patient may have a lot of anxiety about the ability to breathe. Frequently, it is difficult to wean a patient during the late evening or night owing to fatigue. The patient must be physically and mentally ready for the weaning process.

Intermittent Mandatory Ventilation

Intermittent mandatory ventilation (IMV) may be used as a mode of ventilation if the patient is capable of supporting some of his or her ventilatory needs. It allows for the maintenance of muscle tone. It may also be used as a progressive weaning technique. IMV represents an improvement over the earlier T-piece weaning method. IMV is a ventilatory mode that allows the patient to

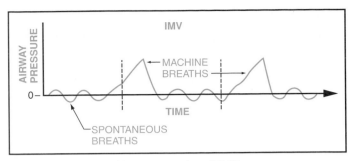

Figure 27-3 *A graphic representation of IMV*

breathe spontaneously between mechanical ventilator breaths. The circuitry required may be assembled externally or, in the case of contemporary volume ventilators, may be an integral part of the ventilator.

By allowing the patient to breathe spontaneously between ventilator breaths, muscle strength and ventilatory drive are preserved. Figure 27-3 graphically depicts IMV. The tall wave forms are the mechanical breaths, and the shallow wave forms are the spontaneous breaths. With nonsynchronized IMV, it is possible to deliver a mechanical breath on top of a spontaneous breath. This is termed *stacking breaths*.

In weaning a patient from IMV, the ventilator (mandatory) breath rate is gradually reduced, forcing the patient to assume more spontaneous respiratory efforts. As the ventilator approaches a rate of approximately 5 or less per minute, or if the patient appears to be physically ready, discontinuance of ventilatory support is possible.

Synchronized Intermittent Mandatory Ventilation

Synchronized intermittent mandatory ventilation (SIMV) is ventilatory mode similar to IMV except that electronic circuitry in the ventilator prevents stacking breaths by sensing the initiation of inspiration for a spontaneous breath. This prevents the delivery of a mandatory breath on top of a spontaneous breath.

SIMV with CPAP

SIMV with CPAP is a weaning modality that incorporates mandatory ventilation of IMV with PEEP during the expiratory phase. During the spontaneous breathing portion of IMV, the patient breaths from a pressurized CPAP system. Positive pressure is maintained on both inspiration and expiration during both mandatory and spontaneous breathing.

Pressure Support

The goal of *pressure support* is to enable the patient to obtain an adequate inspiratory volume by augmenting the patient's effort with positive pressure. It is a spontaneous ventilation mode whereby the patient must trigger or initiate each breath. This mode ensures that the spontaneous breaths are not too shallow. On initiation of a breath, a constant pressure (preset) is delivered until the flow rate reaches approximately 25% of the peak inspiratory flow; then expiration begins. In this mode, flow is variable. Whatever flow is required (within the ventilator's designed limitations) is available to maintain the selected level of pressure.

Frequently this mode is used to wean patients from mechanical ventilation. This mode ensures that the spontaneous breaths are large enough to maintain adequate blood gases and to reverse atelectasis. The delivered volume is not usually as large as that for ventilating a patient using a volume cycle mode. But it is larger than what the patient is capable of obtaining spontaneously.

EMMV and AMV

Extended mandatory minute volume (EMMV) and *augmented minute ventilation (AMV)* may be regarded as specialized forms of IMV. These modes of ventilation guarantee a minimum minute volume that will be adjusted depending on the patient's spontaneous efforts. If the patient's breathing is largely spontaneous, few mandatory breaths will be delivered. The patient is free to breathe in excess of the set minute volume. However, if the patient's spontaneous breathing falls below the set minute volume level, mandatory breaths will be delivered to achieve the set minute volume. The number of mandatory breaths is strictly determined by the extent to which the patient is sustaining ventilation. Some contemporary ventilators have these IMV modes as a feature. These modes are adjusted and monitored electronically and automatically.

These modes are very useful for weaning. If the patient tires and fails to breathe spontaneously enough to maintain blood gases, the ventilator automatically backs up the spontaneous ventilation with mandatory breaths. However, if the patient is principally sustaining adequate ventilation spontaneously, few, if any, mandatory breaths will be delivered.

Flow Triggering

Flow triggering is another method of sensing patient effort or inspiration. Rather than detecting a pressure change, a change in flow (inspiratory flow) initiates a breath. Flow triggering occurs when the ventilator senses a diminished flow level through the circuit (when the patient takes a breath); it then responds by initiating inspiration. The advantage of flow triggering is that work of breathing is reduced when compared with that involved in pressure triggering. There is not a time lag from the time the patient inhales until gas is delivered because the gas flow is already there for the patient.

A continuous flow of gas is maintained through the patient circuit (5 to 20 L/min) by the ventilator. Inspiratory and expiratory flow sensors monitor this continuous flow. When the patient inhales, the inspiratory flow sensor will record more flow than that perceived by the expiratory sensor. This difference in flow is what the ventilator senses as a patient effort; it then initiates inspiration. The flow trigger is adjustable from a minimum of 1 L/min and up to a maximum of ½ the base flow level.

The ventilator may be flow triggered in all modes of ventilation. During CPAP, once a patient effort is sensed, flow increases to meet the patient's inspiratory needs. During SIMV, both spontaneous breaths and ventilator (mandatory) breaths are flow triggered. During pressure ventilation (pressure control and pressure support), when a breath is triggered, flow increases to maintain the set pressure levels.

Airway Pressure Release Ventilation

Airway pressure release ventilation is a mode of ventilation whereby the patient is allowed to breathe spontaneously at two different pressure levels. During inspiration, pressure is at one level; during expiration, the pressure falls to a lower level. The exhalation time period varies from between 1 and 2 seconds.

Mandatory breaths may also be delivered during airway pressure release ventilation. The breath may be pressure or flow triggered. Once the breath is initiated, the pressure rises to the higher level and is maintained throughout inspiration. Once inspiration ends, the pressure falls to the lower level for exhalation.

SPECIALIZED MONITORING PROCEDURES

Shunt Studies

Measurement of the physiologic shunt can be performed while the patient is receiving mechanical ventilation. Shunt can be measured accurately only at two FiO_2 levels, 0.21 and 1.00. The determination of shunt is clinically useful if the patient's PaO_2 has diminished and does not respond to increasing FiO_2 levels. Shunt may be caused by atelectasis, mucous plugging, ARDS, and other pathological conditions.

To calculate the shunt, you must be able to obtain an arterial blood gas sample and a mixed venous blood sample (via Swan-Ganz catheter or CVP line), and you must calculate the alveolar oxygen tension, expressed as P_AO_2. From these values you will calculate the pulmonary arterial, venous, and end-capillary concentrations of oxygen—the CaO_2, the CvO_2, and the CcO_2.

$$CaO_2 = O_2 \text{ saturation } (Hb \times 1.34) + (PaO_2 \times 0.003)$$
$$CvO_2 = O_2 \text{ saturation } (Hb \times 1.34) + (PvO_2 \times 0.003)$$
$$CcO_2 = 1.00 (Hb \times 1.34) + (P_AO_2 \times 0.003)$$
$$P_AO_2 = FiO_2 (PB - PH_2O) - (PaCO_2 \times 1.25)$$

where
Hb is hemoglobin
PB = barometric pressure
PH_2O = partial pressure of water vapor

Once these values have been calculated, they may be arranged to form an equation to calculate the shunt fraction, Q_S/Q_T, where Q_S is cardiac output shunted and Q_T is total cardiac output.

$$Q_S/Q_T = \frac{CcO_2 - CaO_2}{CcO_2 - CvO_2}$$

The result is expressed as a percentage, reflecting the percent of blood flow through the lungs that does not become oxygenated. Once the presence of shunt is confirmed, PEEP or CPAP may be initiated to increase the FRC and reduce the shunt fraction.

V_D/V_T Ratio

The dead space to tidal volume ratio (V_D/V_T) is sometimes helpful in assessing the patient who is difficult to wean from the ventilator. As a patient's physiologic dead space increases, it will require a significant increase in minute ventilation to maintain the same $PaCO_2$. This increase in minute ventilation in the critically ill patient significantly adds to the patient's work of breathing. The V_D/V_T ratio provides a means of comparing dead space and tidal volume. A normal person has a V_D/V_T ratio of between 0.2 and 0.4. As the V_D/V_T ratio increases above 0.4 approaching 0.6, the patient may be unable to sustain spontaneous ventilation. At a V_D/V_T ratio of 0.6, if the patient is spontaneously breathing with a tidal volume of 500 ml, 300 ml of that volume is wasted (0.6×500 ml).

STATIC AND DYNAMIC PRESSURE-VOLUME CURVES

As a routine part of ventilator monitoring, both the static and dynamic pressures are measured and recorded. Clinically, it is also useful to plot these values graphically against volumes once a shift. The steepness of the curves and the distance between them are indicative of changes in compliance and airway resistance (Figure 27-4). As the space between the two curves increases, airway resistance also increases. If the curves flatten out, it is indicative of a decrease in compliance. Compliance may decrease as a result of adult respiratory distress syndrome (ARDS), pneumothorax, pulmonary edema, or severe pneumonia. Because the static and dynamic pressures are routinely monitored, little time is required to include pressure-volume curves as a part of the ventilator monitoring procedure.

CRITERIA FOR WEANING

Generally the criteria to determine weaning readiness are the opposite of the criteria for initiation of mechanical ventilation. Mechanics of ventilation, oxygenation, ade-

quacy of ventilation, and psychological readiness are all considerations prior to weaning. Table 27-1 lists the objective data that may be gathered to evaluate when a patient is ready for weaning.

The measurement of bedside pulmonary function parameters has been discussed in Chapter 5. In assessing a patient requiring or receiving mechanical ventilation, oxygenation of the patient and hyperinflation of the lungs are important steps before and after each maneuver.

Oxygenation and the adequacy of ventilation are easily evaluated by blood gas analysis.

The psychological preparation for weaning may be especially difficult in patients who have been ventilated for an extended period of time. Sleep deprivation, ventilator dependency, disorientation, and anxiety can all contribute to a difficult weaning attempt. Whenever possible,

TABLE 27-1: Weaning Criteria

Mechanics of Ventilation	
Minute volume	<10 L/min
Respiratory rate	12–20 breaths/min
Vital capacity	>15 ml/kg normal body weight
Maximal inspiratory force	> –25 cm H_2O
Oxygenation	
PaO_2	>60 mm Hg with FIO_2 of 0.40
$P(A–a)O_2$	<300–350 mm Hg with FIO_2 of 1.00
Ventilation	
$PaCO_2$	35–45 mm Hg

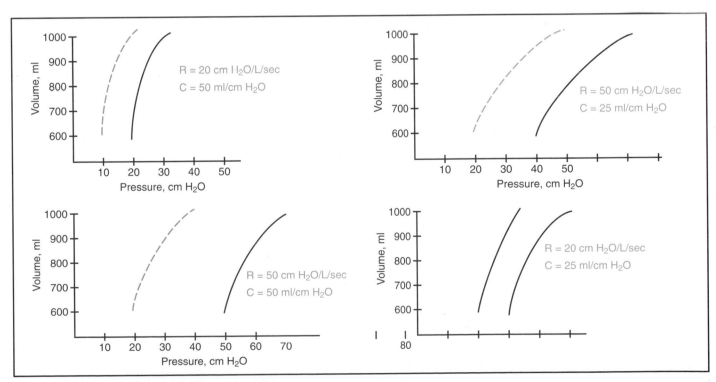

Figure 27-4 *Static and dynamic pressure-volume curves*

careful explanation and psychological preparation should precede any weaning attempts. Psychological support should accompany weaning.

PHYSIOLOGICAL EFFECTS OF WEANING

Effects on PaCO₂

During the initial weaning period, $PaCO_2$ often increases. However as weaning progresses, $PaCO_2$ will return to more normal levels. The initial stages of weaning frequently involve hypoventilation relative to mechanical ventilation. The increase in $PaCO_2$ is more significant early in the weaning process than after 24 hours (Headley-Whyte et al., 1976).

Right to Left Shunt

The presence of right to left shunt may be indicated by an increasing $P(A–a)O_2$. This finding has been attributed to alveolar collapse and atelectasis associated with the early periods of hypoventilation during weaning (Headley-Whyte et al., 1976).

Cardiac Output

Cardiac output may fall during weaning. If the cardiac output drops significantly, hypotension and cardiovascular collapse may result. Blood pressure should be carefully monitored during the weaning attempt. The additional workload on the cardiovascular system may cause this fall in blood pressure.

Oxygen Consumption

The increase in the work of breathing required during spontaneous ventilation may result in a significant increase in oxygen consumption. Frequently during weaning the FiO_2 is increased slightly to help counteract this problem. The increasing use of ear and pulse oximetry is helpful in diagnosing this potential complication.

OBJECTIVES

At the end of this chapter, you should be able to:

* Demonstrate how to assemble, test, and trouble-shoot the following:
  PEEP
  — Water seal
  — Emerson water column
  — Boehringer valve
  — Downs' valve
  CPAP
  — Water seal
  — Emerson water column
  — Boehringer valve
  — Downs' valve
  Diagram the flow of gas through the various PEEP/CPAP systems.
* Demonstrate how to assemble, test, and trouble-shoot the following external ventilator weaning assemblies:
  — Open IMV system
  — Closed IMV system
  — IMV with CPAP
  Diagram the flow of gas through the two systems.
* Identify the baseline data that should be gathered prior to initiation of PEEP, CPAP, or other weaning methods:
  — Cardiovascular
    — Blood pressure
    — Heart rate and rhythm
    — Cardiac output*
    — Central venous pressure (CVP), pulmonary artery wedge pressure (PAWP)*
  — Pulmonary
    — Mechanics of ventilation
    — Arterial blood gases
    — Static and dynamic compliance

* During a proficiency evaluation in the laboratory, demonstrate how to initiate PEEP, IMV, SIMV with CPAP, and CPAP with external circuitry, including the following:
  — Verify the order.
  — Obtain baseline patient data.
  — Auscultate the chest and suction the patient as required.
  — Assemble, test, and troubleshoot the equipment.
  — Monitor the patient.
  — Remove unneeded equipment.
  — Document the procedure on the patient's chart.
* Depending on availability, demonstrate how to initiate the following on the listed ventilators:
  — PEEP
  — SIMV
  — SIMV with CPAP
  — Pressure support
  — CPAP
  — Augmented minute ventilation
  — Flow triggering
  VENTILATORS
  BEAR 1, 2, 3, 5, or 1000
  Bird 8400ST
  Lifecare PLV-102
  Puritan-Bennett MA-1
  Puritan-Bennett 7200ae
  Siemens Servo 900C
  Siemens Servo 300
* Demonstrate how to perform the following:
  — Measure the V_D/V_T.
  — Plot static and dynamic pressure-volume curves.

---

*Information may not be available depending on the patient monitoring being performed.

PEEP and CPAP are frequently incorporated into the design of contemporary ventilators. However, as a respiratory care practitioner, you do not need a sophisticated ventilator to provide quality care with the latest in modalities. The majority of the modalities discussed in this section may be improvised using a few pieces of tubing and a little additional equipment. A good grasp of the concepts underlying these modalities is best obtained by setting up the external circuitry and tracing gas flow rather than by simply changing the position of a switch on the ventilator control panel. Directed practice will involve both external circuitry assembly and operation of the features incorporated into contemporary ventilators. It is recommended that you become proficient in setting up the external circuitry before proceeding to the built-in features of the new ventilators.

POSITIVE END-EXPIRATORY PRESSURE

As defined earlier in this chapter, PEEP is the application of positive pressure on expiration during the mechanical ventilation of the patient. There are several methods employed in the application of PEEP. These include use of the underwater seal, Emerson water column, and Boehringer and Downs' valves.

Underwater Seal

Use of the underwater seal is the easiest and the earliest technique employed in the application of PEEP. To generate PEEP using this technique, the expiratory tubing is submerged under water until the desired PEEP level is reached. Figure 27-5 illustrates this principle. The expiratory tubing is gradually lowered below the surface of the water until the desired PEEP level is indicated on the ventilator manometer. The PEEP level is equivalent to the depth (in centimeters) the expiratory tubing is submerged. The patient must generate sufficient pressure on exhalation to displace the water from the tubing, thus maintaining positive pressure.

This method has its disadvantages. Evaporation of the water, accidental upset of the container, and shifting tube position (tubing depth below the water surface) all may contribute to inconsistencies in PEEP levels. To employ this technique successfully, diligent patient monitoring is mandatory.

Emerson Water Column

Use of the Emerson water column is similar to the underwater seal application of PEEP. A special water column marketed by the Emerson Corporation is employed. Figure 27-6 is a diagram showing a cross sectional view of this device. A flexible diaphragm separates the exhaled gas from the water. The water column is graduated in centimeter increments, facilitating precise levels of PEEP. The diaphragm reduces bubbling and the likelihood of spills. Figure 27-7 illustrates the application of this device and the

gas flow through it. Frequently, these devices are permanently mounted to the side of the ventilator, thus preventing problems associated with spills. However, evaporation remains a problem.

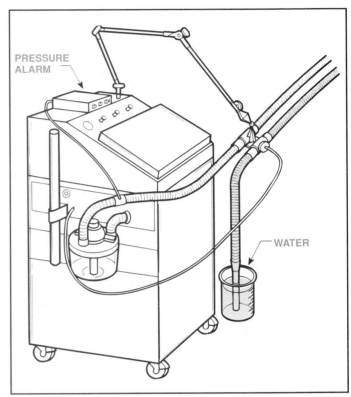

Figure 27-5 *An underwater seal used to generate PEEP. The expiratory limb of the ventilator circuit is typically submerged in water.*

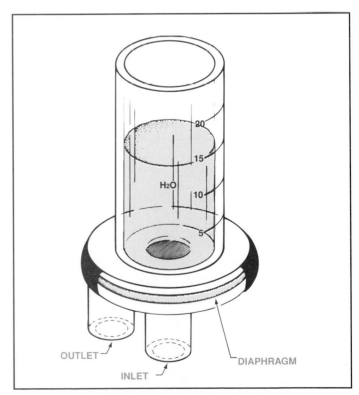

Figure 27-6 *A diagram of the Emerson water column*

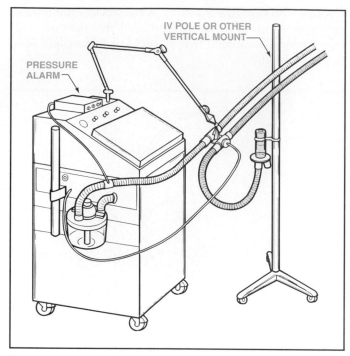

Figure 27-7 *Application of the Emerson water column*

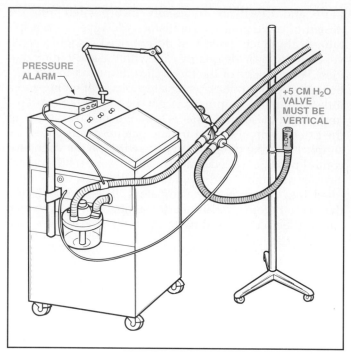

Figure 27-9 *A Boehringer valve incorporated into the ventilator circuit*

Boehringer Valves

Boehringer valves are specially designed valves that incorporate a weighted ball to regulate the PEEP levels. The weight of the ball determines the amount of pressure required to displace it from its valve seat, and the amount of PEEP generated. Figure 27-8 shows a cross section of this valve.

This valve must be used in an upright position. Tipping the valve on its side will result in the loss of PEEP pressure. Frequently these valves are taped or permanently attached

to a vertical surface to prevent them from being inadvertently tipped. As with water seals and the Emerson water column, the expiratory tubing is connected to the Boehringer valve. Figure 27-9 illustrates how this valve is incorporated into the ventilator circuit and the flow of gas through it.

Downs' Valve

The Downs' valve is a spring-type valve that is used to generate PEEP. The internal spring tension of the valve determines the PEEP level. These valves are calibrated in increments of 2.5 cm H_2O up to 15 cm H_2O. Figure 27-10 illustrates a cross section of a Downs' valve. These valves

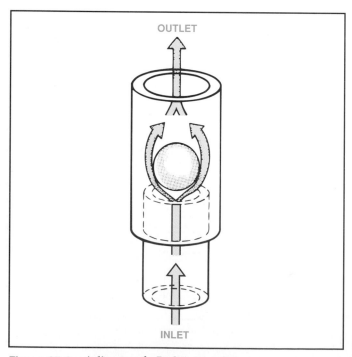

Figure 27-8 *A diagram of a Boehringer valve*

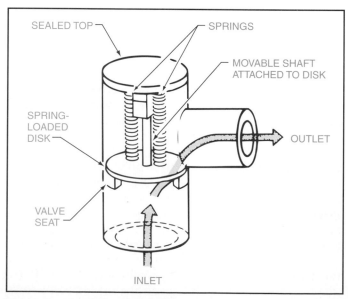

Figure 27-10 *A diagram of a Downs' valve*

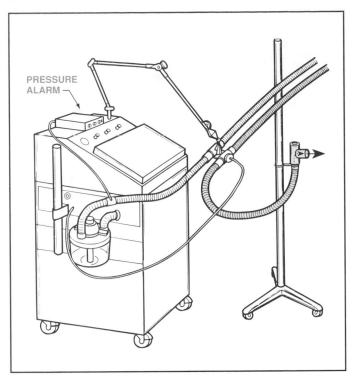

Figure 27-11 *A Downs' valve incorporated into the ventilator circuit*

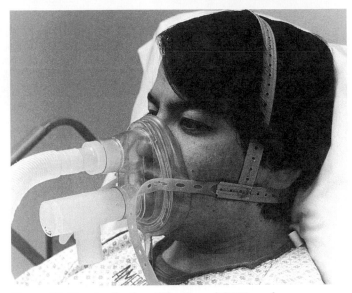

Figure 27-12 *Application of the Downs' CPAP mask*

may be used in any position. Figure 27-11 illustrates how this valve is incorporated into the ventilator circuit and the flow of gas through it.

CONTINUOUS POSITIVE AIRWAY PRESSURE

Continuous positive airway pressure (CPAP) is the application of positive pressure to both inspiration and expiration when a patient is breathing spontaneously. Therefore, some form of pressure generation must be incorporated into both the inspiratory and the expiratory sides of the circuit. To prevent gas from following the path of least resistance between the two sides of the circuit, a Rudolph valve, which is a special one-way valve, is incorporated.

CPAP pressure generation can be accomplished using water seals, Emerson water columns, Boehringer valves, and Downs' CPAP valves. It is important that no matter which device is used, the inspiratory and expiratory pressure values match.

CPAP may be administered to the patient via mask or artificial airway (oral or nasal endotracheal tube or tracheostomy tube). If a mask is used, it must seal tightly and is usually secured with straps. Figure 27-12 illustrates the correct application of a Downs' CPAP mask. If you are using a mask, a clear mask is preferred, especially in the event of vomiting, when early detection is essential. If the patient is having difficulty maintaining a patent airway, an oral airway may be used in conjunction with the mask.

Setup of the CPAP Circuit

Figure 27-13 illustrates how the CPAP circuit is assembled. The blocks labeled "X" are the CPAP-generating devices. These may be water seals, Emerson water columns, Boehringer valves, or Downs' valves. The important point to note is that the inspiratory and expiratory pressures must match. Figure 27-14 is an illustration of how to make a substitute "Rudolph valve" using an aerosol T and two Bird one-way valves. Note that the direction of air flow is the same for both valves. The system-patient interface is at the 15-mm opening (it connects to the mask or artificial airway).

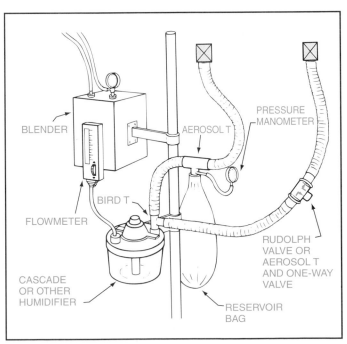

Figure 27-13 *A diagram showing a CPAP circuit. The boxes labeled X can be any device capable of generating PEEP/CPAP such as water seals, Emerson water columns, or Boehringer or Downs' valves.*

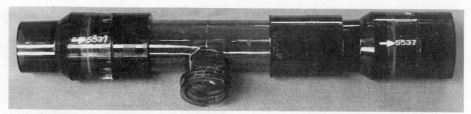

Figure 27-14 *An improvised one-way valve assembly*

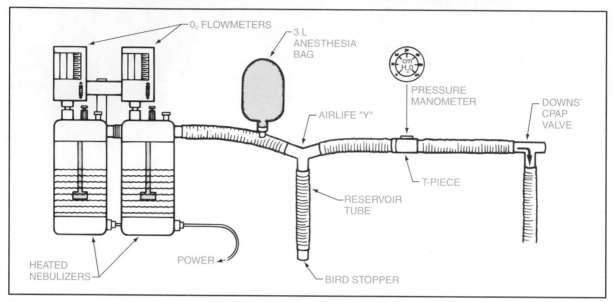

Figure 27-15 *A diagram of the Downs' CPAP circuit*

Figure 27-15 illustrates the assembly of the Downs' CPAP system. It differs slightly from the Rudolph valve system. Only one CPAP valve is utilized with the mask. One-way valves are incorporated into the design of the mask; hence, a Rudolph-type valve is not required. Figure 27-16 illustrates a cross section of the mask–CPAP valve combination and the gas flow through it.

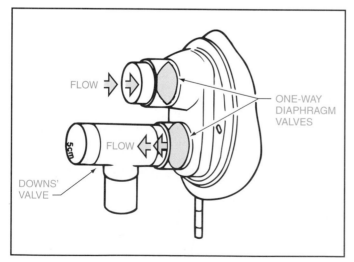

Figure 27-16 *A diagram showing flow through the Downs' CPAP mask*

INITIATION OF CPAP AND PEEP

Verify the Order and Scan the Chart

As with all respiratory care procedures, a written physician's order is required before initiation of CPAP/PEEP therapy. Scan the chart for recent blood gas results, blood pressure, and heart rate and rhythm. Look for any indications of pneumothorax on recent chest x-rays and check whether any chest tubes were inserted.

Gather and Assemble Equipment

Gather and assemble the equipment required to initiate PEEP or CPAP. An additional humidifier may be needed, depending on the mode of therapy the patient is receiving. Assemble all of the equipment and test it for function prior to initiating therapy. It is certainly in the best interest of your patient to discover malfunctions before attachment to the circuitry.

Gather Baseline Data

Because PEEP and CPAP may have deleterious effects on the patient, it is important to assess the patient thoroughly prior to initiation of either of these modalities. The gathering of baseline data will assist you in properly assessing the patient after initiating the modality. Figure 27-17 summarizes the data you should collect prior to initiating PEEP or CPAP.

CARDIOVASCULAR
Blood pressure   * Cardiac output
Heart rate and rhythm   * CVP and PAWP

PULMONARY
Mechanics of ventilation   ** Static and dynamic
Arterial blood gases   compliance

*These items may depend on the monitoring devices in use.
**These are collected only for patients on continuous mechanical
ventilation who are being placed on PEEP.

Figure 27-17   *Baseline data for PEEP and CPAP*

The adverse effects of PEEP/CPAP are usually observed first in the cardiovascular system. That is why it is important to obtain these baseline data.

The mechanics of ventilation include minute volume, tidal volume, frequency, vital capacity, and maximal inspiratory force. PEEP or CPAP is indicated to reduce hypoxemia. Thus, careful attention must be given to preoxygenation, postoxygenation, and hyperinflation for gathering this data.

Position the Patient

When possible, the patient should be in semi-Fowler's position for initiation of this modality.

Auscultate the Chest and Suction if Required

It is important to auscultate the chest and suction prior to initiation of these modalities. The point is to maximize air exchange and ventilation. This cannot occur if the airways are clogged with secretions. Auscultation also provides a point of reference for evaluation of barotrauma should the patient's condition suddenly worsen.

Connect the Patient to the PEEP/CPAP System

Attach the patient to the system. Adjust the PEEP/CPAP devices as required to establish the ordered pressure level. Verify that the system is functioning properly and that the patient's ventilatory needs are being met.

Monitor the Patient's Cardiovascular Parameters

As soon as you have verified that the PEEP/CPAP system is functioning and that the patient's ventilatory needs are being met, monitor the cardiovascular parameters. Monitor the systemic arterial (BP), pulmonary artery pressures, and PAWP pressures. Adverse effects will be observed in these parameters first. It is expected that the blood pressure may fall initially. If the values change significantly, discontinue PEEP/CPAP and notify the physician immediately. Auscultate the chest to assess any changes in ventilation.

Cardiovascular function should be initially monitored every 5 to 10 minutes until parameters stabilize. Once the values are stable, they should be monitored every 15 minutes (Nelson, Hunter, & Morton, 1983).

Monitor the Ventilator or Spontaneous Parameters

PEEP

Monitor and document the ventilator settings after initiation of PEEP. When measuring all pressures, subtract the PEEP level from the measured value. For example:

$$\text{Plateau pressure} - \text{PEEP pressure} = \text{plateau pressure}$$

You may be required to make adjustments in tidal volume or flow rates to maintain ordered levels and adequate inspiratory-expiratory (I:E) ratios. It is especially important to measure static and dynamic compliance because PEEP may cause adverse effects.

CPAP

Once the patient has stabilized, monitor the CPAP pressures and spontaneous parameters on the CPAP system. Depending on the system employed, the patient may need to be disconnected to measure these values. If disconnection is required, you should minimize the frequency with which you measure these parameters.

Measure Arterial Blood Gases

After 15 to 20 minutes, measure arterial blood gases. With the increased usage of pulse and ear oximetry, the need for this blood gas measurement may not be required, depending on your hospital policy.

Remove Unneeded Equipment and Chart

Following initiation of the procedure, remove any unnecessary equipment and document what you have done in the patient's chart. Record all data collected before and after initiating PEEP/CPAP. Record the PEEP/CPAP levels and all spontaneous ventilatory parameters collected.

PEEP TRIAL

A PEEP trial may be ordered to determine the best or optimal level of PEEP. This level of PEEP is defined as the pressure at which cardiac output and total lung compliance are maximized and the dead space–to–tidal volume ratio is minimal (Headley-Whyte et al., 1976). Furthermore, optimal PEEP results in the best PaO_2 and PvO_2 and the lowest $P(A–a)O_2$ (Nelson et al., 1983).

To perform a PEEP trial, pressure is increased in 5 cm H_2O increments. Fifteen minutes following the adjustment of the PEEP level, all of the parameters in Table 27-1 are monitored. The best level of PEEP is found as defined previously. Without performing a PEEP trial, optimal PEEP cannot be determined.

INTERMITTENT MANDATORY VENTILATION

Intermittent mandatory ventilation (IMV) is a ventilation modality that allows the patient to breathe spontaneously between mandatory (machine) breaths. Most contemporary ventilators have IMV as a built-in mode or feature. However, it is possible to deliver IMV by constructing an external circuit.

Open IMV Circuit

An open IMV circuit is one in which the reservoir is open to the atmosphere. Sometimes it is referred to as an ambient reservoir system. Figure 27-18 illustrates how to construct this system.

The most frequent error made by new practitioners is to install the one-way valve incorrectly. An easy way to remember the correct position is that the flow direction is toward the patient or toward the circuit. Note the flow direction arrow in Figure 27-18. This valve should always be inspected for flow direction prior to attachment to the patient.

During spontaneous ventilation, the one-way valve opens and the patient draws gas from the IMV circuit. During mandatory ventilation, the one-way valve closes and the ventilator breath is delivered.

Advantages of this system are twofold. The FiO$_2$ of the nebulizer may be set slightly higher than the ventilator FiO$_2$, giving the patient a little extra reserve. Also, the effort required to open the one-way valve is frequently less than with some demand valve systems.

Closed IMV System

A closed IMV system is similar to an open IMV system except that a closed reservoir is used. Typically, a 3- or 5-liter anesthesia bag is utilized for the reservoir. Figure 27-19 illustrates how this system is constructed. Sometimes this system is referred to as a "pressure reservoir system" because pressure can build in the reservoir. The closed IMV system is used for delivering IMV with CPAP.

CPAP with IMV

CPAP with IMV is a combination IMV system. PEEP is provided during the mandatory (machine) breaths and CPAP is provided during the spontaneous breaths. PEEP/CPAP may be provided using water seals, water columns, or Boehringer or Downs' valves. It is important to match the PEEP and CPAP pressure levels. Figure 27-20 illustrates how this system is assembled. Note the use of a closed IMV system and how the CPAP-generating system is incorporated. Also note that on the expiratory side of the ventilator circuit (distal to the exhalation valve) there is another PEEP pressure generator. Any of the pressure-generating devices mentioned previously may be substituted. This system has advantages similar to those listed for the open IMV system.

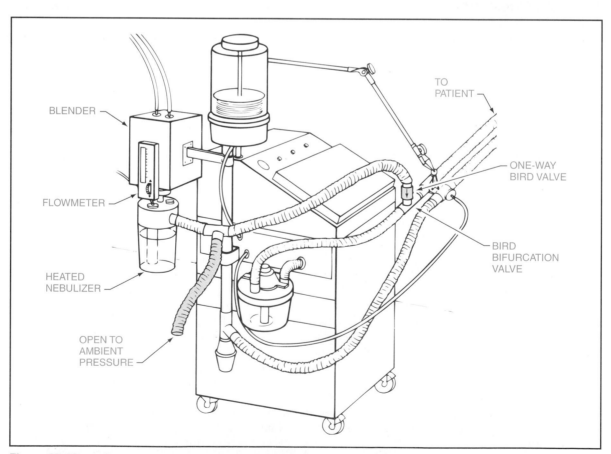

Figure 27-18 *A diagram showing an external open IMV circuit*

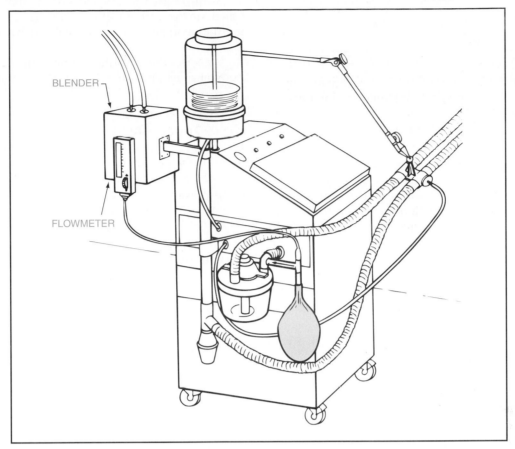

Figure 27-19 *A diagram of a closed IMV circuit*

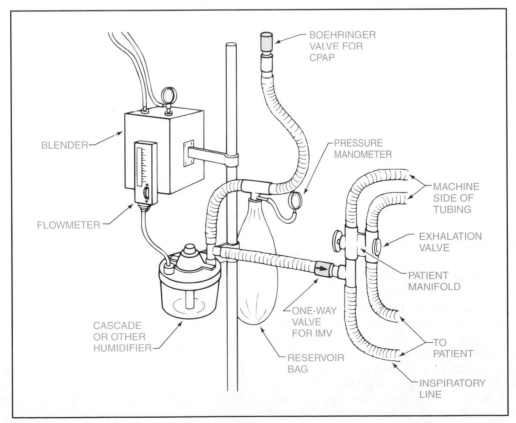

Figure 27-20 *A diagram of a ventilator circuit that will provide IMV with CPAP*

INITIATION OF IMV OR OF IMV WITH CPAP

Verify the Order

Before initiating IMV or IMV with CPAP, verify the physician's order. Also scan the chart for relevant information such as prior blood gas results, blood pressure, heart rate and rhythm, and chest x-ray reports.

Gather and Assemble Your Equipment

Gather the equipment required depending on whether you are initiating IMV or IMV with CPAP. Assemble your equipment and test it for function prior to initiating the procedure on your patient. Adjust the IMV FIO_2 levels to the ordered level prior to initiation.

Obtain Baseline Data

Measure or collect the baseline data listed in Table 27-1. Depending on the monitoring being done, collection of some of the parameters may not be possible. It is essential to gather these data prior to initiation of the modality so that adverse effects may be detected.

Position the Patient and Auscultate the Chest

Position the patient in semi-Fowler's position if possible and auscultate the chest. If required, suction the patient prior to initiating IMV or IMV with CPAP. It is important to maximize ventilation; a clear airway is also helpful.

Attach the Circuit to the Ventilator

Attach the IMV or CPAP with IMV circuit to the ventilator, being careful to verify the direction of flow through the one-way valve.

Adjust the ventilator so that it is operating in control mode. Any spontaneous breaths taken by the patient should be supplied by the IMV system. Observe the patient for excessive work of breathing during spontaneous ventilation.

Measure the FIO_2 supplied by the ventilator and the IMV system. The physician may order that the external IMV system be set at a higher FIO_2 than the ventilator setting. This provides the patient with a slight reserve during spontaneous ventilation.

Monitor the Patient-Ventilator System

Monitor the patient-ventilator system. Record mandatory and spontaneous parameters on the IMV system. Verify that the PEEP/CPAP levels are as ordered.

Measure the corrected mandatory tidal volume and minute volume. If you are initiating IMV with CPAP, subtract the PEEP pressure from the peak inspiratory pressure (PIP) and plateau pressure. Using your watch, time the respiratory rate and verify that it is correct as ordered by the physician. Adjust the tidal volume as required to maintain the ordered tidal volume. To obtain the spontaneous minute volume, subtract the exhaled minute volume from the tidal volume (V_E − [V_t mandatory × rate mandatory]).

Calculate the average spontaneous tidal volume by dividing the spontaneous minute volume by the spontaneous rate.

Measure the minute volume and record the total number of breaths (mandatory and spontaneous).

Monitor Cardiovascular and Pulmonary Parameters

Following the initiation of IMV or IMV with CPAP, monitor the parameters listed in Table 27-1. If the values change significantly, discontinue the modality and notify the physician immediately. Auscultate the chest to assess for any changes in ventilation. Resume the previous ventilatory mode as ordered by the physician.

Remove Unneeded Equipment

Remove any unnecessary equipment and document the procedure in the patient's chart. Document all of the ventilator parameters on the ventilator flow sheet.

PRESSURE SUPPORT

Most ventilators allow the practitioner to use pressure support alone or in conjunction with SIMV. Pressure support augments the patient's spontaneous breathing by applying a low constant pressure. The inspiratory phase is detected by the ventilator as a pressure drop below ambient pressure.

Verify the Order

Before initiation of pressure support, verify the physician's order. You need to ensure that the order specifies the support level, FIO_2, any PEEP/CPAP, and, if it is used in conjunction with SIMV, the tidal volume and mandatory rate.

Obtain Baseline Data

The primary complication of pressure support is hypoventilation. Monitoring of the $PaCO_2$ or capnography can tell you whether the patient is hypoventilating after initiation of pressure support. Pressure support, however, involves the application of positive pressure during inspiration. Therefore, blood pressure, heart rate and rhythm, and if available, CVP or PA pressure and PAWP should be monitored as a baseline.

Auscultate and Suction the Patient As Required

Auscultate the chest and suction the patient before initiation of pressure support. It is important to clear the airways to minimize resistance and maximize gas exchange.

Initiate Pressure Support

Adjust the pressure support to the ordered level. Check to ensure that the trigger sensitivity is low enough so that the work of breathing is minimized. Verify that the ventilator responds when the negative inspiratory pressure is sensed.

Monitor Cardiovascular and Pulmonary Parameters

Monitor the patient's blood pressure, heart rate and rhythm, and PA pressure or PAWP for signs of cardiovascular compromise. Use pulse oximetry, $PaCO_2$ monitoring, and capnography to detect adverse changes in ventilation. If the patient is not tolerating pressure support (is hypoventilating), it may be necessary to resume assist/control or other more supportive ventilatory modes.

AMV AND EMMV

AMV and EMMV, as described earlier in this chapter, provide a guaranteed minute ventilation. The ventilator allows the patient to breathe spontaneously, and if the patient's minute ventilation falls below the preset threshold, the ventilator will augment the patient's spontaneous breathing with mandatory breaths to meet that threshold. AMV and EMMV are "smart" SIMV modes in that the patient is monitored for hypoventilation (reduced minute volume).

Verify the Order

Before initiation of AMV or EMMV, verify the physician's order. You need to ensure that the order specifies the minute volume, FiO_2, tidal volume, and any PEEP/CPAP.

Obtain Baseline Data

As with pressure support, AMV and EMMV are weaning modes of ventilation. Therefore, there is still risk of hypoventilation. When the mandatory breaths are delivered, adverse cardiovascular effects are also possible. Therefore, you should measure as a baseline blood pressure, heart rate and rhythm, PA pressure and PAWP (if available), and $PaCO_2$ (or monitor capnography), with PaO_2 montoring or pulse oximetry.

Auscultate and Suction the Patient As Required

Auscultate the chest and suction the patient before initiation of pressure support. It is important to clear the airways to minimize resistance and maximize gas exchange.

Initiate AMV or EMMV

Adjust the ventilator settings to provide the desired minute volume, tidal volume, FiO_2, trigger sensitivity, and PEEP/CPAP. Monitor the ventilator to ensure that it is operating as you have specified. Monitor the pressure manometer or screen display to ensure that the flow rates are adequate to meet your patient's needs.

Monitor Cardiovascular and Pulmonary Parameters

Monitor the patient's blood pressure, heart rate and rhythm, and PA pressure or PAWP for signs of cardiovascular compromise. Use pulse oximetry, $PaCO_2$ monitoring, and capnography to detect adverse changes in ventilation. If the patient is not tolerating AMV or EMMV (is hypoventilating), it may be necessary to resume assist/control or other more supportive ventilatory modes.

FLOW TRIGGERING

Flow triggering, as described earlier, is a way of triggering the ventilator using inspiratory flow rather than pressure. Flow triggering may reduce the work of breathing to levels lower than are possible with pressure-triggering mechanisms (especially demand valve systems).

Verify the Physician's Order

The physician's order for flow triggering should include the FiO_2, any PEEP/CPAP, and, if it is to be used during SIMV, the SIMV mandatory rate and tidal volume. The trigger sensitivity and base flow are usually left up to the practitioner to adjust according to the patient's inspiratory needs.

Obtain Baseline Data

As with pressure support, flow triggering may result in hypoventilation. When the mandatory breaths are delivered (during SIMV), adverse cardiovascular effects are also possible. Therefore, you should measure as a baseline blood pressure, heart rate and rhythm, PA pressure and PAWP (if available), and $PaCO_2$ (or monitor capnography), with PaO_2 monitoring or pulse oximetry.

Auscultate and Suction As Required

Auscultate the chest and suction the airway before initiation of pressure support. It is important to clear the airways to minimize resistance and maximize gas exchange.

Initiate Flow Triggering

Adjust the ventilator to provide the desired base flow, trigger sensitivity (flow level), FiO_2, PEEP/CPAP, and the mandatory portion of SIMV, if ordered. Monitor the ventilator to ensure that it is delivering gas to the patient as you have adjusted. Monitor the patient for signs of increased work of breathing, and if required, lower the trigger sensitivity value and increase the base flow.

Monitor Cardiovascular and Pulmonary Parameters

Monitor the patient's blood pressure, heart rate and rhythm, and PA pressure or PAWP for signs of cardiovascular compromise. Use pulse oximetry, $PaCO_2$ monitoring, and capnography to detect adverse changes in ventilation. If the patient is not tolerating AMV or EMMV (is hypoventilating), it may be necessary to resume assist/control or other more supportive ventilatory modes.

MEASUREMENT OF V_D/V_T

The measurement of the V_D/V_T ratio involves collection of both a sample for arterial blood gas determination and an exhaled gas sample. The arterial blood gas sample is the easier of the two to obtain. The exhaled gas sample requires special equipment and circuitry to obtain.

Exhaled Gas Collection Circuit

A special circuit is required to prevent the gas contained in the ventilator tubing from mixing with the exhaled gas sample (Figure 27-21). Should the two gases mix, it would lower the P_ECO_2 (partial pressure of exhaled carbon dioxide [mm Hg]), falsely elevating the V_D/V_T ratio. The second exhalation valve in the circuit (proximal to the patient) prevents the collection of compressible volume contained in the ventilator circuit.

Circuit Assembly

To assemble the circuit, you will need an exhalation valve, two lengths of exhalation valve tubing (small diameter), a T fitting to join the exhalation valve tubing together, a collection bag (usually a 100-liter Douglas bag), a one-way valve, and a three-way stopcock to control the flow of gas into the collection bag. Assemble the circuit as shown in Figure 27-21.

Verify the Physician's Order

Verify that the physician has ordered a V_D/V_T ratio determination. Verify that the physician will allow you to obtain a sample of blood gases as a part of the procedure.

Attachment of the Collection Circuit

Open the three-way stopcock so that exhaled gas directed toward the collection valve will vent into the room. Ensure that the one-way valve is oriented so that flow will still be delivered to the patient. Check and double-check the position of the valve. Attach the additional exhalation valve so it is proximal to the patient's airway. Using the T fitting, quickly connect the exhalation valve drive line and the new exhalation valve. When the ventilator delivers a breath, both valves should close. With practice, this part of the procedure should require interruption of only one or two ventilator breaths.

Observe the Patient

Errors in circuit assembly can result in the patient's receiving gas but not being able to exhale it. This could result in a sudden pneumothorax. It is very important that you observe the patient and the ventilator to ensure that both are well.

Collect the Exhaled Gas Sample

Collect an exhaled gas sample over a 3- to 5-minute time frame. Just prior to the end of the collection time, withdraw a gas sample using the sample tube on the Douglas bag and have someone else simultaneously draw an arterial blood gas specimen. Label and send both samples to the blood gas laboratory for analysis. Open the three-way stopcock so that exhaled gas will be directed into the atmosphere.

Disconnect the Circuit

Disconnect the circuit from the patient's ventilator circuit. Remove all unneeded supplies from the room. Monitor the patient and the ventilator to ensure that the settings are correct and that the patient has tolerated the procedure.

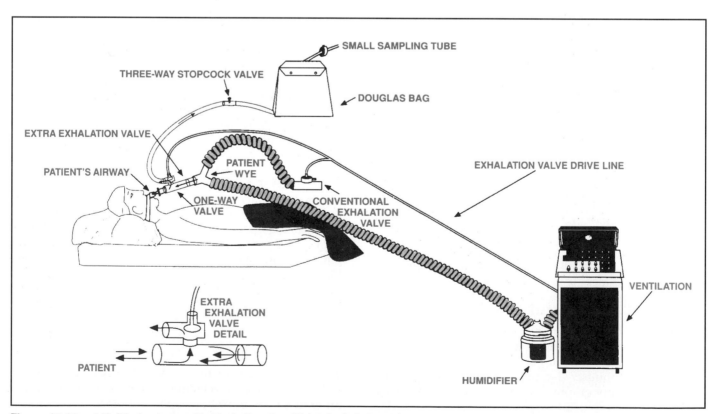

Figure 27-21 *A V_D/V_T circuit assembled including the additional exhalation valve in the circuit*

Calculate the V_D/V_T Ratio

The V_D/V_T ratio may be calculated using the following formulas:

$$P_ECO_{2\ corrected} = \frac{(tidal\ volume\ measured)P_ECO_2}{corrected\ tidal\ volume}$$

$$V_D/V_T = \frac{PaCO_2 - PeCO_{2\ corrected}}{PaCO_2}$$

After you have calculated the V_D/V_T ratio, document the procedure in the patient's chart.

MEASUREMENT OF STATIC AND DYNAMIC PRESSURE-VOLUME CURVES

Measurement and plotting of the static and dynamic pressure-volume curves are useful in the management of critically ill patients. The usual procedure for plotting the static and dynamic pressure-volume curves is to use the patient's ordered tidal volume as the midpoint of the graph.

Verify the Physician's Order

Verify the physician's order for the procedure. In some departments, plotting the static and dynamic pressure-volume curves is routinely performed once each shift.

Auscultate the Patient and Suction If Required

Auscultate the patient's chest and suction the patient if needed. Plotting the static and dynamic pressure-volume curves provides a means of measuring airway resistance. Secretions in the airways can significantly increase airway resistance.

Equipment Required

Graph paper is required to plot the curves. Volume is plotted on the y axis and pressure on the x axis. You may also need a portable respirometer if you are using an older ventilator without real-time exhaled volume monitoring capability.

Plotting the Curves

Decrease the tidal volume by 200 ml. Plot the static and dynamic pressures. Increase the tidal volume by 100-ml increments and plot the static and dynamic pressures for each increment until you have reached a tidal volume 200 ml greater than the ordered tidal volume. Once all values have been obtained, return the patient to the ordered tidal volume.

Monitor the patient during the procedure for adverse effects. A patient who is unstable may not tolerate the decrease in tidal volume. Monitor the blood pressure, heart rate and rhythm, and oximetry readings during the procedure. If the patient's tidal volumes are near the upper limit of acceptable values (12 to 15 ml/kg body weight), further increases in tidal volume may reach the lungs' elas-

tic limits. If pressures increase suddenly, do not increase the volume again because barotrauma may result.

Monitor the Patient

Following the procedure, monitor the patient for any adverse effects. Monitor the ventilator and document all settings. Remove any unneeded supplies from the room. Document the procedure in the patient's chart.

MEASUREMENT OF SPONTANEOUS PARAMETERS

Prior to extubation of the patient, it is important to measure the patient's pulmonary mechanics or spontaneous parameters. The procedure is similar to that described in Chapter 5 for bedside pulmonary function testing. In the intensive care unit, when spontaneous parameters are measured, the respirometer and maximal inspiratory pressure (MIP) meter are interfaced with the patient's artificial airway.

Equipment Required

The equipment you will need includes a respirometer, MIP manometer, a watch, and a manual resuscitation bag and mask. Collect all of your equipment and attach the manual resuscitator to an oxygen source and verify that it functions properly.

Auscultate and Suction the Patient If Required

Auscultate the patient's chest before you begin the procedure. If you can detect the presence of secretions in the airway, thoroughly suction the patient first. It is important to have the airways clear because an increased volume of secretions in the airways increases airway resistance, making the results you obtain less representative of the patient's true effort or ability.

Preoxygenation and Monitoring

In measuring the patient's spontaneous parameters, it is important to remember that the patient is acutely ill and that often the patient's oxygenation or ventilatory status is quite tenuous. Therefore, it is important to preoxygenate the patient before the procedures are performed and to allow rest periods as required by placing the patient back onto mechanical ventilation. When performing this procedure, be certain that the patient has at least electrocardiogram (ECG) and pulse oximetry monitoring in place to assist you in the assessment of the patient during this procedure.

Obtain Your Data

Obtain a minute volume and respiratory rate. Following the measurement of the minute volume, you may connect the patient to an oxygen source to rest, or alternatively, place the patient back onto the ventilator. Be sure to record your findings as you obtain them; often unexpected events can happen, and if your data are not written down, you may not remember your results.

Preoxygenate the patient again, and then obtain a vital capacity. Obtain at least three readings, compare the results, and strive for consistency between the three trials. It may take more than three trials to obtain three vital capacity values that represent the patient's best effort and are consistent with one another. Allow a rest period by connecting the patient to an oxygen source, or alternatively, the patient may be placed back onto the ventilator.

Preoxygenate the patient and obtain an MIP reading. Be sure to explain to the patient that the sensation of not getting any air is only temporary and will last only as long as you are performing the procedure. Watch the MIP manometer, and note the best effort that the patient can provide. Carefully monitor your patient for any adverse effects or intolerance to the procedure.

Return the Patient to Mechanical Ventilation

Unless you have orders that specify to remove the patient from mechanical ventilation if the spontaneous parameters fall within specified ranges, return the patient to mechanical ventilation. Once the previous ventilatory settings have been reestablished, record your findings on the ventilator flow sheet and on the patient's chart.

References

Headley-Whyte, J., Burgess, G. E., III, Feeley, T. W., & Miller, M. G. (1976). *Applied physiology of respiratory care*. Boston: Little, Brown.

Nelson, E. J., Hunter, P. M., & Morton, E. (1983). *Critical care respiratory therapy: A laboratory and clinical manual*. Boston: Little, Brown.

PLV-102 operating manual. (1991). Lafayette, CO: Lifecare.

Scanlan, C. L., Spearman, C. B., & Sheldon, R. L. (1995). *Egan's fundamentals of respiratory care* (6th ed.). St. Louis, MO: Mosby–Year Book.

Additional Resources

Bear 3 instruction manual. (1992). Riverside, CA: Bear Medical Systems.

Bear 1000 Ventilator instruction manual. (1994). Riverside, CA: Bear Medical Systems.

Bi-PAP® Ventilator Support System clinical manual for models S/T and S/T-D. (1990). Murrysville, PA: Respironics.

Demers, R. R., Pratter, M. R., & Irwin, R. S. (1981). Use of the concept of ventilator compliance in the determination of static total compliance. *Respiratory Care, 26*(7), 644.

Eubanks, D. H., & Bone, R. C. (1991). *Comprehensive respiratory care* (2nd ed.). St. Louis, MO: Mosby.

Henry, W. C., West, G. A., & Wilson, R. S. (1983). A comparison of the oxygen cost of breathing between a continuous-flow CPAP system and a demand-flow system. *Respiratory Care, 28*(10), 1273.

Kacmarek, R. M. (1997). Characteristics of pressure-targeted ventilators used for noninvasive positive pressure ventilation. *Respiratory Care, 42*(4), 380–388.

Kacmarek, R. M., Dimas, S., Reynolds, J., & Shapiro, B. (1982). Technical aspects of positive end-expiratory pressure (PEEP): Part I. Physics of PEEP devices. *Respiratory Care, 27*(12), 1478.

Kacmarek, R. M., Dimas, S., Reynolds, J., & Shapiro, B. (1982). Technical aspects of positive end-expiratory pressure (PEEP): Part II. PEEP with positive-pressure ventilation. *Respiratory Care, 27*(12), 1490.

Kacmarek, R. M., Dimas, S., Reynolds, J., & Shapiro, B. (1982). Technical aspects of positive end-expiratory pressure (PEEP): Part III. PEEP with spontaneous ventilation. *Respiratory Care, 27*(12), 1505.

Servo Ventilator 300 — operating manual. (1993). Solona, Sweden: Siemens-Elema AB.

7200 Series Ventilator, options and accessories, operator's manual. (1990). Carlsbad, CA: Puritan-Bennett Corporation.

8400ST Volume Ventilator instruction manual. (1990). Palm Springs, CA: Bird Products Corporation.

IMV and CPAP Practice Activities: The BEAR 1, 2, and 3 Ventilators

CIRCUIT ASSEMBLY, LEAK TESTING, AND TUBING COMPLIANCE

Assemble the circuit, test for leaks, and determine the tubing compliance as outlined in the practice activities for the BEAR 1, 2, and 3 in Chapter 26, "Continuous Mechanical Ventilation."

ACTIVITIES

To complete these practice activities, it is recommended that you use a lung analog/simulator such as a Medishield Lung Ventilator Performance Analyzer or Retec Respirator Teaching Console. Both of these devices or similar devices can alter resistance and compliance, simulating changes in patient condition. If these are not available, a test lung may be used.

SIMV PRACTICE ACTIVITY
Initial Ventilator Settings

Mode	SIMV
Normal Tidal Volume	800 ml
Ventilatory Rate	6 breaths/min
Flow Rate	50 L/min
Normal Pressure Limit	15 cm H_2O > cycling pressure
Low Pressure Alarm	15 cm H_2O < cycling pressure
Sensitivity	2 o'clock position
Wave Form	square
$O_2\%$	21%
Inspiratory Pause	0
Nebulizer	off
Sigh Controls	off
PEEP	0
Inverse Ratio Limit	off
Low Exhaled Volume Alarm	550 ml
Detection Delay	5 breaths (BEAR 2 only)
Apneic Period	20 seconds (BEAR 2 only)
High Rate Alarm	35 breaths/min

For this activity, you must be able to simulate a spontaneous breath by manually manipulating the lung simulator. On some models, this may be accomplished by expanding the bellows. If the lung simulator you have does not permit this, it will be necessary to perform this activity with a laboratory partner.

If you are using a laboratory partner as your patient, attach a mouthpiece to the patient wye. Your patient will breathe on the ventilator using a mouthpiece and a pair of nose clips. It is important for the patient to keep a tight seal on the mouthpiece. Spontaneously breathing on a volume ventilator is not easy and requires some practice for proper technique.

Activity 1: Control Panel and Respiratory Rate

1. Simulate a spontaneous respiratory rate of approximately 12 breaths/min.

2. Observe the control panel during spontaneous breathing.

3. Count the mandatory breaths (machine) and spontaneous breaths (patient) for 1 minute. Simultaneously, measure a minute volume using the minute volume feature.

Questions:

A. What did you observe on the control panel during SIMV?

B. What were the mandatory and the spontaneous respiratory rates?
   1. Add the mandatory and spontaneous rates.

C. Did your respiratory rate (combined) equal the rate the ventilator measured?
   1. If not, verify that the sensitivity control is at the 2 o'clock position and repeat the activity.
   2. Verify that no leaks exist.

Activity 2: Measuring Mandatory and Spontaneous Volumes

1. Adjust the ventilator controls to the values for the previous activity.

2. Simulate a spontaneous respiratory rate of 10 breaths/min.

3. Measure and calculate the mandatory (machine) tidal volume.

Method A

a. Measure a minute volume using the minute volume accumulate feature.

b. Simultaneously, each time the ventilator cycles, record and write down the mandatory tidal volume.

c. At the end of the minute volume period, write down the total minute volume (machine + spontaneous).

d. Determine the average mandatory tidal volume by adding each tidal breath and dividing that number by the mandatory rate. This is the measured tidal volume. Calculate the corrected tidal volume using the following formulas:

Tubing loss = peak inspiratory pressure × tubing compliance

Corrected tidal volume = measured tidal volume − tubing loss

e. Calculate the average spontaneous minute and tidal volume.
   (1) Determine the mandatory minute volume as you did in part d.
   (2) Subtract the mandatory minute volume from the total minute volume. This is the spontaneous minute volume.
   (3) Divide the spontaneous minute volume by the spontaneous rate you counted. This is the spontaneous tidal volume.

Method B

This method is commonly used in clinical practice. However, be certain to check your hospital departmental policy and procedure manual before using this procedure. If your manual does not advocate the use of this procedure, do not use it.

This method involves changing the mode of ventilation from SIMV to assist/control for 10 breaths. Although this time interval is short, it may affect your patient adversely.

a. Turn the mode control to assist/control for 10 breaths. Write down each measured volume. Immediately upon completion, return the patient to SIMV mode.

b. Calculate the average mandatory tidal volume by adding the measured tidal volumes together and dividing by 10.

c. Calculate the corrected tidal volume using the following formulas:

Tubing loss = peak inspiratory pressure × tubing compliance

Corrected tidal volume = measured tidal volume − tubing loss

d. Measure a minute volume using the minute volume accumulate feature. Count the total respiratory rate.

e. Calculate the mandatory minute volume by multiplying the average mandatory tidal volume by the mandatory rate.

f. Calculate the spontaneous minute volume by subtracting the mandatory minute volume from the total minute volume measured in part d.

g. Calculate the average spontaneous minute volume by dividing the spontaneous minute volume by the spontaneous rate.

Questions:

A. Using the following information, calculate the volumes and rates requested.

Total Minute Volume	22 L
Total Respiratory Rate	16 breaths/min
Average Mandatory Tidal Volume	800 ml
Mandatory Respiratory Rate	6 breaths/min
Peak Inspiratory Pressure	28 cm H_2O
Tubing Compliance	3.4 ml/cm H_2O

1. Corrected Mandatory Tidal Volume = _____
2. Mandatory Minute Volume = _____
3. Spontaneous Minute Volume = _____
4. Spontaneous Rate = _____
5. Spontaneous Tidal Volume = _____

B. Using the following information, calculate the volumes and rates requested.

Total Minute Volume	18.4 L
Total Respiratory Rate	18 breaths/min
Average Mandatory Tidal Volume	750 ml
Mandatory Respiratory Rate	4 breaths/min
Peak Inspiratory Pressure	30 cm H_2O
Tubing Compliance	4 ml/cm H_2O

1. Corrected Mandatory Tidal Volume = _____
2. Mandatory Minute Volume = _____
3. Spontaneous Minute Volume = _____
4. Spontaneous Rate = _____
5. Spontaneous Tidal Volume = _____

SIMV with CPAP

SIMV with CPAP is a combination ventilator modality. It is a combination of PEEP with mandatory breaths and CPAP with spontaneous breaths. The BEAR 1 and 2 automatically permit operation in this mode.

Initial Ventilator Settings

Mode	SIMV
Normal Tidal Volume	800 ml
Respiratory Rate	6/min
Flow Rate	50 L/min
Normal Pressure Limit	15 cm H_2O > cycling pressure
Low Pressure Alarm	15 cm H_2O < cycling pressure
Sensitivity	2 o'clock position
Wave Form	square
O_2%	21%
Inspiratory Pause	0
Nebulizer	off
Sigh Controls	off
PEEP	+10 cm H_2O
Inverse Ratio Limit	off
Low Exhaled Volume Alarm	550 ml
Detection Delay	5 breaths (BEAR 2 only)
Apneic Period	20 seconds (BEAR 2 only)
High Rate Alarm	35 breaths/min (BEAR 2 only)
PEEP Alarm	+5 cm H_2O

For this activity, you must be able to simulate a spontaneous breath by manually manipulating the lung simulator. On some models, this may be accomplished by expanding the bellows. If the lung simulator you have does not permit this, it will be necessary to perform this activity with a laboratory partner.

If you are using a laboratory partner as a patient, attach a mouthpiece to the patient wye. Your patient will breathe on the ventilator using a mouthpiece and a pair of nose clips. It is important for the patient to keep a tight seal on the mouthpiece. Spontaneously breathing on a volume ventilator is not easy and requires some practice for proper technique.

Activity 1: Control Panel and Respiratory Rate

1. Simulate a spontaneous respiratory rate of approximately 12 breaths/min.

2. Observe the control panel during spontaneous breathing.

3. Count the mandatory breaths (machine) and spontaneous breaths (patient) for 1 minute. Simultaneously, measure a minute volume using the minute volume feature.

Questions:

A. What did you observe on the control panel during SIMV?

B. What were the mandatory and spontaneous respiratory rates?

C. Did your respiratory rate (combined) equal the rate the ventilator measured?

1. If not, verify that the sensitivity control is at the 2 o'clock position and repeat the activity.

Activity 2: Measuring Mandatory and Spontaneous Volumes

1. Adjust the ventilator controls to the values for the previous activity.

2. Simulate a spontaneous respiratory rate of 10 breaths/min.

3. Measure and calculate the mandatory (machine) tidal volume.

Method A

a. Measure a minute volume using the minute volume accumulate feature.

b. Simultaneously, each time the ventilator cycles, record and write down the mandatory tidal volume.

c. At the end of the minute volume period, write down the total minute volume (machine + spontaneous).

d. Determine the average mandatory tidal volume by adding them and dividing that number by the mandatory rate. This is the measured tidal volume. Calculate the corrected tidal volume using the following formulas:

Tubing loss =
(peak inspiratory pressure − PEEP pressure) × tubing compliance

Corrected tidal volume = measured tidal volume − tubing loss

e. Calculate the average spontaneous minute and tidal volume.

(1) Determine the average mandatory tidal volume using the method outlined in part d above.

(2) Subtract the mandatory minute volume from the total minute volume. This is the spontaneous minute volume.

(3) Divide the spontaneous minute volume by the spontaneous rate you counted. This is the spontaneous tidal volume.

Method B

This method is commonly used in clinical practice. However, be certain to check your hospital departmental policy and procedure manual before using this procedure. If your manual does not advocate the use of this procedure, do not use it.

This method involves changing the mode of ventilation from SIMV to assist/control for 10 breaths. Although this time interval is short, it may affect your patient adversely.

a. Turn the mode control to assist/control for 10 breaths. Write down each measured volume. Immediately upon completion, return the patient to SIMV mode.

b. Calculate the average mandatory tidal volume by adding the measured tidal volumes together and dividing by 10.

c. Calculate the corrected tidal volume using the following formulas:

Tubing loss =
(peak inspiratory pressure − PEEP pressure) × tubing compliance

Corrected tidal volume = measured tidal volume − tubing loss

d. Measure a minute volume using the minute volume accumulate feature. Count the total respiratory rate.

e. Calculate the mandatory minute volume by multiplying the average mandatory tidal volume by the mandatory rate.

f. Calculate the spontaneous minute volume by subtracting the mandatory minute volume from the total minute volume measured in part d.

g. Calculate the average spontaneous minute volume by dividing the spontaneous minute volume by the spontaneous rate.

Questions:

A. Using the following information, calculate the volumes and rates requested.

Total Minute Volume	20 L
Total Respiratory Rate	14/min
Average Mandatory Tidal Volume	800 ml
Mandatory Respiratory Rate	6 breaths/min
Peak Inspiratory Pressure	28 cm H_2O
Tubing Compliance	4.0 ml/cm H_2O
PEEP	+10 cm H_2O

1. Corrected Mandatory Tidal Volume = _____
2. Mandatory Minute Volume = _____
3. Spontaneous Minute Volume = _____
4. Spontaneous Rate = _____
5. Spontaneous Tidal Volume = _____

B. Using the following information, calculate the volumes and rates requested.

Total Minute Volume	23.2 L
Total Respiratory Rate	19/min
Average Mandatory Tidal Volume	900 ml
Mandatory Respiratory Rate	4 breaths/min
Peak Inspiratory Pressure	30 cm H_2O
Tubing Compliance	4 ml/cm H_2O
PEEP	+5 cm H_2O

1. Corrected Mandatory Tidal Volume = _____
2. Mandatory Minute Volume = _____
3. Spontaneous Minute Volume = _____
4. Spontaneous Rate = _____
5. Spontaneous Tidal Volume = _____

CPAP PRACTICE ACTIVITIES

CPAP is a feature incorporated into the design of the BEAR 1 and 2 ventilators. This feature combined with the monitoring and alarm capability simplifies the use of this modality.

Initial Ventilator Settings

Mode	CPAP
Normal Tidal Volume	off
Normal Rate	off
Normal Pressure Limit	off
Sigh Controls	off
Sensitivity	2 o'clock position
Ratio Limit	off
O_2 %	21%
Peak Flow	has no effect
Inspiratory Pause	off
Nebulizer	off
PEEP	+5 cm H_2O
Low Inspiratory Pressure Alarm	off
Minute Exhaled Volume Alarm	300 ml
PEEP/CPAP Alarm	+2 cm H_2O
Detection Delay	5 breaths (BEAR 2 only)

Apneic Period	20 seconds (BEAR 2 only)
High Rate Alarm	35 breaths/min (BEAR 2 only)

Using a laboratory partner as your patient, attach a mouthpiece to the patient wye. Your patient will breathe on the ventilator using a mouthpiece and a pair of nose clips. It is important for the patient to keep a tight seal on the mouthpiece. Spontaneously breathing on a volume ventilator is not easy and requires some practice for proper technique.

Activity 1: Control Panel

1. While breathing spontaneously, carefully observe the control panel. Observe the pressure manometer, expiratory source, exhaled volume/rate monitors, and I:E ratio displays.

2. Measure a minute volume using the minute volume accumulate feature. Simultaneously, count the respiratory rate.

Questions:
A. What event(s) did you observe on the control panel?
B. What were the minute volume and rate you measured? Does the measured respiratory rate coincide with the rate you counted?
   1. If it does not, verify that the sensitivity control is set at the 2 o'clock position.
C. Calculate the average tidal volume by dividing the measured minute volume by the respiratory rate.

Activity 2: Alarm Functions

1. Connect a mouthpiece to the patient wye and breathe, deliberately simulating bradypnea. Observe the control panel.

2. Deliberately simulate hypoventilation by taking very small tidal volumes. Observe the control panel.

3. Remove the mouthpiece from your mouth and observe the control panel.

4. If you are using a BEAR 2, simulate hyperpnea. Observe the control panel.

Question:
A. Describe the event(s) you observed in activities 1, 2, 3, and 4.

Activity 3: CPAP Pressure Variations

1. Repeat activities 1 and 2 using CPAP levels of +10 and +15 cm H_2O.

PRESSURE SUPPORT ACTIVITIES (BEAR 3)

The BEAR 3 ventilator is capable of providing pressure support in SIMV and CPAP modes of ventilation. When pressure support is activated, all spontaneous breaths will be augmented with the level of pressure support established by the practitioner. Pressure support is adjustable between 5.5 and 66 cm H_2O.

SIMV with Pressure Support

1. Set the ventilator to the following settings:

Mode	SIMV
Normal Tidal Volume	800 ml

Respiratory Rate	6/min
Flow Rate	50 L/min
Normal Pressure Limit	15 cm H_2O > peak pressure
Low Pressure Alarm	15 cm H_2O < peak pressure
Sensitivity	2 o'clock position
Wave Form	square
O_2 %	21%
Inspiratory Pause	0.0 seconds
Nebulizer	off
Sigh Controls	off
PEEP	0.0 cm H_2O
Low Exhaled Volume Alarm	550 ml
Detection Delay	5 breaths
Apneic Period	20 seconds
High Rate Alarm	40 breaths/min
PSV	ON
Pressure Support	10 cm H_2O (adjust using right hand button below the pressure manometer)

For this activity, you must be able to simulate a spontaneous breath by manually manipulating the lung simulator. On some models, this may be accomplished by expanding the bellows. You may also perform these activities using a laboratory partner as your patient; however, it is suggested that you decrease the tidal volumes to around 500 ml when doing so. Your "patient" may breathe on the ventilator using a mouthpiece and nose clips.

2. Simulate a respiratory rate of approximately 12 breaths/min.
   a. Observe the control panel during spontaneous ventilation.
   b. Determine the spontaneous and the mandatory rates.
   c. Determine the spontaneous (PSV) and mandatory tidal volumes.

3. Increase the pressure support to 20 cm H_2O.
   a. Observe the control panel during spontaneous ventilation.
   b. Determine the spontaneous and the mandatory rates.
   c. Determine the spontaneous (PSV) and mandatory tidal volumes.

Questions:
A. How did pressure support affect tidal volume when compared with the SIMV exercises without pressure support?
B. How did the increase in pressure support affect tidal volume?

CPAP with Pressure Support

1. Set the ventilator to the following settings:

Mode	CPAP
Normal Pressure Limit	5 cm H_2O > peak pressure
Low Pressure Alarm	5 cm H_2O < peak pressure
Sensitivity	2 o'clock position
O_2 %	21%

Nebulizer	off
Sigh Controls	off
PEEP	10.0 cm H_2O
Low Exhaled Volume Alarm	250 ml
Detection Delay	5 breaths
Apneic Period	20 seconds
High Rate Alarm	40 breaths/min
PSV	ON
Pressure Support	0.0 cm H_2O (adjust using right-hand button below the pressure manometer)

2. Using a mouthpiece and nose clips, have the "patient" breathe from the ventilator.

3. Simulate a respiratory rate of approximately 12 breaths/min.
   a. Observe the control panel during spontaneous ventilation.
   b. Determine the spontaneous rate.
   c. Determine the spontaneous tidal volume.

4. Add pressure support of 10 cm H_2O.
   a. Observe the control panel during spontaneous ventilation.
   b. Determine the spontaneous rate.
   c. Determine the spontaneous (PSV) tidal volume.

Question:

A. How did pressure support affect tidal volume when compared with CPAP without pressure support?

IMV and CPAP Practice Activities: BEAR 5

CIRCUIT ASSEMBLY, LEAK TESTING, AND TUBING COMPLIANCE

Assemble the circuit, test for leaks, and determine the tubing compliance as outlined in the practice activities for the BEAR 5 in Chapter 26, "Continuous Mechanical Ventilation."

ACTIVITIES

To complete these practice activities, it is recommended that you use a lung analog/simulator such as a Medishield Lung Ventilator Performance Analyzer or Retec Respirator Teaching Console. Both of these devices or similar devices can alter resistance and compliance, simulating changes in patient condition.

SIMV PRACTICE ACTIVITIES
Initial Ventilator Settings

Required Settings

Mode	SIMV
Tidal Volume	800 ml
Normal Rate	6 breaths/min
Peak Flow	50 L/min
O_2 %	21%
Sensitivity	–2 cm H_2O

Optional Settings

Compliance Compensation	tubing compensation value
PEEP/CPAP	off
Inspiratory Pause	0
Wave Form	square
Sigh Controls	off
Alarms	select autoset values

For this activity, you must be able to simulate a spontaneous breath by manually manipulating the lung simulator. On some models, this may be accomplished by expanding the bellows. If the lung simulator you have does not permit this, it will be necessary to perform this activity with a laboratory partner.

If you are using a laboratory partner as your patient, attach a mouthpiece to the patient wye. Your patient will breathe on the ventilator using a mouthpiece and a pair of nose clips. It is important for the patient to keep a tight seal on the mouthpiece. Spontaneously breathing on a volume ventilator is not easy and requires some practice for proper technique.

Activity 1: Control Panel and Respiratory Rate

1. Simulate a spontaneous respiratory rate of approximately 12 breaths/min.

2. Observe the control panel during spontaneous breathing.

3. Count the mandatory breaths (machine) and spontaneous breaths (patient) for 1 minute. After 1 minute, measure the values indicated on the CRT screen.

Questions:

A. What did you observe on the control panel during SIMV?

B. What were the mandatory and the spontaneous respiratory rates?
   1. Did this value coincide with the CRT display of BREATH RATE?

Activity 2: Measuring Mandatory and Spontaneous Volumes

1. Adjust the ventilator controls to the values for the previous activity.

2. Simulate a spontaneous respiratory rate of 10 breaths/min.

3. Record the mandatory (machine) tidal volume.

4. Record the spontaneous tidal volumes.

5. Record the accumulated minute volume.

Questions:

A. Using the following information, calculate the volume and rates requested.

Accumulated Minute Volume	8.8 L
Spontaneous Tidal Volume	400 ml
Mandatory Tidal Volume	800 ml
Mandatory Rate	4/min
Total Rate	14/min

   1. Spontaneous Minute Volume   = _____
   2. Mandatory Minute Volume   = _____

B. Using the following information, calculate the volumes and rates requested.

Accumulated Minute Volume	11.7 L
Spontaneous Tidal Volume	350 ml
Mandatory Tidal Volume	900 ml
Mandatory Rate	6/min
Total Rate	24/min

1. Spontaneous Minute Volume = _____
2. Mandatory Minute Volume = _____

SIMV WITH CPAP

SIMV with CPAP is a combination ventilator modality. It is a combination of PEEP with mandatory breaths and CPAP with spontaneous breaths. The BEAR 5 automatically permits operation in this mode.

Initial Ventilator Settings

Required Settings

Mode	SIMV
Tidal Volume	750 ml
Normal Rate	6/min
Peak Flow	50 L/min
O_2 %	21%
Sensitivity	−2 cm H_2O
PEEP/CPAP	+5 cm H_2O

Optional Settings

Compliance Compensation	tubing compensation value
Inspiratory Pause	0
Wave Form	square
Sigh Controls	off
Alarms	select autoset values

For this activity, you must be able to simulate a spontaneous breath by manually manipulating the lung simulator. On some models, this may be accomplished by expanding the bellows. If the lung simulator you have does not permit this, it will be necessary to perform this activity with a laboratory partner.

If you are using a laboratory partner as your patient, attach a mouthpiece to the patient wye. Your patient will breathe on the ventilator using a mouthpiece and a pair of nose clips. It is important for the patient to keep a tight seal on the mouthpiece. Spontaneously breathing on a volume ventilator is not easy and requires some practice for proper technique.

Activity 1: Control Panel and Respiratory Rate

1. Simulate a spontaneous respiratory rate of approximately 12 breaths/min.

2. Observe the control panel and the CRT display during spontaneous breathing.

3. Count the mandatory breaths (machine) and spontaneous breaths (patient) for 1 minute. At the end of the minute interval, compare your values with the CRT display.

Questions:

A. What did you observe on the control panel during SIMV with CPAP?

B. What were the mandatory and the spontaneous respiratory rates?

C. Did your respiratory rate (combined) equal the rate the ventilator measured?

Activity 2: Measuring Mandatory and Spontaneous Volumes

1. Adjust the ventilator controls to the values for the previous activity.

2. Simulate a spontaneous respiratory rate of 10 breaths/min.

3. Record the mandatory (machine) tidal volume.

4. Record the spontaneous tidal volumes.

5. Record the accumulated minute volume.

Questions:

A. Using the following information, calculate the volumes and rates requested.

Total Minute Volume	20 L
Total Respiratory Rate	14/min
Mandatory Tidal Volume	800 ml
Mandatory Respiratory Rate	6/min
Spontaneous Tidal Volume	400 ml
Peak Inspiratory Pressure	28 cm H_2O
PEEP	+10 cm H_2O

1. Spontaneous Minute Volume = _____
2. Spontaneous Rate = _____
3. Spontaneous Minute Volume = _____

B. Using the following information, calculate the volumes and rates requested.

Total Minute Volume	11.1 L
Total Respiratory Rate	19/min
Average Mandatory Tidal Volume	900 ml
Spontaneous Tidal Volume	500 ml
Mandatory Respiratory Rate	4/min
Peak Inspiratory Pressure	30 cm H_2O
Tubing Compliance	4 ml/cm H_2O
PEEP	+5 cm H_2O

1. Corrected Mandatory Tidal Volume = _____
2. Mandatory Minute Volume = _____
3. Spontaneous Minute Volume = _____

CPAP PRACTICE EXERCISES

CPAP is a feature incorporated into the design of the BEAR 5 ventilator. This feature combined with the monitoring and alarm capability simplifies the use of this modality.

Initial Ventilator Settings

Required

O_2 %	21%
Assist Sensitivity	−2 cm H_2O

Optional

PEEP/CPAP	+5 cm H_2O
Alarms	select autoset values

Using a laboratory partner as your patient, attach a mouthpiece to the patient wye. Your patient will breathe on the ventilator using a mouthpiece and a pair of nose clips. It is important for the patient to keep a tight seal on the mouthpiece. Spontaneously breathing on a volume ventilator is not easy and requires some practice for proper technique.

Activity 1: Control Panel

1. Attach a mouthpiece to the patient wye. While breathing spontaneously, carefully observe the control panel. Observe the pressure manometer and the CRT display.

2. Measure a minute volume. Simultaneously, count the respiratory rate.

Questions:
A. What event(s) did you observe on the control panel?
B. What were the minute volume and rate you measured? Does the displayed respiratory rate coincide with the rate you counted?

Activity 2: Alarm Functions

1. Attach a mouthpiece to the patient wye and breathe, deliberately simulating bradypnea. Observe the control panel.

2. Deliberately simulate hypoventilation by taking very small tidal volumes. Observe the control panel.

3. Remove the mouthpiece from your mouth and observe the control panel.

4. Simulate hyperpnea. Observe the control panel.

Question:
A. Describe the event(s) you observed in activities 1, 2, 3, and 4.

Activity 3: CPAP Pressure Variations

1. Repeat activities 1 and 2 using CPAP levels of +10 and +15 cm H_2O.

PRESSURE SUPPORT

Pressure support is a mode that augments the patient's spontaneous efforts. When a patient initiates a spontaneous breath (as sensed by the sensitivity system), a constant pressure is delivered. When the inspiratory flow rate reaches 25% of the peak inspiratory flow, inspiration is terminated.

Modes Available

Pressure support is available in SIMV, CPAP, and augmented minute ventilation (AMV) modes.

Initial Ventilator Settings
Required Settings
Mode	SIMV
Tidal Volume	800 ml
Normal Rate	6 breaths/min
Peak Flow	50 L/min
O_2 %	21%
Sensitivity	–2 cm H_2O

Optional Settings
Compliance Compensation	tubing compensation value
PEEP/CPAP	off
Inspiratory Pause	0
Wave Form	square
Sigh Controls	off
Alarms	select autoset values

Activity 1: Pressure Support with SIMV

1. Select pressure support by depressing the pressure support soft key. Enter +10 cm H_2O using the keypad on the right of the control panel.

2. Repeat the SIMV practice activities using pressure support. Observe the pressure manometer and the CRT display.

3. Increase the pressure support to +20 cm H_2O using the keypad. Observe the control panel and the CRT display.

4. Repeat the SIMV with CPAP practice activities using pressure support.

Activity 2: Pressure Support with CPAP

1. Select pressure support by depressing the pressure support soft key. Enter +10 cm H_2O using the keypad on the right of the control panel.

2. Repeat the CPAP practice activities using pressure support. Carefully observe the control panel and the CRT display.

Questions:
A. What did you observe on the CRT display and the control panel?
B. How did the spontaneous tidal volumes compare to the previous activities without pressure support?
C. What did you observe on the pressure manometer during spontaneous ventilation?

Augmented Minute Ventilation

This is similar to the SIMV mode of ventilation. The exception is that you may select a guaranteed minute ventilation that the patient will receive. If the monitors on the ventilator sense that the patient is breathing less than the guaranteed minute volume, the mandatory breath rate will increase until the minimum level is met.

ACTIVITIES

For this activity, you must be able to simulate a spontaneous breath by manually manipulating the lung simulator. On some models, this may be accomplished by expanding the bellows. If the lung simulator you have does not permit this, it will be necessary to perform this activity with a laboratory partner.

If you are using a laboratory partner as your patient, attach a mouthpiece to the patient wye. Your patient will breathe on the ventilator using a mouthpiece and a pair of nose clips. It is important for the patient to keep a tight seal on the mouthpiece. Spontaneously breathing on a volume ventilator is not easy and requires some practice for proper technique.

Initial Ventilator Settings
Required
Tidal Volume	700 ml
Normal Rate	4 breaths/min
Peak Flow	50 L/min
O_2 %	21%
Assist Sensitivity	–2 cm H_2O
Minimum Minute Volume	8 L/min

Optional
Compliance Compensation	4 ml/cm H_2O
PEEP/CPAP	0
Inspiratory Pause	0
Wave Form	square

Pressure Support	0
Sigh Controls	off
Alarms	select autoset values

Activity 1

1. Simulate a spontaneous respiratory rate of 12 breaths/min. Observe the control panel, pressure manometer, and CRT display.

2. Simulate bradypnea with a rate of 4 breaths/min.

Observe the control panel, pressure manometer, and CRT display.

3. Simulate hyperpnea with a rate of 32 breaths/min. Observe the control panel and CRT display.

Questions:

A. What event(s) occurred during activities 1 through 3?
B. Can you think of a clinical situation in which it would be helpful to use this mode?
C. What are the advantages of this mode?

SIMV, CPAP, and Pressure Support Practice Activities: BEAR 1000

CIRCUIT ASSEMBLY, LEAK TESTING, AND TUBING COMPLIANCE

Assemble the circuit, test for leaks, and determine the tubing compliance as outlined in the practice activities for the BEAR 1000 in Chapter 26, "Continuous Mechanical Ventilation."

To complete these practice activities, it is recommended that you use a lung analog/simulator such as a Medishield Lung Ventilator Performance Analyzer or other device in which resistance and compliance may be easily altered.

Alternatively, you may use a laboratory partner as your patient, with a mouthpiece and nose clips utilized for patient-ventilator interface. In this situation, it is suggested that you decrease tidal volumes to around 500 ml.

SIMV PRACTICE ACTIVITIES

1. Set the ventilator to the following settings:

Mode	SIMV/CPAP (PSV)
Tidal Volume	800 ml
Rate	6/min
Peak Flow	50 L/min
Wave Form	square
O_2 %	21%
Sensitivity	2.0 cm H_2O
PEEP	0.0 cm H_2O
Alarms	adjust as appropriate

2. Simulate a spontaneous respiratory rate of about 12 breaths/min.

3. Observe the control panel and graphics display module.
   a. Determine the spontaneous and the mandatory rates.
   b. Determine the spontaneous and mandatory tidal volumes.
   c. Determine the total minute ventilation, spontaneous minute ventilation, and mandatory minute ventilation.

4. On the basis of your measurements and observations, set the alarms to appropriate settings.

SIMV with CPAP Practice Activities

1. Set the ventilator to the following settings:

Mode	SIMV/CPAP (PSV)
Tidal Volume	800 ml
Rate	6/min
Peak Flow	50 L/min
Wave Form	square
O_2 %	21%
Sensitivity	2.0 cm H_2O
PEEP	5.0 cm H_2O
Alarms	adjust as appropriate

2. Simulate a spontaneous respiratory rate of about 12 breaths/min.

3. Observe the control panel and graphics display module.
   a. Determine the spontaneous and the mandatory rates.
   b. Determine the spontaneous and mandatory tidal volumes.
   c. Determine the total minute ventilation, spontaneous minute ventilation, and mandatory minute ventilation.

4. Breathe on the patient circuit at these settings using a mouthpiece and a pair of nose clips.

SIMV with CPAP and Flow Triggering Practice Activity

1. Add the following to the ventilator settings:

| Base Flow | 8 L/min |
| Flow Trigger | 3 L/min |

2. Simulate a spontaneous respiratory rate of about 12 breaths/min.

3. Observe the control panel and graphics display module.
   a. Determine the spontaneous and the mandatory rates.
   b. Determine the spontaneous and mandatory tidal volumes.
   c. Determine the total minute ventilation, spontaneous minute ventilation, and mandatory minute ventilation.

4. On the basis of your measurements and observations, set the alarms to appropriate settings.

5. Breathe on the circuit using a mouthpiece and a pair of nose clips.

Questions:

A. How did the SIMV and SIMV with CPAP activity differ from one another based upon your observations?
B. As a patient, which would you prefer, pressure or flow triggering? Why?

PRESSURE SUPPORT ACTIVITIES

The BEAR 1000 can provide pressure support in SIMV and CPAP modes, providing pressure augmentation to spontaneous breaths. In this activity set, you will use this ventilator to apply pressure support.

SIMV with Pressure Support

1. Set the ventilator to the following settings:

Mode	SIMV/CPAP (PSV)
Tidal Volume	800 ml
Rate	6/min
Peak Flow	50 L/min
Wave Form	square
O_2 %	21%
Sensitivity	2.0 cm H_2O
PEEP	0.0 cm H_2O
Pressure Support	10 cm H_2O
Alarms	adjust as appropriate

2. Simulate a respiratory rate of approximately 12 breaths/min.
   a. Observe the control panel and graphics display module during spontaneous ventilation.
   b. Determine the spontaneous and the mandatory rates.
   c. Determine the spontaneous (with pressure support) and mandatory tidal volumes.

3. Increase the pressure support to 20 cm H_2O.
   a. Observe the control panel during spontaneous ventilation.
   b. Determine the spontaneous and the mandatory rates.
   c. Determine the spontaneous (PSV) and mandatory tidal volumes.

Questions:

A. How did pressure support affect tidal volume when compared with the SIMV exercises without pressure support?

B. How did the increase in pressure support affect tidal volume?

CPAP with Pressure Support

1. Set the ventilator to the following settings:

Mode	SIMV/CPAP (PSV)
Rate	zero
Sensitivity	2.0 cm H_2O
O_2 %	21%
Nebulizer	off
PEEP	10.0 cm H_2O
Pressure Support	0.0 cm H_2O
Alarms	set as appropriate

2. Using a mouthpiece and nose clips, have your "patient" breathe from the ventilator.

3. Simulate a respiratory rate of approximately 12 breaths/min.
   a. Observe the control panel and graphics display module during spontaneous ventilation.
   b. Determine the spontaneous rate.
   c. Determine the spontaneous tidal volume.

4. Add pressure support of 10 cm H_2O.
   a. Observe the control panel during spontaneous ventilation.
   b. Determine the spontaneous rate.
   c. Determine the spontaneous (PSV) tidal volume.

Question:

A. How did pressure support affect tidal volume when compared with CPAP without pressure support?

IMV and CPAP Practice Activities: Bird 8400ST

CIRCUIT ASSEMBLY, LEAK TESTING, AND TUBING COMPLIANCE

Assemble the circuit, test for leaks, and determine the tubing compliance as outlined in the practice activities for the Bird 8400ST in Chapter 26, "Continuous Mechanical Ventilation."

To complete these practice activities, it is recommended that you use a lung analog/simulator such as a Medishield Lung Ventilator Performance Analyzer or other device in which resistance and compliance may be easily altered.

Alternatively, you may use your laboratory partner as a patient, with a mouthpiece and nose clips utilized for patient-ventilator interface. In this situation it is suggested that you decrease tidal volumes to around 500 ml.

SIMV PRACTICE ACTIVITIES

1. Set the ventilator to the following settings:

Mode	SIMV/CPAP
Tidal Volume	800 ml
Breath Rate	6/min
Peak Flow	50 L/min
Wave Form	square
O_2 %	21%
Sensitivity	2.0 cm H_2O
PEEP	0.0 cm H_2O
Alarms	adjust as appropriate

2. Simulate a spontaneous respiratory rate of about 12 breaths/min.

3. Observe the control panel and the pressure manometer.
   a. Determine the spontaneous and the mandatory rates.
   b. Determine the spontaneous and mandatory tidal volumes.
   c. Determine the total minute ventilation, spontaneous minute ventilation, and mandatory minute ventilation.

4. On the basis of your measurements and observations, set the alarms to appropriate settings.

SIMV with CPAP Practice Activities

1. Set the ventilator to the following settings:

Mode	SIMV/CPAP
Tidal Volume	800 ml
Breath Rate	6/min
Peak Flow	50 L/min
Wave Form	square
O_2 %	21%
Sensitivity	2.0 cm H_2O
PEEP	5.0 cm H_2O
Alarms	adjust as appropriate

2. Simulate a spontaneous respiratory rate of about 12 breaths/min.

3. Observe the control panel and pressure manometer.
   a. Determine the spontaneous and the mandatory rates.
   b. Determine the spontaneous and mandatory tidal volumes.
   c. Determine the total minute ventilation, spontaneous minute ventilation, and mandatory minute ventilation.

4. Breathe on the patient circuit at these settings using a mouthpiece and a pair of nose clips.

SIMV with CPAP and Flow Triggering
Practice Activity

1. Install the special flow sensor onto the ventilator, and change the trigger sensitivity to the following setting:
   Flow Trigger   3 L/min

2. Simulate a spontaneous respiratory rate of about 12 breaths/min.

3. Observe the control panel and graphics display module.
   a. Determine the spontaneous and the mandatory rates.
   b. Determine the spontaneous and mandatory tidal volumes.
   c. Determine the total minute ventilation, spontaneous minute ventilation, and mandatory minute ventilation.

4. On the basis of your measurements and observations, set the alarms to appropriate settings.

5. Breathe on the circuit using a mouthpiece and a pair of nose clips.

Questions:
A. How did the SIMV and SIMV with CPAP activity differ from one another based upon your observations?
B. As a patient, which would you prefer, pressure or flow triggering? Why?

PRESSURE SUPPORT ACTIVITIES

The Bird 8400ST can provide pressure support in SIMV and CPAP modes, providing pressure augmentation to spontaneous breaths. In these activities you will learn how pressure support may be applied with this ventilator.

SIMV with Pressure Support

1. Set the ventilator to the following settings:

Mode	SIMV/CPAP
Tidal Volume	800 ml
Breath Rate	6/min
Peak Flow	50 L/min
Wave Form	square
O_2 %	21%
Sensitivity	2.0 cm H_2O
PEEP	0.0 cm H_2O
Pressure Support	10 cm H_2O
Alarms	adjust as appropriate

2. Simulate a respiratory rate of approximately 12 breaths/min.
   a. Observe the control panel and graphics display module during spontaneous ventilation.
   b. Determine the spontaneous and the mandatory rates.
   c. Determine the spontaneous (PSV) and mandatory tidal volumes.

3. Increase the pressure support to 20 cm H_2O.
   a. Observe the control panel during spontaneous ventilation.
   b. Determine the spontaneous and the mandatory rates.
   c. Determine the spontaneous (PSV) and mandatory tidal volumes.

Questions:
A. How did pressure support affect tidal volume when compared with the SIMV exercises without pressure support?
B. How did the increase in pressure support affect tidal volume?

CPAP with Pressure Support

1. Set the ventilator to the following settings:

Mode	SIMV/CPAP (PSV)
Breath Rate	zero
Sensitivity	2.0 cm H_2O
O_2 %	21%
PEEP	10.0 cm H_2O
Pressure Support	0.0 cm H_2O
Alarms	set as appropriate

2. Using a mouthpiece and nose clips, have your "patient" breathe from the ventilator.

3. Simulate a respiratory rate of approximately 12 breaths/min.
   a. Observe the control panel and graphics display module during spontaneous ventilation.
   b. Determine the spontaneous rate.
   c. Determine the spontaneous tidal volume.

4. Add pressure support of 10 cm H_2O.
   a. Observe the control panel during spontaneous ventilation.
   b. Determine the spontaneous rate.
   c. Determine the spontaneous (PSV) tidal volume.

Question:
A. How did pressure support affect tidal volume when compared with CPAP without pressure support?

SIMV Practice Activities: Lifecare PLV-102

CIRCUIT ASSEMBLY, LEAK TESTING, AND TUBING COMPLIANCE

Assemble the circuit, test for leaks, and determine the tubing compliance as outlined in the practice activity for the Lifecare PLV-102 in Chapter 26, "Continuous Mechanical Ventilation."

ACTIVITIES

To complete these activities, it is recommended that you use a lung analog/simulator such as a Medishield Lung Ventilator Performance Analyzer or Rectec Respiratory Teaching Console. Both of these devices or similar devices can alter resistance and compliance, simulating changes in patient condition.

SIMV Practice Activities

To operate the PLV-102 in the SIMV mode, set the ventilator to the following initial settings:

Mode	SIMV
Tidal Volume	800 ml
Rate	6/min
Flow	40 L/min
Sensitivity	−2 cm H_2O

For this activity, you must be able to simulate a spontaneous breath by manually manipulating the lung simulator. On some models, this may be accomplished by expanding the bellows. If your lung simulator does not permit this, you will need to perform this activity with a laboratory partner as your patient.

Attach a mouthpiece to the patient wye. The "patient" will breathe on the ventilator using a pair of nose clips. It is important for the patient to keep a tight seal on the mouthpiece. Spontaneously breathing on a volume ventilator is not easy and requires some practice for proper technique.

Activity 1: Respiratory Rate

1. Simulate a spontaneous respiratory rate of 12 breaths/min.

2. Observe the control panel during the spontaneous breathing.

3. Count the mandatory breaths and the spontaneous breaths for 1 minute.

Questions:

A. What did you observe on the control panel during SIMV?

B. What were the mandatory and the spontaneous respiratory rates?

C. Record your total minute volume.

4. Increase the mandatory rate to 10/min.

5. Observe the control panel during the spontaneous breathing.

6. Count the mandatory breaths and the spontaneous breaths for 1 minute.

Questions:

A. What did you observe on the control panel during SIMV?

B. What were the mandatory and the spontaneous respiratory rates?

C. Record your total minute volume.

Measuring Mandatory and Spontaneous Volumes

1. Adjust the ventilator controls to the values for the previous activity.

2. Simulate a spontaneous rate of 10 breaths/min.

3. Measure and calculate the mandatory tidal volume. Record at least 10 mandatory breaths and determine an average by attaching an external spirometer.

4. Calculate the corrected tidal volume using the following formulas:

Tubing loss = peak pressures × tubing compliance

Corrected tidal volume = measured tidal volume − tubing loss

Questions:

A. Using the following information, calculate the volumes and rates requested:

Total Minute Volume	8.8 L
Total Respiratory Rate	16/min
Average Mandatory Tidal Volume	800 ml
Mandatory Rate	6/minute
Peak Pressure	28 cm H_2O
Tubing Compliance	3.4 ml/cm H_2O

1. Corrected Mandatory Tidal Volume = _____
2. Mandatory Minute Volume = _____
3. Spontaneous Minute Volume = _____
4. Spontaneous Rate = _____
5. Spontaneous Tidal Volume = _____

B. Using the following information, calculate the volume and rates requested:

Total Minute Volume	10 L
Total Respiratory Rate	18/min
Average Mandatory Tidal Volume	750 ml
Mandatory Rate	4/min
Peak Pressure	30 cm H_2O
Tubing Compliance	4 ml/cm H_2O

1. Corrected Mandatory Tidal Volume = _____
2. Mandatory Minute Volume = _____
3. Spontaneous Minute Volume = _____
4. Spontaneous Rate = _____
5. Spontaneous Tidal Volume = _____

Tidal Volume Control

1. Adjust the ventilator to the following settings:

Mode	SIMV
Tidal Volume	500 ml
Rate	6/min
Flow	40 L/min
Sensitivity	−2 cm H_2O

2. Simulate a spontaneous respiratory rate of 14/min.

3. Measure and calculate the mandatory tidal volume. Record at least 10 mandatory breaths and determine an average by attaching an external spirometer.

4. Calculate the corrected tidal volume using the following formulas:

Tubing loss = peak pressures × tubing compliance

Corrected tidal volume = measured tidal volume − tubing loss

5. Increase the tidal volume to 900 ml.

6. Recalculate the spontaneous and the mandatory tidal volumes and minute volumes.

Questions:

A. What happened to the spontaneous tidal volume before and after the ventilator change?

B. What happened to the mandatory volumes before and after the ventilator change?

Alarm Functions

The low pressure alarm functions during SIMV, sensing the patient's inspiratory effort and resetting the alarm with each spontaneous breath. If the patient fails to initiate a breath within 15 seconds, the alarm will sound.

The pressure limit alarm will function during the mandatory breaths. If the proximal airway pressure increases beyond the alarm setting, the alarm will be activated and the breath will be terminated.

PEEP, IMV, and CPAP Practice Activities: Puritan-Bennett MA-2

CIRCUIT ASSEMBLY, LEAK TESTING, AND TUBING COMPLIANCE

Assemble the circuit, test for leaks, and determine the tubing compliance as outlined in the practice activities for the Puritan-Bennett MA-1/MA-2 in Chapter 26, "Continuous Mechanical Ventilation."

ACTIVITIES

To complete these practice activities, it is recommended that you use a lung analog/simulator such as a Medishield Lung Ventilator Performance analyzer or Retec Respirator Teaching Console. Both of these devices or similar devices can alter resistance and compliance, simulating changes in patient condition.

PEEP PRACTICE ACTIVITIES

PEEP is a feature incorporated into the design of the MA-2 ventilator. PEEP is available in control, assist/control, and IMV modes. It is adjusted using the PEEP/CPAP control and the pressure manometer.

Initial Ventilator Settings

Mode	SIMV
CMV Volume	800 ml
IMV Respiratory Rate	6/min
Peak Flow Rate	50 L/min
O_2 %	21%
Plateau	0
Nebulizer	off
Sigh Controls	off
PEEP	+10 cm H_2O
Sensitivity	−2 cm H_2O

Activity 1: Measuring CMV Volumes

1. Measure and calculate the mandatory (machine) tidal volume.

a. Measure a minute volume using a portable respirometer.

b. Simultaneously, each time the ventilator cycles, record and write down the mandatory tidal volume.

c. At the end of the minute volume period, write down the total minute volume.

d. Determine the average tidal volume by adding the individual volumes and dividing that number by the rate. This is the measured tidal volume. Calculate the corrected tidal volume using the following formulas:

Tubing loss = (peak inspiratory pressure − PEEP pressure) × tubing compliance

Corrected tidal volume = measured tidal volume − tubing loss

Questions:

A. What did you observe on the control panel while using PEEP?

B. Why did you subtract the PEEP pressures from your peak inspiratory pressure?

SIMV PRACTICE ACTIVITIES

Initial Ventilator Settings

Mode	SIMV
CMV Volume	800 ml
IMV Respiratory Rate	6/min
Peak Flow Rate	50 L/min
O_2 %	21%
Plateau	0
Nebulizer	off
Sigh Controls	off
PEEP	0
Sensitivity	−2 cm H_2O

For this activity, you must be able to simulate a spontaneous breath by manually manipulating the lung simulator. On some models, this may be accomplished by expanding the bellows. If the lung simulator you have does not permit this, it will be necessary to perform this activity with a laboratory partner.

If you are using a laboratory partner as your patient, attach a mouthpiece to the patient wye. Your patient will breathe on the ventilator using a pair of nose clips. It is important for the patient to keep a tight seal on the mouthpiece. Spontaneously breathing on a volume ventilator is not easy and requires some practice for proper technique.

Activity 1: Control Panel and Respiratory Rate

1. Simulate a spontaneous respiratory rate of approximately 12 breaths/min.

2. Observe the control panel during spontaneous breathing.
3. Count the mandatory breaths (machine) and the spontaneous breaths (patient) for 1 minute. Simultaneously, measure a minute volume using a portable respirometer.

Questions:
A. What did you observe on the control panel during SIMV?
B. What were the mandatory and the spontaneous respiratory rates?
   1. Add the mandatory and spontaneous rates.
C. Did your respiratory rate (combined) equal the rate the ventilator measured?
   1. If it did not, check the adjustment of the sensitivity control.

Activity 2: Measuring Mandatory and Spontaneous Volumes

1. Adjust the ventilator controls to the values for the previous activity.
2. Simulate a spontaneous respiratory rate of 10 breaths/min.
3. Measure and calculate the mandatory (machine) tidal volume.

Method A

a. Measure a minute volume using a portable respirometer.
b. Simultaneously, each time the ventilator cycles, record and write down the mandatory tidal volume.
c. At the end of the minute volume period, write down the total minute volume (machine + spontaneous).
d. Determine the average mandatory tidal volume by adding the ventilator volumes and dividing that number by the mandatory rate. This is the measured tidal volume. Calculate the corrected tidal volume using the following formulas:

Tubing loss = peak inspiratory pressure × tubing compliance
Corrected tidal volume = measured tidal volume − tubing loss

e. Calculate the average spontaneous minute and tidal volume.
   (1) Determine the mandatory minute volume as you did in part d.
   (2) Subtract the mandatory minute volume from the total minute volume. This is the spontaneous minute volume.
   (3) Divide the spontaneous minute volume by the spontaneous rate you counted. This is the spontaneous tidal volume.

Method B

This method is commonly used in clinical practice. However, be certain to check your hospital departmental policy and procedure manual before using this procedure. If your manual does not advocate the use of this procedure, do not use it.

This method involves changing the mode of ventilation from IMV to assist/control for 10 breaths. Although this time interval is short, it may affect your patient adversely.

a. Turn the mode control to assist/control for 10 breaths. Write each measured volume down. Immediately upon completion, return the patient to IMV mode.

b. Calculate the average mandatory tidal volume by adding the measured tidal volumes together and dividing by 10.
c. Calculate the corrected tidal volume using the following formulas:

Tubing loss = peak inspiratory pressure × tubing compliance
Corrected tidal volume = measured tidal volume − tubing loss

d. Measure a minute volume. Count the total respiratory rate.
e. Calculate the mandatory minute volume by multiplying the average mandatory tidal volume by the mandatory rate.
f. Calculate the spontaneous minute volume by subtracting the mandatory minute volume from the total minute volume measured in part d.
g. Calculate the average spontaneous minute volume by dividing the spontaneous minute volume by the spontaneous rate.

Questions:
A. Using the following information, calculate the volumes and rates requested:

Total Minute Volume	9.8 L
Total Respiratory Rate	16/min
Average Mandatory Tidal Volume	800 ml
Mandatory Respiratory Rate	6/min
Peak Inspiratory Pressure	28 cm H_2O
Tubing Compliance	3.4 ml/cm H_2O

   1. Corrected Mandatory Tidal Volume = _____
   2. Mandatory Minute Volume = _____
   3. Spontaneous Minute Volume = _____
   4. Spontaneous Rate = _____
   5. Spontaneous Tidal Volume = _____

B. Using the following information, calculate the volumes and rates requested:

Total Minute Volume	8.6 L
Total Respiratory Rate	18/min
Average Mandatory Tidal Volume	750 ml
Mandatory Respiratory Rate	4/min
Peak Inspiratory Pressure	30 cm H_2O
Tubing Compliance	4 ml/cm H_2O

   1. Corrected Mandatory Tidal Volume = _____
   2. Mandatory Minute Volume = _____
   3. Spontaneous Minute Volume = _____
   4. Spontaneous Rate = _____
   5. Spontaneous Tidal Volume = _____

IMV WITH CPAP

IMV with CPAP is a combination ventilator modality. It is a combination of PEEP with mandatory breaths and CPAP with spontaneous breaths. The MA-2 automatically permits operation in this mode.

Initial Ventilator Settings

Mode	IMV
CMV Volume	800 ml
IMV Rate	6/min
Flow Rate	50 L/min

CMV Pressure Limit	15 cm H_2O > cycling pressure
Sensitivity	–2 cm H_2O
O_2 %	21%
Inspiratory Pause	0
Nebulizer	off
Sigh Controls	off
PEEP	+10 cm H_2O

For this activity, you must be able to simulate a spontaneous breath by manually manipulating the lung simulator. On some models, this may be accomplished by expanding the bellows. If the lung simulator you have does not permit this, it will be necessary to perform this activity with a laboratory partner.

If you are using a laboratory partner as your patient, attach a mouthpiece to the patient wye. Your patient will breathe on the ventilator using a pair of nose clips. It is important for the patient to keep a tight seal on the mouthpiece. Spontaneously breathing on a volume ventilator is not easy and requires some practice for proper technique.

Activity 1: Control Panel and Respiratory Rate

1. Simulate a spontaneous respiratory rate of approximately 12 breaths/min.

2. Observe the control panel during spontaneous breathing.

3. Count the mandatory breaths (machine) and spontaneous breaths (patient) for 1 minute. Simultaneously, measure a minute volume using a portable respirometer.

Questions:

A. What did you observe on the control panel during SIMV?

B. What were the mandatory and the spontaneous respiratory rates?

C. Did your respiratory rate (combined) equal the rate the ventilator measured?
  1. If it did not, check the setting of the sensitivity control.

Activity 2: Measuring Mandatory and Spontaneous Volumes

1. Adjust the ventilator controls to the values for the previous activity.

2. Simulate a spontaneous respiratory rate of 10 breaths/min.

3. Measure and calculate the mandatory (machine) tidal volume.

Method A

a. Measure a minute volume using a portable respirometer.

b. Simultaneously, each time the ventilator cycles, record and write down the mandatory tidal volume.

c. At the end of the minute volume period, write down the total minute volume (machine + spontaneous).

d. Determine the average mandatory tidal volume by adding the volumes and dividing that number by the mandatory rate. This is the measured tidal volume. Calculate the corrected tidal volume using the following formulas:

$$\text{Tubing loss} = (\text{peak inspiratory pressure} - \text{PEEP pressure}) \times \text{tubing compliance}$$

$$\text{Corrected tidal volume} = \text{measured tidal volume} - \text{tubing loss}$$

e. Calculate the average spontaneous minute and tidal volume.
  (1) Measure the total minute volume.
  (2) Subtract the mandatory minute volume from the total minute volume. This is the spontaneous minute volume.
  (3) Divide the spontaneous minute volume by the spontaneous rate you counted. This is the spontaneous tidal volume.

Method B

This method is commonly used in clinical practice. However, be certain to check your hospital departmental policy and procedure manual before using this procedure. If your manual does not advocate the use of this procedure, do not use it.

This method involves changing the mode of ventilation from IMV to assist/control for 10 breaths. Although this time interval is short, it may affect your patient adversely.

a. Turn the mode control to assist/control for 10 breaths. Write each measured volume down. Immediately upon completion, return the patient to IMV mode.

b. Calculate the average mandatory tidal volume by adding the measured tidal volumes together and dividing by 10.

c. Calculate the corrected tidal volume using the following formulas:

$$\text{Tubing loss} = (\text{peak inspiratory pressure} - \text{PEEP pressure}) \times \text{tubing compliance}$$

$$\text{Corrected tidal volume} = \text{measured tidal volume} - \text{tubing loss}$$

d. Measure a minute volume. Count the total respiratory rate.

e. Calculate the mandatory minute volume by multiplying the average mandatory tidal volume by the mandatory rate.

f. Calculate the spontaneous minute volume by subtracting the mandatory minute volume from the total minute volume measured in part d.

g. Calculate the average spontaneous minute volume by dividing the spontaneous minute volume by the spontaneous rate.

Questions:

A. Using the following information, calculate the volumes and rates requested:

Total Minute Volume	9.6 L
Total Respiratory Rate	14/min
Average Mandatory Tidal Volume	800 ml
Mandatory Respiratory Rate	6/min
Peak Inspiratory Pressure	28 cm H_2O
Tubing Compliance	4.0 ml/cm H_2O
PEEP	+10 cm H_2O

1. Corrected Mandatory Tidal Volume = _____
2. Mandatory Minute Volume = _____
3. Spontaneous Minute Volume = _____
4. Spontaneous Rate = _____
5. Spontaneous Tidal Volume = _____

B. Using the following information, calculate the volumes and rates requested:

Total Minute Volume	10.3 L
Total Respiratory Rate	19/min
Average Mandatory Tidal Volume	900 ml
Mandatory Respiratory Rate	4/min
Peak Inspiratory Pressure	30 cm H_2O
Tubing Compliance	4 ml/cm H_2O
PEEP	+5 cm H_2O

1. Corrected Mandatory Tidal Volume = _____
2. Mandatory Minute Volume = _____
3. Spontaneous Minute Volume = _____
4. Spontaneous Rate = _____
5. Spontaneous Tidal Volume = _____

CPAP PRACTICE ACTIVITIES

CPAP is a feature incorporated into the design of the MA-2 ventilator. This feature combined with the monitoring and alarm capability simplifies patient management when using this modality.

Initial Ventilator Settings

Mode	CPAP
Normal Tidal Volume	off
IMV Rate	0
Normal Pressure Limit	off
Sigh Controls	off
Sensitivity	–2 cm H_2O

O_2 %	21%
Peak Flow	has no effect
Inspiratory Pause	off
Nebulizer	off
PEEP	+5 cm H_2O

Using a laboratory partner as your patient, attach a mouthpiece to the patient wye. Your patient will breathe on the ventilator using a pair of nose clips. It is important for the patient to keep a tight seal on the mouthpiece. Spontaneously breathing on a ventilator is not easy and requires some practice for proper technique.

Activity 1: Control Panel

1. While your patient is breathing spontaneously, carefully observe the control panel. Observe the pressure manometer and the rate control.
2. Measure a minute volume. Simultaneously, count the respiratory rate.

Questions:

A. What event(s) did you observe on the control panel?
B. What were the minute volume and rate you measured? Does the measured respiratory rate coincide with the rate you counted?
C. Calculate the average tidal volume by dividing the measured minute volume by the respiratory rate.

Activity 2: CPAP Pressure Variations

1. Repeat activities using CPAP levels of +10 and +15 cm H_2O.

PEEP, IMV, and CPAP Practice Activities: Puritan-Bennett 7200ae

---

CIRCUIT ASSEMBLY, LEAK TESTING, AND TUBING COMPLIANCE

Assemble the circuit, test for leaks, and determine the tubing compliance as outlined in the practice activities for the Puritan-Bennett 7200ae in Chapter 26, "Continuous Mechanical Ventilation."

ACTIVITIES

To complete these practice activities, it is recommended that you use a lung analog/simulator such as a Medishield Lung Ventilator Performance Analyzer or Retec Respirator Teaching Console. Both of these devices or similar devices can alter resistance and compliance, simulating changes in patient condition.

PEEP PRACTICE ACTIVITIES

PEEP is a feature incorporated into the design of the Puritan-Bennett 7200ae. This feature, combined with the alarm functions available, simplifies patient management when this modality is used.

Using the soft keys and the keypad, input the following settings. When setting the PEEP level, use the pressure manometer to set the PEEP pressure.

Initial Settings

Mode	CMV
Tidal Volume	900 ml
Respiratory Rate	10/min

Peak Inspiratory Flow	50 L/min
O_2 %	21%
Sensitivity	–2 cm H_2O
Plateau	0
Sigh Controls	off

Alarm Settings

High Pressure Limit	10–15 cm H_2O > peak inspiratory pressure
Low Pressure Limit	10–15 cm H_2O < peak inspiratory pressure
Low PEEP/CPAP Pressure	5 cm H_2O
Low Exhaled Tidal Volume	500 ml
Low Exhaled Minute Volume	7 L
High Respiratory Rate	15 L/min

Activity 1: Control Panel

1. Observe the control panel and the pressure manometer during PEEP.
2. Simulate a patient's spontaneous efforts by initiating several breaths. Carefully observe the control panel and pressure manometer.

Activity 2: Measuring Volumes

1. With the same ventilator settings as for activity 1, measure the following volumes:
   (a) Tidal Volume
   (b) Minute Volume

2. Measure peak and plateau pressures.

Question:

A. What event(s) did you observe on the control panel and pressure manometer?

SIMV PRACTICE EXERCISES
Initial Ventilator Settings

Mode	SIMV
Tidal Volume	800 ml
Respiratory Rate	6/min
Peak Inspiratory Flow	50 L/min
O_2 %	21%
Sensitivity	−2 cm H_2O
Plateau	0
PEEP	+10 cm H_2O

Alarm Settings

High Pressure Limit	10–15 cm H_2O > peak inspiratory pressure
Low Pressure Limit	10–15 cm H_2O < peak inspiratory pressure
Low PEEP/CPAP	5 cm H_2O
Low Exhaled Volume	700 ml
Low Exhaled Minute Volume	4 L
High Respiratory Rate	25 breaths/min

For this activity, you must be able to simulate a spontaneous breath by manually manipulating the lung simulator. On some models, this may be accomplished by expanding the bellows. If the lung simulator you have does not permit this, it will be necessary to perform this activity with a laboratory partner.

If you are using a laboratory partner as your patient, attach a mouthpiece to the patient wye. Your patient will breathe on the ventilator using a pair of nose clips. It is important for the patient to keep a tight seal on the mouthpiece. Spontaneously breathing on a volume ventilator is not easy and requires some practice for proper technique.

Activity 1: Control Panel and Respiratory Rate

1. Simulate a spontaneous respiratory rate of approximately 12 breaths/min.
2. Observe the control panel during spontaneous breathing.
3. Count the mandatory breaths (machine) and the spontaneous breaths (patient) for 1 minute. After 1 minute, measure the minute volume using the display.

Questions:

A. What did you observe on the control panel during SIMV?
B. What were the mandatory and the spontaneous respiratory rates?

Activity 2: Measuring Mandatory and Spontaneous Volumes

1. Adjust the ventilator controls to the values for the previous activity.
2. Simulate a spontaneous respiratory rate of 10 breaths/min.

3. Record the mandatory (machine) tidal volume.
4. Record the spontaneous tidal volumes.
5. Record the accumulated minute volume.

Questions:

A. Using the following information, calculate the volume and rates requested:

Accumulated Minute Volume	8.8 L
Spontaneous Tidal Volume	400 ml
Mandatory Tidal Volume	800 ml
Mandatory Rate	4/min
Total Rate	14/min

1. Spontaneous Minute Volume = _____
2. Mandatory Minute Volume = _____

B. Using the following information, calculate the volumes and rates requested:

Accumulated Minute Volume	11.7 L
Spontaneous Tidal Volume	350 ml
Mandatory Tidal Volume	900 ml
Mandatory Rate	6/min
Total Rate	24/min

1. Spontaneous Minute Volume = _____
2. Mandatory Minute Volume = _____

SIMV WITH CPAP

SIMV with CPAP is a combination ventilator modality. It is a combination of PEEP with mandatory breaths and CPAP with spontaneous breaths. The Puritan-Bennett 7200ae automatically permits operation in this mode.

Initial Ventilator Settings

Mode	SIMV
Tidal Volume	750 ml
Respiratory Rate	6/min
Peak Flow	50 L/min
O_2 %	21%
Sensitivity	−2 cm H_2O
PEEP/CPAP	+5 cm H_2O
Plateau	0

Alarm Settings

High Pressure Limit	10–15 cm H_2O > peak inspiratory pressure
Low Pressure Limit	10–15 cm H_2O < peak inspiratory pressure
Low PEEP/CPAP	2 cm H_2O
Low Exhale Volume	700 ml
Low Exhale Minute Volume	4 L
High Respiratory Rate	25 breaths/min

For this activity, you must be able to simulate a spontaneous breath by manually manipulating the lung simulator. On some models, this may be accomplished by expanding the bellows. If the lung simulator you have does not permit this, it will be necessary to perform this activity with a laboratory partner.

If you are using a laboratory partner as your patient, attach a mouthpiece to the patient wye. Your patient will breathe on the ventilator using a pair of nose clips. It is important for the patient to keep a tight seal on the mouthpiece. Spontaneously breathing on a volume ventilator is not easy and requires some practice for proper technique.

Activity 1: Control Panel and Respiratory Rate

1. Simulate a spontaneous respiratory rate of approximately 12 breaths/min.

2. Observe the control panel and the pressure manometer during spontaneous breathing.

3. Count the mandatory breaths (machine) and spontaneous breaths (patient) for 1 minute. At the end of the minute interval, compare your values with those displayed.

Questions:

A. What did you observe on the control panel during SIMV with CPAP?

B. What were the mandatory and the spontaneous respiratory rates?

C. Did your respiratory rate (combined) equal the rate the ventilator measured?

Activity 2: Measuring Mandatory and Spontaneous Volumes

1. Adjust the ventilator controls to the values for the previous activity.

2. Simulate a spontaneous respiratory rate of 10 breaths/min.

3. Record the mandatory (machine) tidal volume.

4. Record the spontaneous tidal volumes.

5. Record the accumulated minute volume.

Questions:

A. Using the following information, calculate the volumes and rates requested:

Total Minute Volume	20 L
Total Respiratory Rate	14/min
Mandatory Tidal Volume	800 ml
Mandatory Respiratory Rate	6/min
Spontaneous Tidal Volume	400 ml
Peak Inspiratory Pressure	28 cm H_2O
PEEP	+10 cm H_2O

   1. Spontaneous Minute Volume = _____

   2. Spontaneous Rate = _____

B. Using the following information, calculate the volumes and rates requested:

Total Minute Volume	11.1 L
Total Respiratory Rate	19/min
Average Mandatory Tidal Volume	900 ml
Spontaneous Tidal Volume	500 ml
Mandatory Respiratory Rate	4/min
Peak Inspiratory Pressure	30 cm H_2O
Tubing Compliance	4 ml/cm H_2O
PEEP	+5 cm H_2O

   1. Corrected Mandatory Tidal Volume = _____

   2. Mandatory Minute Volume = _____

   3. Spontaneous Minute Volume = _____

CPAP PRACTICE ACTIVITIES

CPAP is a feature incorporated into the design of the Puritan-Bennett 7200ae ventilator. This feature combined with the monitoring and alarm capability simplifies patient management when using this modality.

Initial Ventilator Settings

Mode	CPAP
O_2 %	21%
Assist Sensitivity	–2 cm H_2O
CPAP	+10 cm H_2O

Alarm Settings

Low PEEP/CPAP Pressure	5 cm H_2O
Low Exhaled Tidal Volume	200 ml
Low Exhaled Minute Volume	3 L
High Respiratory Rate	30 breaths/min

Using a laboratory partner as your patient, attach a mouthpiece to the patient wye. Your patient will breathe on the ventilator using a pair of nose clips. It is important for the patient to keep a tight seal on the mouthpiece. Spontaneously breathing on a volume ventilator is not easy and requires some practice for proper technique.

Activity 1: Control Panel

1. While breathing spontaneously, carefully observe the control panel. Observe the pressure manometer and the displays.

2. Measure a minute volume. Simultaneously, count the respiratory rate.

Questions:

A. What event(s) did you observe on the control panel?

B. What was the minute volume and rate you measured? Does the displayed respiratory rate coincide with the rate you counted?

Activity 2: Alarm Functions

1. Breathe deliberately simulating bradypnea. Observe the control panel.

2. Deliberately simulate hypoventilation by taking very small tidal volumes. Observe the control panel.

3. Remove the mouthpiece from your mouth and observe the control panel.

4. Simulate hyperpnea. Observe the control panel.

Question:

A. Describe the event(s) you observed in parts 1 through 4.

Activity 3: CPAP Pressure Variations

1. Repeat activities 1 and 2 using CPAP levels of +10 and +15 cm H_2O.

PEEP, IMV, CPAP, and Pressure Support Practice Activities: Siemens Servo 900C

CIRCUIT ASSEMBLY, LEAK TESTING, AND TUBING COMPLIANCE

Assemble the circuit, test for leaks, and determine the tubing compliance as outlined in the practice activities for the Servo 900C in Chapter 26, "Continuous Mechanical Ventilation."

ACTIVITIES

To complete these practice activities, it is recommended that you use a lung analog/simulator such as a Medishield Lung Ventilator Performance Analyzer or Retec Respirator Teaching Console. Both of these devices or similar devices can alter resistance and compliance, simulating changes in patient condition.

PEEP PRACTICE ACTIVITIES

PEEP is a feature incorporated into the design of the 900C ventilator. This feature combined with the monitoring capability simplifies patient management when this modality is used.

Initial Settings

Mode	Volume control
Working Pressure	60 cm H_2O
Preset Minute Volume	6.0 L
Upper Pressure Limit	80 cm H_2O
Breaths per Minute	12 breaths/min
Inspiratory Time	25%
Pause Time	0
Trigger Sensitivity	−2 cm H_2O
O_2 %	21%
Wave Form	square
Upper Pressure Limit	10–15 cm H_2O > peak inspiratory pressure
Inspiratory Pressure above PEEP	off
Inverse Ratio Limit	off
PEEP	+10 cm H_2O

Activity 1: Control Panel and Displays

1. Connect the ventilator to a lung analog.

2. Adjust the PEEP level by adjusting the PEEP control and observing the pressure manometer.

3. Observe the pressure manometer and the control panel for approximately 1 minute.

Activity 2: Measuring Volumes and Pressures

1. Move the parameter selection switch to the expiratory tidal volume position and measure the exhaled tidal volume. Write this number down.

2. Observe the pressure manometer and record the PEEP and peak inspiratory pressures.

3. Count the respiratory rate.

4. Calculate the tidal volume using the following formulas:

$$\text{Tubing loss} =$$
$$(\text{peak inspiratory pressure} - \text{PEEP}) \times \text{tubing compliance}$$

$$\text{Corrected tidal volume} = \text{measured tidal volume} - \text{tubing loss}$$

Questions:

A. What did you observe on the control panel and displays?

B. Calculate the corrected tidal volume for the following examples:

1. a. Measure Tidal Volume — 800 ml
   b. Peak Inspiratory Pressure — 35 cm H_2O
   c. Tubing Compliance — 4 ml/cm H_2O
   d. PEEP — +5 cm H_2O
2. a. Measure Tidal Volume — 1200 ml
   b. Peak Inspiratory Pressure — 50 ml
   c. Tubing Compliance — 4 ml/cm H_2O
   d. PEEP — +10 cm H_2O

SIMV PRACTICE ACTIVITIES

Initial Settings

Mode	SIMV
Working Pressure	60 cm H_2O
Preset Minute Volume	4.8 L
Upper Pressure Limit	80 cm H_2O
Breaths per Minute	6 breaths/min
Inspiratory Time	25%
Pause Time	0
Trigger Sensitivity	−2 cm H_2O
O_2 %	21%
Wave Form	square
Upper Pressure Limit	10–15 cm H_2O > peak inspiratory pressure
Inspiratory Pressure Above PEEP	off
Inverse Ratio Limit	off
PEEP	0

For this activity, you must be able to simulate a spontaneous breath by manually manipulating the lung simulator. On some models, this may be accomplished by expanding the bellows. If the lung simulator you have does not permit this, it will be necessary to perform this activity with a laboratory partner.

If you are using a laboratory partner as your patient, attach a mouthpiece to the patient wye. Your patient will breathe on the ventilator using a pair of nose clips. It is important for the patient to keep a tight seal on the mouthpiece. Spontaneously breathing on a volume ventilator is not easy and requires some practice for proper technique.

Activity 1: Control Panel and Respiratory Rate

1. Simulate a spontaneous respiratory rate of approximately 12 breaths/min.

2. Observe the control panel during spontaneous breathing.

3. Count the mandatory breaths (machine) and the spontaneous breaths (patient) for 1 minute. Simultaneously, measure a minute volume and respiratory rate using the minute volume display and the parameter selection switch.

Questions:

A. What did you observe on the control panel during SIMV?

B. What were the mandatory and the spontaneous respiratory rates?
   1. Add the mandatory and spontaneous rates.

C. Did your respiratory rate (combined) equal the rate the ventilator measured?

Activity 2: Measuring Mandatory and Spontaneous Volumes

1. Adjust the ventilator controls to the values for the previous activity.

2. Simulate a spontaneous respiratory rate of 10 breaths/min.

3. Measure and calculate the mandatory (machine) tidal volume.

   a. Measure a minute volume using the minute volume display.

   b. Simultaneously, each time the ventilator cycles, record and write down the mandatory tidal volume. This may be measured using the parameter selector.

   c. At the end of the minute volume period, write down the total minute volume (machine + spontaneous).

   d. Determine the average mandatory tidal volume by adding the volumes and dividing that number by the mandatory rate. This is the measured tidal volume. Calculate the corrected tidal volume using the following formulas:

   Tubing loss = peak inspiratory pressure × tubing compliance

   Corrected tidal volume = measured tidal volume − tubing loss

   e. Calculate the average spontaneous minute and tidal volume.
      (1) Determine the mandatory volume as you did in part d.
      (2) Subtract the mandatory minute volume from the total minute volume. This is the spontaneous minute volume.
      (3) Divide the spontaneous minute volume by the spontaneous rate you counted. This is the spontaneous tidal volume.

Questions:

A. Using the following information, calculate the volumes and rates requested:

Total Minute Volume	9.6 L
Total Respiratory Rate	16/min
Average Mandatory Tidal Volume	800 ml
Mandatory Respiratory Rate	6/min
Peak Inspiratory Rate	28 cm H_2O
Tubing Compliance	3.4 ml/cm H_2O
1. Corrected Mandatory Tidal Volume	= _____
2. Mandatory Minute Volume	= _____
3. Spontaneous Minute Volume	= _____
4. Spontaneous Rate	= _____
5. Spontaneous Tidal Volume	= _____

B. Using the following information, calculate the volumes and rates requested:

Total Minute Volume	10.6 L
Total Respiratory Rate	18/min
Average Mandatory Tidal Volume	750 ml
Mandatory Respiratory Rate	4/min
Peak Inspiratory Pressure	30 cm H_2O
Tubing Compliance	4 ml/cm H_2O
1. Corrected Mandatory Tidal Volume	= _____
2. Mandatory Minute Volume	= _____
3. Spontaneous Minute Volume	= _____
4. Spontaneous Rate	= _____
5. Spontaneous Tidal Volume	= _____

SIMV WITH CPAP

SIMV with CPAP is a combination ventilator modality. It is a combination of PEEP with mandatory breaths and CPAP with spontaneous breaths. The Servo 900C automatically permits operation in this mode.

For this activity, you must be able to simulate a spontaneous breath by manually manipulating the lung simulator. On some models, this may be accomplished by expanding the bellows. If the lung simulator you have does not permit this, it will be necessary to perform this activity with a laboratory partner.

If you are using a laboratory partner as your patient, attach a mouthpiece to the patient wye. Your patient will breathe on the ventilator using a pair of nose clips. It is important for the patient to keep a tight seal on the mouthpiece. Spontaneously breathing on a volume ventilator is not easy and requires some practice for proper technique.

Initial Settings

Mode	SIMV
Working Pressure	60 cm H_2O
Preset Minute Volume	4.8 L
Upper Pressure Limit	80 cm H_2O
Breaths per Minute	6 breaths/min
Inspiratory Time	25%
Pause Time	0
Trigger Sensitivity	−2 cm H_2O
O_2 %	21%
Wave Form	square
Upper Pressure Limit	10–15 cm H_2O > peak inspiratory pressure
Inspiratory Pressure above PEEP	off
Inverse Ratio Limit	off
PEEP	+5 cm H_2O

Activity 1: Control Panel and Respiratory Rate

1. Simulate a spontaneous respiratory rate of approximately 12 breaths/min.

2. Observe the control panel during spontaneous breathing.

3. Count the mandatory breaths (machine) and spontaneous breaths (patient) for 1 minute. Simultaneously, measure a minute volume using the minute volume display and measure the respiratory rate using the parameter selection switch.

Questions:

A. What did you observe on the control panel during SIMV?

B. What were the mandatory and the spontaneous respiratory rates?

C. Did your respiratory rate (combined) equal the rate the ventilator measured?

Activity 2: Measuring Mandatory and Spontaneous Volumes

1. Adjust the ventilator controls to the values for the previous activity.

2. Simulate a spontaneous respiratory rate of 10 breaths/min.

3. Measure and calculate the mandatory (machine) tidal volume.

   a. Measure a minute volume using the minute volume accumulate feature.

   b. Simultaneously, each time the ventilator cycles, record and write down the mandatory tidal volume.

   c. At the end of the minute volume period, write down the total minute volume (machine + spontaneous).

   d. Determine the average mandatory tidal volume by adding the volumes and dividing that number by the mandatory rate. This is the measured tidal volume. Calculate the corrected tidal volume using the following formulas:

   Tubing loss =
   (peak inspiratory pressure − PEEP pressure) × tubing compliance

   Corrected tidal volume = measured tidal volume − tubing loss

   e. Calculate the average spontaneous minute and tidal volume.

   (1) Determine the mandatory volume as you did in part d above.

   (2) Subtract the mandatory minute volume from the total minute volume. This is the spontaneous minute volume.

   (3) Divide the spontaneous minute volume by the spontaneous rate you counted. This is the spontaneous tidal volume.

Questions:

A. Using the following information, calculate the volumes and rates requested:

Total Minute Volume	12.8 L
Total Respiratory Rate	14/min
Average Mandatory Tidal Volume	800 ml
Mandatory Respiratory Rate	6/min
Peak Inspiratory Pressure	28 cm H_2O
Tubing Compliance	4.0 ml/cm H_2O
PEEP	+10 cm H_2O

   1. Corrected Mandatory Tidal Volume = _____
   2. Mandatory Minute Volume = _____
   3. Spontaneous Minute Volume = _____
   4. Spontaneous Rate = _____
   5. Spontaneous Tidal Volume = _____

B. Using the following information, calculate the volumes and rates requested:

Total Minute Volume	9.6 L
Total Respiratory Rate	19/min
Average Mandatory Tidal Volume	900 ml
Mandatory Respiratory Rate	4/min
Peak Inspiratory Pressure	30 cm H_2O
Tubing Compliance	4 ml/cm H_2O
PEEP	+5 cm H_2O

   1. Corrected Mandatory Tidal Volume = _____
   2. Mandatory Minute Volume = _____
   3. Spontaneous Minute Volume = _____
   4. Spontaneous Rate = _____
   5. Spontaneous Tidal Volume = _____

CPAP PRACTICE ACTIVITIES

CPAP is a feature incorporated into the design of the Servo 900C ventilator. This feature combined with the monitoring and alarm capability simplifies patient management when using this modality.

Initial Ventilator Settings

Mode	CPAP
Working Pressure	+60 cm H_2O
O_2 %	21%
Parameter Selecter	expiratory tidal volume
PEEP	+10 cm H_2O
Upper Pressure Limit	30 cm H_2O
Trigger Sensitivity	−2 cm H_2O
Lower Alarm Limit	3 L
Upper Alarm Limit	8 L

Using a laboratory partner as your patient, attach a mouthpiece to the patient wye. Your patient will breathe on the ventilator using a pair of nose clips. It is important for the patient to keep a tight seal on the mouthpiece. Spontaneously breathing on a volume ventilator is not easy and requires some practice for proper technique.

Activity 1: Control Panel

1. While breathing spontaneously, carefully observe the control panel. Observe the pressure manometer, LED display, and minute volume display.

2. Measure a minute volume using the minute volume display feature. Simultaneously, count the respiratory rate.

Questions:

A. What event(s) did you observe on the control panel?

B. What were the minute volume and rate you measured? Does the measured respiratory rate coincide with the rate you counted?

C. Calculate the average tidal volume by dividing the measured minute volume by the respiratory rate.

Activity 2: Alarm Functions

1. Deliberately breathe, simulating bradypnea. Observe the control panel.

2. Deliberately simulate hypoventilation by taking very small tidal volumes. Observe the control panel.

3. Remove the mouthpiece from your mouth and observe the control panel.

Question:

A. Describe the event(s) you observed in parts 1, 2, and 3.

Activity 3: CPAP Pressure Variations

1. Repeat activities 1 and 2 using CPAP levels of +10 and +15 cm H_2O.

PRESSURE SUPPORT

Pressure support is a feature incorporated into the design of the Servo 900C ventilator. During pressure support, when a patient initiates a spontaneous breath, a constant pressure is delivered (preset) supporting the patient's spontaneous effort. This mode is available by itself or in combination with SIMV, SIMV with CPAP, or CPAP. Inspiration is terminated when the flow decreases to 25% of the peak inspiratory flow.

Initial Ventilator Settings

Mode	Pressure support
Working Pressure	+60 cm H_2O
O_2 %	21%
Breaths per Minute	12 breaths/min
Inspiratory Pressure Level	+12 cm H_2O
Parameter Selector	expiratory tidal volume
PEEP	0
Upper Pressure Limit	30 cm H_2O
Trigger Sensitivity	–2 cm H_2O
Lower Alarm Limit	3 L
Upper Alarm Limit	8 L

Using a laboratory partner as your patient, attach a mouthpiece to the patient wye. Your patient will breathe on the ventilator using a pair of nose clips. It is important for the patient to keep a tight seal on the mouthpiece.

Activity 1: Control Panel

1. Observe the control panel while the patient is spontaneously breathing.
2. Have your laboratory partner describe the experience on pressure support mode.

Activity 2: Volume Measurement

1. Using the minute volume display, measure a minute volume and respiratory rate.
2. Change the parameter selector to the expiratory tidal volume position and measure the average tidal volume.

Questions:

A. What did you observe on the control panel?
B. Describe what your laboratory partner experienced.
C. What were the minute volume and tidal volume?

Activity 3: Pressure Support with IMV and IMV with CPAP

1. Repeat the IMV activities using +5 cm H_2O pressure support.
2. Repeat the IMV with CPAP activities using +10 cm H_2O pressure support.
3. For activities 1 and 2, measure the mean airway pressure.

Questions:

A. What did you observe that was different during these activities?
B. What happened to the mean airway pressure?

SIMV, CPAP, and Pressure Support Practice Activities: Siemens Elema Servo 300 Ventilator

CIRCUIT ASSEMBLY, LEAK TESTING, AND TUBING COMPLIANCE

Assemble the circuit, test for leaks, and determine the tubing compliance as outlined in the practice activities for the Siemens Servo 300 in Chapter 26, "Continuous Mechanical Ventilation."

To complete these practice activities, it is recommended that you use a lung analog/simulator such as a Medishield Lung Ventilator Performance Analyzer or other device in which resistance and compliance may be easily altered.

Alternatively, you may use a laboratory partner as your patient, with a mouthpiece and nose clip utilized for patient-ventilator interface. In this sitation, it is suggested that you decrease tidal volumes to around 500 ml.

SIMV PRACTICE ACTIVITIES

1. Set the ventilator to the following settings:

Range	Adult
Mode	SIMV(Vol. Contr.) + pressure support
Tidal Volume	800 ml
CMV Frequency	18/min
SIMV Frequency	6/min
Inspiratory Time %	25%
Pause Time %	0.0%
Inspiratory Rise Time	1%
O_2 %	21%
Sensitivity	2.0 cm H_2O
PEEP	0.0 cm H_2O
Alarms	adjust as appropriate

2. Simulate a spontaneous respiratory rate of about 12 breaths/min.
3. Observe the control panel and pressure manometer.
   a. Determine the spontaneous and the mandatory rates.
   b. Determine the spontaneous and mandatory tidal volumes.
   c. Determine the total minute ventilation, spontaneous minute ventilation, and mandatory minute ventilation.
4. On the basis of your measurements and observations, set the alarms to appropriate settings.

SIMV with CPAP Practice Activities

1. Set the ventilator to the following settings:

Range	Adult
Mode	SIMV(Vol. Contr.) + pressure support
Tidal Volume	800 ml
CMV Frequency	18/min
SIMV Frequency	6/min

Inspiratory Time %	25%
Pause Time %	0.0%
Inspiratory Rise Time	1%
O_2 %	21%
Sensitivity	2.0 cm H_2O
PEEP	5.0 cm H_2O
Alarms	adjust as appropriate

2. Simulate a spontaneous respiratory rate of about 12 breaths/min.

3. Observe the control panel and graphics display module.
   a. Determine the spontaneous and the mandatory rates.
   b. Determine the spontaneous and mandatory tidal volumes.
   c. Determine the total minute ventilation, spontaneous minute ventilation, and mandatory minute ventilation.

4. Breathe on the patient circuit at these settings using a mouthpiece and a pair of nose clips.

SIMV with CPAP and Flow Triggering
Practice Activity

1. Add flow triggering by turning the sensitivity knob into the green shaded area.

2. Simulate a spontaneous respiratory rate of about 12 breaths/min.

3. Observe the control panel and graphics display module.
   a. Determine the spontaneous and the mandatory rates.
   b. Determine the spontaneous and mandatory tidal volumes.
   c. Determine the total minute ventilation, spontaneous minute ventilation, and mandatory minute ventilation.

4. On the basis of your measurements and observations, set the alarms to appropriate settings.

5. Breathe on the circuit using a mouthpiece and a pair of nose clips.

Questions:
A. How did the SIMV and SIMV with CPAP activity differ from one another based upon your observations?
B. As a patient, which would you prefer, pressure or flow triggering? Why?

PRESSURE SUPPORT ACTIVITIES

The Siemens Elema Servo 300 ventilator can provide pressure support in SIMV and CPAP modes, providing pressure augmentation to spontaneous breaths. In this activity set, you will use this ventilator to apply pressure support.

SIMV with Pressure Support

1. Set the ventilator to the following settings:

Range	Adult
Mode	SIMV(Vol. Contr.) + pressure support
Tidal Volume	800 ml
CMV Frequency	18/min
SIMV Frequency	6/min

Inspiratory Time %	25%
Pause Time %	0.0%
Inspiratory Rise Time	1%
Pressure Support	10 cm H_2O
O_2 %	21%
Sensitivity	2.0 cm H_2O
PEEP	5.0 cm H_2O
Alarms	adjust as appropriate

2. Simulate a respiratory rate of approximately 12 breaths/min.
   a. Observe the control panel and graphics display module during spontaneous ventilation.
   b. Determine the spontaneous and the mandatory rates.
   c. Determine the spontaneous (PSV) and mandatory tidal volumes.

3. Increase the pressure support to 20 cm H_2O.
   a. Observe the control panel during spontaneous ventilation.
   b. Determine the spontaneous and the mandatory rates.
   c. Determine the spontaneous (PSV) and mandatory tidal volumes.

Questions:
A. How did pressure support affect tidal volume when compared with the SIMV exercises without pressure support?
B. How did the increase in pressure support affect tidal volume?

CPAP with Pressure Support

1. Set the ventilator to the following settings:

Range	Adult
Mode	Pressure support/CPAP
CMV Frequency	minimum
Inspiratory Rise Time	1%
Pressure Support	10 cm H_2O
O_2 %	21%
Sensitivity	2.0 cm H_2O
PEEP	5.0 cm H_2O
Alarms	adjust as appropriate

2. Using a mouthpiece and nose clips, have your "patient" breathe from the ventilator.

3. Simulate a respiratory rate of approximately 12 breaths/min.
   a. Observe the control panel and graphics display module during spontaneous ventilation.
   b. Determine the spontaneous rate.
   c. Determine the spontaneous tidal volume.

4. Add pressure support of 10 cm H_2O.
   a. Observe the control panel during spontaneous ventilation.
   b. Determine the spontaneous rate.
   c. Determine the spontaneous (PSV) tidal volume.

Question:
A. How did pressure support affect tidal volume when compared with CPAP without pressure support?

Practice Activities: Special Ventilation Procedures

1. Using a Bennett MA-1 or other volume ventilator, practice assembling, testing for function, and troubleshooting the following external circuits:
   a. PEEP
   b. IMV
   c. IMV with CPAP

2. Practice the assembly and testing of the following CPAP circuits:
   a. CPAP using Boehringer valves, water seals, or water columns
   b. Downs' CPAP circuit and mask delivery

3. In a simulated laboratory exercise, practice initiating the following special ventilation modes:
   a. PEEP
   b. IMV
   c. IMV with CPAP
   d. CPAP
   Include in your practice the following:
   (1) Verify physician's order.
   (2) Obtain the appropriate patient baseline data.
   (3) Auscultate the chest and suction the patient as required.
   (4) Assemble, test, and troubleshoot the equipment.
   (5) Initiate the mode of ventilation.
   (6) Monitor the patient following initiation.
   (7) Monitor appropriate ventilator-patient parameters.
   (8) Remove unneeded equipment and clean up the area.
   (9) Document the procedure appropriately.

4. Use the supplied ventilator check sheet when monitoring the patient-ventilator system in your practice.

5. Complete the practice activities for the ventilator(s) available in your facility or region.

6. In a simulated laboratory setting, practice determining the V_D/V_T ratio.
   a. Assemble the collection circuit.
   b. Correctly attach the collection circuit to the patient's circuit.
   c. Check the circuit assembly for proper function.
   d. Collect an exhaled gas sample.
   e. Remove the collection circuit and monitor the ventilator.
   f. Given simulated values for $PeCO_2$ and $PaCO_2$, calculate the V_D/V_T ratio.

7. In the laboratory setting, plot the static and dynamic pressure-volume curves for the test lung you normally use for practice.

Check List: Special Ventilation Procedures

1. Assemble the equipment required to provide external PEEP, IMV, CPAP, and IMV with CPAP:
   a. One-way valves
   b. Large-bore aerosol tubing
   c. PEEP/CPAP generators:
      (1) Boehringer valves
      (2) Downs' valves
      (3) Emerson water column
      (4) Water seal
   d. Reservoir bag (3- to 5-liter anesthesia bag)
   e. Thermometer for circuit temperature monitoring
   f. Rudolph valve (as required)
   g. Humidifier/nebulizer
2. Assemble, test, and troubleshoot the required circuitry.
3. Position the patient for the procedure:
   a. Semi-Fowler's position
4. Auscultate the patient's chest and suction the patient if indicated.
5. Gather the appropriate baseline data:
   a. Cardiovascular
      (1) Heart rate and rhythm
      (2) Blood pressure
      (3) Cardiac output
      (4) Central venous pressure (CVP) and pulmonary artery wedge pressure (PAWP)
   b. Pulmonary
      (1) Mechanics of ventilation
      (2) Arterial blood gases
      (3) Static and dynamic compliance
6. Initiate ventilation modality.
7. Make any required ventilator adjustments.
8. Monitor the patient for adverse affects.
   a. Cardiovascular
      (1) Heart rate and rhythm
      (2) Blood pressure
      (3) Cardiac output
      (4) CVP and PAWP
   b. Pulmonary
      (1) Mechanics of ventilation
      (2) Arterial blood gases
      (3) Static and dynamic compliance
9. Monitor the ventilator and perform a ventilator check as appropriate for the modality:
   a. Measure the corrected tidal volume.
   b. Count the frequency.
   c. Measure FIO_2 (external circuit and ventilator).
   d. Monitor the inspired gas temperature.
   e. Measure the peak and plateau pressures.
   f. Calculate the static and dynamic compliance.
   g. Measure a minute volume.
10. Monitor blood gases or oximetry as appropriate.

_____ **11.** Measure spontaneous parameters as appropriate.

_____ **12.** Remove unneeded equipment and discard disposable items.

_____ **13.** Document the procedure appropriately on the patient's chart and ventilator flow sheet as appropriate.

Check List: *Spontaneous Ventilation Parameters*

_____ **1.** Verify the physician's order.

_____ **2.** Gather your equipment:

_____   a. Respirometer

_____   b. MIP manometer

_____   c. Watch

_____   d. Manual resuscitator

_____ **3.** Follow standard precautions, including handwashing.

_____ **4.** Auscultate and suction the patient as required.

_____ **5.** Preoxygenate the patient.

_____ **6.** Obtain a minute volume and frequency.

_____ **7.** Oxygenate your patient and allow rest if needed.

_____ **8.** Obtain three consistent vital capacities.

_____ **9.** Oxygenate your patient and allow rest if needed.

_____ **10.** Obtain a maximal inspiratory pressure (MIP).

_____ **11.** Oxygenate your patient and allow rest if needed.

_____ **12.** Appropriately monitor the patient throughout the procedure.

_____ **13.** Resume previous mechanical ventilation orders.

_____ **14.** Clean up the area.

_____ **15.** Record your findings on the patient's record(s).

Check List: *EMMV and AMV*

_____ **1.** Verify the physician's order.

_____ **2.** Follow standard precautions, including handwashing.

_____ **3.** Obtain baseline data:

_____   a. Heart rate and rhythm

_____   b. Blood pressure

_____   c. PA artery and PAWP (if available)

_____   d. $PaCO_2$ or monitor capnography

_____   e. PaO_2 or pulse oximetry

_____ **4.** Auscultate the chest and suction the patient if required.

    5. Initiate EMMV or AMV:

_____   a. Set guaranteed minute volume.

_____   b. Set tidal volume.

_____   c. Set FIO_2 level.

_____   d. Set PEEP/CPAP level.

_____   e. Set the trigger sensitivity.

_____ **6.** Monitor the patient and the ventilator.

_____ **7.** Monitor cardiovascular and pulmonary parameters.

_____ **8.** Follow standard precautions, including handwashing.

_____ **9.** Chart the procedure.

Check List: *Pressure Support*

_____ **1.** Verify the physician's order.

_____ **2.** Follow standard precautions, including handwashing.

_____ **3.** Auscultate and suction the patient as required.

_____ **4.** Obtain baseline data:

_____   a. Heart rate and rhythm

_____   b. Blood pressure

_____   c. PA pressure and PAWP (if available)

_____   d. $PaCO_2$ or monitor capnography

_____   e. PaO_2 or pulse oximetry

    5. Initiate pressure support.

_____   a. Establish ordered pressure support level.

_____   b. Set the FIO_2 level.

       c. If using pressure support with SIMV:

_____   (1) Set mandatory tidal volume.

_____   (2) Set the mandatory rate.

_____   d. Set the trigger sensitivity.

_____ **6.** Monitor the cardiovascular and pulmonary parameters.

_____ **7.** Follow standard precautions, including handwashing.

_____ **8.** Chart the procedure.

Check List: *Bi-level Positive Airway Pressure*

_____ 1. Verify the physician's order for bi-level positive airway pressure support.

2. Assemble your equipment:
_____ a. Bi-level positive airway pressure ventilator
_____ b. Patient circuit
_____ c. Nasal or full-face mask
_____ d. Respirometer, MIP manometer
_____ e. Stethoscope
_____ f. Oximeter

_____ 3. Follow standard precautions, including handwashing.

_____ 4. Introduce yourself and explain the procedure.

5. Assess the patient:
_____ a. Respiratory rate
_____ b. Tidal volume
_____ c. Minute volume
_____ d. Vital capacity
_____ e. MIP
_____ f. Breath sounds
_____ g. SpO_2
_____ h. Use of accessory muscles of ventilation

_____ i. Heart rate
_____ j. Blood pressure

_____ 6. Measure and fit the patient for the mask and strap/support assembly.

_____ 7. Temporarily remove the mask and adjust the ventilator's settings:
_____ a. IPAP
_____ b. EPAP
_____ c. Rate and % IPAP (if required)

_____ 8. Connect the patient to the ventilator by fitting the mask.

9. Monitor the patient:
_____ a. Respiratory rate
_____ b. Heart rate and blood pressure
_____ c. SpO_2
_____ d. Breath sounds
_____ e. Level of comfort or anxiety

_____ 10. Comfort and reassure the patient.
_____ 11. Set any alarms.
_____ 12. Clean up the area.
_____ 13. Chart the procedure.

Check List: V_D/V_T *Ratio Determination*

_____ 1. Verify the physician's order for the procedure.

_____ 2. Follow standard precautions, including handwashing.

3. Gather the required equipment:
_____ a. Collection bag
_____ b. Extra exhalation valve
_____ c. Exhalation valve tubing and "T"
_____ d. Three-way stopcock
_____ e. Large-bore tubing to connect to the collection bag
_____ f. Blood gas collection supplies
_____ g. Large syringe for exhaled gas sample
_____ h. One-way valve

_____ 4. Assemble the circuit, checking the position of the one-way valve.

_____ 5. Attach the collection circuit to the patient's circuit.

_____ 6. Monitor the patient for adverse effects.

_____ 7. Collect an exhaled gas sample and a blood gas.

_____ 8. Disconnect the collection circuit.

_____ 9. Monitor the patient and the ventilator following gas collection.

_____ 10. Calculate the V_D/V_T ratio.

_____ 11. Remove all unneeded supplies from the patient's room.

_____ 12. Follow standard precautions, including handwashing.

_____ 13. Chart your findings in the patient's chart.

Check List: *Static and Dynamic Pressure-Volume Curves*

_____ 1. Verify the physician's order.

_____ 2. Scan the patient's chart to determine the stability of the patient.

_____ 3. Obtain graph paper.

_____ 4. Follow standard precautions, including handwashing.

_____ 5. Auscultate the patient and suction the patient as required.

_____ 6. Plot the static and dynamic compliance below and above the patient's ordered tidal volumes.

_____ 7. Monitor the patient carefully during the procedure.

_____ 8. Return the patient to the ordered tidal volume after the procedure.

_____ 9. Monitor the patient after the procedure.

_____ 10. Follow standard precautions, including handwashing.

_____ 11. Chart your findings.

Self-Evaluation Post Test: Special Ventilation Procedures

1. IMV might be used in which one of the following situations?
   a. To wean a patient from continuous mechanical ventilation
   b. To improve ventilation
   c. To improve oxygenation
   d. To decrease the work of breathing

2. An external IMV device would include:
   I.   a thermometer.
   II. a heated nebulizer.
   III. a dead space tubing.
   IV. a one-way valve.
   V.   a reservoir.
   a. I, IV, V   c. I, II, IV, V
   b. II, IV, V   d. II, III, V

3. When using an external IMV device with the MA-1, you should:
   a. dial out the sigh mode.
   b. increase the oxygen % on the MA-1.
   c. turn off the sensitivity.
   d. increase the pressure limit.

4. Which of the following data should be included in the baseline patient data for weaning?
   I.   Heart rate and rhythm
   II. ABGs
   III. Blood pressure
   IV. CVP
   a. I   c. II, III, IV
   b. I, II   d. I, II, III

5. A complication of IMV is:
   a. pneumothorax.   c. hypocapnia.
   b. atelectasis.   d. hyperventilation.

6. Relevant information on a patient's chart for a CPAP trial would include:
   I.   blood pressure.
   II.   CVP.
   III. ABGs.
   IV.   temperature.
   V.   heart rate and rhythm.
   VI.   respiratory history.
   VII. PAWP.

   a. I, II, IV, V
   b. I, II, III, V
   c. II, III, VI, VII
   d. III, V, VI, VII

7. IMV with CPAP allows:
   I.   positive expiratory pressure during mechanical breaths.
   II. positive pressure during spontaneous breaths.
   III. spontaneous breathing.
   IV. mechanical ventilation only.
   a. I, III
   b. II, III
   c. III, IV
   d. I, II, III

8. When determining the peak airway pressure for using PEEP, you must:
   a. multiply the peak pressure by the PEEP.
   b. add the amount of PEEP to the peak airway pressure.
   c. subtract the amount of PEEP from the peak pressure.
   d. divide the peak pressure by the PEEP pressure.

9. If an equipment malfunction occurs with IMV weaning, you should:
   a. call the doctor immediately.
   b. diagnose and troubleshoot your equipment immediately.
   c. ignore it because it is usually temporary.
   d. remove the patient from the device and manually ventilate the patient.

10. Bi-level positive airway pressure is similar to CPAP, except:
    a. the patient must be intubated.
    b. two pressures are set.
    c. the positive pressure applied is greater.
    d. the patient always exhales to ambient pressure.

PERFORMANCE EVALUATION:
SPONTANEOUS VENTILATION PARAMETERS

Date: Lab _____ Clinical _____ Agency _____

Lab: Pass _____ Fail _____   Clinical: Pass _____ Fail _____

Student name _____ Instructor name _____

No. of times observed in clinical _____

No. of times practiced in clinical _____

PASSING CRITERIA: Obtain 90% or better on the procedure. Tasks indicated by * must receive at least 1 point, or the evaluation is terminated. Procedure must be performed within designated time, or the performance receives a failing grade.

SCORING:
2 points — Task performed satisfactorily without prompting.
1 point — Task performed satisfactorily with self-initiated correction.
0 points — Task performed incorrectly or with prompting required.
NA — Task not applicable to the patient care situation.

TASKS:

			PEER	LAB	CLINICAL
*	1.	Verifies the physician's order	☐	☐	☐
*	2.	Assembles equipment			
	a.	Respirometer	☐	☐	☐
	b.	MIP manometer	☐	☐	☐
	c.	Watch	☐	☐	☐
	d.	Manual resuscitator	☐	☐	☐
	e.	Stethoscope	☐	☐	☐
*	3.	Follows standard precautions, including handwashing	☐	☐	☐
	4.	Introduces self and explains the procedure	☐	☐	☐
*	5.	Auscultates and suctions the patient as required	☐	☐	☐
*	6.	Preoxygenates the patient	☐	☐	☐
*	7.	Obtains a minute volume and frequency	☐	☐	☐
*	8.	Oxygenates patient and allows rest if needed	☐	☐	☐
*	9.	Obtains three consistent vital capacities	☐	☐	☐
*	10.	Oxygenates patient and allows rest if needed	☐	☐	☐
*	11.	Obtains a maximal inspiratory pressure (MIP)	☐	☐	☐
*	12.	Oxygenates patient and allows rest if needed	☐	☐	☐
*	13.	Monitors the patient throughout the procedure	☐	☐	☐
*	14.	Resumes previous mechanical ventilation orders	☐	☐	☐
	15.	Cleans up the area	☐	☐	☐
*	16.	Records findings on the patient's record(s)	☐	☐	☐

SCORE: Peer   _____ points of possible 62; _____%

           Lab   _____ points of possible 62; _____%

           Clinical   _____ points of possible 62; _____%

TIME: _____ out of possible 30 minutes

STUDENT SIGNATURES   INSTRUCTOR SIGNATURES

PEER: _____   LAB: _____

STUDENT: _____   CLINICAL: _____

PERFORMANCE EVALUATION:
PEEP

Date: Lab _____ Clinical _____ Agency _____

Lab: Pass _____ Fail _____   Clinical: Pass _____ Fail _____

Student name _____   Instructor name _____

No. of times observed in clinical _____

No. of times practiced in clinical _____

PASSING CRITERIA: Obtain 90% or better on the procedure. Tasks indicated by * must receive at least 1 point, or the evaluation is terminated. Procedure must be performed within designated time, or the performance receives a failing grade.

SCORING:
2 points — Task performed satisfactorily without prompting.
1 point — Task performed satisfactorily with self-initiated correction.
0 points — Task performed incorrectly or with prompting required.
NA — Task not applicable to the patient care situation.

TASKS:

			PEER	LAB	CLINICAL
*	1.	Verifies the order	☐	☐	☐
	2.	Scans the chart for pertinent informationt	☐	☐	☐
*	3.	Gathers the appropriate equipment	☐	☐	☐
*	4.	Follows standard precautions, including handwashing	☐	☐	☐
*	5.	Auscultates the chest and suctions the patient as required	☐	☐	☐
*	6.	Gathers the appropriate patient data	☐	☐	☐
*	7.	Applies the ordered PEEP level	☐	☐	☐
*	8.	Monitors the patient for adverse effects	☐	☐	☐
*	9.	Monitors the ventilator settings	☐	☐	☐
*	10.	Records all ventilator-patient parameters	☐	☐	☐
*	11.	Monitors blood gases or oximetry	☐	☐	☐
*	12.	Performs a PEEP trial as ordered	☐	☐	☐
	13.	Removes unneeded equipment and cleans up the area	☐	☐	☐
*	14.	Documents the procedure on the patient's chart	☐	☐	☐

SCORE: Peer   _____ points of possible 26; _____%

Lab   _____ points of possible 26; _____%

Clinical   _____ points of possible 26; _____%

TIME: _____ out of possible 25 minutes

STUDENT SIGNATURES   INSTRUCTOR SIGNATURES

PEER: _____   LAB: _____

STUDENT: _____   CLINICAL: _____

PERFORMANCE EVALUATION:
CPAP

Date: Lab _____   Clinical _____   Agency _____

Lab: Pass _____ Fail _____   Clinical: Pass _____ Fail _____

Student name _____   Instructor name _____

No. of times observed in clinical _____

No. of times practiced in clinical _____

PASSING CRITERIA: Obtain 90% or better on the procedure. Tasks indicated by * must receive at least 1 point, or the evaluation is terminated. Procedure must be performed within designated time, or the performance receives a failing grade.

SCORING: 2 points — Task performed satisfactorily without prompting.
1 point — Task performed satisfactorily with self-initiated correction.
0 points — Task performed incorrectly or with prompting required.
NA — Task not applicable to the patient care situation.

TASKS:		PEER	LAB	CLINICAL
*	1. Verifies the order	☐	☐	☐
	2. Scans the chart for pertinent information	☐	☐	☐
*	3. Gathers the appropriate equipment	☐	☐	☐
*	4. Follows standard precautions, including handwashing	☐	☐	☐
*	5. Auscultates the chest and suctions the patient as required	☐	☐	☐
*	6. Gathers the appropriate patient data	☐	☐	☐
*	7. Assembles, tests, and troubleshoots the circuit	☐	☐	☐
	8. Measures the spontaneous parameters			
*	a. Oxygenates the patient	☐	☐	☐
*	b. Measures V_E, V_t, f, VC, MIP	☐	☐	☐
*	9. Establishes the ordered CPAP level	☐	☐	☐
	10. Monitors			
*	a. Inspired gas temperature	☐	☐	☐
*	b. FIO_2	☐	☐	☐
*	c. CPAP level	☐	☐	☐
*	11. Monitors the patient for adverse effects	☐	☐	☐
*	12. Monitors blood gases or oximetry	☐	☐	☐
*	13. Monitors the spontaneous parameters as required	☐	☐	☐
*	14. If required, resumes mechanical ventilation	☐	☐	☐
*	15. Removes unneeded equipment and cleans up the area	☐	☐	☐
*	16. Documents the procedure in the patient's chart	☐	☐	☐

SCORE: Peer _____ points of possible 38; _____%

Lab _____ points of possible 38; _____%

Clinical _____ points of possible 38; _____%

TIME: _____ out of possible 25 minutes

STUDENT SIGNATURES

PEER: _____

STUDENT: _____

INSTRUCTOR SIGNATURES

LAB: _____

CLINICAL: _____

PERFORMANCE EVALUATION:
IMV

Date: Lab _____ Clinical _____ Agency _____

Lab: Pass _____ Fail _____   Clinical: Pass _____ Fail _____

Student name _____   Instructor name _____

No. of times observed in clinical _____

No. of times practiced in clinical _____

PASSING CRITERIA: Obtain 90% or better on the procedure. Tasks indicated by * must receive at least 1 point, or the evaluation is terminated. Procedure must be performed within designated time, or the performance receives a failing grade.

SCORING:
2 points — Task performed satisfactorily without prompting.
1 point — Task performed satisfactorily with self-initiated correction.
0 points — Task performed incorrectly or with prompting required.
NA — Task not applicable to the patient care situation.

TASKS:

			PEER	LAB	CLINICAL
*	1.	Verifies order	☐	☐	☐
	2.	Scans the chart for pertinent information	☐	☐	☐
*	3.	Gathers the appropriate equipment	☐	☐	☐
*	4.	Follows standard precautions, including handwashing	☐	☐	☐
*	5.	Auscultates the chest and suctions the patient as required	☐	☐	☐
*	6.	Gathers the appropriate patient data	☐	☐	☐
*	7.	If using an external circuit, properly assembles, tests, and troubleshoots	☐	☐	☐
*	8.	Performs any required ventilator adjustments	☐	☐	☐
*	9.	Monitors the ventilator settings	☐	☐	☐
*	10.	Monitors and records all ventilator-patient parameters	☐	☐	☐
*	11.	Monitors blood gases or oximetry	☐	☐	☐
	12.	Removes the unneeded equipment	☐	☐	☐
*	13.	Documents the procedure in the patient's chart	☐	☐	☐

SCORE: Peer   _____ points of possible 26; _____%

Lab   _____ points of possible 26; _____%

Clinical   _____ points of possible 26; _____%

TIME: _____ out of possible 25 minutes

STUDENT SIGNATURES

PEER: _____

STUDENT: _____

INSTRUCTOR SIGNATURES

LAB: _____

CLINICAL: _____

PERFORMANCE EVALUATION:
IMV WITH CPAP

Date: Lab _____ Clinical _____ Agency _____

Lab: Pass _____ Fail _____   Clinical: Pass _____ Fail _____

Student name _____   Instructor name _____

No. of times observed in clinical _____

No. of times practiced in clinical _____

PASSING CRITERIA: Obtain 90% or better on the procedure. Tasks indicated by * must receive at least 1 point, or the evaluation is terminated. Procedure must be performed within designated time, or the performance receives a failing grade.

SCORING: 2 points — Task performed satisfactorily without prompting.
1 point — Task performed satisfactorily with self-initiated correction.
0 points — Task performed incorrectly or with prompting required.
NA — Task not applicable to the patient care situation.

TASKS:

			PEER	LAB	CLINICAL
*	1.	Verifies the order	☐	☐	☐
	2.	Scans the chart for pertinent information	☐	☐	☐
*	3.	Gathers the appropriate equipment	☐	☐	☐
*	4.	Follows standard precautions, including handwashing	☐	☐	☐
*	5.	Auscultates the chest and suctions the patient as required	☐	☐	☐
*	6.	Gathers the appropriate patient data	☐	☐	☐
*	7.	If using an external circuit, properly assembles, tests, and troubleshoots circuit	☐	☐	☐
*	8.	Performs any required ventilator adjustments	☐	☐	☐
*	9.	Establishes the ordered PEEP/CPAP level	☐	☐	☐
*	10.	Monitors the ventilator settings	☐	☐	☐
*	11.	Monitors and records all ventilator-patient parameters	☐	☐	☐
*	12.	Monitors the patient for adverse effects	☐	☐	☐
*	13.	Monitors blood gases or oximetry	☐	☐	☐
*	14.	Assesses the spontaneous parameters as required	☐	☐	☐
	15.	Removes unneeded equipment	☐	☐	☐
*	16.	Documents the procedure in the patient's chart	☐	☐	☐

SCORE: Peer   _____ points of possible 32; _____%

Lab   _____ points of possible 32; _____%

Clinical   _____ points of possible 32; _____%

TIME: _____ out of possible 25 minutes

STUDENT SIGNATURES   **INSTRUCTOR SIGNATURES**

PEER: _____   LAB: _____

STUDENT: _____   CLINICAL: _____

633

PERFORMANCE EVALUATION:
PRESSURE SUPPORT

Date: Lab _____ Clinical _____ Agency _____

Lab: Pass _____ Fail _____   Clinical: Pass _____ Fail _____

Student name _____   Instructor name _____

No. of times observed in clinical _____

No. of times practiced in clinical _____

PASSING CRITERIA: Obtain 90% or better on the procedure. Tasks indicated by * must receive at least 1 point, or the evaluation is terminated. Procedure must be performed within designated time, or the performance receives a failing grade.

SCORING: 2 points — Task performed satisfactorily without prompting.
1 point — Task performed satisfactorily with self-initiated correction.
0 points — Task performed incorrectly or with prompting required.
NA — Task not applicable to the patient care situation.

TASKS:		PEER	LAB	CLINICAL
*	1. Verifies the physician's order	☐	☐	☐
*	2. Follows standard precautions, including handwashing	☐	☐	☐
	3. Auscultates and suctions the patient as required	☐	☐	☐
*	4. Obtains baseline data			
	a. Heart rate and rhythm	☐	☐	☐
	b. Blood pressure	☐	☐	☐
	c. PA pressure and PAWP	☐	☐	☐
	d. $PaCO_2$ or capnography	☐	☐	☐
	e. PaO_2 or pulse oximetry	☐	☐	☐
*	5. Initiates pressure support			
	a. Sets the pressure support	☐	☐	☐
	b. Sets the FiO_2 level	☐	☐	☐
	c. If using SIMV:			
	(1) Sets mandatory tidal volume	☐	☐	☐
	(2) Sets mandatory rate	☐	☐	☐
	d. Sets trigger sensitivity	☐	☐	☐
*	6. Monitors cardiovascular and pulmonary parameters	☐	☐	☐
*	7. Follows standard precautions, including handwashing	☐	☐	☐
*	8. Charts the procedure	☐	☐	☐

PERFORMANCE EVALUATION:
EXTENDED MANDATORY MINUTE VENTILATION

Date: Lab _____ Clinical _____ Agency _____

Lab: Pass _____ Fail _____ Clinical: Pass _____ Fail _____

Student name _____ Instructor name _____

No. of times observed in clinical _____

No. of times practiced in clinical _____

PASSING CRITERIA: Obtain 90% or better on the procedure. Tasks indicated by * must receive at least 1 point, or the evaluation is terminated. Procedure must be performed within designated time, or the performance receives a failing grade.

SCORING: 2 points — Task performed satisfactorily without prompting.
1 point — Task performed satisfactorily with self-initiated correction.
0 points — Task performed incorrectly or with prompting required.
NA — Task not applicable to the patient care situation.

TASKS:

			PEER	LAB	CLINICAL
*	1.	Verifies the physician's order	☐	☐	☐
*	2.	Follows standard precautions, including handwashing	☐	☐	☐
*	3.	Obtains baseline data			
	a.	Heart rate and rhythm	☐	☐	☐
	b.	Blood pressure	☐	☐	☐
	c.	PA pressure and PAWP	☐	☐	☐
	d.	$PaCO_2$ or capnography	☐	☐	☐
	e.	PaO_2 or pulse oximetry	☐	☐	☐
*	4.	Auscultates and suctions the patient if required	☐	☐	☐
*	5.	Initiates EMMV or AMV			
	a.	Sets minute volume	☐	☐	☐
	b.	Sets tidal volume	☐	☐	☐
	c.	Sets FIO_2 level	☐	☐	☐
	d.	Sets PEEP/CPAP level	☐	☐	☐
	e.	Sets trigger sensitivity	☐	☐	☐
*	6.	Monitors patient-ventilator parameters	☐	☐	☐
*	7.	Monitors cardiovascular/pulmonary parameters	☐	☐	☐
	8.	Washes hands	☐	☐	☐
*	9.	Charts the procedure	☐	☐	☐

PERFORMANCE EVALUATION:
V_D/V_T GAS SAMPLE COLLECTION

Date: Lab _____ Clinical _____ Agency _____

Lab: Pass _____ Fail _____   Clinical: Pass _____ Fail _____

Student name _____   Instructor name _____

No. of times observed in clinical _____

No. of times practiced in clinical _____

PASSING CRITERIA: Obtain 90% or better on the procedure. Tasks indicated by * must receive at least 1 point, or the evaluation is terminated. Procedure must be performed within designated time, or the performance receives a failing grade.

SCORING: 2 points — Task performed satisfactorily without prompting.
1 point — Task performed satisfactorily with self-initiated correction.
0 points — Task performed incorrectly or with prompting required.
NA — Task not applicable to the patient care situation.

TASKS:		PEER	LAB	CLINICAL
*	1. Verifies the physician's order	☐	☐	☐
*	2. Follows standard precautions, including handwashing	☐	☐	☐
*	3. Gathers the required equipment			
	a. Collection bag	☐	☐	☐
	b. Extra exhalation valve	☐	☐	☐
	c. Exhalation valve tubing	☐	☐	☐
	d. Three-way stopcock	☐	☐	☐
	e. Large-bore tubing	☐	☐	☐
	f. Blood gas supplies	☐	☐	☐
	g. Large syringe	☐	☐	☐
	h. One-way valve	☐	☐	☐
*	4. Assembles the circuit and checks the one-way valve	☐	☐	☐
*	5. Connects the collection circuit to the patient's circuit	☐	☐	☐
*	6. Monitors for adverse effects	☐	☐	☐
*	7. Collects an exhaled gas sample and a blood gas	☐	☐	☐
*	8. Disconnects the collection circuit	☐	☐	☐
*	9. Monitors patient-ventilator parameters following gas collection	☐	☐	☐
*	10. Calculates the V_D/V_T ratio	☐	☐	☐
*	11. Removes supplies and cleans up the patient's room	☐	☐	☐
	12. Follows standard precautions, including handwashing	☐	☐	☐
*	13. Charts the procedure	☐	☐	☐

SCORE: Peer _____ points of possible 40; _____%

Lab _____ points of possible 40; _____%

Clinical _____ points of possible 40; _____%

TIME: _____ out of possible 30 minutes

STUDENT SIGNATURES

PEER: _____

STUDENT: _____

INSTRUCTOR SIGNATURES

LAB: _____

CLINICAL: _____

PERFORMANCE EVALUATION:
STATIC AND DYNAMIC PRESSURE-VOLUME CURVES

Date: Lab _____ Clinical _____ Agency _____

Lab: Pass _____ Fail _____   Clinical: Pass _____ Fail _____

Student name _____   Instructor name _____

No. of times observed in clinical _____

No. of times practiced in clinical _____

PASSING CRITERIA: Obtain 90% or better on the procedure. Tasks indicated by * must receive at least 1 point, or the evaluation is terminated. Procedure must be performed within designated time, or the performance receives a failing grade.

Scoring: 2 points — Task performed satisfactorily without prompting.
1 point — Task performed satisfactorily with self-initiated correction.
0 points — Task performed incorrectly or with prompting required.
NA — Task not applicable to the patient care situation.

TASKS: PEER   LAB   CLINICAL

		PEER	LAB	CLINICAL
*	1. Verifies the physician's order	☐	☐	☐
	2. Scans the patient's chart	☐	☐	☐
*	3. Obtains graph paper	☐	☐	☐
*	4. Follows standard precautions, including handwashing	☐	☐	☐
*	5. Auscultates and suctions the patient as required	☐	☐	☐
*	6. Plots the static and dynamic compliance below and above the ordered tidal volume	☐	☐	☐
*	7. Monitors the patient	☐	☐	☐
*	8. Returns to the ordered tidal volume	☐	☐	☐
*	9. Monitors the patient following the procedure	☐	☐	☐
	10. Follows standard precautions, including handwashing	☐	☐	☐
*	11. Charts the procedure	☐	☐	☐

SCORE: Peer _____ points of possible 22; _____%

             Lab _____ points of possible 22; _____%

             Clinical _____ points of possible 22; _____%

TIME: _____ out of possible 20 minutes

STUDENT SIGNATURES   **INSTRUCTOR SIGNATURES**

PEER: _____   LAB: _____

STUDENT: _____   CLINICAL: _____

CHAPTER 28
WAVE FORM ANALYSIS

INTRODUCTION

The capability to track airway pressures, volumes, and flows graphically during mechanical ventilation of the patient has been available for some time (BEAR, 1987). The most recent acute care ventilators have expanded this graphical monitoring capability beyond pressure, volume, and flow to include combinations of these reflecting air trapping, work of breathing, airway resistance, and other clinical problems and variables relating to ventilation. The method of wave form analysis can be applied for rapid, real-time assessment of the patient-ventilator system, providing important information regarding changes in the patient's status. As a respiratory care practitioner, you must be able to utilize this information at the bedside in the care of your patients.

In this chapter you will learn how to interpret pressure, volume, flow, pressure-volume, and flow-volume wave forms. You will learn how this information can assist you in adjusting ventilator flow, sensitivity, and pressure and in determining the patient's work of breathing, airway resistance, compliance, and other clinical variables.

KEY TERMS

- Air trapping
- Plateau pressure
- Static pressure

OBJECTIVES

At the end of this chapter, you should be able to:

- Differentiate among the following wave forms:
  — Pressure versus time
  — Volume versus time
  — Flow versus time
  — Pressure versus volume
  — Flow versus volume
- Differentiate among the following wave form morphologies:
  — Rectangular
  — Accelerating
  — Decelerating
  — Sinusoidal
  — Oscillating
- Analyze a pressure versus time wave form and identify the following:
  — Inspiration and expiration
  — PEEP
  — Patient effort
  — Peak pressure
  — Plateau or static pressure
  — Inadequate inspiratory flow
  — Spontaneous breaths and inspiratory effort
  — Ventilator or mandatory breaths

- Analyze a flow versus time wave form and identify the following:
  — Inspiratory flow pattern
  — Inspiration and expiration
  — Air trapping
  — Increased airway resistance
- Analyze a volume versus time wave form and identify the following:
  — Inspiration versus expiration
  — Tidal volume
  — Air trapping
  — Spontaneous and ventilator or mandatory breaths
- Analyze a volume versus pressure wave form and identify the following:
  — Inspiration versus expiration
  — Tidal volume
  — Inspiratory work
  — Overdistention
  — Increases or decreases in compliance
  — Increases or decreases in airway resistance
- Analyze a flow versus volume wave form and identify changes in airway resistance.

COMMON WAVE FORMS

Three wave forms are typically presented together on the same screen or page with most acute care ventilators. These wave forms include pressure, flow, and volume (Figure 28-1). All of these wave forms plot the variable—pressure, flow, or volume—versus time. At any point along the time axis, a vertical line can be projected through all three wave forms to analyze what occurred at that moment in time (see Figure 28-1). This information is presented by most ventilators on a real-time, breath-by-breath basis.

Other wave forms are pressure versus volume and flow versus volume wave forms.

The *pressure versus volume* wave form is illustrated in Figure 28-2. Notice that the volume versus pressure wave

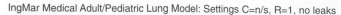

IngMar Medical Adult/Pediatric Lung Model: Settings C=n/s, R=1, no leaks

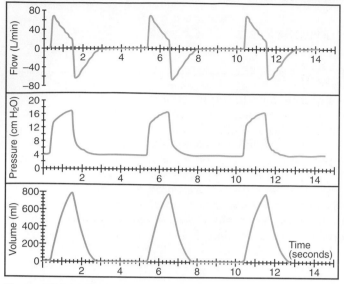

Figure 28-1 *The standard display of pressure, flow, and volume versus time. Note how a vertical line projected through each wave form allows visualization of what occurred at that moment.*

IngMar Medical Adult/Pediatric Lung Model: Settings C=n/s, R=1, no leaks

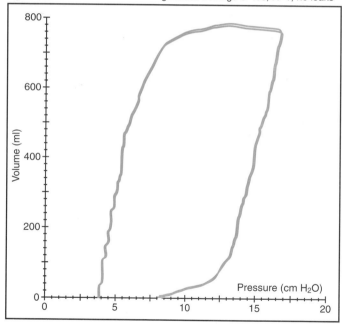

Figure 28-2 *Volume versus pressure wave form. Volume is plotted on the vertical axis, while pressure is plotted on the horizontal axis.*

form makes a loop. This presentation of data is helpful in assessing compliance, airway resistance, and work of breathing. Interpretation of these specifics is described later in this chapter.

The *flow versus volume* wave form also makes a loop, as illustrated in Figure 28-3. Flow-volume loops are common in pulmonary function application. The flow-volume loop is helpful in detecting changes in airway resistance. Changes in this graphical display may be observed before and after administration of bronchodilators.

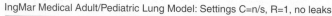

IngMar Medical Adult/Pediatric Lung Model: Settings C=n/s, R=1, no leaks

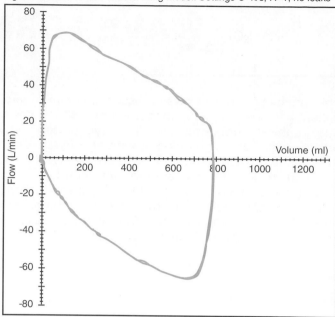

Figure 28-3 *A flow versus volume loop. Flow is plotted on the vertical axis, while pressure is plotted on the horizontal axis.*

WAVE FORM MORPHOLOGIES

The shape of a wave form may be classified as rectangular, accelerating, decelerating, sinusoidal, or oscillating (White, 1999; Chatburn, 1991). These wave form morphologies are illustrated in Figure 28-4. These wave form shapes are usually observed in evaluating the flow versus time graphic. The shape is often determined by the drive mechanism of the ventilator, or the flow pattern setting (White, 1999).

ANALYSIS OF SPECIFIC WAVE FORMS

Pressure versus Time

The pressure versus time graphical display is very helpful in answering many clinical questions. Pressure rises from baseline to the peak pressure value during inspiration and then falls to baseline again during exhalation (Figure 28-5). Addition of positive end expiratory pressure (PEEP) raises the baseline pressure to the PEEP level. Observation of this graphical display allows determination of patient effort, peak and plateau pressures, adequacy of inspiratory flow, and mandatory (ventilator) versus spontaneous breath types.

Patient effort may be evaluated by observing for the pressure to fall below the baseline level (Figure 28-6). With pressure triggering, the ventilator initiates inspiration in response to a pressure drop detected by a transducer (Chatburn, 1991; Nilesestuen & Hargett, 1996). If the pressure drop is large, the sensitivity may be set too high and should be readjusted to reduce the patient's work of breathing. Reduced patient effort will be evident by a smaller pressure drop to initiate inspiration.

Peak pressure and *static* or *plateau pressure* may be evaluated by assessing the pressure versus time graphical

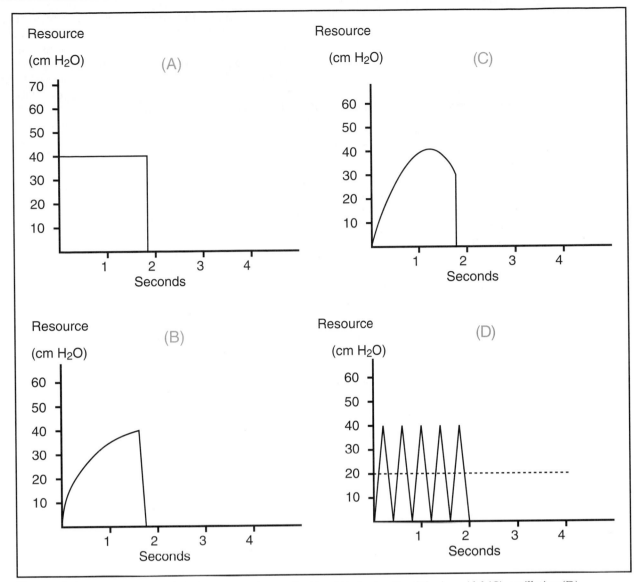

Figure 28-4 *Wave form morphologies: rectangular, accelerating (A), decelerating (B), sinusoidal (C), oscillating (D)*

IngMar Medical Adult/Pediatric Lung Model: Settings C=n/s, R=1, no leaks

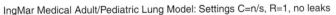

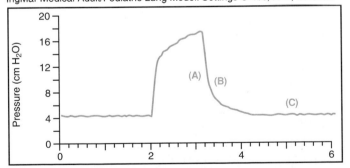

IngMar Medical Adult/Pediatric Lung Model: Settings C=n/s, R=1, no leaks

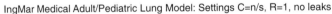

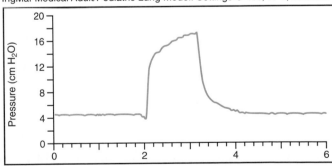

Figure 28-5 *A pressure versus time graphical display. Note inspiration (A) and expiration (B). With the addition of PEEP (C), the baseline pressure changes, reflecting the PEEP level.*

Figure 28-6 *A pressure versus time graphical display illustrating inspiratory effort. Note how the pressure falls below the baseline level.*

display (Figure 28-7). The peak pressure is the highest pressure attained for a given breath during inspiration. By reading the maximum pressure reached on the pressure scale, this pressure may be determined. By adding a slight inspiratory pause, stopping flow at the end of inspiration, the plateau pressure may be measured. The plateau pressure occurs following the peak pressure and is usually lower (see Figure 28-7).

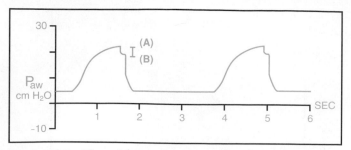

Figure 28-7 *The peak (A) and plateau (B) pressures may be interpreted by assessing the pressure versus time graphical display.*

Adequacy of inspiratory flow may be determined by assessing the rise on the pressure versus time graphical display during inspiration (Figure 28-8). If the pressure rises slowly, or if the curve shows signs of concavity, flow is inadequate for the patient's demand. Flow should be increased, to reduce the patient's work of breathing.

Breath type can be identified by observing the pressure versus time morphology or shape (Figure 28-9). Pressure support breaths may be identified by their rise to a set

IngMar Medical Adult/Pediatric Lung Model: Settings C=n/s, R=1, no leaks

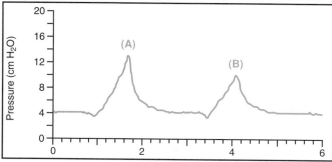

Figure 28-8 *Note how the change in peak flow setting (B) caused the pressure to rise more quickly than it did in (A).*

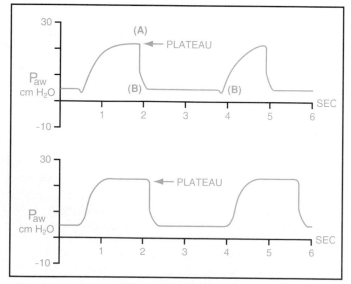

Figure 28-9 *The type of breath may be determined by observing the pressure versus time morphology: pressure-supported breaths (A), pressure-controlled breaths (B).*

plateau pressure with varying inspiratory times. The pressure level (peak value) remains constant, while the inspiratory time varies. Pressure-controlled breaths maintain a constant inspiratory pressure and inspiratory time. Spontaneous breaths without pressure support display smaller variable pressure curves during exhalation and shorter pressure drops during inspiration.

Figure 28-10 shows a combination of mandatory (ventilator) breaths with spontaneous breaths during synchronized intermittent mandatory ventilation (SIMV) without pressure support. Note the variable nature and smaller pressure changes during the spontaneous breaths. The mandatory breaths display a smoother pressure rise to a much higher pressure level.

Flow versus Time

The flow versus time graphical display is helpful in assessing the inspiratory flow pattern, air trapping, and airway resistance. Flow rises above baseline during inspiration and falls below baseline during exhalation (Figure 28-11). Careful study of this wave form will help in assessing many different clinical situations.

The inspiratory flow pattern or morphology may be easily assessed using the flow versus time graphical display. Figure 28-12 illustrates the different types of inspiratory flow patterns. Many of these flow patterns are generated according to the drive mechanism for the particular ventilator (sinusoidal, for example). Most contemporary ventilators allow the operator to select the desired inspiratory flow pattern, and then the microprocessor alters the ventilator's output to match the selected flow pattern.

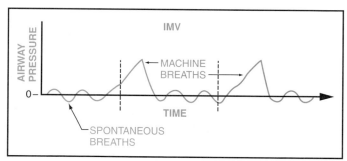

Figure 28-10 *Spontaneous and mandatory breath delivery during SIMV*

IngMar Medical Adult/Pediatric Lung Model: Settings C=n/s, R=1, no leaks

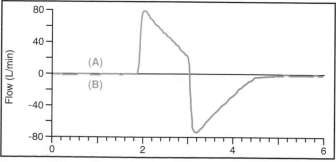

Figure 28-11 *A flow versus time graphical display. Inspiration (A) is above baseline, while expiration (B) is below baseline.*

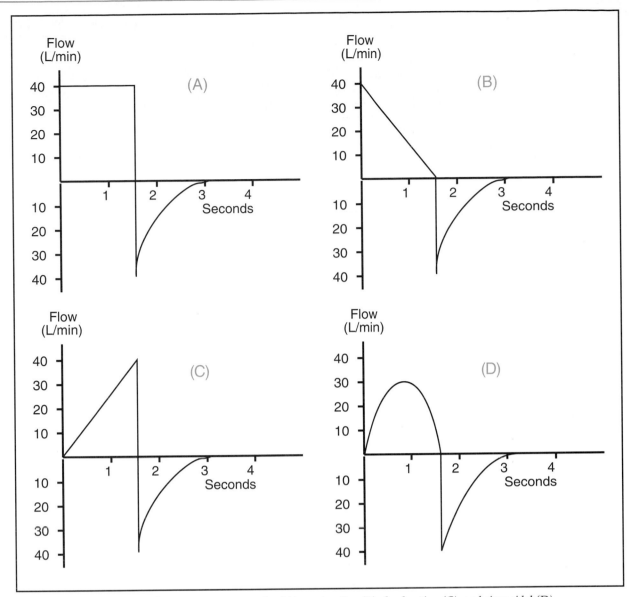

Figure 28-12 *Inspiratory flow patterns: rectangular (A), accelerating (B), decelerating (C), and sinusoidal (D).*

Air trapping, or "auto PEEP," may be detected by failure of the expiratory flow pattern to reach baseline (zero) prior to delivery of the next breath (Figure 28-13). Failure

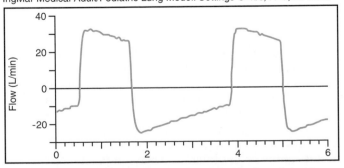

IngMar Medical Adult/Pediatric Lung Model: Settings C=n/s, R=3, no leaks

Figure 28-13 *Air trapping or auto PEEP. Notice how the expiratory flow never reaches zero prior to the next breath being delivered.*

of the lungs to empty prior to delivery of the next breath causes an increased baseline pressure or PEEP. Sometimes, air trapping is intentional—for example, during pressure-controlled inverse ratio ventilation (PCIRV). Other times, the presence of auto PEEP is not intentional. Reducing the ventilatory rate (allowing for more expiratory time) may resolve the air trapping and allow flow to reach zero before the next breath is delivered.

Airway resistance may be assessed by observing the slope of the expiratory flow tracing. A lower slope (smaller angle) is indicative of higher resistance to expiratory flow, while a steeper slope (greater angle) is indicative of lower resistance to expiratory flow (Figure 28-14). The patient's response to bronchodilators may be assessed by observing the flow versus time graphical display before and after bronchodilator administration. If the slope changes (increases) and expiratory time decreases, the patient has responded positively with decreased airway resistance (Puritan-Bennett Corporation, 1990).

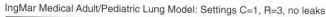

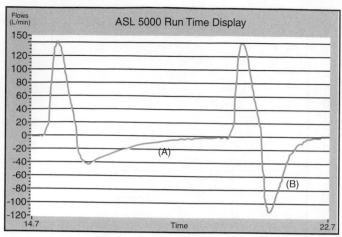

Figure 28-14 *Differences in airway resistance. At (A), the slope is less and expiratory time is greater. The portion of the curve labeled (B) illustrates decreased resistance with a greater slope and shorter expiratory time.*

Volume versus Time

The volume versus time wave form is illustrated in Figure 28-15. Analysis of this graphical display allows the determination of tidal volume, detection of air trapping, and identification of breath type. Tidal volume is the peak value reached during inspiration. By reading the value on the vertical axis in liters, tidal volume delivery may be determined.

Air trapping is evident from failure of the volume wave form to reach zero during exhalation (Figure 28-16). Insufficient expiratory time has been allowed, and gas is trapped in the lungs. Decreasing the ventilatory rate or increasing inspiratory flow may allow for sufficient exhalation time, returning the expiratory volume to zero prior to delivery of the next breath.

Spontaneous and mandatory breath delivery may be assessed by observing the volume versus time wave form. Mandatory breaths have larger volumes than do spontaneous breaths (Figure 28-17).

Combined Wave Forms

Combined wave forms are combination displays of two *scalar* wave forms that form a loop (Nilsestuen & Hargett,

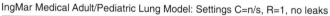

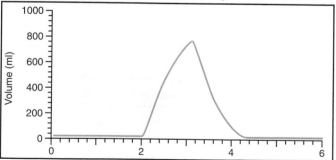

Figure 28-15 *A volume versus time graphical display. Volume is on the vertical axis, while time is on the horizontal axis.*

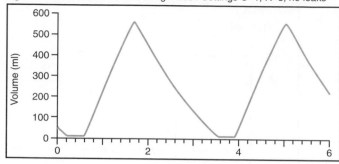

Figure 28-16 *Air trapping, shown by the failure of the volume wave form to reach zero before the next breath is delivered*

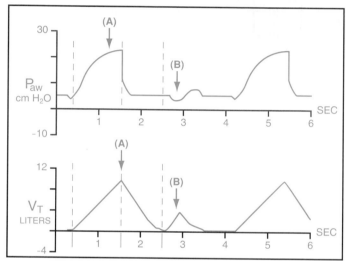

Figure 28-17 *Mandatory breaths (A) have large volumes when compared with spontaneous breaths (B).*

1996). The two most common combined wave forms are pressure versus volume and flow versus volume loops. The graphical display presents information for each scalar relative to each other and to time.

Pressure versus Volume

The pressure versus volume loop is shown in Figure 28-18. Volume is on the vertical axis, while pressure is on the horizontal axis. Positive pressure is displayed to the right of the volume scale, while subambient pressure is displayed to the left of it. Inspiration progresses from the zero point to the right, while exhalation moves from right to left. This graphical display is helpful in determining tidal volume and inspiratory work and in detecting overdistention and changes in compliance and resistance.

Tidal volume delivery during both spontaneous and mandatory breaths is reflected by the maximum value attained on the vertical (volume) axis. Tidal breath delivery may be measured directly using this technique. With spontaneous breath, the graphical loop progresses clockwise from the zero point (moving into subambient pressures) until the tidal volume is reached; with exhalation it continues clockwise, displaying positive pressures (Figure 28-19).

IngMar Medical Adult/Pediatric Lung Model: Settings C=n/s, R=1, no leaks

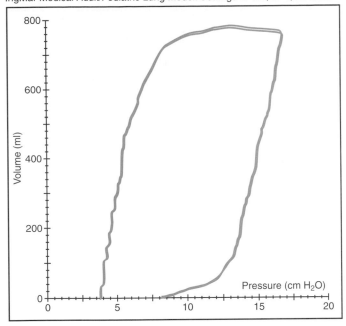

Figure 28-18 *A pressure versus volume graphical display. Volume is displayed on the vertical axis, while pressure is displayed on the horizontal axis.*

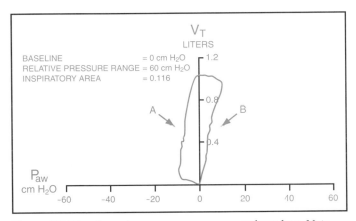

Figure 28-19 *A spontaneous pressure versus volume loop. Note how inspiration is in the subambient pressure range, while expiration is positive. The loop progresses clockwise from left to right.*

IngMar Medical Adult/Pediatric Lung Model: Settings C=n/s, R=1, no leaks

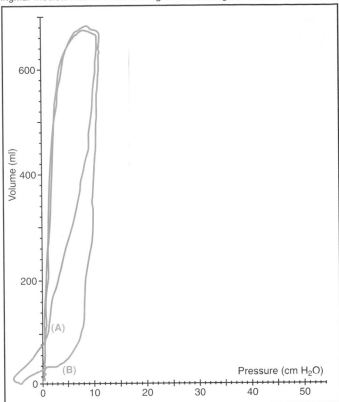

Figure 28-20 *Two different mandatory breaths with differing inspiratory work levels. Loop (A) shows the same volume delivery at a reduced level of work; loop (B) represents greater work (larger area in the subambient range).*

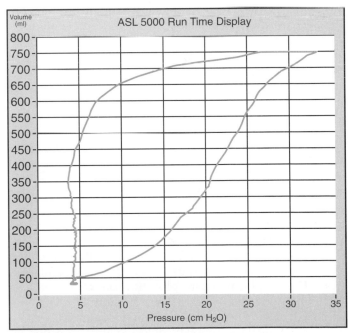

Figure 28-21 *An example of overdistention. Note how pressure rises without continued volume delivery.*

Inspiratory work is reflected by the portion of the loop that remains in the subambient pressure range. Inspiratory work is generated by the primary muscles of ventilation. By making ventilator adjustments to minimize the area of the loop in the subambient pressure range, work may be minimized. Adjustments may include sensitivity (pressure or flow triggering), inspiratory flow, and baseline flow settings. Figure 28-20 illustrates two mandatory breaths delivered at different inspiratory work levels.

Overdistention occurs when pressure continues to rise without concomitant volume delivery (Figure 28-21). This phenomenon results in a graph feature referred to as "beaking" because the curve looks similar to a bird's beak. Overdistention causes the lungs to be stretched, being subjected to higher pressures with little or no change in volume. To minimize this effect, pressure or volume should be

IngMar Medical Adult/Pediatric Lung Model: C=n/s, R=1; and C=1+2, R=1

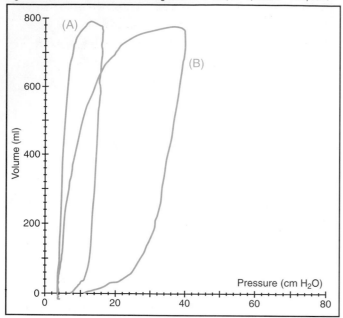

Figure 28-22   *Two pressure-volume loops with differing compliance. Loop (A) represents a higher compliance (more volume change for a given pressure), while loop (B) represents a lower compliance.*

IngMar Medical Adult/Pediatric Lung Model: C=n/s, R=3; and C=n/s, R=1

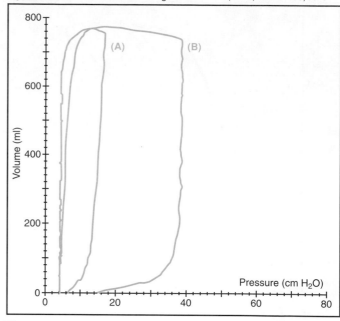

Figure 28-23   *Two pressure-volume loops with different airway resistances. Loop (A) shows the same volume and compliance at a lower resistance; loop (B) displays a greater hysteresis (space between inspiratory and expiratory traces) and resistance.*

lowered (depending on which is a control variable) to match more closely the compliance of the lung/thoracic system.

Changes in compliance may be assessed by observing the slope of the pressure versus volume loop (Figure 28-22). An increased compliance is represented by a steeper slope. More volume is attained at a lower pressure, whereas decreased compliance is represented by a lower slope (smaller volume change for a given pressure).

Changes in airway resistance may be assessed by observing the hysteresis displayed in the loop. *Hysteresis* is the space between the inspiratory and expiratory loops. Two loops of differing airway resistances are shown in Figure 28-23. The loop with greater resistance—loop (B)—is referred to as "bowed"—that is, the inspiratory portion is more rounded and distends toward the pressure axis.

Flow versus Volume

Flow-volume loops are commonly used in the evaluation of spirometry readings (Fitzgerald, Speir, & Callahan, 1996). This graphical display plots flow on the vertical axis and volume on the horizontal axis (Figure 28-24). Flow-volume loops are helpful in assessing changes in airway resistance, which may often be detected after bronchodilator administration. When airway resistance is improved, expiratory flows are greater and the slope of the tracing is also steeper (Nilsestuen & Hargett, 1996).

IngMar Medical Adult/Pediatric Lung Model: Settings C=n/s, R=1; C=n/s, R=3

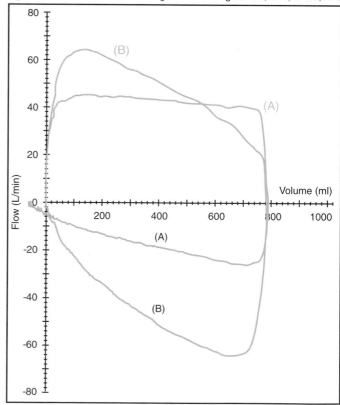

Figure 28-24   *A flow-volume loop display. Part (A) indicates greater R_{AW}, while (B) reflects decrease R_{AW}.*

OBJECTIVES

At the end of this chapter, you should be able to:

- Demonstrate how to select the desired wave form for display:
  — Pressure-time
  — Flow-time
  — Volume-time
  — Pressure-volume
  — Flow-volume

- Demonstrate how to interpret a selected wave form.

- Demonstrate how to select an appropriate wave form to assess:
  — Patient effort
  — Air trapping or auto PEEP
  — Inspiratory flow
  — Airway resistance

Wave form selection will vary depending upon the ventilator being used. Graphics may be selected by depressing soft or hard keys on the display, and function keys on the control panel or by scrolling through menu options. You should learn how to utilize the graphical display monitors for each of the ventilators used in your institution (whether a college or a clinical facility). Graphical analysis is important in patient assessment, and your ability to use these systems quickly and comfortably will enable you to deliver good patient care.

WAVE FORM INTERPRETATION

Once the desired wave form is selected, you must be able to interpret the wave form. Common clinical variables and problems that graphical analysis helps to assess include volume delivery, inspiratory work, overdistention, and compliance and resistance changes. Your laboratory and clinical instructors can assist you in learning how to interpret changes in the wave forms displayed on the ventilator monitor. Using the theoretical concepts presented earlier in this chapter, practice interpreting wave forms every time you are at the bedside caring for patients. Only through repeated practice can you become proficient at this new skill.

CLINICAL CRITERIA FOR APPROPRIATE WAVE FORM SELECTION

Depending on the clinical question, some wave forms are better than others for obtaining the desired information. Clinical scenarios involving patient effort, air trapping, adequacy of inspiratory flow, and changes in airway resistance and compliance are commonly assessed using ventilator graphics.

Patient effort may be determined by observing the pressure-time and pressure-volume graphical displays. Subambient pressure generated by the patient in initiating a breath represents ventilatory work. Both displays show subambient pressure changes during inspiration. Some ventilators use the pressure-volume graphical display and actually measure the area representing the subambient portion of the breath. By comparing changes in this area with different ventilator settings, adjustments can be made to minimize patient work or effort.

Air trapping, or auto PEEP, may be assessed using either the flow-time or volume-time graphical display. For either display, determine whether exhalation (flow or volume) reaches zero prior to delivery of the next breath. If air trapping or auto PEEP is not desired, make ventilator adjustments to minimize it. Your laboratory or clinical instructor can assist you in learning to recognize this, and when it is and is not appropriate for a given patient.

Adequacy of inspiratory flow during mandatory (ventilator) breaths may be assessed using pressure-time, volume-time, and volume-pressure graphical displays. It is important to ensure that the flow setting is adequate for the patient's flow demands. It is not uncommon to observe the patient actively working during a mandatory breath (volume-pressure or flow-time). If you detect this, adjust the flow to meet the patient's needs. Your clinical instructor can assist you in learning how to interpret this event.

Changes in compliance may be assessed using the pressure-volume graphical display. By assessing the slope of the loop, changes in compliance may be determined. Your laboratory and clinical instructors can assist you in learning to interpret these changes. Sometimes they are subtle and require interpretation by an experienced clinician. Experience and practice will help you in learning to assess these changes.

Changes in airway resistance may be assessed using both the volume-pressure and flow-volume graphical displays. Changes in hysteresis (volume-pressure) and peak flow (flow-volume) are indicative of changes in airway resistance. Make it a habit to assess these graphical displays before and after bronchodilator administration. With your clinical instructor, interpret these wave forms and learn to assess these subtle changes.

References

Bear Medical Systems, Inc. (1987). *BEAR 5 ventilator instruction manual*. Riverside, CA: Author.

Chatburn, R. L. (1991) A new system for understanding mechanical ventilators. *Respiratory Care, 36*(10), 1123–1155.

Fitzgerald, D. J., Speir, W. A., & Callahan, L. A. (1996). Office evaluation of pulmonary function: Beyond the numbers. *American Family Physician, 54*(2), 525–534.

Nilsestuen, J. O., & Hargett, K. (1996). Managing the patient-ventilator system using graphic analysis: An overview and introduction to *Graphics Corner. Respiratory Care, 41*(12), 1105–1122.

Puritan-Bennett Corporation. (1990). Waveforms: The graphical presentation of ventilatory data, Form AA-1594. Carlsbad, CA: Author.

White, G. (1999). *Equipment theory for respiratory care* (3rd ed.). Clifton Park, NY: Delmar Learning.

Practice Activities: Wave Form Analysis

1. Using a test lung, set up the ventilator(s) used at your institution and practice selecting the following wave forms:
   a. Pressure-time
   b. Flow-time
   c. Volume-time
   d. Pressure-volume
   e. Flow-volume

2. Using a lung analog (Retec or Manley) in which compliance and resistance may be altered, change the compliance, the resistance, and then both, and observe the changes in the following wave form graphical displays:
   a. Flow-time
   b. Volume-time
   c. Pressure-volume
   d. Flow-volume

3. Using a lung analog (Retec or Manley), establish routine continuous mechanical ventilation settings. Have your laboratory partner change compliance, resistance, or both without your being able to see the lung analog. Assess the ventilator graphics and state what has been changed.

Check List: Wave Form Analysis

_____ 1. Verify the physician's order.
_____ 2. Scan the patient's chart as time permits.
_____ 3. Wash hands before seeing the patient.
_____ 4. Select the desired wave form:
_____   a. Pressure-time
_____   b. Flow-time
_____   c. Volume-time
_____   d. Pressure-volume
_____   e. Flow-volume

_____ 5. Interpret the wave form for:
_____   a. Inspiratory flow
_____   b. Inspiratory work
_____   c. Overdistention
_____   d. Changes in compliance
_____   e. Changes in resistance
_____ 6. Adjust ventilator as required.
_____ 7. Chart appropriately on the patient record.
_____ 8. Wash hands upon leaving the area.

Self-Evaluation Post Test: Wave Form Analysis

1. Which of the following wave form displays are scalars?
   I. Pressure-time
   II. Pressure-volume
   III. Flow-time
   IV. Flow-volume
   a. I, III
   b. I, IV
   c. II, III
   d. II, IV

2. Which of the following wave forms may be used to assess adequacy of inspiratory flow?
   I. Pressure-time
   II. Flow-time
   III. Pressure-volume
   IV. Flow-volume
   a. I
   b. I, II
   c. I, II, III
   d. I, II, III, IV

3. Which of the following wave forms may be used to assess inspiratory work?
   I. Pressure-time
   II. Pressure-volume
   III. Flow-time
   IV. Flow-volume
   a. I, II
   b. I, III
   c. II, III
   d. III, IV

4. In assessing the pressure-volume wave form, which of the following would indicate a change in airway resistance?
   a. Increased hysteresis
   b. Increased slope
   c. Decreased slope
   d. Increased volume

5. In assessing the pressure-volume wave form for changes in compliance, which of the following reflects an increase in lung/thoracic compliance?
   a. Increased hysteresis
   b. Increased slope
   c. Decreased slope
   d. Increased volume

6. In assessing the pressure-volume wave form for changes in compliance, which of the following reflects a decrease in lung/thoracic compliance?
   a. Increased hysteresis
   b. Increased slope
   c. Decreased slope
   d. Increased volume

7. In assessing the flow-time wave form, air trapping is manifested by:
   a. an increased slope.
   b. lower flow rates.
   c. shorter inspiratory times.
   d. flow not reaching zero.

8. Which of the following is indicated when volume fails to reach zero during exhalation in assessing the volume-time graphical display?
   a. Increased compliance
   b. Decreased compliance
   c. Increased resistance
   d. Air trapping

9. "Bowing" of the pressure-volume curve toward the pressure axis is indicative of:
   a. increased compliance.
   b. decreased compliance.
   c. increased resistance.
   d. air trapping.

10. A positive response to bronchodilator therapy is indicated by which of the following changes in the flow-volume graphical display?
    I. Increased slope   a. I, II
    II. Increased peak flow   b. I, III
    III. Decreased slope   c. II, III
    IV. Decreased peak flow   d. III, IV

PERFORMANCE EVALUATION: WAVE FORM ANALYSIS

Date: Lab _____ Clinical _____ Agency _____

Lab: Pass _____ Fail _____   Clinical: Pass _____ Fail _____

Student name _____   Instructor name _____

No. of times observed in clinical _____

No. of times practiced in clinical _____

PASSING CRITERIA: Obtain 90% or better on the procedure. Tasks indicated by * must receive at least 1 point, or the evaluation is terminated. Procedure must be performed within designated time, or the performance receives a failing grade.

SCORING:
2 points — Task performed satisfactorily without prompting.
1 point — Task performed satisfactorily with self-initiated correction.
0 points — Task performed incorrectly or with prompting required.
NA — Task not applicable to the patient care situation.

TASKS:

		PEER	LAB	CLINICAL
*	1. Verifies the physician's order	☐	☐	☐
*	2. Reviews the patient's chart	☐	☐	☐
*	3. Washes hands	☐	☐	☐
	4. Selects the desired wave form			
*	a. Pressure-time	☐	☐	☐
*	b. Flow-time	☐	☐	☐
*	c. Volume-time	☐	☐	☐
*	d. Pressure-volume	☐	☐	☐
*	e. Flow-volume	☐	☐	☐
	5. Interprets the wave form for			
*	a. Inspiratory flow	☐	☐	☐
*	b. Inspiratory work	☐	☐	☐
*	c. Overdistention	☐	☐	☐
*	d. Changes in compliance	☐	☐	☐
*	e. Changes in resistance	☐	☐	☐
*	6. Adjusts ventilator as required	☐	☐	☐
*	7. Charts appropriately on the patient record	☐	☐	☐
*	8. Washes hands upon leaving the area	☐	☐	☐

SCORE: Peer   _____ points of possible 26; _____%

              Lab   _____ points of possible 26; _____%

              Clinical _____ points of possible 26; _____%

TIME: _____ out of possible 15 minutes

STUDENT SIGNATURES   **INSTRUCTOR SIGNATURES**

PEER: _____   LAB: _____

STUDENT: _____   CLINICAL: _____

CHAPTER 29

NEWBORN MECHANICAL VENTILATION

INTRODUCTION

Care of newborn patients being supported by mechanical ventilation is part of the daily responsibilities of many respiratory care departments throughout the United States. Although common goals of oxygenation and ventilation apply in the care of both adults and newborn patients on ventilatory support, the importance of differences in physiology, body size, and equipment needs has been recognized. This recognition has led to the evolution of newborn mechanical ventilation as a subspecialty of respiratory care practice.

In this chapter you will learn the differences between adult mechanical ventilation and newborn mechanical ventilation, the indications for mechanical ventilation of the newborn, some unique concepts regarding mechanical ventilation of the newborn, and hazards and complications associated with this modality.

This chapter serves only as an introduction to mechanical ventilation of the newborn. Further study beyond the scope of this text and extensive clinical practice are required to master this special area of respiratory care practice.

KEY TERMS

- CPAP/IMV
- Pressure limiting
- Time constant
- Time cycling

OBJECTIVES

At the end of this chapter, you should be able to:

- Understand the differences between mechanical ventilation of the newborn and adult patients:
  — Definition
  — Time cycling
  — Continuous flow
- Describe the three common modes of newborn mechanical ventilation:
  — CPAP
  — CPAP with IMV
  — IMV
- State the following indications for mechanical ventilation and the rationale for each:
  — Apnea
  — Hypercapnia
  — Refractory hypoxemia
  — Persistent pulmonary hypertension of the newborn
- List the underlying conditions that may contribute to respiratory failure:
  — Respiratory distress syndrome
  — Drugs administered to the mother during labor
  — Aspiration before, during, or after delivery:
    — Meconium
    — Amniotic fluid
    — Blood
    — Gastric contents
  — Acquired pneumonias
  — Pulmonary hypoplasia
  — Congenital defects
    — Diaphragmatic hernia
    — Cardiac anomalies
- Explain the following concepts with regard to mechanical ventilation of the newborn:
  — Time constants
  — Time cycling
  — I:E ratio and inspiratory time
  — Pressure limiting
  — Flow rate
- Describe the hazards and complications of newborn mechanical ventilation:
  — Barotrauma
  — Retinopathy of prematurity (ROP)
  — Bronchopulmonary dysplasia (BPD)
  — Infection
  — Increased intracranial pressure
  — Reduced cardiac output

CLINICAL PRACTICE GUIDELINES

AARC Clinical Practice Guideline:
Neonatal Time-Triggered, Pressure-Limited,
Time-Cycled Mechanical Ventilation

TPTV 4.0 INDICATIONS:

The presence of one or more of the following conditions constitutes an indication for TPTV.

4.1 Apnea (24–27)

4.2 Respiratory or ventilatory failure, despite the use of continuous positive airway pressure (CPAP) and supplemental oxygen (i.e., FiO_2 > or = 0.60) (24,25,28)

    4.2.1 Respiratory acidosis with a pH < 7.20–7.25 (8,25,29)

    4.2.2 PaO_2 < 50 torr (8,13,25,29,30)

    4.2.3 Abnormalities on physical examination

        4.2.3.1 Increased work of breathing demonstrated by grunting, nasal flaring, tachypnea, and sternal and intercostal retractions (5,27,29,31)

        4.2.3.2 The presence of pale or cyanotic skin and agitation

4.3 Alterations in neurologic status that compromise the central drive to breathe:

    4.3.1 Apnea of prematurity (32)

    4.3.2 Intracranial hemorrhage (33)

    4.3.3 Congenital neuromuscular disorders (34)

4.4 Impaired respiratory function resulting in a compromised functional residual capacity (FRC) due to decreased lung compliance and/or increased airway resistance, (12,35) including but not limited to:

    4.4.1 Respiratory distress syndrome (RDS) (1,2,28,36–39)

    4.4.2 Meconium aspiration syndrome (MAS) (40)

    4.4.3 Pneumonia (41)

    4.4.4 Bronchopulmonary dysplasia (42–44)

    4.4.5 Bronchiolitis (41)

    4.4.6 Congenital diaphragmatic hernia (45)

    4.4.7 Sepsis (41)

    4.4.8 Radiographic evidence of decreased lung volume (27)

4.5 Impaired cardiovascular function

    4.5.1 Persistent pulmonary hypertension of the newborn (PPHN) (46,47)

    4.5.2 Postresuscitation (41)

    4.5.3 Congenital heart disease (48)

    4.5.4 Shock (6)

4.6 Postoperative state characterized by impaired ventilatory function (45,49)

TPTV 5.0 CONTRAINDICATIONS:

No specific contraindications for neonatal TPTV exist when indications are judged to be present (Section 4.0).

TPTV 6.0 HAZARDS/COMPLICATIONS:

6.1 Air leak syndromes due to barotrauma and/or volume overinflation (i.e., volutrauma), (2,11,50–54) including:

    6.1.1 Pneumothorax (16,55–59)

    6.1.2 Pneumomediastinum (55,56,58)

    6.1.3 Pneumopericardium (55)

    6.1.4 Pneumoperitoneum (55)

    6.1.5 Subcutaneous emphysema (55)

    6.1.6 Pulmonary interstitial emphysema (56,60–62)

6.2 Chronic lung disease associated with prolonged positive pressure ventilation and oxygen toxicity (63,64) (e.g., bronchopulmonary dysplasia (42,43,65–68))

6.3 Airway complications associated with endotracheal intubation

    6.3.1 Laryngotracheobronchomalacia (69)

    6.3.2 Damage to upper airway structures (66,69,70)

    6.3.3 Malpositioning of endotracheal tube (ETT) (69,71)

    6.3.4 Partial or total obstruction of ETT with mucus (69,71,72)

    6.3.5 Kinking of ETT (69,71)

    6.3.6 Unplanned extubation (69,71,73)

    6.3.7 Air leak around uncuffed ETT

    6.3.8 Subglottic stenosis (69)

    6.3.9 Main-stem intubation (69)

    6.3.10 Pressure necrosis (74)

    6.3.11 Increased work of breathing (during spontaneous breaths) due to the high resistance of endotracheal tubes of small internal diameter (75)

6.4 Nosocomial pulmonary infection (e.g., pneumonia (76))

6.5 Complications that occur when positive pressure applied to the lungs is transmitted to the cardiovascular system (77,78) or the cerebral vasculature resulting in:

    6.5.1 Decreased venous return (77,78)

    6.5.2 Decreased cardiac output (77,78)

    6.5.3 Increased intracranial pressure leading to intraventricular hemorrhage (27,33,79)

6.6 Supplemental oxygen in conjunction with TPTV may lead to an increased risk of retinopathy of prematurity (ROP) (80,81)

6.7 Complications associated with endotracheal suctioning (82)

6.8 Technical complications

    6.8.1 Ventilator failure (10,83)

    6.8.2 Ventilator circuit and/or humidifier failure (38,70) (Condensate in the inspiratory limb of the ventilator circuit may result in a reduction in V_T (23,84) or inadvertent pulmonary lavage.)

6.8.3 Ventilator alarm failure (10,38,69,83)
6.8.4 Loss of or inadequate gas supply
6.9 Patient-ventilator asynchrony (85,86)
6.10 Inappropriate ventilator settings leading to:
  6.10.1 Auto-PEEP
  6.10.2 Hypo- or hyperventilation
  6.10.3 Hypo- or hyperoxemia
  6.10.4 Increased work of breathing

TPTV 8.0 ASSESSMENT OF NEED:
Determination that valid indications are present by physical, radiographic, and laboratory assessment

TPTV 9.0 ASSESSMENT OF OUTCOME:
Establishment of neonatal assisted ventilation should result in improvement in patient condition and/or reversal of indications (Section 4.0):
9.1 Reduction in work of breathing as evidenced by decreases in respiratory rate, severity of retractions, nasal flaring, and grunting
9.2 Radiographic evidence of improved lung volume (41)
9.3 Subjective improvement in lung volume as indicated by increased chest excursion and aeration by chest auscultation (87)
9.4 Improved gas exchange
  9.4.1 Ability to maintain a PaO_2 > or = 50 torr with FIO_2 < 0.60 (8,30)
  9.4.2 Ability to reverse respiratory acidosis and maintain a pH > 7.25 (8,30)
  9.4.3 Subjective improvement as indicated by a decrease in grunting, nasal flaring, sternal and intercostal retraction, and respiratory rate (31)

TPTV 11.0 MONITORING:
11.1 Patient-ventilator system checks should be performed every 2–4 hours and should include documentation of ventilator settings and patient assessments as recommended by the AARC CPG Patient-Ventilator System Checks (MV-SC) and AARC CPG Humidification during Mechanical Ventilation (HMV) (95,96)
11.2 Oxygen and CO_2 monitoring
  11.2.1 Periodic sampling of blood gas values by arterial, capillary, or venous route (1,24,30) PaO_2 should be kept below 80 torr in preterm infants to minimize the risk of ROP. (6,80,97)
  11.2.2 The unstable infant should be monitored continuously by transcutaneous O_2 monitor or pulse oximeter. (1,90,91)
  11.2.3 The unstable infant should be monitored continuously by transcutaneous (90) or end-tidal CO_2 monitoring. (93,94)
  11.2.4 Fractional concentration of oxygen delivered by the ventilator should be monitored continuously. (38)

11.3 Continuous monitoring of cardiac activity (via electrocardiograph) and respiratory rate (98)
11.4 Monitoring of blood pressure by indwelling arterial line or by periodic cuff measurements (24)
11.5 Continuous monitoring of proximal airway pressures including peak inspiratory pressure (PIP), PEEP, and mean airway pressure (Paw) (1,39,99)
  11.5.1 Increases in Paw may result in improved oxygenation; however, Paw > 12 cm H_2O has been associated with barotrauma. (8,20,41,99–102)
  11.5.2 The difference between PIP and PEEP ($^\wedge$P) in conjunction with patient mechanics determines V_T. As the $^\wedge$P changes, V_T will vary. (16,51,99,100)
  11.5.3 PIP should be adjusted initially to achieve adequate V_T as reflected by chest excursion and adequate breath sounds (8,29,100) and/or by V_T measurement.
  11.5.4 PEEP increases FRC and may improve oxygenation and ventilation-perfusion relationship (PEEP is typically adjusted at 4–7 cm H_2O — levels beyond this range may result in hyperinflation, particularly in patients with obstructive airways disease [e.g., MAS or bronchiolitis] (5,29,35,103–105)).
11.6 Many commercially available neonatal ventilators provide continuous monitoring of ventilator frequency, tI, and I:E. If only two of these variables are directly monitored, the third should be calculated (e.g., the proportion of the tI for a given frequency determines the I:E).
  11.6.1 Lengthening tI increases Paw and should improve oxygenation. (1,2,13,24,41,106,107)
  11.6.2 I:E in excess of 1:1 may lead to the development of auto-PEEP and hyperinflation. (5,20,24,37,105,106,108)
  11.6.3 Frequencies of 30–60 per minute with shorter tI (e.g., I:E of 1:2) are commonly used in patients with RDS. (8,22,41,50,59,85,109–111)
11.7 Depending on the internal diameter of the ventilator circuit, excessive flow rates can result in expiratory resistance that leads to increased work of breathing and automatic increases in PEEP. (17,19,89,98,86,112) Some ventilators are equipped with demand-flow systems that permit the use of lower baseline flow rates but provide the patient with additional flow as needed.

(Continued)

(CPG Continued)

11.8 Because of the possibility of complete obstruction or kinking of the ETT and the inadequacy of ventilator alarms in these situations, continuous tidal volume monitoring via an appropriately designed (minimum dead space) proximal airway flow sensor is recommended. (98,113,114)
11.9 Periodic physical assessment of chest excursion and breath sounds and for signs of increased work of breathing and cyanosis. (3,5,21,87)

11.10 Periodic evaluation of chest radiographs to follow the progress of the disease, identify possible complications, and verify ETT placement (21,27,79)

Reprinted with permission from *Respiratory Care* 1994; 39(8): 808–816. The complete AARC Clinical Practice Guidelines are available from the AARC Web site (http://www.aarc.org), from the AARC Executive Office, or from the *Respiratory Care* journal.

BASICS OF NEWBORN MECHANICAL VENTILATION

Newborn mechanical ventilation, like adult mechanical ventilation, is the support of the respiratory system using positive-pressure ventilation. Ventilatory support will sustain the newborn patient's respiratory needs until pharmacological therapy or maturation of the lungs achieves changes allowing the neonatal lungs to support the body's physiological needs.

Time Cycling

The majority of newborn ventilators are *time-cycled* ventilators. Inspiration is terminated after an operator-selected time interval has passed. Inspiratory time is set directly with an inspiratory time control. This *time cycling* represents a major difference from adult ventilation, which largely uses volume-cycled ventilators.

Volume delivery in a newborn varies. The variables controlling volume delivery are inspiratory time, peak inspiratory pressure (PIP), positive end-expiratory pressure (PEEP), and flow rate.

Continuous Flow

Most newborn ventilators are continuous flow ventilators. Because the inspiratory efforts and volumes of newborns are so small, it is technically difficult to achieve sensitive, accurate patient-sensing mechanisms. A continuous flow of gas past the patient's airway ensures that when the patient needs inspiratory flow, it is already there without the patient's having to activate a demand flow system first. The operator adjusts the level of continuous flow through the circuit by adjusting a flowmeter incorporated into the ventilator's design.

Modes of Ventilation
Continuous Positive Airway Pressure

Continuous positive airway pressure (CPAP) is a spontaneous mode of ventilation used in the support of newborn patients as well as adult patients. A continuous flow of oxygen-enriched gas is provided to the patient's airway at a pressure greater than ambient pressure (zero pressure). This pressure is applied during both inspiration and expiration. A variable resistance at the exhalation valve and the continuous flow of gas provide the pressure for CPAP. As in the adult patient, CPAP helps to increase the newborn's functional residual capacity (FRC), improving gas exchange.

Intermittent Mandatory Ventilation

Intermittent mandatory ventilation (IMV) is typically delivered as a combination of CPAP and IMV modes and is therefore sometimes referred to as *CPAP/IMV*. The mode allows the newborn patient to breathe spontaneously (during CPAP) at a pressure greater than atmospheric pressure between mechanical ventilator breaths (mandatory IMV breaths). During the mandatory breath, the exhalation valve is occluded and the breath is delivered at the inspiratory time, pressure, and oxygen percentage set by the operator. IMV is the mode of ventilation that provides the highest degree of ventilatory support.

INDICATIONS FOR MECHANICAL VENTILATION IN THE NEWBORN

As with adults, neonatal patients must meet certain criteria before mechanical ventilation is initiated. These criteria, as in the adult, are concerned primarily with oxygenation and ventilation.

Apnea

Apnea is a strong indicator for ventilatory support. Newborns in whom manual resuscitation efforts fail are initiated on mechanical support. Apnea may occur because of many factors such as asphyxia, effects of drugs administered to the mother during labor that may pass through the placenta (such as magnesium sulfate), and intracranial disorders (Alone, 1987).

Refractory Hypoxemia

Hypoxemia alone is not an indicator for mechanical support. However, hypoxemia that fails to reverse in spite of more conventional modes of management (oxygen, resuscitation, or CPAP) may indicate a need for mechanical support. There is some controversy regarding the threshold at which mechanical ventilation should be initiated. It is generally accepted that an arterial partial pressure of oxygen (PaO_2) of less than 50 mm Hg or a fraction of inspired oxygen (FIO_2) greater than 0.50 meets the criteria for mechanical ventilation (Koff, 1988).

Hypercapnia (Elevated $PaCO_2$)

Hypercapnia indicates poor ventilatory status. Hypercapnia requiring mechanical ventilation is defined as an arterial partial pressure of carbon dioxide ($PaCO_2$) of greater than 55 mm Hg (Koff, 1988). Hypercapnia may be present in newborns suffering from depression of the central nervous system (CNS), pneumonia, apnea, or other disorders (Alone, 1987). The $PaCO_2$ may be normalized through ventilation of the lungs. Respiratory rate, peak inspiratory pressure (PIP), and, to a lesser degree, CPAP levels are adjusted on the basis of transcutaneous and blood gas monitoring.

UNDERLYING CONDITIONS THAT MAY CONTRIBUTE TO RESPIRATORY FAILURE

In addition to the primary indications for mechanical ventilation, other conditions may contribute to neonatal respiratory distress. These conditions are summarized in Table 29-1.

NEWBORN VENTILATORY SUPPORT CONCEPTS

Time Constants

The lung time constant is calculated by multiplying the airway resistance by the compliance. The *time constant*

TABLE 29-1: Factors Contributing to Respiratory Distress in Newborns
Respiratory distress syndrome (RDS)
Drugs given to the mother during labor

Aspiration
  Meconium
  Amniotic fluid
  Blood
  Gastric contents

Pulmonary hypoplasia

Congenital defects
  Diaphragmatic hernia
  Cardiac anomalies

Persistent pulmonary hypertension of the newborn

provides a reference regarding the lungs' ability to receive or expel gas. A short time constant is present in conditions with a poor compliance and normal resistance (respiratory distress syndrome [RDS], pulmonary hypoplasia) or a normal compliance with decreased resistance. A short time constant is significant in that the expiratory time is very short in duration and abrupt. Pressures are more easily transmitted to the alveoli, and as a result, barotrauma is a common complication.

A long time constant is present in conditions with a normal compliance and high resistance (aspiration, pneumonias). A newborn with a long time constant has an increased expiratory time. Inspiratory pressures are not as easily transmitted, and inspiratory time may need to be lengthened for optimal gas exchange. These patients may present with air trapping if the expiratory time is too short.

Time Cycling

In adults, the majority of the ventilators terminate inspiration following the delivery of a preset volume (volume-cycled). The majority of newborn ventilators terminate the inspiratory phase after an operator-selected time interval has passed (time cycling). Volume delivery in the newborn patient varies depending upon inspiratory time, PIP, PEEP, flow, the patient's compliance, and the patient's airway resistance.

I:E Ratio and Inspiratory Time

The I:E ratio is the ratio of inspiratory time to expiratory time. I:E ratio may be determined by setting inspiratory time and expiratory time controls directly or indirectly by setting a rate and an inspiratory time. An I:E ratio of greater than 1:2 may be required for patients with a long time constant, while a lower I:E ratio may be tolerated by a patient with a short time constant.

Pressure Limiting

During IMV breaths, the ventilator delivers the breath for the specified inspiratory time and builds to the operator-selected pressure. Once the desired pressure is reached, excess circuit pressure is allowed to escape and the pressure is held steady in the airway until the inspiratory time is reached. This *pressure limiting* results in an inspiratory plateau. The duration of the plateau depends upon the flow rate and the inspiratory time.

As in adult ventilation, a safety popoff or limit is also provided to prevent excess pressure within the airways. The pressure popoff helps to prevent barotrauma by minimizing excessive pressures that may occur secondary to tube occlusion or failure of the pressure limit control. The pressure limit feature is also usually operator adjustable in most newborn ventilators.

Flow Rate

As stated earlier, most newborn ventilators provide a constant flow of fresh gas through the patient circuit. The flow rate is operator adjustable, usually by means of a Thorpe tube flowmeter. Flows are typically set between 6 and 10 L/min.

HAZARDS AND COMPLICATIONS OF NEWBORN MECHANICAL VENTILATION

Newborn ventilators are primarily positive-pressure ventilators, applying positive pressure within the thorax to expand the lungs. Because pressure is applied within the chest, some of this pressure is transmitted to the mediastinum, as in adult ventilation. Potential adverse consequences are similar: reduced cardiac output, reduced

venous return, and increased intracranial pressures. In addition, barotrauma to the lungs and mediastinum can occur (Chatburn, 1991).

Because positive-pressure ventilation is dependent upon the placement of an artificial airway, infection is always a concern. Use of careful aseptic technique may help to minimize this complication.

Another complication related to high PaO_2 levels is retinopathy of prematurity (Goldberg & Bancalari, 1986). The risk can be reduced by careful titration of the FIO_2 in relation to the patient's PaO_2. Enough oxygen should be delivered to correct hypoxemia without giving more than is required.

PROFICIENCY OBJECTIVES

At the end of this chapter, you should be able to:

* Demonstrate the ability to recognize a newborn in respiratory distress who requires ventilatory support based upon objective criteria.
* Given a physician's order or a simulated order, demonstrate how to initiate mechanical ventilation, including the following:

— Establish an airway.

— Assemble and test all required equipment.

— Establish ordered ventilator settings.

— Monitor the patient appropriately.

— Document ventilation parameters correctly on the patient's flow sheet.

ASSESSING THE NEED FOR MECHANICAL VENTILATION

Maternal history, the circumstances of delivery, and the infant's condition at birth provide a wealth of information regarding the patient's need for ventilatory support. APGAR scores, resuscitation efforts, evidence of aspiration, signs of asphyxia, physical size, and appearance all provide clues to the skilled respiratory care practitioner regarding the patient's respiratory distress. Laboratory values (for arterial blood gas analysis), chest x-ray reports, and neurological assessment all confirm initial observations regarding the patient's need for support.

Once the need for support has been established by consensus among the physician, members of the nursing team, and the respiratory care practitioner, all efforts must focus on a successful outcome for the patient. An airway must be established and resuscitation efforts continued as required until mechanical support is available.

EQUIPMENT REQUIREMENTS

Many pieces of equipment are required to support a newborn patient on a mechanical ventilator. These include an emergency manual resuscitator, intubation supplies, ventilator, noninvasive monitors, heated humidifier, and the patient circuit.

Ventilator Preparation

The ventilator circuit should be assembled and attached to the ventilator if it is not already prepared for use. Once the ventilator is ready for operation, the humidifier should be

filled, the ventilator's gas sources should be connected, and the ventilator circuit should be pressure-tested. In addition, all alarms should be quickly checked for correct function prior to patient connection.

ESTABLISHING ORDERED VENTILATOR SETTINGS

The initiation of mechanical ventilation is a serious commitment of time, energy, and expense for the support of the newborn patient. It is your responsibility as a respiratory care practitioner to establish the ordered settings and to recommend changes or suggestions when appropriate. The following are some general guidelines useful in establishing ventilatory support.

Mode

The mode selected will depend upon the amount of ventilatory support that the patient requires. Full support would dictate the use of IMV. Some patients require only minimal support through the use of CPAP.

Rate

The respiratory rate is generally set between 30 and 40 breaths per minute. Ultimately, the $PaCO_2$ will dictate what rate is appropriate. Transcutaneous monitoring is very helpful in the titration of ventilator settings without frequent drawing of specimens for determination of arterial blood gases (ABGs). ABGs should be correlated with the monitor, however, to assess how well the monitor is representing the patient's actual condition.

Flow Rate

The flow rate is adjusted using the Thorpe rate flowmeter so that the continuous flow is adequate to meet the patient's inspiratory needs. The flow is generally set between 6 and 10 L/min for most patients.

Inspiratory Time

Inspiratory time is adjusted depending upon the patient's time constant and by observation of the adequacy of chest excursion during inspiration. Generally, inspiratory times of between 0.3 and 0.5 second are typical. Through practice and observation, inspiratory times are adjusted to more closely match the patient's ventilatory requirements.

I:E Ratio

Like the inspiratory time, I:E ratio is largely dependent upon the patient's time constant. Any one I:E ratio is not suitable for all conditions. The patient must be assessed and a judgment made as to what an appropriate ratio is for that patient.

Pressure Limit

The pressure limit is another control in which the adjustment and settings are largely based upon experience and patient observation. The pressure limit is usually set by occluding the patient circuit while depressing the manual breath button. The limit is adjusted until the proximal airway pressure matches the desired pressure level.

The inspiratory pressure is adjusted until adequate chest rise is observed. Once adequate chest expansion is attained, the pressure control is left at that setting. Pressure is then fine-tuned based on noninvasive monitoring techniques.

Oxygen Percent

The oxygen percentage is adjusted according to the patient's needs. Enough oxygen should be provided to correct hypoxemia without giving more than is needed. PaO_2 levels should be maintained between 50 and 80 mm Hg. Excessively high PaO_2 levels may lead to retinopathy of prematurity or brochopulmonary dysplasia. Until a blood gas can be obtained, maintain the FiO_2 to keep the infant "pink."

PEEP/CPAP Level

The PEEP/CPAP level is adjusted to meet the patient's oxygenation status based upon ABG determinations and transcutaneous monitoring. PEEP/CPAP is adjusted by rotating the control until expiratory levels match what is desired. PEEP/CPAP levels may vary from 3 cm H_2O to 20 cm H_2O. PEEP/CPAP levels of between 4 and 7 cm H_2O are most commonly used.

ALARMS

Alarms alert you to changes in the patient's condition and in the ventilator system that may be detrimental. Alarms should always be set and routinely monitored. Larger problems (complications and hazards) may be prevented by paying attention to the smaller details.

Inspiratory or Patient Pressure Alarm

This alarm alerts you to leaks or a patient disconnect. The pressure alarm should be adjusted from between 5 and 7 cm H_2O less than the peak airway pressure.

Low PEEP/CPAP Alarm

This alarm is similar to the low patient pressure alarm except that it alerts you to loss of PEEP/CPAP pressure. The alarm should be adjusted to 1 to 2 cm H_2O less than the PEEP/CPAP level.

Gas Pressure Failure

Many ventilators have alarms that alert you to the loss of oxygen or air pressure. In the event of a gas supply line loss, cylinders may be temporarily used until the supply line problems are corrected.

Ventilator Inoperative Alarms

Some ventilators have a ventilator inoperative alarm. These alarms are not operator adjustable but alert you to serious internal problems that will render the ventilator incapable of supporting the patient. These internal problems include electrical power failures, microprocessor failures, and internal mechanical failures.

PATIENT MONITORING AND ASSESSMENT

The adequacy of ventilation may be assessed through careful monitoring and assessment of your patient. Careful patient monitoring will also alert you to changes in the patient's condition that may require adjustment of the ventilator settings. Newborn monitoring and assessment are most effective if performed in a consistent manner. Variations in technique or observation may result in your missing important information about your patient's condition.

Pulmonary

Auscultation of breath sounds is just as important in the newborn as it is in the adult. Secretions, wheezing, obstruction, and barotrauma all may be initially detected through careful auscultation.

Inspection is also important in the newborn. Volume delivery during ventilatory support varies depending on the patient's physiological status. Observation of chest expansion is important in the peak pressure setting. Use of accessory muscles can easily be observed and provides important information about the proper adjustment of flow and pressures.

Transillumination is a technique employed in the newborn for the detection of a pneumothorax. In newborns on ventilatory support, often a multitude of chest x-rays are obtained. Transillumination is noninvasive and does not carry the hazards associated with repeated x-ray exposure.

ABG determinations and transcutaneous monitoring together provide a consistent picture of oxygenation and ventilation. Transcutaneous monitoring provides you with real-time data, while ABG values allow you to "trend" the monitor with the patient's actual condition.

Cardiac

Blood pressure, heart rate, and general observation are important in assessment for potential harmful effects of mechanical ventilation. Positive-pressure ventilation, while providing patient support, also has its complications and hazards.

Renal

Urine output provides information regarding the adequacy of circulation to the vital organs. A decrease in urine output in response to high airway pressures indicates some impairment of renal function because of the increased intrathoracic pressure. Urine output and daily weights are also an important way to monitor the patient's fluid status.

VENTILATOR MONITORING

Ventilator monitoring consists of verifying the settings and recording any changes in the patient's status. By combining patient assessment with ventilator monitoring, adjustments of the ventilatory support can be intelligently made. It is highly recommended that a ventilator monitor be used in concert with mechanical ventilation of newborns. Ventilator monitors provide the necessary precision in measuring airway pressures and time limits.

Mode

Monitoring the mode setting is simply confirming that the mode the ventilator is operating in is the desired mode. The observation is made and documented on the patient's flow sheet.

FIO_2

The FIO_2 is monitored by checking the control setting, with measurement of the FIO_2 using an oxygen analyzer. Be certain that the analyzer is properly calibrated before measuring the oxygen concentration. Ideally, check the oxygen concentration by breaking the circuit before the humidifier. Newer ventilators allow FIO_2 measurement through a port or flowmeter not connected to the patient circuit.

Airway Pressures

Monitoring airway pressures is important in assessing the adequacy of ventilatory support and to prevent barotrauma and other complications. Several pressures may be monitored, including the peak pressure, mean airway pressure, and CPAP/PEEP levels. All pressure measurements should be taken from the ventilatory monitor.

Respiratory Rate

The ventilator rate (mandatory IMV breaths) and the patient's rate are measured and documented. As ventilatory support decreases, the patient's rate becomes a larger part of the total respiratory rate.

Flow Rate

The continuous flow rate is measured and adjusted to meet the patient's needs. The flowmeter setting is documented on the patient's flow sheet, indicating that the flow rate was assessed.

Inspiratory Time and I:E Ratio

Many neonatal ventilators monitor inspiratory time or I:E ratio and display in real time what the value is. Some ventilators may provide you with both types of information. With some ventilators, the I:E ratio must be calculated from the inspiratory time, expiratory time, and the rate settings.

Pressure Popoff Level

To record the pressure popoff level (above PIP), disconnect the patient and have someone else manually ventilate the patient. Occlude the patient circuit at the patient connection and remove the expiratory line from the expiration valve. Occluding the expiratory line allows the pressure to build in the circuit to the popoff level that is observed on the manometer. The popoff pressure is set at 3 to 5 cm H_2O above the peak pressure.

Temperature

The proximal airway temperature should be maintained between 32 and 34°C. Excessive temperatures can result in damage to the airway and actual burns. Servo-controlled humidifiers are commonly used in newborn ventilation and simplify temperature and humidity delivery.

Alarm Settings

All pressure alarms are monitored and the settings recorded. The function of the alarms should also be periodically checked to prevent potential errors and problems.

References

Alone, C. (1987). *Respiratory care of the newborn: A clinical manual.* Philadelphia: Lippincott.

American Association for Respiratory Care. (1999). AARC clinical practice guidelines: Neonatal time-triggered, pressure-limited, time-cycled mechanical ventilation. *Respiratory Care, 39*(8), 808–816.

Chatburn, R. L. (1991). Principles and practice of neonatal and pediatric mechanical ventilation. *Respiratory Care, 36*(6), 569–595.

Goldberg, R. N., & Bancalari, E. (1986). Bronchopulmonary dysplasia: Clinical presentation and the role of mechanical ventilation. *Respiratory Care, 31*(7), 591–598.

Koff, P. (1988). *Neonatal and pediatric respiratory care.* St. Louis, MO: Mosby.

V.I.P. Bird Infant-Pediatric Ventilator instruction manual. (1991). Palm Springs, CA: Bird Products Corporation.

Additional Resources

Blodgett, D. (1987). *Manual of respiratory care procedures* (2nd ed.). Philadelphia: Lippincott.

Scanlan, C. L., Spearman, C. B., & Sheldon, R. L. (1995). *Egan's fundamentals of respiratory therapy* (6th ed.). St. Louis, MO: Mosby.

Practice Activities: BEAR Medical Systems/BEAR Cub

CIRCUIT ASSEMBLY

When completing this assembly guide, refer to Figure 29-1.

1. Assemble and fill the humidifier and attach it to the ventilator.

2. Connect the inspiratory limb of the patient circuit to the humidifier outlet and the expiratory limb to the exhalation valve.

3. Connect the ventilator outlet to the humidifier inlet.

4. Attach the proximal airway line to the proximal airway nipple on the rear of the ventilator.

5. If the humidifier is servo-controlled, attach the temperature probe to the proximal airway. If the humidifier is not servo-controlled, attach a thermometer to the proximal airway. Heated wire circuits will require an additional temperature probe at the humidifier outlet and attachment of the heated wires to the servo.

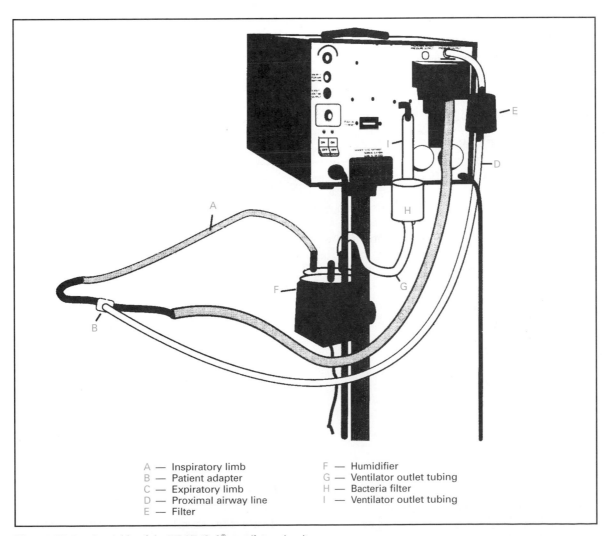

A — Inspiratory limb	F — Humidifier
B — Patient adapter	G — Ventilator outlet tubing
C — Expiratory limb	H — Bacteria filter
D — Proximal airway line	I — Ventilator outlet tubing
E — Filter	

Figure 29-1 *Assembly of the BEAR Cub® ventilator circuit*

6. Connect the ventilator to 50 psi air and oxygen supplies.

7. Connect the ventilator to a suitable 110 V 60 Hz power outlet.

ACTIVITIES

To complete these practice activities, it is recommended that you use an infant lung simulator or tester such as a Biotech VT-2 (Biotech, Winoski, VT), a manufacturer's test lung (BEAR Medical Systems, Inc., Riverside, CA), or a finger cot to simulate a neonate's lung.

Initial Settings

Mode	IMV
Flow Rate	7 L/min
Inspiratory Time	0.5 second
Rate	40/min
FIO_2	0.35
Pressure Limit	25 cm H_2O
PEEP/CPAP	4 cm H_2O

Manipulate only one control at a time and note the result following the change. Answer the questions that follow each of the activities.

INSPIRATORY TIME CONTROL

1. Adjust the inspiratory time to 0.3 second.
   a. Measure the respiratory rate.
   b. Observe the inflation of the test lung or measured tidal volume delivery.
   c. Measure the peak inspiratory pressure.

2. Adjust the inspiratory time to 2.0 seconds.
   a. Measure the respiratory rate.
   b. Observe the inflation of the test lung or measured tidal volume delivery.
   c. Measure the peak inspiratory pressure.

Questions:
A. How was the respiratory rate affected by changes in the inspiratory time?
B. How were peak pressures affected by changes in the inspiratory time?
C. How was volume delivery affected by changes in the inspiratory time?
D. What occurred when the inspiratory time was increased to 2.0 seconds?

VENTILATOR RATE

Adjust the controls to the following settings:

Mode	IMV
Flow Rate	7 L/min
Inspiratory Time	0.5 second
Rate	40/min
FIO_2	0.35
Pressure Limit	25 cm H_2O
PEEP/CPAP	4 cm H_2O

1. Decrease the ventilator rate to 20/min.
   a. Measure the respiratory rate.
   b. Measure the inspiratory time.

2. Increase the ventilator rate to 60/min.
   a. Measure the respiratory rate.
   b. Measure the inspiratory time.

Questions:
A. What effect did the control have on the respiratory rate?
B. What happened to the expiratory time as the control was adjusted?

PRESSURE LIMIT

Return all controls to the following settings:

Mode	IMV
Flow Rate	7 L/min
Inspiratory Time	0.5 second
Ventilator Rate	40/min
FIO_2	0.35
Pressure Limit	25 cm H_2O
PEEP/CPAP	4 cm H_2O

1. Perform the following tasks:
   a. Measure the peak inspiratory pressure.
   b. Observe the inflation of the test lung or measure the delivered volume.

2. Increase the pressure limit to 40 cm H_2O.
   a. Measure the peak inspiratory pressure.
   b. Observe the inflation of the test lung or measure the delivered volume.

3. Decrease the pressure limit to 10 cm H_2O.
   a. Measure the peak inspiratory pressure.
   b. Observe the inflation of the test lung or measure the delivered volume.

Questions:
A. What effect does the pressure limit control have on the delivered volume?
B. What effect does the pressure limit control have on the peak pressure?

PEEP/CPAP CONTROL

Set the controls to the following settings:

Mode	IMV
Flow Rate	7 L/min
Inspiratory Time	0.5 second
Ventilator Rate	40/min
FIO_2	0.35
Inspiratory Pressure	25 cm H_2O
PEEP/CPAP	4 cm H_2O

1. Adjust the PEEP/CPAP control to 10 cm H_2O.
   a. Measure the expiratory pressure using the manometer.

2. Adjust the PEEP/CPAP to zero.

Questions:
A. What effect did the expiratory pressure control have?
B. If the patient is not breathing spontaneously, what did the addition of expiratory pressure provide?

MANUAL BREATH CONTROL

Set the controls to the following settings:

Mode	IMV
Flow Rate	7 L/min
Inspiratory Time	0.5 second
Ventilator Rate	40/min
FIO_2	0.35
Inspiratory Pressure	25 cm H_2O
PEEP/CPAP	4 cm H_2O

1. Depress the manual breath control and observe what happens.

Question:

A. What is the purpose of the manual breath control?

FLOW RATE

Adjust the controls to the following settings:

Mode	IMV
Flow Rate	7 L/min
Inspiratory Time	0.5 second
Ventilator Rate	40/min
FiO_2	0.35
Inspiratory Pressure	25 cm H_2O
PEEP/CPAP	4 cm H_2O

1. Increase the flow to 10 L/min.
   a. Measure the respiratory rate.
   b. Observe the inflation of the test lung or measure the delivered volume.
2. Decrease the flow to 5 L/min.
   a. Measure the respiratory rate.
   b. Observe the inflation of the test lung or measure the delivered volume.

Questions:

A. What effect does the flow rate have on delivered volume?

B. Why does flow affect volume?

C. What effect does the flow have on the respiratory rate?

ALARM FUNCTIONS

Set the controls to the following settings:

Mode	IMV
Flow Rate	7 L/min
Inspiratory Time	0.5 second
Ventilator Rate	40/min
FiO_2	0.35
Inspiratory Pressure	25 cm H_2O
PEEP/CPAP	4 cm H_2O

Low Inspiratory Pressure Control

1. Rotate the patient pressure alarm control to 20 cm H_2O.
2. Disconnect the ventilator from the test lung device.
   a. Observe what happens.
3. Reconnect the ventilator to the test lung device.
   a. Observe what happens.

Questions:

A. What occurred?

B. What is the purpose of this alarm?

Loss of PEEP/CPAP Pressure Alarm

Adjust the controls to the following settings:

Mode	IMV
Flow Rate	7 L/min
Inspiratory Time	0.5 second
Ventilator Rate	40/min
FiO_2	0.35
Inspiratory Pressure	25 cm H_2O
PEEP/CPAP	7 cm H_2O

1. Set the loss of PEEP/CPAP alarm to 5 cm H_2O.
2. Disconnect the patient circuit from the test lung or disconnect the inspiratory limb from the humidifier.
   a. Observe what happens.

Questions:

A. What is the clinical application of this alarm?

B. What factors may cause a loss of PEEP/CPAP pressure?

Practice Activities: V.I.P. BIRD Ventilator

CIRCUIT ASSEMBLY

When completing this assembly guide, refer to Figure 29-2.

1. Attach a heated humidifier to the bracket on the ventilator. Connect the ventilator outlet to the inlet of the heated humidifier.
2. Connect the inspiratory limb of the circuit to the outlet of the humidifier.
3. Connect the proximal airway line to the proximal airway nipple on the front of the ventilator.
4. If the humidifier is servo-controlled, connect its temperature probe to the proximal airway. If the circuit is a heated wire circuit, an additional temperature probe will be required at the humidifier outlet and attachment of the heated wires to the servo unit.
5. Connect the high-pressure hoses to 50 psi air and 50 psi oxygen and the electrical power cord to a suitable alternating current (AC) outlet.

PRESSURE TEST

1. Set the controls to the following settings:

Mode	Time-cycled—IMV/CPAP
Inspiratory Time	1.0 second
Breath Rate	0
Peak Flow	Enough to generate 60–70 cm H_2O
High Pressure Limit	80 cm H_2O
PEEP/CPAP	5 cm H_2O

2. Plug the patient wye and the exhalation valve outlet. Press the Manual Breath button.
3. Pressure should rise and not fall more than 10 cm H_2O during a 2-second period. If pressure falls more than this, check all connections and tighten them, and repeat the pressure test.

TIME-CYCLED — IMV/CPAP

This mode of ventilation is similar to IMV/CPAP modes for other infant ventilators. In this mode you will select an inspiratory time, flow rate, breath rate, pressure limit, PEEP/CPAP level, and oxygen percent.

Connect the ventilator to a test lung or an infant lung simulator. Set the ventilator to these initial ventilator settings:

Mode	Time-cycled—IMV/CPAP
Flow	7 L/min

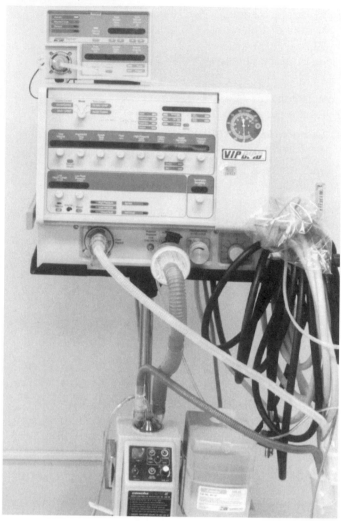

Figure 29-2 *A photograph of the V.I.P. Bird® ventilator (Courtesy of Bird Products Corporation, Palm Springs, CA)*

Inspiratory Time	0.5 second
Breath Rate	40/min
High Pressure Limit	25 cm H_2O
O_2 %	35%
PEEP/CPAP	4 cm H_2O

Manipulate only one control at a time and note the result following the change on a blank piece of paper. Answer the questions that follow each activity. If you need help, ask your laboratory instructor for assistance.

Inspiratory Time Control

1. Adjust the inspiratory time to 0.3 second.
   a. Measure the respiratory rate.
   b. Observe the inflation of the test lung or measure the tidal volume.
   c. Measure the peak inspiratory pressure.

2. Adjust the inspiratory time to 2.0 seconds.
   a. Measure the respiratory rate.
   b. Observe the inflation of the test lung or measure the tidal volume.
   c. Measure the peak inspiratory pressure.

Questions:

A. How was the respiratory rate affected by changes in the inspiratory time?
B. How was peak pressure affected by changes in the inspiratory time?
C. How was volume delivery affected?
D. What occurred when the inspiratory time was increased to 2.0 seconds?

Breath Rate

Set the controls to the following settings:

Mode	Time-cycled—IMV/CPAP
Flow	7 L/min
Inspiratory Time	0.5 second
Breath Rate	40/min
High Pressure Limit	25 cm H_2O
O_2 %	35%
PEEP/CPAP	4 cm H_2O

1. Decrease the ventilator rate to 20/min.
   a. Measure the respiratory rate.
   b. Measure the inspiratory and expiratory time.

2. Increase the ventilator rate to 60/min.
   a. Measure the respiratory rate.
   b. Measure the inspiratory and expiratory time.

Questions:

A. What effect did the control have on the respiratory rate?
B. What happened to the expiratory time as the control was adjusted?

High Pressure Limit

Return the controls to the following settings:

Mode	Time-cycled—IMV/CPAP
Flow	7 L/min
Inspiratory Time	0.5 second
Breath Rate	40/min
High Pressure Limit	25 cm H_2O
O_2 %	35%
PEEP/CPAP	4 cm H_2O

1. Measure the following:
   a. Peak inspiratory pressure.
   b. Observe the inflation of the test lung or measure the delivered tidal volume.

2. Increase the high pressure limit to 40 cm H_2O.
   a. Peak inspiratory pressure.
   b. Observe the inflation of the test lung or measure the delivered tidal volume.

3. Decrease the high pressure limit to 10 cm H_2O.
   a. Peak inspiratory pressure.
   b. Observe the inflation of the test lung or measure the delivered tidal volume.

Questions:

A. What effect does the pressure limit control have on the delivered volume?
B. What effect does the pressure limit control have on the peak pressure?

PEEP/CPAP Control

Set the controls to the following settings:

Mode	Time-cycled—IMV/CPAP
Flow	7 L/min
Inspiratory Time	0.5 second
Breath Rate	40/min
High Pressure Limit	25 cm H_2O
O_2 %	35%
PEEP/CPAP	4 cm H_2O

1. Adjust the PEEP/CPAP control to 10 cm H_2O.
   a. Measure the baseline pressure using the manometer.
2. Adjust the PEEP/CPAP control to zero.
   a. Measure the baseline pressure using the manometer.

Question:

A. What effect did the PEEP/CPAP control have?

Flow Control

Set the ventilator to the following settings:

Mode	Time-cycled—IMV/CPAP
Flow	7 L/min
Inspiratory Time	0.5 second
Breath Rate	40/min
High Pressure Limit	25 cm H_2O
O_2 %	35%
PEEP/CPAP	4 cm H_2O

1. Increase the flow to 10 L/min.
   a. Measure the respiratory rate.
   b. Observe the inflation of the test lung or measure the tidal volume.
2. Decrease the flow to 5 L/min.
   a. Measure the respiratory rate.
   b. Observe the inflation of the test lung or measure the tidal volume.

Questions:

A. What effect does the flow rate have on delivered tidal volume?
B. Why does the flow rate affect the tidal volume?
C. Does the flow rate affect the respiratory rate?

VOLUME-CYCLED ASSIST CONTROL

The V.I.P. Bird ventilator also allows volume-controlled ventilation as well as pressure-controlled, time-cycled ventilation. In this activity set, you will learn how the ventilator functions in the volume-controlled modes.

Tidal Volume Control

1. Set the controls to the following settings:

Mode	Volume-cycled assist/control
Tidal Volume	60 ml
Breath Rate	40/min
Flow	30 L/min
High Pressure Limit	80 cm H_2O
PEEP/CPAP	4 cm H_2O
Assist Sensitivity	3 cm H_2O
O_2 %	35%

2. Measure the following:
   a. Inspiratory time
   b. Tidal volume
   c. Peak pressure
3. Adjust the tidal volume control to 90 ml and measure the following:
   a. Inspiratory time
   b. Tidal volume
   c. Peak pressure
4. Adjust the tidal volume control to 30 ml and measure the following:
   a. Inspiratory time
   b. Tidal volume
   c. Peak pressure

Questions:

A. What effect did the tidal volume control have on volume delivery?
B. What effect did the tidal volume control have on inspiratory time?
C. What effect did the tidal volume control have on peak pressure?

Breath Rate Control

1. Set the controls to the following settings:

Mode	Volume-cycled assist/control
Tidal Volume	60 ml
Breath Rate	40/min
Flow	30 L/min
High Pressure Limit	80 cm H_2O
PEEP/CPAP	4 cm H_2O
Assist Sensitivity	3 cm H_2O
O_2 %	35%

2. Measure the following:
   a. Inspiratory and expiratory time
   b. Peak pressure
   c. Ventilatory rate
3. Set the breath rate control to 80 breaths/min and measure the following:
   a. Inspiratory and expiratory time
   b. Peak pressure
   c. Ventilatory rate
4. Set the breath rate control to 20 breaths/min and measure the following:
   a. Inspiratory and expiratory time
   b. Peak pressure
   c. Ventilatory rate

Questions:

A. What effect did the breath rate control have on inspiratory and expiratory time?
B. What effect did the breath rate control have on peak pressure?
C. What effect did the breath rate control have on ventilatory rate?

Flow Rate Control

Set the ventilator to the following settings:

Mode	Volume-cycled assist/control
Tidal Volume	60 ml

Breath Rate 40/min
Flow .... 30 L/min
High Pressure Limit .... 80 cm H_2O
PEEP/CPAP .... 4 cm H_2O
Assist Sensitivity .... 3 cm H_2O
O_2 % 35%

1. Measure the following:
   a. Inspiratory and expiratory times
   b. Peak inspiratory pressure

2. Set the flow rate control to 15 L/min and measure the following:
   a. Inspiratory and expiratory times
   b. Peak inspiratory pressure

3. Set the flow rate control to 60 L/min and measure the following:
   a. Inspiratory and expiratory times
   b. Peak inspiratory pressure

Questions:
A. What effect did the flow rate control have on inspiratory and expiratory times?
B. What effect did the flow rate control have on peak pressure?

VOLUME-CYCLED SIMV/CPAP AND PRESSURE SUPPORT

The V.I.P. Bird is also capable of volume-cycled SIMV/CPAP as well as pressure-limited SIMV/CPAP. In addition, the ventilator can also provide pressure support in this mode.
Set the ventilator to the following settings:

Mode .... Volume-cycled — SIMV/CPAP
Tidal Volume .... 60 ml
Breath Rate 10/min
Flow .... 30 L/min
High Pressure Limit .... 80 cm H_2O
PEEP/CPAP .... 4 cm H_2O
Assist Sensitivity .... 3 cm H_2O
O_2 % 35%
Pressure Support .... 0.0 cm H_2O

Control Operation

The operation and function of the tidal volume, breath rate, flow, and PEEP/CPAP control are identical to that described in the previous section. Volume-cycled SIMV/CPAP, however, provides a guaranteed volume delivery, unlike the pressure-cycled SIMV/CPAP mode, which delivers a constant pressure breath.

1. Measure the following:
   a. Inspiratory and expiratory times
   b. Peak and baseline pressure
   c. Respiratory rate
   d. Tidal volume delivery

2. Add 10 cm H_2O pressure support by adjusting the pressure support control to that level. Measure and record the following information:
   a. Inspiratory and expiratory times
   b. Peak and baseline pressure
   c. Respiratory rate
   d. Tidal volume delivery

3. Turn the breath rate control to zero, and measure the following information:
   a. Inspiratory and expiratory times
   b. Peak and baseline pressure
   c. Respiratory rate
   d. Tidal volume delivery

Questions:
A. How does the addition of pressure support affect volume delivery during spontaneous breaths?
B. How does pressure support affect peak pressures?
C. What mode is the ventilator operating in when the rate was set to zero?

ALARM SYSTEMS

The V.I.P. Bird has several alarms useful in the management of critically ill patients. These alarms include high pressure limit, low peak pressure, low PEEP/CPAP, and apnea.

High Pressure Limit Alarm

Set the ventilator to the following settings:

Mode .... Volume-cycled assist/control
Tidal Volume .... 60 ml
Breath Rate 40/min
Flow .... 30 L/min
High Pressure Limit .... 80 cm H_2O
PEEP/CPAP .... 4 cm H_2O
Assist Sensitivity .... 3 cm H_2O
O_2 % 35%

1. Set the high pressure limit alarm to 10 cm H_2O greater than the peak pressure.

2. Rapidly squeeze the test lung to simulate a cough and observe what happens.

Questions:
A. What occurred?
B. How could this alarm be clinically useful?

Low Peak Pressure Alarm

Set the ventilator to the following settings:

Mode .... Volume-cycled assist/control
Tidal Volume .... 60 ml
Breath Rate 40/min
Flow .... 30 L/min
High Pressure Limit .... 80 cm H_2O
PEEP/CPAP .... 4 cm H_2O
Assist Sensitivity .... 3 cm H_2O
O_2 % 35%

1. Set the low peak pressure alarm to 10 cm H_2O less than the peak inspiratory pressure.

2. Loosen one of the circuit fittings in such a way as to cause a leak and observe what happens.

Questions:
A. What occurred?
B. What other conditions could cause this alarm to become activated?

Low PEEP/CPAP Alarm

Set the ventilator to the following settings:

Mode	Volume-cycled assist/control
Tidal Volume	60 ml
Breath Rate	40/min
Flow	30 L/min
High Pressure Limit	80 cm H_2O
PEEP/CPAP	10 cm H_2O
Assist Sensitivity	3 cm H_2O
O_2 %	35%

1. Set the low PEEP/CPAP alarm to 5 cm H_2O.
2. Loosen one of the circuit fittings in such a way as to cause a leak and observe what happens.

Questions:

A. What occurred?

B. What other conditions could cause this alarm to become activated?

Apnea

1. With the ventilator set to the settings in the previous exercise, disconnect the test lung and observe what occurs.

Questions:

A. What occurred?

B. How long did it take for the alarm to sound?

C. What might cause this alarm?

Practice Activities: Sechrist IV-100B

CIRCUIT ASSEMBLY

When completing this assembly guide, refer to Figure 29-3.

1. Assemble and fill the humidifier and attach it to the ventilator's mounting pole.
2. Connect the large-diameter tubing between the humidifier inlet and the flowmeter outlet.
3. Connect the inspiratory limb of the patient circuit to the humidifier outlet and the expiratory limb to the exhalation valve.
4. Attach the proximal airway line to the proximal airway nipple on the exhalation valve assembly.

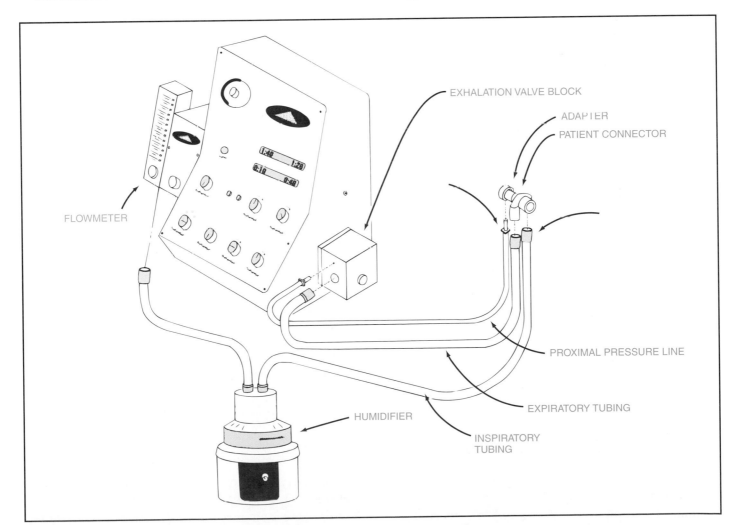

Figure 29-3 *Assembly of the Sechrist IV-100B ventilator circuit*

5. If the humidifier is servo-controlled, attach the temperature probe to the proximal airway. If the humidifier is not servo-controlled, attach a thermometer to the proximal airway.

6. Connect the ventilator to 50 psi air and oxygen supplies.

7. Connect the ventilator to a suitable 110 V 60 Hz power outlet.

ACTIVITIES

To complete these practice activities, it is recommended that you use an infant lung simulator or tester such as a Biotech VT-2, Winoski, VT, a manufacturer's test lung (BEAR Medical Systems, Inc., Riverside, CA), or a finger cot to simulate a neonate's lung.

Initial Settings

Mode	IMV
Flow Rate	7 L/min
Inspiratory Time	0.5 second
Expiratory Time	adjust for a rate of 40/min
FIO_2	0.35
Inspiratory Pressure	25 cm H_2O
Expiratory Pressure	4 cm H_2O

Manipulate only one control at a time and note the result following the change. Answer the questions that follow each of the activities.

INSPIRATORY TIME CONTROL

1. Adjust the inspiratory time to 0.3 second.
   a. Measure the respiratory rate.
   b. Observe the inflation of the test lung or measured tidal volume delivery.
   c. Measure the peak inspiratory pressure.

2. Adjust the inspiratory time to 1.25 seconds.
   a. Measure the respiratory rate.
   b. Observe the inflation of the test lung or measured tidal volume delivery.
   c. Measure the peak inspiratory pressure.

Questions:

A. How was the respiratory rate affected by changes in the inspiratory time?
B. How were peak pressures affected by changes in the inspiratory time?
C. How was volume delivery affected by changes in the inspiratory time?
D. Why do you feel the respiratory rate was affected?
E. What occurred when the inspiratory time was increased to 1.25 seconds?

EXPIRATORY TIME

Set the controls to the following settings:

Mode	IMV
Flow Rate	7 L/min
Inspiratory Time	0.5 second
Expiratory Time	adjust for a rate of 40/min
FIO_2	0.35
Inspiratory Pressure	25 cm H_2O
Expiratory Pressure	4 cm H_2O

1. Rotate the expiratory time control ½ turn clockwise from its current position.
   a. Measure the respiratory rate.
   b. Observe the inflation of the test lung or measured tidal volume delivery.
   c. Measure the peak inspiratory pressure.

2. Adjust the expiratory time control to establish a respiratory rate of 40 breaths/min.

3. Rotate the control ½ turn counterclockwise from its current position.
   a. Measure the respiratory rate.
   b. Observe the inflation of the test lung or measured tidal volume delivery.
   c. Measure the peak inspiratory pressure.

Questions:

A. What effect does expiratory time have on the respiratory rate?
B. What effect does the expiratory time have on delivered tidal volume?
C. What effect does expiratory time control have on the peak pressure?

INSPIRATORY PRESSURE

Return all controls to the following settings:

Mode	IMV
Flow Rate	7 L/min
Inspiratory Time	0.5 second
Expiratory Time	adjust for a rate of 40/min
FIO_2	0.35
Inspiratory Pressure	25 cm H_2O
Expiratory Pressure	4 cm H_2O

1. Perform the following tasks:
   a. Measure the peak inspiratory pressure.
   b. Observe the inflation of the test lung or measure the delivered volume.

2. Increase the inspiratory pressure to 40 cm H_2O.
   a. Measure the peak inspiratory pressure.
   b. Observe the inflation of the test lung or measure the delivered volume.

3. Decrease the inspiratory pressure to 10 cm H_2O.
   a. Measure the peak inspiratory pressure.
   b. Observe the inflation of the test lung or measure the delivered volume.

Questions:

A. What effect does inspiratory pressure have on the peak airway pressure?
B. What effect does the inspiratory pressure have on the delivered volume?

EXPIRATORY PRESSURE

Set the controls to the following settings:

Mode	IMV
Flow Rate	7 L/min
Inspiratory Time	0.5 second
Expiratory Time	adjust for a rate of 40/min
FIO_2	0.35
Inspiratory Pressure	25 cm H_2O
Expiratory Pressure	4 cm H_2O

1. Adjust the expiratory pressure control to 10 cm H_2O.
   a. Measure the expiratory pressure using the manometer.

Questions:

A. What effect did the expiratory pressure control have?

B. If the patient is not breathing spontaneously, what did the addition of expiratory pressure provide?

MANUAL BREATH CONTROL

Set the controls to the following settings:

Mode	IMV
Flow Rate	7 L/min
Inspiratory Time	0.5 second
Expiratory Time	adjust for a rate of 20/min
FiO$_2$	0.35
Inspiratory Pressure	25 cm H$_2$O
Expiratory Pressure	4 cm H$_2$O

1. Depress the manual breath control and observe what happens.

Questions:

A. What is the purpose of the manual breath control?

B. How is the inspiratory time determined?

C. How does the Sechrist manual breath control differ from that of the BEAR Cub?

FLOW RATE

Adjust the controls to the following settings:

Mode	IMV
Flow Rate	7 L/min
Inspiratory Time	0.5 second
Expiratory Time	adjust for a rate of 20/min
FiO$_2$	0.35
Inspiratory Pressure	25 cm H$_2$O
Expiratory Pressure	4 cm H$_2$O

1. Increase the flow to 10 L/min.
   a. Measure the respiratory rate.
   b. Observe the inflation of the test lung or measure the delivered volume.

2. Decrease the flow to 5 L/min.
   a. Measure the respiratory rate.

b. Observe the inflation of the test lung or measure the delivered volume.

Questions:

A. What effect does the flow rate have on delivered volume?

B. Why does flow affect volume?

C. What effect does the flow have on the respiratory rate?

ALARM FUNCTIONS

Set the controls to the following settings:

Mode	IMV
Flow Rate	7 L/min
Inspiratory Time	0.5 second
Expiratory Time	adjust for a rate of 20/min
FiO$_2$	0.35
Inspiratory Pressure	25 cm H$_2$O
Expiratory Pressure	4 cm H$_2$O

Patient Pressure Alarm Control

1. Rotate the patient pressure alarm control to 20 cm H$_2$O.

2. Disconnect the ventilator from the test lung device.
   a. Observe what happens.

3. Reconnect the ventilator to the test lung device.
   a. Observe what happens.

Questions:

A. What occurred?

B. What is the purpose of this alarm?

Alarm Delay Time

Repeat the exercises in the patient pressure alarm section with these additional activities:

1. Adjust the alarm delay to 10.
   a. Observe what happens.

2. Adjust the alarm delay to 45.
   a. Observe what happens.

Question:

A. What is the purpose of the alarm delay control?

Check List: Initiation of Mechanical Ventilation

_____ 1. Verify the order.

_____ 2. Assess the patient:

_____   a. Maternal history

_____   b. Physical assessment

_____   c. Signs of asphyxia

_____   d. Signs of aspiration

_____   e. Laboratory data

_____ 3. Establish an airway.

_____ 4. Assemble required equipment:

_____   a. Ventilator

_____   b. Humidifier

_____   c. Resuscitation bag

_____   d. Patient circuit

_____   e. Noninvasive monitors

_____ 5. Test the ventilator for proper function.

_____ 6. Establish ordered ventilator settings:

_____   a. Mode

_____   b. Inspiratory time

_____   c. Peak pressure

_____   d. Oxygen concentration

_____   e. Rate

_____   f. PEEP/CPAP level

_____ 7. Monitor the patient and the ventilator:

_____   a. Breath sounds

_____   b. Chest rise

_____   c. Appearance

_____   d. Mode

_____   e. Ventilator and patient rates

_____   f. Inspiratory time

_____   g. Peak pressure

_____   h. Flow rate

_____   i. PEEP/CPAP level

_____   j. Oxygen concentration

_____   k. Set all alarms

_____ 8. Set up noninvasive monitors.

_____ 9. Remove any disposable supplies and clean up the patient's area.

_____ 10. Record all information in the patient's chart.

Check List: Newborn Ventilator Monitoring

———— 1. Verify the physician's orders.

———— 2. Wash your hands.

———— 3. Explain the procedure to the patient's parents or other family members if present.

4. Assess the patient:

———— a. Breath sounds

———— b. Inspection

———— c. Noninvasive monitoring

———— d. Heart rate and rhythm

e. Airway

———— (1) Check position.

———— (2) Check security of attachments.

———— 5. Suction the patient as required.

6. Monitor the ventilator:

———— a. Mode

b. Rate

———— (1) Ventilator

———— (2) Patient

———— c. Flow

———— d. Inspiratory time and I:E ratio

e. Airway pressures

———— (1) Peak pressure

———— (2) PEEP/CPAP pressure

———— (3) Mean airway pressure

———— f. Measure the FIO_2.

———— g. Measure the airway temperature.

———— h. Fill the humidifier as required.

———— i. Check all alarm settings.

———— j. Check popoff pressure.

———— 7. Remove any unneeded supplies and clean up the area.

———— 8. Document all information on the patient's flow sheet or chart.

Self-Evaluation Post Test: Newborn Mechanical Ventilation

1. In ventilation of a newborn using a time-cycled ventilator, volume delivery is dependent upon:
   I. inspiratory time.
   II. pressure.
   III. flow.
   IV. expiratory time.
   a. I
   b. I, II
   c. I, II, III
   d. II, III
   e. II, III, IV

2. Which of the following is/are used to assess the adequacy of volume delivery in the newborn?
   I. Chest rise
   II. Patient's time constant
   III. Exhaled tidal volume
   IV. Popoff pressure levels
   a. I
   b. I, II
   c. II, III
   d. II, IV
   e. III, IV

3. During intermittent mandatory ventilation (IMV):
   I. the patient may breathe spontaneously.
   II. the ventilator delivers mandatory breaths.
   III. PEEP/CPAP may be delivered.
   a. I
   b. I, II
   c. I, II, III
   d. II
   e. II, III

4. Indications for mechanical ventilation of the newborn include:
   I. apnea.
   II. PaO_2 <50 mm Hg with an FIO_2 greater than 0.50.
   III. $PaCO_2$ >55 mm Hg.
   a. I
   b. I, II
   c. I, III
   d. II, III
   e. I, II, III

5. Assessment of the newborn for respiratory failure includes:
   I. appearance.
   II. maternal/delivery history.
   III. gestational age.
   IV. APGAR scores.
   a. I
   b. I, II
   c. I, II, III
   d. I, II, III, IV
   e. II, III, IV

6. A newborn with a short time constant should be ventilated with:
   I. a short inspiratory time.
   II. a long inspiratory time.
   III. maximal pressures.
   IV. short expiratory times.
   a. I
   b. I, II
   c. II
   d. II, III
   e. IV

7. The time constant is calculated by:
   a. multiplying the compliance by the airway resistance.
   b. multiplying the compliance times the peak pressure.
   c. multiplying the resistance times the peak pressure.
   d. dividing the peak pressure by the tubing compliance.
   e. dividing the lung compliance by the airway resistance.

8. A newborn patient with a short time constant may not tolerate:
   a. an I:E ratio greater than 1:2.
   b. an I:E ratio lower than 1:2.
   c. a long inspiratory time.
   d. a PEEP/CPAP level of 4 cm H_2O.
   e. a respiratory rate of 40/min.

9. Hazards and complications of mechanical ventilation and oxygen delivery to the newborn include:
   I.   barotrauma.
   II. retinopathy of prematurity.
   III. reduced cardiac output.
   IV. decreased urine output.
   a. I
   b. I, II
   c. I, II, III
   d. I, II, III, IV
   e. II, III, IV

10. The adequacy of ventilation is often established by patient assessment. This assessment may include:
    I.   chest rise.
    II. use of accessory muscles.
    III. noninvasive monitoring.
    IV. breath sounds.
    a. I
    b. I, II
    c. I, II, III
    d. I, II, III, IV
    e. II, III, IV

PERFORMANCE EVALUATION:
INITIATION OF NEWBORN MECHANICAL VENTILATION

Date: Lab _____ Clinical _____ Agency _____

Lab: Pass _____ Fail _____   Clinical: Pass _____ Fail _____

Student name _____ Instructor name _____

No. of times observed in clinical _____

No. of times practiced in clinical _____

PASSING CRITERIA: Obtain 90% or better on the procedure. Tasks indicated by * must receive at least 1 point, or the evaluation is terminated. Procedure must be performed within designated time, or the performance receives a failing grade.

SCORING: 2 points — Task performed satisfactorily without prompting.
1 point — Task performed satisfactorily with self-initiated correction.
0 points — Task performed incorrectly or with prompting required.
NA — Task not applicable to the patient care situation.

TASKS:

			PEER	LAB	CLINICAL
*	1.	Verifies the physician's order	☐	☐	☐
*	2.	Assesses the patient			
	a.	Maternal history	☐	☐	☐
	b.	Physical assessment	☐	☐	☐
	c.	Signs of asphyxia	☐	☐	☐
	d.	Signs of aspiration	☐	☐	☐
	e.	Laboratory data	☐	☐	☐
*	3.	Establishes an airway	☐	☐	☐
*	4.	Assembles required equipment			
	a.	Ventilator	☐	☐	☐
	b.	Humidifier	☐	☐	☐
	c.	Resuscitation bag	☐	☐	☐
	d.	Patient circuit	☐	☐	☐
	e.	Noninvasive monitors	☐	☐	☐
*	5.	Tests the ventilator before use			
*	6.	Establishes ordered settings			
	a.	Mode	☐	☐	☐
	b.	Inspiratory time	☐	☐	☐
	c.	Peak pressure	☐	☐	☐
	d.	Oxygen concentration	☐	☐	☐
	e.	Rate	☐	☐	☐
	f.	PEEP/CPAP level	☐	☐	☐

* 7. Monitors the patient and the ventilator

    a. Breath sounds   ☐ ☐ ☐

    b. Chest rise   ☐ ☐ ☐

    c. Appearance   ☐ ☐ ☐

    d. Mode   ☐ ☐ ☐

    e. Ventilator and patient rates   ☐ ☐ ☐

    f. Inspiratory time   ☐ ☐ ☐

    g. Peak pressure   ☐ ☐ ☐

    h. Flow rate   ☐ ☐ ☐

    i. PEEP/CPAP level   ☐ ☐ ☐

    j. Oxygen concentration   ☐ ☐ ☐

    k. Sets all alarms   ☐ ☐ ☐

* 8. Sets up noninvasive monitors   ☐ ☐ ☐

* 9. Cleans up the patient's area   ☐ ☐ ☐

* 10. Records all information in the patient's chart   ☐ ☐ ☐

SCORE: Peer   _____ points of possible 40; _____%

            Lab   _____ points of possible 40; _____%

            Clinical   _____ points of possible 40; _____%

TIME: _____ out of possible 30 minutes

STUDENT SIGNATURES   INSTRUCTOR SIGNATURES

PEER: _____   LAB: _____

STUDENT: _____   CLINICAL: _____

PERFORMANCE EVALUATION:
MONITORING NEWBORN MECHANICAL VENTILATION

Date: Lab _____ Clinical _____ Agency _____

Lab: Pass _____ Fail _____   Clinical: Pass _____ Fail _____

Student name _____   Instructor name _____

No. of times observed in clinical _____

No. of times practiced in clinical _____

PASSING CRITERIA: Obtain 90% or better on the procedure. Tasks indicated by * must receive at least 1 point, or the evaluation is terminated. Procedure must be performed within designated time, or the performance receives a failing grade.

SCORING:
2 points — Task performed satisfactorily without prompting.
1 point — Task performed satisfactorily with self-initiated correction.
0 points — Task performed incorrectly or with prompting required.
NA — Task not applicable to the patient care situation.

TASKS:		PEER	LAB	CLINICAL
*	1. Verifies the physician's orders	☐	☐	☐
*	2. Follows standard precautions, including handwashing	☐	☐	☐
	3. Explains the procedure to the family members if present	☐	☐	☐
*	4. Assesses the patient			
	a. Breath sounds	☐	☐	☐
	b. Inspection	☐	☐	☐
	c. Noninvasive monitoring	☐	☐	☐
	d. Heart rate and rhythm	☐	☐	☐
	e. Airway	☐	☐	☐
	(1) Position	☐	☐	☐
	(2) Security of connections	☐	☐	☐
*	5. Suctions as required	☐	☐	☐
*	6. Monitors the ventilator			
	a. Mode	☐	☐	☐
*	b. Rate			
	(1) Ventilator	☐	☐	☐
	(2) Patient	☐	☐	☐
	c. Flow	☐	☐	☐
	d. Inspiratory time and I:E ratio	☐	☐	☐
	e. Airway pressures			
*	(1) Peak pressure	☐	☐	☐
	(2) PEEP/CPAP level	☐	☐	☐
	(3) Mean airway pressure	☐	☐	☐

f. Measures the FiO_2 ☐ ☐ ☐

g. Measures the airway temperature ☐ ☐ ☐

h. Fills the humidifier ☐ ☐ ☐

i. Checks all alarm settings ☐ ☐ ☐

j. Checks popoff pressure ☐ ☐ ☐

7. Cleans up the area ☐ ☐ ☐

* 8. Records all data in the chart ☐ ☐ ☐

SCORE: Peer _____ points of possible 50; _____%

Lab _____ points of possible 50; _____%

Clinical _____ points of possible 50; _____%

TIME: _____ out of possible 30 minutes

STUDENT SIGNATURES   INSTRUCTOR SIGNATURES

PEER: _____   LAB: _____

STUDENT: _____   CLINICAL: _____

APPENDIX

ANSWERS TO SELF-EVALUATION POST TESTS

CHAPTER 1
Answers

1. B	3. D	5. B	7. C	9. A
2. C	4. C	6. D	8. A	10. D

CHAPTER 2
Answers

1. C	3. C	5. B	7. B	9. B
2. D	4. C	6. C	8. A	10. B

CHAPTER 3
Answers

1. B	3. D	5. C	7. D	9. D
2. D	4. D	6. D	8. B	10. B

CHAPTER 4
Answers

1. A	3. D	5. D	7. A	9. C
2. B	4. C	6. D	8. C	10. B

CHAPTER 5
Answers

1. B	3. D	5. D	7. C	9. D
2. C	4. D	6. B	8. C	10. C

CHAPTER 6
Answers

1. E	3. D	5. B	7. E	9. C
2. A	4. E	6. D	8. B	10. C

CHAPTER 7
Answers

1. D	3. B	5. B	7. E	9. A
2. D	4. E	6. B	8. B	10. B

CHAPTER 8
Answers

1. B	3. C	5. A	7. C	9. C
2. B	4. B	6. D	8. D	10. B

CHAPTER 9
Answers

1. B	3. A	5. C	7. D	9. A
2. B	4. D	6. D	8. C	10. D

CHAPTER 10
Answers

1. A	3. B	5. C	7. A	9. A
2. B	4. B	6. D	8. B	10. C

CHAPTER 11
Answers

1. D	3. D	5. B	7. D	9. B
2. D	4. D	6. B	8. C	10. D

CHAPTER 12
Answers

1. D	3. C	5. A	7. A	9. B
2. A	4. B	6. D	8. D	10. C

CHAPTER 13
Answers

1. B	3. E	5. C	7. D	9. B
2. B	4. E	6. B	8. E	10. D

CHAPTER 14
Answers

1. C	3. B	5. B	7. B	9. B
2. C	4. B	6. B	8. D	10. C

CHAPTER 15
Answers

1. C 3. B 5. B 7. D 9. D
2. B 4. A 6. C 8. D 10. D

CHAPTER 16
Answers

1. C 3. A 5. A 7. D 9. C
2. C 4. A 6. D 8. D 10. D

CHAPTER 17
Answers

1. B 3. D 5. D 7. E 9. E
2. D 4. C 6. A 8. B 10. B

CHAPTER 18
Answers

1. B 3. A 5. D 7. B 9. D
2. D 4. D 6. D 8. D 10. D

CHAPTER 19
Answers

1. B 3. A 5. B 7. D 9. D
2. B 4. D 6. C 8. B 10. C

CHAPTER 20
Answers

1. D 3. D 5. C 7. D 9. D
2. B 4. C 6. C 8. A 10. D

CHAPTER 21
Answers

1. D 3. D 5. C 7. B 9. D
2. B 4. C 6. C 8. A 10. D

CHAPTER 22
Answers

1. B 3. A 5. C 7. D 9. C
2. C 4. D 6. B 8. A 10. B

CHAPTER 23
Answers

1. E 3. A 5. A 7. E 9. B
2. B 4. D 6. B 8. B 10. D

CHAPTER 24
Answers

1. C 3. A 5. A 7. B 9. B 11. B
2. B 4. B 6. A 8. C 10. D

CHAPTER 25
Answers

1. D 3. D 5. C 7. D 9. D
2. D 4. A 6. C 8. D 10. C

CHAPTER 26
Answers

1. C 3. D 5. C 7. C 9. C
2. D 4. B 6. A 8. B 10. C

CHAPTER 27
Answers

1. A 3. C 5. B 7. D 9. D
2. C 4. D 6. B 8. C 10. B

CHAPTER 28
Answers

1. A 3. A 5. B 7. D 9. C
2. D 4. A 6. C 8. D 10. A

CHAPTER 29
Answers

1. C 3. C 5. D 7. A 9. D
2. A 4. E 6. A 8. A 10. D

GLOSSARY

abnormal breath sounds Abnormal breath sounds, or adventitious breath sounds, are sounds that are produced as a result of abnormal lung pathology (consolidation, edema, fluid, etc.). Abnormal breath sounds include rhonchi, crackles, wheezes, and rubs.

absolute humidity The amount of water vapor contained in a gas at a given temperature and relative humidity. Absolute humidity is expressed in milligrams per liter of gas.

absorption atelectasis An abnormal collapse of lung tissue caused by the administration of high concentrations of oxygen, resulting in the displacement of nitrogen

adjunctive breathing exercises Specific ventilatory exercises designed to increase the overall volume of air inspired or the volume of air to a specific lobe or segment

aerosol Particulate matter suspended in a gas; the particles may be either solid or liquid

afterload The resistance the ventricle must overcome to eject blood. As afterload decreases, ventricular ejection increases.

airborne transmission Transmission of microorganisms (0.5 micrometer or smaller) by air currents

air embolism Blockage of a blood vessel by a bubble of air that has entered the bloodstream

air-oxygen blender A medical device that precisely mixes air and oxygen together

air trapping A respiratory problem in which too much gas remains in the lungs after a complete exhalation (residual volume). In obstructive lung disease, bronchial obstruction causes air trapping distal to the obstruction.

airway resistance (R_{AW}) A measure of resistance to gas flow into and out of the lungs. Normal airway resistance is between 0.6 and 2.4 cm H_2O at a flow of 0.5 L/sec (30 L/min).

alpha receptors Receptor sites located in the peripheral vasculature, heart, bronchial muscle, and bronchial blood vessels. Stimulation of these sites causes peripheral vasoconstriction.

amplitude A measure of vibratory movement or displacement of a sinusoidal wave form about its mean or average value

anatomical dead space The volume of gas comprising the conducting airways. This part of ventilation does not participate in gas exchange.

anatomic reservoir The dead space composed of the nasopharynx and oropharynx, which is approximately 50 ml in volume

anterior mandibular displacement A positional maneuver in which the jaw is displaced anteriorly, separating the tongue from the posterior pharynx. This maneuver may be performed without manipulation of the neck (optimal choice if cervical spine injury is suspected).

anteroposterior (anterior-posterior) Referring to an x-ray view of the chest in which the x-rays pass from anterior to the posterior (front to back) with the film plate resting on the patient's back. This view is common in portable x-ray techniques and tends to magnify the size of the heart.

anticholinergic A class of drugs that block the site of acetylcholine transmission, preventing the action of acetylcholine (bronchospasm) in the lungs

antigen A foreign substance, usually a protein, that causes the body to produce an antibody in response to its presence that reacts specifically to the antigen

antimicrobial agents Drugs used to destroy or inhibit growth or reproduction of microorganisms (bacteria, fungi, protozoans, viruses). These drugs include antibiotics and antiviral, antiprotozoal, and antifungal agents.

antisepsis The application of chemical agents to inhibit microorganisms' ability to reproduce and grow

apical lordotic Referring to an x-ray view of the chest in which the patient is reclined or tilted backward at about 30° to 45° and the x-ray energy passes from anterior to posterior. This view moves the heart shadow and mediastinal structures out of the film plane, allowing a better view of the apices of the lungs.

arterialization Application of a warming pack or hot towel to increase peripheral circulation to an area prior to capillary sampling

arterial sampling The technique of obtaining a blood sample from an artery. Common sites from which samples are obtained are the radial, brachial, and femoral arteries.

asepsis The protection against infection before, during, and after patient contact or patient procedures (surgery, bronchoscopy, intubation, etc.)

assist/control mode A mode of mechanical ventilation that allows the patient's spontaneous efforts to trigger a mechanical breath. In this mode, the patient's respiratory drive will assist in normalizing blood gas values.

ASSS The American Standard Safety System (ASSS) is a safety system designed by the Compressed Gas Association for large medical gas cylinder valve connections. The system prevents the mismatching of regulators or connections with the incorrect cylinder.

atelectasis An airless state of the lung, lobe, or segment

ATPS Ambient temperature pressure, saturated (ATPS) is the condition of ambient temperature and pressure and 100% saturation with water vapor. All spirometry results are measured at ATPS.

atrial fibrillation A nonrhythmic, disorganized, rapid contraction of a group of cardiac muscle cells. This type of contraction is very inefficient and results in poor blood circulation. Fibrillation is usually described as to the specific area of occurrence, such as atrial fibrillation.

atrioventricular node (AV node) A part of the cardiac conduction system located in the septal wall of the right atrium, which conducts the electrical impulse from the sinoatrial node to the bundle of His

augmented minute ventilation A form of synchronized intermittent mandatory ventilation in which the patient is guaranteed a minimum minute volume. If the patient fails to maintain the threshold minute volume, the ventilator augments the patient's efforts to achieve the set minute ventilation.

auscultation The process of listening to the patient's chest using a stethoscope

--------------------------------- B ---------------------------------

bacillus A bacterium that is rodlike in shape

bacteriological surveillance A method by which equipment is routinely cultured and monitored for correct disinfection, sterilization, and handling procedures to identify and resolve sources of contamination

barotrauma Trauma to the thoracic structures resulting directly from the positive pressure (increased intrathoracic pressure) applied in mechanical ventilation. Barotrauma may be manifested as a pneumothorax, pneumomediastinum, subcutaneous emphysema, tracheal rupture, or interstitial emphysema.

barrel chest An abnormal chest conformation characterized by an increase in the anterior-posterior diameter. A barrel chest often accompanies chronic obstructive lung disease in which there is concomitant air trapping.

bedside monitoring Measurement of spontaneous ventilatory mechanics that typically includes minute volume, respiratory rate (frequency), tidal volume, vital capacity, and peak expiratory flow

beta-1 receptors Receptor sites located in the bronchial blood vessels and the heart. Stimulation of these sites results in tachycardia, an increased potential for arrhythmias, and increased cardiac output.

beta-2 receptors Receptor sites located in the bronchial smooth muscle, bronchial blood vessels, systemic blood vessels, and the skeletal muscles. Stimulation of these sites in the lungs causes bronchodilation.

bi-level positive airway pressure A mode of ventilation similar to continuous positive airway pressure except that different pressure levels may be set for the inspiratory and expiratory phases. The inspiratory pressure is greater than the expiratory pressure, offering lower resistance to exhalation.

Biot's respiration An abnormal ventilatory pattern that is characterized by irregular breathing (rate and depth) with periods of apnea

body humidity The maximum absolute humidity at body temperature (100% saturation with water vapor, 37°C, 43.9 mg/L water content, and a partial pressure of water vapor of 47 mm Hg)

bradycardia An abnormally low heart rate

bradypnea An abnormally low respiratory rate

bronchoalveolar lavage (BAL) A technique in which the bronchoscope is wedged and normal saline (0.9%) is instilled and then retrieved for cellular analysis

bronchoscopy A technique or procedure that involves visually examining the tracheobronchial tree with an instrument called a bronchoscope for diagnostic or therapeutic indications

BTPS Body temperature and pressure, saturated (BTPS) is a condition in which the gas present in the lungs is at body temperature and pressure and fully saturated with water vapor

bundle of His A band of fibers in the cardiac conduction system that conducts the impulse from the atrioventricular node to the ventricles. The bundle of His originates at the atrioventricular node and follows the septum of the heart, eventually dividing into the right and left bundle branches.

butterfly catheter A type of intravenous catheter that has a metal needle secured by two plastic tabs resembling a butterfly's wings

butterfly needle A specialized collection needle embedded into a pair of plastic tabs resembling a butterfly's wings. Attached to the butterfly and the end of the needle is a short length of collection tubing that terminates in a female syringe fitting. Syringes are necessary when a butterfly needle is used for phlebotomy collection.

--------------------------------- C ---------------------------------

capacity The maximum amount of water vapor a gas can hold at a given temperature. As the temperature of a gas increases, so does its capacity for water vapor.

capillary sampling Lancing the surface of the skin to obtain an arterialized capillary sample, which is collected in a small capillary tube

capsule A protective membranous shell that surrounds some bacteria, making them more difficult to destroy

cardiac output The amount of blood the heart pumps each minute, expressed in liters per minute. Normal cardiac output for an adult is about 5 L/min.

cardiac phases The four phases of the cardiac cycle: isovolumetric contraction, systolic ejection, isovolumetric relaxation, and diastolic filling

catheter fragment embolism Blockage of a blood vessel that occurs when a portion of an intravenous catheter is cut or broken off and enters the bloodstream

catheter shear The cutting off of a portion of an intravenous catheter. This condition usually occurs when the steel needle stylet is inserted back into the flexible indwelling catheter.

cellulitis Inflammation of the tissue, especially below the skin. This condition is characterized by redness, pain, and swelling.

central venous pressure The pressure measured in the vena cava or right atrium. This pressure reflects the blood volume returning to the heart and also the preload of the right ventricle.

central venous pressure (CVP) catheter A catheter inserted into the vena cava or right atrium to measure the central venous pressure and to provide a convenient route for mixed venous blood sampling or fluid administration

charting by exception A method of documentation in which only information that changes is recorded. Arrows, ditto marks, or other means are used to indicate data that remain constant since the last time the patient was seen.

chest drain A tube placed to remove blood or fluid from a chest cavity. For example, mediastinal chest drains are common postoperatively following coronary artery bypass graft surgery. These drains allow the removal of fluid from residual bleeding or edema following surgery.

chest percussion A technique in which the practitioner claps on the patient's chest wall using a cupped hand to induce vibration throughout the lung parenchyma, facilitating bronchial secretion clearance. The technique may also be performed with the assistance of mechanical devices.

chest tube A tube placed into the pleural space to remove air or fluid. Depending on whether gas or fluid removal is the purpose of the chest tube, it may be placed in an anterior (gas) or a posterior (fluid) location in the chest.

chevron A pattern of taping used in securing an intravenous catheter

Cheyne-Stokes respiration An abnormal ventilatory pattern that is characterized by alternating periods of apnea and an increase in depth and rate of breathing, followed by a tapering of depth and rate leading to another apneic period

cholinergic receptors Receptor sites, located throughout the body, that are stimulated by acetylcholine

clinical goal A desired clinical outcome of a therapy or procedure. Ideally, clinical goals should be objective and measurable.

closed suction system A type of suction catheter that incorporates a protective plastic sheath surrounding the catheter. It is designed to be used multiple times and has the advantage of remaining attached to the artificial airway at all times.

coccus A bacterium that is round or spherical in shape

collarbones Bony structures located on the superior aspect of the anterior chest, generally overlying the first rib. Also called clavicles.

collection chamber The compartment of a chest drainage system located most proximal to the patient. This chamber collects fluid that is removed by the chest drain or chest tube.

computed tomography A radiographic technique in which the body is imaged in many thin slices, typically moving superior to inferior. This imaging modality creates a three-dimensional perspective that other techniques do not provide.

consolidation A condition or process of solidification of the lung tissue. Consolidation may be observed as increased opacification on chest radiographs.

contact transmission Transmission of microorganisms by direct contact (person to person), usually involving the hands

continuous mechanical ventilation The artificial support of a patient's respiratory needs using a mechanical ventilator. Ventilatory support may be total (in the apneic patient) or partial (when some spontaneous breaths are possible but minute ventilation is insufficient to normalize blood gases).

control mode A mode of ventilation in which all breaths are time cycled and delivered at preset intervals (ventilatory rate). In this mode, any spontaneous efforts made by the patient are not recognized by the ventilator; therefore, patient-ventilator asynchrony may occur.

coronary artery disease Obstruction of the coronary arteries, which may be caused by fatty deposits (plaque) or thrombi. The condition can lead to decreased delivery of oxygen to the myocardium, with consequent symptoms.

corticosteroids A class of drugs that act as anti-inflammatory agents, and are typically natural or synthetic hormones

counterpulsation A circulatory assist modality in which the intra-aortic balloon pulses with correct timing so that it is inflated during diastole (dicrotic notch) and deflated before systole (end-diastolic pressure). With this technique, coronary blood flow is improved (increased diastolic augmentation) and afterload is reduced.

CPAP Continuous positive airway pressure (CPAP) is the application of continuous pressure (both inspiration and expiration) in the spontaneously breathing patient. CPAP is similar to positive end-expiratory pressure in that it improves the functional residual capacity.

CPAP/IMV The CPAP/IMV mode is a common ventilatory support mode for neonatal and pediatric patients. In this mode a continuous flow of gas is available for inspiration at all times (CPAP); when mandatory breaths are delivered (IMV), the exhalation valve closes, administering a mechanical breath.

cracking The quick opening and closing of a cylinder valve allowing the high-pressure gas to exit the valve, removing any debris, dust, or dirt

cross-contamination The transmission of microorganisms between places or persons. The most common method of transmission is by direct contact between persons.

Croupette A type of enclosure for infants and toddlers that is used to provide supplemental oxygen and aerosol therapy and is commonly used to treat croup (epiglottitis)

cytology brush A specialized small brush that is designed to pass through the channel of a flexible bronchoscope to obtain tissue samples for analysis

--- D ---

damping An attenuation of the pressure wave form that is most commonly caused by air bubbles in the measuring system

decannulation The removal of the tracheostomy tube from the tracheostomy stoma. With accidental decannulation, if the stoma is not well established, ventilation may be tenuous.

degranulation The lysis of a cell wall, resulting in release of the cell's contents. When mast cells degranulate, histamine, heparin, leukotrienes, and other mediators are released.

depolarization The process of muscle cell contraction in which potassium is exchanged for sodium, resulting in a net negative charge of the cell

diagnostic bronchoscopy A bronchoscopy procedure in which samples of tissue or secretions are taken for further laboratory analysis and workup

diastolic The pressure recorded at the moment of cardiac relaxation, yielding the lower of the paired blood pressure values

diffusion (D_LCO) A pulmonary function parameter measured as the diffusion of gas across the alveolar-capillary membrane. Carbon monoxide is used as a test gas because of its increased affinity for hemoglobin compared with oxygen.

digital clubbing An abnormal enlargement of the distal phalanges, usually caused by chronic hypoxemia

disinfection The process of killing all pathogenic microorganisms (vegetative forms)

DISS Diameter index safety system (DISS) is a safety system designed by the Compressed Gas Association for low-pressure (less than 200 psi) compressed gas fittings.

distal lumen The opening at the tip of the catheter; used to measure the pulmonary artery and pulmonary arterial wedge pressures

downstream Distal to a point in a device, or circuit, in relation to gas or current flow

droplet transmission Transmission of microorganisms by aerosolized droplets (0.5 micrometer or larger) usually produced by coughing or sneezing

dry powder inhaler (DPI) A medication administration device that aerosolizes small particles of dry powder medication. Dry powder inhalers do not require a propellant to operate but rely on the patient's inspiratory flow.

dynamic compliance A measurement of the compliance (distensibility) of the patient's lungs and thorax under conditions of air flow. Therefore, the dynamic compliance reflects not only the compliance of the lungs and thorax but also airway resistance.

--- E ---

endotoxin A toxic compound usually contained in the cell walls of microorganisms. These toxins are released when these organisms die and the body breaks down their cell walls.

endotracheal pilot tube and balloon A small tube that passes the length of an endotracheal tube and connects the pilot balloon with its inflation port to the endotracheal tube cuff. By palpating the pilot balloon and attaching a pressure manometer to the inflation port, endotracheal tube cuff pressures may be assessed.

endotracheal tube An artificial airway that may be passed orally or nasally into the trachea, providing for positive-pressure ventilation and airway protection

endotracheal tube cuff A large inflatable balloon at the distal end of an endotracheal tube that is designed to seal against the tracheal wall when inflated

end-tidal CO_2 monitor A monitor that measures the exhaled partial pressure of carbon dioxide ($PetCO_2$) utilizing infrared technology

ethylene oxide A gas applied with moist heat to sterilize equipment and supplies

eukaryotic bacteria A type of bacteria in which the bacterial cell contains a true nucleus

eupnea A normal breathing pattern

expiratory positive airway pressure (EPAP) In bi-level positive-pressure ventilation, the baseline setting for the expiratory pressure level

expiratory reserve volume (ERV) The maximum amount of air that can be exhaled after a normal tidal exhalation

expiratory retard In mechanical ventilation, the application of resistance to exhaled air flow, usually by means of a variable-orifice type valve. The patient exhales to ambient pressure; however, the expiratory phase is lengthened owing to the increased resistance to gas flow.

exposed Referring to x-ray film that has been subjected to x-ray energy, causing a physical change in the emulsion to create an image.

exposure control policy A specific institutional policy designed to protect caregivers, staff, and patients from exposure to hazardous body fluids or other substances

extubation The process in which the endotracheal tube is removed. Extubation usually follows clinical improvement or accomplishment of therapeutic goals by the patient.

--- F ---

FEF$_{25-75\%}$ The flow rate between 25% and 75% of maximum as measured on a forced vital capacity tracing

FEF$_{200-1200ml}$ The flow rate between 200 and 1200 ml as measured on a forced vital capacity tracing

fenestrated tracheostomy tube A specialized tracheostomy tube in which there is an opening (fene stration) cut into the cannula, permitting passage of air into the upper airway

FEV₁ The amount of air that can be forcefully exhaled in 1 second, usually measured on a forced vital capacity maneuver

fiberoptic bronchoscope A flexible bronchoscope made from fiberoptic bundles that conduct light from the objective (distal end) to the eyepiece

FIO₂ Fraction of inspired oxygen (FIO_2) is the delivered oxygen concentration and is expressed as a decimal fraction.

flash A momentary pulse of blood that enters the syringe when the artery has been punctured. Usually the flash can be first observed at the hub of the needle.

flowmeter A medical gas component that is designed to regulate flow precisely; usually calibrated in liters per minute

flow-volume loop A graphical representation of a pulmonary function study in which flow (y axis) is plotted against volume (x axis). Flow-volume loops allow better characterization of airway obstruction.

forced vital capacity (FVC) The volume of air that can be exhaled forcefully following a maximal inhalation

forceps In bronchoscopy, a specialized miniature grasping instrument designed to be passed through the channel of a flexible bronchoscope to obtain tissue samples for further analysis

frequency The number of times an event occurs per unit of time. In measuring bedside ventilatory mechanics, the frequency is the respiratory rate.

full-face mask A soft-seal mask covering both the nose and mouth, used for resuscitation (bag-mask devices) and for noninvasive ventilation

functional residual capacity (FRC) A combination of expiratory reserve volume and residual volume

funnel chest A chest deformity in which the sternum is depressed (sunken), compressing the lungs. Also called pectus excavatum.

G
---

gamma radiation A very-high-frequency electromagnetic emission of photons from some types of radioactive elements. Gamma radiation is used in the sterilization of newly manufactured medical equipment prior to shipping.

gas dilution technique A method of measuring functional residual capacity by diluting an inspired gas into the lungs. If the initial concentration of a gas, its initial volume, and the final concentration after dilution are known, the final volume may be calculated.

glutaraldehyde A chemical agent (liquid) in which equipment and supplies are soaked to disinfect or sterilize them

Gram stain A technique of staining microorganisms that differentiates between them on the basis of characteristics of their cell wall structure

graphical record A type of documentation in the medical record utilizing graphs. Graphical records are typically used to document vital signs (heart rate, respiratory rate, temperature, blood pressure, etc.).

gt Abbreviation for "drop" (the plural is gtt)

H
---

head box A type of enclosure made of a Plexiglass or acrylic material that encloses only an infant's head, used for administration of supplemental oxygen

head tilt A positional maneuver in which the head is tilted backward, opening the airway by moving the tongue anteriorly away from the posterior pharynx. This maneuver should not be used if head or neck trauma is suspected.

heat and moisture exchanger (HME) A hygroscopic device placed proximal to the patient's artificial airway that captures the exhaled moisture and evaporates it during inspiration, humidifying the airway

heating element In a transcutaneous electrode, a thermostatically controlled heater that arterializes the skin by warming it to 44°C

HEENT An acronym for "head, eyes, ears, nose, and throat." This acronym is commonly dictated by the physician during the physical examination of the patient.

HEPA mask The high-efficiency particulate air (HEPA) filtration mask is a specialized mask that has very small pores that enable it to trap the majority of pathogens and small particles. HEPA masks should be fitted and tested by qualified personnel.

high-flow oxygen delivery system An oxygen delivery system in which all of the patient's inspiratory flow needs are met

high-frequency chest wall oscillation (HFCWO) A means of secretion mobilization (bronchial hygiene) utilizing a specialized vest that oscillates as gas pressure changes within the vest

hilum The center of the mediastinal border where the right and left mainstem bronchi and blood and lymph vessels enter and exit the lungs

histamine A mediator released (from mast cells) in an allergic response, causing capillary dilation and bronchoconstriction in the lungs

humidifier A device that produces water vapor through evaporation, adding water content to the gas that passes through it

humidity Water contained in a gas as a vapor

humpback An abnormal curvature of the upper spine from anterior to posterior, resulting in a humplike appearance of the upper portion of the back. Also called kyphosis.

hydrostatic testing A required test for medical gas cylinders in which the cylinder is filled with water and pressurized to 5/3 the service pressure and then the cylinder's expansion is measured

hyperinflation A state of overinflation or overdistention of the lungs

hyperpnea A deep, rapid ventilatory pattern

hypertension An abnormally high blood pressure

hyperthermia An abnormally elevated body temperature

hypertonic solution An intravenous solution that, by its properties, causes the net movement of fluid from the inside of cells into the vascular space

hyperventilation A ventilatory rate and depth that are greater than normal for metabolic needs, resulting in a decrease in arterial partial pressure of carbon dioxide ($PaCO_2$)

hypopnea A ventilatory pattern of shallow respirations

hypotension An abnormally low blood pressure

hypothermia An abnormally low body temperature (below 35°C)

hypotonic solution An intravenous solution that, by its properties, causes the net movement of fluid from the vascular space into the cells

hypoxemia An abnormally low oxygen tension in the blood (dissolved in the plasma)

———————————— I ————————————

IgE Also called reagin, this antibody is associated with allergic responses. IgE attaches to the mast cell, triggering the release of histamine and other mediators.

incentive spirometer A specific biofeedback device that records volume or flow while the patient breathes, to provide encouragement and feedback data promoting deeper respirations

incentive spirometry The technique of applying biofeedback devices to encourage the patient to take deeper breaths than normal.

infiltrate Abnormally accumulated fluid within lung tissue; observed as an increased opacity of affected lung on chest radiographs.

infiltration Escape of blood or intravenous fluid into surrounding tissues, where it may accumulate. Infiltration occurs when the needle is dislodged from the vein or the vessel is inadvertently punctured in more than one place.

inflation lumen and balloon The lumen is the port used on the pulmonary artery catheter to inflate the balloon located at the distal tip of the catheter

infusion pump A mechanical device used to maintain an infusion at a prescribed rate

inspection The process of observing the patient for color, work of breathing, clubbing of digits, thoracic conformation, ventilatory pattern, and chest wall motion

inspiratory capacity (IC) A combination of tidal volume and inspiratory reserve volume

inspiratory hold A feature of some ventilators that helps to improve distribution of ventilation and alveolar recruitment. After a full tidal breath delivery, the exhalation valve is held closed, and the tidal breath is held within the patient's chest. The inspiratory hold may typically be adjusted between 0.1 and 2.0 seconds, in 0.1-second intervals.

inspiratory positive airway pressure (IPAP) In bi-level positive-pressure ventilation, the setting for the inspiratory pressure level

inspiratory reserve volume (IRV) The maximal amount of air that can be inhaled following a normal tidal inspiration

intermittent positive-pressure breathing (IPPB) therapy The application of positive pressure using a special ventilator to increase the overall volume of air inspired. Additionally, IPPB can provide aerosolized medication delivery simultaneously with hyperinflation.

intra-aortic balloon (IAB) A large-caliber dual lumen balloon catheter that is inserted into the femoral artery, to lie within the aortic arch and proximal to the renal arteries

intra-aortic balloon pump (IABP) A mobile console used to conduct helium into and out of the intra-aortic balloon. The console has electrocardiographic and arterial pressure monitoring equipment to ensure correct timing of the intra-aortic balloon's inflation.

intrapulmonary percussive ventilation (IPV) The application of high-frequency, phased, pulsed gas delivery and the administration of a dense aerosol. This technique is applied using an IPV ventilator.

intubation A technique in which a tube is inserted into the trachea to provide a patent airway for positive-pressure ventilation or airway protection

isolette A type of enclosure for infants usually made of clear Plexiglas or an acrylic material that is primarily used to provide for the infant's thermal environment

isotonic solution An intravenous solution that, by its properties, causes no net movement of fluid from either the vascular space or the cell

———————————— K ————————————

Kussmaul's respiration An abnormal ventilatory pattern that is characterized by abnormally deep and rapid breathing. This is often observed in patients with ketoacidosis (diabetic crisis).

KVO Abbreviation for "keep vein open," referring to a drip rate for intravenous solutions that maintains the patency of the needle

kyphoscoliosis An abnormal curvature of the spine in which both kyphosis and scoliosis are present

kyphosis An abnormal curvature of the upper spine in which the posterior to anterior curve is greater than normal, resulting in a "humpback" appearance

———————————— L ————————————

laryngeal mask airway (LMA) An airway designed to intubate the esophagus while allowing ventilation of the lungs, protecting them from gastric aspiration

laryngeal obstruction Obstruction of the airway at the level of the larynx. This may be caused by laryngospasm, anaphylaxis, foreign body aspiration, or near-drowning.

laryngoscope An instrument that is used to visualize the larynx during intubation

lateral   Referring to a chest x-ray view in which the x-ray energy passes from one side of the body to the other

left anterior oblique   Referring to a chest x-ray view in which the patient is upright and rotated 45° to the right, with the film plate against the patient's back (posteroanterior projection). This view "moves" the heart out of the way for better visualization of other structures.

left heart   A term referring to the left atrium and ventricle, which pump blood through the systemic vasculature. Because the systemic vascular resistance is high, the left heart is a high-pressure system.

leukotrienes   A group of chemical mediators released by the mast cell and causing profound bronchospasm.

lordosis   An abnormal inward curvature of the lumbar spine, causing a swayback appearance

low-flow oxygen delivery system   An oxygen delivery device that meets only part of the patient's inspiratory flow needs, with the rest being made up of room air

——————————— M ———————————

MacIntosh blade   A curved laryngoscope blade that is designed to be inserted into the vallecula and then lifted, exposing the larynx

mainstream monitor   A type of end-tidal carbon dioxide sensor that is placed directly in the stream of the patient's exhaled gas

mast cell   A specialized cell found in the lungs that contains large basophilic granules containing histamine, serotonin, heparin, and bradykinin

maximum absolute humidity   The maximum amount of humidity a gas can contain at any given temperature. As temperature increases, the capacity of a gas to contain water vapor also increases.

maximum voluntary ventilation (MVV)   The maximum amount of air that can be inhaled by breathing as deeply and as rapidly as possible

MDI   A metered dose inhaler (MDI) is a small, compact, self-contained aerosol-dispensing device similar in design to an aerosol spray can

mechanical percussor   A mechanical device designed to aid in effective delivery of percussion. Both electric and pneumatic devices are common.

metabolic acidosis   Acidosis produced as a result of the renal system's not producing enough bicarbonate, thus lowering the blood's pH

Miller blade   A straight laryngoscope blade that is designed to lift the epiglottis, exposing the larynx

minimal leak   Referring to a positive-pressure technique in which the amount of air injected into the cuff of an artificial airway allows for a very small leak during a positive-pressure breath

minimal occlusion volume   The minimum volume of air injected into the cuff of an artificial airway that seals the airway during a positive-pressure breath

minute volume   The amount of air inhaled or exhaled by the patient in 1 minute

MIP   The maximal inspiratory pressure (MIP) is the maximum amount of force that can be generated by a spontaneously breathing patient during inspiration. This is commonly measured using a simple pressure manometer.

modified Allen's test   A test performed prior to the puncture of the radial artery to assess collateral circulation (circulation through the ulnar artery)

mucokinetics   A class of drugs that promote the movement of the mucus blanket by decreasing the viscosity of mucus

muscarinic effect   Vagal (tenth cranial) nerve stimulation resulting in the release of acetylcholine

myocardial contractility   The forcefulness of heart contractions during systole

——————————— N ———————————

nasal cannula   A low-flow oxygen delivery device designed to administer oxygen through the nose, filling the anatomic reservoir with oxygen-enriched gas. This device is used with flows of less than 6 L/min.

nasal mask   A mask that covers the patient's nose only; the mouth is exposed and the patient may speak. Nasal masks are commonly used during bi-level positive-pressure ventilation.

nasogastric tube   A small-diameter tube passed down the esophagus into the stomach to remove gastric contents, thereby decompressing it

nasopharyngeal airway   An artificial airway that passes through the nose and nasopharynx and rests just behind the tongue, where the airway separates it from the posterior pharynx

nebulizer   A device that produces an aerosol

nicotinic effect   Stimulation of the ganglionic nerve endings at the motor nerves of the skeletal muscles

nitrogen washout   A dilutional lung volume technique in which the patient breathes pure oxygen, washing out the nitrogen. Exhaled volume and exhaled nitrogen percentage are measured and used to determine the functional residual capacity.

nonrebreathing mask   A low-flow oxygen delivery device with a small reservoir covering the nose and mouth with an attached reservoir bag and one-way valves that help to limit room air entrainment. The mask should be used with a liter flow sufficient to keep the reservoir bag inflated at all times.

normal breath sounds   The sounds that are produced by normal lung tissue as air passes into and out of the respiratory system. These sounds are divided into tracheal, bronchial, bronchovesicular, and vesicular breath sounds.

——————————— O ———————————

objective data   Data collected by direct observation or measurement. Objective data may be referred to as clinical signs, as opposed to symptoms, which are subjective data.

oropharyngeal airway   An artificial airway that is inserted into the mouth and separates the tongue from the posterior pharynx

over-the-needle catheter A type of intravenous catheter that has a steel needle stylet contained within a flexible catheter. After the vessel is entered, the flexible catheter is advanced into the vessel and remains. The steel stylet is removed.

oxygen analyzer A device used to determine the concentration of oxygen delivered by a device or in an environment (enclosure). With these devices, the oxygen level is usually read as a percentage.

oxygen concentrator A medical device that separates oxygen from room air, supplying up to 95% oxygen at low flow rates; often used in the home

───────────── P ─────────────

palpation A technique in which the patient's body is touched by the examiner's hands. In thoracic evaluation, areas of tenderness, subcutaneous emphysema, symmetry of excursion, tactile fremitus, and tracheal position may be assessed.

partial rebreathing mask A low-flow oxygen delivery device with a small reservoir that covers the nose and mouth with an attached reservoir bag

Pascal's law A law that states that pressure applied within a closed container is equal at all points in the container. The pressure applied against the walls of the container acts perpendicularly to the wall of the container.

Passy-Muir valve A specialized one-way valve that is designed to be placed onto a tracheostomy tube (when the cuff is deflated), which then allows the patient to exhale through the upper airway

pasteurization A hot water bath (77°C) that destroys all vegetative forms of bacteria (disinfection)

patency The condition of an intravenous catheter that remains open and allows for the flow of fluid

pathogen A microorganism capable of producing a disease

patient positioning The technique of positioning the patient different ways to optimize ventilation and perfusion, to promote visualization of structures during imaging studies, and to help to prevent pressure ulcer formation

peak expiratory flow rate The maximal flow rate generated during a forceful exhalation

peak flowmeter A portable medical device that measures a patient's spontaneous peak expiratory flow rate during a forced exhalation

pectus carinatum An abnormal conformation of the lower sternum in which the xiphoid process and lower portion of the sternal body project outward

pectus excavatum An abnormal conformation of the sternum in which it is depressed inward

PEEP Positive end-expiratory pressure (PEEP) is the application of positive pressure during exhalation. This positive pressure increases the patient's functional residual capacity, which improves gas exchange and reduces shunt. PEEP is used in conjunction with continuous mechanical ventilatory support.

percussion A technique in which the examiner taps on the patient's body either directly or indirectly. In examination of the chest, the character (pitch and amplitude) of the resulting sound reflects the density of the underlying tissue.

phlebitis Inflammation of the wall of a vein that can lead to the formation of a thrombus or blood clot

phlebostatic axis The axis located in a plane that is passed through the center of the chest cavity and the heart. It is located at the midaxillary line and in the fourth rib space.

phlebotomy The invasive puncturing of a vein for the purpose of collecting blood

phosphodiesterase inhibitors A class of drugs that inhibit the action of phosphodiesterase, which prolongs the activity of 3',5'-adenosine monophosphate

physician's orders Orders written by the patient's attending or consulting physician. Physician's orders are typically found near the front of the patient's medical record.

pigeon chest A chest deformity in which the sternum projects outward. Also called pectus carinatum.

PISS The pin index safety system (PISS) is a safety system designed by the Compressed Gas Association for small yoke-type cylinder valves (D and E cylinders)

plateau pressure The inspiratory pressure measured when the exhalation valve is temporarily blocked, holding pressure in the lungs. This pressure is measured when there is no gas flow (exhalation valve is held closed).

pneumomediastinum A condition in which air has entered the mediastinal space

pneumothorax Pneumothorax is a condition in which air has entered the pleural space, causing partial or complete collapse of the lung.

Pontoppidan's criteria A set of criteria used to determine the need for mechanical ventilatory support. These criteria may include ventilatory mechanics, blood gases, oximetry, and end-tidal carbon dioxide monitoring.

Positive expiratory pressure (PEP) mask therapy The technique of applying positive-end expiratory pressure during exhalation to assist in mechanically splinting open the airways during exhalation

posteroanterior (posterior-anterior) Referring to an x-ray view of the chest in which the x-ray energy passes from posterior to anterior (back to front) exposing the film plate resting on the patient's anterior chest

postural drainage A technique in which the patient is positioned in specific ways such that gravity assists with the drainage of pulmonary secretions from a lobe or segment

preload The amount of diastolic "stretch" applied to the ventricular myocardium before systole. Preload is important in that too much or too little impedes the efficiency of the ventricular contraction.

premature ventricular complexes (PVCs) A type of cardiac contraction that occurs when the ventricles are stimulated to contract prematurely. PVCs may be caused by stress, acidosis, electrolyte imbalances, hypoxemia, or hypercapnia.

preset reducing valve   A type of reducing valve in which the pressure is not adjustable. These valves are typically set for 50 psi.

pressure control ventilation   A form of mechanical ventilation in which pressure is held constant for the duration of the inspiratory time. The inspiratory flow begins at a high flow rate and then decelerates throughout the inspiratory phase.

pressure limit   The pressure limit is a safety feature used during volume-controlled ventilation. When the pressure limit is reached, inspiration is terminated and exhalation begins (an alarm also usually sounds). This prevents delivery of excessive unwanted pressures to the patient's airways.

pressure limiting   Pressure limiting occurs when pressure is allowed to rise to a preset value and is held at that value during the inspiratory phase. In newborn mechanical ventilation, often pressure plateaus at the pressure limit, until the inspiratory time has been met and the breath ends.

pressure support   A mode of spontaneous ventilation in which the patient's spontaneous efforts are augmented with positive pressure. When the patient initiates a breath, a constant positive pressure is applied to the airways until inspiratory flow decays to 25% of the peak inspiratory flow value. Once inspiratory flow decays to that point, the positive pressure is removed and the patient exhales.

pressure-targeted ventilation (PTV)   Pressure-targeted ventilation is a classification of ventilation in which an inspiratory pressure (pressure target) is administered during inspiration. Volume and flow will vary with changes in compliance and resistance.

prn   "As needed"

progress notes   Notes written by the patient's physician indicating the general medical progress of the patient

prokaryotic bacteria   A type of bacteria in which the bacterial cell lacks a true nucleus and is surrounded by a nuclear membrane

prophylactic   Referring to an agent, substance, or device that prevents an event from occurring, or a disease process from being spread.

prostaglandin   A powerful mediator that causes bronchospasm and increases capillary permeability in the lungs

proximal lumen   The lumen of the pulmonary artery catheter located in the right atrium. This is used for measuring right atrial pressure, for fluid administration, and for injection of cold solution to measure the cardiac output.

pulmonary angiography   A radiographic technique using radiopaque dye to show the pulmonary vasculature. This technique is commonly used for visualization of pulmonary emboli.

pulmonary artery   The vessel that conducts blood from the right ventricle to the lungs

pulmonary artery catheter or **Swan-Ganz catheter**   A catheter that is passed through the right heart (right atrium and ventricle) and rests in the pulmonary artery. It is used to measure the right atrial, pulmonary artery, and pulmonary artery wedge pressures and to measure cardiac output.

pulmonary artery wedge pressure (PAWP)   The pressure obtained when the balloon of the pulmonary artery catheter is inflated, wedging it in the pulmonary artery. This pressure reflects the preload on the left ventricle.

pulmonary vein   The vessel conducting blood from the lungs to the left atrium

pulse oximeter   A medical instrument that allows the measurement of oxygen saturation (SpO_2) noninvasively using the infrared absorption spectra of hemoglobin

Purkinje fibers   A part of the cardiac conduction system originating from the left and right bundle branches and extending into the muscle walls of the ventricles. The Purkinje fibers are last in the cardiac conduction system to receive an electrical impulse.

P wave   The wave on an electrocardiographic tracing that results from the atria depolarizing

Q

QRS complex   The wave on an electrocardiographic tracing caused by the depolarization of the ventricles

quaternary ammonium compound   A liquid containing cationic detergents that are effective disinfection agents

R

radiodensity   Radiodensity refers to a material characteristic of absorbing or passing x-ray energy. A material with high radiodensity absorbs x-ray energy, creating a shadow (white image) on the x-ray film.

rapid-shallow-breathing index   A means of quantitating spontaneous ventilation. The rapid-shallow-breathing index is ventilatory frequency divided by the tidal volume in liters.

receptor sites   A specialized cell that will respond predictably to an external stimulus

reducing valve   A medical gas piping system component that reduces gas pressure from a high pressure to a working pressure (usually 50 psi)

regulator   A combination of a reducing valve and flowmeter in one unit

relative humidity   As a measured quantity, the absolute humidity (actual water content) divided by the capacity (maximum humidity for that temperature) multiplied by 100. This expresses the humidity as a percentage of the gas's capacity at that temperature.

repolarization   The process of exchange of potassium for sodium by the muscle cell, resulting in a net positive charge of the cell

residual volume (RV)   The amount of air remaining in the lungs following a complete exhalation. This volume cannot be measured directly but may only be measured using plethysmography, gas dilution, or radiographic methods.

respirometer   A portable medical device used to measure inspired or expired volumes at the bedside

retinopathy of prematurity   A noninflammatory change in the retinal vessels of newborns' eyes resulting in constriction of the vessels and permanent damage of the retina, caused by increased oxygen tension in the plasma

right and left bundle branches   Two specialized bands of conductive fibers that originate at the lower bundle of His and branch into the left and right ventricles. This part of the cardiac conduction system conducts the electrical impulse from the bundle of His to the ventricles.

right anterior oblique   Referring to an x-ray view in which the patient is upright and rotated 45° to the right, with the film plate against the patient's chest (postero-anterior projection). This "moves" the heart shadow away from the right side.

right heart   A term referring to the right atrium and ventricle, which pumps blood through the pulmonary vasculature. Because pulmonary vasculature resistance is low, the right heart is a low-pressure system.

rigid bronchoscope   A long, rigid, hollow tube that is used to examine the tracheobronchial tree. Rigid bronchoscopy is most often performed in the operating room with the patient under general anesthesia.

riser   A pipe in a medical gas piping system that supplies gas from one floor to the next floor in a multistory structure

---
S
---

scoliosis   An abnormal lateral curvature of the spine

shoulder blades   The bony structures located on the superior aspect of the posterior chest and overlying portions of the second through fifth ribs posteriorly. Also called scapulae.

sidestream monitor   A type of end-tidal carbon dioxide sensor that takes periodic samples away from a patient's airway to measure the $PetCO_2$

sigh mode   A mode of mechanical ventilation in which a larger than normal tidal breath is delivered periodically. A typical sigh tidal volume is 1.5 times the set tidal volume.

simple oxygen mask   A low-flow oxygen delivery device with a small reservoir that covers the nose and mouth

SIMV/IMV mode   Synchronized intermittent mandatory ventilation (SIMV) and intermittent mandatory ventilation (IMV) are modes of mechanical ventilation that allow the patient to breathe spontaneously between mechanical breaths. For SIMV, the ventilator has logic circuits that prevent the delivery of a mandatory breath (ventilator's mechanical breath) simultaneously with a patient's spontaneous breath, which is termed breath stacking.

SIMV with CPAP   Synchronized intermittent mandatory ventilation (SIMV) with continuous positive airway pressure (CPAP) is a combination of positive end-expiratory pressure (mandatory breaths) with CPAP (spontaneous breaths), which elevates the baseline pressure. The goal is to increase the patient's functional residual capacity.

sinoatrial node (SA node)   The part of the cardiac conduction system that functions as the heart's pacemaker. The cardiac conduction cycle begins with electrical impulses from the SA node, resulting in atrial contraction.

soft tissue obstruction   Airway obstruction caused by relaxation of the tongue and posterior pharynx, which obstructs the airway. Soft tissue obstruction is the most common form of airway obstruction.

spacer   A chamber that is attached to a metered dose inhaler to help reduce the velocity of the aerosol and stabilize the particle size by removing larger particles from suspension.

spirilla   A bacterium that is spiral in shape, facilitating motility through fluids

spirometer   A large instrument that is designed to measure accurately lung volumes and flow rates

spontaneous breath   A breath initiated by the patient, in which all volume is attained via the patient's ventilatory muscles

spontaneous combustion   A process in which a substance ignites, often violently, without the addition of significant heat

static compliance   A measurement of the compliance (distensibility) of the patient's lungs and thorax under conditions of no air flow. Therefore, the dynamic compliance reflects the compliance of the lungs and thorax.

station outlet   The connection in a piping system at the point of patient use. These outlets may have either DISS (Diameter index safety system), or quick-connect type attachment fittings.

steam autoclave   A device that applies moist heat (steam) under pressure to sterilize equipment or supplies

steamer   A type of room humidifier that works by boiling water to produce vapor or steam. Steamers are not typically used in the acute care setting owing to the danger posed by a hot water reservoir in close proximity to the patient.

sterility   The absence of microorganisms

sterilization   The complete destruction of all microorganisms

sternal angle   A bony ridge formed at the junction of the manubrium and the body of the sternum

subcutaneous emphysema   The presence of air within the subcutaneous tissues

subjective data   Information provided to the clinician by the patient as a result of asking questions about the patient's current state of health

suction catheter   A small flexible catheter that is used to suction the airway

suction control chamber In a suctioning system, the chamber most distal from the patient. This chamber regulates the vacuum level applied to the chest tube or drain.

suctioning An invasive procedure in which a flexible catheter is inserted into the tracheobronchial tree and vacuum is applied to remove secretions or foreign material

swayback An abnormal inward curvature of the lumbar spine. Also called lordosis.

sympathomimetic A class of drugs that stimulate the sympathetic nervous system, resulting in the formation of cyclic 3',5'-AMP

systolic The pressure recorded at the moment of cardiac contraction, yielding the higher of the paired blood pressure values

---

T

---

tachycardia An abnormally high heart rate

tachypnea An abnormally high respiratory rate

tank factor A constant expressed in liters per psi (pounds per square inch) that is used to determine the duration of oxygen cylinder contents. The tank factor for an H cylinder is 3.14 L/psi, and the factor for an E cylinder is 0.28 L/psi.

therapeutic bronchoscopy A bronchoscopy procedure that is performed to remove secretions, mucous plugs, or foreign bodies

thermistor A temperature-sensitive resistor, located at the distal tip of the catheter, that is used to measure a temperature change in determining the cardiac output

thermistor lumen The lumen of the pulmonary artery catheter that carries the electrical conductors from the thermistor and interfaces with the cardiac output computer on the monitor system

thermocouple An electronic component that acts as a thermostat to control the heating element in a transcutaneous electrode. The thermocouple, when functioning properly, prevents the heating element from becoming too hot and injuring the patient.

thrombus A blood clot that is commonly attached to the interior of a blood vessel wall

tidal volume The amount of air inhaled or exhaled by a spontaneously breathing patient during quiet, resting ventilation

timed breath A breath that is delivered at a set time interval (rate) and is not initiated by the patient's ventilatory efforts

time constant The product of the airway resistance and the compliance. The time constant provides an assessment of the lung's ability to receive gas.

time cycling In mechanical ventilation, a feature in which exhalation begins after a specified time period has passed. In most neonatal ventilators, the practitioner sets an inspiratory flow rate, respiratory rate, inspiratory time, and a CPAP/PEEP level. The inspiratory time determines how long each individual breath will last.

time triggering In mechanical ventilation, a feature in which a mechanical breath is delivered from the ventilator when a set time interval has passed. The ventilatory rate determines the frequency of ventilation.

TKO Abbreviation for "to keep open," referring to a drip rate for intravenous solutions that maintains the patency of the intravenous needle

tomogram An x-ray image in which the chest or body is viewed as a slice or a cut. The x-ray tube is rotated around the body, producing the image.

total lung capacity (TLC) The total gas volume of the lungs (residual volume, expiratory reserve volume, tidal volume, inspiratory reserve volume)

tracheostomy An opening made by surgical incision into the trachea at the second cartilaginous ring, at which point a tracheostomy tube is inserted to maintain a patent airway

tracheostomy button A specialized appliance that is designed to maintain a patent stoma following the removal of the tracheostomy tube

transcutaneous CO_2 monitor A monitor with specialized electrodes that allow measurement of dissolved oxygen and carbon dioxide (PaO_2 and $PaCO_2$) in the plasma noninvasively across the surface of the skin

transcutaneous PO_2 electrode A modified Clark electrode that measures the PO_2 noninvasively across the skin

transducer A device that converts mechanical energy (pressure) to an electrical signal

transillumination The application of a bright light source to illuminate body tissue to identify abnormalities. Transillumination is often used in neonates to identify the presence of a pneumothorax.

transtracheal catheter A specialized catheter that is surgically inserted into the trachea (second cartilaginous ring) for the administration of low-flow oxygen

trocar A blunt instrument inserted into a chest tube, stiffening it and allowing it to be inserted into the chest cavity. Once the tube is inserted, the trocar is removed.

tubing compliance When a mechanical breath is delivered by the ventilator, the tubing stretches or distends slightly during inspiration. The tubing is nonrigid and has its own compliance independent of the patient's lungs and thorax. The compliance of the circuit may be measured by occluding the patient wye and then recording the measured tidal volume and dividing it by the peak pressure (at tidal volumes less than 200 ml).

turning The technique of moving patients from side to side to optimize ventilation and perfusion and to help to prevent pressure ulcer formation

T wave The wave on an electrocardiographic tracing caused by the ventricles repolarizing

---

U

---

unexposed Referring to x-ray film that has not been subjected to x-ray energy. If the film is not exposed, it will appear white when developed.

unilateral chest expansion An adjunctive breathing technique that preferentially expands one side of the chest more than the other.

upstream Located proximal to a point in a device, or circuit, in relation to gas or current flow

V

vacuum collection tubes Specialized collection tubes, similar to test tubes, that contain media for cultures or special anticoagulants in which the air has been removed, creating a vacuum

valvular pathology Valvular disease including such problems as stenosis of the valves, mitral regurgitation, and aortic insufficiency. These pathologic processes result in decreased valvular performance, leakage, and reduction in cardiac output.

vector transmission Transmission of microorganisms via an intermediate host (flea, mosquito, tick, etc.)

vehicle transmission Transmission of microorganisms by an inanimate object, such as equipment used in treating the patient

vena cava The great vessel of the heart that delivers blood to the right atrium

venipuncture A procedure in which a blood vessel is entered through the skin

ventilation-perfusion scan (V/Q scan) A radiographic technique that compares perfusion with ventilation. This is commonly performed to diagnose pulmonary emboli.

ventricular asystole A total absence of any cardiac electrical activity. Ventricular asystole is always life-threatening and requires immediate intervention.

ventricular dysfunction Loss of ventricular performance through hypervolemia, hypovolemia, or loss of contractility.

ventricular fibrillation An unorganized rapid contraction of the ventricles that results in poor circulation and cardiac output. This is very serious, and death often occurs within 4 minutes if ventricular fibrillation is left untreated.

ventricular tachycardia A tachycardia (heart rate faster than 100 beats per minute) that originates in the ventricular Purkinje system

vibration A technique of applying external chest vibration during exhalation, which facilitates the removal of secretions. The technique can be accomplished manually (isometric muscle tensioning) or with the assistance of mechanical devices.

virulence The ability of a microorganism to produce disease. The more virulent an organism is, the greater is its ability to cause disease.

vital capacity (VC) The amount of air that can be exhaled after a full complete inspiration

volume ventilation Mechanical ventilation of a patient in which tidal volume is assured and pressure varies

W

wandering baseline An electrocardiographic tracing that displays an upward and downward displacement of the baseline. This is caused by poor electrical contact between the patient and the electrodes or leads.

Wang needle A special sheathed needle that is used for transbronchial sampling to obtain tissue from areas outside of the tracheobronchial tree

washout volume The amount of gas volume that must pass through a ventilator's circuit to effect a change in FIO_2 once the ventilator's oxygen control has been adjusted

wheal A small, raised area caused by the intradermal injection of a fluid

Z

zone valve A safety shut-off valve that can terminate the supply of gas to a specific area or zone. These values are often activated in the event of fire or when buildings undergo remodeling or construction.

INDEX